NUTRITION
In Perspective

ABOUT THE AUTHOR

Patricia A. Kreutler is Chairperson of the Department of Nutrition at Simmons College, Boston, Mass. Before joining the Simmons faculty, she was a Research Associate in the Department of Nutrition and Food Science at MIT, where she also received her Ph. D. in nutritional biochemistry and metabolism in 1973. She contributed two chapters to R. B. Howard and N. H. Herbold, ***Nutrition in Clinical Care*** (McGraw-Hill, 1978). She has served as Cochairwoman of the Simmons College Project on Women in Science and has been a member of the Executive Board of the Massachusetts Council on Foods, Nutrition, and Health. Her research interests include nutritional effects on growth, development, and oral health.

NUTRITION
In Perspective

Patricia A. Kreutler, Ph. D.
Simmons College, Boston

PRENTICE-HALL, INC., / ENGLEWOOD CLIFFS, NEW JERSEY

Library of Congress Cataloging in Publication Data
Kreutler, Patricia A.
Nutrition in Perspective
Includes bibliographies and indexes.
1. Nutrition. I. Title.
QP141.K69 574.1'3 79-27438
ISBN 0-13-627752-7

Printed in the United States of America

10 9 8 7 6 5 4 3 2 1

PRENTICE-HALL INTERNATIONAL, INC., *London*
PRENTICE-HALL OF AUSTRALIA PTY. LIMITED, *Sydney*
PRENTICE-HALL OF CANADA, LTD., *Toronto*
PRENTICE-HALL OF INDIA PRIVATE LIMITED, *New Delhi*
PRENTICE-HALL OF JAPAN, INC., *Tokyo*
PRENTICE-HALL OF SOUTHEAST ASIA PTE. LTD., *Singapore*
WHITEHALL BOOKS LIMITED, *Wellington, New Zealand*

Credits.
Art Director: Florence D. Silverman; Book Designer: Natasha Sylvester; Cover photo: R. Ustinich/The Image Bank. Part openings, clockwise from upper left: p. 1: *Still Life* by Edouard Manet, Louvre, Jeu de Paume, Cliché des Musées Nationaux, Paris. *Maria de'Medici* by Peter Paul Rubens, The Prado, Madrid; *The Wedding Banquet*, by Pieter Breughel, Museum voor Schone Kunsten, Ghent; *The Snake Dance* by Fred Kabotie, Hopi, Arizona, Museum of the American Indian, New York. p. 393: *Young Corn* by Grant Wood, © estate of Grant Wood. Courtesy of Associated American Artists. *One Hundred Campbell's Soup Cans* by Andy Warhol, Hessische Landesmuseum, Darmstadt, Sammlung Karl Ströher, *Thanksgiving, 1935* by Doris Lee, Courtesy of the Art Institute of Chicago; *Fulton Fish Market, 1953*, woodcut by Antonio Frasconi from *Frasconi Against The Grain*. Chapter openings: p. 2: *The Wedding Banquet* by Pieter Breughel, Museum voor Schone Kunsten, Ghent, p. 38: *Still Life* by Edouard Manet, Louvre, Jeu de Paume, Cliché des Musées Nationaux, Paris. p. 76: *Egg* by Odilon Redon, 8″ × 10″ black and white photograph, Collection, The Museum of Modern Art, New York, Gift of Peter H. Deitsch. p. 120: *Interior of a Butcher's Shop* by David Teniers (the Younger), Bequest of Sidney Bartlett 89.500, Courtesy, Museum of Fine Arts, Boston. p. 168: *Fishing*, old Japanese print, the New York Public Library Picture Collection. p. 216: *Wentworth Street, Whitechapel* by Gustave Dore from *London, a pilgrimage* by Gustave Dore and Blanchard Jerrold, New York: Harper, 1890. p. 254: *The Cook* by Pieter Corneliszen Van Ryck, Museum voor Schone Kunsten, Ghent. p. 312: *Maria de'Medici* by Peter Paul Rubens, The Prado, Madrid. p. 364: *The Snake Dance* by Fred Kabotie, Hopi, Arizona, Museum of the American Indian, New York. p. 398: *Fulton Fish Market, 1953*, woodcut by Antonio Frasconi from *Frasconi Against The Grain*. p. 430: *One Hundred Campbell's Soup Cans* by Andy Warhol, Hessische Landesmuseum, Darmstadt, Sammlung Karl Ströher. p. 462: *Mother and Children*, Baule, Ivory Coast, the British Museum, Webster Plass Collection, Photograph by Eliot Elisofon, Museum of African Art, Washington, D.C., Eliot Elisofon Archives. p. 498: *Baby in Red Chair*, artist unknown, Abby Aldrich Rockefeller Folk Art Center, Williamsburg, Virginia. p. 554: *Thanksgiving, 1935* by Doris Lee, Courtesy of the Art Institute of Chicago. p. 588: *The Potato Eaters* by Vincent Van Gogh, Rijksmuseum, Amsterdam. p. 616: *Young Corn* by Grant Wood, © estate of Grant Wood. Courtesy of Associated American Artists. p. 7 "The Secret Sits" by Robert Frost. From *The Poetry of Robert Frost* edited by Edward Connery Lathem. Copyright 1942, © 1962 by Robert Frost. Copyright © 1969 by Holt, Rinehart and Winston. Copyright © 1970 by Lesley Frost Ballantine. Reprinted by permission of Holt, Rinehart, and Winston, Publishers.

Contents

Chapter 12 Nutrition in Pregnancy and Lactation 462

Chapter 13 Nutrition in the Growing Years 498

Chapter 14 The Adult Years 554

Chapter 15 International Nutrition—Issues, Problems, Strategies 589

Chapter 16 Toward a National Food and Nutrition Policy 616

In Retrospect III 649

Glossary 651

Appendix 657

Index 683

Preface

Nutrition is a relatively young and rapidly growing discipline. Past its infancy and childhood, it can perhaps be likened to the everchanging adolescent period: with almost daily changes as new information is discovered, older information is reinterpreted, and new applications are identified, it is truly a dynamic science.

Nutrition in Perspective has been written to provide students with an understanding of the fundamentals of the science of nutrition; to acquaint students with the issues facing nutritionists, scientific and government leaders, and consumers in contemporary society; to prepare students to evaluate nutritional claims made in the popular media; and to enable students to translate knowledge of the science of nutrition into practices that are compatible with their individual philosophies and lifestyles.

Not merely an issue-oriented text, *Nutrition in Perspective* is suitable for courses meeting science distribution requirements as well as for introductory courses for nutrition, dietetics, home economics, and nursing majors. While the scientific basis of nutrition has not been underplayed, every attempt has been made to present lucid explanations of basic biological and chemical processes central to the study of nutrition. It has been the author's experience that most students, even those without a science background, become interested and excited as they learn how the body works. For those who enroll in an introductory nutrition course with a prior knowledge of biology and chemistry, these discussions will serve as a helpful review.

Within the framework of science, presentation of current nutritional issues is a major concern of this text. In discussing these issues, this book emphasizes that nutritional well-being is determined by both the internal environment of the body and the external environment of the outside world. In the course of their study, students will often be reminded of the importance of diversity in food consumption patterns to nutritional—and therefore overall—health.

This text is scientifically accurate and up-to-date. Reading it, students will become aware that nutrition is a dynamic discipline in which new data and interpretations are constantly emerging; they will learn that change should be anticipated. (Indeed, it has been a challenge for the author to incorporate new information into this manuscript as it appeared almost daily!) But readers should not be discouraged; rather, as they learn to appreciate the principles of the scientific method and the intricacies of the human body within its ecosystem, they will also appreciate the significance of change in theory and knowledge and be able to place new information in perspective.

It is hoped that this introduction to the study of nutrition will encourage further study, whether formal or informal. Readers will also recognize how many and varied the disciplines related to nutrition are. Insights and talents from many fields are needed to advance the research, interpretation, and application of this subject which so strongly influences our everyday lives.

Plan of the Book

Nutrition in Perspective is divided into two major parts. In Part One, "Scientific Principles of Nutrition," the underlying biological, chemical, and regulatory mechanisms of the internal environment are presented, using a systems approach. An understanding of the basic roles of nutrients in the body prepares students to appreciate the continuity of the life cycle with its changing nutritional needs, the implications of political and societal change, consumer concerns, and the need for a diversified diet. These topics are developed in Part Two, "Nutrition for Everyday Living."

Information and ideas presented in both parts of the text will allow students to identify the totality of nutrition and enable them to adopt good personal health practices and to be informed consumers and conscientious and aware voters.

Features

Topics of contemporary concern are presented as "Perspectives" within each chapter. These issues—the saccharin debate, use of megavitamins, drug-nutrient interactions, the politics of iron enrichment and water fluoridation, nutrition for athletes, the Green Revolution, the U.S. Dietary Goals, and more—are placed in the context of current scientific knowledge and should stimulate thought and discussion.

Three brief sections—"In Retrospect"—integrate the content of preceding chapters and stress the continuity and regulation of biochemical and life processes. Thus these sections reinforce the concept of nutrition as a systematic discipline, both as a science and in its application to our lifestyles.

In the opening chapter both the metric system and a definition and discussion of the Recommended Dietary Allowances are presented. This provides the student with an understanding of some of the basic concepts and terminology to be introduced in subsequent chapters of Part One. Inclusion of the 1979 revision of the RDAs throughout the text provides the reader with the most current information on this topic. A summary, bibliography, and list of suggested additional readings conclude each chapter, to encourage the learning process.

In-Text Learning Aids

To reinforce the concepts, facts, and principles presented, a variety of learning aids are used. Visual clarification is enhanced by colored diagrams, margin illustrations, photographs, and material in tabular form. Tables of nutrient composition are expressed in useful portion sizes to enable students more realistically to choose appropriate foods. In addition, most of the tables are subdivided into good, fair, and poor sources of specific nutrients. A single serving that provides more than 25 percent of the RDA is considered a good source; poor sources are identified as foods providing less than 2 percent of the RDA for that nutrient.

Descriptions of relevant biological processes are presented in a step-by-step manner, emphasizing regulatory systems. Although the nature of the subject matter requires technical terminology, language has been kept clear and concise. Terms are set in boldface type when they are introduced, and are defined in the glossary. Frequent use of examples to illustrate scientific principles serves to encourage learning, not by memory, but through understanding. As students gain understanding of systems through the use of examples, they will be encouraged to transfer their conceptual knowledge from one system to another.

Supplements

To facilitate the self-discovery of learning, a Study Guide and an Instructor's Manual including a Test Item File have been prepared to accompany this text. For the student, the Study Guide provides an overview of each chapter, a list of the vocabulary terms introduced in each, and a sample of self-study test questions.

The Instructor's Manual is designed to suggest ideas for lectures, demonstrations, creative projects, and research assignments. Many of the projects are directed toward students whose major interest is in a field other than nutrition. These projects will stimulate continued interest in nutrition within the context of another discipline—and may in turn suggest to the student a further area of intellectual and professional development. The Test Item File included in the Instructor's Manual includes questions in a variety of formats.

Acknowledgments

Nutrition in Perspective reflects the talents, dedication, and enthusiasm of innumerable people. Many of the individuals who have influenced the development of this text will remain anonymous: my teachers and colleagues throughout the years, as well as my students, have guided me in my approach to the study of nutrition and its relationship to the quality of life. But the central figure in my professional development has been Sanford A. Miller, who gave me the opportunity to study nutrition and whose valuable insights have influenced my thinking.

My thanks also go to my colleagues and coworkers who shared ideas and resources with me, and provided much-needed moral support: Dr. Michael C. Alfano, Katherine M. Bevacqua, Nancie Harvey Herbold, Rosanne B. Howard, Dr. Marion Mason, Dr. Rena Mendelson, Charlotte Morocco, and Coral Kenney O'Brien.

My family and friends deserve special recognition; their understanding of my hermit-like existence for the past eighteen months, their encouragement, and their support helped me place this project into perspective in my own life.

The production of this text could not have been realized without the cooperation and expertise of many conscientious people. Special thanks are due to my research assistant, Jane S. Pearlman, whose diligence and enthusiasm throughout this project are most appreciated. Toni Goldfarb and Thomas Adams deserve recognition for their assistance with the preparation of the manuscript. I also wish to thank the reviewers who conscientiously read the manuscript and offered helpful suggestions about content and style throughout: Phyllis B. Acosta, Emory University School of Medicine; Frances E. Andrews, University of Tennessee, Knoxville; Kitty R. Coffey, Carson-Newman College, Jefferson City, Tennessee; Penny Donne, West Valley College, Saratoga, California; Margaret D. Doyle, University of Minnesota at St. Paul; Christine Dupraw, San Diego Mesa College; Jeannette M. Endres, Southern Illinois University, Carbondale; Hazel Fox, University of Nebraska, Lincoln; Gail G. Harrison, University of Arizona; John Hathcock, Iowa State University, Ames; James Heffley, Nutrition Counseling Service, Austin, Texas; Cheryl W. Hutton, University of Alabama; Margaret A. James, University of Wisconsin, Stout; Catherine Justice, Purdue University; Mary K. Korslund, Virginia Polytechnic Institute and State University; M. E. Kraynak, University of Oklahoma; Jane S. Lewis, California State University; Katherine Lewis, Arizona State University; Evelyn Mar, California State University, Chico; Kathleen Newell, Kansas State University, Manhattan; Jean H. Peters, Oregon State University; Robert D. Reeves, Kansas State University, Manhattan; Nell B. Robinson, Texas Christian University; Arnold E. Schaefer, Swanson Center for Nutrition, Inc., Omaha, Nebraska; Roseanne L. Shorey, University of Texas at Austin; Nan Singleton, Louisiana State University; Katherine S. Staples, North Dakota State University; Anita Wilson, University of Wisconsin, Stout; Margy Woodburn, Oregon State University; Bonnie Worthington, University of Washington, Seattle; and Bonita W. Wyse, Utah State University.

The contributions of the Prentice-Hall staff are gratefully acknowledged; their support, expertise, and hard work have contributed greatly to the production of this text: Cecil Yarbrough, director, Book Project Division; Kate Moran, market researcher; Ray Keating, book manufacturing buyer; Nancy Perkus, permissions editor; Bruce Williams and Jeanne Libby, production editors; Martha Goldstein, managing editor; and production assistant Jon Dash. Pamela Kirshen and her assistant Edith Riker coordinated the review and marketing processes, and also deserve my thanks. Technical assistance was also provided by Elaine Luthy, copy editor, and Marjorie Graham, photo researcher.

Much of the heart, mind, and soul of this book is a reflection of the efforts of my development editor, Marjorie P. K. Weiser. Her creativity, writing and editorial skills, and cheery personality are mirrored in these pages. Her tireless ability to deal with the minute details of this project, her sense of humor in difficult times, her gentle prodding to meet deadlines, and her indescribable support throughout this entire endeavor are difficult to convey in a few words. And for her friendship, an invaluable result of this book, I am indeed fortunate.

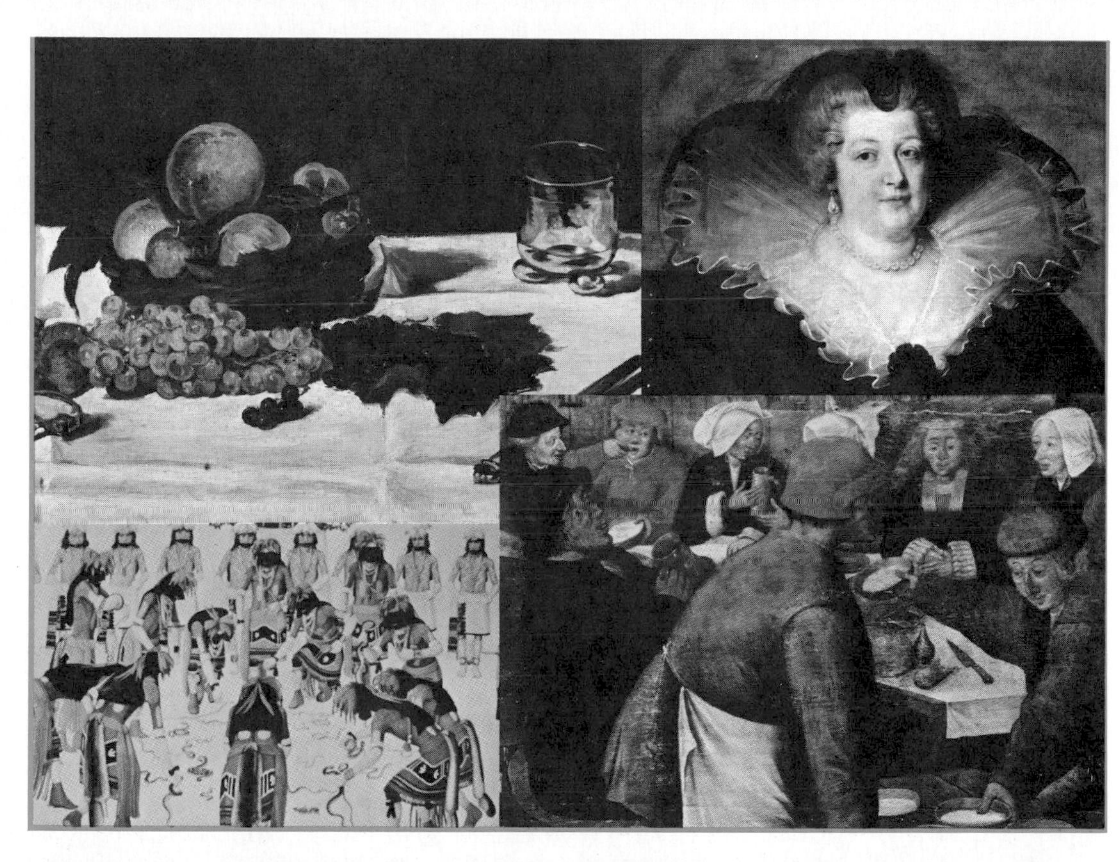

PART ONE SCIENTIFIC PRINCIPLES OF NUTRITION

Chapter 1

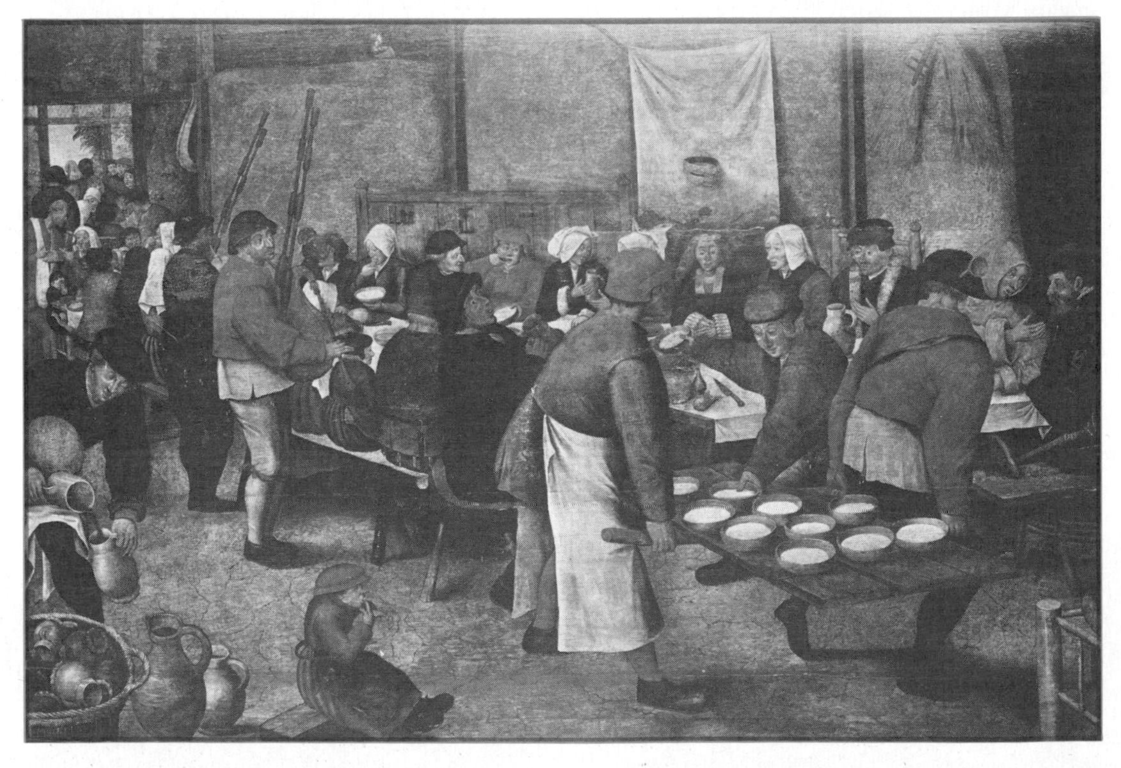

The Wedding Banquet by Pieter Breughel

Introduction to Nutrition

Imagine a lightweight, compact machine, no bigger than a broom closet. A machine containing pumps, processors, valves, conveyor belts, and millions of tiny message-sending and -receiving stations, all working 24 hours a day, 365 days a year, year after year after year, nonstop. Then imagine what it must take to fuel this amazing data processor, ditch digger, cook, and bottle washer—not the Alaska pipeline or the Grand Coulee Dam, but a loaf of bread, a jug of wine, and a bit of companionship.

Bread, wine, and the other foodstuffs we eat, how our bodies process them, and how they affect our health and functioning are the subjects of this book. Discussion of these subjects will present nutrition as a *process*—a process influenced by many external and internal factors. Nutrition is also a *science*. Our introduction begins with a discussion of nutrition as a scientific discipline.

NUTRITION AS A SCIENCE

Science deals with systematically arranged facts that demonstrate the operation of general laws that can be tested. Human nutritional science deals with facts about the consumption and utilization of food by people. These facts have, over many years, been arranged systematically into laws and principles supported by formal, controlled research studies. This controlled testing process is known as the **scientific method.** It is based upon a design developed in the sixteenth century by Sir Francis Bacon, the English philosopher. The basic components of the scientific method are illustrated by what is considered to be the first controlled experiment in nutrition.

The experiment began with the *observation* that many English sailors became ill during long sea voyages and died. Among the explanations and theories proposed to explain this observation was the *hypothesis* that something about the sailors' diet was causing their illness. The **hypothesis** serves to limit the scope of the study. The next step in an experiment is obtaining evidence to corroborate or refute the hypothesis. To support the hypothesis that there was a relationship between sailors' diets and their illness, James Lind, a surgeon of the English fleet, studied 12 afflicted sailors. He gave two of them a quart of cider each day; two, 25 drops of sulfuric acid three times daily; two, vinegar; two, sea water; two, two oranges plus one lemon; and two, some nutmeg, on a daily basis. The *result* was soon apparent: only those sailors given the citrus fruits improved and were again fit for sea duty within a few days. Lind drew a legitimate *conclusion* that something in the oranges and lemons, something not present in the other treatments, cured the men of their ailment. Today, we all know that "something" as vitamin C, ascorbic acid. When Lind performed his study in 1747, he lacked a scientific basis on which to conclude that vitamin C cured scurvy, since the existence of vitamins was unknown. Many years would pass before investigators would identify and isolate vitamins in food.

This long-term progression of research and observation, with many years passing between a discovery and an explanation of it, has often occurred in science. Just as physics progressed step by step from the first discovery of gravity to recent feats of atom splitting, so, too, has the science of nutrition developed one step at a time. Although each step, each experiment, is only a link in the chain of knowledge about nutrition, much care must be taken to make it a strong link. **Controlled experiments** are the foundation on which scientific knowledge is built. In controlled nutrition experiments, a specific food item or diet is often fed to one group of subjects, while a comparable group receives a standard diet; the outcomes for both groups are then compared. Meticulous planning, accurately recorded findings, and careful analysis are the essentials of research and lead to valid and logical conclusions. Scientists are trained in these essentials, but no training can provide the qualities of vision and imagination, courage of convictions, drive, enthusiasm, patience, and persistence necessary to promote scientific discoveries.

Types of Evidence

The end product of experimentation is *evidence*, information that can be used to support the particular hypothesis being investigated. Depending upon the kind of hypothesis, and the methods available to test it, many different types of evidence may be obtained. In studies of nutrition, descriptive, epidemiological, and experimental evidence all have their place.

DESCRIPTIVE EVIDENCE. A collection of facts about a situation that exists in the environment is known as *descriptive evidence*. For example, your casual observation that about one out of ten students in your nutrition class is overweight would be considered descriptive evidence that about 10 percent of college-age individuals are overweight. Casual observations such as this, based on general impressions, are referred to as *anecdotal* evidence. There are obvious limitations to anecdotal reporting. This observation may be an underestimate, because students interested in nutrition may be more likely to control their weight than other students, or your sample may be biased in such a way as to produce an overestimate, if the nutrition course is an adjunct to a campus weight-control workshop. Finally, such casual observations are not supported by written records, and memory may not serve correctly. Despite these limitations, anecdotal evidence can be of value by suggesting hypotheses that can then be tested by more rigorous methods of inquiry, such as the *planned survey*. A survey of all the students at your college, using a specific questionnaire or work sheet on which to record weight and other data, would provide better representation of overweight and normal weight subjects and be more accurate.

EPIDEMIOLOGICAL EVIDENCE. While the survey method would provide more complete information, it may suggest still other questions. For example, do some factors affect overweight students but not others? You would need more than descriptive evidence to answer this question; **epidemiological evidence** would be the next step. Epidemiology is the study of the occurrence and distribution of factors associated with a particular phenomenon in a given population. Thus, epidemiological examination of your descriptive survey may indicate that excess weight is more prevalent in resident students than in students who commute. In scientific terms, you have found an **association** between residency and overweight. But the mere existence of an association does not necessarily indicate a cause-and-effect relationship between the variables. Just as a survey finding that heart attack victims own television sets could not be used as evidence that TV causes heart disease, you could not conclude that residency causes overweight. Despite this limitation, epidemiological evidence is important because, like descriptive evidence, it suggests hypotheses that may deserve further examination. A classic example of epidemiological evidence is the well-known Framingham study, in which several factors, such as overweight and physical inactivity, were found to be associated with the occurrence of coronary heart disease in men in a small town in Massachusetts. (This study and its implications will be discussed at greater length in Chapter 3.)

EXPERIMENTAL EVIDENCE. Scientists are rarely satisfied with associations. They test hypotheses in order to establish proven cause-and-effect relationships. This testing process provides **experimental evidence.** In your study of overweight on campus, you may, for example, hypothesize that resident students have more opportunity than commuting students to take second and third helpings of dessert. To test this hypothesis, you might arrange to limit dessert servings in the residents' cafeteria to one per meal. If, after a long enough period of time, you found that the difference in overweight between residents and commuters had disappeared, you might conclude that extra desserts had indeed caused obesity. Obviously, this experiment would be difficult to perform, because it would be impossible to control other important factors. Your hungry residents may substitute midnight snacks for their usual second dessert helping, or not eat as often in the cafeteria. This difficulty in controlling the behavior of human subjects has produced increased reliance on other types of experimentation.

Experimental Models

Research studies in nonhuman systems are called *experimental models.* Nutritionists use **animal models.** Horses, cows, sheep, pigs, birds, cats, dogs, guinea pigs, and even microorganisms are used, but rats are by far the most popular experimental model. Each year, thousands of rats are used in diet-related studies to determine effects, if any, on health. It is very difficult, if not impossible, to perform such tests on human subjects.

Problems of designing human experiments are many. Foremost is the ethical consideration. It is not ethical to intentionally subject human beings to pain or other health hazards, or to withhold possible cures. Then, there is the problem of availability of sufficient numbers of suitable subjects in a given place. Also, manipulation of only one aspect of a test variable presents problems with human subjects. Finally, there is the problem of time. The human reproductive cycle takes many years. The length of a human life means that young investigators would be of retirement age before they could study effects of an experiment in only one or two generations. Obviously, studies of many generations are more practical in animals. Rats' small size, low maintenance cost, ease of handling, and rapid rate of reproduction have made them particularly useful. And, most important to nutritionists, they are omnivorous, just as humans are, and will eat almost any kind of diet. The disadvantage of using rats is that all of their internal processes are not the same as those of humans. For example, their need for certain vitamins may be different from that of humans. Rat studies may suggest applications to human nutrition, although they cannot prove beyond doubt that results in humans will be exactly the same. Nevertheless, animal models are extremely valuable because ethical, economic, and biological limitations prohibit human testing.

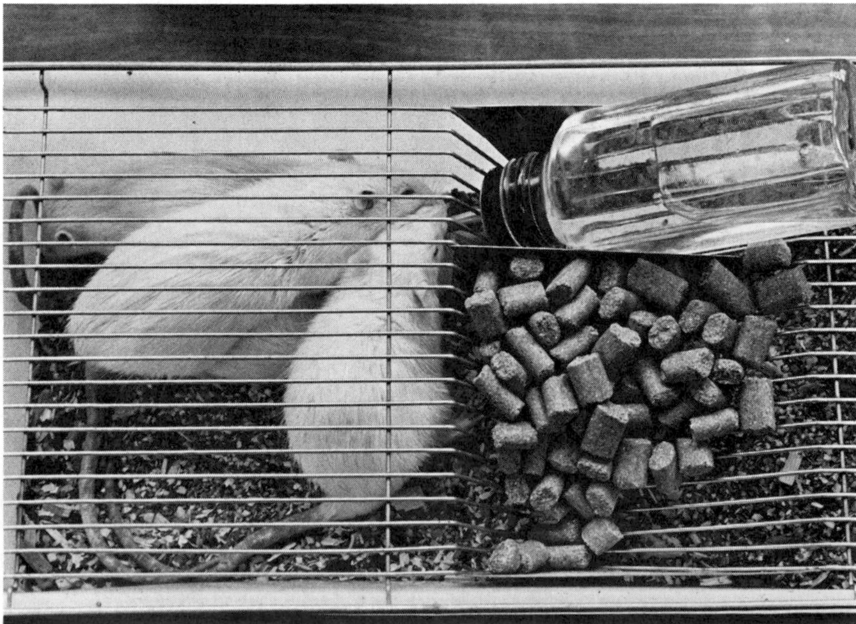

Laboratory rats used in nutrition experiments are given controlled diets. (Hugh Rogers/Monkmeyer)

Although animal models permit precise control of experimental variables, their use does not guarantee attention to other important factors. Experiments are only as good as the researchers who design them, the assumptions they make, and the testing methods they use. Is the experimental hypothesis based on accurate observation? Are the testing methods appropriate? Are important variables well controlled? Do the final conclusions follow from the observed results? Is enough information provided so that another investigator can perform the same study? These are all questions that must be asked in evaluating scientific studies.

Historically, even well-controlled experiments demonstrating supportable conclusions have not always found a favorable reception in the scientific community and in the general population, especially when scientific findings differ from widely held beliefs. It often takes years before the "truth" is accepted, and many more years before long-standing theories and explanations are replaced by laws based on repeated experimentally proven facts. Thus, science is a slow, evolutionary process, a process of step-by-step observation, hypothesis testing, and opinion changing. Although time consuming, science is dynamic. The promise of discovery is forever present. As Robert Frost so aptly put it:

We dance round in a ring and suppose
But the Secret sits in the middle and knows.

—**The Secret Sits,** 1945

HISTORY OF NUTRITIONAL SCIENCE

Nutrition has been called a "twentieth-century science." Indeed, application of many earlier nutritional findings came late in history. James Lind's work on scurvy was performed in 1747 and reported six years later in his book *A Treatise of the Scurvy,* although 48 years would pass before the regular use of citrus juice was enforced in the British Navy.

Of course, communication in Lind's time was not what it is today. Scientific journals were published infrequently and not widely distributed. Thus, sharing of potentially important knowledge was hampered. Nutrition, because it is so directly relevant to the health and functioning of society as a whole, has always been subject to the influences of political, social, economic, cultural, and technological factors. Moreover, important developments in medicine, agriculture, chemistry, physics, and current events often diverted nutrition research from a steady, step-by-step, logical progression. For example, Pasteur's demonstration in the 1850s that bacteria could produce disease probably delayed the discovery of **vitamins.** The idea that illness might stem from a lack of something (**dietary deficiency**) was alien to scientists who had so recently come to associate disease with the presence of something (microorganisms) (Todhunter, 1962).

Time lines are often used to organize the chronology of events, illustrating not only when important discoveries or events occurred, but the related

PERSPECTIVE ON

The Metric System Scientific Measurement

The quantitative language of the science of nutrition and of all other sciences is the **metric system.** Older units of measurement—the quart, the yard, the pound, and so on—have been replaced for research purposes, and are being replaced in the industrial world as well. As the United States moves toward full adoption of the metric system, its usage is becoming more common in everyday life.

Metric measurements are based on units of 10, which facilitates most mathematical calculation. Units of length, volume, weight, and temperature—familiar to us as inches and feet, cubic inches and cubic feet, pints and gallons, ounces and pounds, and degrees Fahrenheit, respectively—all have metric equivalents.

Length: The basic unit of length in the metric system is the *meter*, which was established to represent one ten-millionth part of the distance measured on a meridian from the equator to the pole, or 39.37 linear inches. A meter is just a bit longer than one yard. Using the base-10 units of the metric system, one hundredth of a meter is one centimeter, or 0.394 inches. One tenth of a centimeter (one thousandth of a meter) is a millimeter (mm), or 0.0394 inches. For larger measurements, we use the kilometer (km), one thousand meters, a little more than $^6/_{10}$ mile. These base-10 relationships, and the ease with which one can be converted to another, become apparent when we look at this information in tabular form:

		1 millimeter	=	0.03937	inches
10 millimeters (mm)	=	1 centimeter (cm)	=	0.3937	inches
1000 millimeters (mm)	=	1 meter (m)	=	39.37	inches
1000 meters (m)	=	1 kilometer (km)	=	39370	inches
			=	0.62137	miles

Height: Height is generally expressed in centimeters. Thus:

1 in = 2.54 centimeters (cm)
1 ft = 12 × 2.54 cm = 30.48 cm

Using these equivalents, it is easy to calculate that a person 5 feet 5 inches tall (65 inches) measures 65 × 2.54 = 165 cm.

Weight: The basic metric unit of weight is the gram. There are 28.35 grams to the ounce, a figure usually rounded off to 30 grams to facilitate calculation. Metric weight follows the same base-10 pattern as the millimeters and kilometers we mentioned for length, with a milligram equaling one-thousandth of a gram, and a kilogram equaling one thousand grams. Some weights used in nutrition are so minute that they must be expressed in micrograms (mcg or μg). One thousand micrograms are equal to one milligram.

Body weight is usually expressed in kilograms. Thus:

1 pound = 16 ounces = 454 grams (g)
2.2 pounds = 1000 grams = 1 kilogram (kg)

If you weigh 120 pounds, your weight is:

120 pounds ÷ 2.2 lbs/kg = 54.5 kg,

or, if you prefer multiplication:

developments that may have influenced them either directly or indirectly. A nutrition time line might justifiably begin with the Biblical story of Daniel, who thrived on pulse (legumes) and water while others languished on a diet of the king's meat. But this anecdotal account is not a "nutrition classic." A true classic study presents new ideas or new understandings of older ideas and thereby influences future work in the science of nutrition. Following these criteria, our time line would appear quite bare until the early 1600s, when the first deliberate, scientific nutrition studies were made. That is when Sanctorius, a friend of Galileo, published his studies on body weight and food consumption. Sanctorius was his own best subject. He weighed himself and all the food he ate, and then weighed his excretions. His metabolic studies revealed that food intake, though greater than excretory output, does not necessarily increase body weight. He attributed the lack of weight gain to

$$120 \times 0.454 = 54.5 \text{ kg}$$

Quantities of food are often measured in 100-gram units. Calculations will be easier if you remember that 100 grams is equivalent to approximately 3½ ounces, or a bit less than ¼ of a pound.

Volume: The basic metric unit of volume is the milliliter (ml), also known as a cubic centimeter (cc). There are 28.35 ml to the fluid ounce or, rounded off, about 30 ml. One thousand milliliters equals 1 liter, a common liquid measure just a bit more than 1 quart (1 liter = 1.06 quarts). Other basic volumetric measures are:

1/1000 milliliter (ml)	= 1 microliter (μl)
100 milliliters	= 1 deciliter (dl)
4.7 milliliters (about 5)	= 1 fluid teaspoon
14.2 milliliters	= 1 fluid tablespoon

Solids within Liquids: The concentration of a substance in the blood is usually expressed as a unit of weight within a volume of 100 milliliters of blood, most often written as mg/100 ml (milligrams per 100 milliliters), mg/dl (milligrams per deciliter), or mg% (milligrams percent), which is the same thing. Thus, a concentration of 120 milligrams of glucose in 100 milliliters of blood could be expressed in several ways:

120 mg/100 ml
120 mg/dl
120 mg%

(The blood volume of the average adult is 5000 milliliters or 5 liters; body size, sex, and other factors, however, determine that most individuals have greater or lesser blood volume than average.)

Temperature: In the metric system temperature is expressed in degrees Celsius (C), rather than degrees Fahrenheit (F). In the usual metric base-10 system, freezing is 0°C, as compared to 32°F, while boiling is 100°C, the equivalent of 212°F. To convert Fahrenheit to Celsius, you must subtract 32 and then multiply by 5/9:

$$70°F - 32 = 38 \times 5/9 = 21°C$$
$$212°F - 32 = 180 \times 5/9 = 100°C \text{ (boiling point)}$$

Similarly, to convert Celsius to Fahrenheit, multiply the Celsius temperature by 9/5 and add 32:

$$35° \times 9/5 = 63 + 32 = 95°F$$
$$0°C \times 9/5 = 0 + 32 = 32°F \text{ (freezing point)}$$

Energy: Traditionally, the basic unit of energy in nutrition has been the **kilocalorie** (kcal). The "calorie" is often used when the kilocalorie is really meant. The kilocalorie should properly be written **Calorie.** A kilocalorie is defined as that amount of energy (heat) required to raise the temperature of 1 liter of water from 15 to 16 degrees Celsius. Newer terminology for energy uses the **joule,** a measure of force or capacity to do work, rather than of heat, as its basic unit. Although many nutritionists continue to use calorie (kilocalorie) measurements, the joule and kilojoule are appearing with increasing frequency in writing about nutrition. With this in mind, you should become familiar with the following conversions:

1 calorie = 4.184 joules (J)
1 kilocalorie = 4.184 kilojoules (kJ), where $1 \text{ kJ} = 10^3 \text{ J} = 1000 \text{ J}$

Thus, 100 kilocalories = 418.4 kJ

See also the conversion table, Appendix F.

"insensible perspiration." It was 300 years before metabolic research would offer a full explanation of Sanctorius' finding.

After William Harvey's classic publication on the circulation of blood in 1628, which laid the foundation for the understanding of the transportation of nutrients, Lind's study of scurvy in 1747, and the first measurements of human energy metabolism by Lavoisier in 1789, our time line does not begin to look crowded until the nineteenth century. The first amino acid was discovered in 1810. In 1816, François Magendie demonstrated that nitrogen-containing compounds were essential in the **diet** of dogs. His student, Claude Bernard, investigated sugar formation in the liver.

By 1900, nutrition experiments were well under way. "The Chemical Composition of American Food Materials," United States Department of Agriculture Bulletin 28, was published in 1896. Its author, W. O. Atwater, "father of American nutrition," performed the first extensive analyses of food, which made possible the estimation of dietary intake. In 1907, Elmer V. McCollum began experimenting with rats at the University of Wisconsin to try to determine what constituted the substances that prevented scurvy and beriberi. He was joined by Marguerite Davis, who developed new techniques for using rats in research. In 1913, they published a paper describing a substance they called "Fat Soluble A." In 1912, Casimir Funk coined the term "vitamine," which was changed to "vitamin" when it was discovered that not all vitamins are "amines," or nitrogen-containing substances. By 1921, Robert McCarrison, in *Studies in Deficiency Disease*, cautioned that vitamins were only one link in the chain of essential substances required to maintain the chemical processes in the body.

In 1943 the Food and Nutrition Committee of the National Research Council published the first table of dietary standards. An explosion of technological developments in the last twenty-five years—ultracentrifuges, electron microscopes, and much more—has led to an equivalent explosion of new knowledge.

Hundreds of years of nutritional research have led to discovery, progress, and improvement in the quality of life for millions of people. This historical overview of nutrition discoveries of the past will serve as a prologue to our study of nutrition today.

ECOLOGY OF FOOD AND NUTRITION

The word **nutrition** has several meanings. In popular usage, it conveys ideas of healthy eating and basic food groups. In scientific usage, it has two well defined meanings. First, nutrition is a *process* by which living organisms utilize food to maintain bodily functioning. Second, nutrition is a *field of inquiry*, a science—a systematic collection of facts about the body's chemical processing and biological use of food. Nutrition has other meanings as well, reflecting the special purposes of those who use them. The social scientist and health care provider see it not only as a chemical process but also as a social process involving the availability, acceptability, and need for food.

Our own approach to nutrition combines descriptions of process, science, and social factors. We will define nutrition as "the science of food and its interaction with an organism to promote and maintain health." **Food,** another word of many meanings, is used here as "a collection of nutrients in a form which is eaten, digested, and metabolized to provide energy and materials that build and maintain the structure and regulate the function of the body." We will explore both the scientific and the social aspects of nutrition. Our definition recognizes the constant interaction between the **internal environment** inside the organism, with its precisely regulated physiological systems, and the **external environment** outside the organism, with its many physical, technological, and psychosocial systems that surround the body and determine the availability and choice of foods. We will begin with an examination of these external factors.

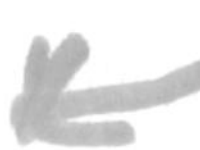

Determinants of Food Behavior: The External Environment

There is an intimate relationship between our lifestyle and what, why, when, and with whom we eat. Food is as much an expression of our lifestyle as our choice of work, clothing, housing, and religious or educational practices. Stylized food habits, known to sociologists as **foodways**, evolved as adaptations to the physical and social environment and are an integral part of our cultural heritage.

In Western society, food is viewed not as a mere necessity of life, but as a glorified, pleasure-filled symbol of love, companionship, and achievement. Food is an integral part of celebrations, the main attraction at holidays, weddings, communion breakfasts, bar mitzvahs, cocktail and dinner parties, and every other kind of get-together, from baptisms to funerals. Entire industries—restaurants, bars, fast-food chains, catering halls—have grown from our food celebrations. Our food overindulgences have swelled the coffers of other businesses, such as manufacturers of indigestion remedies. In our culture, food speaks—of friendship at a kaffeeklatsch, of love between mother and child, of achievement at an expense account business lunch, and even of confrontation during a hunger strike. The language of food in the Western world is the language of plenty.

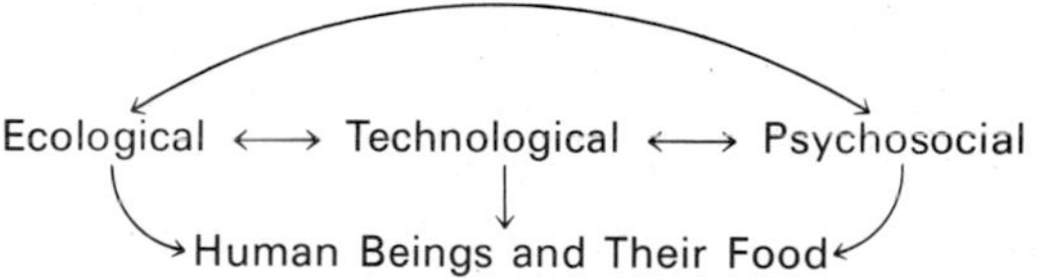

ECOLOGICAL FACTORS. Food must be physically present to be consumed. People can eat only what is available to them. Dry climates foster the production of cereal grains; wet climates, the growing of rice. These environmental facts of life account for the popularity of wheat-based breads and noodles in Central Europe, and for the near-total dependence on rice in most of Asia. In areas of infertile soil, hardy cassava and soybeans become dietary staples. Along coastlines and river shores, fish is plentiful. And where the supply of meat or fish is unpredictable, drying and smoking procedures were developed to preserve enough to last through the lean months. Polish sausages and the concentrated Vietnamese fish sauce nuoc-mam are two pungent examples. All large groups of people—societies—have methods of preserving foods in climates where it is necessary. By accidents of *geography* and *topography*, then, different societies come to favor different foods.

Societal and individual preferences, though, can change. We are all familiar with changes in food habits brought about by the seasons. Winter is the time for thick, hot soups; summer for crisp, refreshing salads.

Seasonal changes affect not only taste buds and appetites, but also the availability of certain foods. In the past many fresh foods were available only in season. The bounty of the fall harvest was the cause for the feast at Thanksgiving, and the limited variety of produce characteristic of winter gave

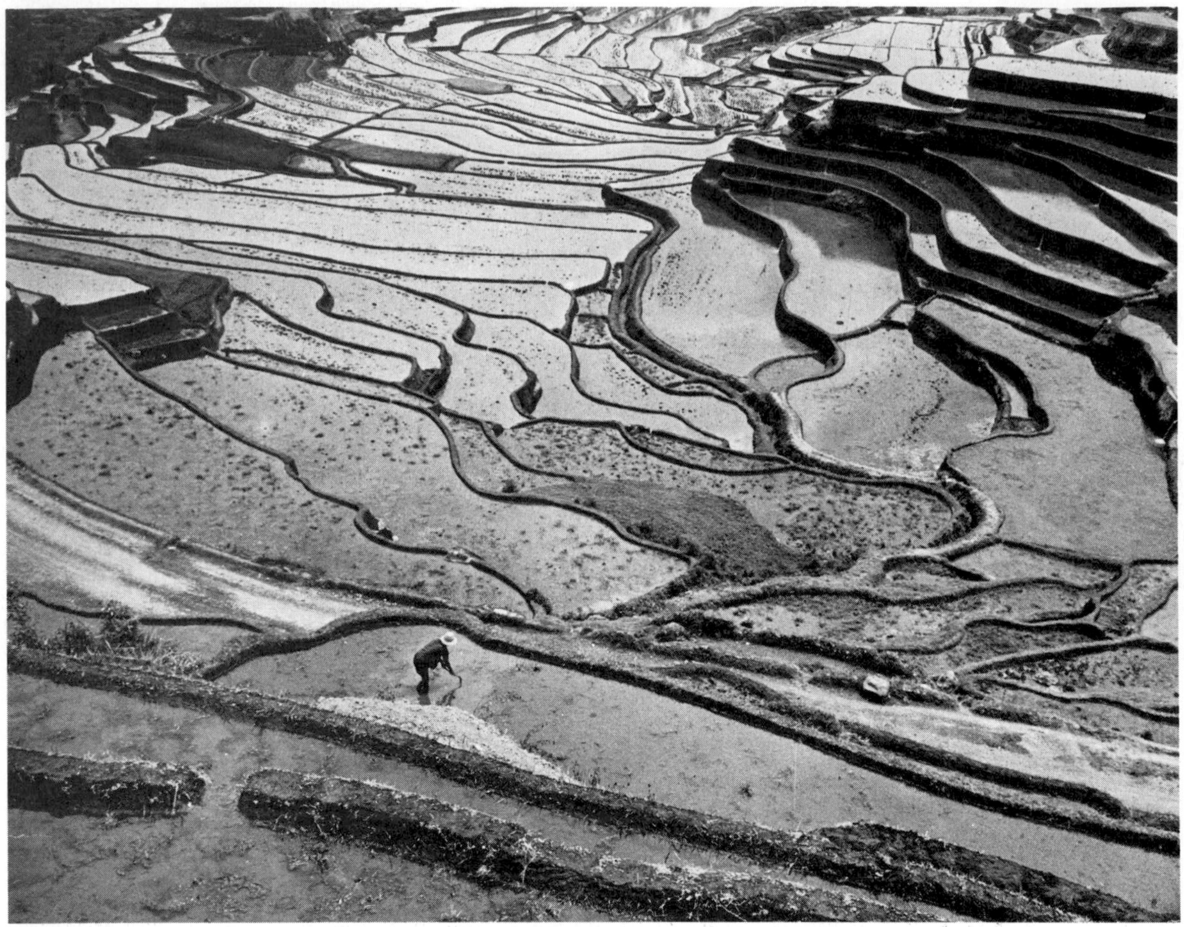

In Indonesia rice is grown on flat terraces cut into the hillside in such a way that a low wall of earth prevents water runoff. (George Holton/Photo Researchers)

reason to look forward to spring with its availability of fresh vegetables. Ways to preserve crops have developed where the growing season is generally short, usually in the cooler, temperate climates. This practical consideration has resulted in canned and pickled fruits and vegetables, dried fruits and beans, English marmalade, Korean kim-chee (pickled cabbage), and American Indian pemmican.

The seasons also affect human needs for certain kinds of foods. For example, sunlight acts on a chemical in the skin to produce vitamin D. In sunny seasons, people spend more time outdoors, and receive more sunlight, reducing their need for vitamin D from food sources. Similarly, climate affects other nutrient requirements. Hot weather diminishes the appetite but, because of excessive perspiration, may increase the need for dietary salt and fluid. Natural disasters—floods, storms, and droughts—also affect the availability and consumption of foods. Drought in the Sahel region of Africa produced widespread famine during the early 1970s. Unfavorable weather conditions in our own country frequently limit the output of farms and orchards and affect the taste, quality, and cost of produce.

TECHNOLOGICAL, ECONOMIC, AND POLITICAL FACTORS. Changing seasons exert other, less direct influences on food consumption. After harvest season, for instance, when many farm workers become unemployed, their limited income and purchasing power alters the quantity and type of food they and their families consume. This illustrates one aspect of the range of economic and technological factors that determine human food behaviors.

Whereas lower animals must accept the natural conditions in which they find themselves, humans have developed the technology to modify their environment in order to increase the production and availability of food. In fact, the tools created by early humans and the development of animal husbandry and agriculture provide the terms—"stone age," "iron age"—by which prehistoric periods are broadly described.

In our own time, *agricultural advances* in irrigation, crop rotation, fertilization, and cultivation have increased crop yields, even while the amount of land being farmed has decreased. Modern methods of *transportation* enable us to move food products across difficult terrain and over large distances in a time brief enough to ensure freshness and wholesomeness when they reach the marketplace. While inhabitants of the Peruvian highlands never receive fish from their coastal countrymen, the most land-locked residents of central United States can feast on seafood from both coasts throughout the year. Modern methods of *refrigeration* and *preservation* enable Americans to indulge a taste for almost every variety of food all year long. Because crops are seasonal, and harvests bring more food than can be consumed immediately, these storage techniques circumvent a "feast or famine" situation.

As our previously agricultural society has become a technological one of large "agribusinesses" and food processing plants, significant changes in food choices and food preferences have taken place. When settlers first arrived in the New World, their dietary staples expanded to include corn, squash, deer, wild turkey and other fowl, fish, cranberries, potatoes, nuts, and a few other locally indigenous foods. Trading ships irregularly supplied expensive tea and spices and a few other luxuries.

By the time our country was founded in 1776, well-to-do colonials were enjoying cultivated crops and readily available imports. Thomas Jefferson, for example, popularized such delicacies as ice cream and French fried potatoes, recipes he brought back from his frequent European travels. Of course, the average person was limited to locally grown foods simply prepared. Today, 200 years later, even average Americans enjoy ice cream and French fries. Whereas only travelers ate outside the home in 1776, by 1976 approximately two million meals per day were served in restaurants. And new, "invented" foods, such as instant pudding, frozen yogurt, and processed cheese, enter our diets almost daily.

Despite our booming technology, nutritious foods are by no means universally available throughout our society. Ready-to-heat TV dinners have little value to the family without a refrigerator or an oven. Poverty sharply restricts the variety and quality of foods available for consumption and ultimately results in a vicious cycle of poor health. Lack of money decreases availability of nutritious food and access to health care, which increases the risk of illness, thus beginning an unfortunate progression: poor health ⟶ decreased work capacity ⟶ loss of income ⟶ decreased purchasing power ⟶ decreased food intake ⟶ worsened nutritional and physical health ⟶ further decrease in work capacity.

The political arena very much influences such socioeconomic food problems. In 1977, about $5.7 billion was expended for the federal food stamp program. Such programs are designed to increase the availability of nourishing and adequate food. Of course, mere availability is no guarantee that individuals will select nutritious diets. A recent survey of hundreds of food-stamp shoppers, however, indicated that, by and large, nutritional foods were frequently chosen, except by the elderly. (*CNI Weekly Report*, 1/5/78).

Government policies have a more directly measurable effect on nutrition during wars and national disasters. Government rationing of available food, ravaging of agricultural land by battle or natural forces, and shift of workers to armed services or disaster relief work all severely limit the food supply. Government influences on the price and availability of food can be seen in peacetime, too. Food supplies increase with government subsidies to farmers; incentives to improve productivity; and credit systems that permit purchases of seed, equipment, and fertilizers. Conversely, government stockpiling of surplus goods, price supports, and foreign commodity sales increase prices and decrease food availability. The consequences of government influence became apparent in this country when sales of surplus wheat to the Soviet Union in 1972 decreased our own supply, thus driving bread prices up to record highs. Consumer actions affect price and supply too: when meat prices rose sharply in 1973, shoppers boycotted meat. Unfortunately, boycotts and cost-conscious shopping tend to impair nutrition particularly among the "nutritionally naive." In one study, researchers found that when food purchases were influenced mainly by cost, the quality of the family diet declined significantly (Schafer, 1978).

Finally, any discussion of technological and economic influences on food choices that did not mention the mass media would be incomplete. Advertising messages on television and radio, and in newspapers and magazines, tell us what is available for consumption and why we should consume it. These messages add a new layer of meaning to each food choice, a meaning relevant not to our nutritional needs, but to our psychosocial needs.

PSYCHOLOGICAL FACTORS. Food nourishes the body and the psyche. While our physiological needs ensure that we eat, our psychological needs determine to a large extent what we choose to eat. Frequently, the choice has little to do with the actual properties of food itself. Instead, food becomes a symbol laden with social and emotional meaning.

Emotional response to food begins on the day of birth. The hungry infant learns to associate food with relief of bodily discomfort, with the warmth of a parent's arm, and with the contented sleep that follows each feeding. Eating soon becomes associated with care, attention, and love. Unfortunately, in adulthood these associations can interfere with good nutrition. Food can become a substitute for emotional gratification or affection. When sleep is elusive, the midnight snack beckons. Reliance on food as a source of emotional satisfaction may result in overweight or obesity. Both overeating and excessive dieting are sometimes used to gain attention.

Food satisfies in many ways. The sensory pleasure associated with food—its appearance, aroma, and taste—do much to ensure that we eat varied dishes in quantities sufficient to meet our nutritional needs. Food fulfills valuable nonnutritional needs, too. Participation in cooking and the artistic creation of dishes are excellent opportunities for self-expression. Slicing, pounding, mixing, and kneading may be good emotional outlets. Careful meal planning satisfies other human needs—the need to care for oneself and to nurture others. Family and personal rituals concerning meals give order and stability to daily life. Even fad diets and health food fanaticism, in leading to predictable food choices, give their adherents a sense of stability (Schafer and Yetley, 1975).

We use food as a reward ("When I finish studying this chapter, I'll have a pizza"), as a punishment ("You didn't eat your vegetables, so you can't have dessert"), and especially as a medical panacea ("Have some chicken soup"). A few years ago a food writer for a major New York City newspaper devoted a column to the foods that were served to her as a child when she was sick and for which she still yearns. All of us can recall foods and even aromas that have a special association of gratification for us.

SOCIAL AND CULTURAL FACTORS. Social aspects of food and nutrition are tied to cultural heritage. A **culture** consists of the patterned sets of reactions, the ways of life learned by and characteristic of a particular group of people. A group with a distinctive culture is a **society**; a society may be a nation, an ethnic group, a village, or a tribe. Societies are defined not by size or complexity but by shared traditions and ways of life. Within a large and complex society, such as our own nation, however, many subcultures with different customs may exist.

All human behavior is influenced by the culture in which the individual is born and brought up, or socialized. While individuals are certainly capable of independent thought and action, most of their actions are guided and influenced by the people around them. In most of the world and most of human history, people have tended to dress similarly, live in the same type of housing, and engage in the same occupations and leisure activities as their parents, grandparents, and great-grandparents before them. Even in our ever-changing modern society, much of how we live and what we eat is determined by the lifestyle and cultural history of our own family.

These cultural habits and traditions influence food behavior. In some cultures, such as the Malayan and the traditional Japanese and Chinese, the father and sons receive their food first while the mother and daughters serve meals and eat later. In parts of Africa and the Middle East, the oldest family members are served first, in reverence for their age. Culturally recognized superstitions and taboos also influence food behavior. Certain Latin-American cultures classify red meats and eggs as "hot foods," unhealthy for children and pregnant women. Though we recognize the potential nutritional harm of this practice, it is adhered to with great conviction by many Latin Americans even after they have migrated to North America (Gifft et al., 1972). Some plants and animals that are considered edible by one group may not be eaten by others, although the plant or animal may be in plentiful supply. In our own culture, who would eat a dog or a cat? However nutritious and plentiful such animals might be, they are considered pets. Eating them would be, for us, like eating our relatives or friends.

Cultural practices and beliefs often follow a kind of "folk logic," which relates food colors and other attributes to their effects in the human body (Shifflett, 1976). For example, Madagascar warriors would not eat ox knees, because the knee joints of oxen are weak, and they feared that their own joints might weaken. Conversely, some foods are eaten in hopes that their qualities will indeed affect the consumer. Some American Indians eat the flesh of certain animals in order to acquire the attributes of those species.

Many religions involve food in rituals or place limitations on the uses of foods. Religious food practices are due to social, economic, and other conditions of long ago.The prohibition against eating pork in Jewish dietary laws has often been ascribed to the health risk of consuming undercooked pork. Historians point out, however, that Egyptians of the nineteenth and twentieth dynasties (about 1341–1085 B.C.) ate great quantities of pork, with no apparent detriment to their health; that the connection between pork and trichinosis was not made until the nineteenth century; and that this disease did not appear on the African continent until our own century (Grivetti and Pangborn, 1974). Another explanation is that the prohibition arose at the time of the Exodus to separate those of Jewish culture from their oppressors, the Egyptians, who at that time not only ate pork but also used it in their sacrificial rites. Modern Egyptians, being Muslims, now share the prohibition against eating pork that originated with the ancient Hebrews. Another explanation for this prohibition is ecologically based. According to anthropologist Marvin Harris, pigs could not be raised efficiently in the hot and arid climate of the Middle East desert regions for a variety of practical reasons. Sheep were much better suited to the **ecosystem** of the ancient Israelites. Thus the keeping of pigs, being both economically and socially unsound, was prohibited (Harris, 1974).

Harris also presents an ecological explanation for another of the best-known religious food taboos—the Hindu prohibition against eating beef. India is a land where cattle are plentiful, yet they are not eaten by devout Hindus and are considered sacred. The cattle native to India are hardy and have an ability to survive on waste products and during drought. These cattle are useful as work animals and valued as producers of dung, which is dried and used for fuel for cooking and heating in this otherwise fuelless land (Harris, 1974).

Other religious food practices have been given other types of explanations. Eating eggs at Easter, for example, is a logical development of the long association of eggs with birth and the continuity of species and, therefore, a symbol of the awakened fertility of the earth in springtime (Shifflett, 1976). The communion wine and wafer of Christianity recall Jewish rituals of blessing bread and wine as symbols of the earth's bounty, given new symbolism as representations of Christ. Buddhists donate food to monks and other holy men in India and Burma as acts of obeisance to the will of Buddha. In Zen Buddhist monasteries, where the cook is almost as important as the Zen master or religious teacher, the right combinations of vegetables and rice are believed to enhance meditation. Food offerings are given to ancestors in Africa, the Pacific, and many other regions; if the living remember the dead, the dead will remember the living.

The social symbolism given to some foods bears little relationship to logic or to the objective attributes of those foods. For example, bread made with

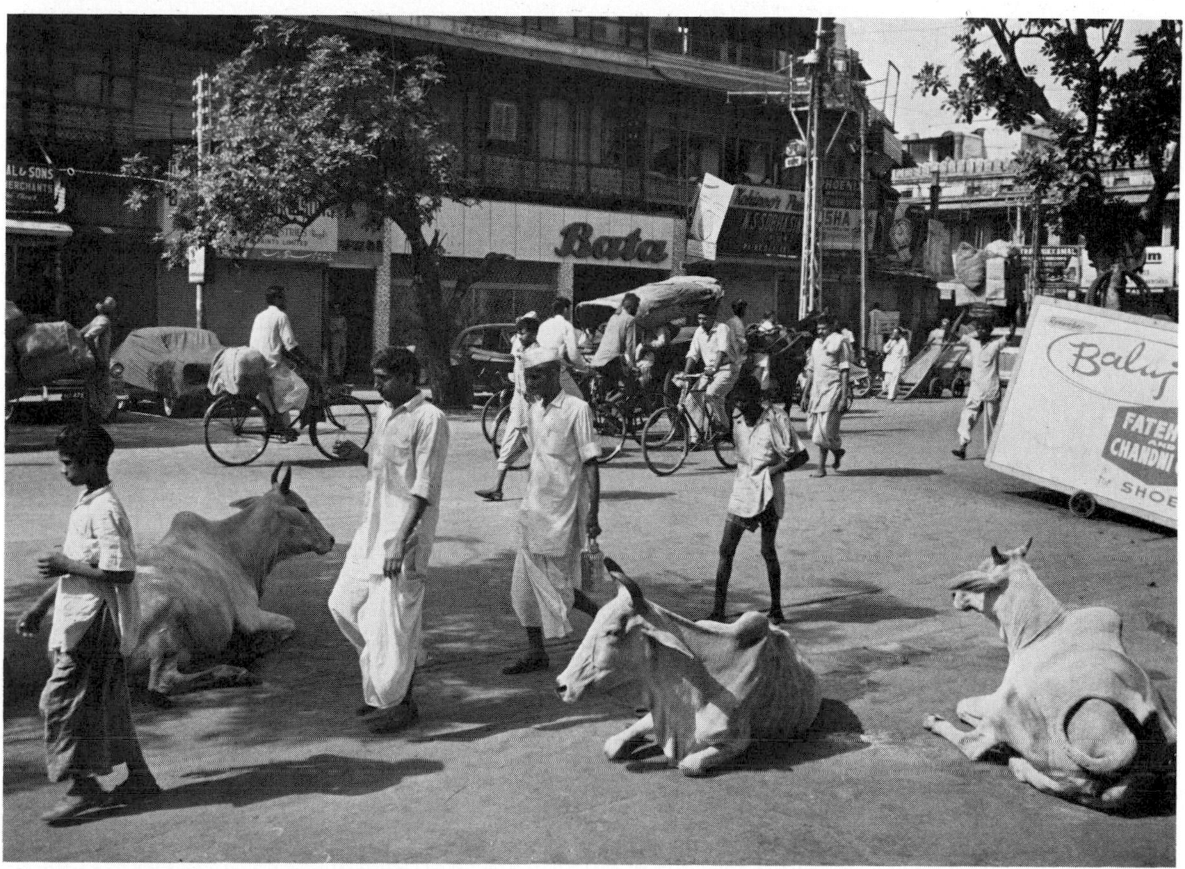

The hardy sacred cows of India wander undisturbed. Here they sit in a Delhi street as people and traffic move around them. (Paul Conklin/Monkmeyer)

bleached white flour and white sugar was a sign of status in the nineteenth century because it was scarce and expensive, and because the poor ate black bread and molasses. Today, white bread has lost status among certain segments of American society because of its ordinariness and bland taste, while dark whole-grain breads have become status foods for "gourmet" and "health" reasons. Of course, advertisers continuously try to convince us that other foods have prestige value, too, as they promote an "expensive spread" or "the taste of luxury." They have created "fun foods" as well: soft drinks ("join the Pepsi generation") and chewing gum ("double your pleasure, double your fun").

While some culturally and socially determined food preferences are harmful, some tradition-based food stereotypes may, in fact, show good nutritional sense. For example, peanut butter sandwiches are often demeaned as "kids' food," but they are excellent sources of the **protein** and energy, as well as other nutrients, needed by growing children. The rice and beans or beans and pasta combinations that used to be thought "starchy" have been shown to be excellent sources of protein—far better than when each is eaten alone. Again, meat and potatoes are often called "masculine foods," in contrast to "feminine foods" such as salads and vegetables.

Research has shown that despite, or perhaps because of, our psychosocial needs, most Americans eat a well-balanced diet. In two studies, investigators found that the family, and specifically the wife and mother, who in most families still bears the primary responsibility for shopping and cooking, is the most important influence on good nutrition. The earlier study reported that advertising was the least influential factor in food choice, being far outweighed by personal preferences and the belief that certain food "is good for you" (Cosper and Wakefield, 1975). In the second study, homemakers who indicated that nutrition education programs had influenced their meal planning did indeed tend to serve better-quality diets than other food preparers (Schafer, 1978).

While these studies say much about family eating habits, what happens to youngsters when they leave the family fold? Do the habits learned at home carry over to the outside world? Do the food practices of college students, for example, reflect their previous eating habits, or are students so involved with academic work and extracurricular activities that they do not make an effort to meet their nutritional needs?

According to two recent studies, there is good news for college students—and their concerned parents. Students, on the whole, have a firm knowledge of good nutrition and meet or exceed the recommended dietary allowances for most nutrients (Stasch et al., 1970; Jakobovits et al., 1977). When researchers compared the nutritional habits of today's college women with those of 30 years ago, they were pleasantly surprised to find that the meal-skipping, snacking, and fad diets attributed to college students in recent years have obviously not been detrimental, and a high level of consciousness of the principles of good nutrition was noted (Jakobovits et al., 1977). However, although the groups studied were in good nutritional condition, some individuals may be less well nourished. Meal skipping and fad diets are definitely ill advised.

This study, of course, does not imply that there have been no significant changes in general American dietary habits during that 30-year period. As indicated in Figure 1-1, the United States Department of Agriculture has identified several nutritional trends in this century. While consumption of meat, poultry, fruits and vegetables has increased notably in the last 30 years, the consumption of cereal products and eggs has declined (Gortner, 1976). The ups and downs of these curves indicate how much our diets are affected by current events and by research. The increase in fruit and vegetable consumption in the early 1940s probably resulted from both the government's encouraging of "victory gardens" while meat and canned goods were rationed, and from the publication of the first nutrition guidelines in the form of recommended allowances for several nutrients. Decreased egg consumption in the 1950s followed widespread publicity given to the scientific finding that an elevated level of **cholesterol** in blood was associated with heart disease; eggs are rich in cholesterol. An increase in potato consumption during the 1960s has been linked to the appearance of dried, instant, and frozen potato products. The popularity of "burger 'n' fries" fast food establishments has helped to maintain this upswing.

FIGURE 1-1 Trends in Consumption in the United States in the Twentieth Century. Source: Data from U.S. Department of Agriculture, Economic Research Service, 1968. Food Consumption, Prices, Expenditures, Agr. Econ. Rept. No. 138 and Supplement for 1975. USDA, Washington, D.C.

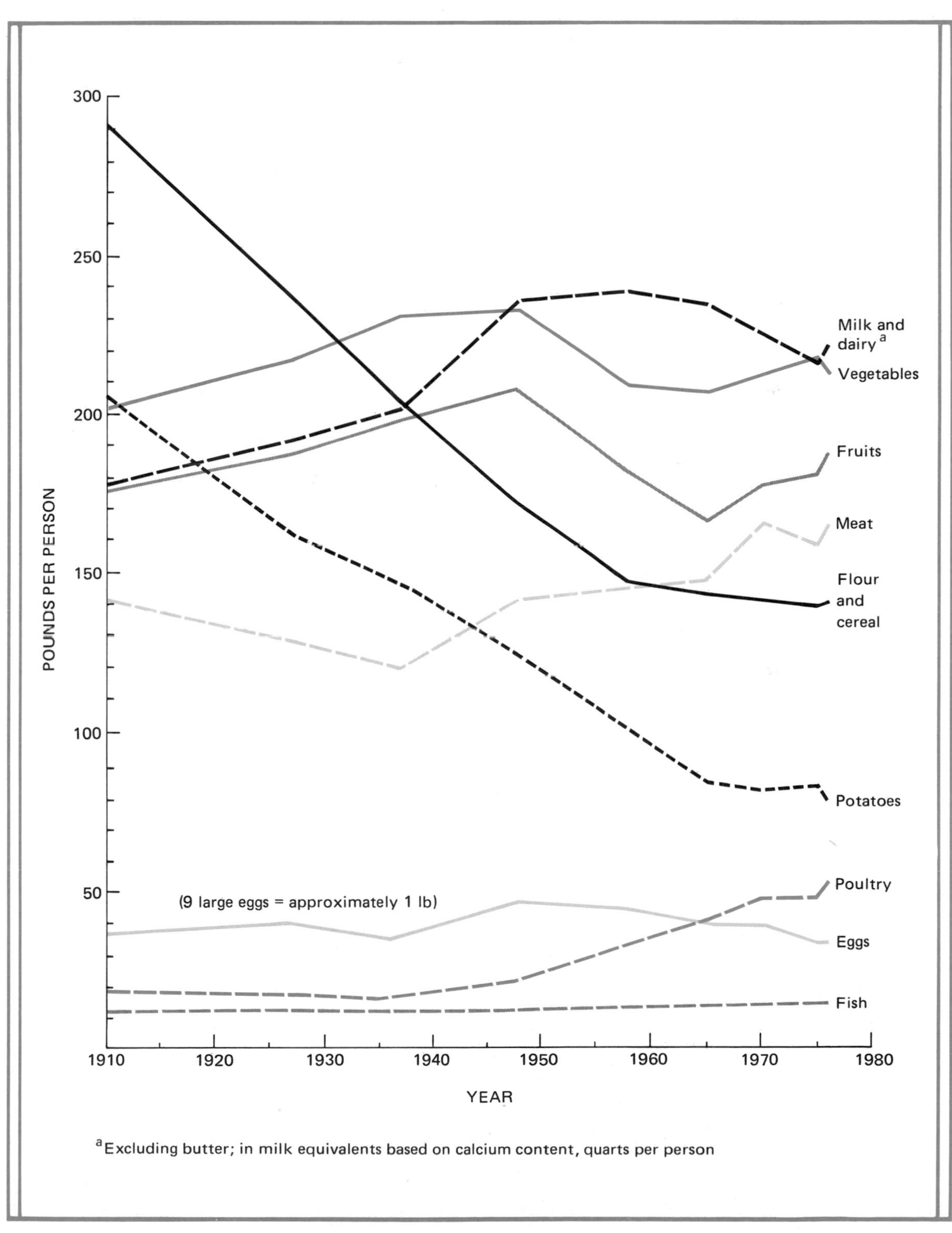

[a]Excluding butter; in milk equivalents based on calcium content, quarts per person

THE INTERNAL ENVIRONMENT

The impact of foods taken in from the external environment depends largely on what happens in the internal environment of the body. This concept of an internal environment and its relationship to food and nutritional health is aptly summarized by the familiar phrase, "Food is not food until it is eaten." In order to understand how food is utilized inside our bodies, we must first consider some basic concepts of chemistry and human biology.

Atoms and Molecules

Chemistry is the study of the composition, structure, and properties of matter, the changes that matter undergoes, and the energy associated with each of these changes. **Matter** is anything that occupies space and has mass or weight, from a drop of water, to a hamburger, to a cow. **Energy** is the capacity to do work; heat, electricity, and movement are familiar forms of energy.

FIGURE 1-2
Hydrogen and Carbon Atoms

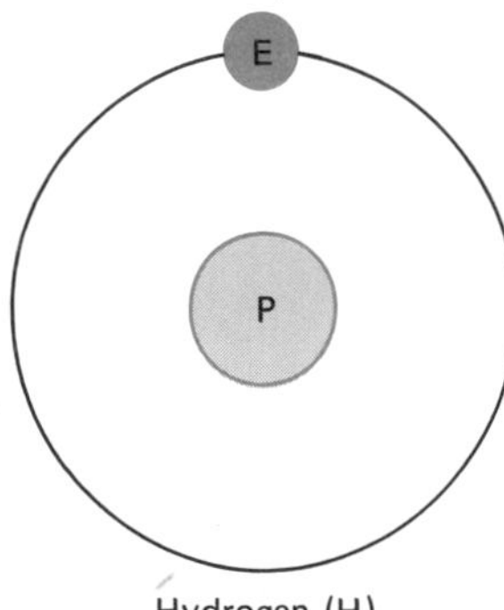

Hydrogen (H)

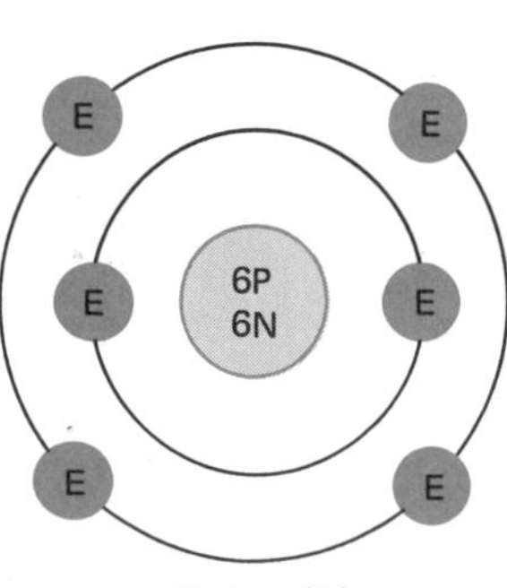

Carbon (C)

The basic building blocks of all kinds of matter—liquid, solid, and gas—are called **atoms.** Although atoms are exceedingly small, they are nevertheless quite complex. Atoms have a central core or **nucleus,** which contains particles with a positive electrical charge, **protons,** and neutral particles having no electrical charge, **neutrons.** Revolving around the nucleus like planets around the sun are negatively charged particles, **electrons.** Any atom—whether it is an atom of metal such as iron, or of a gas such as oxygen—contains the same number of protons as electrons, creating a balance between the positively charged protons and the negatively charged electrons.

The very smallest atom in existence consists of just one proton and one electron, with no neutrons. It is the hydrogen atom (Figure 1-2). Being the smallest, it is also the lightest, weighing only 1.67×10^{-24} grams. It is difficult to work with complex numbers such as this, so scientists have devised a system of atomic weights in which hydrogen is assigned a weight of 1, for its single proton. Because an electron has a mass only $1/_{1,836}$ as large as a proton, its extremely small contribution is disregarded in all calculations of atomic weight. Neutrons, however, have approximately the same mass as protons.

Atoms have a tendency to "lose" and "gain" electrons, thus disrupting their electrical balance or neutrality. When a hydrogen atom, for example, loses its single electron, we say it has an electrical charge of +1. Any charged atom is called an **ion.** A positively charged ion, one which has lost an electron or electrons, is a **cation.** A negatively charged atom, which has gained an electron or electrons, is an **anion.**

The physical properties of matter, such as taste, odor, color, and weight depend upon the composition and arrangement of atoms. Any physical change in matter, such as the melting of ice into liquid water, does not change the composition of its atoms. Other types of changes in matter, called chemical changes, involve rearrangement of atoms. Such rearrangements depend upon the ability of atoms to share electrons. This sharing is known as covalent **bonding.**

Hydrogen	
proton 1	1
electron 1	1
atomic weight	1

Carbon	
protons	6
neutrons	6
electrons	6
atomic weight	12

Iron	
protons	26
neutrons	30
electrons	26
atomic weight	56

A substance composed of only one kind of atom, such as oxygen, iron, and calcium, is called an **element.** When atoms of any one element bond together, the result is a **molecule** of that element. We speak of molecules of oxygen, for example. When atoms of two or more different elements combine, the resulting molecule is a **compound.** Some well-known examples are water, made up of hydrogen and oxygen atoms (see Figure 1-3), and sugar, made up of hydrogen, oxygen, and carbon atoms. A molecule is the smallest particle of any distinct substance, either an element or a compound.

CHEMICAL NOTATION AND BONDING. Only 103 elements have been identified on our planet. Their various combinations, however, produce hundreds of thousands of compounds. Table 1-1 lists the elements that are of greatest interest to the study of nutrition. Note that each element is represented by a **chemical symbol** which chemists use in describing reactions between elements, molecules, and compounds.

A symbol or group of symbols which represents the composition of an element or compound is known as a **chemical formula.** For example, the chemical formula for common table salt is NaCl, representing the bonding of one *atom* of sodium, and one *atom* of chlorine, into one *molecule* of sodium chloride. This bonding is expressed by the **chemical equation:**

$$Na + Cl \longrightarrow NaCl$$

To take another example:

$$4H + C \longrightarrow CH_4$$

That is, four atoms of hydrogen plus one atom of carbon yields one molecule of methane.

By convention, chemical equations are written with the reactants (**substrates**) to the left of the arrow, and the products to the right. Also by convention, no coefficient is indicated when only one atom or molecule of a substance is used or produced. However, when more than one atom or molecule is a reactant or a product, a coefficient is written in front of the

TABLE 1-1
Elements Most Important to the Study of Nutrition

Symbol	Element	Symbol	Element
H	Hydrogen	K	Potassium
C	Carbon	Mn	Manganese
N	Nitrogen	Fe	Iron
O	Oxygen	Co	Cobalt
Ca	Calcium	Ni	Nickel
Na	Sodium	Cu	Copper
Mg	Magnesium	Zn	Zinc
P	Phosphorus	I	Iodine
S	Sulfur	F	Fluorine
Cl	Chlorine	Se	Selenium
		Cr	Chromium

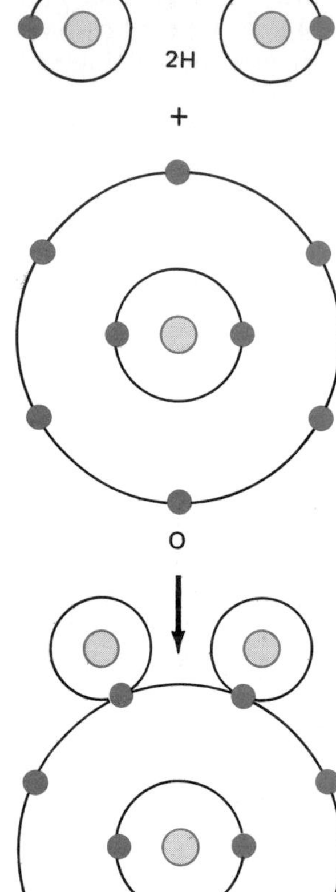

FIGURE 1-3
Water Molecule
Two atoms of hydrogen combine with one atom of oxygen to form a water molecule.

appropriate symbol, as in the four hydrogen atoms above. Subscripts are used to indicate the number of atoms in any particular compound. As with coefficients, no subscript is used if only one atom is involved. Thus, one molecule of methane (CH_4) consists of one atom of carbon and four atoms of hydrogen.

Chemical reactions involve covalent bonding, which is a sharing of electrons. Chemists have developed yet another shorthand system to describe these bonds. It is based on pictorial diagrams representing the outermost ring of electrons in a particular atom. This outer ring, known as the **valence shell,** contains the electrons that are shared in chemical bonds. Carbon, for example, with four electrons in its outermost ring, can share four additional electrons and thus has a valence of 4. It is represented as:

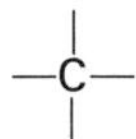

Hydrogen has a valence of 1:

H—

Oxygen has a valence of 2:

—O—

Nitrogen usually has a valence of 3:

```
|
N—
|
```

In a *stable compound,* each of the available electrons is shared, or bonded. Thus, when carbon combines with other elements to form a stable compound, each carbon atom has four chemical bonds.

The bonding of carbon atoms is central to the study of nutrition. In fact, of all the 103 known elements, this one has proven so important that its compounds have been given a science of their own, **organic chemistry.** The number of carbon compounds known today exceeds the number of compounds prepared from all the other 102 elements.

Carbon compounds, usually called organic compounds, are composed of carbon atoms bonded to one another to form what are known as chains and rings. **Hydrocarbons** are the simplest organic compounds, containing only hydrogen and carbons. Methane is a simple example:

```
   H
   |
H—C—H
   |
   H
```

The bonding requirements for both carbon (valence 4) and hydrogen (valence 1) are met in this compound. In more complicated bonding, forms of hydro-

Some Nutritionally Important Functional Groups

Alcohol	$-\overset{\vert}{\underset{\vert}{C}}-OH$
Aldehyde	$-\overset{O}{\overset{\Vert}{C}}-H$
Ketone	$-\overset{O}{\overset{\Vert}{C}}-$
Acid	$-\overset{O}{\overset{\Vert}{C}}-O-H$

A grouping of atoms that imparts characteristic properties to a molecule and to the reactions in which it takes part is known as a **functional group.** Many organic compounds are classified according to their functional group or groups. The double lines connecting the carbon atoms with other atoms in these groups represent a double bond, which is the sharing of two electron pairs.

carbons are produced through the replacement of one or more hydrogen atoms by **functional groups** of atoms. Certain functional groups are particularly important in nutritional compounds, and they will become very familiar in the chapters that follow.

All the foods we eat contain carbon compounds. While their chemical names may be unfamiliar, their everyday names are common household words:

- **Carbohydrates** (sugars and starches) are organic molecules containing C, H, and O, and occasionally N and S.
- **Proteins** are organic molecules containing C, H, O, N and sometimes S.
- **Lipids** (or fats) are organic molecules containing C, H, O, and sometimes N or P.
- **Vitamins** are organic molecules containing C, H, O, and sometimes N, S, and Co.

These four classes of organic compounds present in foods are known as **nutrients.** Vitamins and minerals required in trace amounts are also known as **micronutrients.** Carbohydrates, proteins, and lipids are considered **macronutrients.** Also considered as nutrients are inorganic molecules, such as Na, K, P, S, Ca, Fe, and other elements, better known as the **minerals,** and of **water,** which is a compound of H and O.

Our discussions of nutrition will focus on the composition, structure, and properties of these nutrients and on the changes they undergo, both inside and outside the body. This section should have prepared you to deal with nutrition as a *chemical* science. In the next section, you will learn that nutrition is also a *biological* science.

Organization of the Body

Your body and the foods you eat are made up of atoms and molecules. The process of nutrition involves the transformation of atoms and molecules present in food into the kind of atoms and molecules that make up the body. This transformation occurs inside the cells of all animal bodies.

Cells are the basic structural units ("building blocks") of any living organism. Each cell is like a miniature factory, which processes nutrients for energy, growth, and performance of its particular body-regulating function. Although there is no such thing as a "typical" cell, a representative one can be described, as shown in Figure 1-4.

The body is a highly organized system containing many types of cells, each specifically structured to fulfill a particular function. There are skin (epithelial) cells, blood cells (erythrocytes or red cells and leucocytes or white cells), nerve cells (neurons), fat cells (adipocytes), bone cells (osteocytes), and muscle cells. (Note that the suffix "-cyte" identifies many cells.) Cells are organized into **tissues**—muscle tissue, epithelial (skin) tissue, adipose (fat) tissue, bone tissue, nerve tissue—which, in turn, are organized into **organs**—the digestive

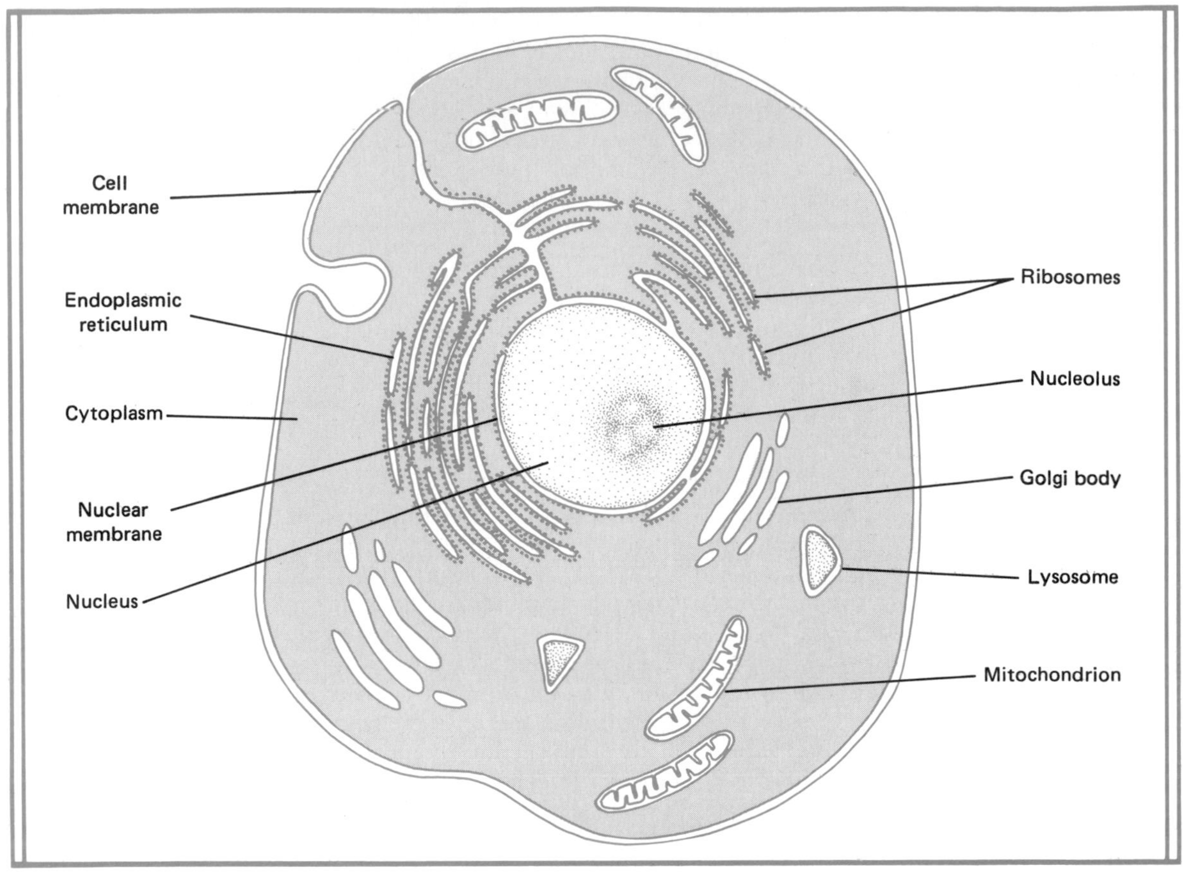

FIGURE 1-4
A Cell

Most cells (with insignificant exceptions) contain the same components or **organelles.**

The cell is enclosed by a double **plasma membrane,** a layered protein-lipid-protein sandwich that determines the shape of the cell and regulates the passage of materials into and out of it. The membrane is filled with a viscous fluid called **cytoplasm.** Cytoplasm provides an optimum environment for the organelles, in which the life functions of the cell are performed.

Within the cytoplasm is a cluster of material, the **nucleus,** which is the "brain" or control center of the cell. In the nucleus are **chromosomes** of deoxyribonucleic acid (DNA), the genetic material that carries the information necessary to create a complete new individual. DNA, which always remains in the nucleus of the cell, determines all cell activities by programming the synthesis of ribonucleic acids (RNA) which can move out of the nucleus to the cytoplasm, where they directly control cellular function. Other RNAs remain in the nucleus, located in a small body, the **nucleolus.**

Mitochondria (singular: *mitochondrion*) are the "powerhouses" of the cell. Mitochondria are responsible for the many chemical reactions related to energy production inside each cell. Some busy cells may contain thousands of mitochondria.

Endoplasmic reticulum is the name given to the system of membranous channels that transport materials throughout the cell. Endoplasmic reticulum (ER) with ribosomes (see below) around its outer surface is referred to as rough ER. Smooth ER has no ribosomes.

Ribosomes are small granules composed of protein and nucleic acid. Some ribosomes float free in the cytoplasm, others are bound to the endoplasmic reticulum. Protein synthesis occurs on the ribosomes.

Golgi bodies make up the system of intracellular membranes contiguous with the ER. Their function is the packaging and storage of various products that the cell will eventually secrete.

Lysosomes are membrane-bound vesicles that contain the enzymes that break down intracellular products and debris.

TABLE 1-2
Distribution of Elements in the Human Body, Percent Body Weight

Element	%	Element	%	Element	%
Oxygen	65.00	Sulfur	0.25000	Iodine	0.0001
Carbon	18.00	Sodium	0.15000	Fluorine	0.0001
Hydrogen	10.00	Chlorine	0.15000	Silicon	0.0001
Nitrogen	3.00	Magnesium	0.05000	Copper	0.0001
Calcium	2.00	Iron	0.00400	Cobalt	0.0001
Phosphorus	1.10	Zinc	0.00020		
Potassium	0.35	Manganese	0.00013		

organs—esophagus, stomach, small intestine, large intestine, pancreas, gall bladder, liver—and others such as the heart, brain, lungs, and reproductive organs. Organs may contain primarily one type of tissue, or they may be a functionally organized collection of several tissue types.

Several organs with related functions together make up larger **organ systems;** for example, the skeletal, respiratory, reproductive, nervous, circulatory, and digestive systems. The integrated product of all these functioning organ systems is, of course, the **organism.**

The organism, with all its component parts, consists entirely of atoms and molecules of chemical elements. Looking at the distribution of elements within the body (Table 1-2), we can see that carbon, oxygen, hydrogen, and nitrogen comprise about 96 percent of body weight. Other elements account for the rest, with the mineral calcium being by far the most abundant.

Anatomy and Physiology of Digestion

Digestion is the mechanical and chemical process by which food is prepared for absorption. Nutrients are absorbed into the circulatory system, which transports them to all the cells of the body.

Obviously, chunks of meat, potatoes, and vegetables don't just float around in the body after a meal. Foods cannot be used without digestion and conversion into simpler substances that can pass through the cells of the small intestine (intestinal mucosa) and then into the blood or lymph. For example, digestion transforms proteins into smaller units known as amino acids, fats into fatty acids and monoglycerides, and starch into glucose.

The transformation of food requires both mechanical and enzymatic means. Both begin in the mouth, as food is chewed and mixed with saliva, meeting the first of many **enzymes** that facilitate its chemical breakdown. Enzymes are specialized protein molecules that catalyze chemical reactions; that is, enzymes speed up the rate of chemical reactions, although they themselves are not part of the product of the reaction. Enzymes increase the rate of chemical reactions by lowering the energy level required to drive these reactions. Enzymes are very specific: Each enzyme can catalyze only one type of reaction. Thus, each of the many chemical reactions occurring in the body employs a different, specialized enzyme. All enzymes can be reused. Some need to be replaced more quickly than others, however.

An enzyme can be visualized as a molecule having specific sites to accept a specific substrate, thereby making the substrate more chemically reactive. As

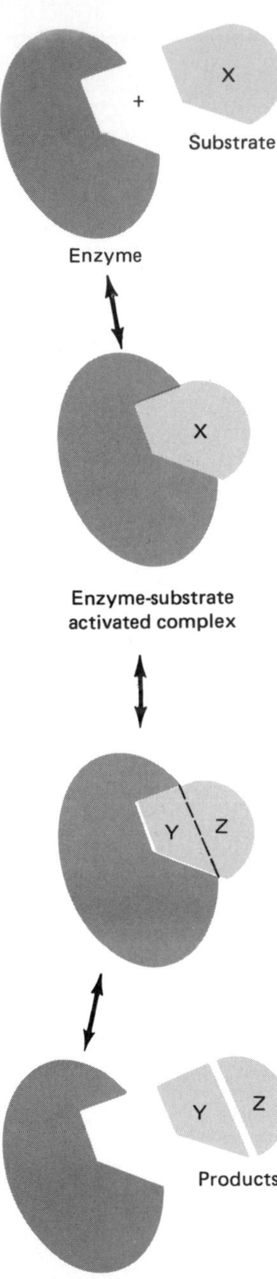

FIGURE 1-5
Model of Enzyme
An enzyme combines with a substrate (the substance to undergo the reaction). A product is produced, after which the enzyme (unchanged) can be used again.

illustrated in Figure 1-5, an enzyme can change compound X into compounds Y and Z, without being changed itself.

Some of the many enzymes of the **digestive system** are manufactured (synthesized) in the cells of the salivary glands (amylase), pancreas (lipase), stomach (pepsin), and small intestine (maltase). (Note that the suffix "-ase" identifies many enzymes.) A complete explanation of the digestive enzymes and their reactions will follow in later chapters. For now, let us examine the digestive system diagrammed in Figure 1-6. The transformation of food begins with mechanical breakdown by the teeth. The mixture of chewed food and saliva (called a bolus) next moves to the **esophagus.** Rythmic contractions of circular muscles in the wall of the esophagus move the bolus down the esophagus to the stomach by the process of **peristalsis.** In the stomach, powerful contractions churn the food and break up large pieces, maximizing their exposure to *gastric juices,* the mixture of hydrochloric acid and digestive enzymes secreted by glands in the stomach lining. Antacid advertising to the contrary, an acid stomach is quite necessary for digestion. Gastric juices work the food into a soupy fluid called **chyme.**

From the stomach, chyme passes through the pyloric valve into the small intestine for its final processing. Here the presence of chyme stimulates the release of many digestive enzymes from the pancreas and the intestinal glands. Each will act upon different nutrients. Proteins are digested by a combination of several pancreatic and intestinal enzymes. Starch digestion is carried out by pancreatic amylase. Another pancreatic enzyme, lipase, acts to split molecules of fat into monoglycerides and fatty acids. The liver produces a fluid called **bile** that also aids in fat digestion. Bile is stored in the gall bladder and released into the small intestine as needed.

The entire small intestine of an adult is 7 or 8 meters (23 feet) long and 2.54 centimeters (1 inch) in diameter. This substantial length is made effectively even greater by numerous folds and ridges. In addition, the mucous lining of the small intestine is covered with small fingerlike projections called **villi** (singular: *villus*). The villi and their surrounding epithelial cells are, in turn, covered with numerous closely packed cylindrical outgrowths called **microvilli.** The microvilli make up the **brush border.** With all these folds, villi, and microvilli, the total surface area of the small intestine is, as one expert estimated, about as large as half a basketball court (Ingelfinger, 1967). These intestinal cells are in a continuous state of turnover and renewal. In fact, the epithelium of the small intestine has the fastest turnover rate of any tissue in the body (Williamson, 1978). Each villus loses one cell per hour from its tip. Calculating the extrusion from all the villi taken together yields a figure of 20 to 50 million cells per minute that are cast off into the lumen (inner space) of the small intestine (Pike and Brown, 1975).These cells may end up being digested and their contents absorbed or excreted from the body.

Large volumes of water are involved in the digestive process and must be recycled to prevent dehydration. In the large intestine, in the next stage of the absorptive process, water is reabsorbed. The large intestine is continuous with the small intestine at the lower right side of the body (as shown in Figure 1-6); then it ascends to the middle of the abdominal cavity, crosses to the left side, and then descends. This pathway forms three sections, called the *ascending, transverse,* and *descending* colons. From the large intestine, water travels back into the bloodstream, and waste matter passes into the rectum, ready for defecation through the anus.

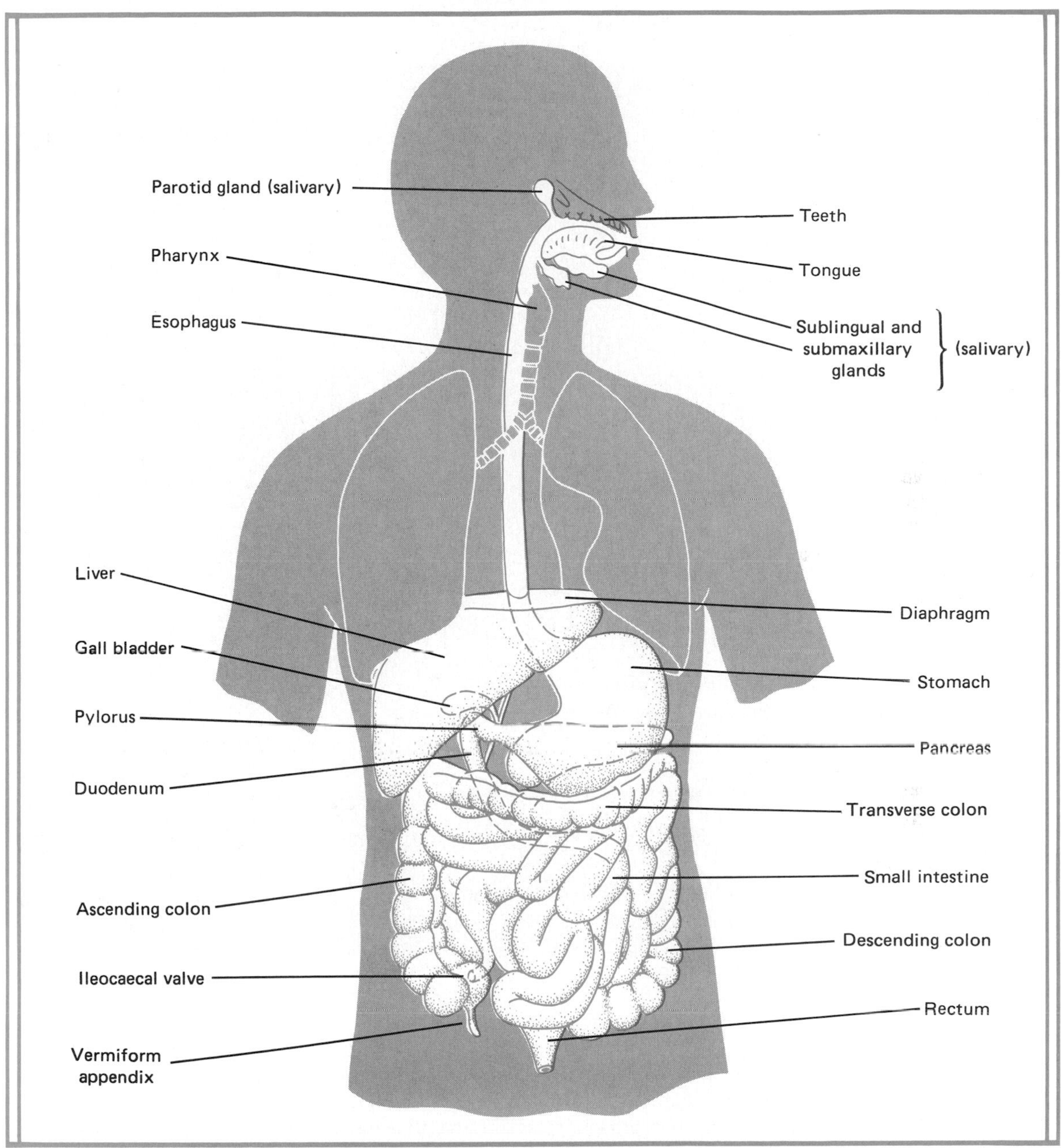

FIGURE 1-6
The Digestive System

ABSORPTION. Digestion is only the beginning of the series of biological events that takes place as food is incorporated into the human body. Eventually, the nutrient materials in some form will reach every cell. Nutrients begin their travels by entering the bloodstream, or circulation, which will carry them to where they are needed. **Absorption** is the passage or transport of digested products into the bloodstream. It occurs in the small intestine and, to a much lesser extent, in the stomach.

Most absorption takes place at the mucosal membrane of the small

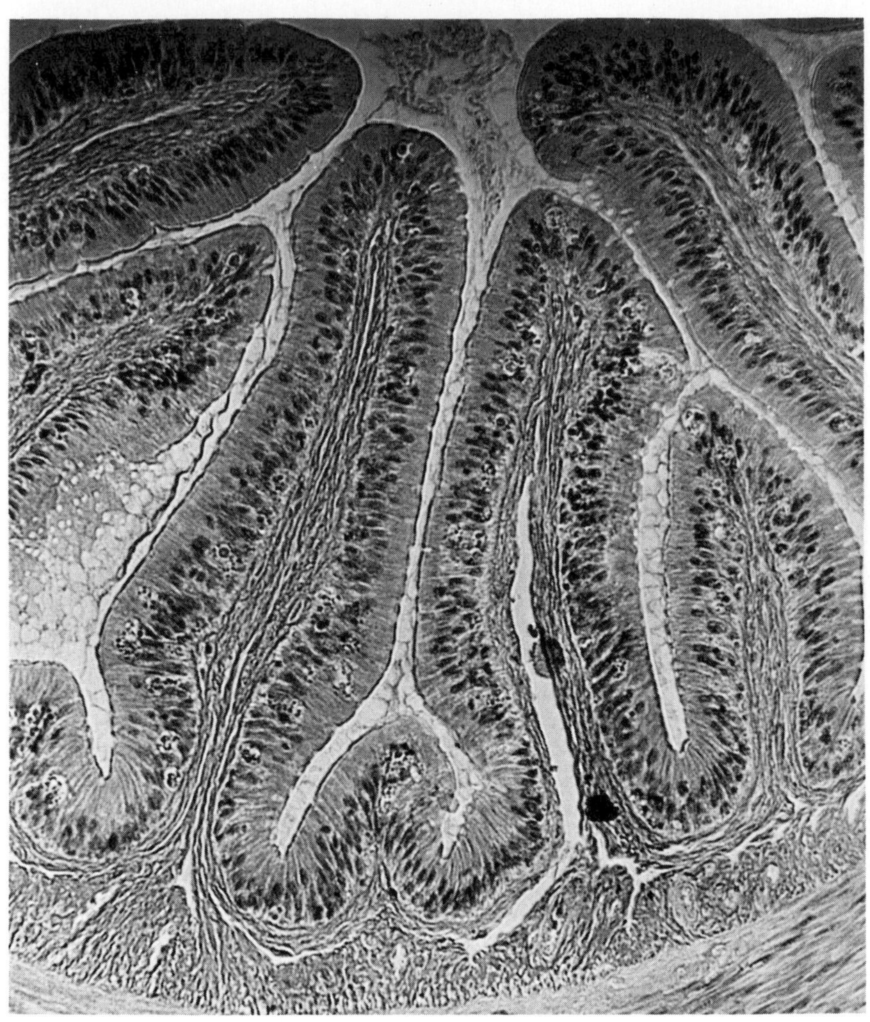

Electron micrograph of a cross section of the small intestine showing the villi. (Photo by Cameron Thatcher from National Audubon Society/ Photo Researchers)

intestine, where the extensive epithelial surface of the villi and microvilli provides a large area to which the nutrients passing through the intestinal lumen are exposed. As you can see in Figure 1-7, the villi are supported by a structure of connective tissue, interlaced with blood vessels and lymph ducts. During absorption, digested nutrients cross the intestinal epithelial layer into the blood vessels and lymph ducts. Because they occupy a central position between the lumen of the small intestine and the blood supply, these epithelial cells act as monitors of what is transported between the two compartments (Ingelfinger, 1967). A variety of transport mechanisms can be broadly classified into *passive* and *active* processes. In one type of **passive transport** thousands of tiny pores in the walls of the microvilli allow water and certain small water-soluble molecules to enter the intestinal cell. Molecules small enough to get through tend to cross the membrane until they are present in equal distribution (concentration) on both sides. In other words, molecules travel from an area of high concentration in the intestinal lumen to an area of lower concentration, until both areas come to have an equal concentration. This passive process is known as **diffusion** down a **concentration gradient.**

You can see diffusion at work if you drop some blue ink into a glass of water. It starts out as a dark, concentrated drop and then slowly diffuses until the water takes on an even, but lighter, blue color. In scientific terms, we say that the ink has diffused from an area of high concentration (the ink drop) to an area of low concentration (the whole glass of water).

The size and shape of epithelial pores are such that only certain molecules can fit through. Many nutrients are chemically unable to flow through these pores. To solve this problem, specific **carrier molecules** combine with these large molecules to permit diffusion through the cell. Transport carriers are proteins that constitute part of the membrane that must be crossed. They can bind themselves to a particular nutrient, help it through the membrane, and release it. Passive transport of this type is known as "carrier-mediated" or *facilitated* diffusion and is analogous to the use of graphite to ease a key into a lock.

Digestion results in a high concentration of nutrients in the intestinal lumen. Through passive diffusion, then, nutrient molecules are carried from

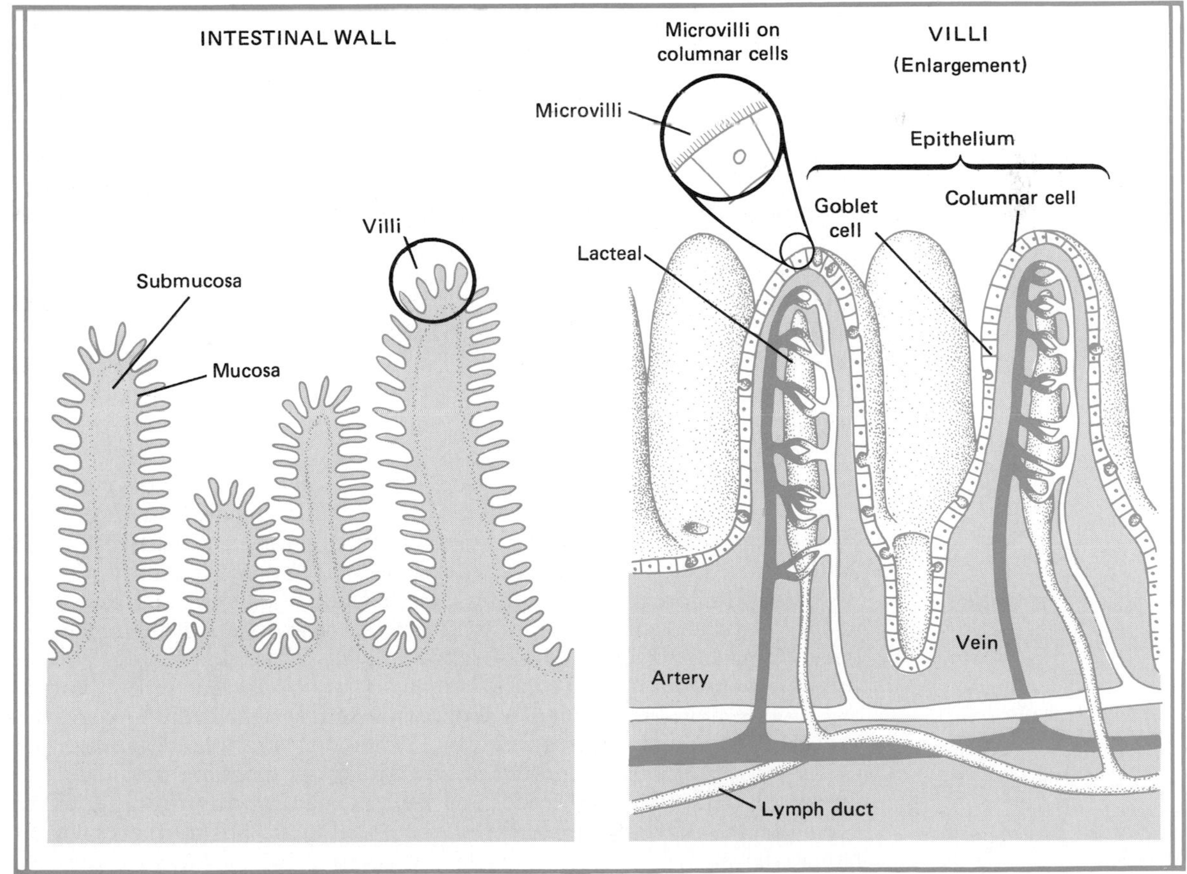

FIGURE 1-7
Intestinal Wall and Villus
The primary site of nutrient absorption is in the mucosa or interior surface membrane of the small intestine, diagrammed at left. It is lined with thousands of projections or villi (singular *villus*), shown in detail at right. Each villus contains blood vessels and a special lymph vessel, the lacteal. The outer surface (epithelium) of each villus consists of columnar cells for absorption and goblet cells for production of mucus. From the columnar cells the microvilli extend, forming the brush border. All of these structures vastly increase the surface area available for nutrient absorption.

their areas of high concentration in the lumen into the blood and lymph vessels. If the body were dependent only on diffusion, absorption would stop once the concentration gradient was equalized on both sides of the membrane. But that would deprive the body of the benefit of the nutrient molecules still remaining in the small intestine. Moreover, the concentration of some molecules is greater in the cell than in the lumen. To transport those molecules from an area of low concentration to high concentration is an **active transport** process requiring energy and a special transport carrier, as a result of which certain nutrients are "pumped" from the lumen into the intestinal cell. This active transport process is responsible for much of the absorption of calcium, iron, glucose, galactose, and amino acids in our bodies.

After the nutrients leave the small intestine, those that are fat soluble and those that are water soluble follow different routes. Water-soluble nutrients enter the bloodstream via nearby veins, which lead into the large portal vein (see Figure 1-8). The portal vein carries the nutrients to the liver, which monitors their passage into the general circulation. The nutrients not removed by the liver cells flow with the blood up through the hepatic vein to the heart. From here, the blood travels to the lungs, where it is oxygenated, and then returns to the heart. Blood, with its nutrient freight, is pumped into arteries that will carry it to small capillaries, present in tissues throughout the body. Nutrients move from the capillaries into the extracellular fluid that bathes all the cells of the body.

Fats and fat-soluble nutrients enter the lymphatic system, another circulatory system for transport of body fluids. The lymphatic system bypasses the liver, releasing its content into the general circulation through the thoracic duct and subclavian vein into the right atrium of the heart.

In digestion and absorption, foods are processed and their nutrients sent throughout the body. Most foods consist of combinations of nutrients. Despite all the different kinds of food humans eat and the different chemical reactions to which each is subjected, eventually all foods are digested and transformed into their component nutrients, and eventually all nutrients enter the general circulation for distribution throughout the body. In a sense, the gastrointestinal tract is a long, convoluted column or space enclosed by walls (sort of like a rubber hose) within the body cavity. Only after the end products of digestion have left the gastrointestinal tract and been absorbed into the blood stream can they really be considered as being "in" the body and accessible to the body's cells.

METABOLISM. **Metabolism** refers to all of the chemical processes that occur in the body from the time nutrients are absorbed until they are either made part of the body, used for energy, or excreted.

Metabolism occurs in two phases: **anabolism,** an **energy-*using*** process by which substances are built up (synthesized); and **catabolism,** an **energy-*releasing*** process by which body substances are broken down into simpler substances. Anabolism and catabolism are dynamic processes, both occurring at the same time, but frequently proceeding at different rates. When anabolism exceeds catabolism, growth occurs. When catabolism predominates, the net effect on the body is deterioration, as in starvation, fever, and certain illnesses. In a healthy adult who is no longer growing, these processes reach an overall steady state in which cellular growth and cellular breakdown are balanced.

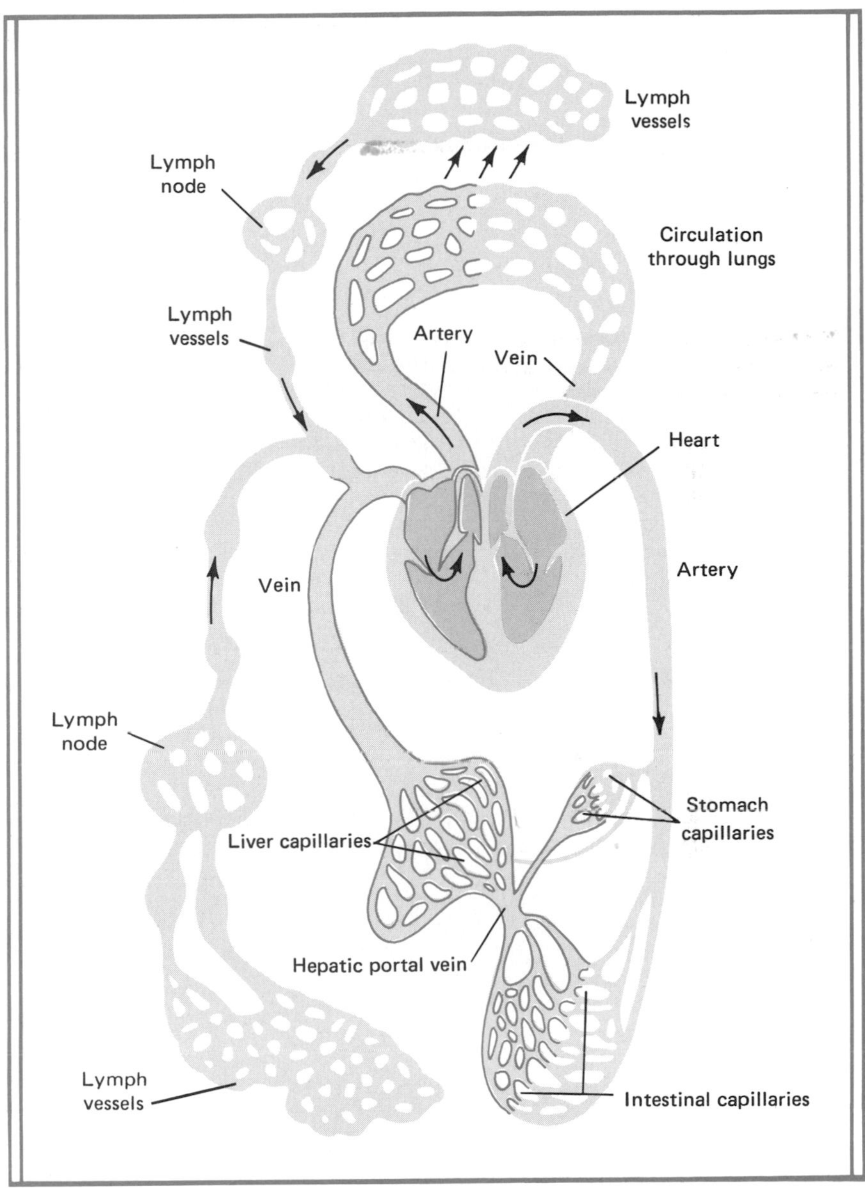

FIGURE 1-8
After absorption in the small intestine, nutrients (except for fats) enter the general circulation through veins which lead to the large portal vein, in which they are carried to the liver. The liver serves as a control system, selectively storing or releasing various metabolites, which enter the hepatic vein and are transported to the heart. Blood is pumped from the heart to the lungs for oxygenation, and returns to the heart for circulation in the arteries. From the arteries blood goes into the capillary network that will carry it, with its nutrient contents, to all body tissues. Fats and fat-soluble substances at first do not go through the liver but are carried by the lymphatic circulation, entering the general circulation through the thoracic duct and subclavian vein, which bring them to the heart.

Metabolic processes occur in every cell of the body. They are regulated by chemicals produced inside the body (endogenous) and also by substances that are supplied from the diet, such as vitamins and minerals (exogenous). Enzymes are part of the metabolic machinery of the internal environment. In addition to the digestive enzymes, hundreds of other enzymes are necessary for anabolism and catabolism. The activity of enzymes, and thus their ability to catalyze reactions, is controlled and influenced by a variety of chemical regulators.

Hormones, for example, are also endogenously produced in body organs

PERSPECTIVE ON
The Recommended Dietary Allowances

The phrase "recommended dietary allowance" (RDA) will appear often in this text as the various nutrients are discussed. To the general public, these numbers seem authoritative. In fact, they are far from absolute, although they are indeed useful.

The RDAs represent levels of nutrient and energy intake thought to be adequate for the nutritional needs of virtually all healthy Americans (Harper, 1974). These levels are set by the Food and Nutrition Board of the National Research Council, and are derived by various statistical procedures from available data. Consequently, RDAs are *not* requirements applicable equally to every individual; they are not even dietary "ideals." They can, perhaps, best be thought of as guidelines, suggested levels of nutrient intake that are likely to keep most of us in good health.

The first version of what would become the RDAs was formulated in 1943, during the Second World War, and was intended to provide information for the development of nutrition programs in connection with national defense. During that period of disruptions and shortages in food supply, it was important to maintain civilian health levels, and public information programs were instituted for this purpose. At the same time, the government had to undertake the most widespread institutional feeding program in its history, in military bases and under battlefield conditions, and guidelines were necessary to ensure the nutritional adequacy of meals served to and specially developed for military personnel. Although national defense is no longer the primary reason for their importance, dietary standards have been revised eight times since they were first issued, and they continue to be useful for practical purposes. Among their most important uses are comparisons of the nutrient intakes of various population groups and as a reference for the nutrient contents of foods.

RDAs are based on several factors: (1) surveys of groups of individuals to determine the relationship of nutrient intake to the presence or absence of disease; (2) controlled feeding experiments with small numbers of individuals; (3) metabolic studies on laboratory animals.

Although average requirements can be determined by these methods, it is recognized that no individual is "average." Human beings vary in body build, internal chemistry, age, life style, and numerous other factors that affect nutrient needs. Some people may require large amounts of particular nutrients, while others maintain equally good health on smaller amounts of the same nutrients.

RDAs represent allowances, not requirements. An allowance implies flexibility. Requirements are actual physiological needs, but they are difficult to measure, differ for every individual, and in practical terms cannot be determined for every individual. Recommendations for nutrient intakes are, therefore, defined as allowances, and have been set high enough to provide a margin of safety so that the actual needs of most healthy individuals are met. The RDA for energy (which is not a nutrient), it should be noted, is determined according to a different procedure, and represents an approximate average requirement with no additional allowance. Since it is an average, the energy allowance will be lower than many people require and higher than many others need. RDA tables (see Appendix Table A) express these calculated numbers in amounts adjusted for age, weight, and sex.

Must we consume the amount represented by the RDA for each nutrient, every day? Probably not, because as we have just seen, the RDAs for nutri-

called glands. They are transported through the blood to *target* organs where they exert a controlling effect. Hormones act as messengers, ordering the increase or decrease of particular metabolic processes in the target organs. Other molecules that contribute to the control of metabolic processes are **coenzymes,** nonprotein substances that assist enzymes in their catalytic action. Coenzymes often contain vitamins, and we shall examine their role in Chapter 7.

The processes of anabolism and catabolism both produce waste products,

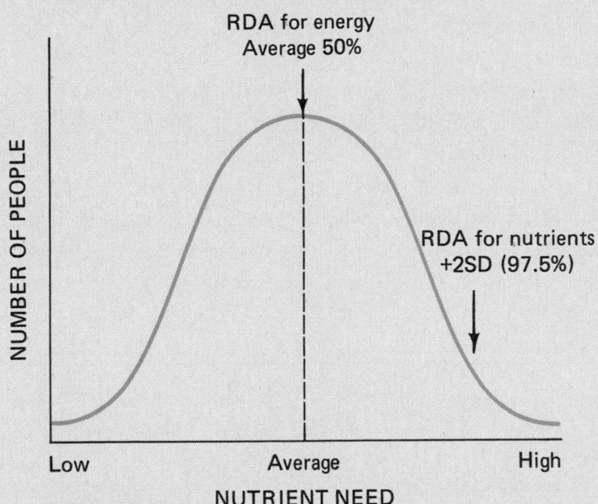

Normal Distribution Graph for RDAs

A graph of the actual nutrient needs of the entire population would be what is known as a *normal distribution curve*. Most healthy individuals cluster about a midpoint (the average), while a smaller number of individuals fall at either extreme. Using a normal distribution curve as a guide, the RDA for most nutrients was established to represent the average requirement *plus* 2 standard deviations. This means that the nutrient RDAs are high enough to meet or exceed the nutrient needs of 97.5 percent of the population of normal, healthy people, and are thus actually higher than the amounts needed by most people.

ents are higher than the amounts required by most healthy people. Nutritional surveys of population groups, however, have shown that intake of less than two-thirds of the RDA value over a prolonged period of time is associated with various symptoms that indicate suboptimal nutritional status within the population. Assessment of the nutritional status of a particular person (as opposed to a population group) must be made on an individual basis using additional information to support a diagnosis of dietary deficiency. (The various methods of dietary assessment are discussed in Chapter 10.) A range of values, rather than a specific number, could be more accurate but less useful in many ways. RDAs have been used to plan diets for groups of people and are used as a measure to evaluate diets. As long as their limitations are recognized, the RDAs currently provide the best standard available for comparison of nutrient intake with needs.

RDAs are not therapeutic recommendations, and cannot be used as guidelines by persons recovering from serious illness or suffering from chronic illness. RDAs do not necessarily take into account the special needs of infants and children, of pregnant and lactating women, or of adolescents or the elderly. Environmental factors such as occupation and climate may also affect an individual's need for and ability to utilize some nutrients.

Still another problem is the lack of adequate data on which to base allowances for many micronutrient elements. It is even possible that some vital nutrients remain to be discovered (Balsley, 1977; Munro, 1977).

Translating RDAs into needs for specific foods, rather than specific nutrients, is more difficult. The nutrient content of a sample of most foods will not be representative of all samples of that food, since nutrient content depends on such variables as climate and soil composition or may be lost in commercial or home processing and preparation (Food and Nutrition Board, 1974, p. 15). Also, interactions among nutrients will affect the nutrient value of foods. For example, the utilization of iron is enhanced if meat and vitamin C are ingested at the same meal, but minimized if they are absent; calcium utilization is negatively affected by increased protein consumption.

The long history and frequent revision of RDAs indicate that, as new data become available, opinions change and interpretations vary. In Chapter 10 the RDAs are examined in conjunction with specific nutrients and food guides.

all of which must be *excreted* from the body. The kidneys and the large intestine are the body's major waste-handling stations, producing urine and feces. The lungs and the skin are also organs for disposal of **metabolic wastes.** Feces consist mainly of materials that cannot be digested and are not, therefore, primarily metabolic wastes. The lungs serve as the main excretory passage for carbon dioxide and a small amount of water. Other waste products are lost through the skin by perspiration. Some nutrients are incorporated into the nails and hair, which are eventually lost. The kidneys, in addition to excreting wastes into the urine, also help the body to retain key nutrients. As needed, glucose, vitamins, minerals, amino acids, and water are reabsorbed into the blood, by way of the kidneys.

Metabolism, then, is vital to all body functions. The structural organization of all body systems and the processes of digestion, absorption, and metabolism constitute the internal environment that enables us to use the food we eat and eliminate that which is no longer useful.

INTERACTIONS BETWEEN THE INTERNAL AND EXTERNAL ENVIRONMENTS

This introduction to the science of nutrition has examined both the external and internal factors that influence the foods consumed and their processing in the human body. Figure 1-9 illustrates the interrelationships of these psychosocial, biological, and chemical variables. It is clear that the internal and external environments influence our nutritional health. In turn, nutritional

FIGURE 1-9
Interaction of Factors Involved in Nutrition

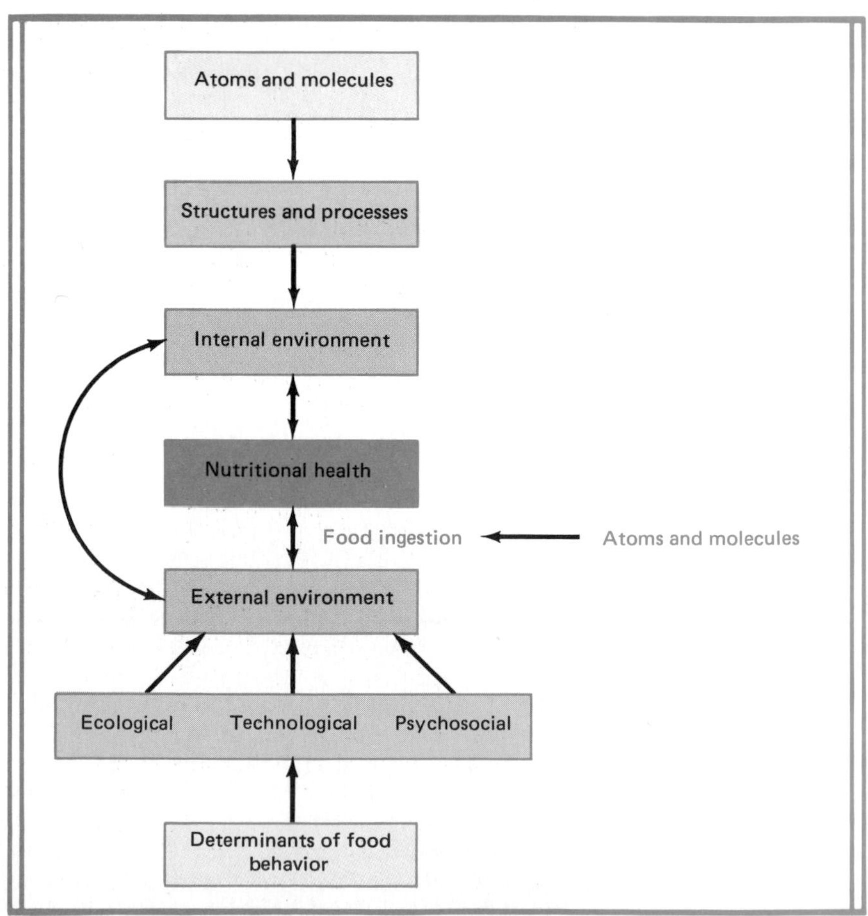

health affects both of these environments. What may not be so obvious is that these environments also influence each other. For example, illness, a disturbance of the internal environment, impinges on the external environment by limiting an individual's work capacity and social activities. Similarly, stressful changes in the external environment may be manifested in the internal environment as increased stomach acidity, perhaps producing ulcers, or as elevated blood pressure, perhaps causing headaches or cardiovascular problems.

Later chapters will explore the interactions between internal and external environments. Chapters 2 through 9 present the basic nutrients required by the body, their functions, and their dietary sources. The watchword in the pages ahead will be *diversity*, the diversity of human needs dictating diversity in diet. Because there is no one perfect food which can supply all needed nutrients, nutritional health is closely tied to diversity.

SUMMARY

Nutrition is both a science and a process. Nutritional science deals with facts and principles derived from research studies. These studies provide descriptive evidence about situations that exist in the environment, epidemiological evidence about the occurrence and distribution of factors associated with particular nutritional phenomena, and experimental evidence about proven cause-and-effect relationships. Because it is difficult to obtain experimental evidence in human subjects, nutritional researchers use animal models, often rats.

Nutrition as a process is influenced by variables in the external and internal environments. External factors, such as geography, topography, technological advances, and culturally transmitted social influences, determine what foods are available to us and which ones we choose to eat. The internal environment exerts other strong pressures. The body and all the foods taken into it are made up of atoms and molecules. These atoms and molecules join together to form compounds. Organic compounds contain carbon. There are four classes of organic compounds in foods: carbohydrates, proteins, lipids, and vitamins. Inorganic molecules of water and of the minerals Na, K, P, S, Ca, and Fe are also considered nutrients.

The process of nutrition involves the transformation of the atoms and molecules of food into the kinds of atoms and molecules that make up the body. This transformation occurs inside the cells. There are many specialized cells in the body, each with a particular structure suited to its particular function. Cells are organized into tissues, which in turn are organized into organs. Organs form larger organ systems.

The digestive system is of obvious importance to nutritionists. Digestive organs perform the mechanical and chemical processes by which food is digested or prepared for absorption into the blood. Specialized protein molecules, enzymes, speed the rate of these chemical reactions; each acts only on a specific nutrient. Molecules of nutrients are absorbed by a variety of mechanisms into the circulatory system, from which they become available to the cells of the body.

Water-soluble nutrients are carried in the blood stream, through the liver and into the heart, where they are pumped throughout the body. Fats and fat-soluble nutrients go from the lymphatic system, a circulatory system that bypasses the liver's regulatory processes, directly to the heart, and then into the bloodstream. From the blood, nutrients enter the individual cells of the body. Here they are metabolized in one of two processes: anabolism, an energy-using process in which substances are made or synthesized; and catabolism, an energy-releasing process in which body substances are broken down into simpler substances. These processes maintain body function, renew body tissue, and produce waste products, which are excreted from the body by the lungs, skin, and kidneys. Solid wastes, representing mainly undigested components of food, accumulate in the large intestine or colon and are eliminated as feces.

Human needs for nutrients vary from one individual to the next, and during the several stages of the life cycle. The best way to provide for adequate intake of all nutrients is to eat a varied diet.

BIBLIOGRAPHY

BALSLEY, M. B. Soon to come: 1978 recommended dietary allowances. *Journal of the American Dietetic Association* 71:149, 1977.

CNI Weekly Report. Study exonerates food stamp shoppers. January 5, 1978, p. 8.

COSPER, B. A., AND L. M. WAKEFIELD. Food choices of women. *Journal of the American Dietetic Association* 66:152, 1975.

FOOD AND NUTRITION BOARD, NATIONAL RESEARCH COUNCIL. *Recommended dietary allowances.* 8th ed. Washington, D.C.: National Academy of Sciences, 1974.

GIFFT, H. H., M. B. WASHBON, AND G. G. HARRISON. *Nutrition, behavior and change.* Englewood Cliffs, N.J.: Prentice-Hall, 1972.

GORTNER, W. A. U.S. dietary trends and implications. *Contemporary Nutrition,* November 1976.

GRIVETTI, L. E., AND R. M. PANGBORN. Origin of selected Old Testament dietary prohibitions. *Journal of the American Dietetic Association* 65:634, 1974.

HARPER, A. E. Recommended dietary allowances: Are they what we think they are? *Journal of the American Dietetic Association* 64:151, 1974.

HARRIS, M. *Cows, pigs, wars, and witches.* New York: Random House, 1974.

INGELFINGER, F. J. Gastrointestinal absorption. *Nutrition Today* 2(1), 1967.

JAKOBOVITS, C., P. HALSTEAD, L. KELLY, D. A. ROE, AND C. M. YOUNG. Eating habits and nutrient intake of college women over a thirty-year period. *Journal of the American Dietetic Association* 71:405, 1977.

MUNRO, H. N. How well recommended are the recommended dietary allowances? *Journal of the American Dietetic Association* 71:490, 1977.

PIKE, R. L., AND M. L. BROWN. *Nutrition: An integrated approach,* 2nd ed. New York: John Wiley, 1975.

SCHAFER, R. B. Factors affecting food behavior and the quality of husbands' and wives' diets. *Journal of the American Dietetic Association* 72:138, 1978.

SCHAFER, R. B., AND E. A. YETLEY. Social psychology of food faddism. *Journal of the American Dietetic Association* 66:129, 1975.

SHIFFLETT, P. A. Folklore and food habits. *Journal of the American Dietetic Association* 68:347, 1976.

STASCH, A. R., M. M. JOHNSON, AND G. J. SPANGLER. Food practices and preferences of some college students. *Journal of the American Dietetic Association* 57:523, 1970.

TODHUNTER, E. N. Development of knowledge in nutrition. I. Animal experiments; II. Human experiments. *Journal of the American Dietetic Association* 41:328, 335, 1962.

WILLIAMSON, R. C. N. Intestinal adaption (first of two parts): Structural, functional and cytokinetic changes. *New England Journal of Medicine* 298:1393, 1978.

SUGGESTED ADDITIONAL READING

BABCOCK, C. G. Attitudes and use of food. *Journal of the American Dietetic Association* 38:546, 1961.

BEATTY, W. K. The history of nutrition: A tour of the literature. *Federation Proceedings* 36:2511, 1977.

BENDER, A. E. Food preferences in males and females. *Proceedings of the Nutrition Society* 35:181, 1976.

CASSEL, J. Social and cultural implication of food and food habits. *American Journal of Public Health* 47:732, 1957.

CRANE, R. K. A perspective of digestive-absorptive function. *American Journal of Clinical Nutrition* 22:242, 1969.

GOLDBLITH, S. A., AND M. A. JOSLYN, eds. *Milestones in nutrition.* Westport, Conn.: AVI Publishing Co., 1964.

GORE, R. The awesome worlds within a cell. *National Geographic,* September 1976, pp. 354–395.

GRIFFITH, W. H. Food as a regulator of metabolism. *American Journal of Clinical Nutrition* 17:391, 1965.

HALEY, M., D. AUCOIN, AND J. RAE. A comparative study of food habits. Influence of age, sex, and selected family characteristics. *Canadian Journal of Public Health* 68:301, 1977.

HOCHBAUM, G. M. Human behavior and nutrition education. *Nutrition News,* February 1977, pp. 1,4.

HOLDEN, P. M. How advertising affects food habits. *Food and Nutrition Notes Review* 28:102, 1971.

INGELFINGER, F. J. Gastric function. *Nutrition Today,* September–October 1971, pp. 2–11.

JALSO, S. B. Nutritional beliefs and practices. *Journal of the American Dietetic Association* 47:263, 1965.

KING, C. G. Notes on the history of nutrition in America. *Journal of the American Dietetic Association* 56:188, 1970.

LEE, D. Cultural factors in dietary choice. *American Journal of Clinical Nutrition* 5:166, 1957.

LOWENBERG, M. E., AND B. L. LUCAS, Feeding families and children—1776–1976. *Journal of the American Dietetic Association* 68:207, 1976.

MCCOLLUM, E. V. *A history of nutrition.* Boston: Houghton Mifflin, 1957.

MEAD, M. The changing significance of food. *American Scientist* 58:176, 1970.

MILLS, E. R. Psychological aspects of food habits. *Journal of Nutrition Education* 9:67, 1977.

OLSON, R. E. Clinical nutrition: An interface between human ecology and internal medicine. W. O. Atwater Memorial Lecture, Boston, 1978. Rpt. in *Nutrition Reviews* 36:161, 1978.

PAARLBERG, D. Food and economics. *Journal of the American Dietetic Association* 71:107, 1977.

TODHUNTER, E. N. The words we use and misuse in nutrition. *Food and Nutrition News,* March–April 1977, p. 1.

TODHUNTER, E. N. Chronology of some events in the development and application of the science of nutrition. *Nutrition Reviews* 34:353, 1976.

TODHUNTER, E. N. Some classics of nutrition and dietetics. *Journal of the American Dietetic Association* 44:100, 1964.

WILLIAMSON, R. C. N. Intestinal adaptation (second of two parts): Mechanisms of control. *New England Journal of Medicine* 298:1444, 1978.

WILSON, M. M., AND M. W. LAMB. Food beliefs as related to ecological factors in women. *Journal of Home Economics* 60:115, 1968.

Chapter 2

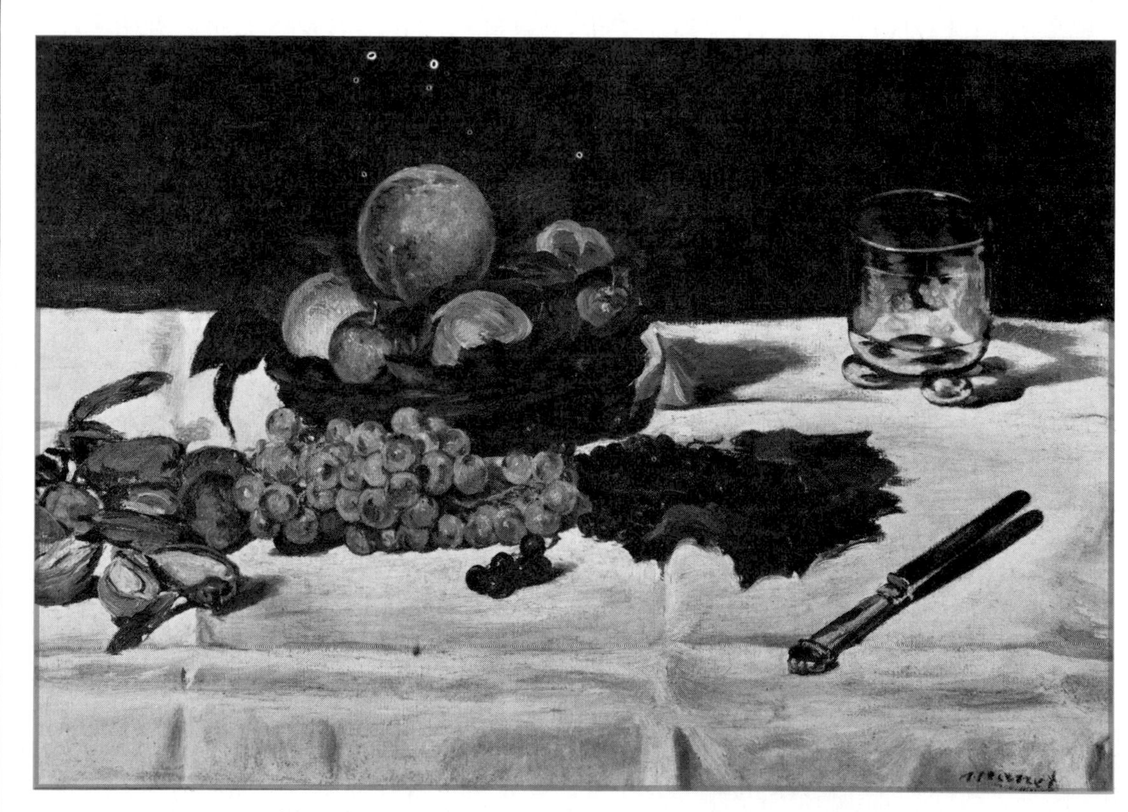
Still Life by Edouard Manet

Carbohydrates

"Quick, what can I eat? I'm famished!" You've probably felt this way many times. Now think back. What kind of food did you reach for? Most probably, it was a soft drink, an apple, a thick slice of bread, a ripe banana, or even a chocolate bar. These foods share an important attribute; they are loaded with carbohydrate. Carbohydrate-rich foods supply quick energy to fuel the body, just what most people feel like having when hunger strikes.

Carbohydrates from grains, fruits, and vegetables account for as much as 80 percent of the energy intake of people in developing countries. In technologically advanced nations, "sweets" often replace grains, fruits, and vegetables as sources of dietary carbohydrate. What makes high-carbohydrate foods so popular? On the practical side, they are usually inexpensive and readily available. On the biological side, carbohydrates are essential to many of the body's metabolic processes.

This chapter examines the biological role of carbohydrates; their composition, molecular structure, and major dietary sources; and their path from ingestion through digestion, absorption, and metabolism. Carbohydrates travel through the circulatory system in the form of simple sugars, and complex mechanisms regulate the sugar levels in the blood. Some of the problems—diabetes, hypoglycemia, and other disorders—associated with disturbances in this regulatory process will be examined along with the significance of dietary carbohydrate in supplying indigestible food remnants called "dietary fiber," which affects the rate at which food residues move through the intestinal tract and which may have other roles as well. Against this biological background, the trends in carbohydrate consumption in the United States, and their significance in the maintenance of good health will be presented.

CARBOHYDRATES: DEFINITION, CLASSIFICATION, SOURCES

Carbohydrates are organic compounds composed of the elements carbon (C), hydrogen (H), and oxygen (O). Generally, the hydrogen and oxygen atoms in a carbohydrate molecule are present in the ratio of 2 to 1, the same proportion in which they occur in a molecule of water. Thus, a carbohydrate molecule, with some modifications, is composed of hydrated carbon atoms.

Monosaccharides

Carbohydrates are classified according to their molecular structure and, in particular, according to the proportion of carbon atoms to the H—OH group. **Monosaccharides,** or simple sugars, contain one carbon atom for each group of two hydrogens and one oxygen. This relationship is expressed as $C_n(H_2O)_n$. (In chemical terminology, the subscript—here designated by "$_n$"—is used to represent the number of atoms or molecules of the element or compound immediately preceding it—in this case, carbon atoms and water molecules.) Different classes of monosaccharides are distinguished by the number of carbon atoms; for example, 5-carbon sugars are called **pentoses** (from *penta-*, five, and *-ose,* carbohydrate).

The monosaccharides of most importance in nutrition are the **hexoses** or 6-carbon sugars, expressed in the general formula $C_6(H_2O)_6$, or simply $C_6H_{12}O_6$. Examples of hexoses are **glucose, fructose,** and **galactose.** Even though all hexoses have the same *empirical* (chemical) *formula,* they are distinguished from one another by differences in **chemical structure,** that is, by the arrangement of C, H, and O atoms in the molecule. The differences in arrangement of the H and O atoms around the carbons in these three sugars can be seen in their structural formulas, illustrated in Figure 2-1. Although the structural differences among these three hexose molecules are slight, they are responsible for significant differences in properties. Glucose, galactose, and fructose differ in taste, in degree of sweetness, and in their metabolic roles. Although other hexose molecules exist, the three shown are the most important in the study of nutrition.

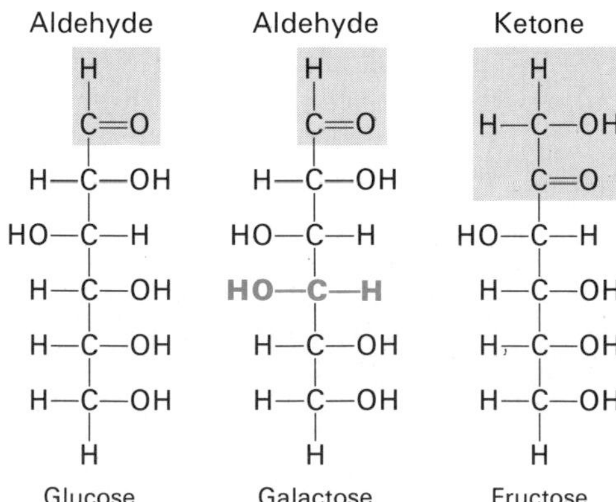

FIGURE 2-1

Structural Formulas of Three Hexoses

These three hexoses differ from each other because their H and OH groups are arranged differently about the carbon atoms. Glucose and galactose both have aldehyde groups and are called aldoses; fructose has a ketone group and is called a ketose.

Ring Structures of Three Hexoses

Ring structures show details of molecular arrangement and bonding that are not apparent in Figure 2-1. Note that an oxygen "bridge" connects the first (*) and fifth (•) carbons in the aldoses and that a similar bridge between the second and fifth fructose carbons forms a five-membered ring.

Two of these monosaccharides are widely found in foods. Glucose—also known as dextrose or corn sugar—is present in sweet fruits, such as berries, grapes, pears, and oranges, and in certain vegetables, notably corn and carrots. Relatively large amounts occur in honey as well. Dextrose from corn syrup is often used commercially as a sweetener in prepared foods. Fructose—sometimes called levulose or fruit sugar—is also found in most fruits and vegetables. Galactose is not found free in foods, although it is a major constituent of the principal carbohydrate in milk, lactose.

Because the details of molecular structure are significant in organic chemistry, several ways have been devised to represent them diagrammatically. Often used is a diagram called a **ring structure,** which is especially convenient for illustrating large, complex molecules.

Disaccharides and Their Food Sources

Disaccharides are formed when two monosaccharides are chemically bonded together by means of a **condensation reaction.** This reaction is characterized by the release of a molecule of water, as shown by the general equation for a condensation reaction between two monosaccharides:

$$C_n(H_2O)_n + C_n(H_2O)_n \longrightarrow C_{2n}(H_2O)_{2n-1} + H_2O$$

The condensation of two hexoses is written:

$$2C_6(H_2O)_6 \longrightarrow C_{12}(H_2O)_{11} + H_2O$$

The condensation product of glucose and fructose is sucrose—sometimes called table sugar—which is shown using ring structures in Figure 2-2(a). Table sugar comes mainly from either sugar cane or sugar beets. Found in most fruits and vegetables, sucrose is also the major component of brown sugar, maple sugar, and molasses. Many processed foods are sweetened with sucrose.

The condensation product of glucose and galactose is the disaccharide **lactose** shown in Figure 2-2(b), the only significant dietary carbohydrate of animal origin. Produced solely by the mammary glands of lactating mammals, including humans, lactose—known also as milk sugar—is found only in milk and milk products. **Maltose,** another important disaccharide, is the result of a condensation reaction between two identical glucose units. See Figure 2-2(c). An intermediate product of starch breakdown during human digestion, maltose is found also in germinating seeds, in some breakfast cereals, and in fermented products, such as beer.

Polysaccharides

The word **polysaccharide** means "many sugars," a logical name for a molecule in which a number of monosaccharides are combined. Polysaccharides are often referred to as **complex carbohydrates,** as contrasted with the **simple carbohydrates**—the mono- and disaccharides discussed in the preceding

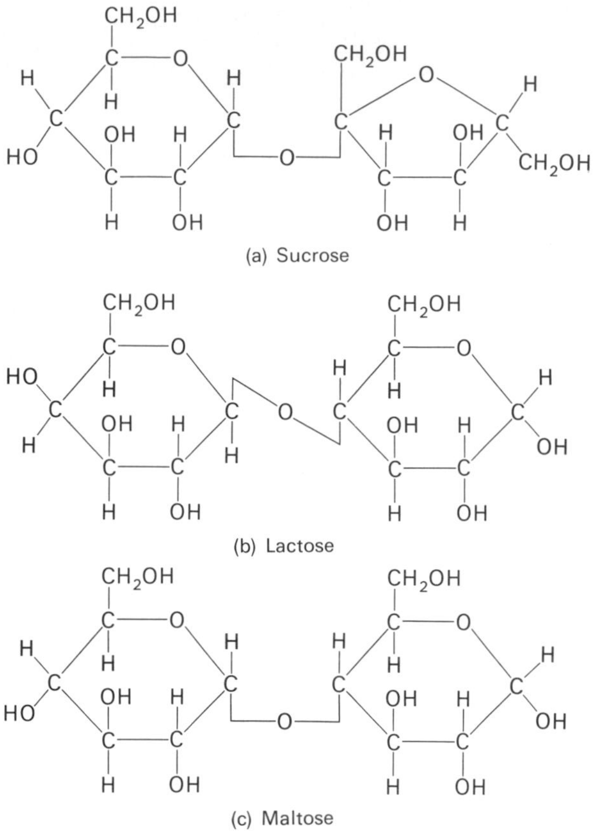

(a) Sucrose

(b) Lactose

(c) Maltose

FIGURE 2-2
Ring Structures of the Major Disaccharides

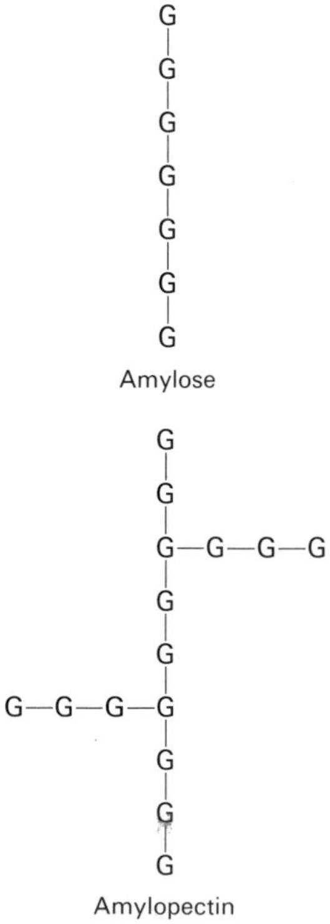

Amylose

Amylopectin

Structure of Two Plant Starches

sections. A polysaccharide molecule is represented by the general empirical formula of, for example, a polyhexose: $(C_6H_{10}O_5)_n$. Monosaccharides become linked through successive condensation reactions, and one molecule of water is lost as each hexose unit is added to the molecule. The combination of from three to ten monosaccharide units in this way is sometimes known as an **oligosaccharide** (from *oligo-*, few). True polysaccharides are **polymers,** large molecules built up through the linking together of many molecular units, which may or may not be identical.

Most polysaccharides of plant origin are commonly known as **starches,** of which there are several types. Different carbohydrate-containing foods—corn, wheat, and apples, for example—have different starches, each of them genetically determined. For example, amylose is a plant starch in which hundreds of glucose units are combined in a sequence of condensation reactions to form one long straight chain. Amylopectin is another plant starch, also composed solely of glucose units, but arranged in branched chains. Various plants contain both amylose and amylopectin, although in different proportions.

The most abundant polysaccharide (and probably the most common organic molecule on earth) is cellulose, a component of plant cell walls.

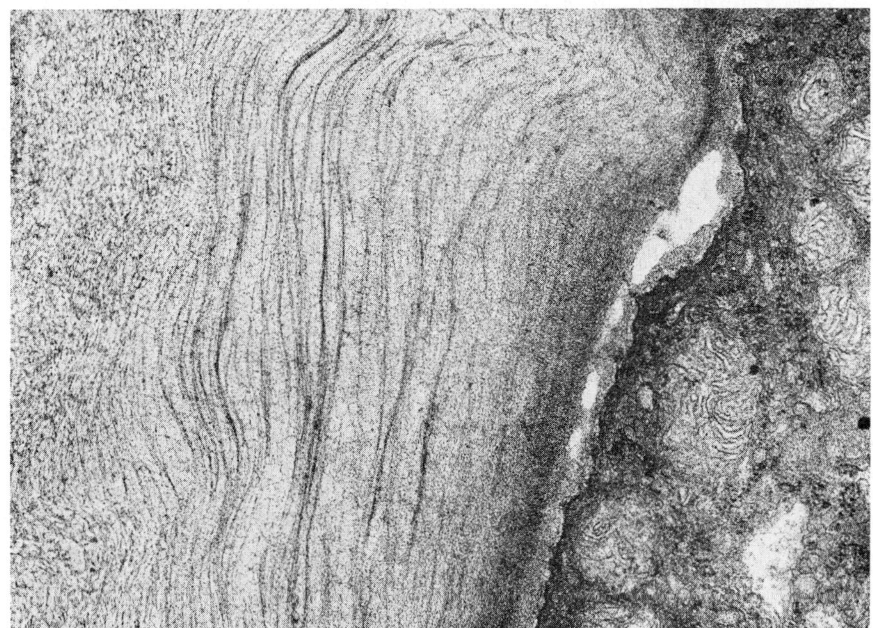

Electron micrograph showing parallel bundles of cellulose fibers in the cell wall of wheat, magnified 34,000 times. (Myron Ledbetter, Brookhaven National Laboratory)

Cellulose resembles amylose in that it, too, is made up of glucose units arranged in a straight chain, but there the resemblance stops. The key difference is in the way the glucose units are linked together, as shown in Figure 2-3. Because of the difference in linkage structure, these two polysaccharides have strikingly different chemical and physical properties and are utilized by the body in different ways. Most significant is that the human

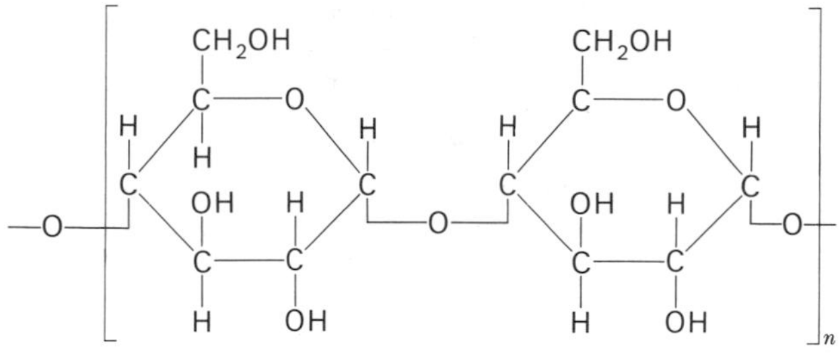

Amylose

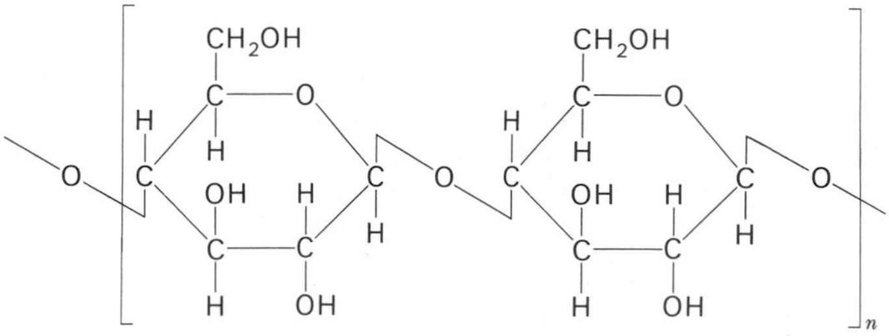

Cellulose

FIGURE 2-3

Ring Structures of Amylose and Cellulose

body cannot digest cellulose because the human digestive system does not have the capacity to break the cellulose linkage structure. The amylose structure, however, is readily digested. Small structural distinctions, then, make all the difference in how each molecule behaves and is utilized.

The one animal polysaccharide, **glycogen,** is not present in the food supply to an appreciable extent. Although it is stored as an energy source in some animal tissue (muscle and liver), it disappears with the death of the animal, leaving only negligible amounts in such foods as liver and fresh shellfish. The significance of glycogen for humans is its manufacture by the body during the course of glucose metabolism.

PROPERTIES OF CARBOHYDRATES

Despite basic similarity in chemical structure, the various carbohydrates differ markedly in their physical properties. The simple sugars—monosaccharides and disaccharides—have a distinctively sweet taste and are readily soluble in water. Polysaccharides, however, are not sweet, but often bland or tasteless, and are relatively insoluble. These properties make flour, cornstarch, and other such polysaccharides good thickening agents in food preparation. Their bland taste also accounts for the nearly universal culinary popularity of adding flavorful gravy and sauces to such starch-laden foods as potatoes, spaghetti, rice, and beans.

Carbohydrates in Our Diet

The carbohydrate composition of some common foods is shown in Figure 2-4. These are average figures, since individual samples of any food item can vary widely. Foods are listed according to the predominant type of carbohydrate that each contains, ranging from complex (mainly polysaccharides) at the top of the graph to simple (mainly sugars) at the bottom. The main dietary carbohydrates that we obtain from cereals and potatoes, for example, are starches, while the main dietary carbohydrates in dried fruits and sweeteners are sugars. Baked goods and beer, with both grain and sugar components, are intermediate.

The proportion of a food listed as carbohydrate depends on the water content of the sample. Dried legume seeds (peas and beans) contain relatively little water until they are cooked; consequently, their carbohydrate content is concentrated and proportionately high. Milk, fresh vegetables, and fresh fruits generally have a high water content and, therefore, contain much less carbohydrate per 100-gram sample. Generally, frozen and canned fruits to which sugar has not been added have as much natural sugar as fresh fruits. Because water has been removed, the sugar in dried fruits is more concentrated and therefore greater on a weight-for-weight basis than in fresh fruits.

Tables of food composition provide information for specific food items, usually on a per-serving basis. Data on the total carbohydrate content of foods also appear on some package labels.

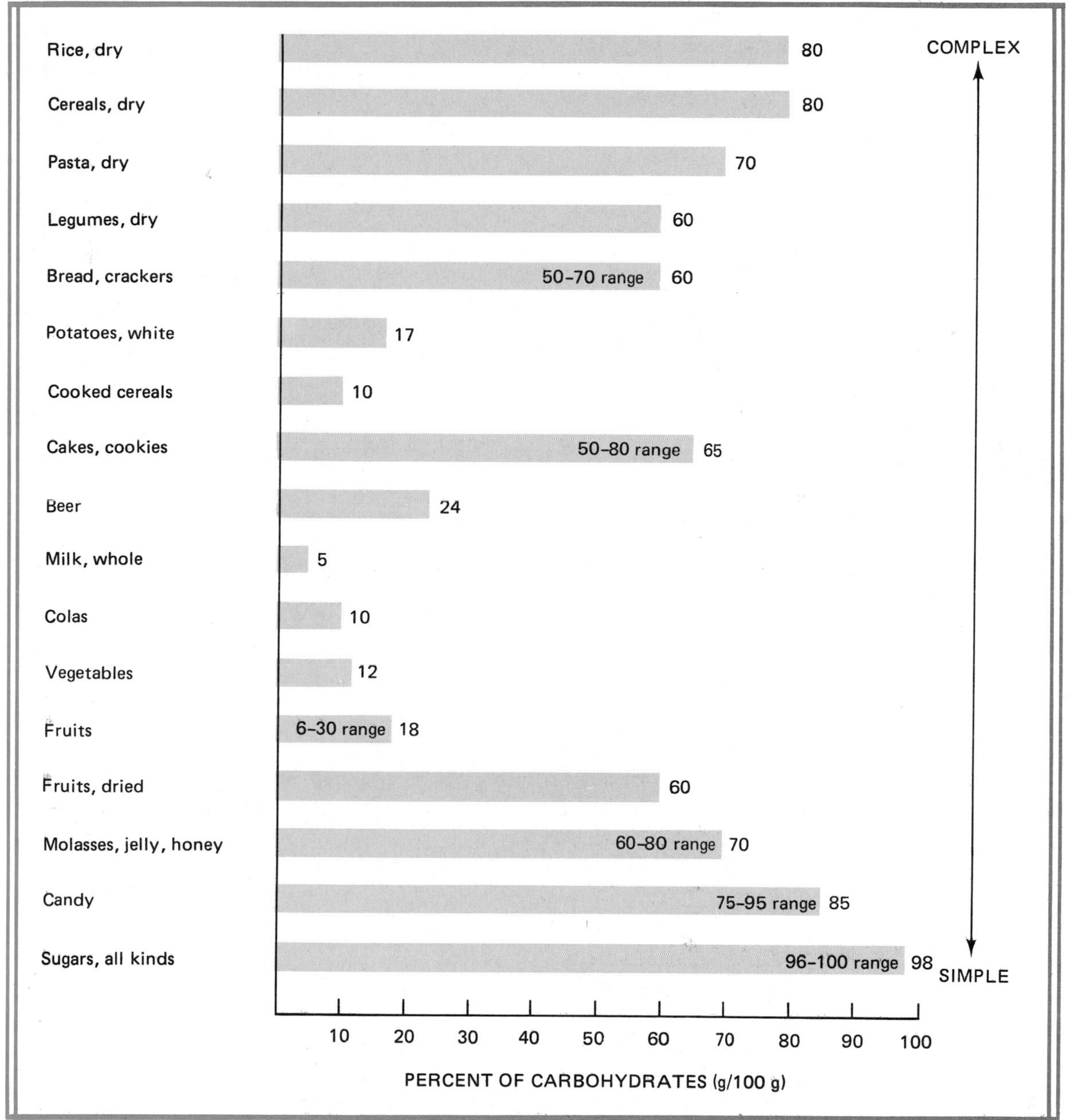

FIGURE 2-4

Carbohydrate Composition of Selected Foods

Note that milk is the only food of animal origin shown; lactose, or milk sugar, is the only sugar of animal origin.

PERSPECTIVE ON
Sugars in Foods

Sugar, particularly in its refined forms, has long been used not only for its flavor, but as a preservative. Fruits, for example, in the form of jams, jellies, marmalades, and candies last far longer than in their natural state. Sugar syrup acts as a bacteriostatic agent and has made it possible to have a wide range of fruits available at all seasons. Consumers have thus come to expect sugars in such foods. Candy bars, sugar added to tea or coffee, and sweet desserts are also obvious sources of sugar.

But sugar is used far more than most consumers realize to flavor and preserve processed foods in which one might not normally expect a high sugar content. Bottled salad dressing, for example, may contain as much as 30 percent sugar. Barbecue-flavored oven-dry breading mix may have more than 50 percent sugar, and hamburger extenders are about 23 percent sugar. The percentage of sugar in such foods as presweetened breakfast cereals may also be much higher than consumers expect. Because of recent studies linking high intakes of refined sugar to heart disease, as well as to dental caries and diabetes, the sugars hidden in foods where consumers do not expect to find them may be cause for concern. The high percentages of sugar in a few prepared foods are shown in the table. Generally, the sugar content of such

SUGAR IN SELECTED PROCESSED FOODS

Product	Percent Sugar[a]	Serving Size	Grams Sugar/ Serving
Coffee creamer	60.0	1 tsp = 2 g	1.2
Presweetened cereal	57.0	1 oz = 28 g	16.0
Chocolate bar	51.0	1 oz = 28 g	16.0
Catsup	30.0	1 tbsp = 15 g	4.5
Ice cream (10% fat)	20.0	1 c = 133 g	27.0
Blueberry yogurt (low fat)	14.0	1 c = 245 g	33.5
Plain low-fat yogurt	5.3	1 c = 245 g	13.0

[a] *Consumer Reports*, March 1978, pp. 136–142.

products is not apparent to the average buyer. Manufacturers are not required to and, therefore, usually do not list on the label the actual percentage of each ingredient in a product. They *are* required to list the principal ingredients in descending order of the amount of each; so the presence of "sugar words" (such as corn syrup and dextrose in addition to sugar itself) at or near the beginning of a list of ingredients is the only clue the consumer is given. Consumer activists and health professionals are working for a law that would mandate the percentage labeling of food ingredients. If they are successful, consumers may become more aware of the "hidden sugars" in foods.

It is, however, important to note that expressing sugar as a percentage of ingredients may be deceiving. The reason can be understood by examining the last two columns of the table, which indicate the amount of each food in an average serving, and the amount of sugar that would actually be consumed. With this in mind the high percentage of sugar in coffee creamer does not seem quite so bad; a cup of low-fat yogurt will contribute more sugar to the diet than a teaspoon of creamer. Informed consumers must make diet decisions based on the real meaning of all data available.

Nevertheless, of the nearly one quarter of our energy needs being filled by sugar, only about 6 percent comes from the natural sugars in fruits, vegetables, and milk. Of the total caloric intake of the average American diet 18 percent comes from sugars added to food (*Consumer Reports*, 1978). Does this extra sugar serve a useful purpose? We have all often heard that sugar is "quick energy," or "an inexpensive source of energy." Sugar is not the only source of energy, however, and normal food intake probably provides an adequate supply of energy for most individuals.

Sugar as we know it—the white, slightly gritty, sweet powder that usually sits in a handy container on the dining table—is not a "natural" food for human beings, or for any other beings for that matter. It is the final product of the commercial processing of plants such as sugar beets or sugar cane. The cultivation and processing of sugar goes back more than 2,000 years, but until the sixteenth century sugar was both a rarity and a luxury. With the settlement of the Americas, however, sugar cane

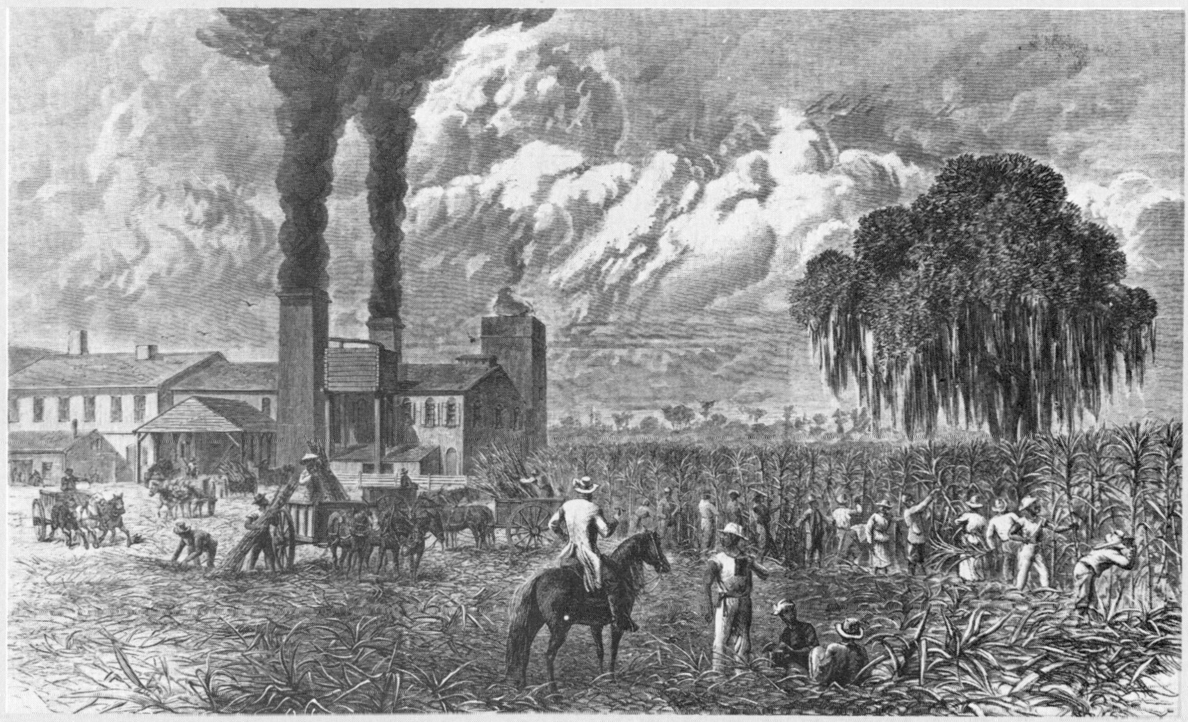

Growing, harvesting, and processing sugar cane on a Louisiana plantation. Wood engraving from an American newspaper of 1875. (The Granger Collection)

production became big business and an essential component of a complex transoceanic trade network. The commercial cultivation of beet sugar began in France in the early nineteenth century, when the Napoleonic wars prevented the transport of Caribbean sugar (*Consumer Reports*, 1978). While sugar cane is still an important crop in subtropical and tropical regions, most sugar production in the United States is from beets.

According to a recent report, 65 percent of the national production of sucrose is used by the food processing industry; 11 percent by large food serving organizations, such as the government and the restaurant and hotel industry; and only 24 percent is directly purchased by consumers (*Consumer Reports*, 1978). The sugar industry has, in fact, been so productive that there was a worldwide surplus of 6 million tons in 1978. Plans to utilize sugar's potential energy as a source of fuel for industrial combustion, rather than human combustion, are under way and a sucrochemical industry is developing to convert sugar into biodegradable raw materials for textiles, cosmetics, and other industries (*Business Week*, 10/15/78).

Some of the influences that television is alleged to exert on children are related to nutrition. Interspersed through most programs is a constant barrage of messages extolling the virtues of highly sugared breakfast foods, drinks, and candies. No provision exists for equal time for discussion of the possible risks involved in eating too much sugar. Young children are a particularly susceptible class of consumers and are easily led by television sales techniques to form eating habits that are nutritionally detrimental. Dental caries, obesity, and limited intake of more nourishing foods are probable consequences. Children whose television and food fare are supervised by informed parents will be less likely to be misled into poor nutritional habits.

Trends in Carbohydrate Consumption

American eating habits have changed considerably during this century, especially in regard to the quantity and patterns of our use of carbohydrate-containing foods. Although total caloric intake has remained about the same, a moderate but steady decrease occurred in overall carbohydrate consumption with a corresponding increase in the proportion of calories derived from fats. The changes in the composition of our carbohydrate intake are shown in Figure 2-5. Note the striking decrease in consumption of starch (grains and potatoes) and the corresponding increase in the consumption of sugars. Starch consumption decreased from 68.3 percent of total carbohydrate intake early in the century to 47.1 percent in 1976; in the same period, sugar intake increased from 31.7 percent to 52.9 percent (Brewster and Jacobson, 1978). Several factors are involved in these trends.

As countries throughout the world develop technologically and economically, the carbohydrate proportion of total energy intake tends to decrease. Carbohydrate consumption is, apparently, inversely proportional to economic status. The high-carbohydrate, predominantly vegetarian diet common to the poor almost everywhere is gradually replaced by a higher-fat diet containing more food items from animal sources. Production and distribution of grains and food products derived from them (cereal, pasta) are less costly than the production and distribution of foods that are better sources of other energy

FIGURE 2-5

Trends in Carbohydrate Consumption*

* Shown as a percent of 1909–1913 per capita civilian consumption.

Source: USDA Agricultural Research Service.

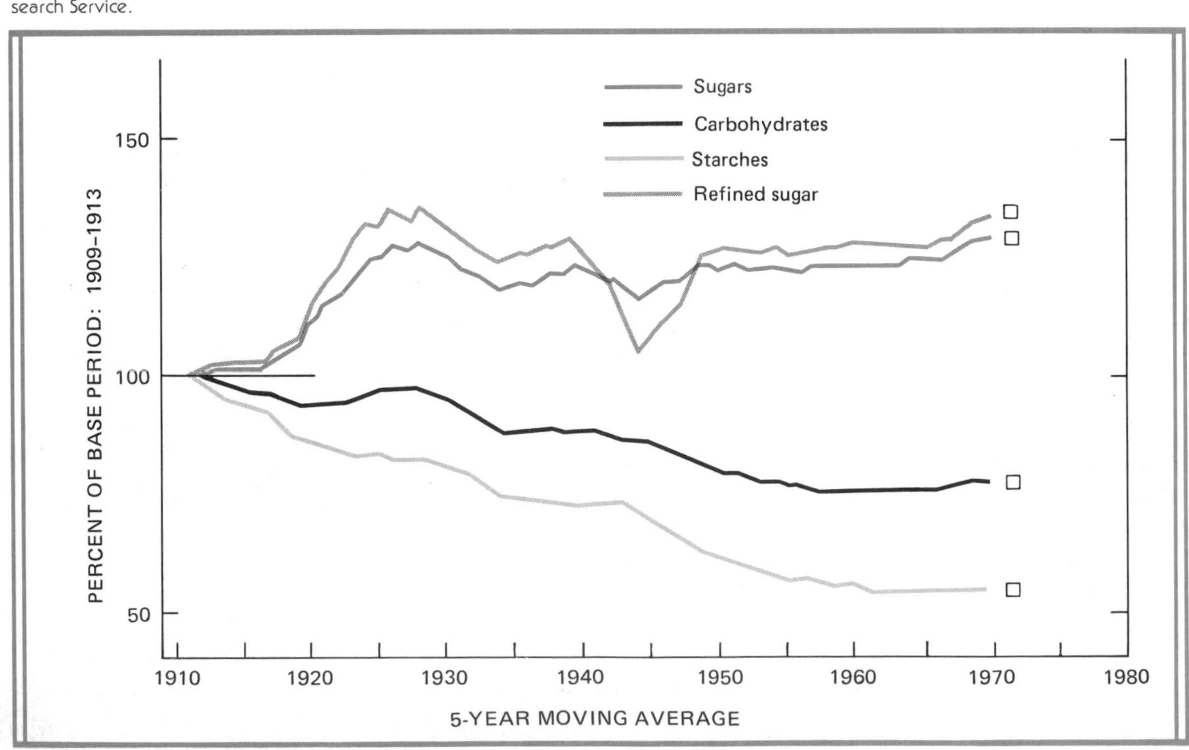

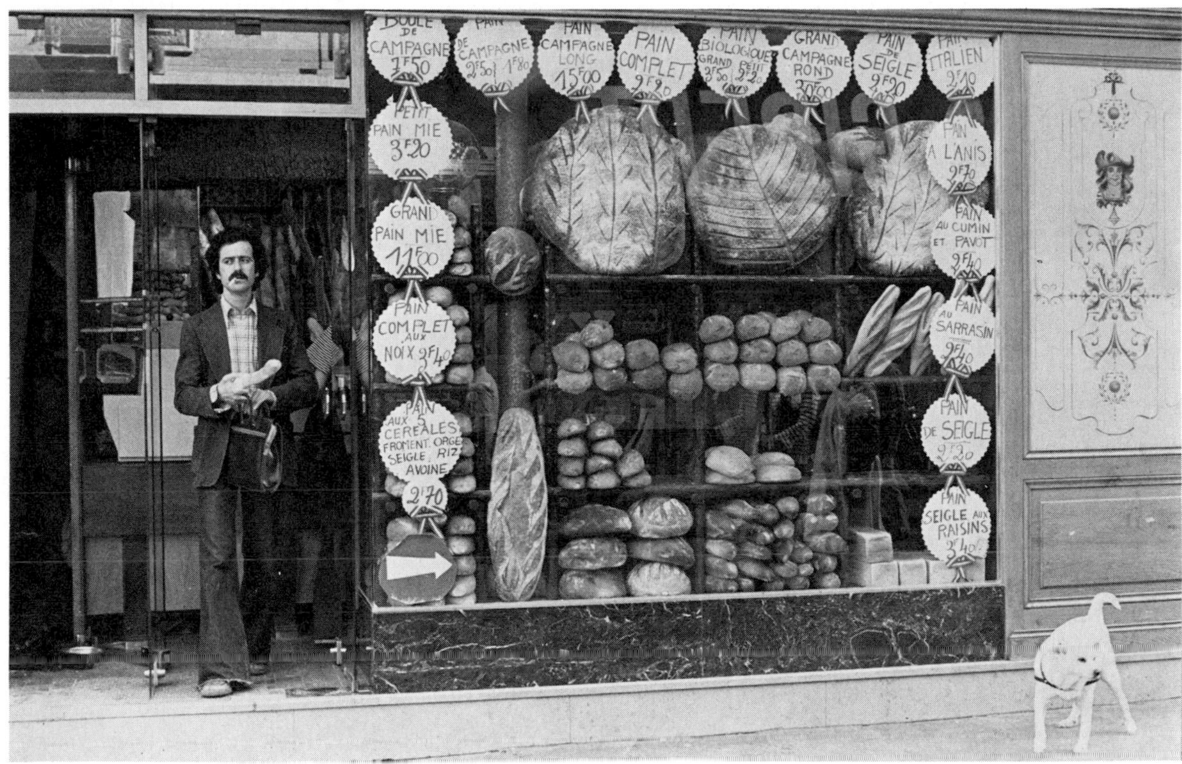

Several different varieties of bread are displayed in the window of a Paris bakery. (Mario Rossi Photo Researchers)

nutrients (proteins and fats), such as meat; consequently, meats are status foods almost everywhere.

Similarly, it has been observed that as economic status improves there is a shift away from foods containing mainly complex carbohydrates—grains, potatoes, legumes—and toward those with more sugar. Instead of fresh fruits, we eat fruits canned in sugar syrup; instead of whole-grain cereal, we eat a "breakfast bar." This pattern is associated with the movement of people from rural to urban areas; with more people attending schools or working in offices and factories and having lunch hours and coffee breaks; and with a number of

TABLE 2-1
Dietary Sources of Sugar

Dietary Source	1909–1913		1971	
	*Pounds**	*Percent*	*Pounds**	*Percent*
Sugar added by consumer	52.1	68.2	24.7	24.3
Commercially prepared foods and beverages	19.3	25.3	70.2	69.2
Other	5.0	6.5	6.6	6.5
Total	76.4	100.0	101.5	100.0

*L. Page and B. Friend. Level of use of sugar in the United States. In *Sugars in nutrition,* ed. H. L. Sipple and K. W. McNutt (New York: Academic Press, 1974).

related socioeconomic factors, which will be considered in several chapters in Part Two of this book.

An important change has occurred in the dietary sources of sugars that we eat. A greater amount now comes from processed foods and correspondingly less is added in the kitchen or at the table (see Table 2-1). Sweeteners produced predominantly for the food processing industry—dextrose and corn syrup—represented more than one quarter of all sweetener use in 1976, whereas in the early years of the century, they contributed only 7 percent of sugar consumption (Jacobson and Moreland, 1977) (see Figure 2-6).

Since it is not possible to tabulate all the sugar actually measured into our cooking pots and coffee cups, and to subtract that lost when we spill a soft drink or throw away stale cake, the figures in such tables are considered "disappearance data"; they reflect the "disappearance" of sugar when it is distributed either through retail channels or to commercial food processors. For this reason they may not reflect actual or real consumption, and should be used with this limitation in mind.

These per capita figures, moreover, represent an average, useful for com-

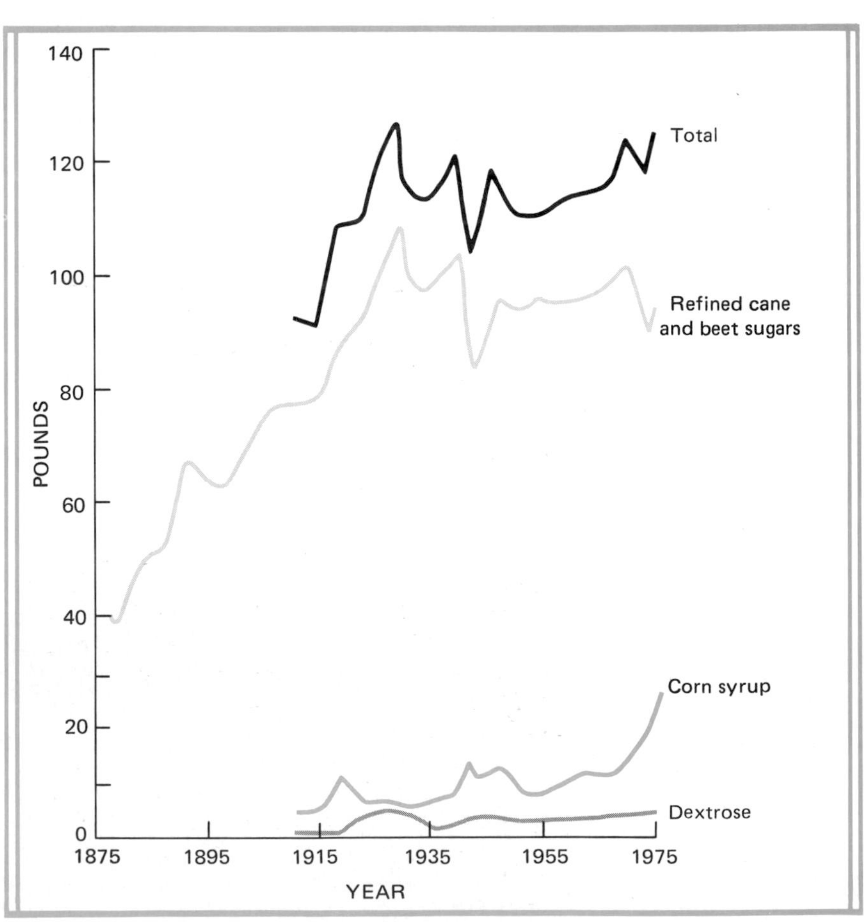

FIGURE 2-6

Trends in Per Capita Sugar Consumption in the United States

Sources: For 1875–1909 data; U.S. Bureau of the Census, *Historical statistics of the United States—Colonial times to 1959* (1960). For 1910–1965 data: USDA Rep. 138 (1968). For 1966–1976 data: Sugar and Sweetener Report (May 1977).

parison of overall national consumption at different periods in time, but do not take personal differences into account. A person who eats two desserts a day, snacks on soft drinks, and drinks heavily sweetened coffee is surely consuming proportionately more than the average; another, who scrupulously avoids adding sugar to food and eats only fresh fruit for dessert, is consuming significantly less.

A gradual but steady increase has occurred in sugar consumption over the last 25 years. As Figure 2-6 shows, sugar consumption in the last quarter of the nineteenth century was less than half of what it is now. Per capita sugar consumption today, however, is nearly as great as it was in 1930, when it reached a high of 128.7 pounds (58.5 kg) per person.

In sum, Americans are consuming a smaller proportion of their calories in carbohydrate form; and within this smaller carbohydrate intake there is a marked decrease in foods that contain complex carbohydrates (especially starches) and an increase in sugars. Direct use of table sugar appears to be declining, but this is compensated for by a striking increase in the sugars eaten, often in concealed form, in processed foods. The long-term effects, if any, of these changing patterns, which appear to accompany increasing affluence, are not known at present. Many authorities, however, consider these changes to represent at least a risk and, possibly a real threat to individual health and well-being.

DIGESTION AND ABSORPTION OF CARBOHYDRATES

Carbohydrates contained in food are not available for metabolic use by the body until after they are changed into simple sugars and absorbed into the blood stream. Some dietary carbohydrate is, of course, already in this form. But complex carbohydrates must be broken down into simple sugars. Specific enzymes present in the mouth and in certain cells of the pancreas and the small intestine play an important part in these chemical processes.

Digestion: Enzymatic Hydrolysis

The digestive reactions of carbohydrates are hydrolytic reactions; **hydrolysis** occurs when a larger molecule is split into two smaller ones and a water molecule is added to the broken ends. The water molecule is itself split into H^+ and OH^-, one ion being added to each of the products of hydrolysis. By many successive repetitions of the hydrolytic reaction occurring at the oxygen bridges between two simple sugars, even very large molecules of such complex carbohydrates as starch are eventually broken down into monosaccharides.

The first chemical step in carbohydrate digestion starts as soon as food enters the mouth. Here a salivary enzyme called amylase (or **ptyalin**) is mixed with the bolus of food and begins to hydrolyze starch. The polysaccharides are progressively broken down by amylase into smaller disaccharide units. Hydrolysis of polysaccharides can take place only in the catalyzing presence of amylase.

Salivary amylase will not effectively hydrolyze all or even very much of the starch in the bolus, because food stays in the oral cavity for a relatively short time. As food is swallowed, it is propelled by peristaltic action down the esophagus and into the stomach. Here the amylase mixed with the bolus is inactivated by gastric acid and the hydrolysis of starch is temporarily halted.

A limited amount of carbohydrate digestion, however, does occur in the stomach. Some hydrolytic reactions, notably those transforming sucrose into its components, glucose and fructose, occur spontaneously in an acid environment, such as that provided by gastric hydrochloric acid; such reactions need no enzyme catalysis.

Since only a small fraction of the carbohydrate is usually hydrolyzed in the stomach, the most important site of carbohydrate digestion is the small intestine, into which food passes from the stomach. At its junction with the stomach the small intestine is joined by a duct from the pancreas, which releases pancreatic amylase into the lumen of the small intestine (see Figure 1-6). This amylase, produced in certain pancreatic cells, has a slightly different structure from salivary amylase and functions under a different set of conditions, although both act to hydrolyze starches. Pancreatic amylase reduces starch to a specific disaccharide, maltose. Here the hydrolytic process catalyzed by amylase is virtually completed.

The cells of the brush border of the small intestine contain a group of enzymes—the **disaccharidases.** (Enzymes are often named by combining the name of their substrate with the suffix *-ase*.) Each member of this group—sucrase, maltase, lactase—catalyzes the hydrolysis of just one disaccharide—sucrose, maltose, or lactose—to its component simple sugars:

$$\text{sucrose} \xrightarrow[\text{sucrase}]{H_2O} \text{glucose and fructose}$$

$$\text{lactose} \xrightarrow[\text{lactase}]{H_2O} \text{glucose and galactose}$$

$$\text{maltose} \xrightarrow[\text{maltase}]{H_2O} \text{two glucose}$$

Although three different enzymes are involved, the chemical reaction is identical: Water is added to the bond between components of the disaccharide and two monosaccharides are produced from each hydrolytic reaction.

Because glucose, fructose, and galactose are monosaccharides, no further digestion is needed. As shown in Figure 2-7, all of the dietary carbohydrates that can be digested are hydrolyzed in the small intestine to these three monosaccharides.

LACTOSE INTOLERANCE. Many people have difficulty digesting lactose, the disaccharide in milk. Some individuals produce the enzyme **lactase** only in limited quantity, while others fail to synthesize it at all. Unable to digest most or all of this sugar, they experience a variety of digestive problems when they consume milk or milk products.

Lactose intolerance affects many adults and even some children and infants. It is, however, only very rarely present at birth, and virtually all babies are born with an adequate lactase-synthesizing capacity. In some cases, however, this capacity begins to diminish in early childhood, occasionally as early as after weaning.

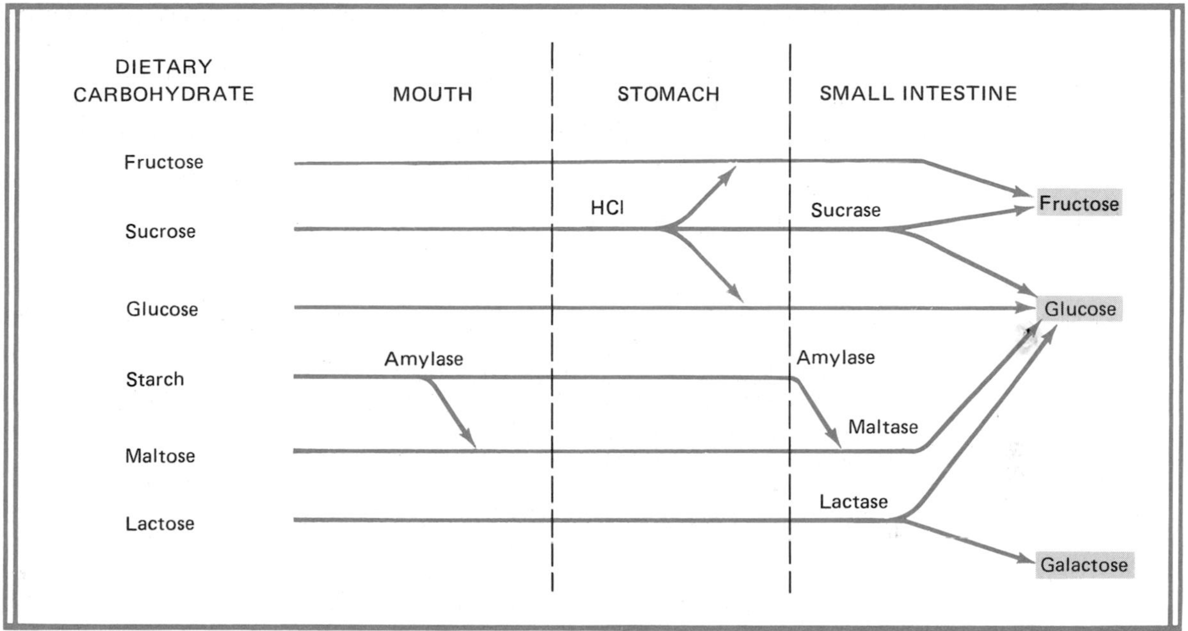

FIGURE 2-7
Schematic Diagram of Carbohydrate Digestion

Lactose intolerance is usually of genetic origin, and may become increasingly severe with age. Individuals able to digest lactose readily are most likely to be of northern European and North African descent. It has been estimated that 70 to 90 percent of non-Caucasians may be lactose intolerant (Latham, 1977). Temporary or even permanent intolerance can also result from gastrointestinal disease, heavy medication, surgery, or malnutrition.

The symptoms of lactose intolerance are varying degrees of abdominal distress; this may include bloating, cramps, flatulence, and/or diarrhea. Because the lactose ingested cannot be hydrolyzed, it cannot be absorbed. It remains in the small intestine and draws water, which results in bloating. As the undigested lactose eventually continues along the gastrointestinal tract, passing to the large intestine, it is fermented by intestinal bacteria to organic acids and gases, causing the characteristic discomforts.

Lactose intolerance is diagnosed by a test that measures the blood glucose level after the subject has been given a measured oral dose of lactose. Lactose intolerance is present if the blood glucose level does not rise at a defined rate that indicates digestion and absorption of the test sugar into the bloodstream. The general observation has been that all non-European populations display a variable but high percentage of intolerance by this definition (*Nutrition Reviews*, 1978). This test, which requires a dose of lactose equivalent to drinking more than a liter of milk, has been criticized as being unrealistically strict, however, and some authorities even question whether it has any practical significance (*Nutrition Reviews*, 1978; Latham, 1977). According to the Committee on Nutrition of the American Pediatric Society, even children of lactose-intolerant populations should be able to drink milk in normal quantities without showing distress (*Nutrition Reviews*, 1978). In one study, for example, black American children who were diagnosed by the standard test as lactose intolerant had no difficulty digesting 1 cup (240 ml) of milk (Garza and Scrimshaw, 1976).

Most lactose-intolerant individuals are easily able to digest such milk products as cheeses, yogurt, and ice cream. For children with a severe form of this condition, ordinary milk can be treated with a commercial lactase that will hydrolyze the lactose so that it can be absorbed. Milk can be treated with this preparation during pasteurization or drying, but the lactase is also available in powdered form to be added to milk immediately before consumption.

INDIGESTIBLE CARBOHYDRATES. The most widely occurring of all carbohydrates is cellulose which, along with some other complex polysaccharides, is not digestible because the human body has no enzyme capable of hydrolyzing it into its component glucose units. Because it is not hydrolyzed, cellulose simply passes through the small intestine into the colon and is eventually excreted. We have seen (Figure 2-3) that cellulose and amylose (starch) are very similar in structure, except that the chemical bonds connecting the glucose units are arranged differently in each of these polysaccharides. Each linkage requires its own enzyme for hydrolysis to take place and, although amylase can hydrolyze amylose, it is ineffective in dealing with the very similar cellulose. This indigestibility of cellulose in humans emphasizes the specificity of enzymes.

Enzymes that can hydrolyze cellulose do exist, however, and are produced by many microorganisms, including some normally found in the digestive tracts of various animals. Indirectly, by means of these bacterial enzymes, such animals can digest cellulose and other carbohydrates indigestible in humans. Some slight digestion of this sort is thought to be carried on by the human intestinal flora, but it is not enough to be of any practical significance. Cellulose and other indigestible carbohydrates are of nutritional interest as components of **fiber**, which will be discussed later in this chapter.

Absorption of Carbohydrates

To be utilized, the mix of monosaccharides resulting from the action of digestive enzymes must be absorbed into the blood through the cells lining the intestine. The absorptive process, occurring mostly in the jejunum (middle portion) of the small intestine, is a complex one. The simple sugars must be transported through the cells and across capillary walls into the portal vein. This movement occurs both by passive diffusion and by active transport.

Fructose is absorbed predominantly by diffusion, as are glucose and galactose when their concentrations are higher in the intestine than in the blood. When the gradient of glucose or galactose is reversed, with more of these sugars in the blood than in the intestine, active transport takes place. This process requires energy and a specific carrier system.

Several factors influence the rate of monosaccharide absorption. Concentration gradients are important and hormones, specifically thyroxine and insulin, also appear to play a role. Studies have indicated that galactose and glucose are absorbed somewhat more rapidly than fructose; however, the efficiency of absorption of all three monosaccharides is quite high and may approach 98 percent of the digestible carbohydrate in a diversified American diet.

FUNCTION OF CARBOHYDRATES: INTERMEDIARY METABOLISM

The portal vein transports all monosaccharides directly to the liver, where fructose and galactose are enzymatically converted to glucose. Thus, in studying the metabolism of carbohydrates, we are really discussing the metabolism of glucose.

The liver is the principal organ that regulates glucose metabolism, although other organs have important roles in maintaining homeostatic glucose levels. **Homeostasis** is the maintenance of a constant internal environment. Glucose metabolism is a state of dynamic equilibrium, so that cells receive an adequate supply of glucose over a period of time. Glucose metabolism ultimately produces the ATP (**adenosine triphosphate**) that provides energy for all cell functions. Although glucose metabolism is described as a separate process, it always occurs in conjunction with the metabolism of other nutrients.

Maintenance of Blood Glucose

Tracing glucose as it leaves the liver, we might locate it in the following sources.

BLOOD GLUCOSE. Glucose circulating in the blood provides all the body cells with an energy source and with a substrate for the synthesis of other compounds. The blood glucose level is regulated by several elegant mechanisms. In the fasting state (that is, before breakfast, or at least 12 hours after eating), glucose concentration normally ranges between 70 and 100 mg/dl. After a meal containing carbohydrates, blood glucose may rise to about 140 mg/dl, but it returns to its former level in an hour or two. Values of 70 to 110 mg/dl (fasting) are generally considered to reflect **normoglycemia** (the normal level of glucose in the blood). Abnormal functioning of the regulatory mechanisms may result in persistent **hyperglycemia** (higher than normal levels) or **hypoglycemia** (lower than normal levels).

MUSCLE AND LIVER GLYCOGEN. Glucose molecules are enzymatically condensed in muscle and liver cells to **glycogen,** the storage form of carbohydrate in animals. This process is called **glycogenesis.**

LIPIDS. By the process of **lipogenesis,** glucose can be converted to fat (see Chapter 3).

AMINO ACIDS. Carbohydrate derivatives can be **aminated** (by the addition of an amino, or nitrogen-containing, molecular group) to produce nonessential **amino acids,** so called because the body can synthesize them as needed. (**Essential** amino acids must be supplied as such in the diet; see Chapter 4.)

SPECIAL METABOLITES. These include **nucleic acids** (the building blocks of DNA and RNA), heparin, and the components of cell membranes and connective tissues, all of which contain glucose derivatives or metabolites.

CELLULAR ENERGY-PRODUCING SYSTEMS. Body cells and tissues must have a constant supply of energy for the synthesis and catabolism (breakdown) of cell compounds, for active transport of materials across cell membranes, and for the activation of muscle and nerve cells. This energy is provided mainly by glucose.

The interactions of these functions become clear if the entire system is viewed in terms of the regulation and utilization of blood glucose. Figure 2-8 depicts the processes that raise and lower the blood glucose level.

Maintenance of the level of glucose in the blood is the central element regulating the movement of glucose throughout the system. With very minor fluctuations, a constant level is maintained every hour of every day, despite the fact that dietary carbohydrate is ingested only at irregular intervals. Homeostasis is accomplished by a series of mechanisms that control the rates at which glucose is converted into glycogen or fat for storage, released from storage, reconverted into glucose, and returned to the circulation. Hormones play a key role in regulating these processes by controlling the rate and direction of the enzymatic reactions involved and by influencing the rates of active transport processes. Table 2-2 lists the sources, sites of action, and effects on blood glucose levels of several of these hormones.

When the blood glucose level falls to a "triggering" value (less than 70 mg/dl), hormonal mechanisms immediately begin functioning to restore it to normal. Glycogen stored in the liver is broken down into glucose for release to the blood. In addition, some amino acids can be **deaminated** by removal of an amino group, leaving a carbon chain fragment, which is then metabolized

FIGURE 2-8

Maintenance of Glucose Homeostasis

Levels of glucose in the blood are *raised* by ingestion of dietary carbohydrate, by release of fructose and galactose from storage in the liver, and by glycogenolysis and gluconeogenesis. Blood glucose levels are *reduced* as glucose is diverted to the energy and biochemical needs of all body tissues. After these body needs have been met, glycogenesis and lipogenesis transform glucose into glycogen and lipids, respectively, for storage. If serum levels of glucose rise higher than 160 to 180 mg/dl, the excess is excreted in the urine.

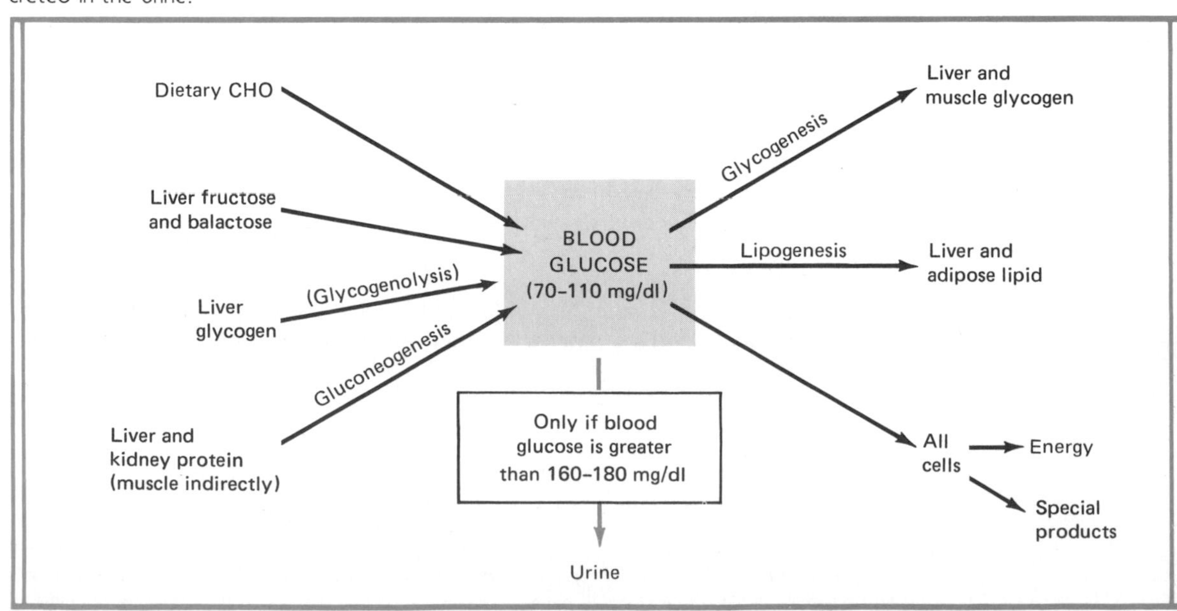

TABLE 2-2
Hormones that Influence Blood Glucose Levels

Hormone	Secreted by	Target Tissue and Effect	Net Effect on Blood Glucose
Insulin	Pancreas	Muscle: ↑ glucose transport	↓
Thyroid hormone	Thyroid	Gastrointestinal tract: ↑ glucose absorption	↑
Glucagon	Pancreas	Liver: ↑ glycogenolysis	↑
Epinephrine	Adrenal glands	Liver and muscle: ↑ glycogenolysis	↑
Steroid hormones	Adrenal glands	Muscle; liver: ↑ gluconeogenesis	↑

Key: ↑ increase ↓ decrease

to glucose. The glycerol part of a fat molecule can similarly be converted. These latter pathways are normally used only when dietary intake of carbohydrates is not available to replace blood glucose as it is utilized, and they become especially important during starvation or other severe stress conditions.

The precise functioning of the mechanisms for maintaining glucose homeostasis and the fact that more than one mechanism exists emphasize the great importance to health, and even to life itself, of the maintenance of a stable blood glucose level. The cells of the body must have this energy and substrate source for function and survival. Any interference with glucose supply through malfunction of these mechanisms (or simply through continued lack of food) is extremely serious and may be ultimately life-threatening.

PERSPECTIVE ON

Diabetes and Hypoglycemia: Disorders of The Blood Glucose Level

The importance of glucose homeostasis will be emphasized by a description of two conditions in which the blood glucose level falls more or less consistently outside the normal range.

Diabetes or Hyperglycemia. Although there are several possible reasons for hyperglycemia (high levels of blood glucose) by far the most common is the condition called **diabetes mellitus.** It takes its name from the Greek words *diabetes*, meaning "siphon" (originally referring to the large volume of urine excreted in the uncontrolled diabetic state), and *mellitus*, "honey-sweet," from the honeylike odor and taste of the urine in this condition.

Diabetes, as it is commonly called, is an ancient disease, known and described at least 3,000 years ago. Today, about 10 million Americans have diabetes in one form or another. Until recently, diabetics had a greatly shortened life expectancy, but in the last half-century improved methods of diagnosis and treatment have changed the status of diabetes from an acute and life-threatening disease to a chronic and partially controllable disorder, resulting in an extended life span for diabetics. This disease and its complications, however, are a major cause of fatalities in this country, accounting for as many as 300,000 deaths a year (American Diabetes Association, 1976). The following brief discussion of the **etiology** (origins or causes of disease) and clinical symptoms of this complicated syndrome shows the role of glucose homeostasis.

Diabetes: Etiology and Symptoms. Of all the hormones listed in Table 2-2, **insulin** is probably the most involved in overall glucose metabolism. The symptoms of diabetes result from some disturbance in the production and functioning of this hormone—decreased synthesis by the pancreas, decreased body response to insulin, or the production of hormones antagonistic to insulin. In fact, recent theories propose that disturbances in growth hormone secretion and **glucagon** (a pancreatic hormone that triggers glycogenolysis) are important in the etiology of diabetes.

Interference with insulin production and functioning can have dramatic consequences. The normal functions of insulin are: to stimulate entry of blood glucose into body cells, to increase the use of glucose for energy, and to stimulate the synthesis of glycogen, fat, and protein. When insulin function is diminished, for whatever reason, glucose movement from the blood into the cells is retarded, resulting in high blood sugar. Glycogen storage is then reduced and breakdowns of body fat and protein develop. These biochemical malfunctions lead to the characteristic signs and symptoms of the diabetic condition—polyuria (excessive volume of urine), polydipsia (thirst), polyphagia (hunger), and weight loss. Such a relationship between biochemistry and clinical symptoms will be observed repeatedly throughout our study—biochemical abnormalities underlie and indeed precede, symptoms. Let us look in more detail at how the relationship works in this instance.

When the blood glucose level rises above 180 mg/dl the kidneys cannot keep glucose from spilling over into the urine. Normally, the kidneys are able to reabsorb the usual low levels of glucose. Whenever glucose goes into the urine in large amounts, much of it is, of course, excreted. A symptom of this loss is polyuria, caused by the osmotic (water-attracting) properties of the glucose in the urine. This, in turn, upsets the normal water balance of the body, resulting in polydipsia as an attempt to restore that balance (see Chapter 9). Meanwhile, even though there is an excess of glucose in the blood, it is not able to enter the cells in amounts adequate for cellular energy needs. Feelings of hunger accompany the "glucose-starved" state. Eventually there is also loss of weight accompanied by debilitation from the loss of muscle protein.

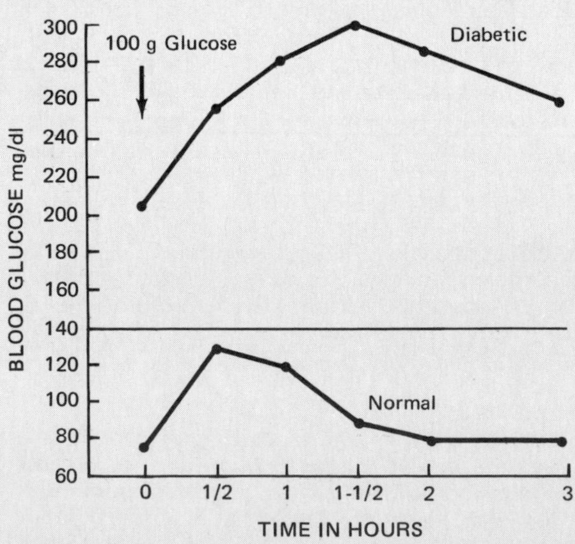

Results of oral glucose tolerance test in a normal person and a diabetic.

These clinical signs and symptoms of the diabetic condition can be confirmed by several diagnostic tests that measure the levels of glucose in the blood and urine. In another test, the oral glucose tolerance test, a standard amount of glucose (usually 100 grams for adults) is ingested in a fasting state; blood glucose is then measured repeatedly at standard intervals. The graph compares the results of the glucose tolerance test in a normal individual with those of a diabetic.

Factors in Diabetes Incidence. Researchers generally agree that a major factor in the development of diabetes is heredity, but the genetic mechanism is complex and not yet fully understood. Also, diabetes is strongly associated with obesity, although again the precise mechanism involved is not clear. The incidence of diabetes increases, however, with increasing obesity, and it doubles with every 20 percent of overweight (American Diabetes Association, 1976). Although obesity may predispose an individual to diabetes, it is not directly causative.

Age is, however, a major factor. Among the progressive body changes during the adult years is the loss of some ability to remove glucose from the blood. Diabetes is much more likely to occur in those 40 years or older than in younger people. Two major forms of this disease are, indeed, categorized according to the usual age of incidence, although this is not a hard and fast rule.

Most frequent is adult-onset diabetes, which may occur at any time, but is usual in the sixth and seventh decades of life. This form is very often associated with obesity; it is characterized by diminished insulin production (relative to metabolic need), or relative insensitivity of cells to the insulin that is produced. Adult-onset diabetes can usually be controlled by dietary management alone, sometimes accompanied by minimal medication.

Juvenile-type diabetes, developing generally before age 20, is characterized by a total lack of insulin production. It is a severe condition, often leading to serious complications including atherosclerosis, blindness, nerve damage, and kidney disease. Juvenile-type diabetes is treated with insulin therapy as well as dietary management.

Because the precise cause of diabetes is unknown and because medical science has not yet discovered a way to increase human insulin production or efficiency, treatment now centers on controlling the levels of glucose in the blood, preventing early complications, and mitigating symptoms. Diet management, weight control, and sometimes insulin therapy or other drug therapy are used to keep blood glucose levels as nearly normal as possible, thus reducing the chances for complications to develop. Diabetics are advised to have frequent medical examinations and to test themselves daily for glycosuria (the presence of extra sugar in the urine).

A number of studies in different parts of the world have aroused suspicions that the prevalence of diabetes may coincide with changing dietary patterns. In particular, as Western foods and food habits have replaced traditional foodways in Africa, Japan, the Pacific Islands, and elsewhere, the incidence of diabetes has increased (West, 1976). The marked increase in its prevalence in the United States also has led to the suggestion that high diabetes incidence correlates with increasing consumption of simple carbohydrates (sugars), while low diabetes incidence has been noted in places where complex carbohydrate (starch) intake is high (West, 1976). There is presently no definitive evidence that sugar consumption causes diabetes in humans. The studies suggesting a relationship are epidemiological; such studies may suggest, but do not conclusively demonstrate, the existence of causative relationships.

When the incidence of a disease in a given population shows an apparent increase, it is essential to examine all possible associations before one can be singled out. Is there a true increase in the incidence or have more sophisticated testing methods, more broadly applied, identified a larger proportion of diabetics in the population—especially those with mild symptoms who might not otherwise have been noticed? Again, as treatment methods have improved, the life expectancy of diabetics has increased; they are, thus, more likely to reproduce, thereby increasing the proportion of the population with a genetic predisposition to the condition. Finally, because early fatalities from smallpox, diphtheria, and other infectious diseases have been largely prevented, people have more years in which to develop a disease that mostly appears after middle age. All of these and other possible influences must be carefully analyzed before a relationship suggested by epidemiological studies is shown to have causal significance. At present, we are able to say with assurance only that, while at least some evidence suggests an association between sugar intake and diabetes, the most likely relationships have to do with the role of sugars in producing obesity and the association of obesity with diabetes (West, 1976).

Hypoglycemia: Etiology and Symptoms. In recent years, hypoglycemia (low blood sugar) seems to have acquired popular status as a "disease." Most alleged cases of this ailment are self-diagnosed, and not clinically verified. Only a series of blood glucose tests taken over a period of time can provide an accurate diagnosis.

True hypoglycemia is a symptom of an underlying biochemical disorder. Associated symptoms are weakness, excessive perspiration, faintness, nervousness, and headache—all of which are probably caused by the excessive secretion and release of **epinephrine** as a reaction to low levels of blood sugar. Treatment depends on the reason for chronic low blood sugar.

The most common form of hypoglycemia is **nonfasting reactive hypoglycemia.** Symptoms typically appear two to five hours after eating, and last for less than 30 minutes. Most patients have normal blood sugar levels and insulin production after an oral glucose test, with no glandular or other disease to account for the hypoglycemic symptoms. For some reason insulin is oversecreted in response to elevated blood sugar levels after eating. This causes a sudden and exaggerated drop in the blood glucose level, accounting for the observable symptoms.

Carbohydrate intake of those with this type of hypoglycemia should be restricted to 75–125 grams per day, and it should be primarily in the form of complex carbohydrates. Such a diet can be maintained most easily by eating three light but regular meals per day, with three snacks at two- to three-hour intervals after each meal.

Reactive hypoglycemia accounts for 70 percent of all cases. Low blood sugar may result from other causes as well. Fasting (that is, nonreactive) hypoglycemia may result from conditions that interfere with maintenance of glucose homeostasis, such as tumors of the pancreas, liver disease, medication, and surgery. Hypoglycemia can also result from an excessive dose of insulin taken by a diabetic. Accurate diagnosis through laboratory analysis is essential for appropriate treatment. For example, hypoglycemia originating with liver disease must be treated with carbohydrate supplements rather than with a low-carbohydrate diet.

Self-diagnosis can be dangerous because it may prevent the discovery and treatment of such underlying disorders.

CARBOHYDRATE STORAGE

Glucose, transported from the blood into the tissues, may be needed immediately, either to supply energy or as a substrate for synthesis of various products. If it is not immediately needed, however, it can be stored in the form of glycogen or fat for future use. Glycogenesis occurs first, assuming that the body's limited capacity for glycogen storage is not yet saturated: The liver can store only about 110 grams of glycogen; muscle tissue can hold perhaps 245 grams. These figures are averages, and there may be considerable individual variation according to body size and conformation. Glycogen synthesis is facilitated by insulin.

When the glycogen storage capacity is fully utilized, excess glucose will be converted into body fat, since the body has a much larger capacity for its storage. Lipogenesis (the synthesis of fat) is also facilitated by insulin.

In addition to these storage mechanisms, some glucose is used for the synthesis of various essential carbohydrate derivatives, such as heparin (produced in the liver and which affects blood clotting). Because these derivatives are functioning molecules, however, they are not considered storage products in the same sense that glycogen and fat are.

Energy Production

Cells can survive only with a fairly constant and adequate supply of energy for their life processes. This energy is normally obtained from glucose, primarily by two reaction sequences or "pathways." (Although other pathways exist, the two we shall discuss here are more significant.) The **anaerobic pathway** can proceed in the absence of oxygen or under conditions of limited oxygen supply, such as might occur during vigorous exercise. This series of reactions takes place in the cytoplasm of the cell, and is called the **Embden-Meyerhof pathway,** or simply **glycolysis.** The **aerobic pathway** requires oxygen and functions in the mitochondria (cell organelles specialized for energy exchange). This pathway is also known as the tricarboxylic acid (TCA) cycle, the citric-acid cycle, and the **Krebs cycle.** The latter name recognizes Sir Hans Krebs, an English biochemist who contributed significantly to the understanding of this metabolic cycle.

These two sequences of reactions are interrelated. Some of the reactions are also common to protein and lipid metabolism, and vitamins and minerals have their places in these reactions as well. Taken together, the interactions of substrates, enzymes, and coenzymes in these pathways are as intricate as the set of delicate parts in the mechanism of a fine watch, and as precisely controlled.

These two major pathways are diagrammed in Figure 2-9, which shows the conversion of glucose, first to various intermediates, and ultimately to energy. The essential and primary function of these reaction sequences is the production of energy. There are in the body certain chemical compounds, known as high-energy compounds, that can trap and hold large amounts of energy. One of the most important of them is *adenosine triphosphate,* or ATP. High-energy compounds such as ATP can "trap" energy, much as a

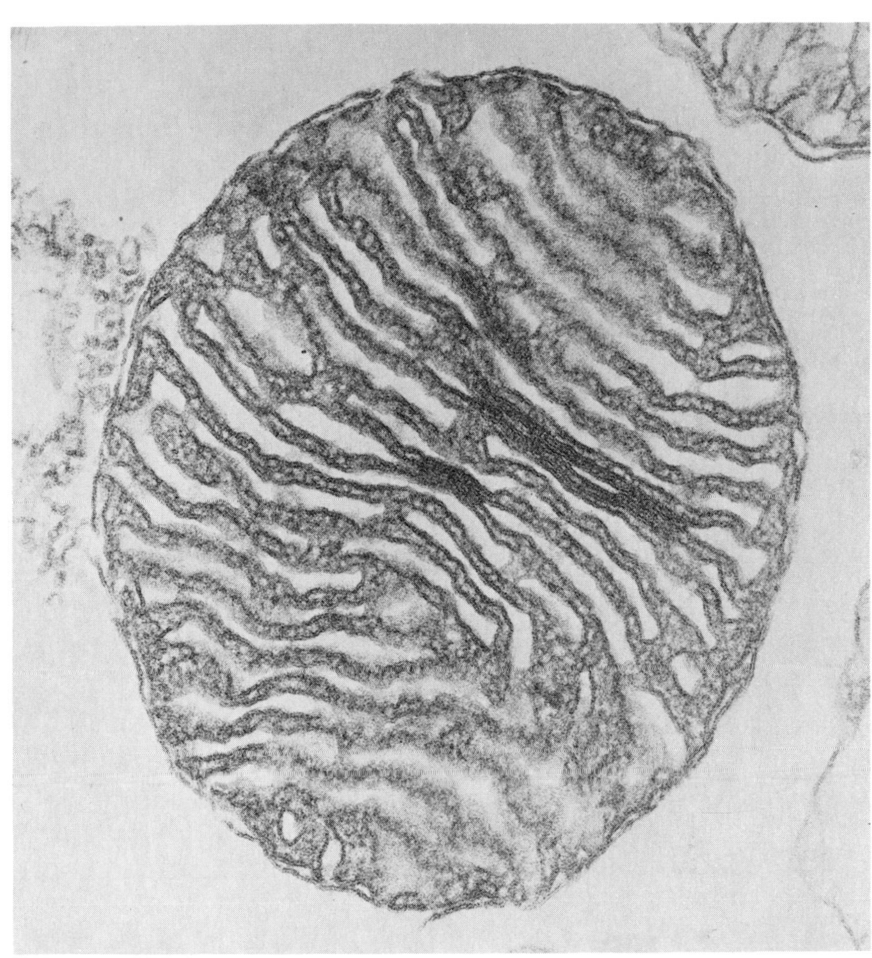

Electron micrograph of an isolated heart mitochondrion from a beef heart, magnified 110,000 times. (Dr. Sidney Fleischer and Akitsugu Saito)

storage battery does, and release it as needed to power essential cell reactions that would not occur, or would not occur fast enough, without this energy. The ATP molecule is composed of adenine (a nitrogen compound), ribose (a pentose), and three phosphate groups. Two of these phosphates are attached to the rest of the molecule by so-called "high energy bonds." The energy in these bonds can be trapped by the cell and used to power muscle and nerve impulses for transport of materials, for heat production, and for essential biochemical reactions. Glycolysis and the Krebs cycle both result in the generation of ATP, but in markedly differing quantities.

GLYCOLYSIS. The net result of this sequence is the production of two molecules of ATP and two molecules of hydrogen for every glucose molecule that enters the sequence. The glucose molecule itself is converted into two 3-carbon molecules of pyruvate, which enter the Krebs cycle. Specific enzymes and coenzymes must be present to catalyze these reactions. When the cell's oxygen supply is limited, some pyruvate is enzymatically converted to lactic

FIGURE 2-9
Glycolysis and the Krebs Cycle

In *glycolysis*, glucose crosses the cell membrane into the cytoplasm, where it is converted into two 3-carbon molecules of pyruvate with the release of two ATP and two hydrogens (2H) for every molecule of glucose.

In the *Krebs cycle*, the pyruvate enters the mitochondrion and is decarboxylated to acetyl CoA. The acetyl CoA molecule condenses with oxaloacetate to form a 6-carbon compound citric acid (from which one name of the cycle is derived). In the following stages of the cycle, two additional molecules of CO_2 are released as a result of reactions that use the carbons derived from acetyl CoA; several pairs of hydrogens (2H) are released; and another high-energy compound, guanosine triphosphate (GTP, similar to ATP), is produced. At the completion of the cycle, a molecule of oxaloacetate is regenerated, ready for combination with acetyl CoA on the next turn of the cycle.

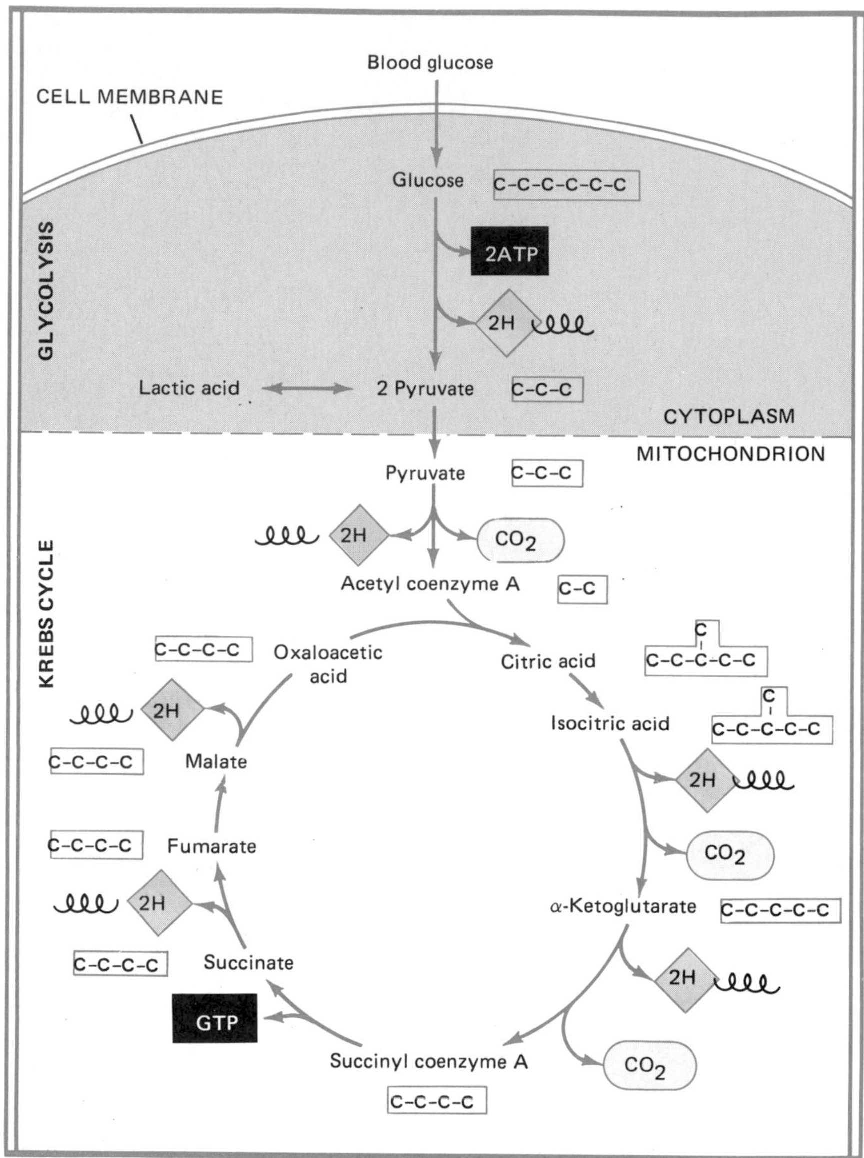

acid, utilizing the hydrogen molecules produced during the reaction sequence.

KREBS CYCLE. Under aerobic conditions, pyruvate can be further oxidized with a much greater production of ATP. First, the 3-carbon pyruvate molecule crosses the mitochondrial membrane, where its initial reaction takes place. This involves the removal of a single carbon atom, in the form of a carbon dioxide (CO_2) molecule. This reaction is known as **decarboxylation.**

The remaining 2-carbon fragment is a molecule of "active acetate," or **acetyl coenzyme A (acetyl CoA)**, which plays a pivotal role in intermediary metabolism.

Through the series of reactions diagrammed in Figure 2-9, the two carbons in acetyl CoA become carbon dioxide. Energy is produced as the hydrogen ions released in the Krebs cycle enter and proceed through the electron transport system. This energy eventually becomes "trapped" in the high-energy compound ATP—note that much more of the energy in the original glucose molecule is captured via the Krebs cycle than during glycolysis. Oxygen is important to the cell because it makes possible the efficient energy production of the aerobic Krebs cycle. Substrates other than glucose, primarily fats and amino acids, can also power the Krebs cycle.

THE GENERATION OF HIGH-ENERGY BONDS. Most of the potential energy produced during glycolysis and the Krebs cycle becomes trapped as ATP through the electron transport system. This is a series of reactions that occurs inside the mitochondria of the cells, using vitamins and minerals as cofactors required for the reaction but not consumed in it.

Each set of two hydrogen atoms generated in glycolysis and the Krebs cycle passes through the electron transport system (described in Chapter 7), eventually combining with oxygen to form a molecule of water. At the same time, phosphate is joined to adenosine diphosphate (ADP) by a high-energy bond, thereby producing a molecule of ATP (see Figure 2-10).

Glycolysis yields two molecules of ATP for each molecule of glucose. Complete oxidation through the Krebs cycle and the passage of hydrogen ions through the electron transport system generates another 34 ATP molecules. Complete oxidation of one glucose molecule will therefore supply 36 ATP, plus a total of 6 molecules of CO_2. This CO_2 diffuses out of the cell into the blood, which carries it to the lungs where it is released and exhaled. The overall reaction of glucose metabolism is therefore:

$$C_6H_{12}O_6 + 6O_2 \longrightarrow 6CO_2 + 6H_2O + 36ATP \text{ (chemical energy)}$$

FIGURE 2-10
The Formation of ATP

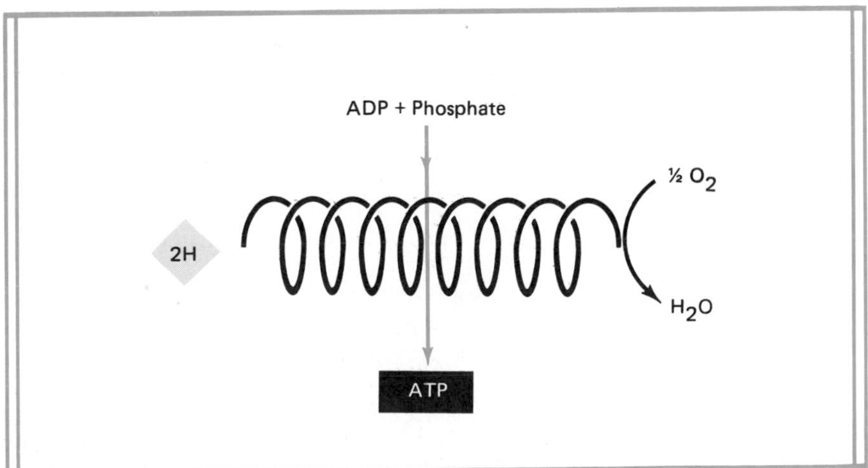

Green plants, by the process of photosynthesis, use CO_2, H_2O, and the energy of sunlight to produce carbohydrate and to release oxygen:

$$6CO_2 + 6H_2O + \text{(light energy)} \longrightarrow C_6H_{12}O_6 + 6O_2$$

Animals, in turn, utilize the carbohydrate in plant food sources to produce chemical energy, CO_2, and water through the processes just described. These different but interacting plant and animal energy cycles are at the heart of the food chain.

DIETARY REQUIREMENTS: HOW MUCH AND WHAT KIND

The precise requirement of the human body for carbohydrate in the diet is not known. The Food and Nutrition Board has recommended that a minimum of 50 to 100 grams be eaten every day. Eating less than 50 grams for an extended period of time could result in potentially harmful fat and protein catabolism, as we will see in later chapters. Most Americans need not worry: The average diversified diet consumed in this country provides three to four times the recommended minimum of carbohydrates. Many fad diets, however, do not. The whole question of the necessary amounts and types of carbohydrate is the subject of continuing debate and research, much of it concerned with consumption of refined sugars. The remainder of this chapter will examine several issues related to carbohydrate consumption.

Sugar and Disease

On the average, Americans have been increasing their sugar intake in recent years, with greater amounts incorporated into commercially processed foods than ever before. Much evidence suggests that our high sugar intake does us little good, and that it may be potentially harmful. Excessive consumption of sugar has been implicated in the etiology of several chronic diseases and as a factor in obesity, although its role in different situations is not always clear. It is, however, generally agreed that sugar contributes to dental caries since sucrose nourishes the bacteria that cause tooth decay. This problem affects 95 percent of the population and constitutes a significant component of our national dental costs of almost $5 billion a year.

Sucrose has also been implicated in the etiology of heart disease, especially for the 10 percent of the population who are classified as carbohydrate-sensitive because they respond to ingestion of dietary carbohydrate (especially sucrose and fructose) with increased blood lipid levels, which have been strongly associated with the development of atherosclerosis. Yudkin and Morland (1967) report evidence from a wide variety of studies that cardiovascular disease is associated with high sugar intake. Some researchers consider that the effect of sugar on blood lipids, however, is not well established and hold that the major influence of sugar probably results from excess energy intake and its consequence, obesity, which in turn puts excess stress on the cardiovascular system (Connor and Connor, 1976). The relationship of diet to heart disease is a complicated issue and will be discussed at length in the following chapter. Hypertension and diabetes may also be related to sugar intake but, again, primarily through the obesity effect (Mayer, 1978). The role of sugar in diabetes has been discussed above.

Although the body must have sugar to maintain the supply of energy for its cells and their functions, that sugar does not have to be eaten in the form of sucrose. We have seen that blood sugar or glucose can be obtained through digestion and enzymatic conversion from other sources as well. Fructose in fruit and lactose in milk are both converted to glucose. The starch molecules in cereals, potatoes, grains, and legumes are long chains or polymers of glucose units, which are converted to glucose in the course of the digestive process.

Sweets, table sugar, and other "quick-energy" foods can indeed be used to provide the energy boost sometimes needed by athletes or for strenuous physical work, because this is the fastest way to increase the blood sugar supply. But sugar taken in this way is used up quickly, and such sugar intake usually displaces other foods that have significant nutritional value in addition to energy content. In particular, the proportion of complex carbohydrates ingested is decreased. Table sugar, and such foods as candy and soft drinks, are sources of nothing except kilocalories. The Senate Select Committee on Nutrition and Human Needs has recommended that total consumption of carbohydrates should be increased, with emphasis on complex carbohydrates; that consumption of sugars be decreased; and that these goals can best be accomplished by the substitution of grains, legumes, and fresh fruit for empty-caloric desserts and snacks (Select Committee, 1977). Foods rich in complex carbohydrates supply vitamins and minerals as well as some protein.

Nonsucrose Sweeteners

Most of us have a "sweet tooth." In an effort to reduce sugar intake without eliminating the pleasures of eating sweet foods, many people have been turning to alternative sweeteners. Some of these are natural nonsucrose sources of sweetness and some are of chemical origin. Although this emphasis is recent, there is nothing new about many of these products.

NATURAL SWEETENERS. Brown sugar, molasses, and honey, for example, are old standbys that have been glamourized by new claims that they are more nutritious than refined white sugar. As Table 2-3 indicates, these sweeteners do contain several nutrients not found in white sugar. Comparison of these nutrient amounts with the RDA demonstrates that none of the sweeteners in the diet is likely to be a significant source of anything except kilocalories. Even the relatively higher iron, calcium, and phosphorous values shown for blackstrap molasses are minimal fractions of the RDAs for those nutrients (and many would consider this particular sweetener to be an acquired taste!). Furthermore, the nutrient content of these sweeteners tends to vary with climate and soil conditions during the growing season and with manufacturing conditions during the production and packaging process, so that these substances are not only poor but also unreliable nutrient sources.

TABLE 2-3 **Nutrient Content of Various Sweeteners (per tbsp)**

Sweetener	kcal	(kJ)	Protein g	Fat g	CHO g	Ca mg	Fe mg	P mg	K mg	Thiamin mg	Riboflavin mg	Niacin mg
Corn syrup, light and dark	58	(244)	0	0	15	9.0	0.8	3.2	0.8	0	0	0
Honey, strained	65	(273)	0	0	17	1.0	0.1	1.3	10.7	0	0.01	0.10
Maple syrup, pure	53	(223)	0	0	14	21.8	0.2	1.7	37.0	0	0	0
Molasses, light	50	(210)	0	0	13	33.0	0.9	9.0	183.0	0.01	0.01	0.04
Molasses, blackstrap	45	(189)	0	0	11	137.0	3.2	17.0	585.0	0.02	0.04	0.40
Sugar, brown	50	(210)	0	0	13	12.0	0.5	2.7	48.0	0	0	0
Sugar, table	45	(189)	0	0	12	0	0	0	0.4	0	0	0
RDA: Males 23–50 years	—		56	—	—	800.0	10.0	800.0	—	1.40	1.60	18.00
Females 23–50 years	—		44	—	—	800.0	18.0	800.0	—	1.00	1.20	13.00

Source: C. F. Adams, *Nutritive value of American foods in common units.* Agriculture Handbook No. 456. Agricultural Research Service USDA (Washington, D.C.: U.S. Government Printing Office, 1975).

Sugars found naturally in fruits, vegetables, cereals, grains, and milk are accompanied by other nutrients important for good health and are provided in less concentrated form than in refined sugars. In addition, degrees of sweetness vary with the type of sugar. The relative sweetness of several sweeteners is shown in Table 2-4. Honey has more "sweetening power" than table sugar, but it is not a "calorie-saver."

ARTIFICIAL SWEETENERS. For many years, calorie-free, nonnutritive sweeteners have been widely used by the weight-conscious, as well as by those wanting to avoid sugar for other reasons, as in diabetes. Saccharin and cyclamate are chemical compounds that are much sweeter than sugar; saccharin is 350 times as sweet. Minimal amounts are necessary for desirably sweet taste. Both of these, however, have been implicated as possible carcinogens, and the use of cyclamate was prohibited in 1970 by the Food and Drug Administration (FDA). In June 1979 the FDA announced plans to reopen the investigation of cyclamate.

TABLE 2-4
Relative Sweetness of Different Sweeteners

Sweetener	Equivalent Sweetness	kcal	(kJ)
Honey	¾ tsp	16	(67)
Table sugar	1 tsp	15	(63)
Brown sugar	1⅛ tsp	19	(80)
Molasses	1½ tsp	25	(105)
Corn syrup	1½ tsp	29	(122)
Saccharin (¼ grain)	1 tablet	0	(0)

Source: Adapted from J. C. Gates, *Basic foods* (New York: Holt, Rinehart & Winston, 1976), p. 475.

The safety of saccharin was questioned as long ago as the 1880s, shortly after its discovery. Some years ago it was believed that 1 gram per day was probably a safe dose for humans. (In its usual commercial powdered form, saccharin is bulked with glucose. The most readily available packets contain a total of 1 gram of powder, of which 4 percent, or 40 milligrams is saccharin, equivalent in sweetening power to 2 teaspoons of sugar.) A 1967 National Academy of Sciences report, undertaken at the request of the FDA, while not disagreeing with the earlier conclusion, stated that the evidence from previous studies was inadequate and called for additional research. The first evidence that saccharin might be carcinogenic appeared in 1971, in a study conducted by the Wisconsin Alumni Research Foundation (WARF), showing that 7 of 15 rats who ingested saccharin as 5 percent of their diet for two years developed bladder cancer (Wightman, 1977). Soon afterward the Canadian government began a larger-scale test of saccharin, and the results became available in 1977: Of 200 rats fed saccharin at a level of 5 percent of their diets, 21 developed bladder tumors, while only one of the controls (who received no saccharin) was so afflicted. Tumor incidence was particularly high in the second generation of rats indicating that saccharin intake during fetal and early postnatal development had even more serious consequences (Pines and Glick, 1977).

An officer of the corporation that markets the biggest-selling artificial sweetener stands beside one and a half million packets of the product in March, 1977, after the Food and Drug administration proposed a ban on sales of saccharin. The marketing firm maintains that a human would have to ingest this much saccharin in a year, to consume the equivalent of the amount fed to rats in the study that led to the FDA proposal. (Wide World Photos)

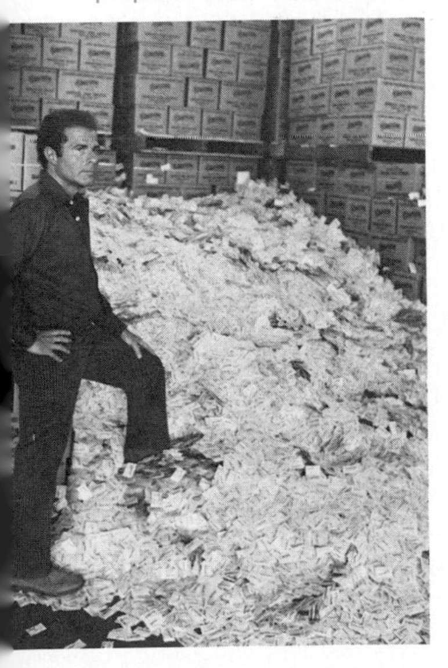

In March 1977, the FDA announced its intention to ban saccharin from use in food and beverages, and to prohibit table use as well. The public outcry against the proposed ban, unprecedented in its breadth and intensity, was notably greater than the protest against the cyclamate ban less than ten years earlier. Among the reasons for this strong reaction was the fact that, because cyclamate had already been prohibited, there would now be no alternative calorie-free sweetener available (Parham, 1978). Artificial sweeteners had gained wide acceptance with consumption up to about 5 million pounds a year (Pines and Glick, 1977), much of it added, as is sugar, to commercially processed foods, such as soft drinks and snacks. Not only the food industry but large numbers of consumers were also affected.

Opponents of the 1977 ban pointed out that the test doses were far higher in relation to body size and weight than the amounts of saccharin that human users would be likely to ingest (equivalent, according to some, to drinking 800 cans of diet soft drink every day for a lifetime). Some questioned the validity of animal, and especially nonprimate, tests. Many argued that, assuming the validity of the tests, the danger of sugar was greater than that of saccharin, while others felt that consumers were entitled to determine relative risk for themselves (Parham, 1978).

The FDA had no choice but to ban the use of saccharin. The Delaney Amendment (1958) to the Food, Drug and Cosmetics Act requires that the FDA prohibit the use of *any* food additive shown to cause cancer in test animals or in humans. In response to the public reaction, however, Congress voted for a moratorium on the ban, requiring only that saccharin and foods containing it be accompanied at the point of sale by a label or sign indicating possible carcinogenicity. A result of this action was to allow consumers to make their own appraisal of the risks involved. Some saw the whole episode as an opportunity to review, and perhaps revise, the Delaney Amendment (Galbraith, 1977).

How valid is the testing procedure used in the Canadian study? In Chapter 1 the rationale for large dose/short-term animal tests was examined.

Such tests have proved particularly fruitful in cancer research, because the incidence of cancer is proportionate to the dose rate or exposure. Thus, the incidence resulting from a relatively mild carcinogen would be both low and slow in appearing under normal use conditions. In such cases, a high dose over a short period of time tells us what would presumably happen with a low dose over a long time. If such tests produce cancer, we can be sure the substance tested is a carcinogen. A substance that is not a carcinogen—and this is the crucial point—will never produce cancer, no matter how high the dose rate.

Of course, doubts would probably subside if epidemiological studies unequivocally confirmed the results of animal studies. A number of epidemiological studies have now been made, but conclusions are not in complete agreement. In a Canadian study of patients hospitalized with bladder cancer, men who had used saccharin in tablet form were shown to have a 60 percent greater risk than controls, while men who ingested saccharin-containing foods and beverages, and women who used all forms of saccharin showed no significant risk (Howe et al., 1977). Before the results of the Canadian rat study were known, a similar epidemiological study in an American city was initiated. The controls generally had not consumed significantly smaller amounts of nonnutritive sweeteners in any form than had those with bladder cancer and, thus, neither cyclamate nor saccharin usage was shown in this study to be associated with increased risk (Kessler and Clark, 1978). A recent report by the National Academy of Sciences concluded that saccharin is "a potential carcinogen in humans, but one of low potency in comparison to other carcinogens. . . . Even low risks, applied to a large number of exposed persons, may lead to public health concerns" (*CNI Weekly Report*, 11/9/78).

In June 1979 a Congressional committee voted to extend the moratorium on the saccharin ban until June 30, 1981. Obviously, the last word on this subject is yet to come, and evidence from additional animal and epidemiological studies is being awaited.

In the meantime, alternative artificial sweeteners are being developed, and some natural products look promising too. Pending its approval by the FDA, the product aspartame might be a useful sweetener. The "miracle fruit," *Synsepalum dulcificum*, actually causes sour foods to taste sweet and apparently has no harmful effects (Wightman, 1977). Monellin, extracted from "serendipity berries," *Dioscoreophyllum cumminisii*, is a protein said to taste 2,500 times as sweet as sucrose. Xylitol is one of a group (including mannitol and sorbitol) of sweet-tasting alcohols distilled from wood and is already in limited use in products such as chewing gum. Although it has nearly as high a caloric value as sucrose, xylitol does not promote, and in fact apparently protects against, dental caries; however, a recent study has implicated xylitol, too, as a carcinogen. With all natural sweeteners, however, the actual carbohydrate and caloric content will have to be taken into account by diabetics and others on special diets. As yet, little is known about the mechanism of taste, or why substances do or do not taste sweet.

RECOMMENDATIONS. Many consumers face a sometimes difficult choice. Some diabetics and extremely carbohydrate-sensitive or obesity-prone individuals would probably prefer the relatively low level of risk of bladder cancer indicated by the animal studies, to the demonstrably greater risk, for them, of sugar consumption. Moderation in the use of any sweetening agent, natural or

PERSPECTIVE ON
Dietary Fiber

The popular press has paid much attention in recent years to the roles of fiber in the maintenance of human health. Here, we shall separate fad from fact, and discuss the functions and sources of what is indeed an important, if nowadays sometimes overemphasized, dietary component.

Concern with fiber is not a contemporary innovation. Popular writers and healers have long urged that special attention be paid to the inclusion of "roughage" in the diet. In the fifth century B.C., the Greek physician Hippocrates recommended that bread be made from unrefined flour. In nineteenth-century America, Sylvester Graham traveled the country advocating, among other practices, the ingestion of bran. He gave his name to the Graham cracker, a bran-containing cracker that is a staple on grocery shelves even today. The role of fiber has until recently been relatively overlooked by the scientific community, probably because fiber is not a nutrient (Burkitt et al., 1974). While studies contributing to the modern understanding of fiber date back to the 1930s, only in the last two decades have sophisticated methodology and analysis been applied to this dietary component.

Components of Fiber. Some carbohydrates are not hydrolyzed by human digestive enzymes. The indigestible remnant, known as dietary fiber, passes through the gastrointestinal tract and is eliminated in the feces. Fiber consists of the walls of plant cells, which are composed mostly of three polysaccharides, (cellulose, pectic substances, and hemicellulose), as well as of the noncarbohydrate, lignin (Spiller and Amen, 1975). Fiber is a component of plant foods only; it is not found in foods of animal origin.

Fiber has the capacity to absorb water readily and in quantity. Cellulose is the most abundant component of dietary fiber. The hemicelluloses are polymers of several hexoses and pentoses. Pectic substances are complex polymers originating in cell walls and fibrous parts of fruits, vegetables, and other land plants. Some of them can be chemically converted to pectinic acid, a water-soluble substance from which pectin, used to bind fluid in making jellies, is derived. Most commercial pectin comes from the pulp of apples and citrus fruits.

Dietary tables frequently show "crude" fiber content of foods; this term is older than "dietary fiber," and refers to the residue left after foodstuffs have been subjected to extreme laboratory procedures. These processes destroy some fiber that is indigestible in the human body and do not distinguish between the different chemical structures making up plant cell walls (each type of plant has its own type of cell-wall composition). "Crude fiber," then, underestimates total fiber content by as much as 80 percent of the hemicellulose, 50 to 90 percent of the lignin, and 20 to 50 percent of the cellulose (Spiller and Amen, 1975). The table provides crude and dietary fiber data for some common foods. These crude fiber figures, which may be only one-fifth to one-half of the actual dietary fiber content, represent largely cellulose and lignin (Kelsay, 1978).

More accurate is the modern method of analyzing the fiber content of foods, a detergent process which separates the different carbohydrate components in sequence. This results in a more precise determination of the quantity of each component, and is expressed as a total called *neutral detergent fiber* (NDF) which better approximates the total fiber content of foods (Spiller and Amen, 1975).

Problems of Low Fiber Intake. It has been suggested that lack of fiber in the diet may be associated with coronary heart disease, diabetes, cancer of the colon, diverticulosis, irritable bowel syndrome, hiatus hernia, and other diseases of the gastrointestinal system. Many observers have noted that these problems occur far less frequently among non-Westernized, nonurban peoples who consume traditional diets high in fiber materials, and that their incidence increases in populations consuming a Western-style diet. For example, 70,000 new cases of cancer of the colon and rectum are diagnosed every year in the United States. In Africa this ailment is very rarely encountered. Similarly, heart disease, which kills an estimated 30 percent of American men and 15 percent of American women, is virtually unknown in Africa, although it is beginning to make its appearance in African cities, presumably as Western lifestyles, including diet, are adopted (Burkitt et al., 1974). These comparisons, however, result from epidemiological studies; conclusive experimental data on the role of fiber, and of other factors inherent in Western civilization, such as stress, are not yet available.

Functions of Fiber. A significant role of fiber derives

APPROXIMATE FIBER CONTENT OF SELECTED FOODS

Product	Serving Size	Crude Fiber[a] g/serving	Dietary Fiber[b] g/serving
Cereals, Breads, and Flours			
Bran	1 oz	—	14.4
Whole grain flour	½ c	—	13.2
White flour	½ c	—	4.0
All bran	½ c	2.3	—
Bran flakes	¾ c	1.0	—
Raisin bran	½ c	0.7	—
Oatmeal, cooked	1 c	0.5	—
Cornflakes	1 c	0.2	3.08
Cream of wheat, cooked	1 c	0.1	—
Bread, "high fiber" type	1 slice	2.1	—
Bread, whole wheat	1 slice	0.4	2.0
Bread, pumpernickel	1 slice	0.4	—
Bread, white, enriched	1 slice	trace	0.6
Fruits and Vegetables			
Peas, green	⅔ c	2.0	7.2
Pear	1 medium	—	3.9
Carrots	⅔ c	1.5	3.8
Banana	1 medium	—	3.1
Cabbage, cooked	⅔ c	—	2.8
Apple with skin	1 medium	2.0	2.6
Strawberries	½ c	1.0	1.6
Tomato, raw	1 medium	—	1.4
Plum	1 medium	—	1.1
Potato	3¼" diam.	0.9	—
Orange	3" diam.	0.8	—
Corn, canned	½ c	0.7	—
Raisins, dried, seedless	½ c	0.7	—
Beans, fresh green	½ c	0.6	—
Spinach	½ c	0.5	—
Celery, stalk	1 large	0.4	—
Grapes, green seedless	18–20	0.2	—
Fruit juice	1 c	0.2	—
Legumes			
Chick peas	½ c	5.0	—
Beans, navy	½ c	4.3	—
Lentils	½ c	3.9	—
Meat and Dairy Products	—	0	—
Nuts and Seeds			
Sunflower seeds	3½ oz	3.8	—
Sesame seeds	3½ oz	2.4	—
Walnuts, English	½ c	2.1	—
Peanuts, roasted, with skin	1 tbs	0.5	1.4
Pistachio nuts	30	0.3	—
Cashews, roasted	6–8	0.2	—

[a] C. T. Church and H. N. Church *Food values of portions commonly used*, 12th ed. (Philadelphia: Lippincott, 1975).
[b] D. A. T. Southgate, B. Bailey, E. Collinson et al., A guide to calculating intakes of dietary fiber, *Journal of Human Nutrition* 30:303, 1976.

from the water-binding capacity of cellulose and pectin. This contributes weight, bulk, and softness to fecal matter, allowing it to move through the gastrointestinal tract more rapidly and with regularity. A diet low in fiber will result in a small quantity of fecal matter; in addition, dry stools remain in the intestine longer and are passed with more difficulty.

With low fiber intake, large intestine action will be sluggish. The pressure of accumulated wastes on the walls of the colon may lead to a pouching or ballooning of pockets of those walls through weak areas in the surrounding musculature. This is *diverticulosis*. When infection occurs in these pockets *diverticulitis* results. It is estimated that diverticular disease affects 40 percent of all Americans over 40 years of age. Hard fecal matter may also contribute to the development of appendicitis and of hemorrhoids and other vascular problems. These conditions, however, are caused by other factors as well.

In fiber-poor diets, the bowel contents become more concentrated and remain in the body longer. Thus, according to one hypothesis, there is more time for food substances and bile acids to be acted upon by intestinal bacteria that may produce carcinogenic substances and for any dangerous byproducts to damage the colon (Leveille, 1976).

Evidence suggests that low blood cholesterol levels are correlated with diets of high fiber content. The evidence of the connection between dietary fiber intake and atherosclerosis or colon cancer, however, is by no means absolute or generally accepted.

Not all of the materials composing dietary fiber are likely to have identical effects on the human system. Differences in the action of some fiber components have been recorded (Mendeloff, 1977) and other differences undoubtedly remain to be discovered.

Recommendations and Reservations. No specific requirement has been established for dietary fiber, but it has been suggested that Americans should increase their crude fiber intake from its present level of about 4 or 5 grams per day to 12 to 20 grams (McNutt, 1976). Most fiber in the American diet comes from wheat, potatoes, fruits, and vegetables. More concentrated sources of fiber are bran, prepared cereals with high bran content, and high-fiber whole-grain breads. It is not necessary, however, to consume large quantities of such foods to add fiber to the daily menu; all whole grains, such as brown rice and millet, as well as dried beans, peas, and nuts are good sources of dietary fiber. Bran is perhaps the most concentrated source, and can absorb up to 200 times its dry weight in water. It is dangerous to consume dry bran, which can cause intestinal blockage. Increased fluid intake should accompany increased fiber intake.

It has also been suggested that fiber-rich diets with their brief transit time through the body can contribute to weight loss by lessening the time in which digested material can be absorbed. Depending on this action as a significant component of a weight loss program could be dangerous, however, since the more rapid transit period would sidetrack not only calories but also key vitamins and minerals at the same time (Beyer and Flynn, 1978). Nevertheless, a moderately higher fiber intake can probably contribute to weight loss in two ways: First is the sense of fullness that comes from eating complex carbohydrate foods, which appease the appetite, thus reducing extra food intake. Second is the relatively lower caloric value of these foods, which would replace sugars and fats, both of which have been implicated in the etiology of obesity and heart disease.

Decreased bowel transit times due to increased fiber intake should affect diverticular disease by lessening pressure on the bowel wall. Formerly, the standard treatment for this condition was a low-fiber diet to avoid irritation and reduce the amount and frequency of stools; but there has been a complete reversal, and high-fiber diets are now often prescribed, with good results reported (Leveille, 1976). Until further research is done to define both the potential benefits and hazards of high-fiber diets, it seems prudent to increase intake of dietary fiber moderately, relying primarily on whole-grain breads and cereals, fresh fruits, and vegetables.

A high-fiber diet is closer to the foods available to early humans. Many believe that the human digestive system has not evolved to accommodate the kinds of diets eaten by most Westerners today, and that a wide range of health problems is the consequence. If this is true, we should seriously consider readjusting our food habits and returning, at least in part, to a diet such as that consumed by our ancestors containing greater carbohydrate content from unrefined plant food sources. Such a diet might come much closer than most present-day menus to being "natural."

artificial is a good guideline to follow. The effects of long-term use of nonnutritive sweeteners are not truly known or understood. According to an estimate by the FDA, daily consumption by every American of only one large diet soft drink containing saccharin might result in 1,200 additional cases of bladder cancer every year (Pines and Glick, 1977). It is clear that there is some risk to the use of saccharin for adults. Allowing children to drink the diet sodas consumed by weight-conscious parents presents additional risks, because exposure even to a weak carcinogen, beginning so early and continuing for prolonged periods that may extend for a lifetime, increases the hazard considerably.

While adequate carbohydrate intake is important, and while our bodies require glucose, they do not need table sugar. There is nothing wrong with having an occasional sweet, but it should not be at the expense of complex carbohydrates and natural sources of sugar. Decreased consumption of sucrose tends to improve overall nutritional status. In a sugar-restricted diet as for diabetics and the obese, it would be prudent to use artificial sweeteners in moderate amounts only. For nutritional adequacy, four servings of whole grain or enriched breads and cereals (not presweetened) should be eaten daily, along with such other natural sources of carbohydrate as fruits and vegetables. All of these contain additional nutrients as well as nonnutritive fiber. It would surely be beneficial if we could wean ourselves away from our national sweet tooth.

SUMMARY

Carbohydrates, compounds of carbon, hydrogen, and oxygen in the proportions of one carbon atom to one water molecule ($C_n(H_2O)_n$), are the primary energy source in the average human diet. The two main types of carbohydrates are simple carbohydrates, or sugars, and complex carbohydrates, or starches. The names of many sugars contain the suffix *-ose* and have a prefix that defines the number of carbon atoms present in a molecule of that sugar —for example, hexoses are 6-carbon sugars, with the formula $C_6(H_2O)_6$ (or $C_6H_{12}O_6$).

Sugars may be monosaccharides (one simple sugar molecule) or disaccharides (two monosaccharides bonded together). In the bonding process, known as a condensation reaction, a molecule of water is released; therefore, the general formula for disaccharides is $C_{12}(H_2O)_{11}$. Glucose, galactose, and fructose are three different 6-carbon monosaccharides; sucrose, lactose, and maltose are three disaccharides.

Similar bonding of additional sugar units produces polysaccharide molecules (complex carbohydrates). Different arrangements of the chemical bonds within the sugar molecule (as in the monosaccharides) or between the sugar molecules (as in di- and polysaccharides) result in the formation of compounds with correspondingly different chemical and physical (for example, taste) properties.

Simple sugars are found primarily in fruits and vegetables. Sugars are commonly added to many kinds of processed foods. Complex carbohydrates are found in grains, legumes such as peas and peanuts, tubers such as potatoes, and other plant products. Lactose (milk sugar) is the only important dietary carbohydrate of animal origin.

Average consumption of sugars has been increasing, but complex carbohydrate consumption has decreased. Expansion of the food processing industry, the widespread use of convenience foods, and other changes in food habits are among the factors involved in this shift, which has health implications that are causing concern. Dental caries and obesity are definitely related to sugar intake; heart disease and other serious illnesses may be related as well.

Disaccharides and polysaccharides in food must be converted to monosaccharides in order to be absorbed into the blood. In the process of digestion, they undergo hydrolytic reactions. The opposite of the condensation reaction, hydrolysis incorporates a water molecule to split a complex molecule into its simpler components. A specific enzyme is required to catalyze the hydrolytic reaction of each carbohydrate. If a particular enzyme is missing for any reason, its substrate cannot be digested. Lactose intolerance, for example, is a condition in which lactase, the enzyme necessary to digest lactose, is not produced in adequate quantity.

Glucose is the primary form in which digested carbohydrate enters the blood circulation. The maintenance of a constant level of glucose in the blood is of critical importance, and several body mechanisms interact to regulate that level. Diabetes and hypoglycemia are disturbances of blood glucose level regulation. From the blood, glucose enters the body cells. There it is used to produce energy by glycolysis and the Krebs cycle, or to function in the synthesis of various essential compounds. Excess glucose may also be converted into glycogen or fat and stored in that form for future availability.

The Food and Nutrition Board recommends that a minimum of 50 to 100 grams of carbohydrate (about $\frac{1}{8}$ to $\frac{1}{4}$ pound) be ingested daily, most of which should derive from grains, fruits, and vegetables. These sources contain naturally occurring simple sugars and complex carbohydrates as well as vitamins, minerals, and nonnutritive dietary fiber. Some processed foods contain excessive amounts of sugar, supplying only "empty calories" accompanied by little other nutrient content. Use of such foods as a substantial portion of total energy intake deprives the body of the important nutrients in other foods.

Some polysaccharides cannot be digested because the human body lacks appropriate enzymes. Known as dietary fiber, undigested carbohydrates pass through the digestive tract and are excreted in the feces. Fiber content of foods is usually expressed as "crude fiber," but this is a significant underestimation of total fiber content; new methods of measuring dietary fiber accurately are being developed. Although dietary fiber contains no usable nutrients, it serves an important function in the regulation of the passage of fecal wastes. Lack of fiber in the diet may be related to such chronic ailments as diverticulosis, and also to atherosclerosis and cancer of the colon. Although questions about the role of fiber in health maintenance remain, increased consumption of high fiber foods, especially whole-grain breads and cereals, fresh fruits, and vegetables, may be beneficial.

BIBLIOGRAPHY

American Diabetes Association. *What you need to know about diabetes.* New York: American Diabetes Association, 1976.

Beyer, P. L., and M. A. Flynn. Effects of high- and low-fiber diets on human feces. *Journal of the American Dietetic Association* 72:271, 1978.

Brewster, L., and M. Jacobson. *The changing American diet*. Washington, D.C.: Center for Science in the Public Interest, 1978.

Burkitt, D. P., A. R. P. Walker, and N. S. Painter. Dietary fiber and disease. *Journal of the American Medical Association* 229:1068, 1974.

Business Week. Sugar: A troubled industry turns to energy uses. September 25, 1978, p. 72.

CNI Weekly Report. NAS warns against saccharin. November 9, 1978, p. 1.

Connor, W. E. and S. L. Connor. Sucrose and carbohydrate. In *Present knowledge in nutrition*, 4th ed., ed. D. M. Hegsted, Washington, D.C.: The Nutrition Foundation, Inc., 1976.

Consumer Reports. Too much sugar. 43:136, March 1978.

Galbraith, A. L. A.D.A. testimony on the ban of saccharin. *Journal of the American Dietetic Association* 70:526, 1977.

Garza, C. and N. S. Scrimshaw. Relationship of lactose intolerance to milk intolerance in young children. *American Journal of Clinical Nutrition*. 29:192, 1977.

Howe, G. R., J. D. Burch, A. B. Miller, et al. Artificial sweeteners and human bladder cancer. *Lancet* 2:578, 1977.

Jacobson, M., and G. Moreland. Settling a sugar controversy. *Nutrition Action*, August 1977, pp. 8–9.

Kelsay, J. L. A review of research on effects of fiber intake on man. *American Journal of Clinical Nutrition* 31:142, 1978.

Kessler, I. I., and J. P. Clark. Saccharin, cyclamate, and human bladder cancer. *Journal of the American Medical Association* 240(4): 349, 1978.

Latham, M. C. Public health importance of milk intolerance. *Nutrition News* 40(4):13, 16, 1977.

Leveille, G. A. Dietary fiber. *Contemporary Nutrition*, 1976.

Mayer, J. Sugar: Taking the bitter with the sweet. *Family Health* 10(3):26, 1978.

McNutt, K. W. Perspective: Fiber. *Journal of Nutrition Education* 8(4):150, 1976.

Mendeloff, A. I. Dietary fiber and human health. *New England Journal of Medicine* 297(15):811, 1977.

Nutrition Reviews. Nutritional significance of lactose intolerance. 36(5):133, 1978.

Parham, E. S. Comparison of responses to bans on cyclamates (1969) and saccharin (1977). *Journal of the American Dietetic Association* 72(1):59, 1978.

Pines, W. L., and N. Glick. The saccharin ban. *FDA Consumer* 11(4):10, 1977.

Select Committee on Nutrition and Human Needs, U.S. Senate. *Dietary Goals for the United States*, 2nd ed. Washington, D.C.: U.S. Government Printing Office, 1977.

Spiller, G. A., and R. J. Amen. Dietary fiber in human nutrition. *Critical Reviews in Food Science and Nutrition*, November 1975, p. 39.

West K. M. Prevention and therapy of diabetes mellitus. In *Present Knowledge in Nutrition*, 4th ed., ed. D. M. Hegsted. Washington, D.C.: The Nutrition Foundation, Inc., 1976.

Wightman, N. Perspective saccharin: Are there alternatives? *Journal of Nutrition Education* 9(3):106, 1977.

Yudkin, J., and J. Morland. Sugar intake and myocardial infarction. *American Journal of Clinical Nutrition* 20(5):503, 1967.

SUGGESTED ADDITIONAL READING

Ahrens, R. A. Sucrose, hypertension, and heart disease: A historical perspective. *American Journal of Clinical Nutrition* 27:403, 1974.

Bing, F. C. Dietary fiber: A historical perspective. *Journal of the American Dietetic Association* 69(5):489, 1976.

Burkitt, D. P. The role of dietary fiber. *Nutrition Today* 11(1):6, 1976.

CNI Weekly Report. USDA researchers hit sugar report. April 16, 1978, p. 7.

Food and Nutrition Board, National Research Council. *Recommended dietary allowances*. 8th ed. Washington, D.C.: National Academy of Sciences, 1974.

Food Technology. Dietary fiber. January 1979, p. 35.

Gortner, W. A. U.S. dietary trends and implications. *Contemporary Nutrition*, November 1978.

Guthrie, D. W., and R. A. Guthrie. Diabetes in adolescence. *American Journal of Nursing* 75:1740, 1975.

Hardinge, M. G., J. B. Swaner, and H. Crooks. Carbohydrates in foods. *Journal of the American Dietetic Association* 46:197, 1965.

Harland, B., and A. Hecht. Grandma called it roughage. *FDA Consumer* 11(6):18, 1977.

Kraus, B. *Calories and carbohydrates*. New York: Signet (NAL), 1975.

Lenner, R. A. Specially designed sweeteners and food for diabetics: A real need? *American Journal of Clinical Nutrition* 29:726, 1976.

McMichael, H. Intestinal absorption of carbohydrates in man. *Proceedings of the Nutrition Society* 30:248, 1971.

Mendeloff, A. I. Dietary fiber. In *Present Knowledge in Nutrition*, 4th ed., ed. D. M. Hegsted. Washington, D.C.: The Nutrition Foundation, Inc., 1976.

Nisbet, I. C. T. The bitter problem of sweets. *Technology Review*, October–November 1977, p. 6.

Page, L., and B. Friend. Level of use of sugar in the United States. In *Sugars in Nutrition*, ed. H. L. Sipple, and K. W. McNutt. New York: Academic Press, 1974.

Paige, D. M., et al. Lactose hydrolyzed milk. *American Journal of Clinical Nutrition* 28:818, 1975.

Select Committee on GRAS Substances. *Evaluation of the health aspects of sucrose as a food ingredient*. Bethesda, Maryland: Federation of American Societies for Experimental Biology, 1976.

Shannon, I. L. *Brand name guide to sugar: Sucrose content of over 1000 common foods and beverages*. Chicago: Nelson-Hall, 1977.

Shen, S. W., and R. Bressler. Hypoglycemia. *Rational Drug Therapy* 11(5):1, 1977.

Sipple, H. L., and K. W. McNutt, eds. *Sugars in nutrition*. New York: Academic Press, 1974.

Solomon, G. L. Sugar may be harmful to your rat's health. *CNI Weekly Report*, August 8, 1977, p. 7.

Walker, A. R. P. Health implications of fiber depleted diets. *South African Medical Journal* 52(10):767.

West, K. M. Prevention and therapy of diabetes mellitus. *Nutrition Reviews* 33:193, 1975.

Yudkin, J. Sugar and disease. *Nature* 239:197, 1972.

Chapter 3

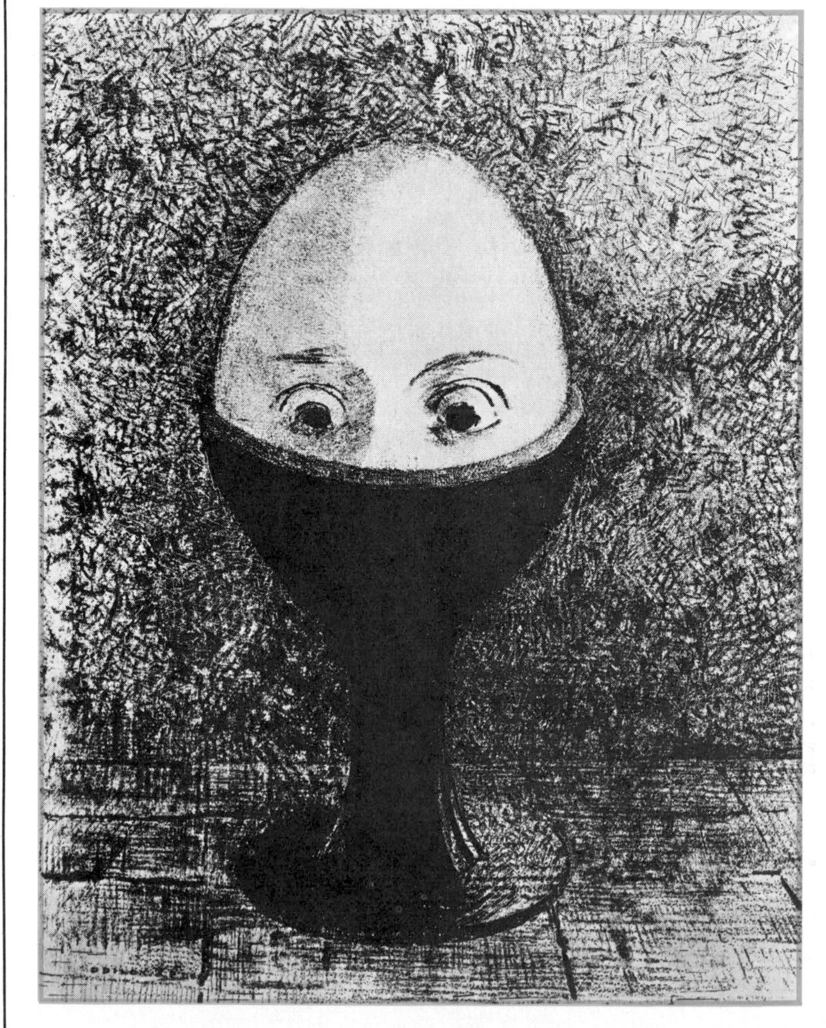

Egg, lithograph by Odilon Redon, 1885

Lipids

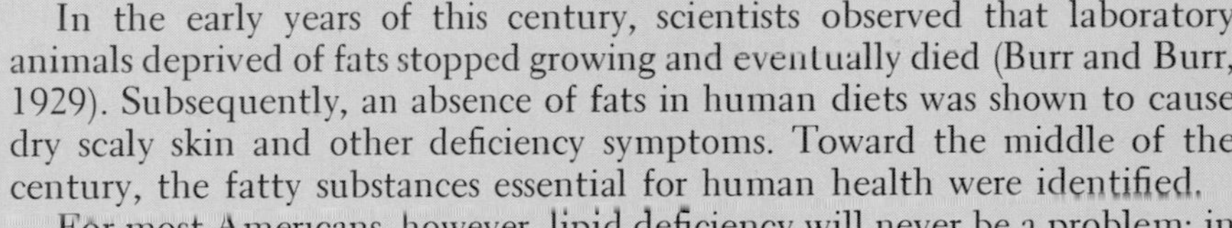

In the early years of this century, scientists observed that laboratory animals deprived of fats stopped growing and eventually died (Burr and Burr, 1929). Subsequently, an absence of fats in human diets was shown to cause dry scaly skin and other deficiency symptoms. Toward the middle of the century, the fatty substances essential for human health were identified.

For most Americans, however, lipid deficiency will never be a problem; in fact, the current intake of dietary fats far exceeds nutritional needs. Average individual fat consumption in the United States has risen by nearly one-third since the early years of the twentieth century. As much as 42 percent of our energy intake now comes from fats—more than is provided by either of the other two **macronutrients**, proteins and carbohydrates (Brewster and Jacobson, 1978). Moreover, the human body, as we shall see, readily synthesizes fats from other nutrient sources—as some of us know all too well.

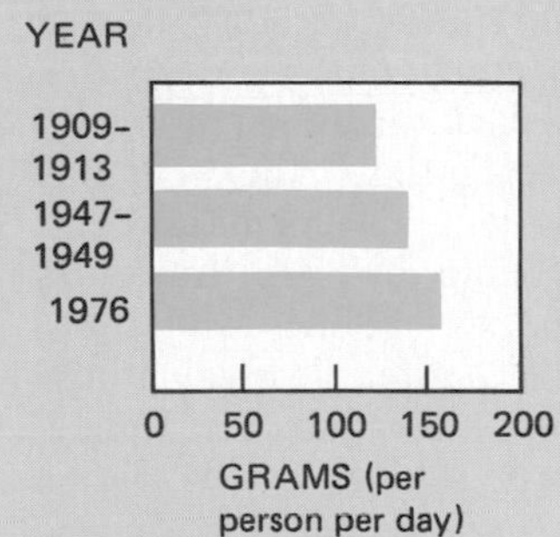

Total Fat Consumption in the United States

Source: L. Brewster and M. F. Jacobson, *The changing American diet* (Washington, D.C.: Center for Science in the Public Interest, 1978). p. 60, Figure 30.

Fat deficiency, then, is not a significant health problem in this country. The problem is, rather, an overabundance of dietary lipids. Excessive fat intake has been cited as a possible cause of heart disease and cancer, and the suspected relationship between dietary fats and chronic illness continues to generate considerable research as well as many controversial articles in both professional and popular publications. The dietary importance of fats, however, tends to be forgotten amid all the controversy.

Many body functions depend on fats. They provide an excellent source of energy, enhance transport of fat-soluble vitamins, insulate and protect internal tissues, and contribute to vital cell processes. In this chapter we shall examine these roles. We shall look also at the structures of different lipids and how they relate to their roles and functions. Finally, we shall discuss the suspected relationship between fats and chronic diseases.

WHAT ARE LIPIDS?

Lipid molecules differ in chemical composition, and therefore in chemical and physical properties, from the two other macronutrients. The elements found in carbohydrates—carbon, hydrogen, and oxygen—also occur in lipid molecules, but in different proportions and with different structural arrangements. In particular, lipids contain a much lower proportion of oxygen atoms than do carbohydrates; some lipids contain nitrogen and phosphorus as well.

Because of their chemical composition, lipids do not dissolve in aqueous (water) solutions, but they do dissolve in organic solvents, such as chloroform, ether, and benzene. This can be illustrated from firsthand experience. If some butter is dropped into water it will remain, identifiably, a glob of butter; even if the water is warmed so that the butter melts, still the butter may be seen clearly. If butter melts into your shirt, plain water will not remove it; only benzene or other solvents, like soap, will do the job.

The chemical composition of lipids also determines their gross, or obvious, appearance. Strictly speaking, **fats** are lipids that are solid at room temperature (butter or beef fat, for example), although as a practical matter the term fat is often used interchangeably with lipid. **Oils** are lipids with melting points so low that they are liquid at room temperature (corn oil or olive oil, for example). Lipids with much higher melting points also exist but have little nutritional significance; we commonly refer to them as **waxes.** The generic term lipid properly includes waxes as well as fats and oils, although our discussion will be concerned only with the nutrient, or edible, lipids.

CLASSIFICATION OF LIPIDS

The different structures and functions of various lipids have been the basis for a number of classification systems. Most useful for nutritional purposes is a system based on the amount of a specific lipid present in the human body. In such a scheme lipids are generally organized according to whether they are major or minor constituents of our internal environment. The major lipids of nutritional interest are listed in Table 3-1. This table does not, however, include all lipids, or even all those of nutritional significance. The major lipids will be the subject of most of the discussion in this chapter. Prostaglandins, which are synthesized in the body from certain fatty acids, will be mentioned later in this chapter; **fat-soluble vitamins** will be the subject of Chapter 6.

TABLE 3-1
Classification of Lipids

I. Major Constituents
   A. Fatty acids
   B. Fatty-acid derivatives
      1. Glycerol esters: Mono-, di- and triglycerides, phospholipids
      2. Cholesterol esters
      3. Glycolipids
   C. Sterols and sterol derivatives: Cholesterol, bile acids, steroids
II. Minor Constituents
   A. Fat-soluble vitamins: A, D, E, K
   B. Prostaglandins

Source: Adapted from R. Montgomery et al., *Biochemistry: A case-oriented approach* (St. Louis: C. V. Mosby, 1974), p. 306.

CHEMICAL ORGANIZATION AND STRUCTURE

CH_3
Methyl group

COOH
Acid or
Carboxyl group

The basic structural unit of many lipid molecules is a **fatty acid.** A fatty acid is a chain of hydrocarbons with a methyl group at one end and an acid or carboxyl group attached at the other. As Table 3-1 indicates, some lipids are simple fatty acids and some are derivatives of fatty acids in combination with other substances. Other lipid molecules contain no fatty acid groups.

Fatty Acids

The general chemical formula for a fatty acid is

$$CH_3(CH_2)_nCOOH,$$

where n is usually a multiple of two. In most fatty acids of nutritional significance, the hydrocarbon chain consists of an even number of carbon atoms ranging from 4 to 6 carbons for the so-called short-chain fatty acids, 8 to 12 carbons for medium-chain fatty acids, and 14 to 26 carbons for long-chain fatty acids. Butyric acid, for example, a 4-carbon fatty acid present in butter and other dairy products, can be written chemically either as

$$CH_3\text{-}CH_2\text{-}CH_2\text{-}COOH, \text{ or as } CH_3(CH_2)_2COOH.$$

The value of the shorthand formula is obvious when long-chain fatty acids, such as the 14-carbon myristic acid, are considered: $CH_3(CH_2)_{12}COOH$ versus

$$CH_3\text{-}CH_2\text{-}CH_2\text{-}CH_2\text{-}CH_2\text{-}CH_2\text{-}CH_2\text{-}CH_2\text{-}CH_2\text{-}CH_2\text{-}CH_2\text{-}CH_2\text{-}CH_2\text{-}COOH.$$

Generally, each carbon in a hydrocarbon chain is attached by electrochemical bonding (explained in Chapter 1) to two hydrogen atoms and to each of two adjacent carbon atoms. You will remember that a carbon atom has the potential for forming four such bonds; thus, the valence requirement of carbon is 4:

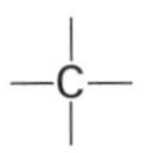

$$\begin{array}{c} | \\ -C- \\ | \end{array}$$

A fatty acid in which the valence requirements of all carbon atoms is met in this way

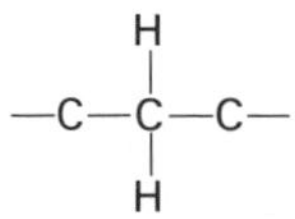

$$\begin{array}{c} H \\ | \\ -C-C-C- \\ | \\ H \end{array}$$

is classified as a **saturated fatty acid.**

TABLE 3-2
Major Naturally Occurring Fatty Acids

Number of C Atoms	Number of Double Bonds				
	0	1	2	3	4
4	Butyric				
6	Caproic				
8	Caprylic				
10	Capric				
12	Lauric				
14	Myristic				
16	Palmitic	Palmitoleic			
18	Stearic	Oleic	Linoleic	Linolenic	
20	Arachidic				Arachidonic

Certain important fatty acids are classified as **unsaturated;** that is, some of their constituent carbon atoms are bound to only a single hydrogen atom. To fill the remaining gaps in their valence requirement, these carbon atoms are joined by a double bond to an adjacent atom. Thus, in oleic acid, which has a total of 18 carbons, there is a double bond between the ninth and tenth carbon atoms:

$$CH_3(CH_2)_7\overset{\displaystyle H}{\overset{|}{C}}{=}\overset{\displaystyle H}{\overset{|}{C}}(CH_2)_7COOH.$$

(Carbon atoms are numbered from the carbon in the COOH group at the right of the chemical formula and continuing to the last carbon in the methyl group on the left.) Oleic acid, with only one double bond, is a **monounsaturated fatty acid.** A fatty acid having two or more double bonds is a **polyunsaturated fatty acid** (PUFA).

Table 3-2 groups the naturally occurring fatty acids according to the number of carbon atoms and type of bonds between them. Note that four different fatty acids each contain 18 carbon atoms. The structural differences between these four fatty acids can most simply be expressed as 18:0, saturated stearic acid; 18:1, monounsaturated oleic acid; 18:2, polyunsaturated linoleic acid; and 18:3, polyunsaturated linolenic acid.

These numerical formulas are a convenient way to express the molecular structures of fatty acids. The number to the left of the colon indicates the total number of carbon atoms in the molecule, while the number following the colon indicates the number of double bonds. This formula can be expanded to show the location of the double bonding as well. For example, oleic acid can be expressed as 9–18:1 meaning that the only double bond in the molecule comes after the ninth carbon atom in the chain. The chemical and numerical structural formulas for linoleic acid are

$$CH_3(CH_2)_4\overset{H}{C}{=}\overset{H}{C}{-}CH_2{-}\overset{H}{C}{=}\overset{H}{C}(CH_2)_7COOH \text{ and } 9,12\text{–}18{:}2.$$

Linolenic acid is expressed as

$$CH_3CH_2\overset{H}{C}{=}\overset{H}{C}{-}CH_2{-}\overset{H}{C}{=}\overset{H}{C}{-}CH_2{-}\overset{H}{C}{=}\overset{H}{C}{-}(CH_2)_7COOH \text{ and } 9,12,15\text{–}18{:}3.$$

Depending, then, on the number of hydrogen atoms in proportion to the carbon atoms on the hydrocarbon chain of their molecules, fatty acids may be saturated or unsaturated; and unsaturated fatty acids may be monounsaturated or polyunsaturated. The differences between these forms may have dietary and health implications, as we shall see below.

Although these molecules must be diagrammed in two dimensions on a book page, in reality they exist in three-dimensional form. The double bonds between some carbon atoms have more flexibility than do single bonds. Consequently, the other parts of the hydrocarbon chain are able to rotate, bend, or otherwise take different positions around the double bond. Unsaturated fatty acids generally can take one of two geometric shapes. A molecule that is more or less stretched out is known as the **trans form,** and a molecule that is folded back on itself is known as the **cis form.** (The terms are derived from Latin prefixes, with *cis* meaning "on this side," and *trans* meaning "on the other side.") Each form of a molecule that exists in more than one configuration is known as an **isomer.** The *cis* and *trans* forms of oleic acid (18:1) are shown below, along with the general structural formulas for fatty acid isomers.

Generally, the *cis* isomer is more flexible and often has a zigzag shape, important in membrane structure and function. Most naturally occurring unsaturated fatty acids are *cis* isomers. Under certain conditions, such as heat or hydrogenation (see below), these natural *cis* forms may be converted to the less flexible *trans* forms. This transformation often takes place during commercial processing of foods, as a result of which the melting points of some

General structural formulas of fatty acid isomers

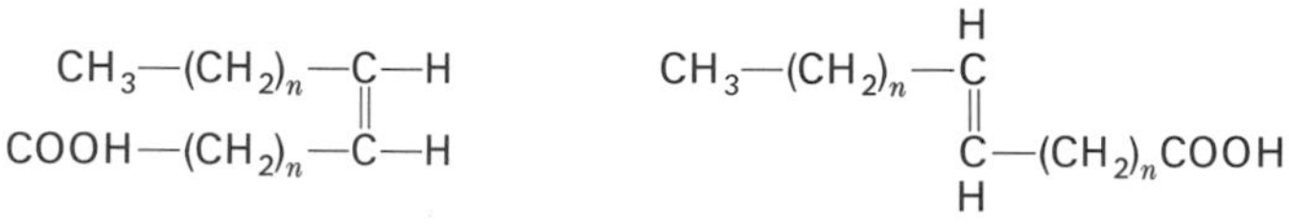

$$\begin{array}{l} CH_3{-}(CH_2)_n{-}C{-}H \\ \qquad\qquad\quad \| \\ COOH{-}(CH_2)_n{-}C{-}H \end{array} \qquad \begin{array}{l} \qquad\qquad\quad H \\ CH_3{-}(CH_2)_n{-}C \\ \qquad\qquad\quad \| \\ \qquad\qquad\quad C{-}(CH_2)_nCOOH \\ \qquad\qquad\quad H \end{array}$$

Cis form — Trans form

Isomers of oleic acid (18:1)

$$\begin{array}{l} HC{-}(CH_2)_7COOH \\ \ \ \| \\ HC{-}(CH_2)_7CH_3 \end{array} \qquad \begin{array}{r} HC{-}(CH_2)_7COOH \\ \| \qquad\qquad\quad \\ H_3C(CH_2)_7{-}CH \qquad\qquad\quad \end{array}$$

Cis form — Trans form

dietary fats may increase. The energy value of fats, however, is not altered by such changes.

Fatty Acid Derivatives

The compound that results from the combination of one or more fatty acids with an alcohol is called an **ester.** Two categories of lipids are derived from fatty acids in this manner, *glycerol esters* and *cholesterol esters.*

GLYCEROL ESTERS. **Glycerol,** an important molecule derived in the body from glucose metabolism, contains three carbon atoms, each of which is attached to an alcohol group (—OH). A condensation reaction between the carboxyl group of a fatty acid and the alcohol group of glycerol results in the formation of a **glyceride.** Depending upon the number of fatty acids and alcohol groups that take part in the reaction, **mono-, di-,** or **triglycerides** are formed (see Figure 3-1).

This condensation reaction is similar to the one in which a disaccharide is formed from two monosaccharides (as we saw in Chapter 2), with a molecule of water being released in the process. Remember, however, that every chemical reaction that takes place in the body must be catalyzed by a specific enzyme. Thus, each of these two reactions involves distinctive enzymes, as well as different substrates.

Successive condensation reactions incorporating the same original glycerol molecule result in the formation of diglycerides and triglycerides. Triglycerides, the most abundant type of lipid in food, result from the catalyzed reaction of glycerol and three fatty acids, a reaction which may be expressed

$$\text{glycerol} + 3 \text{ fatty acids} \longrightarrow \text{triglyceride} + 3H_2O.$$

In a simple triglyceride, all three combining fatty acids are identical. In a mixed triglyceride, however, two or three different fatty acids have condensed, or esterified, with the alcohol groups of the glycerol molecule, as shown in Figure 3-2. Most dietary triglycerides are mixed.

Phospholipids are constructed like triglycerides, except that a phosphate-containing group replaces the third fatty acid. **Lecithin** is a phospholipid (see Figure 3-3).

CHOLESTEROL ESTERS. These esters are formed through condensation reactions involving the sterol (alcohol lipid) cholesterol (discussed below),

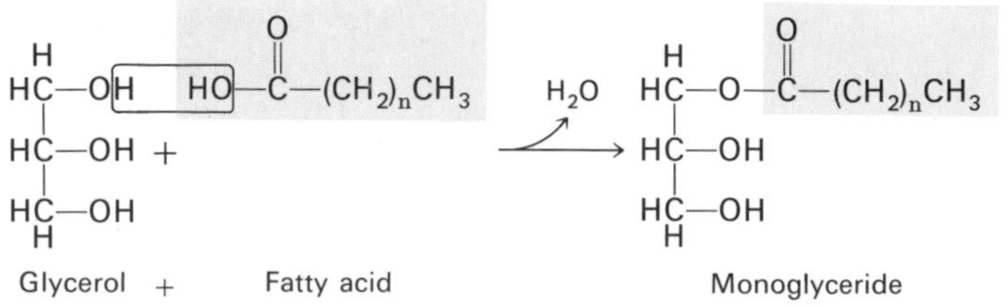

FIGURE 3-1
Formation of a Monoglyceride

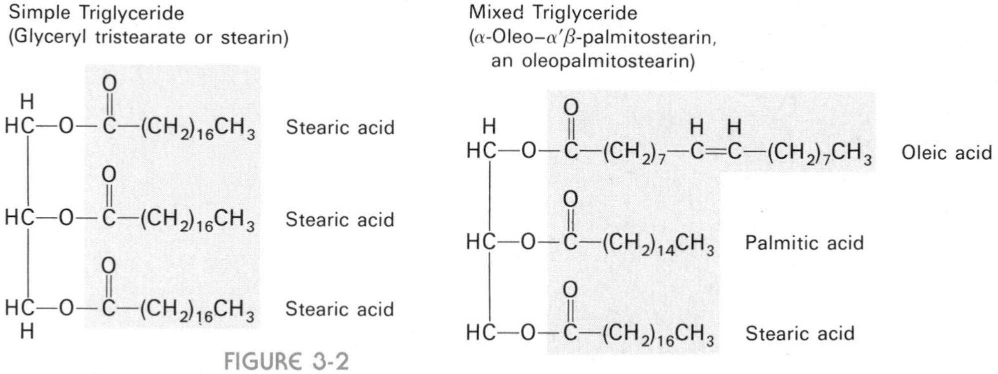

Simple Triglyceride
(Glyceryl tristearate or stearin)

$H_2C-O-C(=O)-(CH_2)_{16}CH_3$ Stearic acid
$HC-O-C(=O)-(CH_2)_{16}CH_3$ Stearic acid
$H_2C-O-C(=O)-(CH_2)_{16}CH_3$ Stearic acid

Mixed Triglyceride
(α-Oleo–$\alpha'\beta$-palmitostearin, an oleopalmitostearin)

$H_2C-O-C(=O)-(CH_2)_7-CH=CH-(CH_2)_7CH_3$ Oleic acid
$HC-O-C(=O)-(CH_2)_{14}CH_3$ Palmitic acid
$HC-O-C(=O)-(CH_2)_{16}CH_3$ Stearic acid

FIGURE 3-2
Examples of Simple and Mixed Triglycerides

with the fatty acid attaching to the alcohol (—OH) group shown in Figure 3-4. Only a small quantity of dietary cholesterol is in this esterified form; by far the greatest amount is in the form of cholesterol without a fatty acid component, that is, free cholesterol.

GLYCOLIPIDS. Compounds of one or more sugar molecules (usually glucose or galactose) with a fatty acid and nitrogen are called glycolipids. These complex molecules have the physical properties of lipids. Cerebrosides are a group of glycolipids present in large quantities in the brain and in lesser amounts in other tissues such as the liver, spleen, and kidneys.

Sterols

Sterols, which constitute the third major dietary lipid category, are fat-soluble alcohols. The most familiar sterol is, of course, cholesterol, which has figured in extensive controversy regarding its possible contribution to the etiology of atherosclerosis and coronary heart disease. A number of other important sterols are found in food as well.

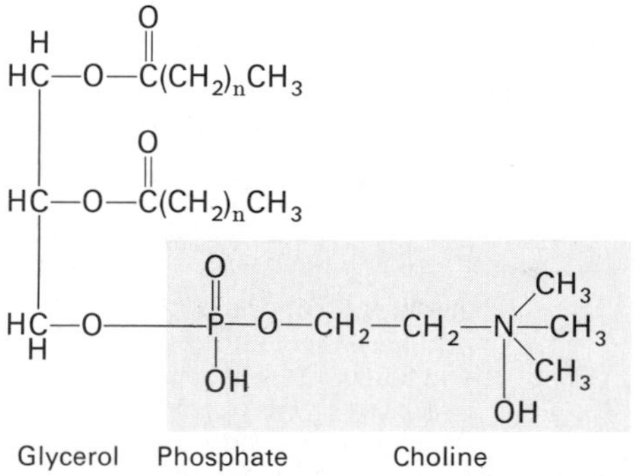

$H_2C-O-C(=O)(CH_2)_nCH_3$
$HC-O-C(=O)(CH_2)_nCH_3$
$H_2C-O-P(=O)(OH)-O-CH_2-CH_2-N(CH_3)_3OH$

Glycerol Phosphate Choline

FIGURE 3-3
Lecithin

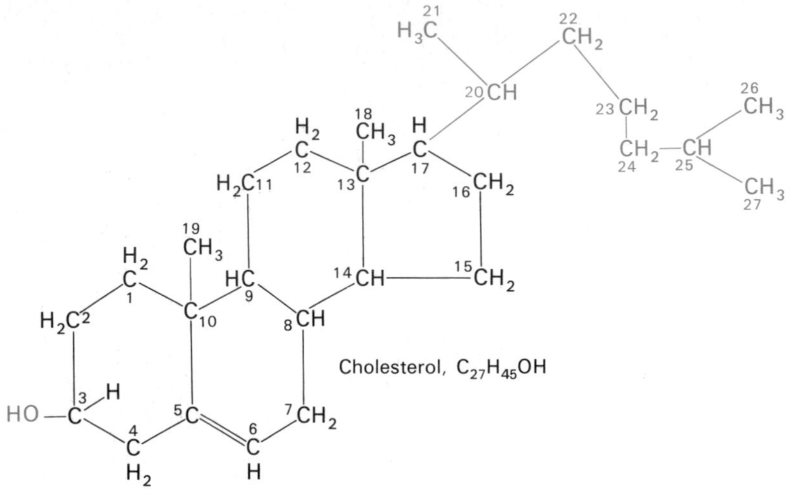

FIGURE 3-4

Cholesterol Molecule

Sterols differ from other lipids in having a ring structure. Typically, sterols have a nucleus of four interlocking rings, of which three contain six carbon atoms each and the fourth contains five. An alcohol (—OH) group is attached to carbon number 3 of the first ring, and a chain of eight or more carbon atoms is attached to carbon number 17 of the fourth ring. The valence requirement of all carbon atoms is met through single or double bonding to adjacent carbon atoms and through attachment to one or more hydrogen atoms. These linkages can be clearly seen in the diagrammatic representation of cholesterol in Figure 3-4. Another way of illustrating the chemical structure is depicted in Figure 3-5.

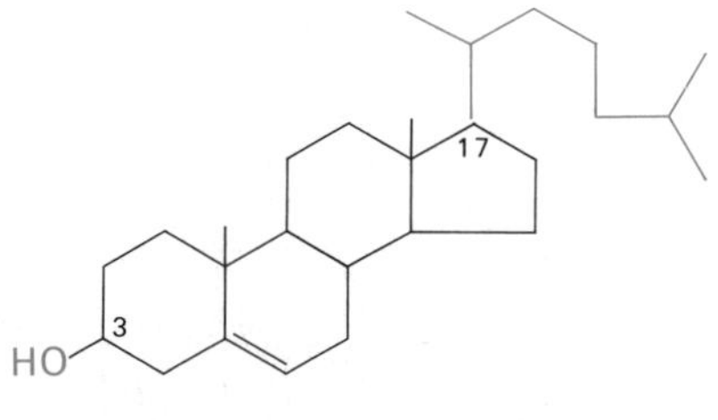

FIGURE 3-5

Structural Diagram of a Cholesterol Molecule

Another way of illustrating chemical structure is depicted above. A comparison of Figures 3-4 and 3-5 will show that each angle in Figure 3-5 represents a carbon atom with the number of hydrogen atoms needed to satisfy valence requirements. Note that a single line represents single bonding, and a double line represents double bonding. The hydroxyl group at carbon number 3 provides the attachment for a fatty acid in the ester linkage (or condensation reaction) that results in a cholesterol ester. The hydrocarbon chain is shown attached to carbon number 17 of the steroid nucleus.

Although the role of cholesterol in disease is being debated, there is no question about the necessity for this lipid in the human body. Cholesterol is essential as a precursor of several important compounds, particularly the steroid hormones (which include cortisone and the sex hormones); cholesterol is also required for the body's production of vitamin D and bile salts.

LIPIDS IN FOODS

Although lipids are relatively tasteless, their chemical structure enables them to trap pleasurable flavors. The oil in tomato sauce lets it cling not only to your spaghetti, but also to your taste buds. Poultry cooked without its skin, and so without its natural blanket of fat, would be almost flavorless (and, therefore, is often cooked in a flavored oil or sauce).

Different fats and oils have distinctive flavors, because of their different chemical structures. Olive oil tastes different from peanut oil, and both taste

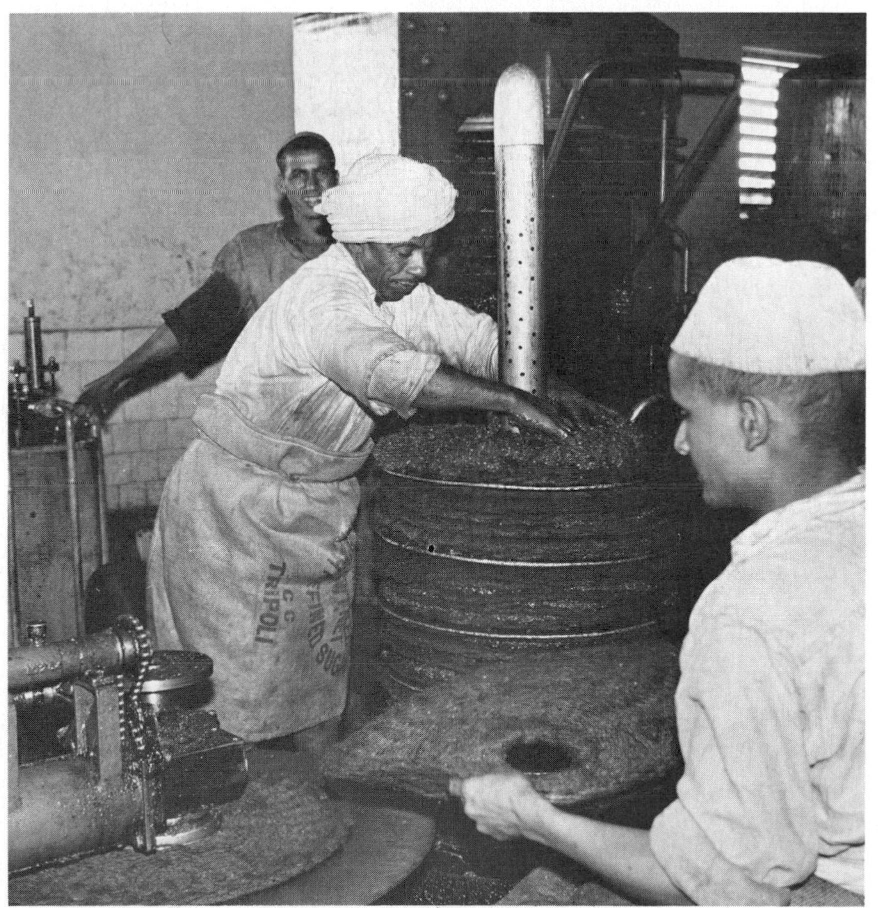

At an olive oil plant in Libya, the olives are crushed in large drums. Then the olive pulp is put through a machine which presses it out onto circular mats. The olive mash next goes into a steam press and the oil produced is put through centrifuges to become clarified. Here the circular mats covered with olive pulp are piled up ready to go into the steam press. (FAO photo by A. Defever)

different from sesame oil. Every region, and every ethnic group has its characteristic cooking oil, which gives the cuisine its distinctive flavor. Corn oil prevails in Mexico (and throughout the Americas); olive oil throughout the Mediterranean, from Greece to Italy to Spain; peanut and coconut oils in Africa; butter and lard in northern Europe; clarified butter (ghee) in India; and seal and whale oils among the Eskimo.

Functions of Fats

The palatability of fats and the greater taste appeal fats give to other foods help to ensure that our overall intake is adequate. The fat component of a meal is responsible for our feeling satisfyingly full after we have eaten. Fats and oils are digested and leave the stomach more slowly than carbohydrates or proteins, and are absorbed more slowly as well. For these reasons, the inclusion of some fatty foods in every meal will leave the eater feeling more satisfied for a longer period of time, an important consideration in the design of weight reduction diets (see Chapter 5).

The primary function of dietary lipid is to provide a concentrated source of energy in relatively low bulk. The caloric density of fat is more than twice as great as that of either carbohydrate or protein. One gram of fat produces 9 kilocalories (37.8 kJ), while one gram of carbohydrate produces only 4 (16.8 kJ). Perhaps the efficiency with which fat provides the body's fuel can best be appreciated when one compares the caloric content of various food portions; one-half cup of rice (carbohydrate) contains 112 kilocalories, while a single tablespoon of butter contains 100 kilocalories.

Another major role of dietary fats is to transport fat-soluble vitamins. Absorption of vitamins A, D, E, and K will not occur very efficiently in the absence of lipid.

Finally, dietary lipids are the source of an essential nutrient. "Essential" has a special nutritional meaning; it refers to a substance that cannot be synthesized by the body at all, or cannot be synthesized in adequate amounts, and whose lack results in specific deficiency symptoms. Certain fatty acids are essential in this special nutritional sense, and these must be supplied from dietary sources.

Linoleic acid, a PUFA, has been identified as an essential nutrient, necessary for normal growth and health maintenance. In its absence, specific deficiency symptoms develop. It is also a precursor for the synthesis of the prostaglandins, 20-carbon fatty acids that have hormonelike functions.

When essential fatty acid (EFA) deficiency was initially described, it was thought that linolenic (18:3) and arachidonic (20:4) acids were essential also. However, subsequent studies have shown that, although linolenic acid is necessary for growth, it can be synthesized from linoleic acid. Arachidonic acid, which is about three times more effective than linoleic acid in promoting growth, is synthesized by the body from linoleic acid as well (Wene et al., 1975). Linoleic acid, then, because it cannot be synthesized by the body, is in every sense *the* essential fatty acid. Fortunately, it is present in a large number of edible vegetable oils, including corn, peanut, cottonseed, safflower, and soybean oils, as well as from other sources, and deficiency is rare.

Lipid Content of Foods

Most people are aware of the "visible" fats of butter, oils, bacon, and the layer surrounding most cuts of meat but may not realize that homogenized milk, nuts, avocados, cheese, and egg yolk, as well as pie crusts and most cakes contain "invisible" fat in substantial quantities. In general, however, fruits, grains, and vegetables contain very little fat.

Everyone has noticed that the appearance and texture of visible fats vary from one food to another. For example, beef fat is whiter and firmer than that of poultry, which is in turn more solid than that found in fish. The appearance and texture of beef fat varies with the age of the animal; fat of mature beef is whiter and harder than the fat of young beef which is soft and translucent. The difference between the lipids contained in butter and those in corn oil is also obvious.

TRIGLYCERIDES. Virtually all—about 90 percent—of the fat in our food is in the form of triglycerides. The remaining tenth of our fat intake is primarily in the form of cholesterol and phospholipids. The length of the carbon chains and the degree of saturation of the fatty acids in the triglycerides account for the different textures, appearance, and other properties of the various dietary fats.

In general, those triglycerides containing short- and medium-chain fatty acids, as well as those containing unsaturated long-chain fatty acids, are liquid at room temperature (peanut oil). But fatty foods containing a high proportion of saturated long-chain fatty acids will be solid under the same conditions (beef fat). A single food may contain many different triglycerides, and the composite mixture of fatty acid length and degree of saturation will determine not only the physical properties, but also the important biological effects of a particular dietary lipid.

The fatty acid composition of various substances is listed in Table 3-3. Most food fats consist predominantly of long-chain fatty acids (16 or more carbons), with butter, milk (including human milk) and milk products, and, particularly, coconut oil, containing significant amounts of short- and medium-chain fatty acids as well. Animal products generally contain significant amounts of saturated (palmitic and stearic) and monounsaturated (oleic) fatty acids, with lesser amounts of PUFA. Vegetable products, on the other hand, except for coconut oil, contain higher proportions of the long-chain unsaturated oleic and linoleic acids and lesser amounts of saturated fatty acids. Although coconut oil is largely saturated, it consists for the most part of medium- or short-chain fatty acids containing 12 or fewer carbon atoms, and is therefore liquid. People who, for health reasons or by choice, want to modify their fat intake by switching to polyunsaturated vegetable oils, should be aware that coconut oil is the exception to the vegetable oil–PUFA rule.

Detailed analyses of the fatty acid content of specific foods have been presented in a series of articles in the *Journal of the American Dietetic Association* (1975–1977). (See the Suggested Additional Reading section for a list of these articles.) One study, for example, focused on the lipid composition of more than twenty species of shellfish. Generally, shellfish were found to have a low total lipid content of less than 3 percent, and a relatively high

TABLE 3-3 **Major Fatty Acid Content of Selected Animal-origin and Plant-origin Fats**

	Saturated							Unsaturated					
	4–8	*Capric 10:0*	*Lauric 12:0*	*Myristic 14:0*	*Palmitic 16:0*	*Stearic 18:0*	*Arachidic 20:0*	*Palmit-oleic 16:1*	*Oleic 18:1*	*Linoleic 18:2*	*Linolenic 18:3*	*Arachi-donic 20:4*	*Other Polyenoic Acids*
Animal-origin Fats													
Lard				1.5	27.0	13.5		3.0	43.5	10.5	0.5		
Chicken			2.0	7.0	25.0	6.0		8.0	36.0	14.0			
Egg					25.0	10.0			50.0	10.0	2.0	3.0	
Beef				3.0	29.0	21.0	0.5	3.0	41.0	2.0	0.5	0.5	
Butter	5.5	3.0	3.5	12.0	28.0	13.0		3.0	28.5	1.0			
Whole cow's milk[a]	6.5	2.5	3.0	11.0	28.0	12.5		2.5	26.5	2.5	1.5	trace	
Yogurt, fruit-flavored, low-fat[a]	6.0	3.0	4.0	10.5	28.0	10.0		2.0	24.0	2.0	1.0	trace	
Cheddar cheese[a]	6.0	2.0	2.0	10.5	31.0	13.0		3.0	25.0	2.0	1.0	trace	
Human milk		1.5	7.0	8.5	21.0	7.0	1.0	2.5	36.0	7.0	1.0	0.5	
Human adipose[b]			0.1–2	2–6	21–25	2–8		3–7	39–47	4–25			2–8
Plant-origin Fats													
Corn					12.5	2.5	0.5		29.0	55.0	0.5		
Peanut					11.5	3.0	1.5		53.0	26.0			
Cottonseed				1.0	26.0	3.0		1.0	17.5	51.5			
Soybean					11.5	4.0			24.5	53.0	7.0		
Olive					13.0	2.5		1.0	74.0	9.0	0.5		
Coconut	7.0	6.0	49.5	19.5	8.5	2.0			6.0	1.5			

[a]Consumer and Food Economics Institute, *Composition of foods . . . dairy and egg products . . . raw, processed, prepared,* USDA Agriculture Handbook No. 8-1 (Washington, D.C.: U.S. Government Printing Office, 1976).

[b]Adapted from E. S. West et al.: *Textbook of biochemistry,* 4th ed. (New York: Macmillan, 1966).

Source: Food and Nutrition Board, *Dietary fat and human health,* Pub. 1147 (Washington, D.C.: National Academy of Sciences–National Research Council, 1966), p. 6.

Note: Composition is given in weight percentages of the component fatty acids as determined by gas chromatography. The number of carbon atoms and the number of double bonds is indicated under the common name of the fatty acid. These data were derived from a variety of sources, and considerable variation is to be expected in individual samples.

proportion of polyunsaturates was found in such popular shellfish as oysters, crabs, mussels, shrimp, and scallops (Exler and Weihrauch, 1977). (However, a favorite method of cooking these foods—deep frying—will add considerably to the lipid content of a seafood dinner!)

Interestingly, it has been found that by changing the fatty acid composition of feed, livestock with a higher PUFA content in their tissues can be produced. These findings have nutritional implications for humans. Similarly, recent studies have shown that the fatty acid content of the adipose tissue of human infants reflects the dietary fats received in formula or breast milk (Widdowson et al., 1975).

HYDROGENATION. We have seen that vegetable oils are liquid at room temperature because of their high proportion of polyunsaturated fatty acids. How, then, do we account for the fact that margarine, which consists of vegetable oils, is solid at room temperature? Food technologists found that, by the process of **hydrogenation,** (chemically adding hydrogen atoms to polyunsaturated fatty acids), vegetable oils could be solidified and made more spreadable. As the hydrogen atoms become attached to the carbon atoms of the molecule, the number of double bonds is reduced, and the linoleic acid content is decreased. If hydrogenation is complete, the resulting fat will be saturated.

Hydrogenation may be terminated before complete saturation is achieved, resulting in a product that is only partially hydrogenated and that contains a proportionately greater quantity of monounsaturated oleic acid. Margarine, then, consists of vegetable oils that have been hydrogenated so that they have a higher proportion of saturated and monounsaturated fatty acids than the original product, and it is therefore solid at room temperature. Because the chemical nature of the lipid has been changed, its physical properties—appearance, taste, melting point—have been altered also.

When margarine was first introduced commercially as a butter substitute, consumer acceptance of the new product was poor. It did not, after all, look like butter (it was a pasty white color) nor did it taste like the "high-priced spread." Food technologists went back to their laboratories to create today's margarines, which not only have color, flavorings and preservatives added to them, but also are fortified with vitamins A and D to give them nutritive value and taste as similar as possible to those of butter. Margarine even has the same calorie count as butter, approximately 100 per tablespoon, and must, by law, contain at least 80 percent fat (as must butter). Exceptions are the "imitation" or diet margarines which have less then 80 percent fat and contain more water than regular margarines. The fat composition of different kinds of margarine is shown in Table 3-4. Most margarines cost somewhat less than butter, although the price differential has narrowed in recent years as consumer demand for polyunsaturated fats has grown. As one might expect, the highest-priced margarines are those with the highest PUFA content.

Hydrogenation is also used to improve the keeping qualities of liquid oils. Exposure to the oxygen in air causes the double bonds in unsaturated fats to break down. This **oxidation** leads to the production of undesirable odors and flavors characteristic of rancidity. It is accelerated by exposure to light, air, and heat, and through contact with certain metals such as iron, copper, and

TABLE 3-4
Fat Composition of Margarine Types (g/tbsp)

Margarine[a]	Total Fat	Saturated Fat	PUFA	Energy Content (kcal, rounded)
Stick (soybean oil)	11	2	1	100
Soft (soybean oil)	11	2	3	100
Soft (corn oil)	11	2	5	100
Soft diet (corn oil)	6	1	2	50

[a]Single brand, comparing various types.
Source: Adapted from *Medical Newsletter*, September 24, 1976.

nickel. Partial hydrogenation, which makes oil less susceptible to oxidation, is one solution to the problem of spoilage. Other solutions include the addition of chemicals, such as BHT (butylated hydroxytoluene) and BHA (butylated hydroxyanisole), that act as **antioxidants** because they are preferentially oxidized instead of the PUFA; vitamin E is a natural antioxidant. Air-tight, dark, and cool storage conditions also retard the oxidation process.

PHOSPHOLIPIDS AND CHOLESTEROL. Our discussion of dietary lipids has thus far concentrated on the triglycerides which account for 90 percent of our fat intake. The remaining important components of dietary lipid are phospholipids and cholesterol.

Phospholipids are found in significant quantities in egg yolk and soybeans and in marginal amounts in a number of other foods. Lecithin is a major phospholipid.

Cholesterol is a natural body substance, required for several vital processes. The greater portion of the human cholesterol requirement is met by synthesis within the body. Table 3-5 shows both the fat and cholesterol content of a

TABLE 3-5 **Total Fat and Cholesterol Content of Selected Foods**

Food	Fat Content g/100 g	Cholesterol Content mg/100 g	Serving Size	Fat Content g/serving	Cholesterol Content mg/serving
Beef liver, raw	3.2	300	$3\frac{1}{2}$ oz	3.2	300
Whole eggs	11.2	548	1 large	5.6	274
Egg yolk	32.9	1602	1 large	5.6	274
Shrimp, canned, drained	1.1	150	1 c	1.4	192
Lobster, cooked, meat only	1.5	85	1 c	2.2	123
Crabmeat, canned	2.5	101	$\frac{1}{2}$ c	2.0	80
Beef, lean, cooked	14.7	91	3 oz	13	77
Chicken breast, cooked	3.4	80	1, meat and skin (92 g)	3.1	74
Haddock, flesh only	0.1	60	$3\frac{1}{2}$ oz	0.1	60
Oysters, meat only	2.0	50	$\frac{1}{2}$ c	2.4	60

TABLE 3-5 **Total Fat and Cholesterol Content of Selected Foods (Continued)**

Food	Fat Content g/100 g	Cholesterol Content mg/100 g	Serving Size	Fat Content g/serving	Cholesterol Content mg/serving
Tuna, in water	0.8	63	3¼ oz	0.73	58
Clams, raw, meat only	1.6	50	½ c	1.8	57
Chicken drumstick, cooked	3.4	91	1, meat and skin (52 g)	1.8	47
Macaroni and cheese, home recipe	11.1	21	1 c	22.2	42
Hot dog, cooked	27.2	62	1 (8 per lb)	15	34
Whole milk	3.3	14	1 c	8	33
Yellow cake with chocolate frosting	13.0	44	1/16 of 9-in cake	10	33
Ice cream, 10% fat	10.8	45	½ c	7.1	30
Process American cheese	31.2	94	1 oz	8.9	27
Swiss cheese	27.4	92	1 oz	7.8	26
Brownie with nuts (homemade)	31.3	83	1 (20 g)	6	17
Cream cheese	35.2	111	1 tbsp	5	16
Yogurt, plain, low fat	1.6	6	8 oz	3.5	14
Butter	81.0	2.9	1 pat	4.1	11
Cottage cheese, 1% fat	1.0	4	1 c	2.3	10
Margarine, ⅔ animal, ⅓ vegetable	81.0	50	1 tbsp	12	7
Skim milk	0.1	2	1 c	0.4	4
Angel food cake	0.2	0	1/12 of 10-in cake	trace	0
Apple, raw with skin	0.6	0	1 medium	0.6	0
Banana	0.2	0	1 small	0.2	0
Bread, white	5.0	0	1 slice (22 per lb)	1	0
Corn oil	100.0	0	1 tbsp	14	0
Egg white	0	0	1 large	0	0
Margarine, vegetable	81.0	0	1 tbsp	12	0
Peanut butter	45.0	0	1 tbsp	10	0
Red kidney beans, cooked	1.7	0	1 c	1.0	0
Sweet potatoes	0.9	0	1 medium	1.0	0

Note: Generally, animal products are the food sources which contain significant amounts of cholesterol. Organ meats and eggs have the highest concentration, with the yolk containing *all* of the cholesterol found in whole eggs. Fat content is not necessarily indicative of cholesterol content, as can be seen in the values for beef liver, eggs, corn oil, and margarine.

Source: Compiled from C. F. Church, and H. N. Church, *Food values of portions commonly used*, 12th ed. (Philadelphia: J. B. Lippincott, 1975); and R. M. Feeley, et al., Cholesterol contents of foods, *Journal of the American Dietetic Association* 61: 134–149, 1972.

Source: L. P. Posati and M. L. Orr. *Composition of foods—Dairy and egg products—Raw, processed, prepared,* USDA Agriculture Handbook No. 8-1 (Washington, D.C.: U.S. Government Printing Office, 1976).

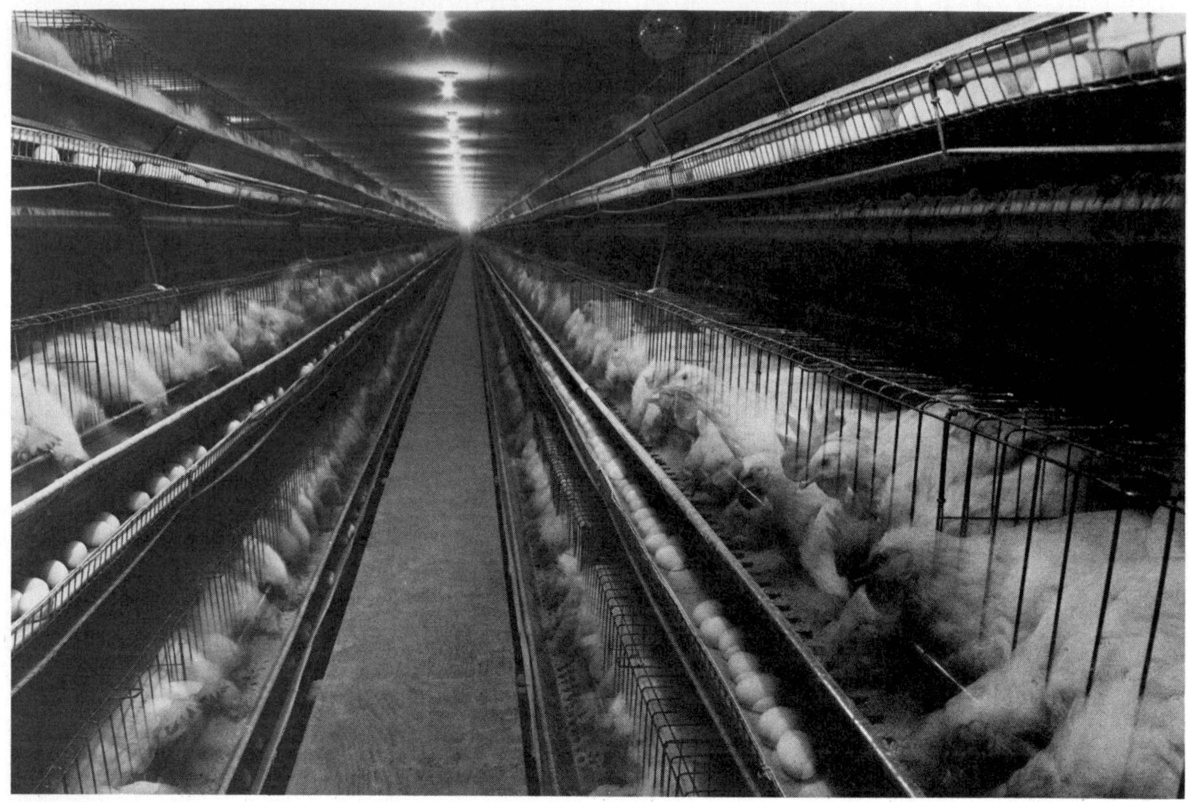

Cages line 3 tiers on either side of a walkway in the laying house of this modern egg farm. (Grant Heilman)

number of foods. It will be noted that fat content is not an indicator of cholesterol content: corn oil, for example, is 100 percent lipid but has no cholesterol. Cholesterol occurs only in foods of animal origin, including all meats. Organ meats such as liver and brains, and egg yolks, have the highest concentration. Egg yolks, in fact, contain the entire cholesterol content of the egg; there is no cholesterol in egg white. Fish and shellfish have a relatively low total lipid content and, with the exception of shrimp, have moderate amounts of cholesterol. Although low in fats, shrimp contain large amounts of cholesterol and should be eaten only infrequently by persons following a cholesterol-restricted diet. The concern over dietary cholesterol and its possible implication in the development of atherosclerosis will be examined later in this chapter.

DIGESTION AND ABSORPTION

Before examining some of the specific physiological functions of lipids, we shall consider the processes by which lipids in foods are transformed into lipids having structural and functional significance in the body. Although the basic principles of preparing food chemicals for entry into the blood and cells of the body are the same for lipids as they are for carbohydrates, certain important differences exist.

Because lipids are insoluble in water—which comprises the medium of cells, interstitial fluids, and the circulatory system—they must be rendered more water soluble before they can be biologically useful. This is achieved by two major mechanisms: **emulsification,** and the use of specialized transport systems.

Emulsification

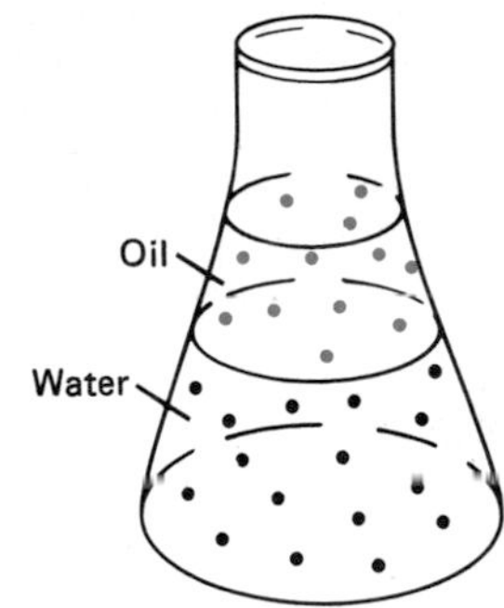

Lipid molecules must be emulsified in order to be able to mix with water. An emulsifier is a molecule that contains both a water-soluble and a lipid-soluble group. Emulsification takes place when the water-soluble group of such a molecule interacts with a water-based substance, and the lipid-soluble group interacts with a lipid-based substance. The emulsifier acts as a bridge between two substances that would otherwise be immiscible (unblendable).

Bile acids and lecithin are two major biochemical emulsifiers. They disperse fat into small globules within the gastrointestinal tract, thereby increasing the surface area available to interact with digestive enzymes.

Emulsification can also be effected mechanically through a physical process in which fat globules are broken into smaller particles so that they may be dispersed in a watery medium. The homogenization of milk is an example of mechanical emulsification.

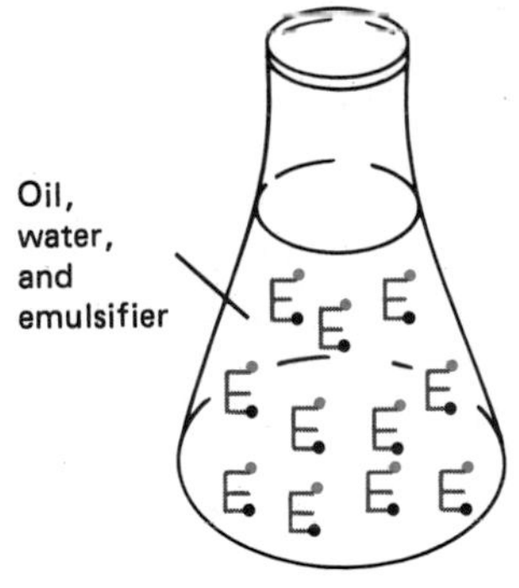

• Fat molecules

• Water or water-soluble molecules

E Emulsifier

Lipid Transport

Lipids are carried through plasma in the form of **lipoproteins.** Because plasma is an aqueous medium, lipids cannot be transported without the mediation of this group of substances—proteins that tend to combine with lipids—specialized for lipid transport.

Each of the four major classes of lipoproteins performs a specific physiological function, and each differs in the proportions of its protein and lipid components. Because pure fat is lighter than water, as the proportion of lipid to protein increases the density of the lipoprotein decreases. Thus, the lipoprotein with the greatest amount of lipid in proportion to protein will be lightest, or least dense. This makes it possible for the various lipoproteins to be separated in the laboratory by techniques, such as ultracentrifugation, that depend on the relative density of each kind of molecule. A comparison of the composition of these molecules is presented in Table 3-6.

Chylomicrons, the least dense type of lipoprotein, transport primarily triglycerides but also carry some cholesterol. *Very low density lipoproteins* (VLDLs), synthesized in the liver, also transport primarily triglycerides, carrying them from the liver to other tissues, especially to adipose tissue for storage. *Low density lipoproteins* (LDLs) transport mainly cholesterol, somewhat over half of it in the form of cholesterol esters. *High density lipoproteins* (HDLs) transport phospholipids and cholesterol esters.

TABLE 3-6 **Composition and Synthesis of Lipoproteins**

Lipoprotein (in order of increasing density)	Components (percent)						Synthesized in
	Protein	*Lipid*				*Carbohydrate*	
		Triglyceride	*Cholesterol & Cholesterol esters*	*Phospholipid*	*Total*		
Chylomicrons	1	90	7	2	99	trace	Intestine
VLDLs	10	60	15	14	89	1	Liver
LDLs	25	10	44	20	74	1	Liver and intestine
HDLs	50	3	16	30	49	1	Liver

In rare instances, individuals are unable to synthesize certain of the lipoproteins, resulting in abnormalities of lipid metabolism. These conditions, genetic in origin, are manifested by a variety of digestive and other severe symptoms.

Lipid Digestion

No significant chemical digestion of fat occurs before dietary lipid enters the duodenum. The mouth merely provides mechanical lubrication and mastication. Mechanical action is continued during peristalsis in the esophagus and during churning in the stomach. In the stomach, however, the enzyme gastric lipase initiates hydrolysis of such highly emulsified dietary fats as those in egg yolk and milk and has some small effect on triglycerides containing short- and medium-chain fatty acids. In hydrolysis the ester bond holding the fatty acid to glycerol is broken in the presence of a facilitating enzyme, with the addition of a water molecule.

When it leaves the stomach, most fat is still in the form of large globules. Because of its low density, the fat floats on top of the chyme and is the last nutrient component to leave the stomach. As with carbohydrates, most lipid digestion takes place in the small intestine.

As dietary triglycerides leave the stomach and enter the duodenum, cells of the small intestine release the hormone *cholecystikinin.* This substance is then transported in the blood to the gall bladder, where it stimulates the release of stored bile. Bile is composed of cholesterol derivatives known as bile salts, along with water and other compounds. It is synthesized by cells in the liver and stored in the gall bladder until needed for lipid digestion. (The enterohepatic circulation of bile will be described later in the chapter.) Bile is the major emulsifying agent for dietary lipids. This substance makes it possible for digestive enzymes, which are water-soluble protein molecules, to interact with a larger surface area of the lipid particles and thus increases their effectiveness.

The presence of fat in the duodenum also stimulates release of *enterogastrone*. This hormone appears to regulate the rate at which fat enters the duodenum, so that it will correspond with the rate of secretion of the fat-digesting enzymes from the pancreas.

Pancreatic juice, which enters the duodenum by way of the pancreatic duct, contains three enzymes which affect lipid digestion: pancreatic lipase, phospholipase, and cholesterol esterase.

Pancreatic lipase acts on long-chain triglycerides. As almost all dietary triglycerides are of this type this enzyme is responsible for a substantial portion of lipid digestion. (Triglycerides containing medium-chain fatty acids do not usually require hydrolysis.) In the presence of pancreatic lipase, the ester bonds of long-chain triglycerides are broken and two molecules of water are incorporated, forming a 2-monoglyceride and two fatty acids. (The 2-monoglyceride is so called because the fatty acid is attached to the second carbon of the glycerol unit.)

Similarly, *phospholipases* hydrolyze some dietary phospholipids; however, some dietary phospholipid is left intact. And *cholesterol esterase*, in the presence of bile, hydrolyzes dietary cholesterol esters, breaking them down into cholesterol and fatty acid. However, most dietary cholesterol is in the free sterol form and does not undergo digestive action at this point.

Absorption

The end products of lipid digestion in the small intestine are monoglycerides, fatty acids, and cholesterol; in addition, some phospholipids and short- and medium-chain triglycerides remain in essentially dietary form.

In the lumen of the small intestine, the monoglycerides, fatty acids, cholesterol, and phospholipids combine with bile to form specialized aggregates called **micelles.** Acting as an emulsifier, the bile attaches to the fatty components and enables them to become distributed through a watery medium. In this case, the digested lipids are attached to bile and suspended in the form of infinitesimal particles in the contents of the small intestine, ready to be absorbed. It has been estimated that, in the formation of a micelle, the diameter of individual lipid particles is decreased 100 times and surface area increased 10,000 times (Johnston, 1968).

The primary site of lipid absorption is the surface of the jejunum or middle section of the small intestine. The intestine has an extremely large surface area because of the presence of villi or projections. Each villus contains blood vessels and a special lymph vessel called a **lacteal.**

Micellar lipids and short- and medium-chain triglycerides are absorbed directly into the mucosal cells of the jejunum by a process as yet unknown. As the lipid contents of the micelle move on their way, the bile salts are removed; they will remain in the lumen, to be reabsorbed from the ileum, or terminal portion of the small intestine.

In the mucosal cells, several reactions take place, depending on the type of fat to be absorbed. Medium- and short-chain triglycerides are hydrolyzed by **intestinal lipase** to glycerol and short- and medium-chain fatty acids. These products, along with short- and medium-chain fatty acids that have been produced as a result of previous intestinal hydrolysis, leave the mucosal cells and enter the capillaries directly, from which they are transported by the portal vein to the liver. Fatty acids transported into the blood are bound to the protein, **albumin,** which enhances their solubility.

In the meantime, long-chain fatty acids are re-esterified with glycerol to produce long-chain triglycerides. Together with the cholesterol and phospholipids in the mucosa, the newly synthesized long-chain triglycerides are combined with a protein to form the lipoprotein chylomicron, a fat-rich particle which accounts for the transport of a substantial portion of dietary lipid. If a blood sample is taken a few hours after a high-fat meal has been eaten, a creamy layer will be noticed rising to the top. This layer consists of the fat-bearing chylomicrons and is a convincing demonstration indeed of their low density.

Chylomicrons enter the lymphatic system through the lacteals in the villi. Lymph vessels generally deposit their contents into the blood stream through the thoracic duct, the pathway by which chylomicrons join the general circulation. Eventually they are carried by the hepatic artery to the liver. The liver is also the destination of the glycerol and the short- and medium-chain fatty acids which were transported directly through the capillaries and portal vein. Any excess lipid content not needed by cells in the liver will be transported to other tissues, including adipose tissue, by lipoproteins. The digestion and absorption of dietary lipids are diagrammed in Figure 3-6. Table 3-7 summarizes these processes.

BILE. The **enterohepatic circulation** is the mechanism by which bile becomes available for its role in lipid digestion. Bile is released from storage in the gall bladder in response to the presence of fat at the entrance to the small intestine. Then, by means of the bile duct, it enters the duodenum, where it forms micelles with dietary lipids. As the lipid particles enter the mucosa of the jejunum, the bile salts detach from the micellar complex. Most of the bile salts are reabsorbed in the ileum, from which they enter the portal vein, which carries them back to the liver.

This enterohepatic circulation is so efficient that the relatively small total pool of bile salts, amounting to about 3 to 5 grams, is recycled many times during a day, and only a small amount (approximately 0.5 g) is lost and excreted in the feces. The lost bile salts are promptly replaced through synthesis from cholesterol, which takes place in the liver. From the liver the bile goes to the gall bladder for storage until, once again, the presence of lipid in the duodenum signals its release.

DISTURBANCES OF LIPID ABSORPTION. Lipid absorption is extremely efficient, with about 95 percent of total lipid intake being absorbed. Normal adults can absorb up to as much as 300 grams of fat a day. Under certain circumstances, however, absorption is disrupted and lipids may appear in excessive amounts in the stool. This condition, known as **steatorrhea,** may be caused by any of several different factors.

In diarrhea, for example, lipids move through the intestine so rapidly that they cannot be efficiently hydrolyzed by the various enzymes. Consequently, most of the dietary fat is not absorbed and is excreted.

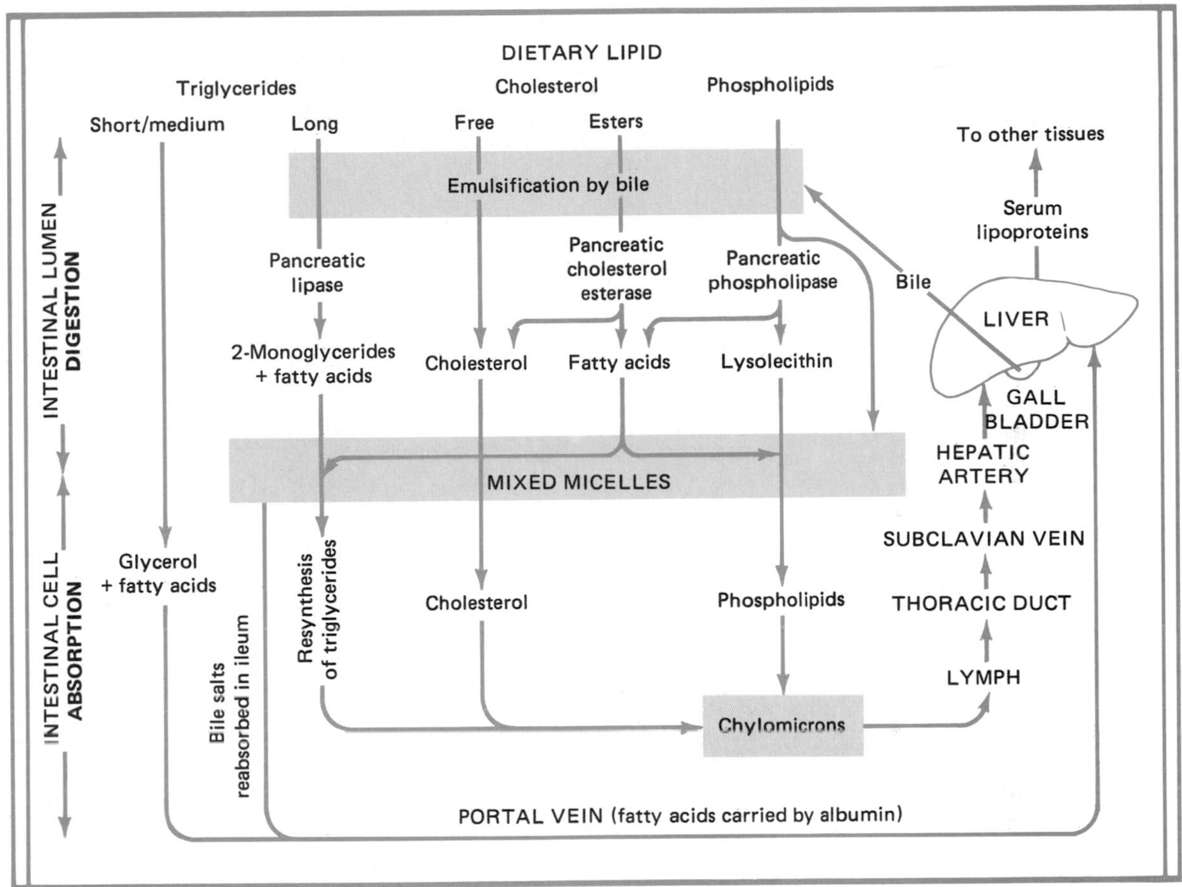

FIGURE 3-6
Digestion and Absorption of Dietary Lipids

An obstruction of the gall bladder duct, or removal of the gall bladder itself, will decrease the amount of bile available for action in the duodenum and jejunum. After removal of the gall bladder, however, adaptive mechanisms take over. Many people who have had this operation gradually become able to tolerate normal, or nearly normal, amounts of fat in their diets. This happens because, even though bile can no longer be stored, the liver synthesizes it in adequate quantity, and the bile then enters the small intestine directly from the liver.

Other causes of steatorrhea are pancreatic disease or blockage of the pancreatic duct. Decreased levels of pancreatic enzymes in the intestinal lumen will prevent adequate hydrolysis of long-chain triglycerides or cholesterol esters, and these lipids, which are not in a form which can be absorbed, will be excreted. For people with these and similar conditions, medium-chain triglyceride (MCT) oil with 8:0 and 10:0 chain fatty acids has been useful. Prepared by distillation from coconut oil, the short- and medium-chain fatty acids of MCT do not require hydrolysis before absorption, nor do they need to be solubilized with bile. Instead they are hydrolized by intestinal lipase in the mucosa and then absorbed directly into the blood vessels of the villi. Use

TABLE 3-7 **Summary of Lipid Digestion and Absorption**

Dietary Lipid	Acted on by	Digested Products	Preparation for Absorption	Absorption	In Mucosa	Product
Long-chain triglycerides	Pancreatic lipase	2-monoglyceride + 2 fatty acids	Form micelles with bile	Absorbed into mucosa of the small intestine	Long-chain fatty acids reesterified with glycerol; all other components are unchanged	Long-chain triglycerides and other components
Phospholipids	Pancreatic phospholipase	Fatty acids, glycerol, phosphate-containing group				
Cholesterol esters	Pancreatic cholesterol esterase	Cholesterol + fatty acid				
Cholesterol						
Medium- and short-chain triglycerides	⟶			Absorbed directly into mucosa of small intestine	Hydrolyzed by intestinal lipase	Glycerol + short- and medium-chain fatty acids

of MCT oil, therefore, reduces the fat loss of chronic steatorrhea, and the excessive energy loss that accompanies it.

Ingestion of mineral oil can also cause steatorrhea. Mineral oil is sometimes taken as a laxative, or used instead of salad oil by persons on weight-loss diets. Because mineral oil does not contain any oxygen, it is not a true lipid. It cannot be digested and absorbed, but merely passes through the digestive tract, accounting for its laxative action. On its way, however, it solubilizes fatty materials, including fat-soluble vitamins, and carries them along so that they cannot be absorbed. Potentially serious deficiencies of some of these substances may result from frequent ingestion of mineral oil. It is not generally advisable to use mineral oil for a laxative effect. If mineral oil is prescribed for a specific condition, it should be taken some time after eating, never during a meal.

METABOLISM OF LIPIDS

Having been digested and absorbed, lipids are now available for use by all tissues of the body, to which they are transported by lipoproteins. When the circulating lipids are needed for cell functions, an enzyme (lipoprotein lipase, which is bound to capillary and cell membranes) releases the lipid portion from its protein carrier and hydrolyzes the constituent triglyceride into glycerol and fatty acids. The lipid molecules are ready to enter cells for further utilization.

The metabolic needs of the organism determine the particular metabolic process that will take place. Fat breakdown or **lipolysis,** and fat synthesis or **lipogenesis,** are the dynamic processes of lipid metabolism. These processes

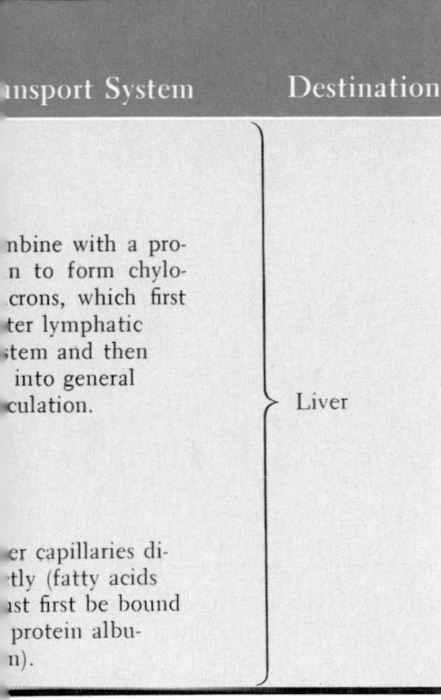

ansport System	Destination
nbine with a pro- n to form chylo- crons, which first ter lymphatic stem and then into general culation.	Liver
er capillaries di- tly (fatty acids ast first be bound protein albu- n).	

are not merely the reverse of each other; each involves different pathways, reactants, and enzymes. Before examining these processes in detail, we shall consider the functions of the liver and of adipose tissue, the primary regulators of lipid metabolism.

Role of The Liver

The cells of the liver constitute a complex internal biochemistry laboratory where a number of different processes occur as they are needed. The body's requirements are signalled by hormones and enzymes that regulate the lipid metabolic processes.

Within the liver, fatty acids are synthesized by lipogenesis into new triglycerides. These are normally transported out of the liver by the lipoproteins, especially the VLDLs, which carry them to adipose tissue for storage until otherwise needed. Lipogenesis and subsequent transport are triggered by lipotropic (from Greek *tropos*, turning or changing) factors such as choline and methionine, thereby preventing excessive accumulation of fat in the liver. Carbohydrates (as well as lipids) also provide the raw materials for lipogenesis: fatty acids and glycerol synthesized from carbohydrates follow the same pathway as the triglycerides synthesized directly from digested lipid. This process is the reason excess intake of kilocalories from carbohydrate adds to our fat reserves.

Also in the liver, long-chain fatty acids are made even longer and are desaturated, which transforms them into different fatty acids. For example, stearic acid (18:0) becomes oleic acid (18:1), and linoleic acid (18:2) becomes arachidonic acid (20:4).

But lipolysis is also occurring in the liver at the same time, as triglycerides are hydrolyzed to form fatty acids and glycerol. The triglyceride reactions are reversible and occur in response to the needs of the organism at a particular time. If there is an oversupply of lipid in the liver, lipogenesis will convert it into a form for transport and storage. If the energy needs of the organism require available lipid, on the other hand, lipolysis will occur to produce accessible lipid products for circulation. Triglycerides, then, can be hydrolyzed and resynthesized, used for energy, or used in the synthesis of other lipids, such as phospholipids and cholesterol (processes which also take place in the liver and which we will examine in greater detail below).

In the liver, cholesterol is synthesized from 2-carbon fragments of acetyl CoA. The liver also removes cholesterol from the circulation. Cholesterol from both sources is converted to bile acids, which enter the gall bladder for storage as a component of bile.

Role of Adipose Tissue

Adipose tissue, which serves as a reservoir of stored energy, is located not only under the skin, but also in the abdominal cavity and within muscle tissue. Lipids are stored primarily in the form of triglycerides. Contrary to popular belief, adipose tissue doesn't just "sit" there; it is metabolically active. Fat cells (**adipocytes**) contain both lipogenic and lipolytic enzymes. When energy

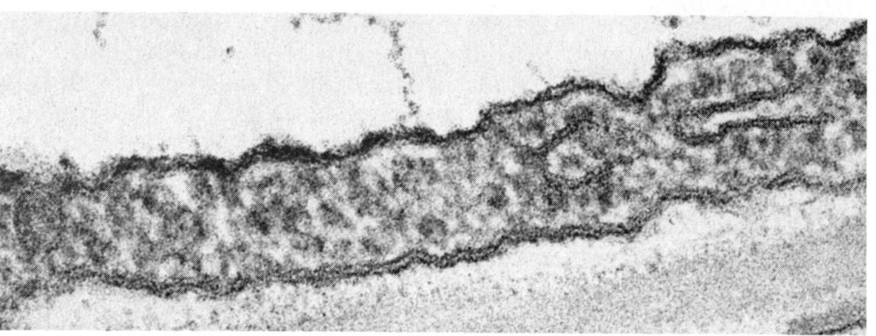

Electron micrograph showing a plasma membrane and vacuolar membrane. Each of these membranes (darkest lines) consists of a double layer of lipid molecules "sandwiched" between two protein layers. (Myron C. Ledbetter, Brookhaven National Laboratory)

intake equals energy output, enzymes and processes are in equilibrium. However, when energy intake exceeds output, lipogenesis (facilitated by the hormone insulin) predominates, and triglycerides are synthesized from fatty acids and glycerol.

When energy is in demand, the reverse process takes place. The stored triglycerides are hydrolyzed, releasing **free fatty acids** (FFA) from adipose tissue into the blood stream. Bound to albumin, the FFA travel to other tissues to provide energy.

At any one time, the amount of FFA circulating in the plasma is normally very low, accounting for only about 5 percent of total blood lipids. The contribution of circulating FFA to energy production, however, is high. Many cells of the body, particularly muscle, preferentially use fatty acids as a source of energy, and their rapid flux throughout the circulation is vital. FFAs are a dynamic pool of potential energy, and can be removed from the blood within minutes.

Several hormones influence the hydrolysis of triglycerides and the rate of release of FFA from adipose tissue—epinephrine, growth hormone, and glucagon among others. The various enzymes that catalyze lipolysis—lipases—are sensitive to these hormones and are triggered by them to catalyze the process of lipolysis in the adipocytes. Each hormone is released in response to specific metabolic conditions—stress or hypoglycemia, for example—but the net effect is to mobilize stored energy.

When there is no dietary energy source, adipose tissue is stimulated by hormones to release more fatty acids. As might be expected, blood levels of FFA will be higher during fasting than following a meal.

Biochemistry of Lipid Metabolism

We have discussed the regulatory role of the liver and of adipose tissue in fat metabolism. We shall now examine these processes in greater detail from a biochemical point of view.

FATTY-ACID SYNTHESIS. Fatty acids are synthesized in a complex process that requires the presence of two B vitamins, involves energy in the form of adenosine triphosphate (ATP), and uses a CO_2-containing compound, malonyl CoA. This series of reactions requires the presence of several different enzymes and several coenzymes and cannot proceed if any of these are absent. It can be thought of as a kind of molecular assembly line for the orderly building up of fatty-acid chains. Acetic acid (CH_3COOH), which is a breakdown product of nutrient metabolism, is the primary raw material, and the 16-carbon fatty acid, palmitic acid, is a major end product.

TRIGLYCERIDE SYNTHESIS. In triglyceride synthesis, fatty acids are combined or **esterified** with a glycerol molecule. The fatty acids that react with this glycerol molecule to form triglycerides may be newly synthesized, or they may have resulted from earlier triglyceride breakdown (hydrolysis). Three fatty acids react with glycerol to form a triglyceride; two fatty acids and a phosphate-choline group react with glycerol to produce phospholipids (see Figure 3-3).

β-OXIDATION. The process by which fatty acids are broken down for transformation into energy is known as β-oxidation (Beta-oxidation). Coenzyme A is a key participant in this reaction, first activating, and then aiding in the oxidation of the fatty acids. A number of other enzymes and cofactors are involved as well. During each step in the process, the enzymes remove a 2-carbon fragment (acetyl CoA) from the fatty acid, leaving the fatty acid two carbons shorter. The process is repeated until complete. Thus, after seven turns of the cycle in the case of palmitic acid (illustrated in Figure 3-7), eight molecules of acetyl CoA have been produced. In this manner, the complete oxidation of a fatty acid is achieved.

Acetyl CoA condenses with oxaloacetate in the Krebs cycle; ultimately, mediated by the electron transport system, the end products of β-oxidation are CO_2, H_2O, and ATP. (The interrelationship of these several biochemical processes is shown in Figure 3-8.)

Energy production from lipids is significantly higher than that from glucose; one molecule of glucose yields 36 molecules of ATP, while one molecule of palmitic acid produces 130 molecules of ATP. Even 3 molecules of glucose (which contains 18 carbons, the same number as in stearic acid) yield only 108 molecules of ATP, while β-oxidation of stearic acid yields 152.

Even those fatty acids having an odd number of carbon atoms can be metabolized by β-oxidation, releasing acetyl CoA and finally a single 3-carbon

Palmitic acid (16:0)
→Myristic acid (14:0) + Acetyl CoA
→Lauric acid (12:0) + Acetyl CoA
→Capric acid (10:0) + Acetyl CoA
→Caprylic acid (8:0) + Acetyl CoA
→Capriotic acid (6:0) + Acetyl CoA
→Butyric acid (4:0) + Acetyl CoA
→2 Acetyl CoA

Net: Palmitic acid produces 8 Acetyl CoA.

FIGURE 3-7
Breakdown of Palmitic Acid by β-oxidation

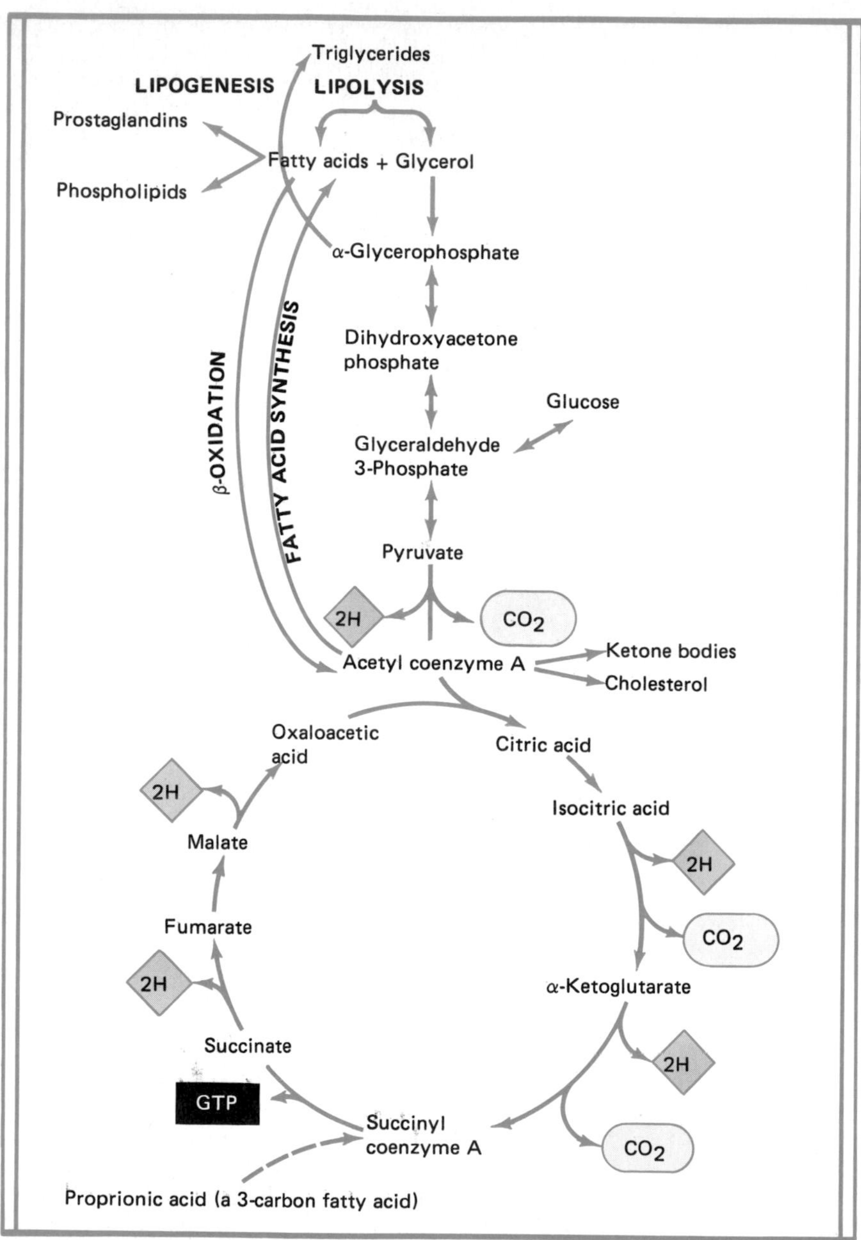

FIGURE 3-8
Lipid Metabolism and the Krebs Cycle

molecule of proprionic acid. Proprionic acid can also produce energy through a reaction that depends on the presence of vitamin B_{12}. This reaction converts the 3-carbon molecule to an intermediate of the Krebs cycle, succinyl CoA. Here, then, is yet another route of energy production.

In addition to providing energy, the acetyl CoA produced by oxidation can also be utilized as the immediate source of malonyl CoA required for the synthesis of fatty acids. It is also involved in the synthesis of cholesterol and other important compounds.

The entire set of interactions is extremely efficient, and no component of a compound goes to waste. The glycerol unit released during the hydrolysis of triglycerides can also be converted to energy. Glycerol enters the Embden-Myerhof pathway and is metabolized to **pyruvate.**

Glycerol can also be converted to glucose. The synthesis of glucose from a precursor of noncarbohydrate origin is called **gluconeogenesis.** Glycerol, while not a major contributor to gluconeogenesis (because only a small part of the triglyceride molecule is glycerol), should not be overlooked as a contributing factor in the elevation of blood glucose levels. Fatty acids, unlike glycerol, are not gluconeogenic; that is, they cannot be converted to glucose.

The cells of adipose tissue, adipocytes, are metabolically active; within these cells, lipogenesis and lipolysis occur in dynamic equilibrium. It is also important to remember that fat can be synthesized from carbohydrates; fatty acids are synthesized from acetyl CoA, which is a product of glucose metabolism as well as of lipid metabolism. When the energy needs of the body have been met, the remaining acetyl CoA is converted to fatty acids and esterified with glycerol to produce a triglyceride. In this form, it can be stored in the adipose tissue. This set of processes occurs in a positive energy state—that is, when the supply of energy exceeds the demand for it.

KETONE BODIES. Most cells of the body can utilize free fatty acids for energy production. Until recently, it was believed that brain cells could not metabolize anything other than glucose to meet their energy needs. It is now known that brain cells can, after a period of adaptation, convert the so-called **ketone bodies** to ATP. The ketone bodies are three derivatives of fatty acids, produced when there is an excessive rate of fatty acid breakdown in the body. In the absence of carbohydrate, as in starvation or high-protein weight-reduction diets, there will be an imbalance between lipogenesis and lipolysis in adipose tissue, with the release of excess fatty acids into the blood. Some of these fatty acids are used for energy production, but some are oxidized only partially to the ketone bodies.

The condensation of two molecules of acetyl CoA results in the formation of acetoacetate or β-hydroxybutyrate, two of the ketone bodies. The third is acetone, resulting from the decarboxylation of acetoacetate. The reasons for this incomplete oxidation are not definitely known; the diminished supply of oxaloacetate in starvation may cause a "slowdown" of the Krebs cycle.

The liver cannot utilize ketone bodies for energy because it does not have specific enzymes to do so. Normally, the body's small production of ketones, primarily acetoacetate, is transported to skeletal and cardiac muscle. These cells produce enzymes that facilitate the oxidation of acetoacetate with acetyl CoA, providing a minor energy source for these tissues. The normal concentration of ketones in the blood is less than 2 mg/dl. When ketones are produced in excess of the capacity of the heart and skeletal muscles to oxidize them, they remain in the circulatory system, causing an increase in the level of plasma ketones.

Excessive accumulation of ketone bodies, a reflection of an imbalance between their production and utilization, is known as **ketosis.** Starvation and diabetes mellitus can produce ketosis; the lack of insulin prevents carbohydrate oxidation, and ketone production is a result. Excessive levels of ketones in the blood (ketonemia) and in the urine (ketonuria) are measurable symptoms of a disturbance of carbohydrate metabolism and/or excessive lipolysis.

CHOLESTEROL METABOLISM. Cholesterol is synthesized in the body primarily by the cells of the liver, intestine, and adrenal glands, although all cells have the capacity to produce this sterol. Through a complicated series of reactions, the simple 2-carbon fragment, acetyl CoA, is converted to 1 or 2 grams of cholesterol daily (see Figure 3-5). In the body, endogenous (synthesized) and exogenous (dietary) cholesterol are indistinguishable.

Cholesterol is needed for the synthesis of steroid hormones, bile salts, and vitamin D—all vital substances. It is transported between tissues bound to lipoproteins, primarily the chylomicrons and LDLs. The precise requirement of the body for cholesterol is not known, but scientists agree that even the small amount produced by the body is greater than the need. Unneeded cholesterol is eliminated in the feces, about half of it in the form of bile salts and the remainder as neutral steroids. Some individuals may have substantial amounts of cholesterol in their circulation, however. Elevated levels of cholesterol in the blood have been linked with atherosclerosis and heart disease.

PHOSPHOLIPID METABOLISM. Phospholipids are constituents of cell membranes throughout the body and play a role in cholesterol synthesis. Because of their emulsifying properties, they act as carriers of fatty acids in the blood. All cells contain phospholipids, but the cells of such metabolically active tissues as the brain, liver, and nerve tissue have particularly high concentrations. Although some phospholipids are present in the diet, the body is capable of synthesizing them in adequate amounts, and they are not considered essential in a nutritional sense. The lecithins, the most widely distributed phospholipids, are synthesized in the liver (see Figure 3-3). Phospholipids are transported primarily by HDLs. The interrelationships of the tissues involved in lipid metabolism are summarized in Figure 3-9.

ESSENTIAL FATTY ACIDS. As we mentioned earlier in this chapter, although it was once thought that linolenic and arachidonic acids were essential fatty acids, linoleic acid is now considered to be the only truly essential fatty acid (EFA) since the others can be synthesized from it. Its absence from the diet produces several symptoms in both laboratory animals and humans, including skin lesions, growth retardation, liver and kidney degeneration, and increased susceptibility to infection. Adults usually have adequate stores of linoleic acid in adipose tissue; deficiency symptoms have not been reported in otherwise healthy adults. Symptoms, particularly eczema, have been identified in infants and in adults receiving long-term, fat-free intravenous feedings (Caldwell et al, 1972; Wene et al., 1975). Infants maintained on skim milk for long periods of time have also displayed symptoms of EFA deficiency (Hansen et al., 1958). These deficiencies are easily corrected by ingestion of small amounts of linoleic acid.

The biochemical reasons for these deficiency symptoms are still being investigated, but it is believed that EFA plays a role in the regulation of cholesterol metabolism, transport, and excretion, acting to lower blood

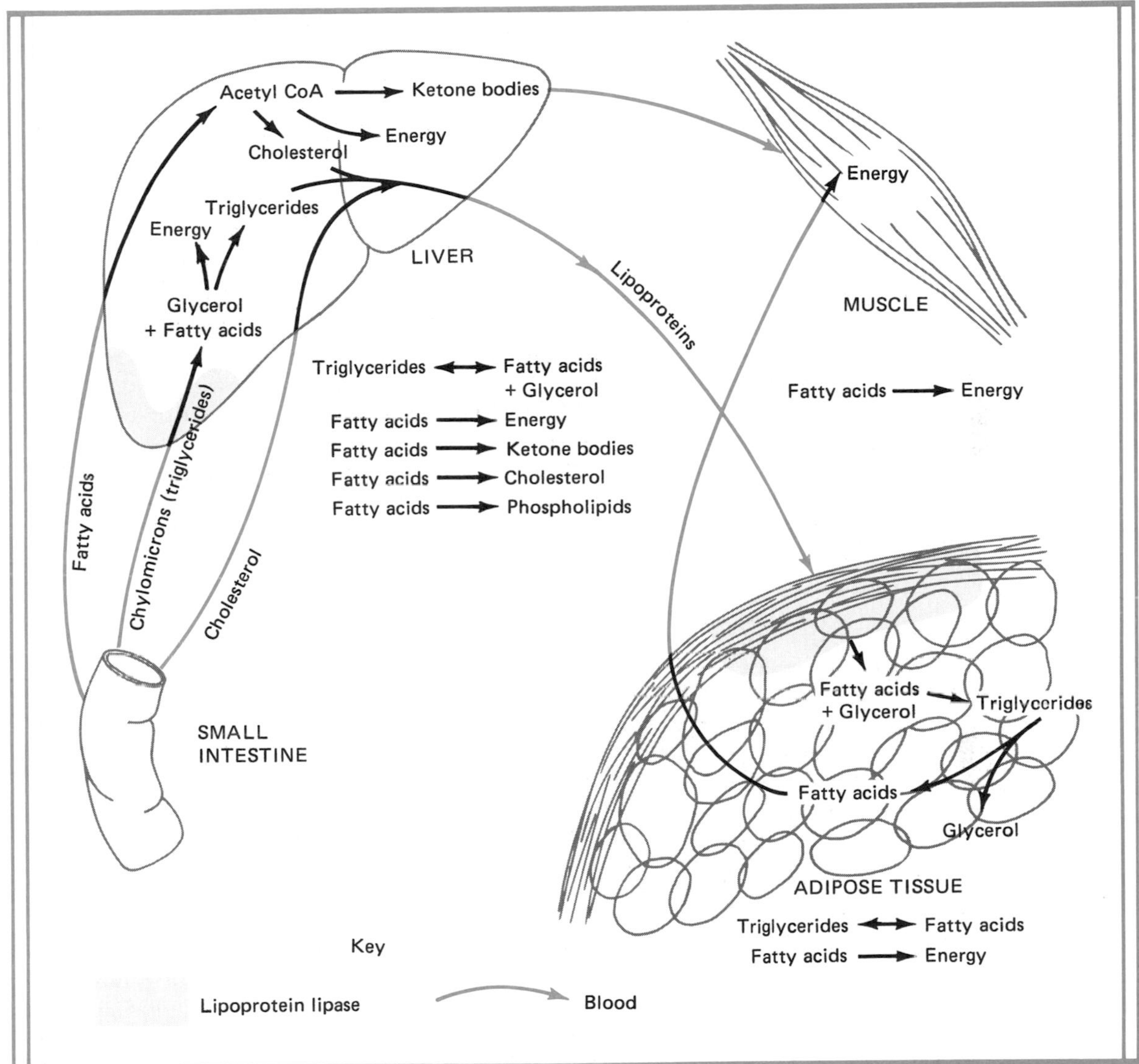

FIGURE 3-9
Interrelationships of Body Tissues in Lipid Metabolism

cholesterol levels, although the fate of the removed cholesterol is unclear. In addition, as components of phospholipid molecules, EFA constitutes an important part of all cell membranes. A major role for linoleic acid is its conversion to arachidonic acid (20:4), the first step in the formation of hormonelike compounds, the prostaglandins, which are derived from the 20-carbon fatty acid. Although their exact action is unclear, the prostaglandins apparently perform such diverse physiological functions as the stimulation of smooth-muscle contraction, the lowering of blood pressure, and, in conjunction with a variety of hormones, the regulation of intermediary metabolism (Pickles, 1969; Vergroesen, 1977; Mattson, 1976). Prostaglandins have been used therapeutically to induce uterine contractions and abortion and have been proposed for other clinical uses as well.

Functions of Fat in the Body

The importance of fat derives from its structural role as a component of cell membranes and its functional roles as a source of energy and a factor in the snythesis of cholesterol and its derivatives as well as of lipids, prostaglandins, and other body substances. In addition, body fat, in the form of adipose tissue, serves two other important needs. First, it acts as an insulator to help to maintain body temperature at an appropriate level by conserving heat when the external temperature is low. (The insulating effect of fat in persons with an overabundance of subcutaneous adipose tissue is well known and can present a problem in hot weather.) Second, fat deposits act as a protective cushion surrounding the kidneys, heart, and other vital organs.

Because of their important roles in the maintenance of health and well-being, dietary fats should not be avoided. They are necessary for many vital body functions, contribute energy, and add to the flavor and aroma of our foods, as well as to our feelings of satisfaction after dining.

DIETARY REQUIREMENTS FOR FATS

The Food and Nutrition Board has not established a Recommended Dietary Allowance for fat, but suggests that adequate lipid be ingested to provide the body with essential fatty acids and carriers of fat-soluble vitamins (Food and Nutrition Board, 1979). It has been estimated that ingesting between 15 and 25 grams of fat per day will normally meet this requirement. Studies with both animals and human subjects indicate that the necessary requirement for EFA is fulfilled when 1 to 2 percent of the total caloric intake is provided by linoleic acid (Hansen et al., 1963; Holman, 1964). A diet of 1,800 calories per day should provide 2 to 4 grams of linoleic acid. This is readily accomplished; many vegetable oils used in cooking and salad dressings are good sources of this essential nutrient. A single tablespoon of mayonnaise or any of several oils will more than meet the requirement of most people. (See Table 3-8).

TABLE 3-8
Sources of Linoleic Acid (EFA)

	Linoleic Acid g/tbsp
Safflower oil	10
Corn, soy, and cottonseed oil	6–8
Mayonnaise	6
Peanut oil	5
Margarine	1–5
Olive oil	1

FATS IN THE AMERICAN DIET

Average Daily Lipid Intake of Americans

Year	Total Fat g/day
1909–1913	125
1925–1929	135
1935–1939	133
1947–1949	141
1957–1959	143
1965	145
1970	157
1974	158
1976	159

Sources: Adapted from G. V. Mann, Diet-heart: End of an era, *New England Journal of Medicine* 279(12):644, 1977 (Table 3); and T. Brewster and M. Jacobson, *The Changing American Diet,* (Washington, D.C.. Center for Science in the Public Interest, 1978).

Since the beginning of this century, consumption of fats by Americans has been increasing. The nearly 30-percent rise in our national fat intake since 1910 is largely attributable to three categories: edible fats and oils, ice cream, and red meat. During this period, consumption of certain kinds of fats—cooking fats such as lard and shortening combined—remained about the same, while the consumption of butter and margarine combined actually declined, from 19.9 pounds per person per year in 1910, to 16.9 pounds in 1976 (see Figure 3-10).

Particularly notable are the sharp increases related to improved food technology and marketing. Edible fats are found in almost every supermarket aisle, bottled as cooking oil and salad dressing or hidden in such foods as "all natural" health cereals, frozen pizzas, and cake mixes. Thanks to refrigerated transport and commercial freezers, ice cream is available everywhere.

The increase in consumption of high-fat foods of animal origin such as meat results from economic prosperities. For reasons of status as well as taste more high-fat animal foods seem to be preferred over less-expensive high-carbohydrate, plant-origin foods. Fat consumption generally increases at a time of affluence, when there is more money to be spent on food (consumption of nearly all fats dipped somewhat in the Depression years; Americans ate only 38.6 pounds of beef per person in 1930). The economic situation has other effects as well: at a time of rising prices, people try to economize by substituting lower-price alternatives—vegetable margarine for butter, corn oil for olive oil, chicken for sirloin.

Our changing lifestyles are another result of increased individual and national affluence in the last few decades. The entry of more women into the work force and the greater mobility that removes many individuals from the

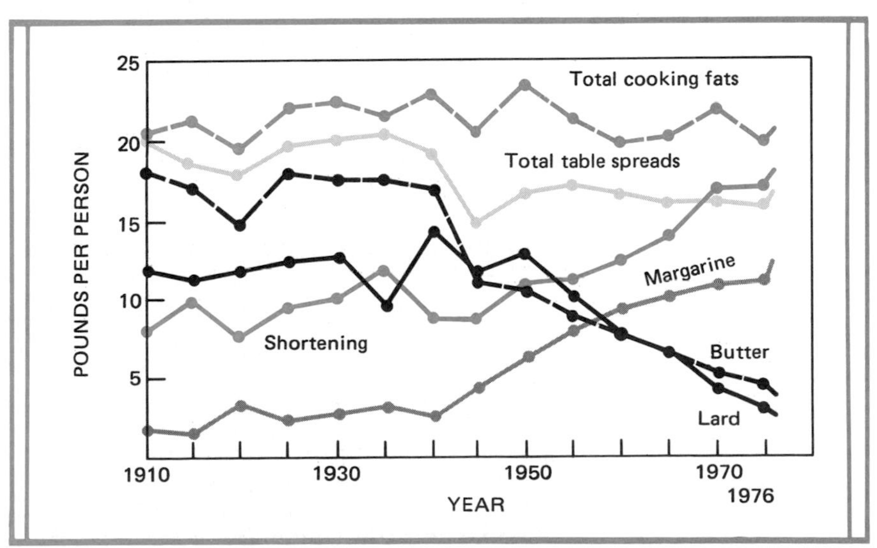

FIGURE 3-10

Consumption of cooking fats and table spreads, 1910–1976.

Source: T. Brewster, and M. Jacobson, *The changing American diet,* (Washington, D.C., Center for Science in the Public Interest, 1978).

family home and kitchen have resulted in greater dependence on convenience foods. The same factors, along with greater leisure and more frequent travel, account for our increasing reliance upon restaurant, including fast-food, meals. (Many convenience and fast foods are notably higher in fat content than similar foods prepared "from scratch," and their use is associated with decreased consumption of whole-grain and vegetable materials.)

Still other factors affect fat consumption. Cultural dietary patterns determine which fat is used within a people's cuisine and how much: Japanese foods are prepared with far less fat than are, for example, the foods of Mediterranean peoples. (National dietary patterns are, of course, directly related to the availability of certain food items, as well as to cultural preferences.)

One increase in fat consumption in the United States has occurred in the shift to vegetable fats for cooking and in salad dressings (shortening, margarine, corn oil), which accounted for only 16 percent of dietary fat intake in 1909 to 1913 but reached a high of 43 percent in 1976 (Brewster and Jacobson, 1978). Meanwhile, the use of animal fats (butter, lard) decreased slightly overall. This shift is partially related to the idea that vegetable fats are "better for you" than animal fats. Recently, fats have been assigned "good" reputations if they have a high proportion of PUFAs, and vegetable fats generally fall into this category. Exceptions are nuts and olives, which contain high levels of monounsaturated fatty acids rather than PUFAs. Also, many margarines have been partially hydrogenated for firmness and palatability, a process that lowers their PUFA content.

The public has been made aware of studies linking fat consumption to heart disease, some types of cancer, and obesity. Many authoritative sources, including the American Heart Association, recommend that the current American pattern of fat consumption should be altered. The Senate Select Committee on Nutrition and Human Needs has summarized the recommendations: total fat intake should be reduced from its present level of 42 percent of energy intake to 30 percent, and no more than 10 percent of total caloric intake should be derived from saturated fats, with the balance to be about evenly distributed between PUFAs and monounsaturates. Dietary cholesterol intake, it was suggested, should not exceed 300 milligrams daily (Select Committee, 1977). Many nutritionists believe, however, that this level is unrealistically and unnecessarily low.

The public responds, apparently, with great selectivity to such advice. Since the possible linkage between cholesterol and heart disease was first announced in the 1950s, consumption of eggs, including eggs used in processed foods such as mayonnaise and cake mixes, has dropped sharply, from a high of 403 per person in 1945 to a low of 276 per person in 1976. Similarly, consumption of butter, implicated because of its saturated fat content, also decreased in the same period, reaching an all-time low of 4.4 pounds per person in 1976 (Brewster and Jacobson, 1978). Beef consumption, however, continued to climb, and one might tentatively conclude that affluence and status considerations take precedence for most people over health needs.

Eggs on the market today contain from 252 to 274 milligrams of cholesterol. One laboratory analysis found that the eggs of Araucana chickens, which have been promoted as being lower in cholesterol, and even cholesterol-free, actually contained more cholesterol on a per weight basis than did commercial eggs (Peterson et al., 1978). Recent reports of experiments with chickens fed on a special feed supplement, however, indicate a reduction of about 30 percent in egg cholesterol (Sullivan, 1978); the resulting eggs have not yet been made commercially available. Similarly, the cholesterol content of meat is related to the type of meat, and not to whether it was organically produced.

It is not difficult to effect the dietary changes—reducing overall lipid intake and shifting to polyunsaturates—called for by the Senate Select Committee and the American Heart Association. Use of corn and safflower oils in salad dressings and cooking, substitution of margarine, especially highly unsaturated varieties, for butter in most cooking uses; broiling or baking instead of sautéing or deep frying; more frequent servings of vegetarian, poultry, and fish main courses; drinking skim instead of whole milk and eating ice milk in preference to ice cream—all are easily accomplished. It will not be as easy to convince all manufacturers to substitute unsaturated for saturated oils in processed foods. Nor will it be easy to achieve accurate labels stating the amount and kind of fat contained in a product . . . for those who wish to modify their fat intake, either to lose or maintain weight or as part of a preventive or therapeutic program to reduce serum cholesterol.

PERSPECTIVE ON
Diet and Heart Disease

Coronary heart disease (CHD) is the leading cause of death in affluent countries. Half of all deaths in the United States in 1977 were related to major cardiovascular disease, with heart attacks and strokes heading the list. [The next highest cause of death, all forms of cancer, was not even a close second, accounting for 20 percent of all fatalities (National Center for Health Statistics, 1978).] It is estimated that one out of every four American males between the ages of 40 and 65 will develop some form of heart disease (McGill and Mott, 1976). Until menopause, women are at substantially less risk than their male contemporaries; in later middle age, however, women are increasingly susceptible. This differential suggests some protective role for the female sex hormones. Epidemiological studies showing that CHD is less prevalent in some cultures than in the contemporary United States has led to considerable hypothesizing regarding the role of environmental factors in general and diet in particular. Despite extensive research, however, the entire subject remains controversial, with relationships strongly suggested but not definitively proved.

Atherosclerosis, the disease process that leads ultimately to CHD, develops from the accumulation of fatty deposits, primarily plaques of cholesterol and its esters in the inner walls of the arteries, probably beginning early in life. As fat deposits increase, they become surrounded by the growth of smooth muscle and connective tissue (fibrous plaques and other lesions). In this process (popularly called hardening of the arteries), the arterial passages become narrowed, interfering with effficiency of circulation and putting great stress upon the heart, which must work harder in order to accomplish less. In severe cases, the arterial lumen can suddenly close (occlude), resulting in a sharp decrease in blood circulation to tissues (ischemia), which directly causes the heart or the brain to cease functioning (Strong et al., 1973). The clinical names for these events are myocardial infarction, when heart vessels are affected, and stroke (or cerebrovascular accident), when the brain is involved.

Fatty streaks have been observed in the walls of the aorta, or main artery, of very young children, and these fat deposits become increasingly frequent and extensive in the second and third decades of life. This is true for people everywhere. Fatty streaks, however, do not necessarily progress to the more complicated lesion stage. Fatty streaks tend to develop into lesions in distinctive popula-

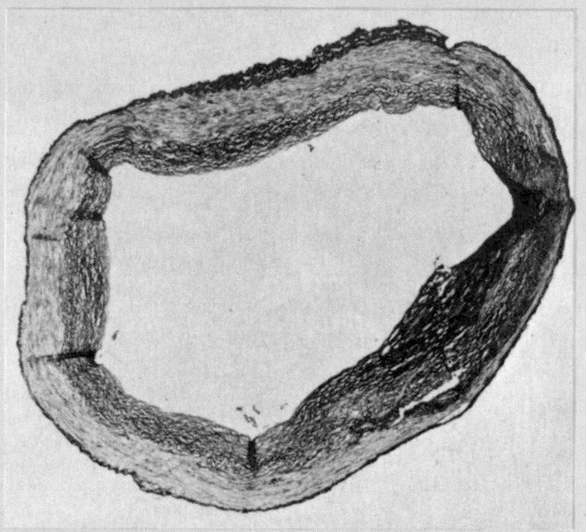

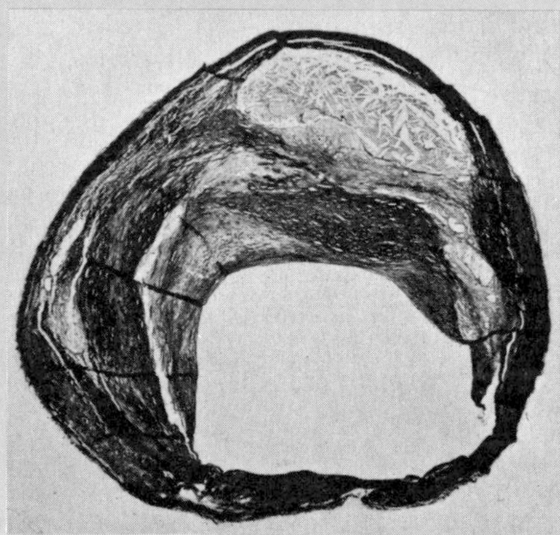

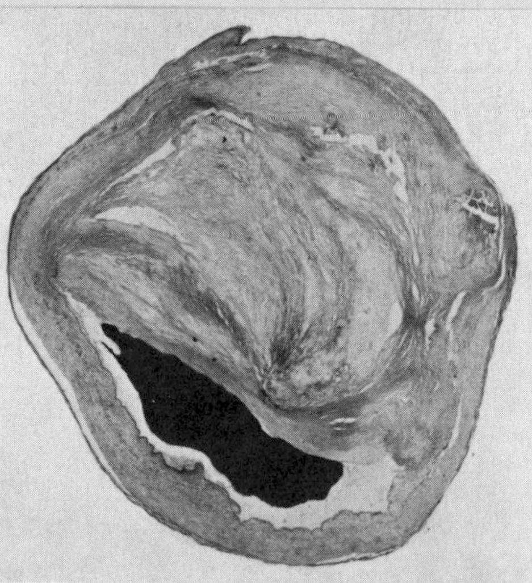

Three stages in the development of atherosclerotic deposits: ***Top***, cross section of a normal coronary artery. ***Center***, deposits form in inner lining and begin to harden. ***Bottom***, arterial channel is narrowed and blocked by a blood clot. (American Heart Association)

tion patterns that correlate with the incidence of CHD. Lesions are formed earlier and are more extensive, for example, in urban, industrialized societies than among such peoples as rural Mexicans and Guatemalans or nonurbanized Africans.

Recognizable symptoms of CHD were described as far back as the eighteenth century and perhaps even earlier. Early in this century, work with experimental animals resulted in observations that rabbits fed a pure cholesterol diet developed arterial lesions resembling human atherosclerosis (McGill and Mott, 1976). Although a relationship between diet and heart disease continued to be suspected and supported by occasional animal or epidemiological studies, the role of diet in the etiology of CHD remained for many years an untested hypothesis.

In 1949 the U.S. Public Health Service began a large-scale study, the Epidemiologic Investigation of Cardiovascular Diseases in Framingham, Massachusetts. More than 5,000 healthy men and women aged 30 to 62 were examined every other year for evidence of CHD and other atherosclerotic conditions. Living habits as well as medical findings prior to the study and in the more than 30 years since it began have been analyzed. Among the results to date of the Framingham Study was the identification of a number of risk factors clearly associated with the development of CHD. A risk factor increases the probability of an event but does not imply or predict that the event will occur. For example, it was found that men who were overweight had a significantly higher incidence of CHD; those whose lifestyles included extensive physical activity had a lower incidence of CHD. Elevated levels of serum cholesterol were found consistently in association with other high-risk factors.

Dietary Factors in CHD The Framingham Study indicated that persons with serum cholesterol levels in excess of 225 mg/dl are at risk of developing CHD and that at higher levels, the risk increases markedly. The blood content of this lipid is derived both from endogenous and exogenous sources. Typically, Americans ingest from 600 to 900 mg of cholesterol per day. It has been shown that there will be a predictable elevation of serum cholesterol levels if the dietary intake of cholesterol is increased from 0 to 400 mg, but cholesterol intakes in larger amounts raise serum cholesterol levels higher in some individuals than in others (McGill and Mott, 1976). These studies seem to indicate the importance of factors other than dietary intake in determining serum cholesterol levels. The Framingham Study corroborates this. It was found, for example, that men's serum cholesterol increased sharply with weight gains of 7 percent or more (Kannel, 1971).

It is now believed by most researchers that the high dietary cholesterol intake of most Westernized peoples is directly related both to high serum cholesterol levels and to high CHD rates. There are, however, enough exceptions to the high-intake, high-serum level rule to generate controversy. Among some African groups, for example, the diet of meat and milk is as cholesterol-rich as that of any American, yet these people have virtually no CHD. Possible explanations include a high-fiber diet, much more physical activity than most Americans experience, and a genetic factor (McGill and Mott, 1976; Mann, 1977).

To achieve even a slight decrease in serum levels, dietary cholesterol must be sharply reduced. The National Diet-Heart Study of 1960 found that, after a year, men who were put on low-cholesterol diets of 350 to 450 mg per day and who increased the ratio of PUFA to saturated fats in their diets (ratio of 1.5–2.0) had reduced serum cholesterol levels by an average of 11 percent, to "safe" levels slightly over 200 mg/dl. A control group put on a diet resembling the "typical" American fare (650–750 mg cholesterol, PUFA to saturated fat ratio 0.4), experienced a 4-percent reduction in serum cholesterol levels, suggesting that their prestudy intake had been much higher (National Diet-Heart Study Research Group, 1968).

Serum cholesterol levels seem to be sensitive, however, not only to cholesterol intake but to other components of lipid intake and metabolism as well. Saturated fat raises the level of plasma cholesterol; monounsaturated fat has no significant effect; and PUFA actually lowers blood cholesterol levels. When serum cholesterol is lowered by PUFAs, we do not always know whether the excess cholesterol has been excreted from the body or has shifted from the blood into tissues. There is some evidence that increasing PUFA intake may have some potentially negative effects as well (Reiser et al., 1959; Melchior et al., 1974). The mechanisms for all of these observations have not yet been fully explained and must be studied further.

Lipid intake is not the only dietary factor that may have an impact on CHD. There is some evidence that high dietary fiber intakes are associated with lower rates of CHD. It is postulated that dietary fiber lowers serum cholesterol levels by increasing the excretion of bile acids, which are products of cholesterol metabolism, and by generally reducing the time in which cholesterol and other substances are in transit in the digestive tract, thereby decreasing the amount absorbed by the body.

Other nutrients may also have an effect on the development of CHD. Mineral imbalances, especially of copper, have been implicated. A number of studies suggest that reductions in animal protein intake with the substitution of vegetable protein result in lower serum cholesterol (Carroll, 1978). Sucrose has also been held to be a risk factor, and Yudkin (1969) claims that sucrose is more responsible for atherosclerosis than is animal fat. It has been suggested that sucrose, by raising the level of triglycerides in the blood, increases serum cholesterol and, consequently, the likelihood of developing CHD. This mechanism, however, apparently occurs in only a small fraction of the population. For these individuals, restriction of sucrose may be warranted. Hypertriglyceridemia (elevated serum triglycerides) by itself, however, is not a strong risk factor for CHD.

Recent studies suggest that the form in which cholesterol is carried in the blood may influence the appearance of CHD. It has been observed that the level of cholesterol carried by HDLs (as opposed to the other lipoproteins; see Table 3-6) is inversely related to the prevalence of CHD. Nonsmokers, people who are physically fit, and those who are not obese appear to have more HDL cholesterol than do smokers, the obese, and inactive people (Truswell, 1978). Clearly, additional research is needed to answer the many dietary questions raised by these findings.

Other Factors in CHD Etiology Nondiet factors that have been associated with CHD include genetic predisposition; hypertension; such aspects of lifestyle as cigarette smoking, stress, and lack of exercise; the use of oral contraceptives; diabetes; obesity; and psychological factors.

Most cases of hypertension or high blood pressure

have no specifically known cause, although heredity and obesity apparently predispose people to it. Elevated blood pressure is easily diagnosed and responds readily to treatment. Persons who are aware of being genetically predisposed and those in whom hypertension has been diagnosed should certainly decrease consumption of salt; those who are overweight would be well advised to reduce their weight and their salt intake (these aspects of hypertension control will be discussed further in Chapters 5 and 8).

It has been suggested that there is a strong psychological component in the origin of hypertension and of CHD. In particular, persons who exhibit "type A" behavior patterns—competitive, overachieving, always-on-the-go types—are said to be more prone to heart attacks, the calmer "type B" personality being less so. The evidence is not at all clear, however; and this must be ranked as a hypothesis, not yet proved. The role of stress is often cited by those who claim that it, no less than a diet high in animal fat, characterizes Western civilization but is lacking in the lives of nonurbanized peoples. Others claim that not stress itself, but our pattern of reacting to it, is the real culprit. A review of the evidence for psychological and social factors influencing the onset of coronary heart disease can be found in Jenkins (1976).

Another lifestyle factor often cited in CHD is the sedentary life led by most Americans in contrast to the greater physical activity required of people in simpler societies. The Framingham results indicate that men who are least active physically have three times the risk of developing CHD as those who are most active (Kannel, 1971). Low levels of physical activity have certainly been shown to be concomitants of high serum cholesterol and of CHD, but the effects of exercise and physical activity may operate in a number of ways. First of all, those who are physically active are not likely to be obese. Second, there is evidence that the preventive effect of exercise comes from its stimulation of the circulatory mechanism—the heart and lungs operate, it is claimed, more efficiently in a well-exercised body. There is no indication that exercise alone reduces serum cholesterol, however.

Cigarette smoking is clearly associated with increased risk of CHD in all forms for both men and women. Smoking, moreover, has a synergistic effect, multiplying the influence of any other risk factor present. With only one other risk factor, smoking one pack of cigarettes per day nearly doubles the risk for men; with two or more other risk factors present, cigarette smoking increases the risk by almost a third (Kannel, 1971). The combinations of smoking and hypertension, or smoking and oral contraceptive use for women, are particularly dangerous; all of these risks can, however, be readily controlled. Coffee and moderate alcohol drinking, both often indicted, have been found to have no significant effect.

The Diet-Cholesterol Controversy Of all possible factors in the onset of CHD, the relationship of dietary cholesterol to serum cholesterol has most captured public attention. Sensing a sizable market, the food industry has developed cholesterol-free egg substitutes, as well as other no-cholesterol, low-saturated-fat products, such as cream and sausage substitutes, for example. The egg substitute largely contains egg white, corn oil, nonfat dry milk, emulsifiers, vitamins, and artificial color, simulating the characteristics of egg yolk without its cholesterol content. Consumer acceptance has so far been low, and may reflect the higher cost of such products, the lack of information about their value, or simply a preference for the natural product (Ostrander et al., 1977).

Whether or not diet can have a significant effect on serum cholesterol and whether or not a change in serum levels can affect CHD incidence and mortality are highly controversial issues.

Kannel (1978) addresses the first part of the question when he says, "Given the same overconsumption of saturated fat, cholesterol and energy, there is a fairly wide range of serum cholesterol values in the United States." Mann (1977) charges that modification of diets because of public concern about cholesterol has not substantially reduced serum levels.

Hundreds of studies have been carried out to demonstrate the effects of modifying lipid intake. Often cited is a study of vegetarians whose levels of serum cholesterol and triglycerides were lower than those of control subjects (Sacks et al., 1975). Cholesterol intake in itself was not measured in this study, and reduced animal fat consumption was only one of several possible factors in the lower serum cholesterol levels. Others included lower total energy consumption, recent weight loss, and higher intake of vegetable protein, complex carbohydrate, and dietary fiber, which have all been advocated as cholesterol-lowering agents.

Mann (1977), among others, cites studies showing a lack of relationship between dietary and serum cholesterol. He shows that the Framingham data indicated that serum cholesterol levels were about the same in individuals with greater than the median cholesterol intake and in individuals with lower than median intake. In Mann's opinion, high levels of serum cholesterol are due to an impairment in the mechanism for converting cholesterol to bile acids.

In a recent survey, more than 200 atherosclerosis researchers agreed overwhelmingly that there was indeed a connection between diet and CHD and that present knowledge is sufficient to recommend dietary changes for the population in general (Norum, 1978).

While some studies have apparently demonstrated that serum cholesterol can be controlled by dietary and pharmacological means, the more important question is whether dietary modification to reduce cholesterol in the blood actually decreases the incidence of heart disease. Such studies are under way. Walker (1977), for example, has noted a sharp decline in CHD mortality dating from 1964 and correlates it with a decrease in per capita consumption of tobacco, animal fat, eggs, and dairy products. While noting other contributing factors, Walker emphasizes that "reduced smoking and change in diet seemed to turn the tide and reverse the trend in coronary mortality." Decreased mortality, while suggestive, is not the same as decreased rate of heart disease and may reflect such factors as improved emergency and surgical procedures.

Determining the precise role of cholesterol in CHD is obviously complex. A study of the Tarahumara Indians of Mexico points up the dilemma. This population group has a low incidence of CHD. They have very low serum cholesterol levels, and moderate triglyceride levels. Their diet is low in cholesterol, low in total fat, and low in saturated fat (the ratio of polyunsaturated to saturated fats, is greater than 2). The Tarahumara also have low sugar intake, high fiber intake, and high vegetable-protein intake. They are in exceptionally good physical condition, have virtually no obesity, have low blood pressure, and are genetically fairly homogeneous (Conner et al., 1978).

The Tarahumara then, add little that is new to the diet-heart controversy, since no single dietary (or other) factor can be isolated to account for their low rate of CHD. In fact, this example serves to emphasize the multiplicity of factors that are involved in the etiology of atherosclerosis and heart disease.

Recommendations What, then, should we do? Despite all the uncertainties, it would probably be advisable to attempt to reduce or eliminate as many risk factors as possible from our lives. (Factors such as age, sex, and heredity are, of course, beyond our control!)

Total fat intake should be decreased to between 30 and 35 percent of total energy intake. Overweight individuals should achieve desirable weight. The ratio of PUFAs to saturated fats in our diets should be increased to approximately 1.5 to 2.0. The table shows the PUFA-to-saturated fat ratio of selected foods. We should also, particularly if there is a family history of hypertension, reduce our intake of sodium, especially table salt. We should try to change our patterns of reaction to stress, through relaxation and other techniques. It would be prudent also to increase physical exercise in moderation, to ingest more dietary fiber, and to stop smoking. Moderation, but not fanaticism, is probably the best answer.

RATIO OF POLYUNSATURATED TO SATURATED FATTY ACIDS (P/S) OF VARIOUS FOODS

Group A: P/S more than 2.5	
Almonds	Safflower oil
Corn oil	Sesame oil
Cottonseed oil	Soybean oil
Linseed oil	Sunflower oil
Margarine, soft	Walnuts
Mayonnaise	
Group B: P/S 1.5–2.5	
Chicken breast	Fish (freshwater)
Chicken skin	Margarines, semisolid
Chicken thigh	Peanut oil
Chicken fat (?)	
Group C: P/S 0.5–1.5	
Beef, heart and liver	Hydrogenated or hardened vegetable oils
Chicken heart	Peanut butter
Fish (saltwater)	Pecans
	Margarines, solid
Group D: P/S 0.1–0.5	
Chicken liver	Olive oil
Lard	Pork, all cuts
Group E: P/S less than 0.1	
Beef, both lean and fat	Egg yolk
Butter	Milk and milk products
Coconut oil	Mutton, both lean and fat

A. K. Katchadurian: Hyperlipoproteinemia, Dietetic Currents 4(4):19, 1977 (Table 1).

Our expectations of results from such measures should not be unrealistic. Even a reduction in dietary cholesterol that succeeds in decreasing serum cholesterol is no guarantee against the development of a stroke or heart attack. Because heart disease usually develops in the later years of life, it is possible that, no matter how many adjustments in living and eating habits are made, the predisposition to CHD is determined by factors of earlier years. A good prospective study is needed to answer such questions, and it will be many years before we have the answers.

Since the groundwork for CHD may well be laid early in life, dietary modifications may be useful in protecting the very young—less beef and more fish and poultry, skim instead of whole milk, occasional instead of daily egg consumption—all may help to reduce the development of fatty streaks in young arteries, and result in fewer deposits of plaques and lesions, as well as lowered serum cholesterol levels throughout life. In families where there is a high risk of CHD, the American Heart Association recommends that children be examined early and regularly for hyperlipidemia (*Journal of the American Dietetic Association*, 1978). During the growing years especially, physical exercise and weight control should be stressed.

To make such changes in eating habits, it is necessary to know the nutrient content of the foods we buy and eat. Some manufacturers are now labeling their products to indicate the amount and kinds of fat per serving; some list cholesterol, saturated fat, and PUFA content. But even where detailed nutritional labeling is absent, a conscientious consumer can learn how to be adequately informed. Because ingredients must be listed in descending order of their content in the product, labels listing liquid corn oil, for example, as a first ingredient will be relatively high in polyunsaturates, while "partially hydrogenated soybean oil" indicates less PUFA content, and coconut oil, of course, is largely saturated.

Other sources of information include the American Heart Association, which has branches in major cities across the country and offers data relating to the fat content of various foods, as well as specific suggestions for modifying dietary fat intake. Nutritionists in community health clinics can also provide information. Many food companies have consumer relations departments that will provide information about specific products as well.

In view of present knowledge there is certainly no disadvantage to following the dietary recommendations (although there remain questions about how effective such changes in food habits actually are in preventing heart disease), and there may be important advantages.

SUMMARY

The most controversial of the major nutrients, lipids have important body functions which are often overlooked. American consumption of fats has increased by more than a third since the beginning of the century, and 42 percent of daily caloric intake, on the average, is derived from fats.

At the molecular level, lipids consist of carbon, hydrogen, and oxygen in proportions that differ from those of other nutrients. Some lipids also contain nitrogen and phosphorous. Lipid molecules are relatively insoluble in water and can be dissolved only in organic solvents. Some dietary lipids (fats) are solid at room temperatures and some are liquid (oils). A useful classification of lipids depends on their proportion in the human body. Major constituents include fatty acids, several fatty acid derivatives, and sterols and sterol derivatives. Minor constituents include the fat-soluble vitamins A, D, E, and K, and the hormonelike prostaglandins.

The basic structural unit of most lipid molecules is a fatty acid, a chain of hydrocarbons with an acid (carboxyl) group at one end. In a saturated fatty acid, every carbon atom is joined by a single electrochemical bond to each of two hydrogen and two other carbon atoms. In unsaturated fatty acids, some carbon atoms are joined to only one hydrogen atom, and by a double bond to one adjacent carbon atom. A fatty acid with one double bond is monounsaturated; with two or more, it is polyunsaturated.

Triglycerides are an important fatty acid derivative, formed by a reaction between the carboxyl groups of three fatty acids and the three alcohol (—OH) groups of glycerol. Phospholipids are formed in the same way, except that a phosphate-containing group becomes attached to one of the three alcohol groups; lecithin is an important phospholipid.

Sterols, of which cholesterol is the most important, are fat-soluble alcohols. Although high levels of cholesterol in the blood serum have been implicated in the etiology of atherosclerosis and coronary heart disease, cholesterol is an important body substance, which is created by the body daily.

The body's sources of fat are both exogenous (dietary) and endogenous (synthesized within the body), and the supply is often far in excess of need. Of all lipids, only linoleic acid cannot be synthesized; when it is not supplied in the diet, deficiency symptoms occur. For this reason linoleic acid is an essential fatty acid (EFA), necessary for growth and health.

Among the functions of dietary fat are its contribution to the palatability of food, and to our feelings of satiety for several hours after we have eaten. The primary function of fat, however, is to provide a concentrated source of energy. In addition, fat makes possible the transport and utilization of the fat-soluble vitamins.

Virtually all lipid digestion and absorption takes place in the small intestine. Most digested lipid enters the lymphatic and subsequently the blood circulation and ultimately goes to the liver, which uses each lipid for a different process and prepares the excess for storage in adipose tissue.

The various kinds of fats are transported in the body by one or another of the four lipoproteins. Lipids become attached to emulsifiers, molecules with water-soluble and lipid-soluble components, which enable them to mix with body fluids. Bile, produced by the liver and stored in the gall bladder, is a key emulsifier, necessary for lipid digestion.

High concentrations of cholesterol in the blood have been found in association with coronary heart disease. The precise relationship between dietary fat and the development of CHD is still not clear and has generated a great deal of controversy.

At present there is sufficient evidence to warrant a modified dietary approach in the management and prevention of CHD processes. But diet alone is not the complete answer. Many risk factors have been linked to CHD. General recommendations include an end to smoking, reduction of stress, weight loss, higher fiber intake, and more exercise, in addition to lower cholesterol and higher polyunsaturated fat intake. Americans have been urged to reduce fat consumption to about 30 percent of daily energy intake.

BIBLIOGRAPHY

BREWSTER, L., AND M. F. JACOBSON. *The changing American diet.* Washington, D.C.: Center for Science in the Public Interest, 1978.

BURR G. O. AND M. M. BURR. A new deficiency disease produced by the rigid exclusion of fats from the diet. *Journal of Biological Chemistry* 82:345, 1929.

CALDWELL, M., H. T. JONSSON, AND H. B. OTHERSEN, JR. Essential fatty acid deficiency in an infant receiving prolonged parenteral alimentation. *Journal of Pediatrics* 81:894, 1972.

CARROLL, K. K. Dietary protein in relation to plasma cholesterol levels and atherosclerosis. *Nutrition Reviews* 36(1):1, 1978.

CONNER, W. E., M. T. CERQUEIRA, R. W. CONNER, R. B. WALLACE, M. R. MALINOW, AND H. R. CASDORPH. The plasma lipids, lipoproteins, and the diet of the Tarahumara Indians of Mexico. *American Journal of Clinical Nutrition* 31:1131, 1978.

EXLER, J., AND J. L. WEIHRAUCH. Comprehensive evaluation of fatty acids in foods. XII. Shellfish. *Journal of the American Dietetic Association* 71:518, 1977.

FOOD AND NUTRITION BOARD, NATIONAL ACADEMY OF SCIENCES. *Recommended dietary allowances,* 9th ed. Washington, D.C.: National Academy of Science, 1979.

HANSEN, A. E., H. F. WIESE, A. N. BOELSCHE, M. E. HAGGARD, D. J. D. ADAM, AND H. DAVIS. Role of linoleic acid in infant feeding: Clinical and chemical study of 428 infants fed on milk mixtures varying in kind and amount of fat. *Pediatrics* 31 (supplement), 1963.

HANSEN, A. E., M. E. HAGGARD, A. E. BOELSCHE, D. ADAM, AND H. F. WIESE. Essential fatty acid in infant nutrition, clinical manifestations of linoleic acid deficiency. *Journal of Nutrition* 66:565, 1958.

HOLMAN, R. T., W. O. CASTER, AND H. F. WIESE. The essential fatty acid requirement of infants and the assessment of their dietary intake of linoleate by serum fatty acid analysis. *American Journal of Clinical Nutrition* 14:70, 1964.

JENKINS, C. D. Recent evidence supporting psychologic and social risk factors of coronary disease. *New England Journal of Medicine* 294:987, 1033, 1976.

JOHNSTON, J. M. Mechanics of fat absorption. *Handbook of physiology,* vol 3. Washington, D.C.: American Physiological Society, 1968.

Journal of the American Dietetic Association. Diet for children with hypolipidemia—A.H.A. recommendation. Vol. 72:394, 1978.

KANNEL, W. B. Status of coronary heart disease risk factors. *Journal of Nutrition Education* 10(1):10, 1978.

KANNEL, W. B. The disease of living. *Nutrition Today* 6(3):2, 1971.

MANN, G. V. Diet-heart: End of an era. *New England Journal of Medicine* 297:644, 1977.

MATTSON, F. H. Fats. In *Present knowledge in nutrition,* 4th ed., ed. D. M. Hegsted: Washington, D.C.: Nutrition Foundation, Inc., 1976.

MCGILL, H. C., AND G. E. MOTT. Diet and coronary heart disease. In *Present knowledge in nutrition,* 4th ed., ed. D. M. Hegsted. Washington, D.C.: Nutrition Foundation, Inc., 1976.

MELCHIOR, G. W., H. B. LOFLAND, AND D. C. JONES. Influence of dietary fat on cholelithiasis in squirrel monkeys. *Federation Proceedings* 33:626, 1974.

NATIONAL CENTER FOR HEALTH STATISTICS. *Monthly Vital Statistics Report* 27(1), 1978.

NATIONAL DIET-HEART STUDY RESEARCH GROUP. *National diet-heart study final report. Circulation* 37 (Supplement 1): 1-419, 1968.

NORUM, K. R. Some present concepts concerning diet and prevention of coronary heart disease. *Nutrition Reviews* 36:194, 1978.

OSTRANDER, J., C. MARTINSEN, J. MCCULLOUGH, AND M. CHILDS. Egg substitutes: Use and preference—with and without nutritional information. *Journal of the American Dietetic Association* 70:267, 1977.

PETERSON, D. W., A. LILYBLADE, C. K. CLIFFORD, R. ERNST, A. J. CLIFFORD, AND P. DUNN. Composition of and cholesterol in Araucana and commercial eggs. *Journal of the American Dietetic Association* 72:45, 1978.

PICKLES, V. S. Prostaglandins. *Nature* 224:221, 1969.

REISER, R., M. F. SORRELS, AND M. C. WILLIAMS. Influence of high levels of dietary fats and cholesterol on atherosclerosis and lipid distribution in swine. *Circulation Research* 7:833, 1959.

SACKS, F. M., W. P. CASTELLI, A. DONNER, AND E. H. KASS. Plasma lipids and lipoproteins in vegetarians and controls. *New England Journal of Medicine* 292:1148, 1975.

SELECT COMMITTEE ON NUTRITION AND HUMAN NEEDS, U.S. Senate. *Dietary goals for the United States,* 2nd ed. Washington, D.C.: U.S. Government Printing Office, 1977.

STRONG, J. P. Pathology and epidemiology of atherosclerosis. *Journal of the American Dietetic Association* 62:262, 1973.

SULLIVAN, J. F. Hen's feed reduces cholesterol in eggs. *The New York Times,* December 26, 1978. p. C3.

TRUSWELL, A. S. Diet and plasma lipids: A reappraisal. *American Journal of Clinical Nutrition* 31:977, 1978.

VERGROESEN, A. J. Physiological effects of dietary linoleic acid. *Nutrition Reviews* 35:1, 1977.

WALKER, W. J. Changing United States life-style and declining vascular mortality: Cause or coincidence? *New England Journal of Medicine* 297:163, 1977.

WENE, J. D., W. E. CONNER, AND L. DENBESTEN. The development of essential fatty acid deficiency in healthy men fed fat-free diets intravenously and orally. *Journal of Clinical Investigation* 56:127, 1975.

WIDDOWSON, E. M., M. J. DAUNCEY, D. M. T. GAIRDNER, J. H. JONXIS, AND M. PELIKAN-FILIPOVA. Body fat of British and Dutch infants. *British Medical Journal* 1:653, 1975.

YUDKIN, J. Sucrose and heart disease. *Nutrition Today* 4(1):16, 1969.

SUGGESTED ADDITIONAL READING

ANDERSON, B. A. Comprehensive evaluation of fatty acids in foods. 7. Pork products. *Journal of the American Dietetic Association* 69:44, 1976.

ANDERSON, B. A., J. E. KINSELLA, AND B. K. WATT. Comprehensive evaluation of fatty acids in foods. 2. Beef products. *Journal of the American Dietetic Association* 67:35, 1975.

ANDERSON, B. A., G. A. FRISTROM, AND J. L. WEIHRAUCH. Comprehensive evaluation of fatty acids in foods. 10. Lamb and veal. *Journal of the American Dietetic Association* 70:53, 1977.

Dairy Council Digest. Biological effects of polyunsaturated fatty acids. Vol. 46(6):32, 1975.

BEARE-ROGERS, J. L., L. M. GRAY, AND R. HOLLYWOOD. The linoleic acid and *trans* fatty acids of margarines. *American Journal of Clinical Nutrition.* 32:1805, 1979.

BRIGNOLI, C. A., J. E. KINSELLA, AND J. L. WEIHRAUCH. Comprehensive evaluation of fatty acids in foods. 5. Unhydrogenated fats and oils. *Journal of the American Dietetic Association* 68:224, 1976.

EXLER, J., AND J. L. WEIHRAUCH. Comprehensive evaluation of fatty acids in foods. 8. Finfish. *Journal of the American Dietetic Association* 69:243, 1976.

EXLER, J., R. M. AVENA, AND J. L WEIHRAUCH. Comprehensive evaluation of fatty acids in foods. 11. Leguminous seeds. *Journal of the American Dietetic Association* 71:412, 1977.

FEELEY, R. M., P. E. CRINER, AND B. K. WATT. Cholesterol content of foods. *Journal of the American Dietetic Association* 61(2):134, 1972.

Flemine, C. R., L. M. Smith, and R. E. Hodges. Essential fatty acid deficiency in adults receiving parenteral nutrition. *American Journal of Clinical Nutrition.* 29:976, 1976.

Flynn, M. A. The cholesterol controversy. *Contemporary Nutrition* 3(3), 1978.

Fristrom, G. A., and J. L. Weihrauch. Comprehensive evaluation of fatty acids in foods. 9. Fowl. *Journal of the American Dietetic Association* 69:517, 1976.

Fristrom, G. A., B. C. Stewart, J. L. Weihrauch, and L. P. Posati. Comprehensive evaluation of fatty acids in foods. 4. Nuts, peanuts, and soups. *Journal of the American Dietetic Association* 67:351, 1975.

Glueck, C. J., F. Mattson, and E. L. Bierman. Diet and coronary heart disease: Another view. *New England Journal of Medicine* 298(26):1471, 1978.

Greenberger, N. J., and T. G. Stillman. Medium-chained triglycerides. *New England Journal of Medicine* 280(19):1045, 1969.

Hausman, P. Fatty encounters of the worst kind. *Nutrition Action* 5(2):8, 1978.

Hennekens, C. H., M. E. Drolette, M. J. Jesse, J. E. Davies, and G. B. Hutchison. Coffee drinking and death due to coronary heart disease. *New England Journal of Medicine* 294:633, 1976.

Herrick, J. B. Clinical features of sudden obstruction of the coronary arteries. *Journal of the American Medical Association* 59:2015, 1912.

Hill, P., and E. L. Wynder. Dietary regulation of serum lipids in healthy, young adults. *Journal of the American Dietetic Association* 68:25, 1976.

Klevay, L. M. Coronary heart disease—The zinc/copper hypothesis. *American Journal of Clinical Nutrition* 28:764, 1975.

McCollum, E. V. *A history of nutrition.* Chapter 3. Boston: Houghton Mifflin Company, 1957.

Nichols, A. B., C. Rarencroft, and D. E. Lamphiear. Daily nutritional intake and serum lipid levels: The Tecumseh study. *American Journal of Clinical Nutrition* 29:1384, 1976.

Nutrition Reviews. Long-term effects of diets prescribed in coronary prevention programs. Vol. 35: 140, 1978.

Nutrition Reviews. Prevention of coronary heart disease. Vol. 34:220, 1976.

Nutrition Reviews. Composition of human fat from different sites. 30(40), 1972.

Paulsrud, J. R., L. Pensler, C. F. Whitten, S. Stewart, and R. T. Holman. Essential fatty acid deficiency in infants induced by fat-free intravenous feedings. *American Journal of Clinical Nutrition* 25:897, 1972.

Porter, M., W. Yamarake, S. Carlson, and M. Flynn. Effects of dietary egg on serum cholesterol and triglyceride of human males. *American Journal of Clinical Nutrition* 30:490, 1977.

Posati, L. P., J. E. Kinsella, and B. K. Watt. Comprehensive evaluation of fatty acids in foods. 1. Dairy products. *Journal of the American Dietetic Association* 66:482, 1975.

Posati, L. P., J. E. Kinsella, and B. K. Watt. Comprehensive evaluation of fatty acids in foods. 3. Eggs and egg products. *Journal of the American Dietetic Association* 67:111, 1975.

Potter, M. J., and J. P. Nestel. The effects of dietary fatty acids and cholesterol on the milk lipids of lactating women and the plasma cholesterol of breast fed infants. *American Journal of Clinical Nutrition* 29:54, 1976.

Pratt, D. E. Lipid analysis of a frozen egg substitute. *Journal of the American Dietetics Association* 66(1):31, 1975.

Reiser, R. The three weak links in the diet-heart disease connection. Nutrition Today. 14 (4):22, 1979.

Ross, R., and J. A. Glomset. Pathogenesis of atherosclerosis. *New England Journal of Medicine* 295:369, 1976.

Shorey, R., L. Brewton, R. D. Sewell, and M. O'Brien. Alterations of lipids in a group of free-living adult males. *American Journal of Clinical Nutrition* 27:268, 1974.

Shurtleff, D. Some characteristics related to the incidence of cardiovascular disease and death: The Framingham study, 18-year followup. Washington, D.C.: U.S. Department of Health, Education and Welfare, National Institutes of Health, Framingham study, section no. 30, DHEW publication no. (NIH) 74-599, 1974.

Weihrauch, J. L., J. E. Kinsella, and B. K. Watt. Comprehensive evaluation of fatty acids in foods. 6. Cereal products. *Journal of the American Dietetic Association* 68:335, 1976.

Chapter 4

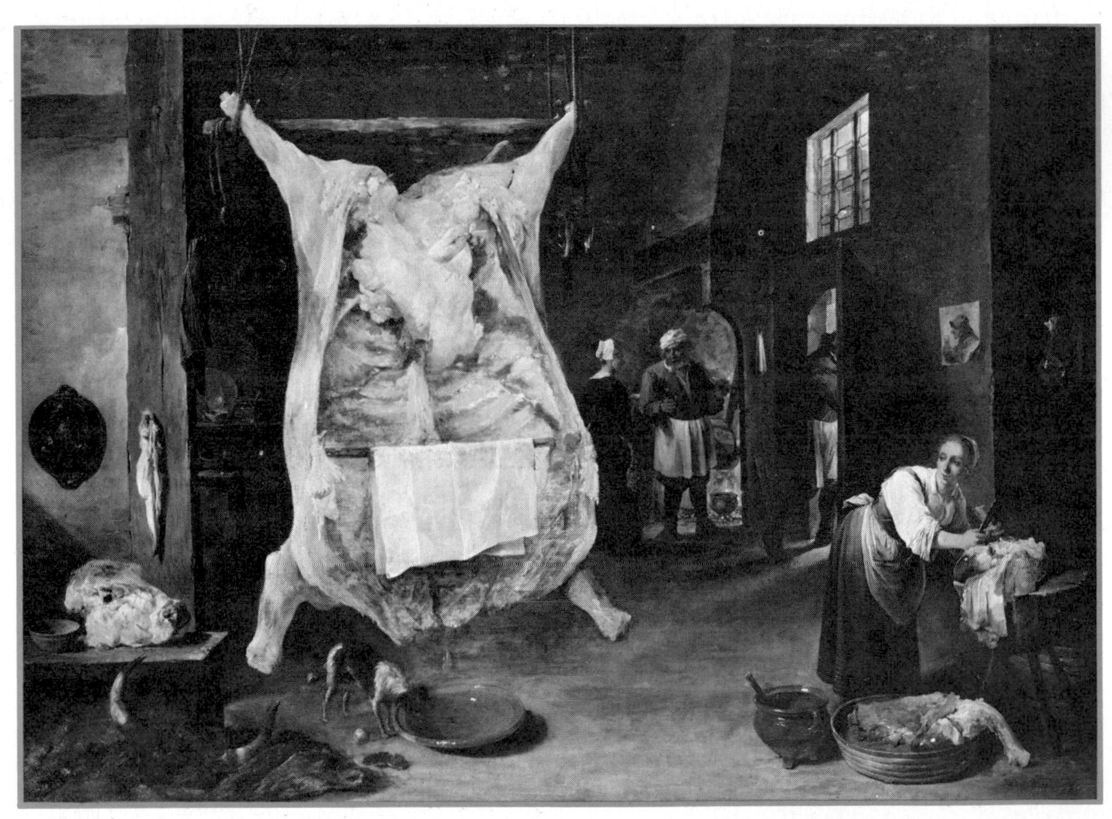

Interior of a Butcher's Shop by David Teniers (The Younger)

Proteins

Archeological evidence shows that even in prehistoric times an "animal principle" was recognized as being essential for human diets. Not, however, until the early nineteenth century was a group of substances which acted as the "animal principle" identified. At that time, two scientists applied the word "protein" (from the Greek *proteios*, meaning "of the first rank") to this "principle." The Swedish chemist Jöns Jakob Berzelius had first proposed the word in a communication to the Dutch agricultural chemist Gerard Johannes Mulder. Mulder first used the word in published papers in 1838 to describe what he thought was a single substance that was a component of all living matter.

Although research since Mulder's time has shown that protein is not one but a multiplicity of substances, it has confirmed that proteins are truly "of the first rank" in importance to all life. We know now, too, that protein molecules are complex, and consist of smaller entities known as amino acids. Some amino acids had been chemically identified as far back as 1810, even before proteins were described, but others were still being identified more than a hundred years later. Investigations of how they function are among the most exciting biochemical inquiries of our time.

Amino acids are essential for every body process, from transmission of the genetic information necessary to perpetuate every species, to the growth and maintenance of the cells of the individual organism. And this is as true of one-celled microorganisms as it is of *Homo sapiens.* Body cells are able to build their own proteins from amino acids, and carry out many essential functions by means of proteins. Although under certain circumstances, proteins can also serve as a source of energy, this is not their primary function.

Ever since proteins were identified, controversy has raged over dietary requirements. Although most Americans already consume amounts far in excess of any known need, numerous advertisements for protein-enriched products imply that we as a nation are a protein-deprived people. **Protein-energy malnutrition** is, however, of critical importance in a number of developing nations, where inadequate food supplies lead to both protein and energy undernutrition. (We shall examine this situation in Chapter 15.)

In this chapter we shall consider the various roles of protein in the economy of the human body, examine sources of dietary protein, and the routes by which it supports physiological function. The interactions of protein with other nutrients, trends in protein consumption, and the nature and amount of protein necessary for health will be discussed. Finally, we shall take a close look at vegetarianism and some special concerns about diets that include little or no animal protein.

CLASSIFICATION, STRUCTURES, AND SOURCES OF DIETARY PROTEIN

Classification of Amino Acids

Essential	
Neutral Aliphatic:	
Threonine	Thr
Isoleucine	Ile
Leucine	Leu
Valine	Val
Neutral Cyclic:	
Phenylalanine	Phe
Tryptophan	Try
Neutral Sulfur-containing:	
Methionine	Met
Cysteine (infants?)	Cys
Basic:	
Histidine	His
Lysine	Lys
Nonessential	
Neutral Aliphatic:	
Glycine	Gly
Alanine	Ala
Serine	Ser
Neutral Cyclic:	
Tyrosine	Tyr
Proline	Pro
Hydroxypro-line	Hyp
Neutral Sulfur-containing:	
Cystein	Cys
Acidic:	
Aspartic acid	Asp
Glutamic acid	Glu
Basic:	
Hydroxylysine	Hyl
Arginine	Arg

Proteins are organic compounds that always contain the elements carbon, hydrogen, oxygen, and nitrogen. Frequently, they contain sulfur and phosphorus as well, and less frequently they may contain other elements such as iron, copper, and iodine.

Proteins are indeed complex molecules. The structure of each protein molecule is an assembly of amino acids, subunits whose name is derived from their chemical composition: Each has an amino (NH_2) group and a carboxyl (COOH) group, both attached to the same carbon atom. Also attached to this carbon are a hydrogen atom and a radical (R) group. The radical is different for each of the different amino acids and determines the characteristics and functions of each. The radical may be only a single hydrogen, as in glycine, or it may be a complex chemical structure, as in tryptophan. Some R groups include an additional carboxyl or amino group, a sulfur-containing group, or cyclic arrangements of carbon and other atoms. Nitrogen is the element characteristic of all amino acids and, therefore of proteins. Most protein molecules contain from 12 to 19 percent nitrogen (usually considered 16 percent on average), a reflection of the amino acid nitrogen content.

Proline is technically an **imino acid** (having NH in a cyclic form instead of a free NH_2 group), but it is included with the amino acids because its role in protein structure is similar to theirs. Hydroxyproline and hydrosylysine contain an additional hydroxyl (—OH), added only after the parent compound (proline or lysine, respectively) has been incorporated into a protein.

Twenty-two amino acids are commonly found in foods; a few others, not present in foods, are synthesized in the body from other amino acids.

Classification of Amino Acids

Amino acids are classified in several different ways. From a functional viewpoint, those amino acids that are synthesized in the human body in adequate amounts are termed *nonessential.* Those that cannot be synthesized at all in the body, or that are synthesized in inadequate amounts, are termed *essential* because they must be supplied by exogenous food sources.

Normally, the body synthesizes all of the nonessential amino acids it needs, as long as it is provided with an adequate supply of nitrogen to use for this purpose. A carbon "skeleton" around which the amino acid forms is derived from various substrates; an amino group, often transferred from other amino acids, becomes attached; and the whole process must be facilitated by a specific enzyme. In the case of essential amino acids some of the enzymes

Basic Structure of Amino Acids

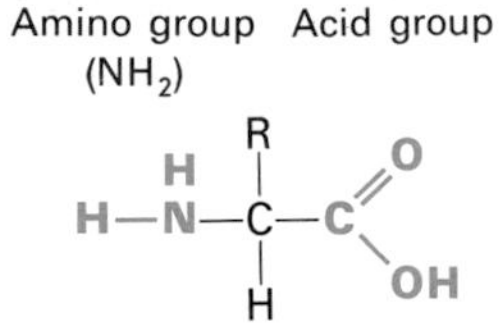

Amino group (NH_2) Acid group

$$H-\underset{H}{N}-\overset{R}{\underset{H}{C}}-C\!\begin{smallmatrix}//O\\ \backslash OH\end{smallmatrix}$$

Chemical Structures of Representative Amino Acids

Neutral aliphatic:

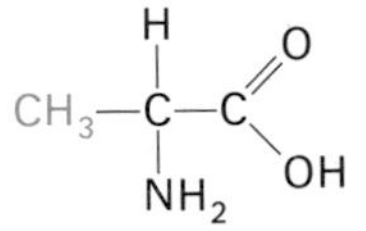

$$CH_3-\overset{H}{\underset{NH_2}{C}}-C\!\begin{smallmatrix}//O\\ \backslash OH\end{smallmatrix}$$

Alanine Ala

Neutral Cyclic:

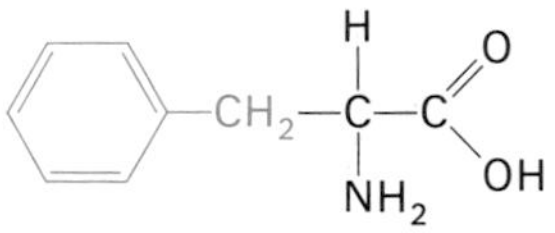

$$C_6H_5-CH_2-\overset{H}{\underset{NH_2}{C}}-C\!\begin{smallmatrix}//O\\ \backslash OH\end{smallmatrix}$$

Phenylalanine Phe

Neutral Sulfur-containing:

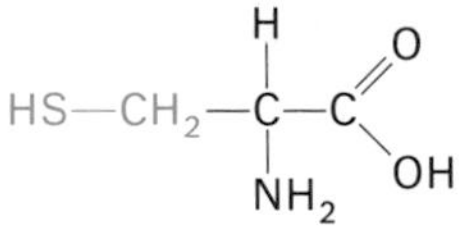

$$HS-CH_2-\overset{H}{\underset{NH_2}{C}}-C\!\begin{smallmatrix}//O\\ \backslash OH\end{smallmatrix}$$

Cysteine Cys

Acidic:

$$HO\overset{O}{\overset{\|}{C}}-CH_2-\overset{H}{\underset{NH_2}{C}}-C\!\begin{smallmatrix}//O\\ \backslash OH\end{smallmatrix}$$

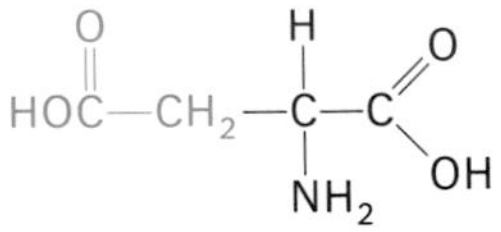

Aspartic acid Asp

Basic:

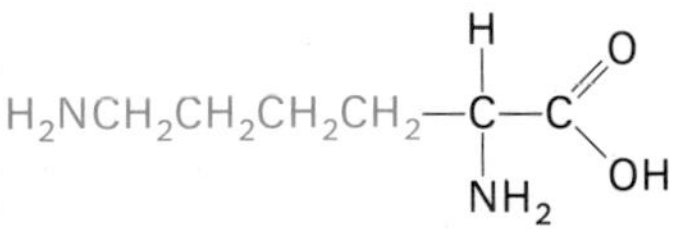

$$H_2NCH_2CH_2CH_2CH_2-\overset{H}{\underset{NH_2}{C}}-C\!\begin{smallmatrix}//O\\ \backslash OH\end{smallmatrix}$$

Lysine Lys

Imino acid:

H₂C——CH₂ H / H₂C C——C(=O)OH / N–H

$$\text{(ring: } H_2C-CH_2-C(H)-N(H)-CH_2\text{)}-C\!\begin{smallmatrix}//O\\ \backslash OH\end{smallmatrix}$$

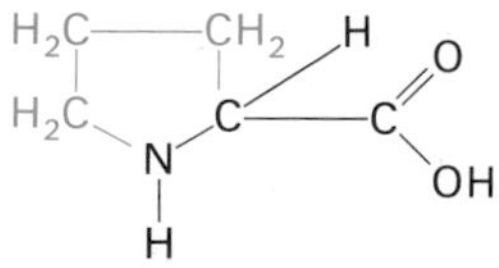

Proline Pro

required for this synthesis are either lacking or are not present in sufficient quantity.

The essential amino acids for human adults are *isoleucine, leucine, lysine, methionine, phenylalanine, threonine, tryptophan,* and *valine.* All others, with the possible exceptions of *histidine* and *cysteine,* are nonessential. Until recently histidine was thought to be essential only for infants, but recent evidence suggests that adults also may require exogenous histidine (Kopple and Sweinseid, 1975). Also, it has been suggested that newborn infants require exogenous cysteine until they mature sufficiently to produce the enzyme required for cysteine synthesis (Gaull et al., 1972).

Under certain circumstances, cysteine and *tyrosine,* too, may have to be considered essential for humans. Normally, the body meets its requirement for cysteine by synthesizing it from methionine, and for tyrosine by converting phenylalanine. But in certain disease states when these conversions cannot take place, cysteine and/or tyrosine must be supplied from dietary sources and are, therefore, considered essential amino acids.

Another classification of the amino acids is based on the chemical composition of their radicals or "side chains." Remember that all amino acids have both carboxyl and amino groups, which can be thought of as balancing each other, producing an overall neutral state of the amino acid molecule as a whole. There may, however, be additional carboxyl or amino groups present as part of the radical. If the radical contains an additional amino group, the amino acid is classified as *basic;* if it contains an additional carboxyl group, it is classified as *acidic.* And if the side chain contains no additional acidic or basic groups, the amino acid is *neutral.*

"Basic" and "acidic" have specific meanings in chemistry, referring to the presence of hydrogen ions (H^+). An **acid** substance will release hydrogen ions in a solution, while a **base** will combine with hydrogen ions. The chemical term **pH** measures relative acidity. By definition, a pH of 7 is neutral, with the number of hydrogen ions (H^+) equal to the number of hydroxyl ions (OH^-) as in water itself (H_2O). If the pH is greater than 7, the substance is basic, and tends to combine with hydrogen ions; if the pH is less than 7, the substance is acidic and tends to release hydrogen ions. The pH of most physiological fluids is about 7.4.

The presence of $-NH_2$ or -COOH in the side chains of individual amino acids gives them their *net* basic or acidic character. For instance, in the basic amino acid lysine, the side chain NH_2 group acquires an H^+ and is ionized to NH_3^+; in aspartic acid the additional COOH gives up its hydrogen and is ionized to COO^-. These charged groups contribute to the overall structure and characteristics of the various protein molecules of which they are a part.

Neutral amino acids can be further classified according to whether they are *aliphatic,* with a straight side chain, or *aromatic* or *cyclic,* with a side chain containing a ring structure; or according to whether or not they contain sulfur. The various classifications of the amino acids are shown in the table at the left.

Structure of Proteins

Protein molecules are composed of amino acids bonded together in a particular way, known as a *peptide linkage* or *peptide bond.* The central NH_2 group of one amino acid is joined to the central COOH group of another amino

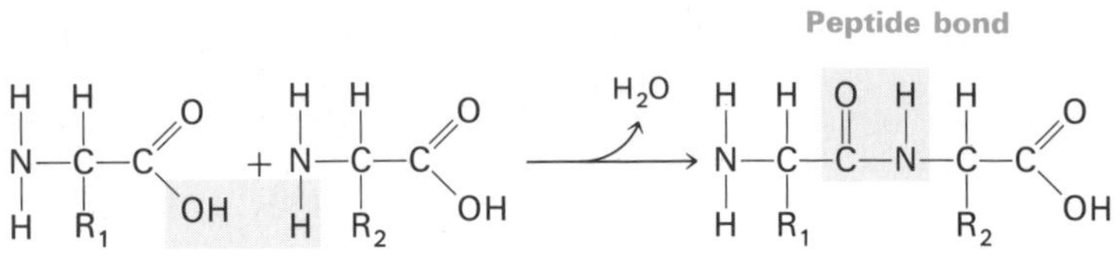

Peptide bond

Amino acid + Amino Acid ⟶ Dipeptide

FIGURE 4-1
Formation of a Dipeptide

acid through a condensation reaction, similar to that which occurs when a monosaccharide is added to a polysaccharide, or when a fatty acid is added to a glycerol molecule: the carboxyl group gives up an —OH and the amino group an —H to release a molecule of water.

Figure 4-1 shows the formation of a dipeptide, that is, two amino acids joined by a peptide bond. If three amino acids are joined, there will be two peptide bonds and the result is a tripeptide. Most protein molecules, however, consist of at least 50 and frequently hundreds of amino acids, and are known as **polypeptides.** But no matter how many amino acids comprise the protein molecule, they are joined together in the same peptide bonding. As a result, at one end of the protein molecule there will be a free amino group; that is, an NH_2 that has not participated in the peptide condensation reaction. This is known as the amino or N-terminal end of the protein. Similarly, the other end of the protein chain has a free carboxyl group and is known as the C-terminal end.

PRIMARY STRUCTURE. The polypeptide chain has a natural tendency to coil and become folded back on itself. This creates a complex structure, which can be described on several different levels. The primary structure of proteins depends on two factors: the sequence in which the amino acids are joined in the polypeptide chain (or chains—some proteins have more than one), and the presence of disulfide bonds.

The amino acid sequence is specific for each protein; thus, hemoglobin, collagen, the hundreds of enzymes, and all other protein molecules each consists of a specific and unique sequence. Most protein molecules contain from 15 to 20 different amino acids, and the number of possible, chemically meaningful sequences of 50 or more units that can be constructed from them is, for all practical purposes, infinite. It has been calculated that there are 10^{65} possible ways in which 20 amino acids could be arranged to form protein sequences of only 50 amino acid units (Strand, 1978)—and most proteins contain more than 100 such units. Estimates indicate there are more than 100,000 distinct proteins, and therefore more than 100,000 different amino acid sequences, in the human body. (Other life forms, of course, contain other proteins.)

But primary structure also involves the presence of disulfide bonds, which are cross-links formed between the sulfur components of two cysteine units in the polypeptide chain. Cysteine has a sulfhydryl (—SH) group at one end. When two cysteine units come together to form cystine, the two sulfhydryl groups are oxidized, giving up their H atoms and leaving a strong link between the two sulfides, known as a *disulfide bond* (—S—S—). Whenever cysteines appear in a polypeptide chain they tend to form these disulfide bonds, causing the chain to fold back on itself so that sulfhydryl groups meet and become linked. If this happens between cysteine units of two or more

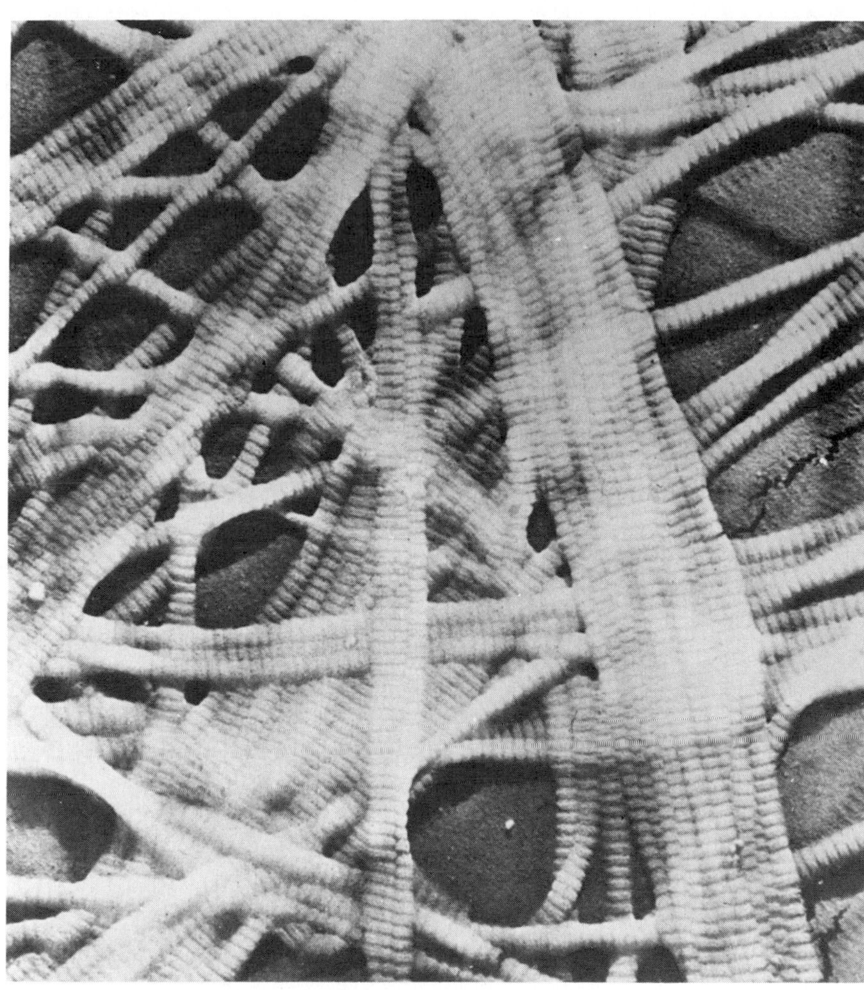

Fibrils of collagen from human skin, magnified 31,000 times. (Courtesy of Dr. Jerome Gross)

chains making up a single protein molecule, the bonds between those two chains are strengthened. The insulin molecule, for example, consists of two polypeptide chains linked together by two disulfide bonds; one of the chains is also linked internally by a disulfide bond (see Figure 4.2).

SECONDARY, TERTIARY, AND QUATERNARY STRUCTURE. Secondary, tertiary, and quaternary structures refer to the three-dimensional shape of the protein molecule. *Secondary structure* results from hydrogen bonding between different amino acids within the polypeptide chain and is manifested in the characteristic coiled or helical shape of the molecule. A hydrogen atom has a tendency to share its electron and seems to "look for" an oxygen atom to share it with. This creates a weak attraction between the hydrogen of an amino group in a peptide and an oxygen of the carboxyl group of neighboring amino acids. While each of these hydrogen bonds is, in itself, weak, the many hydrogen bonds between amino acids of the same chain give stability to the coiled form of the polypeptide chain. The result is a fairly regular secondary

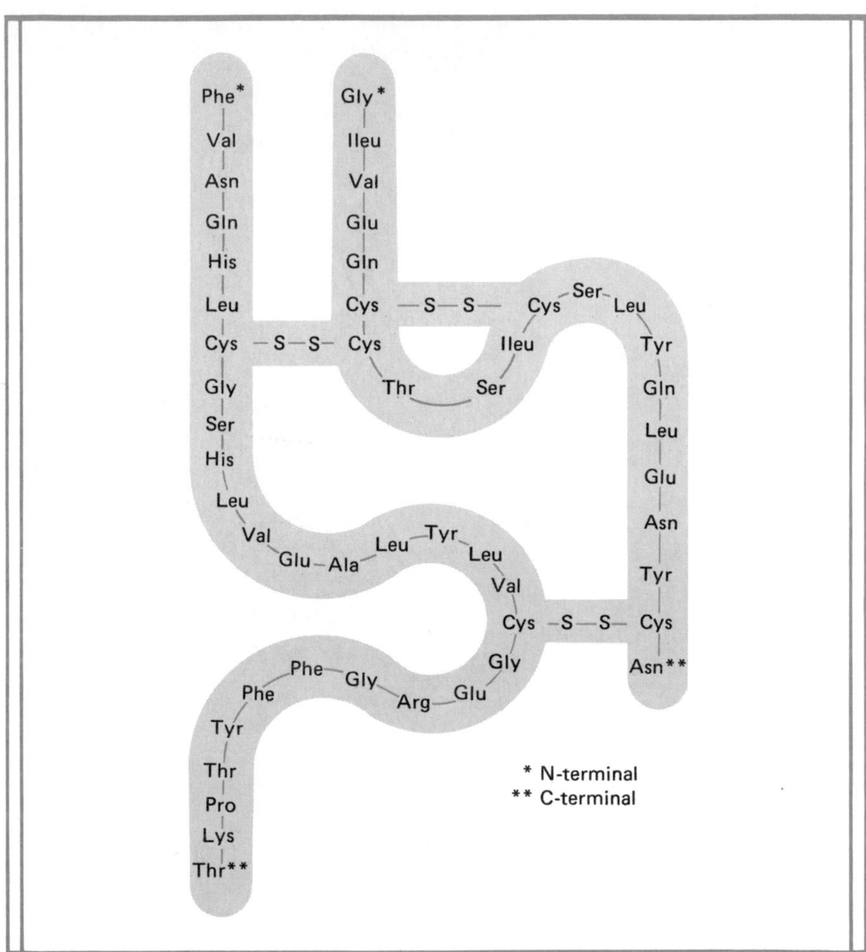

FIGURE 4-2
Polypeptide Chains of Human Insulin

structure called the α-helix, which contains about 3.6 amino acids in each coil or turn. This particular helical pattern can be discerned in many protein molecules; other patterns of secondary structure have also been identified.

Tertiary structure reflects the chemical relationship of amino acids that are more distant from one another in the linear structure. Electrostatic bonding (electron sharing), hydrogen bonding, and other types of bonding mechanisms link amino acids in a variety of spatial configurations.

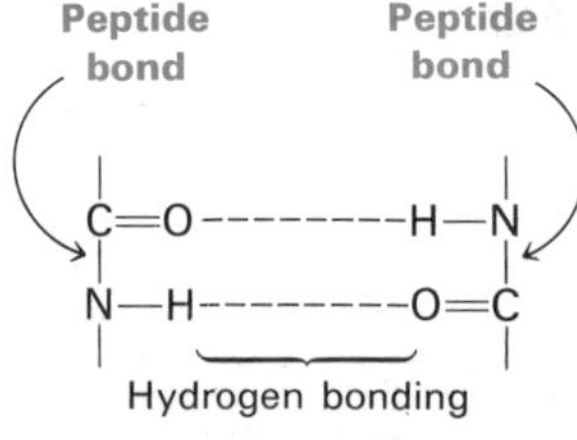

Hydrogen Bonding

We have been emphasizing the roles of two particular kinds of bonding—disulfide and hydrogen—in determining the architecture of the protein molecule. It must be kept in mind that it is the chemical organization of the component amino acid units, and with its two reactive ends and side chain, that facilitates the different kinds of bonding (as well as the other reactions into which the resulting molecules will enter). When there is limited bonding *within* the polypeptide chain, there is a greater possibility of the formation of cross-links *between* different polypeptide chains, both within the same molecule (as in the case of insulin), or between different molecules.

Both secondary and tertiary structures allow two different basic shapes of protein molecules. *Fibrous proteins* are polypeptides that are "stretched out" so that the molecule has a relatively linear shape. There is less internal bonding and, consequently, less coiling, leaving more side chains available to enter into cross-linkages with side chains of other similar molelcules. Fibrous proteins are therefore able to provide support and structure for cells and tissues and are relatively insoluble in water. They are found, for example, in muscle (myosin), connective tissue (collagen), and hair (keratin).

Globular proteins, on the other hand, are polypeptide chains that are very much folded and crumpled up to form rounded or elliptical molecules. They have a substantial amount of internal bonding, along with many exposed side chains. This structure makes globular proteins relatively soluble in body fluids. Not surprisingly, enzymes, albumin, hemoglobin, and most other plasma proteins are globular.

Finally, the *quaternary structure* of a protein is formed by the joining together of two or more similar protein subunits into a single large molecule, held together primarily by electrostatic forces. Hemoglobin, for example, is composed of two pairs of subunits, making four in all. While all proteins have primary, secondary, and tertiary structure, only some have quaternary structure.

Under some circumstances, the structural arrangement of a protein molecule can be disrupted. Heat, acids, or mechanical action are among the forces that break the hydrogen, disulfide, or other bonds and produce this disruption or **denaturation.** A well-known example of protein denaturation is the transformation of albumin (egg white) when it is cooked. Although in some cases denaturation is reversible, the coagulation of egg white totally alters the structure of its component polypeptide chains and cannot be reversed.

It is important to recognize that the function of proteins is a reflection of every aspect of their structure: the unique and specific amino acid composition and sequence, how the polypeptide chain is folded by internal bonding, and how subunits are combined. Even a brief introduction to the enormously complex structure of proteins leads to the conclusion that these are, in every way, complex and fascinating molecules.

Other Ways of Classifying Proteins

Another structural classification of proteins depends on whether or not a nonprotein component is incorporated into the molecule. Because of the readiness with which some polypeptides are able to react with other molecules, proteins have a notable tendency to form combinations in which they are part of a larger aggregate. In Chapter 3 we discussed lipoproteins, macromolecules with both a lipid and a protein component. Proteins that do not combine with nonprotein substances are *simple*, while those in combination are *conjugated*. Table 4-1 lists conjugated proteins according to their nonprotein components.

Finally, proteins can be classified on the basis of their *physiological functions*, according to which there are six classes:

1. Enzymes, which catalyze body processes.
2. Some hormones, which regulate body processes.

TABLE 4-1
Structural Classification of Proteins

Class of Proteins	Nonprotein Component	Example
Simple	None	Albumin, collagen
Conjugated		
Nucleoproteins	Nucleic acid (DNA, RNA)	Chromosomes
Lipoproteins	Lipids	Chylomicrons
Glycoproteins	Carbohydrate	Immunoglobulin
Metalloproteins	Metal ions (Zn, Cu, Fe)	Ferritin, carboxypeptidase
Chromoproteins	Heme, retinal	Hemoglobin, rhodopsin

Source: Adapted from R. Montgomery, R. L. Dryer, T. W. Conway, and A. A. Specter, *Biochemistry: A case-oriented approach* (St. Louis: C. V. Mosby, 1974), page 49.

3. Antibodies or immunological substances.
4. Structural proteins, which constitute cartilage, skin, nails, and hair.
5. Contractile proteins, which make up the skeletal muscle.
6. Blood proteins such as hemoglobin and albumin.

Proteins in Foods

You will remember that it is the essential amino acids that the body must obtain from food for constructing its own proteins; as long as all are provided in appropriate quantity, the particular food form in which they are ingested is of no significance. While protein can be obtained from both plant and animal food sources, the latter generally contain all of the essential amino acids in amounts that will support human growth and maintain physiological functioning. These are called, somewhat incorrectly, **complete proteins.**

Incomplete proteins contain suboptimal amounts of certain essential amino acids. Except for a few in which one or more essential amino acids are totally absent, they are not literally incomplete. But they are "less" complete than most animal-derived proteins. Zein, for example, found in corn, is not capable of sustaining life if it is the sole protein being fed. Corn, however, contains other proteins that increase the usefulness of zein.

The protein content of various foods is shown in Table 4-2. A high protein content does not, however, necessarily indicate a high **protein quality** for a given food; the essential amino acid pattern is what counts. For this reason, two foods with comparable protein content will not necessarily be of equal value to the organism. For example, 1 tablespoon of gelatin has about as much protein as 8 ounces (240 ml) of skim milk (9 g), but because gelatin is an incomplete protein, the protein quality of these two foods is not the same. Since most proteins of vegetable origin are incomplete, it is also important to know the biological value of given foods, especially in determining dietary protein requirements and the adequacy of vegetarian diets, topics to be discussed later in this chapter.

It will be noted that virtually all the foods of high protein content in Table 4-2 are of animal origin: milk and milk products, meat, fish, and shellfish. The only exceptions are legumes—nuts and beans and their derivatives, such as peanut butter and tofu (soybean curd). Note also that the protein content of milk and yogurt products varies, depending upon the addition of milk solids to the low-fat varieties.

Worldwide, per capita protein availability ranges widely, from about 55 grams per day in the Far East to 93 grams in the United States and Canada. In general, people in developing countries consume less protein (an

TABLE 4-2
Protein Content of Selected Foods

Food	Serving Size	Protein Content g/Serving
Cottage cheese, uncreamed	1 c	34
Round steak, lean & fat	3½ oz	29
Swordfish, broiled	3½ oz	28
Tuna fish in water	3½ oz	28
Scallops	3½ oz	23
Chickpeas	½ c	21
Haddock, fried	3½ oz	20
Soybeans, boiled	1 c	20
Yogurt, nonfat milk + milk solids	8 oz	13
Yogurt, low-fat + milk solids, plain	8 oz	12
Yogurt, low-fat + milk solids, fruit-flavored	8 oz	10
Milk, low-fat or skim, + milk solids	1 c	9–10
Almonds, roasted	⅓ c	9.5
Gelatin, dry	1 tbsp	9
Milk, whole	1 c	8
Milk, low-fat or skim	1 c	8
Yogurt, made with whole milk	8 oz	8
Cashews, roasted	⅓ c	8
Peanut butter	2 tbsp	8
Cheddar cheese	1 oz	7
Egg, whole	1 medium	6
Kidney beans	½ c	6
Broccoli, cooked	⅔ c	3
Rice, brown, cooked	⅔ c	3
Tofu (soybean curd)	1 oz	2.5
White bread, enriched	1 slice	2
Bean sprouts, raw	½ c	2
Rice, white milled, enriched	⅔ c	2
Gelatin dessert, plain	½ c	2
Carrots, cooked	⅔ c	1
Bouillon cube	1 cube	trace
Butter	1 tbsp	trace
Margarine, oils	1 pat	0

Sources: Consumer and Food Economics Institute, *Composition of foods—Dairy and egg products—Raw, processed, prepared,* USDA Agricultural Handbook No. 8-1 (Washington, D.C.: U.S. Government Printing Office, 1976); and C. F. Adams, *Nutritive value of American foods in common units,* USDA Agricultural Handbook No. 456 (Washington, D.C.: U.S. Government Printing Office, 1975).

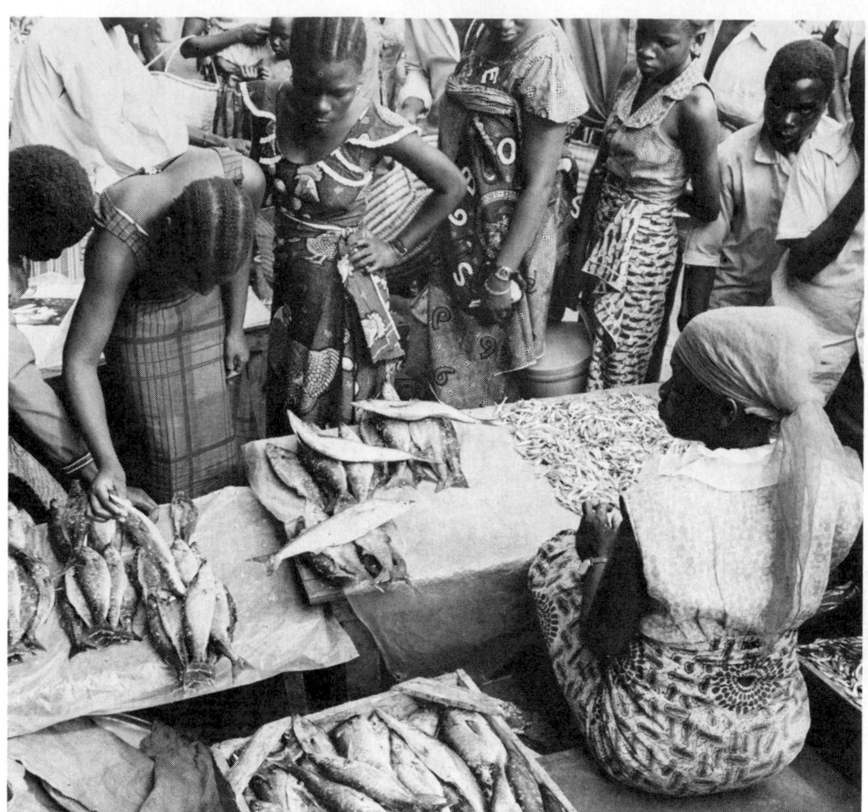

Fish from Lake Tanganyika being sold at the central fish market of Bujumbura, Burundi. (FAO photo by F. Botts)

Protein Consumption in the United States and Canada

Protein Type	Percent of Total Protein Consumption
Animal Proteins, Total	69.9
Meat	36.3
Milk	24.9
Eggs	5.8
Fish	2.9
Vegetable Proteins, Total	30.1
Cereals	17.6
Fruits and vegetables	5.2
Legumes, nuts, seeds	4.6
Starchy roots, tubers	2.6

Source: Adapted from R. A. Lawrie, *Protein as human food* (Westport, Conn.: Avi Publishing Co., 1970), Table 2.

average of 57.6 g per capita per day) than in developed regions (89.1 g) (Lawrie, 1970). In developing regions, too, most protein—over 80 percent—is derived from plant food sources, compared to only about 45 percent from plant sources in developed nations (Lawrie, 1970). (Figures represent estimated available protein, not necessarily consumption, and are for the years 1963–1965.)

That protein consumption is tied to availability is underscored by the figures for certain categories of protein in some places: In South and East Asia, fish consumption accounts for about 15.5 percent of all protein intake, with meat consumption in the 6–7 percent range; people in West and Central Africa get a substantially greater proportion of their protein (14.8 percent) from starchy roots and tubers than do people anywhere else in the world; and Brazilians receive more than a quarter of their protein from legumes, nuts, and seeds (Lawrie, 1970).

The major influences on availability of plant versus animal sources of protein foods are economic and technological and have to do with such factors as methods of production (irrigation, fertilization, mechanized tilling, and slaughtering methods), storage facilities, transportation, and distribution (village markets versus supermarkets, for example). Traditional religious and cultural preferences (many of which also derive ultimately from technological factors) surely have some influence as well. Consumption of protein, perhaps even more than of the other major nutrients, is tied to socioeconomic factors. As a nation's or a family's socioeconomic status improves, protein, and especially animal-derived protein, will form a greater proportion of the diet.

DIGESTION AND ABSORPTION

The significance of protein in foods will become clearer as we examine its functions in the body—growth, maintenance of tissues, regulation of physiological processes and, under certain conditions, a source of energy. During digestion and absorption, proteins are transformed into their constituent amino acids which are then delivered to body cells for all of these purposes.

Enzymatic Hydrolysis

In protein digestion, the peptide bonds linking amino acids in the polypeptide chain are broken down, releasing smaller peptide fragments and individual amino acids. This is a hydrolytic reaction, similar to those we have already examined for the digestion of carbohydrates and lipids, and the reverse of the condensation reaction by which the peptide bonds were formed. In hydrolysis of peptide bonds (proteolysis), which requires action by specific proteolytic enzymes, a water molecule is added at each bond.

Peptide bond

$$-\mathrm{N(H)}-\mathrm{C(H)(R_1)}-\mathrm{C(=O)}-\mathrm{N(H)}-\mathrm{C(H)(R_2)}-\mathrm{C(=O)}- \xrightarrow[\text{Enzyme}]{H_2O} -\mathrm{N(H)}-\mathrm{C(H)(R_1)}-\mathrm{C(=O)}-\mathrm{OH} + \mathrm{H}-\mathrm{N(H)}-\mathrm{C(H)(R_2)}-\mathrm{C(=O)}-$$

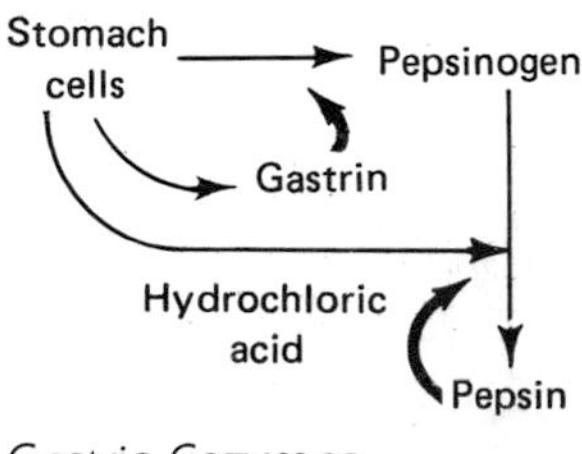

Gastric Enzymes

The initial phase of protein digestion takes place in the stomach. There is no chemical action on protein in the mouth or esophagus, although lubrication, mastication, and peristaltic action prepare protein food mechanically for chemical attack. In the stomach, specialized cells release hydrochloric acid, which begins the denaturation of dietary protein. This loss of structure makes protein more susceptible to subsequent action by digestive enzymes. Hydrochloric acid acts also as a primer to convert the inactive precursor enzyme *pepsinogen* to **pepsin.** Pepsinogen is produced by specific cells of the stomach under the influence of the gastrointestinal hormone gastrin. Pepsin hydrolyzes large proteins into smaller polypeptides and also accelerates its own production from pepsinogen. This is, indeed, a complicated and elegantly interconnected sequence of biochemical events!

As is characteristic of the proteolytic enzymes, pepsin is selective, hydrolyzing only those bonds in which the nitrogen is provided by either phenylalanine or tyrosine. Consequently, only a minimal amount of protein hydrolysis is accomplished in the stomach. Most occurs within the lumen of the small intestine, under the influence of intestinal and pancreatic enzymes. But gastric hydrolysis is the important first step.

As soon as stomach contents enter the duodenum, the intestinal hormone *pancreozymin* stimulates the cells of the pancreas to release their complement of proteolytic enzymes (as well as other enzymes needed for carbohydrate and lipid digestion). These inactive precursor enzymes—*trypsinogen, chymotrypsinogen, proelastase,* and *procarboxypeptidase*—are secreted into

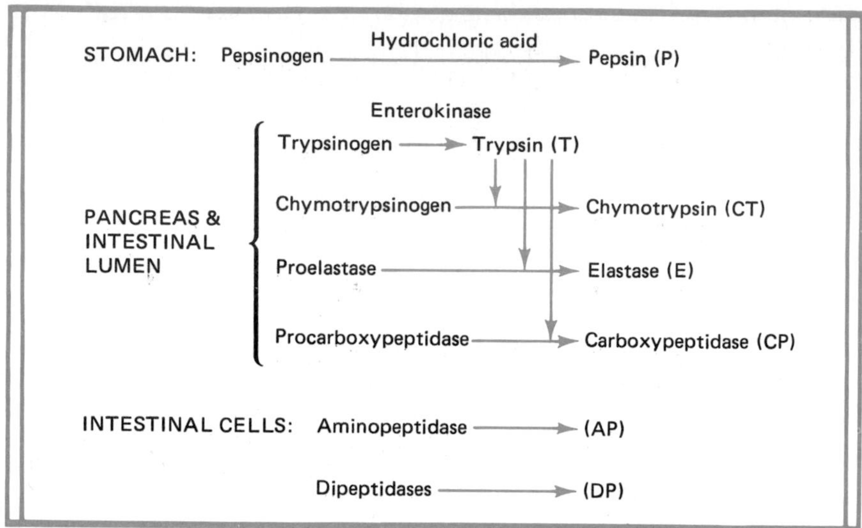

FIGURE 4-3
A Summary of Enzymes in Protein Digestion

the duodenum where they are transformed into active participants in the digestive process. By means of *enterokinase*, an enzyme present in the duodenum, a fragment is split from the trypsinogen molecule to produce the active enzyme *trypsin*. The presence of trypsin initiates a "cascade" of further conversions, as it activates the precursor forms of *chymotrypsin*, *elastase*, and the *carboxypeptidases*. Figure 4-3 diagrams this cascade effect. These enzymes are released by hydrolysis of a fragment from the polypeptide chain of their respective precursors. Now active, each of these enzymes acts only on specific peptide bonds.

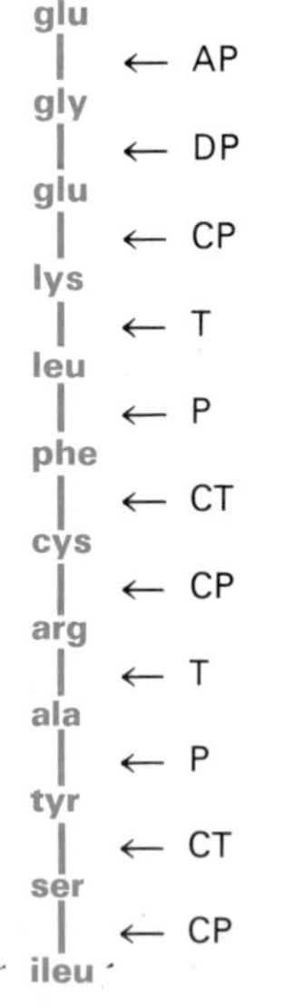

Enzyme Action on Polypeptides

Trypsin selects only those bonds whose carboxyl groups are provided by arginine and lysine residues. Chymotrypsin similarly attacks only those peptide bonds where the carboxyl group is contributed by tyrosine, phenylalanine, and tryptophan. Elastase acts on a number of different amino acid residues, but is the only enzyme able to hydrolyze the protein elastin, found in muscle meats. Because they attack interior peptide bonds only, and not those adjacent to the ends of the polypeptide, these three enzymes are known as **endopeptidases.** Through their action, the polypeptide chains of large protein molecules become progressively more fragmented into shorter peptide chains.

The two carboxypeptidases, on the other hand, hydrolyze the peptide bonds at the C-terminals of the peptides. Amino peptidase hydrolyzes amino acids from the N-terminal end. These *exopeptidases* release free amino acids.

The digestibility of some proteins may be affected by other substances present in particular foods, as well as by certain processing and preparation methods. Soybeans, lima beans, and peas, for example, contain a factor that has been associated with growth failure in laboratory animals. This factor, which is destroyed by heat, probably acts as an inhibitor of trypsin and perhaps chymotrypsin. The clinical and practical significance of this discovery for human nutrition is not yet clear, but it indicates these foods should probably not be eaten raw.

Excessive heating of proteins sometimes creates enzyme-resistant linkages between amino acid units (severe denaturation), which will interfere with digestion and subsequent absorption. Moderate heating, such as occurs in normal preparation and cooking, may, on the other hand, split natural cross-linkages and facilitate enzyme action. Overcooking, however, does not increase digestibility.

In some instances, pancreatic deficiency or inherited diseases will interfere with efficiency of protein digestion. The result is loss of protein via the feces.

Not all of the protein in the small intestine is derived from food. The digestive enzymes, for example, are themselves proteins. Moreover, protein-containing cells of the intestinal mucosa are continually being sloughed off at the outer ends of the villi, as they are replaced by new cells formed at the villi bases. Together, these and other endogenous sources may provide as much as 70 grams of protein per day, in addition to the average American dietary intake of 90 to 100 grams (Crim and Munro, 1976). Since daily fecal losses of protein are only about 10 grams, total absorption in the intestine must approximate 160 grams per day.

While most proteolysis takes place in the lumen of the small intestine, there are some enzymes in the brush borders and the intracellular fluid surrounding the mucosal cells. These dipeptidases act on the smaller peptides that are released during intestinal digestion. As soon as small peptides cross from the lumen into the mucosa (see below), the brush border and intracellular peptidases begin to hydrolyze them, a process which results in the production of free amino acids.

Amino Acid Absorption

From the lumen of the small intestine, amino acids are transported to the mucosal cells by means of special carriers in an energy-dependent process. Several different carrier systems have been identified, specific for neutral, basic, or acidic amino acids, or for dipeptides. Amino acids enter the general circulation through the portal vein.

Protein absorption is extremely efficient, with more than 90 percent of dietary protein absorbed as amino acids. Proteins of animal origin are digested and absorbed with even greater efficiency—97 percent—than are those in cereals, legumes, fruits, and vegetables (78–85 percent).

Infants are born with the ability to absorb proteins intact, without their being broken down completely. This ability, retained for a short time only, serves an important protective function. It enables antibodies, which are proteins, to be absorbed from the mother's milk, and thus confers a temporary immunity against certain contagious diseases.

Except for the first month of life, however, dietary proteins cannot be absorbed in intact form but are always broken down into their component amino acids. Thus, the frequent commercial claims that certain foods contain *essential proteins* that *must* be consumed for good health cannot be reconciled with what we know of the physiology of digestion. No *protein* is essential; it is the individual amino acids contained in dietary proteins and hydrolyzed during digestion that actually enter into the body's physiological processes.

METABOLISM

The body's access to amino acids is regulated primarily by the liver. Following digestion of a protein-containing meal, the amino acid concentration in the portal vein increases severalfold. The liver, then, must deal with sharp fluctuations in the supply of amino acids several times a day, day after day, throughout the life of the organism. By catabolizing essential amino acids, synthesizing amino acids into proteins for use in its own processes as well as for transport through the blood to body cells, and by synthesizing nonessential amino acids, the liver keeps the amino acid levels in body tissues in dynamic equilibrium.

Amino acids are thus involved in a whole range of anabolic and catabolic processes which take a number of different pathways, each influenced by many factors. We shall examine the major reactions involving amino acids, beginning with protein synthesis, which is by far the primary function of amino acids in all living organisms.

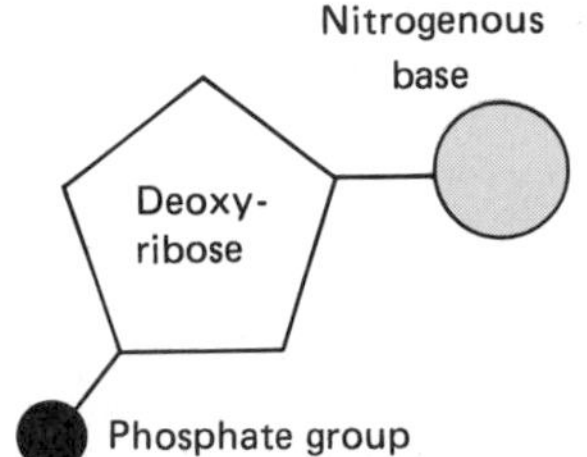

Diagram of Nucleotide Structure

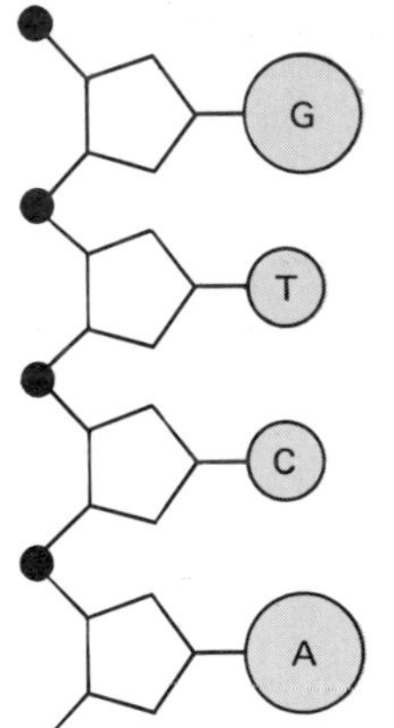

Segment of a Nucleotide (DNA) Chain

Each nucleotide consists of deoxyribose (a 5-carbon sugar), phosphate, and a nitrogen-containing base. There are four different bases (adenine, guanine, cytosine, and thymine), and therefore four different kinds of nucleotides, usually expressed as A, G, C, and T. The sugar of one nucleotide is always attached to the phosphate group of the next, forming the "backbone" of the DNA molecule, with the different bases branching off as side chains.

Protein Synthesis

All life depends on the synthesis of new protein molecules by body cells. Of the vast number of different protein structures possible, each cell synthesizes only the ones needed for its own purposes, and produces them in precisely required amounts; this is true of every cell of every living organism, be it bacterium, bat, or human being. In every individual, all cellular chemical activities are programmed by a genetic code unique to that individual. The genetic code itself is contained within the chromosomes inside every cell nucleus.

"BREAKING" THE GENETIC CODE. It had long been known that the chromosomes were responsible for duplicating and transmitting the genetic message, and that the actual units of heredity were a component of the chromosomes known as **deoxyribonucleic acid** (DNA). But the actual molecular structure and behavior of DNA remained a mystery until 1953, when Watson and Crick unraveled its chemical organization and proposed a model for its biochemical action. These scientists determined that the DNA molecule was an elongated double helix, whose two twisting and intertwined strands were composed of linked subunits called **nucleotides.**

Watson and Crick proposed that the two strands of a DNA molecule were held together by hydrogen bonds between specific nucleotide bases. The specificity of nucleotide bonding means that a new DNA molecule can be constructed from a single strand of the old DNA molecule: the single strand serves as a pattern to define a complementary strand. Thus, the information contained in a given pair of nucleotide chains is duplicated precisely, and hereditary information is transmitted from generation to generation. The cell-duplicating mechanism is so perfect that every cell in an individual contains identical nucleotide sequences in its DNA.

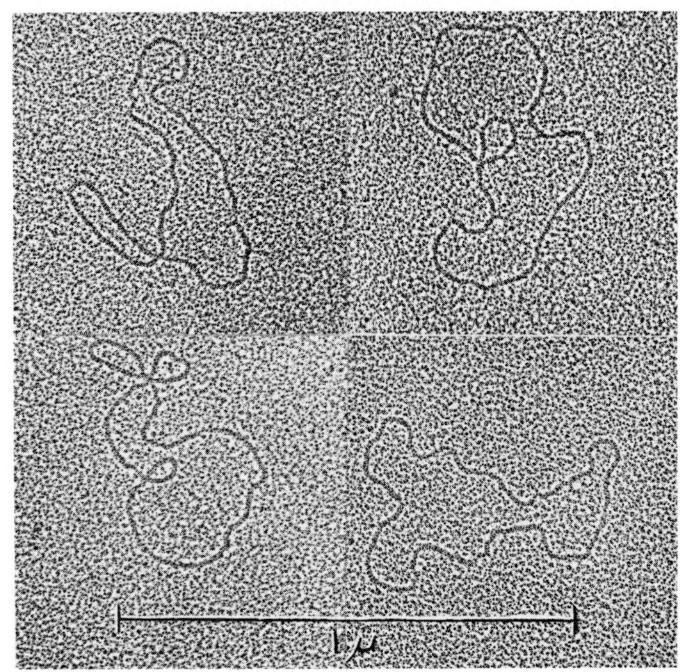

Electron micrograph of loops of DNA. Each loop is a complete double helix, and contains about 5,5000 pairs of bases. This DNA is from molecules of the bacterial virus Øx174. (Professor Arthur Kornberg, Stanford University School of Medicine)

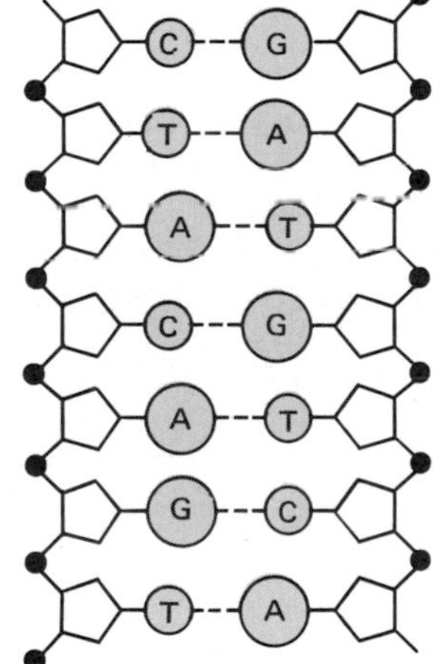

Hydrogen Bonding of DNA Nucleotide Strands

Hydrogen bonds form between the side-chain bases that "face" each other as they extend from opposite nucleotides. Crick and Watson determined from various measurements that hydrogen bonds could exist only between adenine and thymine and between guanine and cytosine. Thus, where one strand has A, the opposite strand must have T, and so on.

The genetic code itself consists of the sequences of nucleotides within the DNA molecule, which act by programming the synthesis of the specific proteins that make up each species and individual. The actual genetic code is different for every species and for every individual within a species.

The DNA and its nucleotide sequences are located in the nucleus of the cell, however, while protein synthesis occurs in the cytoplasm. The genetic information, therefore, must somehow be carried from the DNA, which never leaves the cell nucleus, to the scene of the action. This is accomplished by another macromolecule, **ribonucleic acid** (RNA), which exists in both the nucleus and the cytoplasm of the cell. RNA is very similar to DNA except that it consists of a single strand of nucleotides instead of a double strand, its 5-carbon sugar is ribose instead of deoxyribose (from which the names of the two molecules are derived), and it contains uracil (U) instead of thymine.

Actually, several kinds of RNA are required to carry out the instructions of the DNA. Messenger ribonucleic acid (mRNA) is produced in the nucleus of the cell, modeled by a single strand of DNA, which separates from its mate for this purpose. The completed mRNA molecule then moves through the nuclear membrane and enters the cytoplasm. Here it encounters the ribosomes, the parts of the cell that actually synthesize proteins. Ribosomes are able to synthesize every protein, but must be given specific "instructions" in order to "know" which proteins to produce in a given cell.

The functioning unit of protein synthesis, and thus of heredity, is a sequence of three nucleotides called a **codon.** Each codon is identified by the three letters standing for its component nucleotides. There are 64 different possible codons from the combinations of the four different nucleotides (4^3). We now know that each of 61 of them codes for only one specific amino acid: for example, AAG for lysine, AGA for arginine, GAA for glutamic acid. But there are only 22 amino acids, and so some may be called for by more than one codon: lysine, for example, is coded by either AAG or AAA, and serine by UCU, UCC, UCA, or UCG. The remaining three codons are chain-terminating (or "nonsense") codons, which signal the end of a particular message sequence.

THE MAKING OF A POLYPEPTIDE. In the bloodstream, ready to enter the cytoplasm at an instant's notice, is a pool of amino acids that have resulted both from digestion of dietary protein and from the breakdown of existing protein. Waiting in the cytoplasm are relatively small molecules of transfer ribonucleic acid (tRNA). Each tRNA molecule contains a single 3-nucleotide sequence that "fits" a similar sequence on the mRNA strand, and each tRNA molecule is also able to attach to a particular amino acid from the cellular amino acid pool.

Once the mRNA enters the cytoplasm, ribosomes cluster along its length. The mRNA and its attached ribosomes are known as a polyribosome complex. Each ribosome moves along the strand of mRNA, touching two codons at a time. Codon by codon, a tRNA molecule and its amino acid arrive on the scene. Enzymes in the ribosome form a peptide bond which attaches the new amino acid to the growing peptide chain. The tRNA molecule is released, and the ribosome moves along the mRNA to the next codon, where instructions for the next amino acid in the sequence are received. As each appropriate tRNA molecule carrying its amino acid responds, the polypeptide chain grows longer (Fig. 4-4).

Actually, many ribosomes move at the same time along a single strand of mRNA, each producing a protein molecule in the course of its journey. Thus, a single molecule of mRNA can direct the synthesis of many identical protein molecules. The whole process occurs very quickly, within seconds. This amazingly complex set of reactions is still being actively studied.

Some of the most intriguing questions related to protein synthesis deal with the regulation of the process: How is it initiated? How is it limited to

FIGURE 4-4
Polypeptide Synthesis

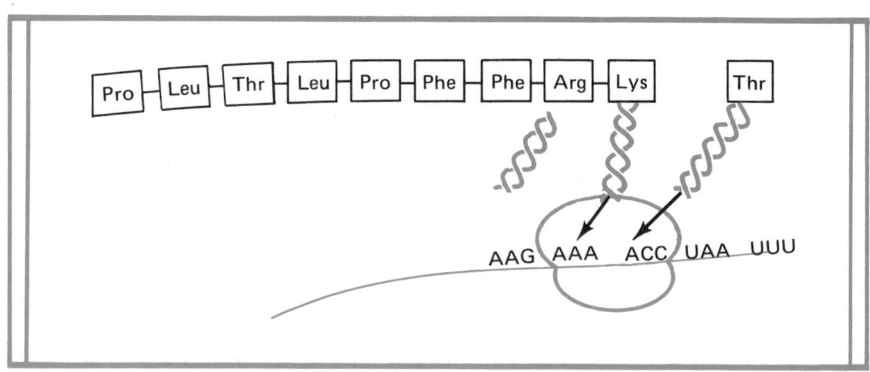

specific proteins? All cells in the body have the same DNA information, but they obviously don't all do the same thing. Somehow, in all cells, part of the total coded information is "turned off" so that only those parts specific to the functioning of each type of cell are operative. How this "turning off" is effected is not as yet clearly understood. But in every cell, the necessary combination of appropriate amino acids is "strung together" in a particular sequence, as programmed by the genetic code unique to that individual, via a series of elegant enzymatic reactions.

Several factors are involved in keeping this vital and intricate mechanism functioning smoothly. The first requirement is an adequate supply in every cell of all amino acids. This is truly an "all-or-nothing" situation: If even one of the amino acids called for by an mRNA codon is missing, synthesis of the whole polypeptide chain comes to a halt. This, then, is the reason why the "essential" amino acids must be provided by dietary protein; there is no other way for them to be available within the cell.

Energy, in the form of ATP, is the second requirement; it is needed both to initiate and continue the process of protein synthesis. ATP activates the amino acids in the cytoplasm so that they become attached to their tRNA molecules; it moves the mRNA, tRNA, and the ribosomes in their appointed courses; and it is necessary at several other stages. If there is insufficient energy, the process cannot proceed.

Protein synthesis is regulated by a number of other factors as well—so many other factors, and with functions so intricate, that description of their interactions is beyond the scope of this book.

FUNCTIONS OF SYNTHESIZED PROTEINS. All cells synthesize protein by the mechanism that has just been described. These proteins are used as constituents of a number of essential body substances for growth and for maintenance of all tissues. The growth of the body depends on incorporation of newly synthesized protein into bone, muscle, skin, hair, nails, and other tissues. Most growth, of course, takes place during the earlier years of the individual's life; however, skin, nails, and hair continue to grow throughout life.

Throughout life, too, the protein in body tissues is continually being broken down into amino acids, which become part of the amino acid pool in the cells. When tissue proteins are broken down, they must be replaced by new proteins. This tissue maintenance requires a constant supply of amino acids. The amino acids that result from tissue breakdown, along with amino acids from dietary protein, are used for synthesis of new proteins and special molecules, and for energy. This breakdown and replacement is known as **protein turnover.** Without an adequate supply of amino acids from both dietary and endogenous sources, protein turnover could not be accomplished.

Proteins are also important for regulation of the body's water balance. This role will be discussed more fully in Chapter 9, but here we should note that plasma proteins, such as albumin, serve the important function of maintaining **osmotic pressure** in the blood. Thus, they help to effect a proper distribution of fluid between blood and body tissues. If plasma protein levels decrease, as in protein deficiency situations, fluid accumulates in the tissues, causing the condition known as edema.

TABLE 4-3 **Amount of Protein Synthesis**

Age Group	Body Weight (BW) kg	Total Body Protein Synthesis		Protein Synthesis g/g Protein Intake
		g/kg BW/day	*g/day*[a]	
Newborn (premature)	1.94 ± .59	17.4 ± 7.9	33.8	5.4
Infants (10–20 mos.)	9.0 ± .5	6.9 ± 1.1	62.1	5.3
Young adults (20–23 yrs.)	71 ± 15	3.0 ± 0.2	213.0	5.2
Elderly (69–91 yrs.)	56 ±	1.9 ± 0.2	106.4	4.5

[a]Calculated from Young's data.

Source: V. R. Young, W. P. Steffee, R. B. Pencharz, J. C. Winterer, and N. S. Scrimshaw, Total human body protein synthesis in relation to protein requirements at various ages, *Nature* 253:192, 1975.

Proteins also regulate the acid-base balance (pH) of body fluids. The acidic and basic side groups of the various amino acids constituting protein molecules enable them to act as buffers and to neutralize acids and bases in the body so that the generally neutral pH level is maintained. Maintenance of pH neutrality is vital; several different regulatory mechanisms exist to preserve it.

Finally, some functional proteins are antibodies, which destroy infectious organisms and thereby fight disease.

It has been estimated that as much as 300 grams of protein per day may be synthesized in the body of an average adult male weighing 70 kilograms. Recent experiments suggest that the quantity of protein synthesized is related to body size and to age (see Table 4-3), as well as to overall energy expenditure. Data from Young et al. (1975) indicate that a single gram of dietary protein supports the synthesis of 4 to 5 grams of protein, regardless of age. Differences in protein needs, as expressed in grams per kilogram of body weight per day, result from the differences in the rate of protein synthesis (that is, the amount of protein synthesized in a given period of time).

Synthesis of Nonessential Amino Acids

About half of the more than 20 amino acids found in the human body can be synthesized in the liver from other compounds. Formation of an amino acid requires the attachment of an amino or nitrogen group to a "carbon skeleton," which contains the distinctive radical or side chain that will characterize the resulting amino acid. The carbon skeleton is a keto acid, such as pyruvate or α-ketoglutarate, which is a product of carbohydrate or fat metabolism. The nitrogen group is provided by other amino acids present in larger quantity, through the processes of transamination or deamination.

Keto and amino acids exist in pairs, related by similar structure of the carbon chain; several pairs exist. In **transamination,** an amino group is transferred from an amino acid of one pair (alanine–pyruvate) to the keto acid of another pair (α-ketoglutarate–glutamic acid). Transamination requires the assistance of specific enzymes known as transaminases and must be accompanied by pyridoxine (vitamin B_6), which serves as a coenzyme (Figure 4-5).

PERSPECTIVE ON
PKU, An Inborn Error of Protein Metabolism

Despite its amazing complexity, the protein synthesizing process functions to perfection in virtually every individual. There are, however, a few conditions in which a key component of the mechanism fails to work. These inborn errors of metabolism are due to inherited defects that result in biochemical abnormalities, often with serious clinical symptoms; some of them may even threaten survival. We shall consider here one of the most familiar of such diseases, phenylketonuria or PKU.

Extensive research has been undertaken to clarify the etiology of many inherited diseases. Usually, such defects are the result of damage to a single gene, the unit by which hereditary traits are considered to be transmitted. In the light of today's knowledge, genes can be described as the set of nucleotide codons on a DNA molecule that direct the formation of a particular protein from its component amino acids. However, it is convenient to refer to genes in terms of their net effect, as has been traditional since Gregor Mendel first suggested their existence a century ago. Every DNA molecule in every chromosome contains a multiplicity of genes.

A damaged gene is known as a mutant. Mutations result from factors, such as exposure to radiation, that interfere with the replication of the DNA molecule. If even a single nucleotide were missing, or if an incorrect nucleotide were to replace a correct one, the mRNA strand would be transmitting the "wrong" information and keying the addition of an incorrect amino acid at the level of the ribosome. If the resulting protein were a metabolic enzyme, the metabolic process for which it was necessary would not be able to take place.

This is precisely what happens in PKU. For some reason, an incorrect nucleotide is present in the DNA strand that codes for the structure of the hepatic enzyme (a protein) necessary for metabolizing phenylalanine. Since phenylalanine is an essential amino acid, a certain amount must be obtained from dietary sources; the genetic defect does not interfere with the utilization of this necessary amount. But the excess phenylalanine is normally converted by the enzyme into the nonessential amino acid tyrosine, which is used for growth and other protein functions. If this pathway is blocked because the key enzyme is missing, phenylalanine is forced to be metabolized by alternate pathways and accumulates, along with its abnormal metabolites, in body fluids. At the same time, there is an inadequate supply of tyrosine. The combination of excessive phenylalanine and its byproducts, and inadequate tyrosine, results in the symptoms found in untreated phenylketonuric patients.

The symptoms, which appear in infants between 6 and 18 months of age, include irritability, hyperactivity, convulsive seizures, lighter skin and hair color than other family members, moderate to severe mental retardation, and a general slowdown of physical growth and development. Untreated individuals have a markedly shortened life expectancy, with only a 25-percent chance of surviving past the third decade.

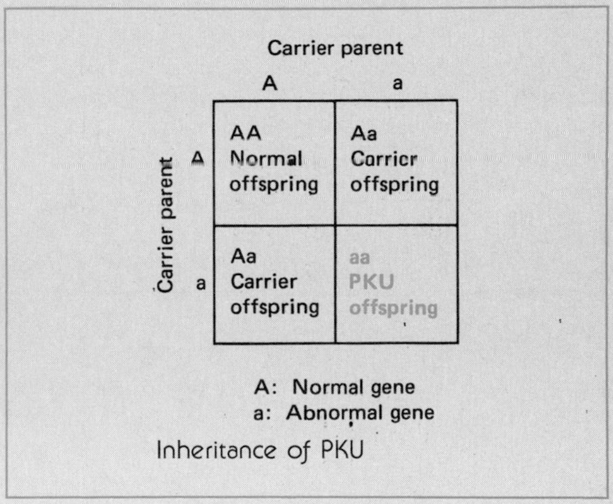

Inheritance of PKU

It is estimated that the mutant gene that accounts for PKU exists in about 1.5 percent of the population. However, because an individual acquires chromosomes equally from each of two parents, and because a normal gene will "overrule" or be dominant over the effects of a mutant, almost all of these individuals have normal or near-normal phenylalanine metabolism. They are, however, "carriers" of the recessive mutation. And if two such carriers should marry, the outcome of *each* pregnancy can be expressed as a statistical probability. Their offspring may have two normal genes for production of the necessary enzyme (25%), may be a carrier like the parents (50%), or may have two recessive genes and therefore be afflicted with PKU.

Fortunately, PKU can now be detected by a simple blood test performed on newborn infants. In this way, the one individual in every 20,000 born with PKU can be identified and immediately treated through careful dietary management. PKU screening of newborns is now mandated in most states.

Dietary management consists of a carefully controlled food plan containing only enough phenylalanine for essential purposes, and an adequate intake of energy, other amino acids, and all other nutrients. Phenylalanine is present in a great many foods of both animal and vegetable origin and is especially plentiful in milk, the basic food in the first months of life. Infants with PKU receive a special formula (Lofenelac, from which phenylalanine has been removed) supplemented by small amounts of cow's milk to provide only as much phenylalanine as necessary. As the child grows older, other foods containing some phenylalanine, mainly fruits and vegetables, are introduced. Animal foods contain excessive amounts and must generally be avoided. Regular blood tests monitor the levels of phenylalanine in the child's blood, and the diet is adjusted accordingly. Near-normal growth and intellectual development can be expected if such a regime is instituted in the earliest weeks of life. Treatment initiated after the first year will eliminate behavioral problems, but will be too late to correct mental retardation.

Current research is concerned with the question of when, or even whether, the PKU diet can be safely discontinued. One study reported no serious consequences following termination at age 6 (Holtzman et al., 1975). However, evidence has also been presented showing that children who were taken off the diet at age 5 or 6 subsequently had lower IQ scores than when they were on the diet, and perhaps some brain damage as well (Cooke, 1978). In the absence of conclusive evidence to the contrary, it would seem prudent to continue dietary management.

With present knowledge we can only hope to alleviate the effects of genetically determined metabolic diseases such as PKU. The protein-synthesizing process is so precise that a single error in one nucleotide sequence can have truly devastating effects. Extensive investigations have been conducted to understand the etiology of such diseases; but much remains to be done to develop adequate screening tests, methods of treatment, and, perhaps in the not-too-distant future, a means of prevention.

(Students interested in a detailed discussion of the nutritional management of PKU should refer to therapeutic nutrition textbooks for additional information. Those interested in inborn errors of metabolism will find a compilation of current knowledge in Stanbury et al., 1978.)

In **deamination,** nitrogen is released from glutamine, a basic amino acid, in the form of ammonia. A new amino acid is produced by the addition of the ammonia to a keto acid (Figure 4-6).

A steady supply of nonessential amino acids for use in protein synthesis depends upon the efficient functioning of these conversion reactions. It is important to remember that these reactions are reversible. Although nonessential amino acids can be synthesized in the body, diet is still the usual source. If, however, the diet fails to provide them in adequate amounts, this process of endogenous synthesis must take up the slack. This fail-safe mechanism ensures that the nonessential amino acids needed for protein synthesis will always be available to the cells.

FIGURE 4-5
Transamination

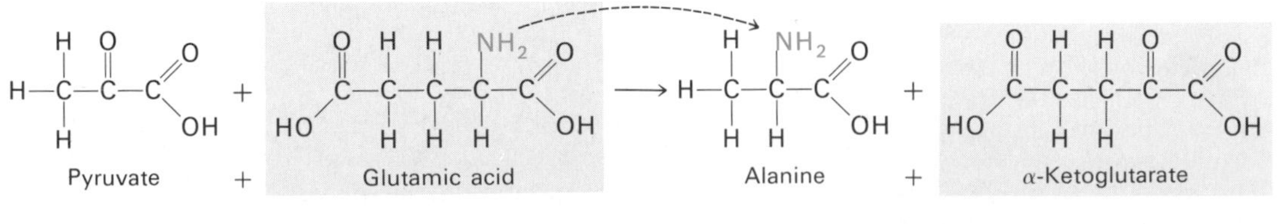

Pyruvate + Glutamic acid → Alanine + α-Ketoglutarate

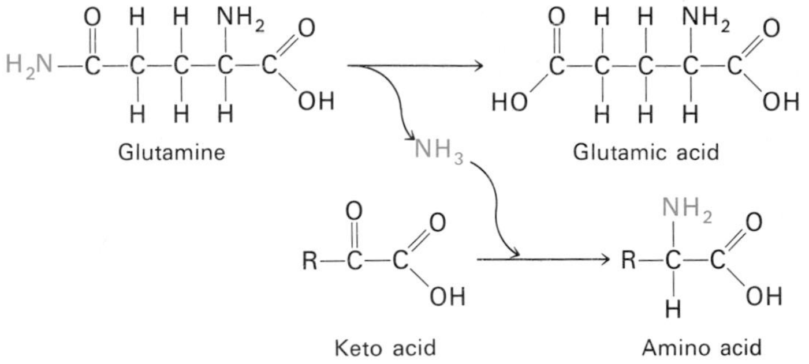

Glutamine → Glutamic acid + NH_3

Keto acid + NH_3 → Amino acid

FIGURE 4-6
Deamination

Gluconeogenesis and Energy Metabolism

When carbohydrate and lipid intake or reserves are insufficient, body proteins and amino acids can be utilized for energy needs. The same amount of energy can be obtained from protein as from carbohydrates—1 gram yields 4 kilocalories. Some amino acids can be converted to glucose by the process gluconeogenesis. Protein that cannot be used immediately is generally metabolized to fat for storage. In all of these processes, the participating amino acids are deaminated to provide the carbon skeleton that takes part in the particular metabolic pathway, releasing ammonia which will be disposed of by the body in the form of urea. These processes are interrelated; we shall discuss first the pathways by which excess protein is converted to glucose, then the circumstances which result in nitrogen loss, and finally the synthesis of lipids from protein.

DISPOSAL OF THE CARBON SKELETON. Once amino acids have lost their nitrogen groups, the remaining carbon skeletons enter the Krebs cycle at various points. Most amino acids are **glycogenic;** that is, their carbon skeletons are degraded to pyruvate or other intermediates (oxaloacetic acid, fumaric acid, succinyl CoA, α-ketoglutarate) that can be transformed into glucose. A few amino acids cannot be converted to glucose; tryptophan and leucine are purely **ketogenic,** being metabolized only to acetoacetyl CoA and acetyl CoA, which enter the Krebs cycle for the production of ATP, CO_2, and water. A few amino acids are both ketogenic and glucogenic and can be converted to acetyl CoA or to glucose.

The process of gluconeogenesis is virtually a reversal of the Embden–Meyerhof pathway (by which glucose is converted to pyruvate). The direction followed along this pathway depends on the metabolic needs of the body at a given time. Amino acids may thus be used to raise blood glucose levels, which subsequently are oxidized for energy.

DISPOSAL OF NITROGEN: THE UREA CYCLE. Humans and other terrestrial vertebrates excrete their nitrogenous wastes (ammonia, NH_3) in the form of urea. Ammonia is highly toxic and must be removed from the blood before it can build up to dangerous concentrations. (It is important to note

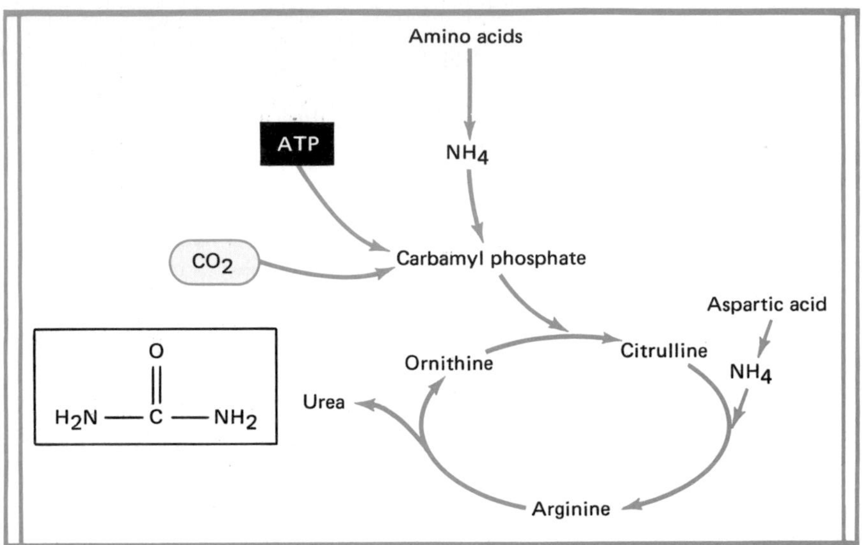

FIGURE 4-7
The Urea Cycle

that transamination alone does not release nitrogen; deamination must follow.) The liver removes ammonia from circulation and converts it to urea in the urea cycle. In the form of urea, the nitrogenous wastes return to the kidney, which dilutes the urea with water and adds other substances prior to excretion.

In the urea cycle, the amino acid ornithine receives ammonia from amino acid deamination and an additional amount from the amino acid aspartic acid. Adding these two nitrogenous components to its amine group, the ornithine is converted to arginine. The enzyme arginase then splits off urea from the arginine, leaving ornithine which continues to circulate (Figure 4-7). The urea cycle requires, in addition to specific enzymes, energy in the now-familiar form of ATP, along with CO_2. Figure 4-8 illustrates the production of urea and energy from the amino acid alanine.

LIPID SYNTHESIS. After the body's amino acid needs for protein synthesis have been met, the amino acid surplus is metabolized to fat and stored in that form. This is accomplished by conversion of the amino acids to pyruvate and acetyl CoA, which are then synthesized to fatty acids. These then combine with a molecule of glycerol to form a triglyceride.

SUMMARY OF PROTEIN METABOLISM. Because of the intricate interactions between protein anabolism and catabolism, we say that these processes are in dynamic equilibrium; that is, the balance between them tips one way or another depending on the immediate need of the individual. Figure 4-9 summarizes protein metabolism. The interaction between and regulation of these pathways depend on various factors that together determine body needs at a given time. These factors include the organism's stage in the life cycle, hormonal balance, energy status, presence of disease, and the availability of appropriate substrate (the specific amino acids needed for a given process). The normal turnover of body protein, by normal degradation processes, provides much of the supply in the amino acid pool.

FIGURE 4-8
Summary of Amino Acid Catabolism

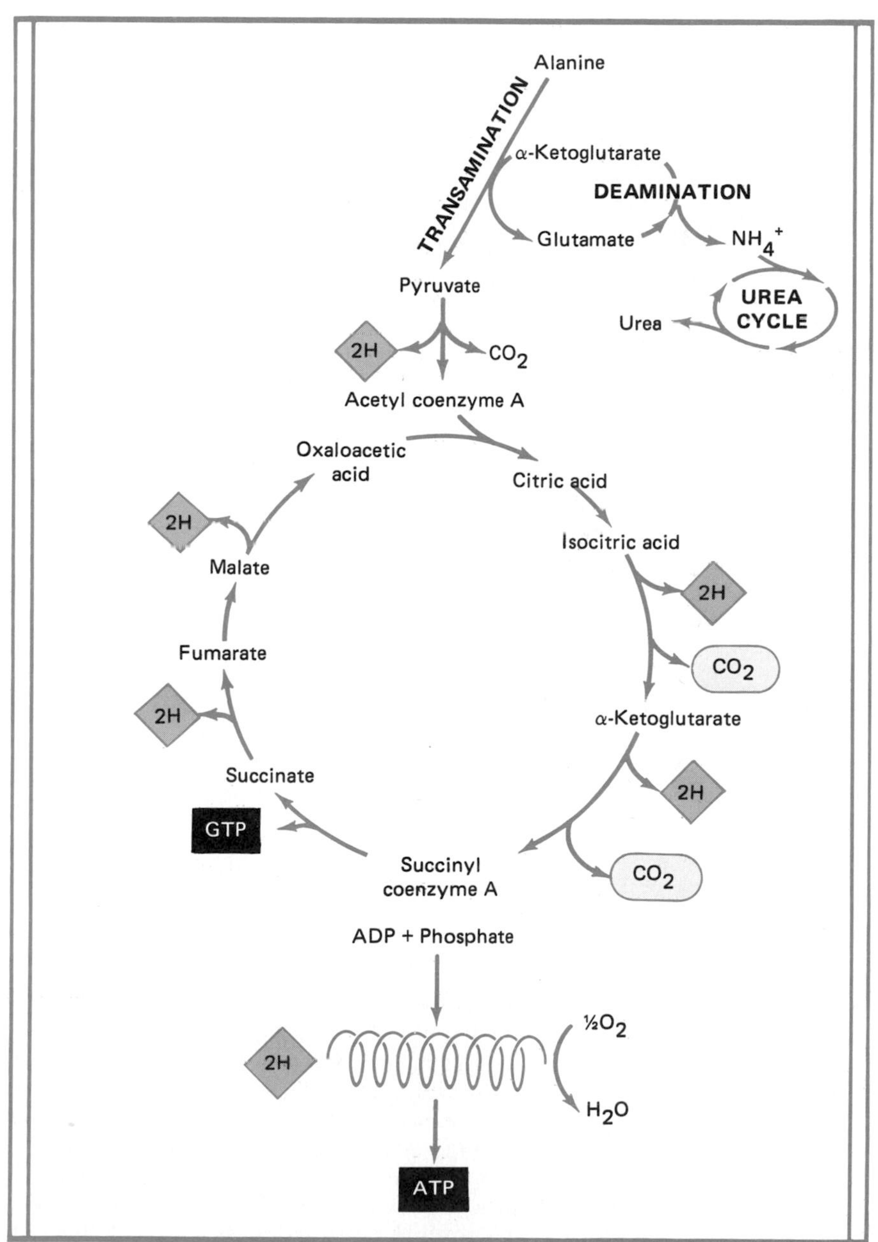

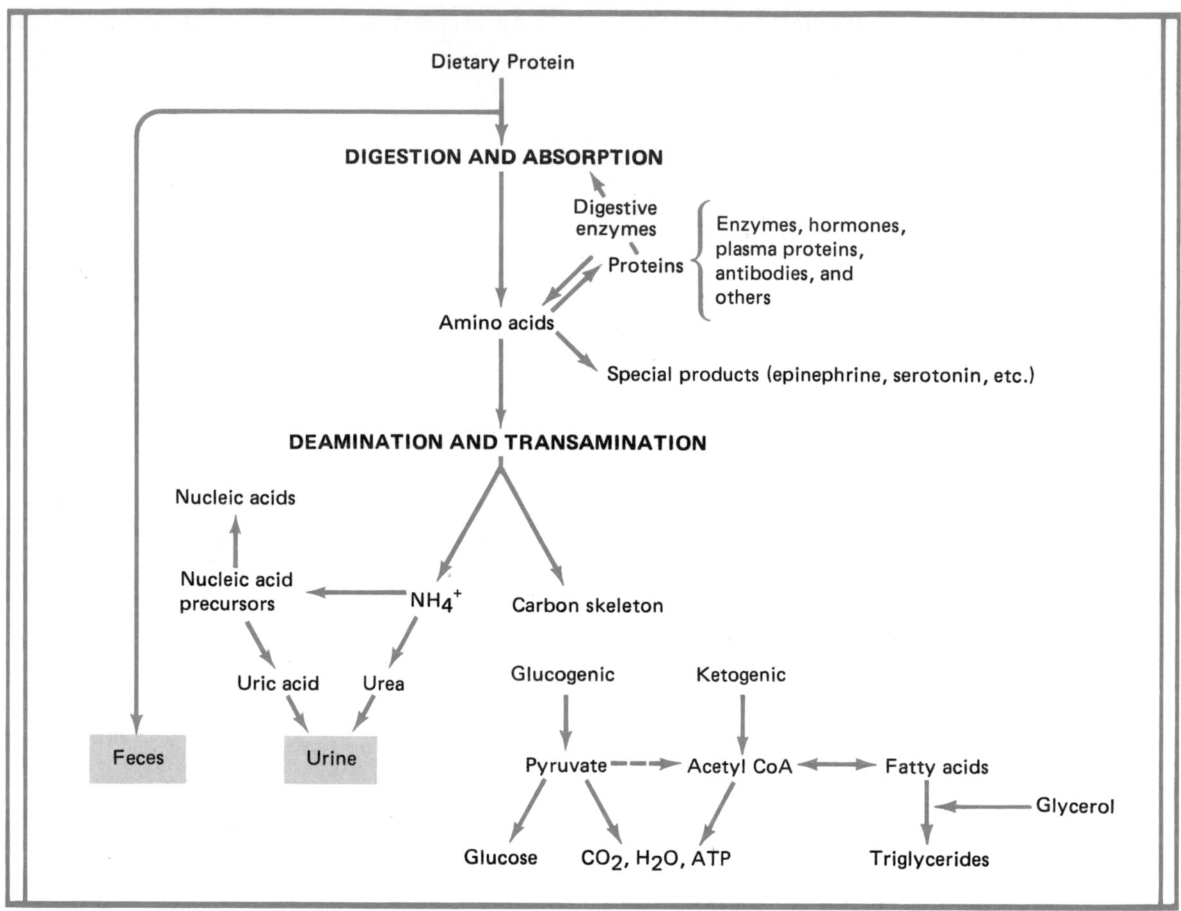

FIGURE 4-9
Summary of Protein Metabolism

PROTEIN REQUIREMENTS

There is no storage of protein in the body; and because protein is constantly being depleted, there is a need to replenish the supply through diet every day. Estimates of the amount of protein that must be provided in the diet have varied widely. In the late nineteenth century, the German physiologist Carl Voit concluded, after a statistical analysis of the diets of his countrymen, that an average adult man doing moderate physical work needed 118 grams of dietary protein per day, or 1.5 grams per kilogram of body weight. In the early twentieth century, however, in a series of meticulous experiments, the American Russell H. Chittenden showed that 40 to 60 grams per day, from a varied food selection, were enough to maintain health and nitrogen balance. Later, work pioneered by William Rose (1949) demonstrated that there were requirements for individual essential amino acids as well as for overall protein intake.

Nitrogen Balance Studies

Traditionally, protein requirements have been determined through nitrogen balance studies, which compare intake and excretion of that element. Significant discoveries have been made in this way, despite the fact that precise measurements of nitrogen content of dietary protein and excretory products (urine, feces, and wastes from the skin) are time consuming, subject to error, and, especially for human subjects, expensive. It is, of course, essential to control all conditions of such experiments.

Nitrogen balance data are conveniently expressed as actual protein gained or lost over a period of time. Because approximately 16 percent of protein consists of nitrogen, it is possible to obtain a valid estimate of total protein by multiplying grams of nitrogen by 6.25. Thus, 2 grams of nitrogen would be roughly equivalent to 12.5 grams of protein. However, protein requirements can be validly estimated by the nitrogen balance method only when energy intake is adequate. Otherwise, dietary protein will be diverted to make up any energy deficit, and protein requirements will be overestimated.

COMPONENTS OF NITROGEN LOSS. As we have seen, the predominant nitrogen compound excreted in urine is urea. Certain nonprotein compounds containing nitrogen, such as creatinine and uric acid, make smaller contributions. Whenever protein intake exceeds the amount the body can use immediately, the nitrogen content of the urine increases. As protein intake decreases, the nitrogen content of the urine correspondingly decreases. However, even with very low protein intake (or none at all), a small amount of nitrogen continues to be excreted. This is known as the obligatory urinary nitrogen loss.

Nitrogen from undigested protein, both dietary and endogenous, is also excreted in the feces. On average, fecal nitrogen excretion of an adult is about one gram per day, but the actual amount for any individual depends on the efficiency of digestion and absorption, and possibly also on the specific dietary proteins consumed. Persons with malabsorptive disorders will have increased levels of nitrogen in the feces.

Nitrogen is also lost from the skin, principally in sloughed-off epidermal cells, lost hair and nails, and in perspiration. Small as these contributions to overall nitrogen losses may be, they are not insignificant. In fact, profuse sweating can increase nitrogen loss substantially. However, with acclimatization to a warm environment, such losses are reduced (FAO/WHO, 1973). Loss of blood through hemorrhage will also add to nitrogen loss and may even be heavy enough to place an individual in negative nitrogen balance, in which nitrogen loss exceeds intake.

Determination of Protein Quality

Early in the twentieth century, a series of classic experiments led to the development of the concept of *protein quality*, which is an important factor in determining protein requirements. Studies with growing rats showed that growth, as measured in weight gain, was supported by the milk protein casein but not by wheat protein, and that an actual loss of weight resulted when the corn protein zein was the sole dietary protein. Further investigations made it clear that the differences in ability of these proteins to support growth were due to differences in their amino acid composition. A number of indices have since been developed for measuring protein quality, several of which are based on the nitrogen balance principle.

BIOLOGICAL VALUE. **Biological value** is an index of protein quality that reflects the percentage of absorbed nitrogen from dietary protein actually utilized (retained) by the body, measured under standard conditions. The derived figure is an estimate of the adequacy of a given protein to meet body needs. The basic formula for biological value is

$$BV = \frac{N_{retained}}{N_{absorbed}} \times 100.$$

To determine the biological value of a given protein food source, that food must be fed (usually to rats) exclusively during the test period. Nitrogen content of diet, urine, and feces is measured, and numerical values are derived for use with the following equivalent formula:

$$BV = \frac{\text{Dietary N} - (\text{Urinary N} + \text{Fecal N})}{\text{Dietary N} - \text{Fecal N}} \times 100$$

The greater the proportion of nitrogen retained, the higher is the biological value, or quality, of the protein being tested. Protein foods containing optimal quantities and proportions of all the essential amino acids, as well as adequate supplies of nonessential amino acids, will have the highest biological values. Eggs, for example, top the list with a biological value ranging from 87 to 97, a near-perfect score; cow's milk, at 85–90, is a close second. Note that these are animal protein sources; no plant protein even approaches these values, although rice and tofu, a soybean product, have biological values of 75. But, with the exception of gelatin, no animal protein has a BV lower than 72. Generally speaking, and provided that caloric intake is adequate to meet energy needs, proteins with a biological value of 70 or more are capable of supporting growth.

When a diet consisting of mixed proteins is analyzed, the biological value of the mixture is usually greater than the average of the biological values of its component proteins. This complementary effect is due to the fact that particular amino acids deficiencies in one protein source are often made up by another source, thus increasing the usefulness of the otherwise "incomplete" proteins to the body.

The timing of ingestion is crucial to this synergistic effect of mixed proteins. Because tissues must have all the necessary amino acids present at the same time for protein synthesis to occur, complementary proteins should be eaten in the same meal for optimal effect. Otherwise, some dietary amino acids will be wasted, since an excess of one kind absorbed on one day cannot be held over for use on the next.

NET PROTEIN UTILIZATION. Even the best mix of amino acids will be less available for use if it is packaged in a protein that is only partially digested.

Net protein utilization (NPU) is an index that takes into account the relative digestibility of proteins. It is, simply, biological value multiplied by digestibility, expressed as a percent; NPU is determined by the following formulas:

$$\text{NPU} = \frac{N_{\text{retained}}}{\text{Dietary N}} \times 100$$

$$= \frac{\text{Dietary N} - (\text{Urinary N} + \text{Fecal N})}{\text{Dietary N}} \times 100$$

Proteins are generally easy to digest, however, with most being 90 percent or more digestible. Thus, in most cases, NPU approximates the BV.

PROTEIN EFFICIENCY RATIO. Unlike the indices previously discussed, the **protein efficiency ratio** (PER) is not based on nitrogen balance studies. For this reason, it is somewhat less precise than biological value and NPU, but it is technically easier to derive and use. The protein efficiency ratio is defined as the change in body weight relative to the amount of protein eaten. It is usually measured in laboratory rats kept under standardized conditions. If a rat receives 2 grams of casein per day as the sole dietary protein in an otherwise standard diet, and gains 5 grams of weight per day, the PER of casein would be determined as 2.5:

$$\text{PER} = \frac{\text{Weight gain in grams}}{\text{Dietary protein in grams}}$$

Whole egg has a PER of 3.8, while at the other extreme gelatin has a PER of 0. PER values are used in labeling foods to show the nutritional value of the protein they contain.

AMINO ACID SCORE. Another index of protein quality, the **chemical score,** is based on chemical analysis, not on a biological test. It compares the content of essential amino acids in a protein or protein mixture with that found in a standard reference protein, defined by the FAO/WHO (1973). The amino acid score is determined by the following formula:

$$\text{Amino acid score} = \frac{\text{Milligrams of amino acid per gram of test protein}}{\text{Milligrams of amino acid per gram of reference protein}} \times 100$$

The score of the test protein is determined by the amino acid that is lowest in proportion to its amount in the reference protein. In soybeans, for example, the sulfur-containing amino acids methionine and cystine are the essential amino acids present in the smallest proportion to their level in the reference protein. Since soybean protein has only 74 percent as much of these amino acids as the reference protein, the amino acid score of soybean protein is 74. The sulfur-containing amino acids are then the limiting amino acids in soybean protein. Generally, lysine, threonine, and the sulfur-containing amino acids are the limiting amino acids in most foods. Importantly, measurement of protein quality by this method corresponds quite well to biological testing methods, emphasizing the accuracy and usefulness of all of these indices.

Provisional Amino Acid Scoring Pattern

Amino Acid	Suggested Level mg/1 g of Protein
Isoleucine	40
Leucine	70
Lysine	55
Methionine + cystine	35
Phenylalanine + tyrosine	60
Threonine	40
Tryptophan	10
Valine	50
Total	360

Source: FAO Nutrition Report Series No. 52, *Energy and protein requirements*, WHO Technical Report Series No. 522 (Rome: Food and Agricultural Organization, 1973), p. 63.

The significance of this concept of limiting amino acids was demonstrated when rats, whose growth had halted when they were fed on wheat protein, resumed growing when they were given supplementary lysine. Lysine is the limiting amino acid in wheat protein; supplementary amounts enabled the organism to make greater use of the other amino acids in the wheat protein. Similar results were observed when rats fed on corn protein were provided with a lysine and tryptophan supplement. Here, then, is experimental evidence for the "all-or-none" amino acid requirement previously discussed at the molecular level. (Remember, if even one of the several amino acids required for synthesis of a specific protein molecule is not available in the amino acid pool when it is summoned to the ribosomes by RNA, synthesis of that protein is halted.)

This concept of limiting amino acids has a number of practical applications. It is, for example, important in the dietary planning of informed vegetarians. Since every plant-origin food is low in one or more essential amino acids, vegetarians must try at every meal to include foods providing complementary proteins (Figure 4-10). In another application, food engineers are developing special products, such as mixtures of plant proteins in which the limiting amino acid of one protein component is provided by an amino acid found in greater amounts in another. Incaparina is an example of a plant protein food developed especially for child feeding programs in Guatemala. Such foods provide a high-quality protein mix in a relatively inexpensive and easily stored form, making them as nutritious but less expensive and more readily available than animal food sources (Scrimshaw, 1959).

There have been other attempts to increase the chemical scores of foods, especially plant foods. Agricultural research has, for example, already produced new strains of wheat with increased levels of lysine and tryptophan (the limiting amino acids in traditional varieties). Direct fortification of wheat flour with lysine has also been practiced in some developing countries.

Protein-enriched products are also appearing on supermarket shelves in the United States. One recent addition is a wheat-and-soy-flour spaghetti, which also contains corn germ and added lysine. It contains 13 grams of protein per 2-ounce serving (compared to 8 grams in ordinary spaghetti), and the quality

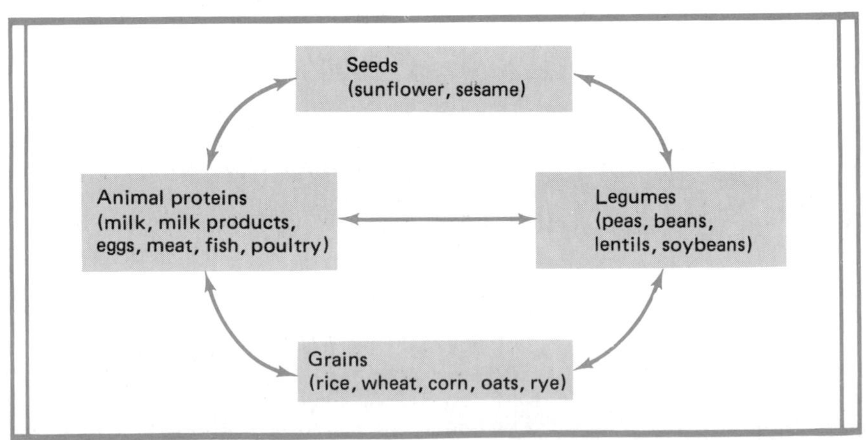

FIGURE 4-10
Food Combinations Providing Complementary Proteins
Combinations of foods represented in groups connected by arrows should be eaten together.

of the protein, moreover, is improved by the additional complementary amino acids. It is also more expensive than ordinary spaghetti: In a recent supermarket check, 12 ounces of the new product cost as much as 16 ounces of the standard version. However, the new product is being marketed as a meat alternative, and it is notably less expensive per serving than most animal protein sources.

Fortified foods used in conjunction with a generally low protein diet can result in an amino acid imbalance. Experiments with laboratory animals have shown that excesses of certain amino acids can create an increased need for the next most limiting amino acid, leading to diminished appetite, growth failure, and other metabolic abnormalities. That overfortification may have similar effects in humans, while not yet ascertained, should be considered a possibility (Harper, 1973).

Protein and Amino Acid Requirements

The body's needs for essential amino acids and nitrogen require dietary protein of optimal quality and adequate quantity. Obviously, the bodies of different individuals will have different needs, which are governed by a variety of factors including genetic variation, sex, age, overall health status, and perhaps climate and occupation.

In the first month of life, a stage of rapid growth, infants require at least 2 grams of protein per kilogram of body weight per day. This amount is, of course, provided in milk. Protein requirements fall gradually as the child's growth rate slows, dropping to 1.5 grams per kilogram at 6 months, and continues falling even more gradually throughout life.

Pregnancy substantially increases the protein requirement for women, to provide for the growth of the fetus and additional tissues in the mother. Some evidence suggests, furthermore, that efficiency of protein utilization is lowered during pregnancy, thereby increasing the need for dietary sources. During lactation, also, protein needs are markedly increased, since the milk produced by the mother must supply the protein for the infant's growth needs (National Academy of Sciences, 1979).

Illness and other physiological, and perhaps psychological, stresses lead to increased nitrogen loss and thus increase protein requirements. Although profuse sweating increases nitrogen loss and therefore the protein requirement, only a slight increase in protein intake will adjust for all but the most active sports or heaviest physical labor. Any period of nutritional inadequacy, whether from dieting or disaster, will also increase needs for protein, since available supplies will be diverted to energy needs, leaving less for protein functions.

On the basis of various nitrogen balance studies, the basal protein requirement for an average adult male has been estimated at 0.47 grams per kilogram body weight. This figure, however, is not the same as a recommendation or dietary allowance, which must take into account the greater-than-average needs of about half of the population. To allow for individual variations, the basal estimate is increased by 30 percent (which also provides a margin for error), to 0.61 g/kg. A correction is also made for 75-percent efficiency of utilization, on the assumption that the average American diet contains protein with average biological values of 75. This results in an adjusted protein recommendation of 0.8 g/kg body weight per day.

For a man weighing 70 kilograms, the protein allowance is thus 56 grams per day; for a woman of 55 kilograms, it is 44 grams per day. Protein allowances have also been issued by the Food and Nutrition Board to cover the special needs of pregnant and lactating women, to distinguish between the needs of males and females at every age, and to account for greater requirements in the younger years (see Appendix, Table A). Generally, these allowances will meet all amino acid needs if half of the daily intake is of high quality protein providing all the essential amino acids in optimal balance.

Other indices of protein quality have also been used to determine protein requirements, and a vast literature has developed detailing the requirements of human beings under various circumstances; a review of this literature (Irwin and Hegsted, 1971) can be consulted by interested students. Some of the factors that must be considered in research on protein requirements have been outlined in a recently published lecture (Scrimshaw, 1977).

PROTEIN EXCESS AND PROTEIN DEFICIENCY

Excessive intake of proteins, unlike that of other major nutrients, is not a significant dietary hazard for healthy people. A few problems have been noticed, but normal individuals can apparently tolerate large amounts of amino acids as long as all essential amino acids are included in a well-balanced pattern. In an early study, human subjects subsisted exclusively on meat, with intakes of 100 to 140 grams of protein per day, for a year without showing evidence of adverse effects (McClellan and Dubois, 1930, cited in Draper, 1977).

Essential Amino Acid Content of an Egg

Amino Acid	Milligrams per Egg
Tryptophan	97
Threonine	298
Isoleucine	380
Leucine	533
Lysine	410
Phenylalanine	343
Valine	437
Methionine	196
Total protein	12.1%

Source: Consumer and Food Economics Institute, *Composition of foods—Dairy and egg products—Raw, processed, prepared,* USDA Agricultural Handbook No. 8-1 (Washington, D.C.: U.S. Government Printing Office, 1976).

High Protein Intake and the Arctic Eskimo

The Eskimo people constitute a particularly interesting natural laboratory for studying the effects of a predominantly protein diet. Traditionally, approximately 82 percent of the protein intake of Eskimos in Alaska was provided by meat and fish alone, with the remainder derived from all other sources; just under a third of total calories were provided by protein. (Lipids accounted for nearly all the remaining energy intake, with carbohydrate making a negligible contribution; Draper, 1977). Although these levels were considerably higher than those found in other populations, no adverse effects were associated with this diet pattern (Heller and Scott, 1967).

A predominantly meat and fish diet, however, raises concern about calcium, which most populations derive from milk and other dairy products, and which is needed for bone development and maintenance. Apparently Eskimos ingest just enough soft bone and cartilage, especially of fish and sea mammals, to prevent noticeable calcium deficiencies. However, additional

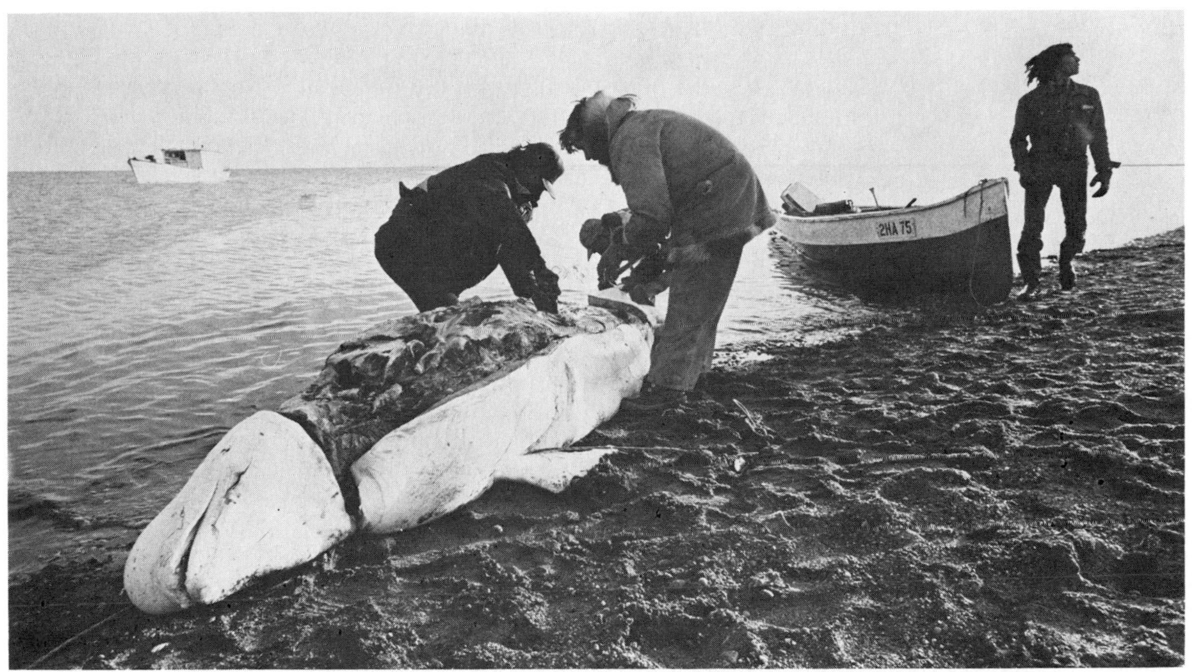

A Beluga whale being cut up by Eskimos at their whaling camp near Kittigasuit, Beaufort Sea (Artic Ocean), Northwest Territories, Canada. (Paolo Koch/-Photo Researchers).

concern has been raised about the Eskimo diet because high protein intakes increase urinary calcium loss (see Chapter 8). High rates of bone loss have indeed been observed among older Eskimos in northern Alaska, and there is a good possibility that this condition may be associated with their high protein and relatively low calcium intake (Draper, 1977).

Surprisingly, the Eskimo have been found, despite their high-protein, high-fat diet, to have normal cholesterol levels. This is attributed to the high levels of polyunsaturated fats in the fish and lean mammals they consume (Draper, 1977). High excretion levels of nitrogenous wastes from amino acid metabolism are associated with consumption of a great deal of water and are apparently tolerated without difficulty (Draper, 1977).

Eskimos have been genetically adapted to their traditional diet. However, those who have moved to towns and cities are being exposed to, and are acquiring some of the food habits of other Americans. Dietary acculturation is being accompanied by obesity, cardiovascular diseases, hypertension, and tooth decay—problems all too familiar in the "lower forty-eight" but seldom encountered with the traditional diet (Draper, 1977).

Most humans are not quite as well adapted to high protein intakes as are the Eskimo, and it is known that liver and kidney damage can result from prolonged and markedly excessive intakes. This indicates that regulation of a variety of metabolic processes is undermined when those organs must process excessive quantities of amino acids and remove large amounts of nitrogenous wastes. For this reason, too, kidney damage may result from high-protein weight-loss diets. Because kidney function is not fully developed in infants, substantial protein intake is not recommended in the early months of life, and protein foods should be introduced gradually.

Protein Deficiency

Kwashiorkor, the disease resulting from a deficit of protein relative to energy intake, was first noted in Africa and described by Cicely Williams (1935) and has subsequently been noted in Latin American and Asian populations as well. It was considered of sufficient importance that, at its first meeting in 1949, the FAO/WHO Expert Committee on Nutrition called for a study of kwashiorkor etiology in Africa (Brock and Autret, 1952).

Kwashiorkor (the name of the disease is derived from a West African word which means "sickness of the child when a second baby is born") generally appears shortly after weaning. In traditional societies this usually occurs between 1 and 4 years of age and is precipitated by the arrival of a new baby who must receive the mother's milk. The young child is suddenly put on a traditional diet, consisting almost exclusively of grains and other carbohydrates. Such a diet provides adequate energy but very little vegetable protein and no animal protein. Kwashiorkor is sometimes found in adults, but children are more frequently afflicted because of their higher protein and energy requirements in proportion to body weight. Adults can consume enough rice or other grains to meet their protein needs, but the sheer bulk of such foods necessary to approach the protein needs of children would be simply too much for them to eat.

Children of Biafra suffering from kwashiorkor. (Daily Telegraph Magazine Woodfin Camp & Associates)

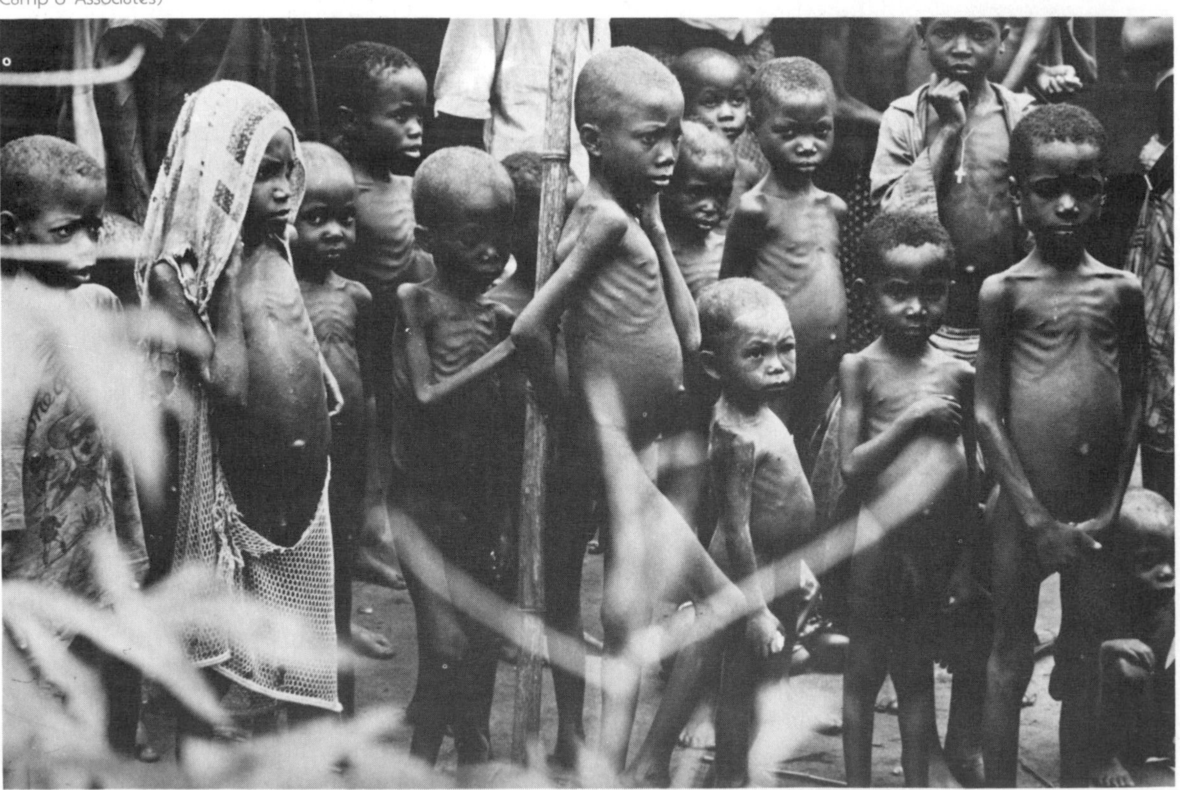

The first symptoms may well go unnoticed. The child seems listless and loses appetite and may develop a sudden attack of diarrhea or other infection due to lowered resistance. Edema, the accumulation of interstitial fluid, especially in the legs and abdomen, follows shortly—and is often misinterpreted, since the puffiness and apparent weight gain due to fluid retention give the child a healthy and well-fed appearance for a while. Often, the first symptoms noted by the family are the loss of pigmentation in the hair and skin, the loss of some hair itself, and the development of patchy, discolored and/or sore areas on the body. Clinical symptoms also include decreased amino acid levels in blood plasma, decreased serum albumin, fat accumulation in the liver, decreased production of pancreatic enzymes (which results in malabsorption of what little nourishment is available), and marked retardation of physical and mental growth, along with increased susceptibility to infection.

The interaction of malnutrition and infection is synergistic. Even a moderate protein shortage weakens the body's resistance. Infection makes greater demands for protein and thus sets up a vicious cycle in which the protein deficit is ever greater and malnutrition more severe, causing the individual to deteriorate more rapidly. In many cultures, this interaction is aggravated by the belief that food should be withheld when a person, and particularly a child, is ill. Usually it is infection, and not specific symptoms of kwashiorkor, that leads to the child being brought for treatment.

If recognized at an early stage, kwashiorkor responds readily to feedings of skim milk and animal protein, with vegetables and fat added gradually. At the beginning of treatment, only 2 to 3 grams of protein and 61 kilocalories per kilogram body weight are given, increasing to 6 or 7 grams protein and 100 to 120 kilocalories per kilogram of body weight within 10 days to two weeks (Mayer, 1972). In advanced cases, however, irreversible damage, especially to growth and the digestive system, may have already occurred. Even where treatment has been successful, the child is most likely to return home to the same inadequate diet that caused the condition in the first place, so that relapse within a matter of months is common. Mortality following repeated episodes of kwashiorkor is high (Mayer, 1972).

Kwashiorkor is now being considered as but one form of protein-energy malnutrition (PEM). Another form is marasmus, the disease condition reflecting deficits of energy and due to a generally inadequate food supply; it will be discussed in Chapter 15.

Recently, the incidence of kwashiorkor has increased in populations that have accepted bottled formula instead of mother's milk for infant feeding. Because of poverty, inadequate amounts of formula are extended with plain water (which is often unsanitary as well), and the infant receives fewer rather than more, nutrients.

In the United States and other developed countries, kwashiorkor is not likely to be a problem. Occasional instances, however, have been reported. Lozoff and Fanaroff (1975), for example, saw two cases in which milk was removed from the diets of two infants in Cleveland, and typical symptoms of kwashiorkor developed. In both cases, misconceptions on the part of the mothers were the cause. Both infants responded to appropriate therapy, and the mothers were instructed in the importance of milk. Because American physicians are generally unfamiliar with this syndrome, and are unlikely, due to its rarity, to suspect the absence of milk from an infant's diet, diagnosis is likely to be delayed.

Generally, protein deficiency is nonexistent in the United States. However, certain subgroups—pregnant and lactating women of low socioeconomic levels and their children, elderly persons on a limited budget, the chronically ill—may have subclinical protein deficiencies and serum levels may be low, due to suboptimal intakes. Certainly the social, economic, educational, and other factors responsible for such instances should be corrected. But American protein intake is typically higher, not lower, than allowances.

TRENDS IN U.S. PROTEIN CONSUMPTION

The protein content of the American diet has remained essentially the same for most of this century, but the sources of that protein have changed considerably. The most striking changes are the increase of 40 percent in meat consumption and the decrease of 50 percent in the consumption of flour and cereal grains, which formerly constituted fully half of our protein intake (Rensberger, 1978; Brewster and Jacobson, 1978). But overall, protein consumption has not varied much over the years, with little difference between the 1910 and 1976 figures of 102 and 101 grams respectively. The low of 88 grams in 1945–1946 was still well above recommended allowances (Rensberger, 1978; Chopra et al., 1978).

The dramatic increase in meat consumption reflects an increase in consumption of virtually every category of animal protein—beef, veal, poultry, fish, and shellfish (see Figure 4-11). Of all animal protein sources, only pork, lamb, egg, and dairy product consumption have not increased significantly (Brewster and Jacobson, 1978). (It should be remembered that consumption statistics are derived from "disappearance data," discussed in Chapter 2, which tally the sources available in the marketplace, but may not accurately reflect actual consumption.)

Reasons for this strong trend are interrelated and not hard to find. Meat in general, and beef in particular, have always been viewed as "status" foods, and increased protein, meat and beef consumption have been observed to accompany increased prosperity in virtually all times and places. Americans are not alone in this trend: Meat consumption in Taiwan and South Korea has doubled in the last 20 years, and in Japan it has increased ninefold (Rensberger, 1978). Increased meat consumption is everywhere associated with improved economic conditions, suggesting that any people able to afford a high-meat diet will eat one.

But in some ways the American emphasis on beef is unique. From the time the continent was opened up for settlement, cattle raising has been a dominant force both in folklore (with its songs and stories concerning cowboys and life "on the lone prairie") and as big business. Increased industrialization of every aspect of meat production, from cattle breeding to chicken plucking, along with improved marketing practices, greatly increased availability. The more recent "fast-food" phenomenon, with its emphasis on burgers and fried chicken, has made ever more animal protein available on every street and superhighway. Even the growth of suburbia and the development of tract

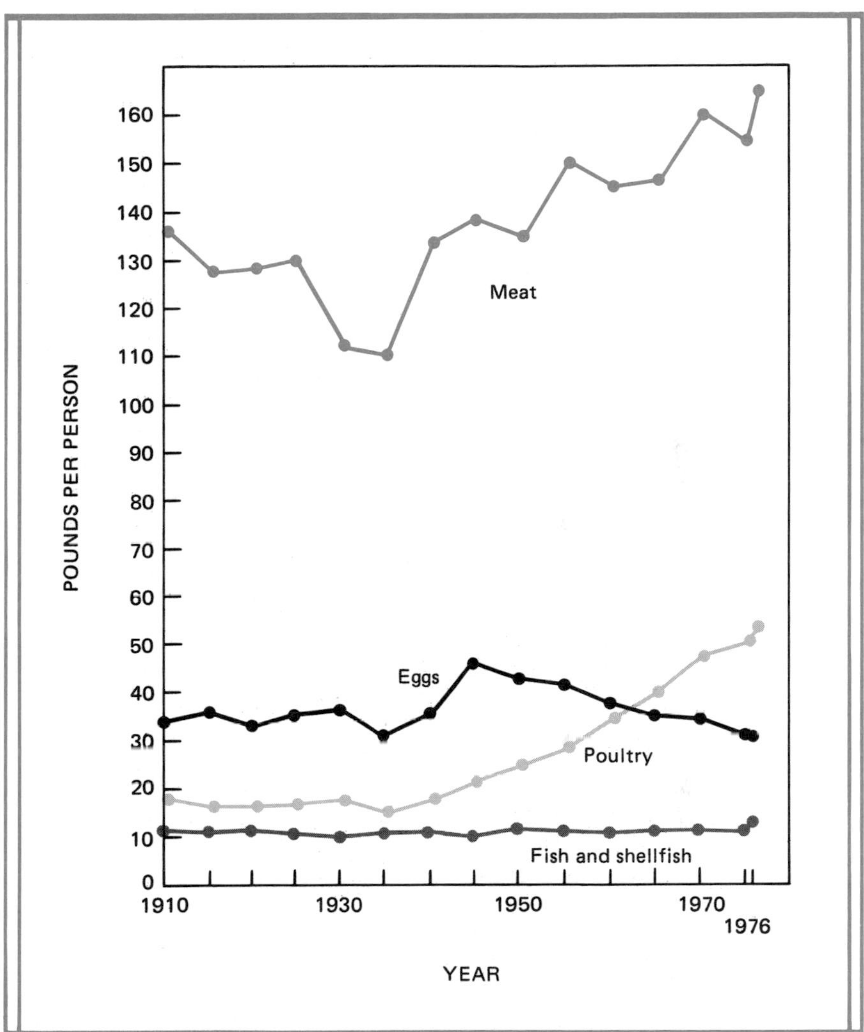

FIGURE 4-11

Consumption Trends for Primary Sources of Protein in the American Diet

Source: adapted from L. Brewster and M. Jacobson, *The changing American diet* (Washington, D.C.: Center for Science in the Public Interest, 1978).

housing had an effect, as the backyard barbecue became a way of life (Rensberger, 1978). To these influences must be added those which at the same time decreased our consumption of vegetarian sources of protein: the disappearance of the small farm and the home vegetable garden, the sharp decline in home baking and other time-consuming methods of food preparation, and substitution of the "eat-and-run" breakfast for the traditional morning meal of hot cereal.

Whether this trend is desirable from a nutritional viewpoint does not relate to problems of protein excess (which is not dangerous for most people) but, rather, to the high levels of saturated fats, cholesterol, and kilocalories in animal food. Each of these may be involved in the development of heart disease.

In any event, despite statements to the contrary from some segments of the food industry, we in the United States are far from being a protein-malnourished nation. In several studies it has been shown that even most low-income individuals consume well over the RDAs for protein. Among the few exceptions are some low-income teenage girls, pregnant and lactating women, and elderly men and women, in all of whom moderate (not major) protein deficits are related to suboptimal food intake generally (Chopra et al., 1978). Although all such individuals would benefit from increasing their total food consumption, hardly anyone in the United States would benefit from protein supplements. Misconceptions are at the root of what Hegsted calls the "protein mystique" that would make everything, from baby food to snack food, "high protein" (Hegsted, 1976).

While the cost of beef and most other meats and fish is high and going higher, top-quality proteins are available at reasonable prices for most people. Table 4-4 shows the cost per 14-gram protein serving of a number of good sources of this nutrient. Eggs, beef liver, beans, peanut butter, American cheese, chicken, and dry milk are all protein "bargains." Since four such servings would meet daily protein requirements for just about everyone, even in these inflationary times, a good supply of dietary protein can be had for less than a dollar a day.

TABLE 4-4
Cost per 14-gram Protein Serving of Selected Foods

Food	Serving Size to Provide 14 Grams Protein	Cost of 14 Grams Protein
Dry beans	1 c, cooked	$ .09
Peanut butter	$3\frac{1}{2}$ tbsp	.12
Eggs	2 eggs	.15
Bologna	4-5 slices (if 18 slices/lb)	.56
Beef liver	(6-7 servings/lb)	.22
Milk	$1\frac{3}{4}$ c	.19
Dry milk	9 tbsp	.12
Cottage cheese	(4-5 servings/lb)	.16
Hamburger	(5-6 servings/lb)	.32
Haddock fillets	(5-6 servings/lb)	.35
Tuna fish	2 oz	.39
American process cheese	$2\frac{1}{2}$ slices (if 16-18 slices/lb)	.26
Chicken, whole	(4 servings/lb)	.22
Ham, whole	(4-5 servings/lb)	.57
Pork sausage links	6 links (if 16 links/lb)	.69
Frankfurters	about $2\frac{1}{2}$ (if 10/lb)	.37
Pork chops with bone	(4 servings/lb)	.33
Bacon, sliced	$5\frac{1}{2}$ slices (if 20 slices/lb)	.60
Sirloin steak, choice-grade	($4\frac{1}{3}$ servings/lb)	.73
Rib roast of beef	(4-5 servings/lb)	1.04
Round pot roast	(6-7 servings/lb)	.36

Source: Prices in a Boston supermarket, May 31, 1979.

PERSPECTIVE ON
Vegetarianism

In recent years, **vegetarianism** has become increasingly widespread, particularly among young adults who often adopt this eating pattern out of philosophical and/or religious conviction. There is nothing new about this phenomenon; in Ancient Greece and Rome vegetarianism was advocated, both as a protest against the dietary excesses of the upper classes and for its alleged health benefits and moral purity. For that matter, most of the world's human beings normally obtain their nutrients primarily from plant foods. This is, however, not from choice, but because meat has been unobtainable for individuals in most parts of the world for most of human existence. Although the cave dwellers of the ice age are often envisioned as clubbing and tearing into mammoths and other beasts, there is evidence that much of the diet of earliest times was of plant origin. This should not be surprising, since most primates are herbivores.

In the United States, however, people have become vegetarians by choice. A particular influence in recent years has been the new interest in the religions of the East, Hinduism and Buddhism, both of which have attracted large numbers of adherents among young Americans. These religions prohibit consumption of meat, a consequence of their belief in reincarnation and reverence for all life. Some religious groups in the West also espouse vegetarianism: For Trappist monks it is part of their vow of poverty and their generally abstemious lifestyle, and for Seventh Day Adventists it is recommended, although optional. Philosophical and even politicoeconomic reasons advanced by American vegetarians who are not "into" Eastern religions include concern over the world food supply and the three-to-one proportion of grain feed required to produce beef. Many find the slaughter of animals for food abhorrent; others are emulating such hero figures as Thoreau; and some are motivated by health concerns such as reducing cholesterol and saturated fat intake.

The types of vegetarianism are as diverse as the motivations of their adherents. Some individuals abstain only from red meat, or from red meat and poultry, while continuing to eat fish. Lacto-ovo-vegetarians will generally eat no animal flesh but include eggs, milk, and dairy products in their menus. Some people have chosen to be only lacto-vegetarians, eating milk and cheeses but not eggs, or to be ovo-vegetarians, eating eggs but no dairy products. Strict or pure vegetarians, or **vegans** as they are often called, consume no foods of animal origin at all. (Interestingly, one study of food intake of vegetarians found that, in every category, some individuals included fish as part of their diet—as many vegans ate fish as did not; Brown and Bergan, 1975.)

Adherents of Zen macrobiotic diets may fall into several categories on the basis of actual food habits, since the Zen program consists of a ranked series of ten dietary plans. At the beginning level, some animal foods are included along with fruits, vegetables, and cereal grains. A particular mark of the Zen system is its division of foods into two opposing categories of Yin (foods that are light, sweet or sour, hot) and Yang (heavy, salty, bitter, red). Five parts Yin to one part Yang is considered the ideal balance, and brown rice allegedly is the most ideally balanced food. At the "highest" Zen level, the foods allowed are extremely restricted and consist almost solely of brown rice and green bancha tea. Fluid intake is progressively limited along with the range of permissible foods, and resulting problems include kidney disorders.

Historically, the major nutritional concern has focused on the protein content of vegetarian diets. Those vegetarians who include fish, eggs, and/or dairy products in their menus will not have any problems. But strict vegetarian programs require careful planning to provide adequate supplies of proteins from plant sources. Nonanimal protein foods should be eaten in combinations that provide a balance between lysine, tryptophan, and the sulfur-containing amino acids, the amino acids that are generally lacking in foods of plant origin. Vegetarian diets depend heavily on four groups of plant foods: legumes (including beans and peas); grains and cereals; fruits and vegetables; and nuts and seeds. By including something from each of these food groups at every meal, essential amino acids will be assured. Legumes are a good source of lysine but are low in tryptophan and the sulfur-containing amino acids; nuts and seeds and, generally speaking, cereal grains are good sources of tryptophan and sulfur-containing amino acids but are low in lysine. An exception is wheat germ, a cereal product which is a good source of lysine and more akin to legumes in amino acid composition. Many peoples have food patterns that combine these effectively: the beans and rice of Cuba, the corn, beans, and rice of Mexico, and the soybean products and rice of Asian countries are good examples and have, indeed, been emulated by many American vegetarians. The food industry is also making available soybean-based substitutes, or analogs, for many meat products (meat loaf, sausage, and the like).

While amino acid balance may not, then, be a significant problem for most vegetarians, other more important considerations are often overlooked; these concern a number of key vitamins and minerals. Deficiencies of vitamin D, riboflavin, and calcium (especially for children), and iron for women of childbearing age, are potential problems. Zinc and iodine deficiencies are possible as well. A particularly serious problem for pure vegetarians is deficiency of vitamin B_{12}, found only in animal-origin foods and some fermented soybean products. However, a few packaged cereals have recently been fortified with this vitamin.

Adequate riboflavin, iron, and calcium can be provided by generous servings of most green leafy vegetables. Zinc can be obtained from nuts, legumes, and wheat germ, and iodine from use of iodized salt and seaweed. Those vegetarians, and especially those on macrobiotic diets, who use soy sauce and sea salt instead of commercial iodized salt face a potential iodine insufficiency problem. Fortified soy milk and/or exposure to sunlight will provide vitamin D. Nuts and seeds, whole grains, dried fruits, and green vegetables contribute iron; however, women, especially during pregnancy and lactation, should have a supplemental source of this mineral.

On all vegetarian diets, and especially the more strict versions, energy consumption is quite low. For most adults this is not unhealthful, and for many it is probably a distinct advantage. In one study, for example, vegetarian subjects weighed an average of 20 pounds less than omnivorous controls, who averaged 12 to 15 pounds above their ideal weights (Hardinge and Stare, 1954). But evidence is accumulating that infants and children raised on vegetarian diets do not reach their growth potential. A major reason is that the foods they do eat provide more bulk in proportion to energy and nutrients; with relatively small stomach capacity, infants and children are unable to consume the sheer quantity of plant-origin foods that would be necessary to provide nutrient adequacy. In a study of preschool vegetarian children, height, weight, and general development were lower than for nonvegetarian controls, and below standards for their age. The discrepancies became increasingly pronounced after six months of age. There was also some correlation between degree of underdevelopment and the strictness of the vegetarian regime (Dwyer et al., 1978).

A major concern for vegetarian children is vitamin B_{12} deficiency. A recent report described an infant who had been exclusively breast-fed by a strict vegetarian mother. At six months, growth and muscle development were severely retarded, the infant had severe anemia, was in coma, and had other major symptoms as well. Response to intramuscular injections of the vitamin was dramatic (Higginbottom et al., 1978). This case emphasizes the need for B_{12} supplementation for the pregnant and nursing mother on a strict vegetarian diet, the infant, or, preferably, both.

With careful planning to meet the requirements for amino acids, and allowances for calcium, riboflavin, iron, and vitamin B_{12} in particular, a vegetarian diet can be perfectly safe and may even confer some health benefits by reducing obesity and high cholesterol levels. With any diet, and especially with those limited to plant food sources, diversity is the key to success. As we have seen, a combination of protein sources often raises the biological value of "incomplete" proteins. No one food contains all nutrients. When any group of foods is entirely eliminated from the diet, special care must be taken to ensure that nutrient requirements are met from acceptable food categories. Unless supplemented, strict vegan and higher levels of macrobiotic diets are potentially harmful.

SUMMARY

Proteins, the largest and most complex molecules known, are organic compounds that always contain carbon, hydrogen, oxygen, and nitrogen; frequently they contain sulfur, phosphorus, and/or other elements as well.

Proteins are catalysts (enzymes) and regulators (hormones) of body processes; they are antibodies; they are components of the body's structure itself (cartilage, skin, nails, hair), of skeletal muscle, and of substances in the blood. Proteins are required for growth and for maintenance of all tissues.

Protein molecules consist of subunits, the amino acids, which are linked together by peptide bonds. All amino acids have an amino (NH_2) group, a radical (R) group, which differs for each and gives each its distinctive properties, and a carboxyl (COOH) group. Twenty-two amino acids are found in foods; a few others, not present in foods, are synthesized in the body from other amino acids. Many of those found in foods can be synthesized as well. These are the nonessential amino acids. Essential amino acids are those that cannot be synthesized in the body, or cannot be synthesized in adequate amounts, and so must be supplied in adequate amounts from dietary sources.

Complete proteins provide all the essential amino acids in optimal amounts; incomplete proteins generally contain a smaller amount of some of these. Most foods of animal origin contain complete proteins, but foods of plant origin have incomplete proteins and should be consumed in combinations that will make up for the amino acid deficiencies.

During digestion and absorption, the peptide bonds joining amino acids are hydrolyzed by various enzymes from the stomach, pancreas, and small intestine.

Amino acids are made available for use in the construction of the protein molecules needed by the body. This process of protein synthesis is programmed by hereditary material in DNA, a component of all cell nuclei. Actual protein synthesis takes place outside the cell nucleus, in bodies known as ribosomes. Protein synthesis is exceedingly complex and is regulated at several stages by various hormones. It also requires energy. As much as 300 grams of protein may be synthesized daily in the body of an adult male.

When carbohydrate and fat intake or reserves are inadequate for energy needs, proteins can be utilized instead. Amino acids not needed for body processes are generally metabolized to fat for storage. Some amino acids can be converted to glucose by the process of gluconeogenesis. Carbon skeletons for these conversions are derived from deamination of amino acids, which produces nitrogenous waste in the form of ammonia.

The liver removes ammonia, which is highly toxic, from circulation and converts it to urea, which is ultimately excreted in the urine. Protein synthesis and protein breakdown are always in dynamic equilibrium or balance, depending on the needs of the individual at any given time.

Protein requirements are greatest in infancy, a period of rapid growth, at 2 grams per kilogram of body weight per day. Requirements fall gradually as growth slows and then ceases in adulthood; for average adult males it is estimated at 0.47/kg body weight per day. Intake recommendations, set higher to allow for individual variation and inefficiency utilization are 0.8/kg, or 56 grams per day for the reference adult man, 44 grams per day for the reference adult woman.

Kwashiorkor is a protein deficiency disease, first described in Africa in 1935, that may occur despite adequate energy intake. It typically occurs in very young children who have been suddenly weaned and placed on a predominantly starchy diet.

Protein consumption in the United States has not changed significantly in this century, averaging in the neighborhood of 100 grams per person per day. There has been a marked increase in the amount of protein derived from animal sources, especially beef, and a corresponding decrease in the amount from grains and cereals. Increased meat consumption is apparently correlated with increased affluence, since it occurs in other developed nations as well.

Vegetarianism has become increasingly popular in recent years. Those vegetarians who consume no foods of animal origin at all should choose from vegetable foods providing complementary amino acids and eat a variety of foods. Supplementation, particularly of vitamin B_{12} and soy milk fortified with vitamin D for children, and of iron for pregnant and lactating women, is advisable for strict vegetarians and those on the higher levels of Zen macrobiotic diets. Vegetarians who consume some animal protein in the form of fish, eggs, and/or dairy products are not at nutritional risk.

BIBLIOGRAPHY

Brewster, L., and M. Jacobson. *The changing American diet.* Washington, D.C.: Center for Science in the Public Interest, 1978.

Brock, J. F., and M. Autret. Kwashiorkor in Africa. *Bulletin of the World Health Organization* 5:1, 1952.

Brown, P. T., and J. G. Bergan. The dietary status of "new" vegetarians. *Journal of the American Dietetic Association* 67:455, 1975.

Chopra, J. G., A. L. Forbes, and J. P. Habicht. Protein in the U.S. diet. *Journal of the American Dietetic Association* 72:253, 1978.

Cooke, R. IQ dip feared if kids go off disease diet. *Boston Globe* August 4, 1978.

Crim, M. C., and H. N. Munro. Protein. In D. M. Hegsted, ed., *Present knowledge in nutrition,* 4th ed. Washington, D.C.: Nutrition Foundation, 1976.

Draper, H. H. The aboriginal Eskimo diet in modern perspective. *American Anthropologist* 79:309, 1977.

Dwyer, J. T., R. Palumbo, H. Thorne, I. Valadian, and R. B. Reed. Preschoolers on alternate life-style diets. *Journal of the American Dietetic Association* 72:264, 1978.

FAO Nutrition Report Series No. 52. *Energy and protein requirements.* WHO Technical Report Series, No. 522, 1973.

Gaull, G., J. A. Sturman, and N. C. R. Raiha. Development of mammalian sulphur metabolism: Absence of cystathionase in human fetal tissues. *Pediatric Research* 6:538, 1972.

Hardinge, M. G., and F. J. Stare. Nutritional studies of vegetarians. 1. Nutritional, physical, and laboratory findings. *American Journal of Clinical Nutrition* 2:73, 1954.

Harper, A. E. Amino acids of nutritional importance. In *Toxicants occurring naturally in foods,* ed. Committee on Food Protection, Food and Nutritional Board, National Research Council, 2nd ed. Washington, D.C.: National Research Council, 1973.

Hegsted, D. M. Protein needs and possible modifications of the American diet. *Journal of the American Dietetic Association* 68:317, 1976.

Heller, C. A., and E. M. Scott. *The Alaska dietary survey* (*1956–1961*). Public Health Service Publication No. 999-AH-2. Anchorage: U.S. Department of Health, Education, and Welfare, Arctic Health Research Center, 1967.

Higginbottom, M. C., L. Sweetman, and W. L. Nyhan. A syndrome of methylmalonic aciduria, homocystinuria, megaloblastic anemia and neurologic abnormalities in a vitamin B_{12}-deficient breast-fed infant of a strict vegetarian. *New England Journal of Medicine* 299:317, 1978.

Holtzman, N. A., D. W. Welcher, and E. D. Mellits. Termination of restricted diet in children with PKU: A randomized controlled study. *New England Journal of Medicine* 293:1121, 1975.

Irwin, M. I., and D. M. Hegsted. A conspectus of research on protein requirements of man. *Journal of Nutrition* 101:385, 1971.

Kopple, J. D., and M. E. Swendseid. Evidence that histidine is an essential amino acid in normal and chronically uremic men. *Journal of Clinical Investigation* 55:881, 1975.

Lawrie, R. A. *Protein as human food.* Westport, Conn.: Avi Publishing Co., 1970.

Lozoff, B., and A. A. Fanaroff. Kwashiorkor in Cleveland. *American Journal of the Diseases of Children* 129:710, 1975.

Mayer, J. *Human nutrition.* Springfield, Ill.: Chas. C Thomas, 1972.

McClellan, W. S., and E. F. DuBois. Clinical calorimetry. XLV. Prolonged meat diets with a study of kidney function and ketosis. *Journal of Biological Chemistry* 81:651, 1930.

National Academy of Sciences, Food and Nutrition Board. *Recommended dietary allowances,* 9th ed. Washington, D.C.: National Academy of Sciences, 1979.

Rensberger, B. The American way of eating: For most, beef is the staple. *The New York Times,* May 24, 1978, p. C1.

Rose, W. C. Amino acid requirements for man. *Federation Proceedings* 8:546, 1949.

Scrimshaw, N. S. Progress in solving world nutrition problems. *Journal of the American Dietetic Association* 35:441, 1959.

Scrimshaw, N. S. Through a glass darkly: Discerning the practical implications of human protein-energy interrelationships. *Nutrition Reviews* 35:321, 1977.

Stanbury, J. B., D. Fredrickson, and J. F. Wyngaarden, eds. *Metabolic basis of inherited disease,* 4th ed. New York: McGraw-Hill, 1978.

Strand, F. L. *Physiology: A regulatory systems approach.* New York: Macmillan, 1978.

Williams, C. D. Kwashiorkor: A nutritional disease of children associated with a maize diet. *Lancet* 2:1151, 1935.

Young, V. R., W. P. Steffee, P. B. Pencharz, J. C. Winterer, and N. S. Scrimshaw. Total human body protein synthesis in relation to protein requirements at various ages. *Nature* 253:192, 1975.

SUGGESTED ADDITIONAL READING

Adibi, S. A. Intestinal phase of protein assimilation in man. *American Journal of Clinical Nutrition* 29:205, 1976.

Altschul, A. M. *Proteins—Their chemistry and politics.* New York: Basic Books, 1965.

Barness, L. A. Nutritional aspects of vegetarianism, health foods, and fad diets. *Nutrition Reviews* 35:153, 1977.

Beckner, A. S., W. R. Centerwall, and L. Holt. Effect of rapid increase of phenylalanine intake in older PKU children. *Journal of the American Dietetic Association* 69:148, 1976.

Carroll, K. K. Dietary protein in relation to plasma cholesterol levels and atherosclerosis. *Nutrition Reviews* 36:1, 1978.

Clark, H. E., M. A. Kollenlark, and J. D. Halvorson. Ability of 6 grams of nitrogen from a combination of rice, wheat, and milk to meet protein requirements of young men for 4 weeks. *American Journal of Clinical Nutrition* 31:585, 1978.

Crosby, W. H. Can a vegetarian be well nourished? *Journal of the American Medical Association* 233:898, 1975.

ERHARD, D. The new vegetarians. Part 1: Vegetarianism and its medical consequences. *Nutrition Today* 8(6):4, 1973.

ERHARD, D. The new vegetarians. Part 2: The Zen macrobiotic movement and other cults based on vegetarianism. *Nutrition Today* 9(1):20, 1974.

GRAY, G. M., AND H. L. COOPER. Protein digestion and absorption. *Gastroenterology* 61(4):535, 1971.

LAPPE, F. M. *Diet for a small planet*, rev. ed. New York: Ballantine, 1975.

LEWIS, H. B. Fifty years of study of the role of protein in nutrition. *Journal of the American Dietetic Association* 28:701, 1952.

LOZY, E., AND D. M. HEGSTED. Calculations of the amino acid requirements of children at different ages by a factorial method. *American Journal of Clinical Nutrition* 28:1052, 1975.

Nutrition Reviews. Human protein deficiency—Biological changes and functional implications. Vol. 35:294, 1977.

RAND, W. M., N. S. SCRIMSHAW, AND V. R. YOUNG. Determination of protein allowances in human adults from nitrogen balance data. *American Journal of Clinical Nutrition* 30:1129, 1977.

REGISTER, U. D., AND L. M. SONNENBERG. The vegetarian diet. *Journal of the American Dietetic Association* 62:253, 1973.

ROBERTSON, L., K. FLINDERS, AND B. GODFREY. *Laurel's kitchen: A handbook of vegetarian cookery and nutrition*. New York: Bantam, 1977.

VICKERY, H. B., AND C. L. SCHMIDT. The history and discovery of the amino acids. *Chemical Reviews* 9(1):169, 1931.

VYHMEISTER, I. B., U. D. REGISTER, AND L. M. SONNENBERG. Safe vegetarian diets for children. *Pediatric Clinics of North America* 24(1):203, 1977.

WHITE, P. L., AND D. C. FLETCHER. *AMA nutrients in processed foods—Proteins*. Littleton, Mass.: Publishing Sciences Group, 1974.

WILLIAMS, F. L., AND C. L. JUSTICE. A ready reckoner of protein costs. *Journal of Home Economics*, March 1975.

In Retrospect I

SUMMARY OF MAJOR NUTRIENT METABOLISM

In the preceding chapters, the energy-yielding nutrients—carbohydrates, lipids, and proteins—have been examined. Although each macronutrient was discussed as a distinct entity, our bodies do not consider them apart from one another. The digestion, metabolism, and excretion of each of these nutrients is directly influenced by the digestion, metabolism, and excretion of every other nutrient.

As we eat them, foods contain more than one nutrient. The macronutrients do not segregate themselves in separate corners of our mouths. They are chewed together, swallowed together, and processed together throughout the digestive tract. Although each macronutrient is acted upon by different enzymes, proceeding on different time schedules, all of these enzymatic processes are occurring simultaneously. This is true also of absorption, metabolism, and excretion, thus ensuring the simultaneous distribution, utilization, and elimination of all digested nutrients.

As the previous chapters have emphasized, the digestive processes are well coordinated. Figure I-1 illustrates this efficient coordination. Hydrolysis is the first process to occur. All nutrients are hydrolyzed by digestive enzymes. In the case of carbohydrates, proteins, and the triglycerides that contain short- and medium-chain fatty acids, the end products of hydrolysis (monosaccharides, amino acids, glycerol, and fatty acids) are ready for absorption. These products enter the portal vein, either by diffusion or active transport, and are then carried directly to the liver. There, they are either metabolized or passed directly into the general circulation.

Triglycerides containing long-chain fatty acids undergo a more complicated absorption process. Their hydrolysis products are transported into the cells of the intestinal mucosa, where they are reesterified. These "new" triglycerides combine with a transport molecule, a protein, which permits them to enter the lymph system. Cholesterol esters and phospholipids also require preparation for absorption and transport. They are first packaged into chylomicrons and VLDLs, and then absorbed into the lymph system.

As Figure I-1 illustrates, digested nutrients are carried from the lymph and general circulatory systems to all the cells of the body. Depending on the current needs of the organism, these nutrients will enter metabolic pathways which channel them into growth, maintenance, or energy-producing processes.

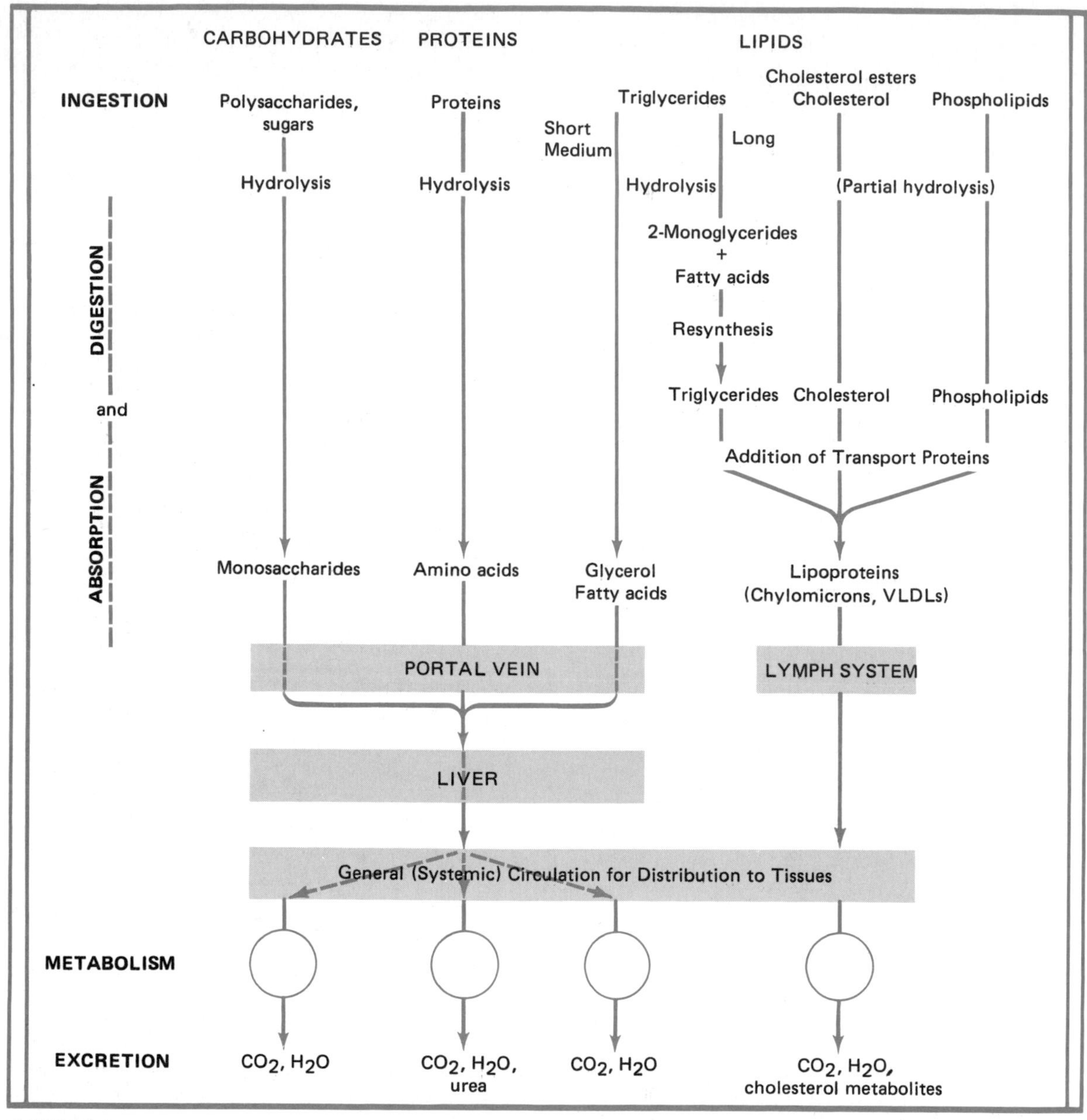

FIGURE I-1

Schematic Diagram of Macronutrient Metabolism.

Metabolic wastes will be excreted as CO_2, H_2O, and, in the case of amino acids, urea. Products of cholesterol metabolism will be excreted as bile salts, bile acids, and bile pigments.

As the four empty circles in Figure I-1 imply, this overview has not yet included the numerous metabolic processes occurring between the absorption and excretion of digested nutrients. This information is presented in Figure

I-2. Many cyclical or reversible processes integrate the metabolic pathways we have studied thus far. The processes going on within each of these pathways are regulated by specific enzymes. Of the many regulatory enzymes, those that control only one or perhaps two key reactions in any one pathway still have an influence on the overall flow along the entire pathway. And, because the metabolic pathways are interconnected, each regulatory interaction may create a chain-reaction effect along the entire metabolic system.

In the glycolytic pathway, shown in the center of Figure I-2, glucose is metabolized to pyruvate. Decarboxylation to acetyl CoA is followed by complete oxidation to CO_2 through the Krebs cycle. The hydrogen ions produced during glycolysis and the Krebs cycle are passed through the electron transport system, in which both H_2O and the high-energy compound ATP are produced.

But glucose can follow other pathways as well. It can be polymerized to the polysaccharide glycogen, which is stored in liver and muscle tissue as an energy reserve. It can be stored as fat through conversion to fatty acids and glycerol. And (not shown in the diagram) glucose can also be converted to other important structural and functional compounds, such as heparin. Still another pathway of glucose metabolism, the hexose monophosphate shunt (also known as the pentose pathway), generates the 5-carbon sugars ribose and deoxyribose, which are components of the nucleic acids. One final pathway represents the release of glucose units from glycogen and other sources. When the level of glucose in the blood falls, these new glucose molecules are channeled directly into the blood, primarily by the liver and the kidneys.

Amino acids also follow specific metabolic pathways, separate from but related to those of glucose metabolism. For example, glucose-derived metabolites can be aminated to produce the nonessential amino acids. Similarly, amino acids in excess of the body's immediate metabolic needs are deaminated. Their nitrogen is metabolized to urea in the liver and then excreted in the urine. The remaining carbon skeletons can be stored as energy reserves. When energy is needed, some carbon skeletons enter the metabolic cycle at the levels of pyruvate, α-ketoglutarate, succinyl CoA, fumarate, or oxaloacetate. Other carbon skeletons follow a different pathway for synthesis to glucose. This process of gluconeogenesis involves a reversal of the glycolytic pathway, with some modifications. It is an excellent example of the interrelationships we have been discussing.

Of course, glucose is not the metabolic destination of all amino acids. Usually, most are synthesized into protein molecules that play important structural and functional roles in the body, for example, enzymes, hormones, collagen, hemoglobin, antibodies, and plasma proteins. Some of these are utilized in nucleic acid synthesis. Others are **precursors** for epinephrine, norepinephrine, and serotonin. Still other amino acids, the ketogenic type mentioned above, are ultimately degraded to acetyl CoA. Following the condensation of acetyl CoA with oxaloacetate in the Krebs cycle, its two carbons are released as CO_2. Thus, there cannot be any synthesis of glucose from the ketogenic amino acids, or from acetyl CoA itself.

Lipid metabolism is also intimately connected with amino acid and glucose metabolism. The hydrolysis of triglycerides to glycerol and fatty acids has already been discussed. Dynamic utilization of these lipids involves the

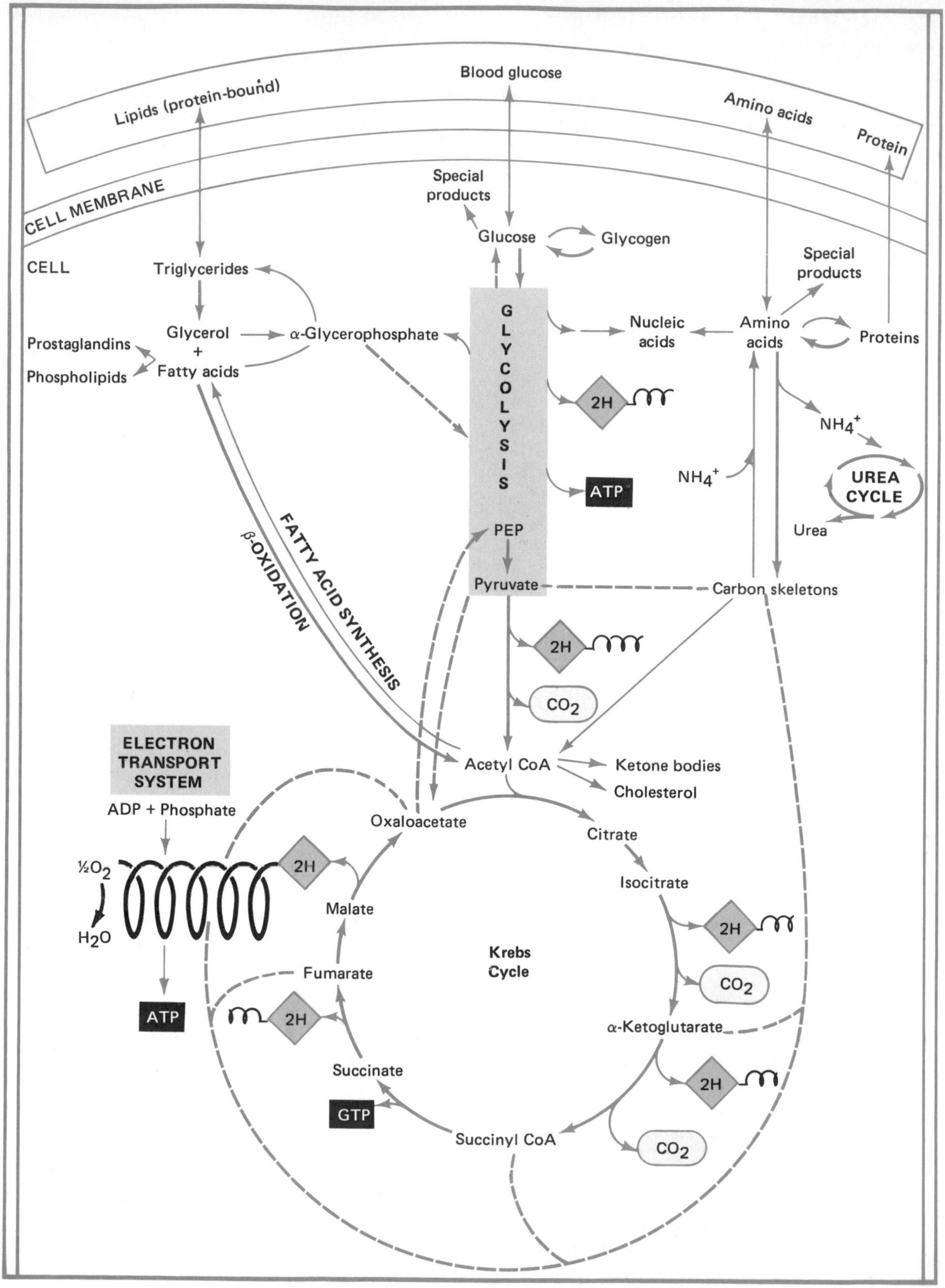

Blood glucose
Lipids (protein-bound)
Amino acids
Protein
CELL MEMBRANE
Special products
Glucose
Glycogen
CELL
Triglycerides
Special products
Glycerol + Fatty acids
α-Glycerophosphate
Prostaglandins
Phospholipids
GLYCOLYSIS
Nucleic acids
Amino acids
Proteins
2H
ATP
NH_4^+
NH_4^+
UREA CYCLE
Urea
PEP
Pyruvate
Carbon skeletons
FATTY ACID SYNTHESIS
β-OXIDATION
2H
CO_2
ELECTRON TRANSPORT SYSTEM
ADP + Phosphate
Acetyl CoA
Ketone bodies
Cholesterol
Oxaloacetate
Citrate
½O_2
H_2O
2H
Isocitrate
Malate
2H
Krebs Cycle
Fumarate
CO_2
ATP
2H
α-Ketoglutarate
Succinate
2H
GTP
Succinyl CoA
CO_2

FIGURE I-2 (facing page). Pathways and Processes of Intermediary Metabolism.

β-oxidation of fatty acids, producing acetyl CoA. Acetyl CoA can be reutilized for the synthesis of fatty acids, cholesterol, or ketone bodies. Glycerol can enter the glycolytic pathway for use as energy in two ways: It can be converted to pyruvate and enter the Krebs cycle, or it can be converted to glucose.

From these many examples, you should now have a better idea of the complex interrelationship of the macronutrients and their metabolic pathways. Notice in Figure I-2 that the metabolism of carbohydrate, lipid, and protein intersects at acetyl CoA, which we referred to early in this book as the pivotal point of metabolism. The importance of this compound in the overall metabolic scheme cannot be overstated.

Finally, as you view the figure, try to imagine the many different metabolic products moving busily within a cell along their assigned pathways, first in one direction, and then around, or back again to their starting point. Coordinating so many reactions requires numerous biological "traffic lights." They take the form of certain key enzymes and hormones that determine whether the net result of metabolism will be anabolic or catabolic. The availability of necessary nutrients at any particular time acts to control the release of hormones and the activity of the key enzymes.

An example will help to clarify the workings of this complex system. Consider carbohydrate metabolism. After a meal, the hormone insulin is normally secreted. It causes circulating glucose to enter the body's cells, increases lipogenesis, and increases protein synthesis. This assumes the availability of normal dietary levels of carbohydrates. But when normal carbohydrate availability is disrupted by starvation or disease, the relative amount of insulin decreases, and there follows a corresponding increase in secretion of glucagon, glucocorticoids, and other hormones. These hormones have opposite effects to those of insulin: glucagon increases lipolysis and glycogenolysis; glucocorticoids increase amino acid catabolism and gluconeogenesis. By shifting from one kind of process to the other, the body attempts to maintain a constant level of vital metabolites. Of course, this coordinated maintenance system can only go so far. Prolonged starvation or radical weight loss, for example, tax the control system to a point at which balance becomes impossible.

Enzymes are the key to all of the interrelated processes of digestion, absorption, metabolism, and excretion. We say that hormones regulate certain reactions, as in the carbohydrate example above, but what is really happening is that hormones control the actions of key enzymes involved in these reactions. Thus, the explanation of carbohydrate metabolism might be restated, thus: Under conditions of normal availability of carbohydrates, the enzymes involved in the utilization of glucose are all activated, and the enzymes responsible for producing glucose by the pathway of gluconeogenesis are all depressed. The term "depressed" emphasizes the fact that metabolism along any one pathway never stops completely; it merely speeds up or slows down, as required by the body.

If you are interested, you can find a more detailed explanation of pathway regulation in any biochemistry textbook. As you read the chapters that follow, try to fit each newly introduced process into the neat, coordinated scheme diagrammed in Figures I-1 and I-2. And remember . . . everything depends on the enzymes!

Chapter 5

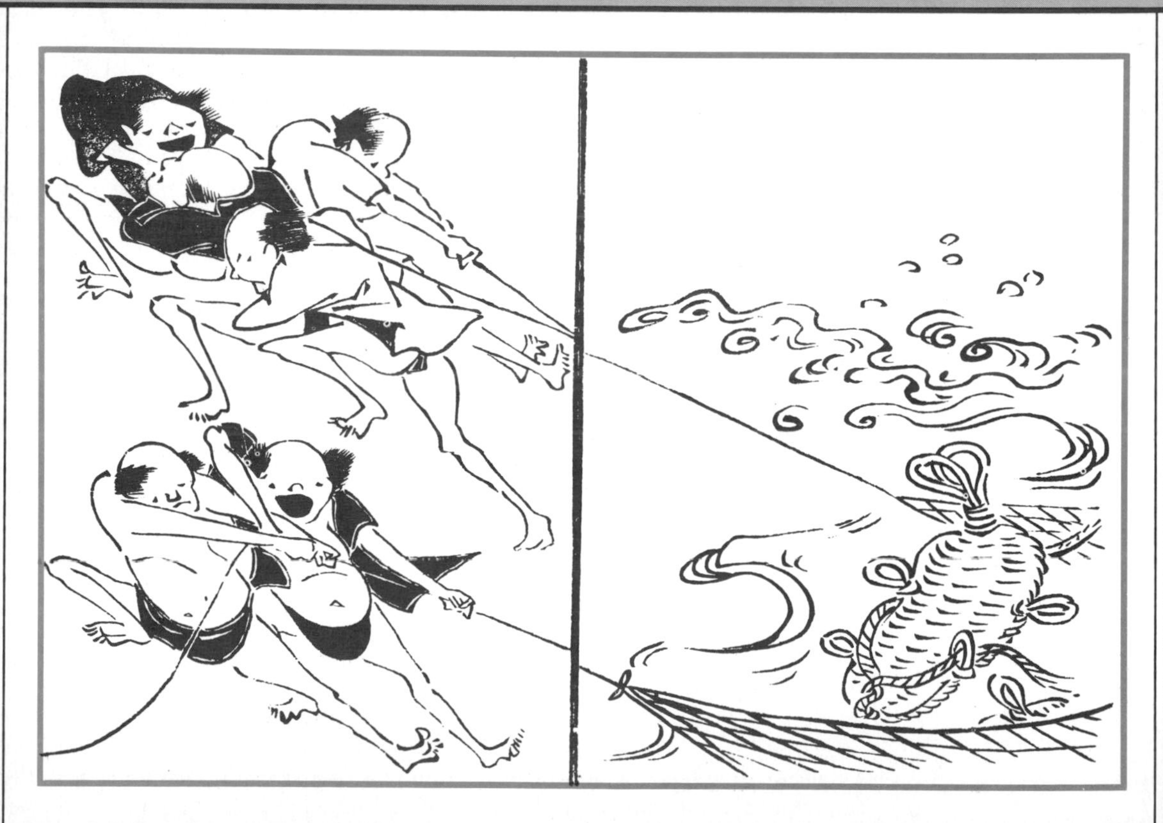

Fishing, old Japanese print

Concepts of Energy Balance

Whether we are running or sleeping, thinking or watching television, our bodies are using energy. We require energy to function, to grow, and to be physically active. In every cell, energy makes possible the synthesis of various compounds. Energy is necessary for fetal and childhood growth, during pregnancy and lactation, and for the rehabilitation of body systems following the stress of illness and injury. Surprisingly, all of these anabolic processes together consume only 30 to 40 percent of the energy our bodies derive from metabolizing food nutrients (Hegsted, 1974). The greatest portion of available energy is used to support still another vital function, the maintenance of body temperature. To do this, energy is transformed to heat, much of which is dissipated from the body surface. Maintenance of body temperature is essential because it provides the optimal conditions for all of the biochemical reactions that take place within our internal environment. The high proportion of energy assigned to this task is an indication of its importance.

We saw in the preceding chapters how oxidation of the energy-producing nutrients—carbohydrate, amino acids, fatty acids, and glycerol—yields water, CO_2, and high-energy phosphorylated compounds such as ATP. This chapter will focus on the ways in which these oxidation products are used to achieve an energy balance. We shall consider the concept of the energy measure, the kilocalorie, and its counterpart the kilojoule, and discuss the components of energy requirements. Aberrations in energy balance, both positive and negative, will be examined.

ENERGY: FORMS AND MEASUREMENT

Energy is defined as the capacity to do work. Although different aspects of this capacity are emphasized in the study of physics, chemistry, and nutrition, the essential meaning of energy is basic to all disciplines.

Energy Transformations

The concept of energy as a capacity may seem somewhat abstract. Although we can't actually see a capacity, we can, however, see work being done, the result of energy being expended. In the work process, energy doesn't get used up and then vanish; it is transformed. Electrical energy, for example, can be transformed into light and heat; just look at and touch a light bulb. The First Law of Thermodynamics states this well-known fact succinctly: Energy can neither be created nor destroyed. Thus, energy can be thought of as constituting a vast, eternal cycle.

The central point of the energy cycle is the sun. The sun shines on growing plants which, by the process of photosynthesis, use solar energy to convert carbon dioxide from the air and water from the soil to glucose. Carbohydrate is stored by the plants, along with nutrients taken up from the soil and air. Animals, including humans, consume the plants and thus obtain nutrients that will provide the energy required for their own life processes.

The energy provided by plant and animal foodstuffs is called *potential* energy; until it is actually used for work, it exists in storage form. Potential energy must be transformed by metabolic reactions before it can do work in the body. It is changed into several different kinds of working energy: electrical for conduction of nerve impulses, mechanical for muscle contraction and movement, chemical for anabolism and catabolism, and heat for maintenance of normal body temperature.

Energy released from the body in these various forms must be replaced; in fact, replacement of expended energy is the primary need of adults. We rely, therefore, on the potential energy supplied by food for the continual replacement of energy utilized by our cells and tissues. When the amount of energy supplied is equal to the amount of energy expended in physiological processes, *equilibrium* is achieved; the organism is in a state of energy balance. If the energy supplied by foods exceeds that which is utilized, potential energy is stored by the body as glycogen or fat; this is a *positive* energy state. Conversely, when utilization exceeds supply, potential energy is released from storage sites and transformed into the energy forms required by the body; this is a *negative* energy state.

Units of Measurement

Nutritional scientists measure energy as heat, a concept that reflects nutrient oxidation within the body. The traditional unit of heat measurement is the kilocalorie (Calorie, kcal). A *kilocalorie is defined as the amount of heat required to raise the temperature of 1 kilogram (kg) of water by 1°C* (generally measured from 15°C to 16°C).

The pre-eminence of the kilocalorie has recently been challenged by the Seventh International Congress of Nutrition meeting in Prague in 1969, and by the American Institute of Nutrition in 1970. These groups recommended the adoption of a different standard, the *joule,* the nonheat unit of energy measurement in the metric system. This change would bring nutritional terminology into accord with the measurements used in physics, chemistry, and the other disciplines on which the basic principles of nutrition are founded (Ames, 1970).

The metric system, which is the international measurement terminology of science, includes several similar units for specific kinds of energy: the ampere (A) for electrical current, the kelvin (K) for thermodynamic temperature, and the candela (cd) for light intensity. These, along with the more familiar meter (m) for length, kilogram (kg) for mass, and second (s) for time, serve as the bases from which all other metric units are derived. The newton (N), for example, is the metric unit of force. By definition, a *joule is the amount of energy expended when 1 kilogram is moved a distance of 1 meter by a force of 1 newton.* By this definition, energy is a force, quite different from the concept of the kilocalorie, which expresses energy only in terms of one of its forms, heat. In metric terms, the joule is the *mechanical* (that is, work-producing) equivalent of heat.

Even though converting traditional caloric measurements into their metric equivalents is cumbersome, nutritionists recognize that failure to follow universally accepted scientific terminology would isolate the nutritional sciences from advances in related fields. In fact, the mathematical conversion of kilocalories to kilojoules is not complex. James Prescott Joule, the English physicist for whom the unit is named, determined that 1 kilocalorie is equivalent to 4,184 joules (J), or 4.184 kilojoules (kJ), where $10^3 J = 1{,}000 J = 1 kJ$. Thus, the conversion of kilocalories to kJ involves multiplication of the value in kilocalories by 4.184 or, more speedily but a little less precisely, by 4.2.

1 kilocalorie (kcal)
= 4,184 joules
= 4.184 kJ
1 kilojoule (kJ)
= 1,000 joules
= 0.240 kcal
1 megajoule (MJ)
= 1,000 kJ
= 240 kcal

Despite the ease of mathematical conversion, practical and psychological problems still remain. Tables of food composition listing energy content of various foods, and tables of energy requirements, now expressed in kilocalories, must be revised. Professionals and the public alike will have to adjust to the new terminology. To make the transition easier, journals and other publications for the specialist have decided to use the familiar nonmetric units, with their metric equivalents in parentheses; for example, "55 kcal (230 kJ)." It is anticipated that, at one time in the future, the sequence will be reversed: "230 kJ (55 kcal)," and eventually the values will be given only in kilojoules (Harper, 1970).

Energy Value of Foods

The change from kilocalories to kilojoules will not change the methods by which food energy values are determined. The most common method involves the use of a **bomb calorimeter** (shown in Figure 5-1), a device that determines the amount of heat produced after a dried, weighed sample of food is oxidized. The food sample is placed within the well-insulated bomb, which is then filled with pure oxygen and placed in a measured quantity of water. The sample is then ignited by an electrical spark, and the temperature increase in the surrounding water is carefully measured. Because the quantity of heat needed to raise the temperature of a given volume of water is known,

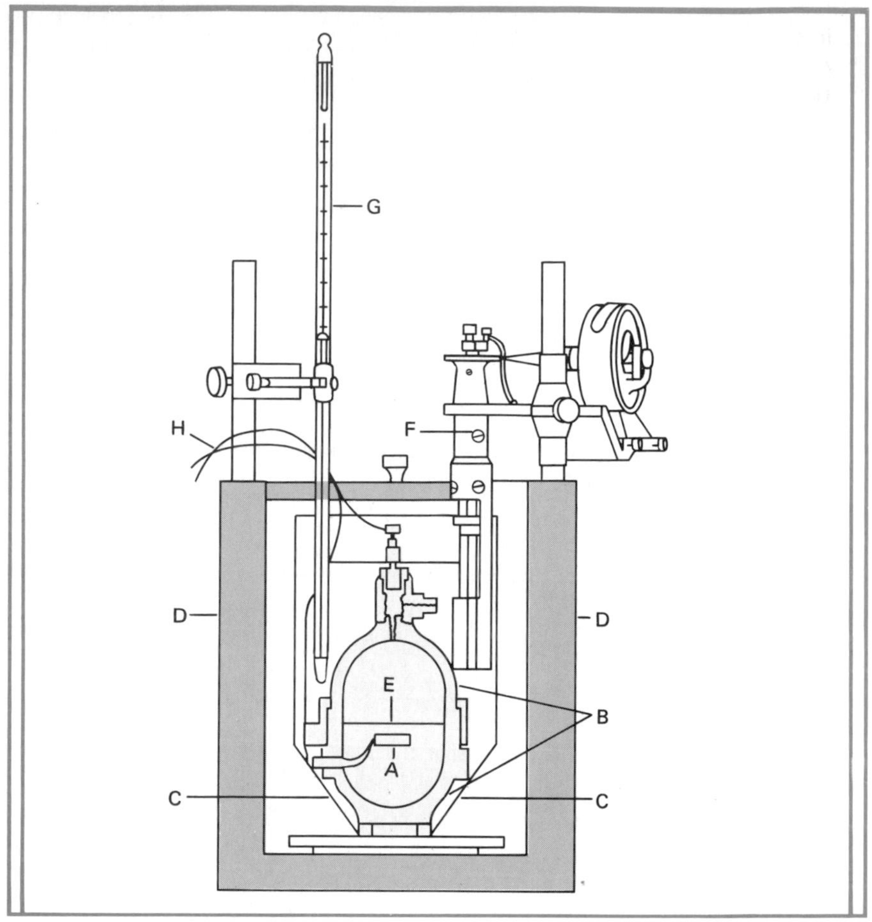

FIGURE 5-1

Diagram of a Bomb Calorimeter with Bomb in Position

(A) Platinum dish holding weighed food sample: (B) Bomb filled with pure oxygen enclosing food sample; (C) Can holding water of known weight in which the bomb is submerged; (D) Outer double-walled insulating jacket; (E) Fuse, which is ignited by an electric current; (F) Motor-driven water stirrer; (G) Thermometer calibrated to $\frac{1}{1,000}$ °C; (H) Electric wires to send current through fuse.

the energy value of the food (its heat of combustion) can be calculated. The energy values determined by burning 1 gram of pure protein, carbohydrate, and fat are shown in the first column of Table 5-1.

Values for ethanol, commonly known as grain alcohol, are also included in this table. Ethanol, the "active" ingredient in alcoholic beverages, is metabolized primarily in the liver, by the enzymes ethanol dehydrogenase and acetaldehyde dehydrogenase, both of which require a cofactor containing the vitamin niacin (Figure 5-2). Further oxidation of acetaldehyde via acetyl CoA proceeds through the Krebs cycle. Ethanol, which will be discussed more fully

TABLE 5-1
Estimation of Physiological Fuel Value

	Heat of Combustion kcal/g	Coefficient of Digestibility (%)	Urinary Loss kcal/g	Physiological Fuel Value	
				kcal/g[a]	*kJ/g*[b]
Protein	5.6	92	1.25	4	17
Carbohydrate	4.1	99	—	4	17
Fat	9.4	95	—	9	38
Ethanol	7.1	100	negligible	7	29

Note: The use of the physiological fuel value (also known as the Atwater coefficient) tends to overestimate the number of Calories that can be obtained from foods containing large amounts of undigestible carbohydrate (dietary fiber). Newer tables of food composition also consider the fact that different proteins contain different percentages of nitrogen, rather than the 16 percent that was generally assumed in the past. Appropriate correction factors have been applied in recent tables.

[a]Heat of Combustion × Coefficient of Digestibility − Urinary Loss

[b]Calculated as kcal/g × 4.2 = kJ/g

in Chapter 14, is not usually considered a nutrient, but it contributes significantly to total energy intake in many individuals.

Ethanol does not require digestion and is very efficiently absorbed from the stomach and the rest of the gastrointestinal tract. This fact is reflected in the 100 percent coefficient of digestibility of ethanol, listed in the second column of Table 5-1. The coefficient of digestibility is used to correct for the inefficiency of human digestion and absorption, which is ultimately reflected as the production of less energy in the body than in the bomb calorimeter.

The energy value of dietary protein must be corrected for a factor in addition to digestibility. Pure protein is completely oxidized in the calorimeter. In the human body, however, the urea and other nitrogenous wastes produced by amino acid catabolism are not converted to energy; thus, they represent a decrease in the total energy value of consumed protein-containing food. This appears in Table 5-1 as a urinary loss of 1.25 kcal per gram of protein. The *actual* physiological fuel values (Atwater coefficients) of the energy-producing nutrients are the familiar 4 kcal/g of carbohydrate and protein, 9 kcal/g of fat, and 7 kcal/g of ethanol.

FIGURE 5-2
Metabolism of Ethanol

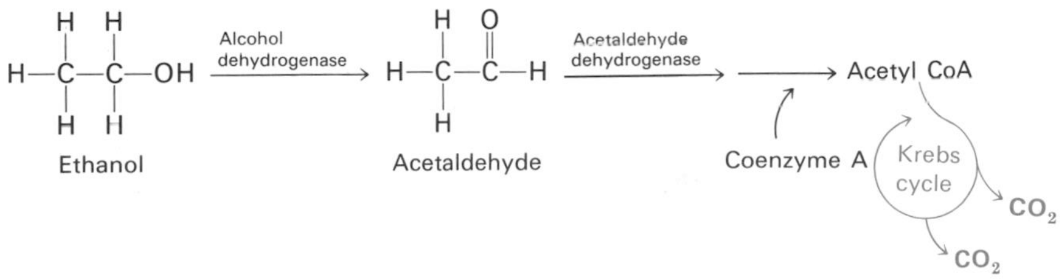

To calculate the approximate energy value of each of the foods we eat, nutritionists determine its percentage composition of carbohydrate, protein, fat, and ethanol, and then multiply by the appropriate Atwater coefficients. Since different samples of the same food may differ slightly in their exact proportions of carbohydrate, protein, and fat, and since individuals differ in their efficiency of digestion, the energy provided by any single serving of a particular food can never be known precisely. Recognizing this, laboratories analyze many samples of each food, and calculate an average, to ensure a reasonably accurate estimate of energy value.

ENERGY REQUIREMENTS

Methods of Determination

Determination of energy requirements is a time-consuming and expensive task. In order to know how much energy-producing food an individual requires each day, that person's daily energy expenditure must be calculated. This is the amount of energy that must be replaced to keep the body at equilibrium.

Obviously, different individuals have different energy requirements, and total energy expenditure varies from day to day even for the same individual. But by averaging the requirements of many individuals in a given group—growing children, pregnant women, adult males—the energy requirements of a typical member of that population group can be estimated.

Energy expenditure is measured as heat released. The body "combusts" foodstuffs in the same way, essentially, as the bomb calorimeter does—although no electric spark is needed to initiate the process, and it doesn't happen quite as rapidly!

Several methods of measuring energy expenditure have been developed. One technique, **direct calorimetry,** utilizes the principle that heat released by the body is a product of energy expended. Measurements of the heat given off by an individual can therefore be used to calculate that individual's energy expenditure. This technique involves placing the person in a *respiratory calorimeter*, a large ventilated and well-insulated chamber whose exterior surface is lined with water-filled coils. Heat given off by the individual raises the temperature of the water in the coils, providing a measurement that can be converted to kilocalories or kilojoules. As you may recognize, the respiratory calorimeter is quite similar in principle to the bomb calorimeter; it can also be used to measure carbon dioxide production as well as oxygen consumption.

Oxidation of glucose

$$C_6H_{12}O_6 + 6O_2 \longrightarrow 6CO_2 + 6H_2O + \text{heat}$$

$$\text{R.Q.} = \frac{6CO_2}{6O_2} = 1.00$$

Oxidation of stearic acid

$$CH_3(CH_2)_{16}COOH + 26\,O_2 \longrightarrow 18CO_2 + 18H_2O + \text{heat}$$

$$\text{R.Q.} = \frac{18CO_2}{26O_2} = 0.70$$

The ratio of the volume of CO_2 produced to the volume of O_2 consumed is known as the **Respiratory Quotient** (R.Q.). Studies have shown that the R.Q. varies with the type of food ingested. Foods that contain greater relative proportions of oxygen require less molecular oxygen for biochemical oxidation; these foods have a higher R.Q. Glucose, the nutrient with the highest proportion of oxygen, has an R.Q. of 1. Stearic acid, with a lower proportion

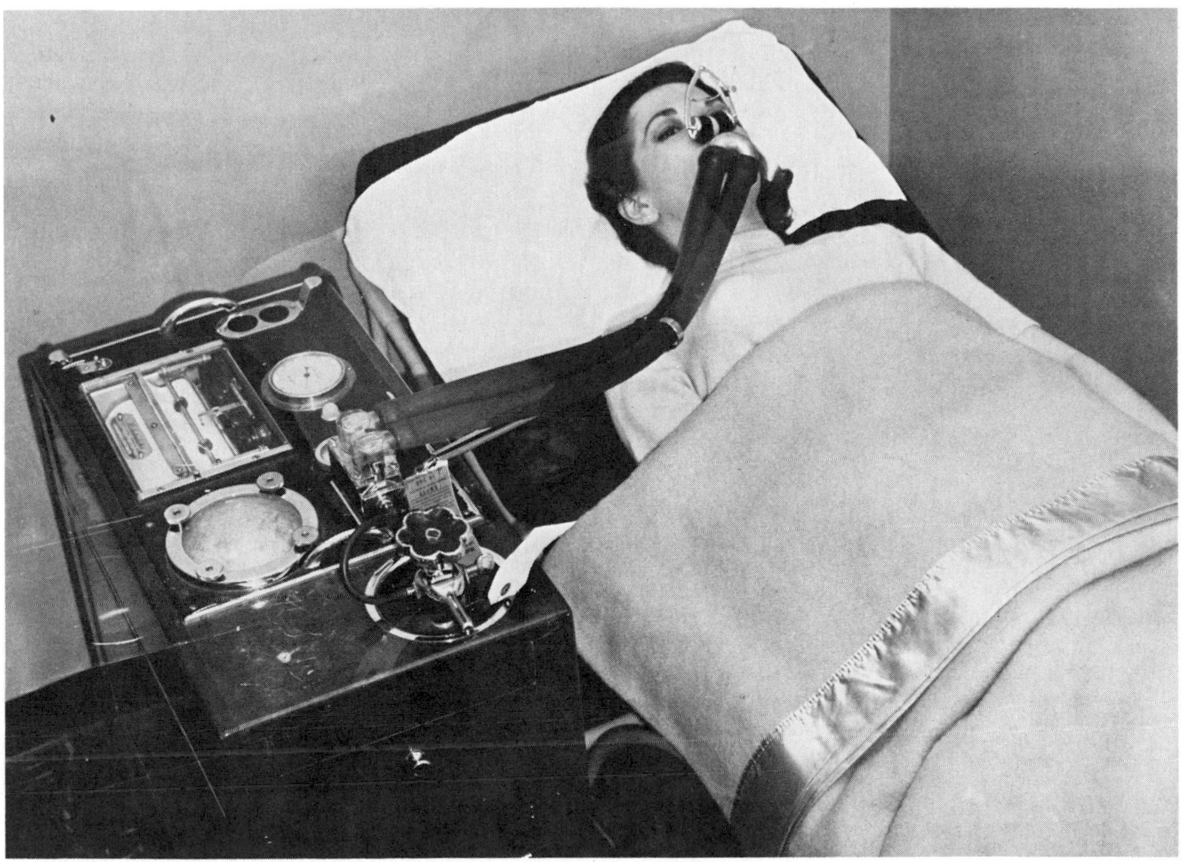

Measurement of basal metabolic rate by the indirect calorimetry method (see p. 176). (Lester V. Bergman & Assoc.)

of oxygen, therefore requiring more molecular oxygen for metabolism, has a lower R.Q. Protein, with an oxygen content intermediate between glucose and fatty acids, has an R.Q. of approximately 0.8.

The R.Q. of a diet of mixed nutrients is approximately 0.85. In fasting and uncontrolled diabetes, where lipolysis and subsequent fatty acid oxidation is greatly accelerated, the measured R.Q. approaches 0.70. Administration of insulin, which accelerates glucose metabolism, produces an R.Q. greater than 0.85.

Because respiratory calorimeters are expensive and complicated to operate, they are not practical for routine use. Methods of **indirect calorimetry** have been devised, and are both more convenient and lower in initial and operating costs. These methods depend on the fact that the amount of oxygen consumed during any activity is in direct proportion to the amount of energy liberated as heat. Calorimetric studies on many different subjects have shown that 1 liter of oxygen is required when approximately 4.8 kilocalories are liberated under basal (resting) conditions. Many experiments have confirmed this relationship.

From these figures, energy expenditures under a variety of experimental conditions can be readily calculated. All that is required is a respirometer, a lightweight apparatus that measures oxygen used and carbon dioxide exhaled. The resulting data are used to determine equivalents in kilocalories.

Factors Related to Energy Requirements

Using these techniques, the energy requirements of many individuals, under many different circumstances, have been determined. Several factors contribute to the amount of energy required by an individual at a given time: **basal metabolic rate** (BMR), physical activity, and, to a lesser extent, the **specific dynamic effect** (SDE) of foods.

BASAL METABOLIC RATE. Energy is needed just to keep body systems working. Nerves firing, blood circulating, involuntary movements of muscles in the heart and diaphragm—these and other activities go on continuously in each individual, even when the body is at rest.

Researchers have studied the involuntary work of the brain, heart, muscles, and digestive organs to determine the amount of energy required for these processes. This energy requirement is known as the *basal metabolic rate* (BMR). BMR measurements may be obtained by indirect calorimetry under carefully controlled conditions. Subjects are instructed not to eat for 12 to 16 hours before BMR testing to ensure that they are in a postabsorptive state. They must be relaxed, calm, and fully rested. Thus, testing is most frequently scheduled for early morning. The test consists of measuring oxygen consumption for six minutes with the subject at rest but awake. Standard calculations estimate the daily at-rest or basal energy requirement. If, for example, a subject consumes 1.4 liters of oxygen (1400 ml) during the six-minute test, daily energy requirements are calculated as

$$1.4 \text{ liters } O_2 \times \frac{60 \text{ min/hr}}{6 \text{ min}} \times 24 \text{ hr/day} \times \frac{4.8 \text{ kcal}}{1 \text{ liter } O_2}$$

$$= 1{,}615 \text{ kcal/day } (1{,}612.8 \text{ rounded off})$$

Through extensive testing of many healthy men and women, nutritionists have defined a useful rule of thumb: The BMR for adults is approximately 22 to 24 kilocalories per kilogram body weight per day (101 kJ/kg/day). Alternatively, for women of average body build, an approximation of BMR is 0.9 kcal (3.8 kJ) per kg per hour; for men, it is 1.0 kcal (4.2 kJ) per kg per hour.

To estimate your BMR, convert your body weight to kilograms (pounds ÷ 2.2); then multiply by 22 (women) or 24 (men). This gives some idea of the energy required for minimal metabolic functioning.

Basal metabolic rate is influenced by many factors, including age, sex, hormonal status, body size, nutritional state, and other factors. Considering age, for example, basal metabolism is high during periods of rapid growth. Infants and adolescents have the highest BMR and elderly people, the lowest. Women have a 6 to 10 percent lower metabolic rate than men. This sex difference has been attributed to women's higher proportion of adipose tissue and to hormonal differences. Hormones, the secretions of the endocrine glands, affect metabolism in many ways. Oversecretion of thyroxine by the thyroid gland (hyperthyroidism), for example, may speed up metabolism by as much as 75 to 100 percent. Conversely, undersecretion (hypothyroidism) may reduce metabolism by 30 to 40 percent. Thus, the pituitary gland, which stimulates thyroxine secretion by the thyroid, obviously exerts strong control on metabolism. Thyroxine acts slowly but maintains its effectiveness over long periods. Another important hormone, epinephrine (adrenalin), secreted by the adrenal glands, has a quick but transitory effect on metabolism. The sudden rush of energy you feel during excitement, fear, or emotional stress is the result of epinephrine secretion.

Body size and body composition also affect BMR. Bodies composed of a greater percentage of fatty tissue have a lower basal metabolism than bodies with a greater percentage of muscle tissue. This difference is due to the active oxidative processes that take place in muscle tissue, which continuously expend more energy than the processes occurring in fatty tissue. As we mentioned before, men, who typically have a larger amount of lean body tissue than women, also have a higher BMR.

Most of the body's energy is lost through the skin as heat. Thus, a tall thin person, having a greater surface area than a short person of the same weight (who would obviously be fatter!), would also have a higher basal metabolism. The greater the skin surface area, the greater the loss of heat, and the greater will be the amount of heat that must be produced to equal the heat lost.

What effect does body temperature have on the BMR? Temperature elevation increases the BMR by 7 percent for each degree Fahrenheit (0.55°C) above 98.6° (37°C). Thus, a fever of 103.6°F, which is 5°F (2.8°C) above normal, would increase basal metabolism by 35 percent. This effect applies to internal temperature changes only. Although climate influences basal metabolism somewhat, the significance of this factor has been reduced primarily because clothing and climate-control systems moderate the effects of temperature extremes.

Nutritional status also has an important effect on BMR. The metabolism of chronically malnourished individuals is lower than that of comparable normal individuals. The more severe the state of malnutrition, the lower the BMR. This decrease is due to the loss of muscle tissue, which begins to be metabolized as fat stores are depleted, and also to a general decrease in the metabolic rate per unit of body weight. Underweight individuals who are not malnourished, however, often have a *higher* BMR per unit of body weight; this has been attributed to their relatively greater proportion of muscle mass to adipose tissue.

Obviously, so many factors influence BMR that predictions of energy requirements based on standardized tables are merely approximations. For most people, however, no matter what their actual BMR may be, more than half of daily energy needs are devoted to continuing the vital processes of growth, regulation, and maintenance of physiological function.

PHYSICAL ACTIVITY. Any kind of physical activity will increase the body's energy requirement above the basal level. Of course, some activities require more energy than others. Interestingly, a heavy individual will require more energy than a slim one engaged in the same activity because more energy is needed to move the greater mass of the heavier body (Passmore and Durnin, 1955).

The average individual spends about one-third of a normal day in sleep, an activity that doesn't greatly increase energy expenditure. Nevertheless, sleep may account for as much as one-fourth of the total daily energy requirement. Obviously, this figure varies from individual to individual. Some people enjoy relatively long periods of absolute rest during sleep, while others toss, turn, and move about for much of the night.

Walking, climbing, and running are necessary functions in our daily lives, and so are recreational activities. The energy cost of these activities varies according to the speed involved, the gradient and surface of the ground covered, and the weight of the individual performing the activity. Predictably, the greater the speed, the steeper the level walked or the stairs climbed, the rougher the surface, or the heavier the individual, the greater will be the energy expenditure. Similar relationships hold for more strenuous activities, such as bicycling, skiing, and playing tennis.

For some of us, recreational time is far exceeded by work time. Obviously, strenuous physical work carries with it energy demands just as great as those required for strenuous recreation. But what of mental labor? It may be a surprise for students to learn that their exhaustion after studying or concentrating during an examination is all psychological. Research conclusively demonstrates that mental work requires insignificant increases in energy expenditure. The energy you use in studying comes from muscle tension, opening and shutting books, or in writing notes—but not from thinking!

Most adults engage in an activity mixture that is largely determined by their occupations. The Joint Food and Agriculture Organization/World Health Organization Committee on Energy and Protein Requirements (1973) has classified occupations according to the level of physical activity they involve. Most office and professional work is listed as "light" activity, in contrast to the "moderate" activity of light industry and the "exceptional" activity of construction work. Because people in industrialized nations are engaged primarily in light or moderate occupational activity and in spectator, rather than active, sports, the Food and Nutrition Board (1974) has issued energy guidelines tailored to the lower activity level of today's population. FNB tables for men indicate an average energy expenditure (in kilocalories per kilogram per hour) for very light work (seated and standing activities) of 1.5, increasing to 8.4 for heavy activities (tree felling, working with pick and shovel). The average range of energy expenditure for women is listed as 1.3 (light activity) to 8.0 (heavy activity).

SPECIFIC DYNAMIC EFFECT OF FOOD. Digestion itself is known to increase energy expenditure. Several explanations for this increase have been advanced. It was originally attributed to the "work" involved in digestion and absorption. However, experiments in which nutrients were administered intravenously (bypassing the digestive system) or provided orally in the form of glucose and amino acids still produced an increase in the body's metabolic rate.

This thermogenic effect, known as the specific dynamic effect (SDE) of food, is particularly noticeable following protein ingestion. Protein increases metabolic rate by as much as 30 percent, compared with an increase for carbohydrate and fat of only 5 or 6 percent. Krebs (1964) suggested that protein ingestion increases the body's energy requirements by stimulating urea synthesis. Ashworth (1969) proposed, however, that it is protein *synthesis* that increases the metabolic rate. Recently, Hegsted (1974) has suggested that the specific dynamic effect of food results from "wasted energy" generated at the cellular level when the potential energy in food is converted to the free energy (usually ATP) required by the organism. The metabolic efficiency of this conversion process is 40 percent at maximum, varying with different metabolic pathways and with the nutritional status of the organism. Hegsted postulated that food ingestion further decreases the efficiency of energy transformation, resulting in the heat loss known as the specific dynamic effect.

Whichever of the many explanations is correct, the SDE is recognized as a relevant variable in any precise calculation of energy requirements. It has been estimated to represent approximately 6 percent of the body's total energy needs, a minor contribution in comparison with the energy required for basal metabolism and physical activity.

Recommendations for Energy Allowances

Precise energy requirements are difficult to establish for any one individual. Although the basal metabolic rate remains relatively stable in each person, activity patterns may vary, often on a daily basis. Tables of suggested energy allowances obviously cannot consider each of these variables as they affect every individual. As a practical compromise, the Food and Nutrition Board (1974) made several assumptions in devising its RDA tables:

1. The average activity level of an adult (age 23 to 50) engaged in a light-activity occupation, in an environment with a mean temperature of 20°C (68°F), consists of 8 hours of sleep, 12 hours of very light activity, 3 hours of light activity, and 1 hour of moderate activity.
2. The energy expenditure during sleep is approximately 90 percent of an individual's resting basal metabolic rate. In contrast to the rigid experimental requirements of morning testing after 14 hours without eating in determining strict basal metabolism, the resting BMR is taken in the course of a day, with the subject at rest. Because it is not a fasting BMR, the calculation includes a correction for the SDE of foods. The resting BMR thus represents an average of the metabolic rate during a pause in the day's occupation.
3. In contrast to allowances for *nutrients*, which are set at a level above the estimated average requirement (see Chapter 1), the recommended allowance for *energy* is set at the average value thought to be consonant with good health.

Note that the energy/weight/day calculation figures in Table 5-2 compare reasonably well with the quick rule of thumb for adult BMR (22 or 24 kcal/kg body weight/day) plus 40 to 50 percent for activity.

For those who are not appreciably over or under ideal body weight, individual energy requirements can be determined with more precision from

TABLE 5-2 **RDA for Energy for Adults**[a]

	Body Weight (BW)		Energy Allowance			
	kg	*lb*	*kcal/day*	*kJ/day*	*kcal/kg BW/day*	*kJ/kg BW/day*
Males						
19–22 yrs	70	154	2,900	12,200	41	174
23–50 yrs	70	154	2,700	11,340	39	162
Females						
19–22 yrs	55	120	2,100	8,820	38	160
23–50 yrs	55	120	2,000	8,400	36	153

Source: Food and Nutrition Board, National Research Council, *Recommended dietary allowances*, 9th rev. ed. (Washington, D.C.: National Academy of Sciences, 1979).
[a]For energy recommendations for all ages see Appendix, Table A.

the energy-activity guidelines of the Food and Nutrition Board (1974). After determining how much time is spent at light, moderate, and heavier work, in other activities, and in sleep, it is possible to more closely approximate just how much energy an individual usually expends per day. Table 5-3 illustrates the method of estimating energy needs from total daily activities.

Those individuals whose weight is more than about 10 percent above or below the ideal should calculate their energy *needs* based on their ideal, not actual, weights. For overweight people, these estimations will usually dictate a decrease in food consumption, though still within the energy level required for efficient growth and body maintenance.

But what of the overweight individual who is consuming an energy level appropriate for his or her ideal body weight, sex, and age? The Food and Nutrition Board does not recommend starvation, which would be necessary to achieve energy intakes *below* minimal need. They suggest, instead, increased *activity* to achieve the desired weight balance and to avoid degenerative arterial diseases that have been associated with a sedentary lifestyle and obesity.

Most individuals do not need to rely on extensive calculations of energy requirements. The most practical way to monitor your own energy balance state is to watch the scale. It will tell you whether you are matching your intake to your daily needs! Energy allowances for persons at different stages of the life cycle, and during pregnancy and lactation, will be discussed in the appropriate chapters in Part 2 of this text.

OBESITY: POSITIVE ENERGY BALANCE

A certain amount of body fat is desirable and necessary to protect against starvation and, as mentioned in Chapter 3, to protect the internal organs and provide insulation for the body. Normal energy intake and energy expenditure maintain this necessary level of body fat. Excessive energy intake and deficient energy expenditure result in a positive energy balance, causing unused potential energy to be stored as fat. There is virtually no limit to the amount of fat that can be stored by the human body.

Definition and Diagnosis of Obesity

The accumulation of excess body fat to such a degree that actual body weight is 20 percent or more greater than ideal body weight is termed **obesity.** It is *the* most prevalent nutritional disorder in the United States. Estimates indicate that more than 30 percent of the adult population in this country is obese. Increasing concern over the number of obese children, adolescents, and adults has stimulated considerable research into the causes of overweight, ways to "cure" it and, most importantly, educational campaigns to prevent it.

Obesity, however, is not simply a problem of "overweight," but of "overfat." Because bone and muscle also contribute importantly to body weight, athletes or others may well be 10 percent or more above the average

TABLE 5-3
Estimation of Energy Needs for a 23-Year-Old Female, 65 Inches (165 cm) Tall, 120 Pounds (54 kg)

A. Calculation of BMR:

22 kcal/kg BW/day = 22 × 54 = 1,188 kcal/day

B. Adjustment for physical activity:

Activity	Time hrs	Energy Expenditure	
		kcal/kg/hr	*kcal*
Sleeping	8	—	—
Dressing	0.5	0.7	18.9
Driving car	1	0.9	48.6
Eating	1.5	0.4	32.4
Typing (electric typewriter)	5	0.5	135.0
Bicycling	1	2.5	135.0
Housework (making bed, 10 mins.; washing dishes, 20 mins.; vacuum cleaning, 30 mins.)	1	1-3	113.4
Sitting	5.5	0.4	118.8
Sewing by hand	0.5	0.4	10.8
Walking upstairs (2 flights)		0.036[a]	3.9
Walking downstairs (2 flights)		0.012[a]	1.3
Total			618.0

C. Subtotal for basal metabolism plus physical activity:

1,188 + 618 = 1,806

D. Specific dynamic effect (+6%):

1806 × .06 = 108.36

E. Total Energy Requirement:

1,806 + 108 = 1,914 kcal/day

[a]Allowance per kg for 15-step staircase, disregarding time.

weight for their height and yet not be fat. The percentage of an individual's weight accounted for by muscle and bone is known as **lean body mass.** Precise ways of determining lean body mass exist and are used primarily in experiments in which it is desired to determine body composition. These methods are, however, too cumbersome and expensive for routine clinical use.

Fortunately, they are not necessary. Most of us have simpler methods of determining when we have gotten heavier than we should be. Accumulation of adipose tissue is the best clue. When the body looking back at you from the mirror shows unmistakable bulges and folds, no ultrasophisticated technology is required. *Physical appearance* is the best indicator of "overfat."

Weekly weighing provides another check and should be part of every health maintenance routine. Weight increases are normal during the growth years, but for adults over 25 years of age rising scale readings are the early warning signals of obesity. Weight gain *per se* is not necessarily a problem; athletes often gain weight without increasing their fat stores, and many underweight individuals could benefit from increased fat deposition and the extra few pounds that go with it. Problems arise when weight gain is out of proportion to body build. And sudden, sharp increases in weight are a danger signal at any age.

Height-weight tables categorizing adults by height, sex, and body frame—small, medium, or large—are compiled from life insurance company statistics (see Appendix Table D). While determinations of body frame size are inexact, the validity of categorizing weight by body build is supported by mortality statistics. These figures show that adults who maintain their weight at a level appropriate for a 25-year-old of their height and body build tend to live longer. The customary assumption that weight gain with increasing age is normal and desirable is simply not so. This fallacious viewpoint grew from surveys of *actual*, rather than desirable, weights of typical men and women in each group. Although our sedentary life style may contribute to a yearly weight gain even in normal, healthy individuals, mortality figures prove that this "real" standard is not consistent with the "ideal" of overall good health.

Recently, the National Center for Health Statistics published growth charts for children and adolescents. Children throughout the country were studied to calculate growth curves showing percentile levels of normal development by sex and age, from early infancy through 18 years of age (see Figures 13-1, 13-2, 13-4 and 13-5). Growth charts do not correct for body build and body composition; they are a means of comparing a given child's development in terms of height and weight with that of other children. The pattern of development shown by the child over a period of time can also be checked against the normal curves. An overfed infant, for example, might be in the 50th percentile for height, but the 99th percentile for weight. A large-boned child who falls at the 85th percentile for height may well be at the 85th percentile for weight with no sign of obesity. However, a consistent pattern of increasing percentile measures of weight, with increased age, would signal obesity in a growing child.

Estimation of **skinfold thickness** is another way to identify excess adiposity. Can you "pinch an inch"? If the fold of skin and underlying subcutaneous fat on the side of your lower chest, or the back of your arm, is greater than an inch in thickness, you are probably obese. This "pinch test" may be performed more scientifically with a calibrated measuring instrument known as calipers. Using calipers to make measurements at carefully specified body sites, researchers have established age and sex norms for skinfold thickness (see Appendix Table E). Girls and women have greater skinfold thickness than boys and men, and young people have lower values than older people. Calipers may never replace the tape measure, however. Some researchers find significant variability in caliper measurements both from day to day and from observer to observer. They recommend a return to circumference measurements of chest, waist, hips, and biceps, which are easy to obtain and more reliable (Bray et al., 1978).

Ultimately, then, the surest indicator of obesity is fat accumulation, not total weight. When clinical analysis is not feasible, charts and tables may help the individual to identify fat accumulation. These are used in many large clinics and in most "self-help" groups such as Weight Watchers, and by many physicians as well. In the final analysis, however, each individual is the best judge of her or his own condition. Look in the mirror, weigh yourself, check your weight against statistical tables, try to pinch an inch. Are you obese?

Prevalence of Obesity

If you are obese, you have lots of company. More than 70 million Americans are overweight and more than 7 million adults are severely obese. According to the National Center for Health Statistics, severe obesity—defined as 30 percent or more above desirable weight for men and 50 percent or more for women—afflicts 2.8 million American men and 4.5 million women (*New York Times*, 12/12/78). Another study which confirmed that women are more likely than men to be overweight was the Ten State Nutrition Survey of 1968–1970 (Garn and Clark, 1976). By race, white men tend to be fatter than black men; and white females are fatter than black females through adolescence, but significantly thinner from age 18 through 70.

The postadolescent reversal in incidence of obesity in black and white females has been attributed to socioeconomic factors. Before puberty, girls of lower socioeconomic status are thinner (as are lower-class boys), no matter what their skin color. After mid-adolescence, working-class women get heavier while more affluent women get slimmer. Current research has corroborated these socioeconomic differences, suggesting that they are not caused by hidden biological factors or by childhood feeding practices. For example, researchers find that women of low educational status who marry into high-income families are significantly thinner than their low-income-group peers. Obviously, social factors are implied (Garn et al., 1977).

Socioeconomic influences, however, do not always remain constant. In the past, large girth has often been considered a symbol of high status because it signified wealth and the ability to obtain generous amounts of food. Today, however, being slim is "in," as more and more educated and higher-income level people have been limiting intake of saturated fats, working out at the health clubs, or jogging in the park. The slimness trend may soon affect even those socioeconomic and ethnic groups who until now have continued to find plumpness acceptable or even desirable.

Concerns About Obesity

If so many people are obese, can it be that bad? Unfortunately, the answer is yes. The medical, psychological, and economic costs of obesity are extremely high.

MEDICAL CONCERNS. At every age, mortality rates for people who are obese exceed those for people of normal weight. The Build and Blood Pressure Study (Society of Actuaries, 1959) found that people who were 20 percent overweight had a corresponding increase in mortality of 25 percent for males and 21 percent for females. At 30 percent overweight, men had mortality rates 42 percent above normal, and women 30 percent. And when obesity exceeded these levels, the risk of premature death was even greater. Estimates indicate that for every 10 percent above normal weight, life span is decreased by one year—and it has been shown that return to normal weight is accompanied by a return of normal life expectancy (Yudkin, 1978).

Not only are obese people more likely to die at earlier ages, but they are also more likely to become seriously ill. Conditions in which obesity may be implicated include coronary heart disease, hypertension (high blood pressure), diabetes mellitus, osteoarthritis, renal (kidney) disease, cirrhosis of the liver, pulmonary (lung) disease, and even surgical complications and proneness to accidents (Yudkin, 1978). Why is this so? Research suggests that being overweight places a physical burden on the respiratory, circulatory, and digestive systems of the body. The increased synthesis and transport of fat caused by overeating may clog blood vessels and further burden these systems. Reduction of weight to desired levels may often arrest or even reverse these disease processes. For example, a recent report indicates that weight reduction alone, without medication, can reduce blood pressure in hypertensive patients who are overweight (Reisin et al., 1978).

PSYCHOLOGICAL CONCERNS. As great as the physical costs of obesity may be, the psychological costs for many individuals can be even greater. In fact, since health warnings are notoriously poor motivators (as the continuing prevalence of cigarette smoking shows), psychological factors are more likely than physical ones to motivate people to lose weight.

Our land of plenty shows a surprising readiness to revile those who show signs of enjoying that plenty. Americans view obesity as a repulsive sign of self-indulgence, of lack of willpower, and even of immorality. Fat people are stigmatized, as if they were totally responsible for their deviation from the accepted norm. This attitude toward fatness is inculcated very early in life. In one study, when boys aged 6 to 10 were asked to comment on silhouettes of fat, muscular, and thin people, responses to the muscular bodies were always favorable. But the fat silhouettes drew uniformly negative comments related not only to appearance, but also to imputed social and personality characteristics. Being fat was equated with being lazy, sloppy, naughty, ugly, dirty, stupid, and forgetful (Stofferi, 1967).

These prejudices against fat people also translate into actions. Obese youngsters are less likely to gain admission to college, and subsequently less likely to achieve high earning power. Career opportunities are also limited, and job bias against employing or promoting overweight individuals is openly acknowledged. Some corporations insist upon physical examinations that few obese people can pass. The *Wall Street Journal* (1973) found that one-third of the people in a weight-reducing organization had experienced job discrimination—and this was probably only the tip of that iceberg. Appearance *counts.*

The overweight share society's views and, as a result, develop negative self-images. From distaste for their own appearances it is but a short step to disregard. Too often those who have "let themselves go" in weight also let themselves go where grooming is concerned. And often, the psychological negativism associated with being overweight becomes a vicious cycle: As people eat to console themselves for their real losses of self-esteem as well as of social and economic opportunities, they become even more obese. As we have noted, however, our society's disdain for the heavy is not universal; plumpness has been much admired at other times and places, and even in the United States some ethnic groups continue to reject the mainstream ideal of slenderness.

ECONOMIC CONCERNS. Society is not only a harsh critic of obesity, but a frequent victim as well. Obesity is costly to society as well as to the individual. Consider the loss of working days and expenses incurred for medical services by those with obesity-related illness. Consider the expenses involved in staffing hospital obesity clinics, and the cost to the community of caring for dependents of those who die prematurely from such illnesses. Consider the $200 million spent annually for diet pills and liquid diet aids (Berland, 1978). Consider too the cost to the individual who cannot find or hold a job, and the further cost to society from the loss of tax revenues as well as the additional expenses of providing supplemental income and services. Finally, add in the cost of growing, processing, and distributing the superfluous food eaten by obese individuals.

The current energy shortage and scarcity of food in many areas of the world make obesity a pressing socioeconomic problem. According to estimates by scientists at the University of Illinois, the overweight men and women in the United States carry a grand total of 2.3 billion extra pounds. By dieting for six months, they would save the equivalent of 5.676 *trillion* kilocalories, and about 3.430 trillion kilocalories more would be conserved if these formerly obese people ate only enough to maintain their new weight. Translating these kilocalories into fossil fuel energy, the Illinois researchers estimated energy savings equivalent to 1.3 billion gallons of gasoline annually (*New York Times,* 11/4/78).

Etiology of Obesity: Biochemical Factors

Recognition that obesity is related to excessive food intake is ages old, and so is advice to the overweight. But obesity is more complex than simple overconsumption of food. Socrates, for example, had this advice for the overweight in 399 B.C.:

> *Beware of those foods that tempt you to eat when you are not hungry and those liquors that tempt you to drink when you are not thirsty.*

And the connection between food intake in excess of energy expenditure was addressed by the famed French gourmet Brillat-Savarin in 1825:

> *Any cure for obesity must begin with the three following and absolute precepts: discretion in eating, moderation in sleeping, and exercise on foot or on horseback.* [*Quoted in Jordan, 1973*]

If following such advice were the sole answer, millions of people would not be obese. The origins of obesity are unclear and, it seems, the more we learn, the more questions are raised. A number of biological factors in the etiology of obesity have been proposed.

Heredity is one such factor. In some animal strains, obesity is an inherited trait, but there is little evidence that the same holds true for humans. Fat parents do tend to have fat children, and thin parents to have thin children. However, obesity in families is probably due more to their shared environment and lifestyle, including eating patterns, than to heredity (Garn and Clark, 1976).

Studies of twins, on the other hand, provide some support for a genetic role: Identical twins raised in different homes have been shown to reach more similar weights than do fraternal twins raised in the same home. Another possible genetic factor is body build or somatotype, an inherited characteristic. Ectomorphs, thin individuals with long fingers, arms, and legs, rarely get fat. In contrast, endomorphs, who are rounder individuals with larger abdomens than chests, have a greater likelihood of becoming obese.

Other biological factors may contribute to obesity. In rare cases, obesity may be correlated with disturbances of the **endocrine system.** An underactive thyroid gland is the usual culprit, a situation which is easily treated by hormone replacement therapy. However, the thyroid gland has been blamed out of all proportion to the actual incidence of this problem. Only a very small percent of obesity is due to hormonal abnormalities. Some hormonal abnormalities, moreover, are the *consequences* of weight gain, not the *causes*, and disappear following weight loss.

Metabolic disturbances have also been cited as factors in obesity. Some research suggests that enzymes, especially those required for lipid synthesis (lipogenesis), act differently in obese than in normal individuals. As yet, there is little supporting evidence for a metabolic explanation of obesity.

There is more agreement for another biological explanation, the so-called *adipose cell theory*. Winick's demonstration that varying food intake in rats during their early development influenced the number and size of cells of various organs (Winick et al., 1972) led to a number of investigations relating the timing of excess food intake to the development of obesity. Hirsch and Knittle (1970) presented evidence that both the number and size (a reflection of the amount of accumulated lipid) of adipose cells in obese children exceeded those of nonobese children. Confirmation of this finding in rats strengthened the hypothesis that overfeeding early in life resulted in an increased number of adipocytes, a condition that persisted throughout life.

Additional studies led to the statement of the adipose cell theory: During the early developmental years, overfeeding causes excessive growth of adipose tissue, resulting in a greater number of cells and an increased amount of lipid within those cells. In other words, more *cells* contain more *lipid.* If weight reduction is achieved later, lipid is lost from the cells; but the cells remain, to be refilled with fat when energy intake exceeds expenditure.

Several investigations have attempted to determine whether, in fact, infant obesity persists to become adult obesity, whether moderate food consumption during infancy would prevent obesity in adulthood, whether adult-onset obesity is characterized by an increase in size but not number of adipocytes, and whether weight loss indeed represents a loss of lipid but not of cells.

This theory has been surrounded by much controversy, and it has not been universally accepted. Questions about the methodologies used to test the hypothesis have been raised (Winick, 1975), and the Working Group of the British Department of Health and Social Security and the Medical Research Council (James, 1976) have pointed out that the number of cells is not fixed during infancy but continues to increase at least until adolescence.

At the present time, the adipose cell theory has been neither accepted nor rejected as important in the etiology of human obesity, but current research suggests that adipose cell studies will continue to be an intriguing topic for some time to come.

OTHER PHYSIOLOGICAL FACTORS IN OBESITY. Of course, not only fat cells but all body cells are affected by food intake. Some biological explanations of obesity propose a complex interaction of body cells and systems that results in metabolic balance for the organism. These theories emphasize the transmission within the body of "hunger" and "full" signals. **Hunger** is a strictly physiological feeling, and appears to be controlled by internal mechanisms. **Appetite,** on the other hand, is cued by external stimuli—taste, smell, and social and numerous other cues—that make us feel we want—or don't want to—eat. All of us often eat when appetite is aroused, even if we are not particularly hungry at that moment. It has been theorized that many obese individuals respond more readily to appetite cues and may not even experience hunger, possibly because the biochemical mechanisms producing hunger or satiety are malfunctioning.

Mayer has speculated that special receptors in the part of the brain known as the hypothalamus are sensitive to changes in the blood glucose levels. After food is eaten, blood reaching the hypothalamus contains high levels of glucose which, according to this theory, stimulate these receptors to send a "stop eating" message to the rest of the brain. A few hours later, the blood glucose level falls to a critical triggering point, the hypothalamus receptors receive less glucose in the blood, and a message of hunger is transmitted (Mayer, 1966).

More recent research has proposed that the key control mechanism is located in the liver, where biochemical signals activate the release into the blood stream of metabolites and enzymes which are then carried to the brain (Friedman and Stricker, 1976). Additional candidates for hunger regulators have been proposed, including serum amino acids, lipid release from adipose stores, and a variety of hormonal and other control mechanisms.

According to theories of biochemical regulation of appetite, an imbalance in the control mechanism or process results in scrambled messages that set off eating binges. But no theory so far proposed has won widespread acceptance as a complete explanation of eating behavior. Many people are able to adjust energy intake to needs automatically, but some individuals, for reasons that are still unclear, seem to lack such a built-in control mechanism. These individuals, especially if they have been obese for many years, may have to learn to adjust their intake needs by using portion size and meal frequency, rather than appetite, as regulators. It does seem curious, at this late date in human development, that we still do not know for certain either how appetite is regulated or how appetite regulation relates to obesity. We do know that the relationship is complex.

Etiology of Obesity: Social and Psychological Factors

We all have times when we continue to eat despite the lack of hunger or appetite. We may eat because the clock says it is "lunchtime," because others are doing so, or because "it's good for us"—and for dozens of other reasons completely unrelated to our physiological state.

Some of these reasons are environmental and social. Our technologically advanced society has provided a plentiful supply of tasty food and has increased our opportunities to consume it. Our ancestors had to forage for or raise their own food supply, but we just hop into the car or walk down the street and buy whatever we choose at an amply stocked supermarket or fast-food emporium.

Then, too, our workday activities have changed. From a nation of active food producers, we have become a nation of sedentary paper pushers. The shift in activity patterns is a key contributor to the growth of our national girth. Labor-saving devices and "automobility" save time and energy expenditure and allow the kilocalories to accumulate in fat storage. Habits of inactivity develop early: Today's children play outdoors less than did children of previous generations.

While much of our lifestyle has changed, one tradition has continued: the American way of hospitality. Food traditionally accompanies social occasions, and this pattern has now been extended to sports events (at which we are usually observers, not participants) and even to the working day. Coffee breaks, business lunches, and office parties are common occupational hazards. After work we go home, where we may entertain at cocktails and dinner, or "get the munchies" while watching television.

Cultural and socioeconomic factors also influence the tendency toward obesity. Many Americans are members of ethnic groups in which plumpness is considered desirable for esthetic reasons or as a sign of prosperity. To these groups, the American preoccupation with slimness is subversive rather than healthy.

Perhaps the most important influence of society on body configuration is socioeconomic. We have already seen that women of low-income groups and older men of greater prosperity are often overweight. The reasons for these phenomena involve both economics and status. Meals in nonaffluent homes are high in sugar, starch, and fat content. Fresh fruits and vegetables and lean meats and seafoods are rarely served. And as for the increased girth of older and prosperous men—there is a good reason why the characteristic protruding tummy is often referred to as a "corporation"! Until recently, the expansion of the belt and of the bank balance were equally prized. However, it is now fashionable to be slim and fit, and men of all ages have started watching their weight and exercising. And as increased opportunities for paid employment and upward mobility reach women of all social groups, the start of a shift away from obesity is being observed among those formerly less well off.

Social customs influence habits and patterns of eating. The increased tendency toward snacking and "grabbing a bite" has deemphasized the traditional pattern of "three square meals a day." Some experimental work with animal models suggests that this may be beneficial for those with a tendency toward obesity. In one study, rats were allowed to eat as much food as they wanted, but only for two hours a day, while controls were allowed to nibble their food all day long (the normal rat eating pattern). After a few weeks, the meal-fed rats were gaining weight as rapidly as the controls, even though their food intake was 15 percent lower. They had apparently become more efficient metabolically when ingesting energy in excess of immediate needs. Fat deposits therefore increased (Leveille and Romsos, 1974). Similarly, in a study of elderly men in Czechoslovakia, there was a 58 percent incidence of obesity among those who ate three or fewer meals per day, while men who ate more frequently (five or more meals per day) had a 30 percent likelihood of becoming obese. Other researchers have found that subjects who eat less frequently have abnormal glucose tolerance (Leveille and Romsos, 1974).

While these experimental findings may give comfort to snackers, they must be tempered with caution in regard to the *quantity* of food eaten. Frequent meals are valuable because they spread energy intake over time. But if additional meals only increase the amount of food eaten, there would be no benefit.

Frequent snacking may be a product of our speeded-up lifestyle, but it may also have psychological and emotional roots. We are most likely to start nibbling when we are bored or tense. Psychologists believe that the pleasantly full sensations we get from eating take us back to the security of infancy, when our needs were fulfilled by an all-providing mother. However, the sense of satisfaction and fulfillment derived from eating is reinforced daily throughout life. Constant pairing of the act of eating with the satisfaction of biological and psychological needs is similar to the close association of other stimuli and responses in our lives. Just as we learn that turning a knob will open the door, or that carrying an umbrella will protect us from rain, so we learn that eating leaves us feeling satisfied.

As growth proceeds, the baby's response to a bottle of milk extends to a bowl of oatmeal, to a cookie, to a full meal. By the time adulthood is reached, the number of stimuli that are associated with contentment may be sufficient to fill a refrigerator or an entire supermarket. The frequent use of food as a reward for a child complicates these associations even more. From a parent's offer of a cookie for good behavior it is only a small step to adults rewarding themselves with chocolate cake. A home environment in which a child is made to feel guilty for not eating everything on the plate may be responsible for setting a lifelong pattern of overeating. In these and other ways food is used to manipulate behavior, and children often learn to view food not as a source of sustenance or gustatory enjoyment, but as a manipulative device. And, despite the adult's ability to learn other associations—between over-

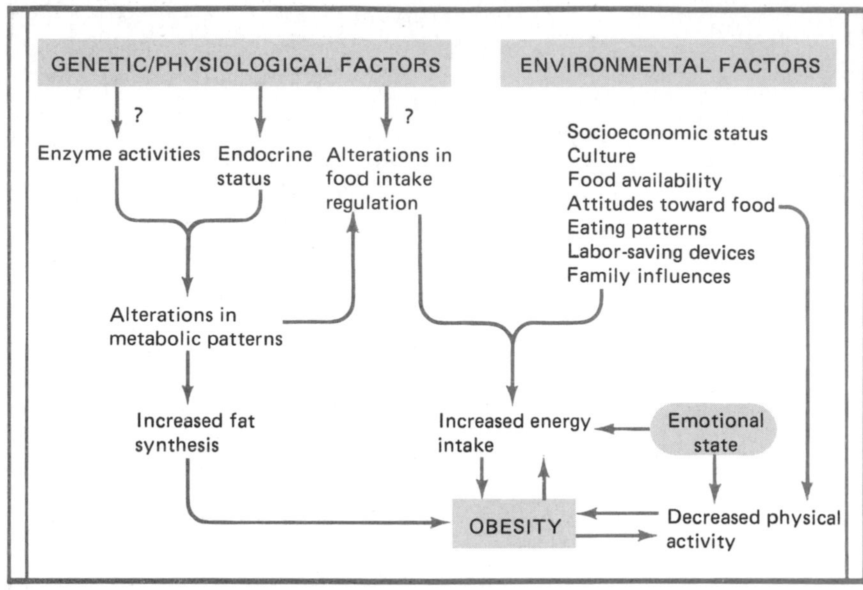

FIGURE 5-3

Possible Causes of Obesity

Factors in both the internal and external environments can contribute to a state of positive energy balance resulting in obesity. The relative importance of each of these influences is not known and probably varies for each individual.

eating and indigestion, between overeating and obesity, between obesity and social ostracism—it may be impossible to counteract the pleasurable or manipulative associations learned in early life. The more unpleasant the consequences of obesity, the more unloved and worthless the individual feels, and the more comfort is sought from food. (The complex interactions between such emotional factors and obesity are discussed by Bruch, 1973).

All the factors discussed so far—heredity, endocrine changes, metabolic alterations, activity level, environmental and social influences, psychological needs—interact to produce a continuous pattern of increased energy intake and decreased energy expenditure (see Figure 5-3). Of course, not every obese person is affected by every factor. For some people, cultural influences are overriding; for others, genetic factors take precedence; and for many, the psychological influences predominate. The crucial factor for *all* cases of obesity, however, is the critical ratio of energy intake to energy expenditure. Whenever intake exceeds expenditure, weight gain follows inexorably.

From a mathematical point of view, an intake of 100 "extra" kilocalories (420 kJ) per day will produce a 10-pound weight gain in just a year's time! One hundred kilocalories may seem like a lot, but translated into two small chocolate chip cookies, one fried egg, or a glass of low-fat milk it becomes a mere "snack." Any food, even a recognized "low-calorie" food, has the potential to contribute to obesity, if it is eaten in addition to foods that meet normal daily energy requirements. As can be seen in Table 5-4, eating just one extra apple (87 kcal) each day will add one pound of body fat in 34 days. That one-pound gain will take only 7 days if the extra is a 12-ounce milkshake (420 kcal) (Konishi and Harrison, 1977).

Treatment of the Overweight Condition

The Last Chance Diet, the Calories-Don't-Count Diet, the Dupont Diet, the Air Force Diet, the Drinking Man's Diet, the Doctor's Quick Weight-Loss Diet, the Diet Revolution, Doctor's Quick Inches-Off Diet, the Scarsdale Diet, Weight Watchers, "rainbow" diet pills, Metrecal, Relaxacisor, body wrap, hormones, laxatives, diuretics, fasting, intestinal bypass, liquid protein—this plethora of weight-loss approaches is testimony to the difficulty of the task.

Despite all the hard-sell promises, there is no magic way to lose pounds and inches. Diets and weight-reducing treatments that sound unbelievable are just that: unbelievable. There are several satisfactory approaches to weight loss, but all require energy intake to be lower than energy expenditure. Any sustained decrease in energy intake, with energy expenditure held constant or, better, increased, will produce weight reduction.

It should be remembered that even in this context, the word **diet** doesn't

TABLE 5-4
Weight Gain Equivalents of Selected Foods When Eaten in Addition to Daily Needs

Food Item and Portion Size	Weight g	Energy kcal	Body Weight Gain			
			1 lb days	*25 lb weeks*	*1 kg days*	*25 kg weeks*
Apple, medium, 2½″ diam.	150	87	34	121	75	267
Beef roast, 1 slice 4″ × 2½″ × ½″	53	150	20	70	43	155
Brandy, cognac, 1 pony	30	75	39	140	87	310
Bread, 1 slice with 1 pat butter	28	96	31	110	68	242
Bread, peanut butter, and jam: 1 slice; 1 tbsp; 1 tsp	38	195	15	54	33	119
Brownie with nuts 2″ × 2″ × ¾″	30	146	20	72	44	159
Cookies, chocolate chip, 2	22	100	30	105	65	232
Ice cream cone, ½ c dip	72	160	18	66	41	145
Martini, 3½ fluid oz	100	140	21	75	46	166
Milk, whole, 8 fluid oz	240	160	18	66	41	145
Milk, skim, 8 fluid oz	240	88	34	120	74	264
Milkshake, 12 fluid oz	345	420	7	25	15	55
Orange juice, 4 fluid oz	120	54	55	195	120	430
Peanuts, 1 oz	30	170	17	61	38	136
Pizza, ⅛ of 14″ diam. pie	75	190	16	55	34	122
Potato chips, 10	20	115	26	92	56	202

Source: Adapted from F. Konishi and S. L. Harrison, Body weight-gain equivalents of selected foods, *Journal of the American Dietetic Association* 70:365, 1977 (Table 1).

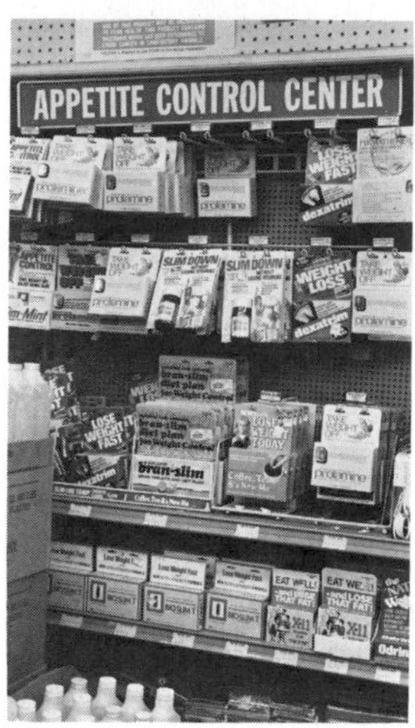

(William H. Graham)

necessarily imply a weight-loss regimen. There are diets that promote weight gain, diets that restrict salt or fats, diets free of roughage, and diets designed to detect allergies. A diet is, simply, a prescribed regimen of eating and drinking. Most people, however, do mean "weight reduction" when they say diet. There are a number of accepted, nutritionally sound principles that apply to all weight-control regimens. These principles will be considered first, and then some efficient diet programs will be examined.

Principles of Weight Reduction: Balanced Deficit Dieting

As noted above, even a small daily excess of energy intake over expenditure accumulates slowly but steadily as adipose tissue. The expectation that the pounds that went on slowly should be able to come off rapidly is probably the greatest diet fallacy, and leads to rapid dissatisfaction and discouragement on the part of dieters. Another fallacy is the expectation that, once desired weight is achieved, prediet eating habits can be resumed. After all, those habits put the weight on in the first place. For weight reduction to be lasting, balanced intake patterns and regular eating habits must be established. Unfortunately, the vast majority of dieters are unable to maintain their weight loss. They return to their former eating patterns and, soon, to their former weights. (Johnson and Drenick, 1977).

The regaining of weight may be partially explained by studies demonstrating that starved rats convert food to body fat more efficiently than nonstarved rats eating the same amount of food. A similar principle may be at work in some humans who have dieted. After a period of restricted intake their bodies adapt, like those of the meal-fed rats, to retain energy more efficiently. Then, even when desirable weight is achieved and normal intake patterns resumed, the rate of lipid synthesis continues at the higher adaptive level, and weight gain follows. Maintaining regular eating patterns while reducing overall food intake may unwind this dietary "yo-yo" (Leveille and Romsos, 1974).

In addition to the hazard of developing increased lipogenesis, diet methods that call for omission of breakfast and lunch are likely to fail for another reason: People who skip meals often more than make up for it at the next meal. Whether it's because they "owe it to themselves" or because they are ravenous (and no wonder!), meal skippers are rarely as successful at dieting as meal trimmers.

More important than learning *when* to eat, however, is determining *how much* to eat. It is difficult to determine precisely the level of kilocalorie reduction necessary to produce a specified weight loss for a given individual. But there are several workable approximations. They are derived primarily from the fact that, in order to lose 1 pound of fat, a 3,500-kilocalorie deficit must be achieved. Thus, to lose 1 pound per week, a dieter must have a deficit of 500 kcal per day; to lose 2 pounds (4.4 kg) per week, the deficit must be 1,000 kcal per day.

To determine the desired level of reduced caloric intake, it is first necessary to estimate the number of kilocalories needed to maintain present weight, then subtract 500 (to lose 1 pound per week) or 1,000 (to lose 2 pounds per week). For a quick approximation multiply present weight in pounds by 15 (assuming a moderate activity level, 15 kilocalories per day will maintain 1 pound of body weight). A young woman who weighs 150 pounds and wishes to reach her ideal weight of 130 pounds can maintain her present weight on 2,250 kcal per day (150 × 15); to lose 1 pound per week she must reduce intake to 1,750 kcal per day, and to lose 2 pounds per week intake should be reduced to 1,250 kcal per day.

Obviously, to continue losing weight at the same rate, intake levels should be readjusted downward as weight loss occurs. For example, after the 150-pound woman loses 10 pounds, she should refigure her caloric intake; her weight is now 140 pounds, and a daily intake level of 2,100 kcal (140 × 15) will maintain that weight. To continue losing weight at the rate of 1 pound per week, therefore, she should consume 1,600 kcal per day; to continue losing at the rate of 2 pounds per week intake should be reduced to 1,100 kcal per day.

Alternately, the would-be dieter could resort to another nutritionists' rule of thumb: Multiply the ideal weight by 10 and consume that level of kilocalories per day. This, too, will surely take pounds off. Using this method, the young woman in the example given above would plan a diet consisting of 1,300 kcal per day. Her weight loss at the start would be about the same as she would achieve on a 1,000-kcal daily deficit, but the *rate* of weight loss would slow as she approached her ideal weight. However, she would get there—and would then be able to adjust intake upward to the level needed to maintain her ideal weight, approximately 1,950 (130 × 15) kilocalories per day.

In all weight-reduction programs, there comes a time when weight loss slows and then appears to stop altogether. This plateau is notoriously difficult for dieters. Until that time, weight loss has been a true loss of fat. During the plateau period, however, loss of fat apparently continues, but it does not show up (on the scales) because, for reasons that are not clearly understood, water is accumulated by the body. After a period of one to three weeks, *if reduced kilocalorie intake is maintained*, the water will be eliminated and weight will suddenly drop. But even on a markedly lowered caloric intake, the last few pounds often do not come off. An additional reduction of intake and/or a slight increase in physical activity should help dieters to reach their goal.

Perhaps the easiest approach of all is to follow tables of recommended energy intake appropriate to sex and age. This will result in an automatic reduction in energy intake for most overweight individuals. However, it will not be enough of a reduction to achieve ideal body weight.

Nutritionists rarely recommend a weight loss greater than 3 pounds per week (Fineberg, 1972). Beyond this level, the body begins to metabolize body protein producing weakness and metabolic imbalances. Ideally, weight loss occurs because of the loss of fat, not of lean body mass (muscle) or water. On an energy-restricted diet, the energy required to support basal metabolism and physical activity in excess of that provided by food must come from the body's fat stores, which are released and burned as metabolic fuel.

But, although the total food intake is drastically reduced in energy-restricted diets, all necessary nutrients must be provided—adequate amounts of vitamins and minerals, enough protein and carbohydrate, and a limited amount of fat. Thus, these are nutritionally *balanced* deficit diets. Diets of less than 1,000 kcal (4,200 kJ) per day are seldom advised, no matter how great the weight loss desired, because it is difficult to ingest the necessary nutrients in adequate amounts. Whenever a diet of 1,000 or fewer kilocalories per day is followed, a vitamin and mineral supplement providing RDA levels should be taken daily. Remember that nutritional adequacy is always related to the diversity of the diet; as intake of certain categories of food is drastically reduced or eliminated altogether, achievement of nutrient balance becomes more and more difficult. In addition, most people cannot adhere to a severe energy-restricted diet; they feel deprived and, instead of developing sound eating habits, tend to starve one day and "binge" the next.

Dieters should make a particular effort to choose foods that have a high nutrient content in proportion to energy content, that is, foods that have a high "nutrient density." The "empty calories" found in candy bars, alcoholic beverages, and chocolate cake are not accompanied by significant nutrients; these and similar foods should be on the "seldom if ever" list of every dieter. If you do have a small piece of chocolate cake, something else must go. Dieters must learn to adjust portion sizes of high-energy foods—and even so, empty calorie foods should not be eaten regularly on a weight-loss diet. When energy intake is limited to 1,000 or 1,500 kilocalories daily, it is particularly important to make those calories count in terms of their nutritional value. You may have heard that "calories don't count"—but they do!

Because fat-rich foods are "high calorie" foods, they should be eaten in moderation by dieters. But they should not be omitted altogether. Butter, margarine, salad dressings, cold cuts, and other fatty foods provide essential fatty acids and fat-soluble vitamins. They also add appetite appeal and reduce boredom. Fortunately for dieters, fat also has a satiety-producing effect. Thus, the inclusion of some fat in each meal will satisfy nutritional needs and leave the dieter feeling fuller longer.

Potatoes and grain products have similar hidden benefits, despite the widespread notion that bread, pasta, and other grain-based foods are "fattening." A check of the energy content of a piece of bread (70 kcal, 294 kJ), even with a pat of butter (35 kcal = 147 kJ) added, shows it to be a better dinnertime addition than a second 3-ounce serving of lean roast beef (165 kcal = 693kJ). This is not to say that protein is "fattening" either. Foods themselves are not fattening when taken in moderation; it is the energy we consume in excess of our daily needs that is fattening. Eating "low-calorie" foods is just as damaging as eating "high-calorie" foods, if we are consuming more energy than our bodies require. It doesn't matter in what form the kilocalories are provided; too much from any nutrient source—whether carbohydrate, protein, and/or fat—will lead to weight gain.

What about other grain products, such as pizza or beer and hard liquor? Pizza is a good source of nutrients, but, depending on the "extras," can be a significant energy source. Alcoholic beverages are sources of kilocalories, but not of nutrients. (Beer and wine do have slight amounts of some vitamins and minerals, but in proportion to energy content these are negligible.) Obviously, a 1,000 kilocalorie diet doesn't leave much room for beer. Does that mean that dieters can *never* drink? No, but it does mean that careful planning will be necessary. When it's going to be a long evening, they can sip club soda or mineral water with a lemon or lime wedge. Highball drinkers can make it a tall one rather than a short one (the added ice and water don't add calories), and compensate with a decrease in bread and fat intake for that day. Since having more than one may make it difficult to obtain sufficient nutrients without going over one's energy allowance, unlimited drinking of alcoholic beverages is not a way to lose weight.

Meals for weight-reduction diets can be planned in several ways. Food composition tables (see Appendix Table H) list energy content as well as nutrient values. These can be used by themselves to plan a day's eating, or they can be used in conjunction with the two most useful food grouping systems. The Food Group system (see Chapter 10) can be used to plan meals that include two servings each from the milk and the meat/alternate groups, four servings of grains/breads, and four servings of fruits/vegetables (including one citrus fruit or juice for vitamin C and one dark green or yellow vegetable for vitamin A). These choices, if prepared without additional sugar or fat, will provide about 1,200 kilocalories. Exchange Lists (also explained in Chapter 10) are also helpful for many who find it tedious to actually count calories. Table 5-5 indicates suggested distribution of exchange groups for diets at various energy intake levels. Consult the lists in the Appendix for foods and amounts included in each of these categories.

Noting the approximate amount of kilocalories in an average serving from each of the Exchange Lists or basic food groups is an easy way for weight-conscious individuals to make substitutions in accord with their personal likes and dislikes. It is important that no complete group of foods be eliminated from the diet. By including foods from all groups, an adequate supply of essential vitamins, minerals, and fatty acids, as well as necessary carbohydrate and protein will be likely.

Portion sizes described in these lists may be distributed throughout the

TABLE 5-5 Distribution of Exchange Groups for Diets at Various Energy Intake Levels

Exchange List	Serving Size	Kcal per Serving	Number of Exchanges at Different Energy Levels (kcal)						
			1,000	1,200	1,400	1,600	1,800	2,000	2,200
Milk, skim	1 c	80	2	2	2	2	2	3[a]	3[a]
Vegetables	½ c	25	2	2	2	2	3	3	3
Fruit	1 small apple or equivalent	40	2	3	3	3	5	4	5
Bread/grains (cereals and starchy vegetables)	1 slice bread or equiv.	70	4	5	6	8	9	9	9
Meat/alternate (medium-fat)[b]	1 oz	75	4	5	6	7	7	8	9
Fat	1 tsp margarine or equivalent	45	3	3	4	4	5	7	8

[a]To substitute whole milk for skim milk, decrease the number of fat exchanges by 2 for each milk exchange to keep equivalent kilocalorie content.

[b]To simplify the table, medium-fat meat exchanges have been used. Lean meats (55 kcal/oz) should be stressed in low energy diets. High-fat meats provide 100 kcal per ounce.

Source: Exchange lists for meal planning (American Diabetes Association, and the American Dietetic Association, Chicago, 1976). (See Appendix Table G.)

day. For example, two cups of milk may include ½ cup eaten with breakfast cereal, another ½ cup taken in three cups of coffee, and a glass drunk as a snack. Options such as this, and the choices provided by the food groups or lists, allow variety in meal planning. If diets are boring, people don't stick with them. And when an individual develops a diet plan most compatible with his or her own likes and eating habits, the chances for successful weight loss are tremendously increased. Also, making choices during a diet is good preparation for the choices that must be made when dieting is completed. Remember, the goal is not only short-term weight loss but the long-term dietary change, necessary to maintain ideal weight.

Snacking can help reduce boredom and prevent the empty feeling between diet meals. Low-calorie snacks such as plain tea, bouillon, an apple, raw crunchy vegetables, tomato juice, or skim milk are good choices. Snacks should provide nutrients as well as calories. Peanut butter or cheese and crackers are nutritious snacks that can be eaten in moderation during a weight-loss program, and are often more satisfying than a stalk of celery.

Another way to make choices easier while limiting energy intake is to control portion size. A dieter who can't "live" without ice cream may survive quite well on smaller portions of this favorite. Portion size assumes particular importance with high-calorie foods. Although we can't eliminate them from our diets, we can limit our intake. Three ounces of lean meat, for example, contain 165 kcal; a double-sized portion will therefore contain 330 kcal, twice as many. This may sound obvious but it's something dieters often forget. "Calorie counting" is only accurate when portion size is considered. And for many people, a reduction in portion size *alone* will produce weight loss.

Dieters often substitute "dietetic foods" for other foods. Is there any reason to buy these special foods which are also more expensive than the regular products? Generally speaking, no. Foods are labeled "dietetic" for various reasons; they may be low in salt, but not in kilocalories. Careful label reading will distinguish these products from true low-calorie items, such as water-packed fruits, which have fewer kilocalories than those packed in heavy syrup, and can be used when fresh fruits are not available.

The advantages of a balanced deficit diet are as follows: Weight loss is steady, foods eaten are nutritionally adequate, bizarre eating patterns are avoided, ordinary and readily available foods are utilized, and there is no medical risk. Too, there is maximal opportunity to learn new eating patterns, which are the key to continued weight maintenance. The major disadvantage of balanced deficit diets is that, although weight loss is steady, it is relatively slow. Most dieters want to lose their excess weight fast, forgetting that it accumulated slowly in the first place. Even two pounds a week seems too slow to most overweight individuals. So they go on highly publicized diets in which the initial weight loss is rapid but alas, impermanent. Before we discuss some of these "popular" diets, we shall examine the important role of physical exercise in losing weight.

Physical Exercise

For most people, basal metabolic needs account for the greatest portion of total energy expenditure. However, individuals engaged in hard physical labor or strenuous recreational activity will have very different energy utilization patterns. A lumberjack, or an athlete in training, may expend 4,500 or even more kilocalories in one day. Since energy intake must match energy expenditure, that individual must consume at least 4,500 kilocalories in order to maintain his or her weight (Konishi, 1965). On the other hand, energy expended in sedentary activity patterns may not significantly increase energy requirements and will therefore be insufficient to counterbalance an intake of even 1,400 kcal per day. Particularly in middle age, as metabolism slows, many individuals find that the levels of energy intake that once kept them trim now produce an uncomfortable layer of fat around the midsection. The choice is clear: Increase activity or decrease intake.

So, which would you prefer: running, or not eating? Table 5-6 may help you to decide. This table translates the energy content of various foods into activity equivalents. Note that these equivalents are calculated by time. Thus, it would take you six minutes of running to "pay" for eating one serving of potato chips (ten chips). If you prefer swimming, you can work off two strips of bacon in nine minutes. And if you start bicycling for a half-hour each day *and* eliminate just one slice of bread and butter from your daily diet, you will be achieving the same effect as if you had eliminated three slices of bread and butter.

But why exercise, dieters ask, when I'm already "starving" myself? Contrary to popular notions, moderate exercise actually *decreases* appetite. Also on the positive side, exercise provides many health benefits, such as improved muscle tone (which all by itself can make the dieter *look* slimmer) and increased circulatory efficiency. It may also make people feel better psychologically. Finally, exercise can be enjoyable. Calisthenics and "diet exercises" are widely considered boring, but tennis, swimming, jogging, and even rope jumping are frequently more fun.

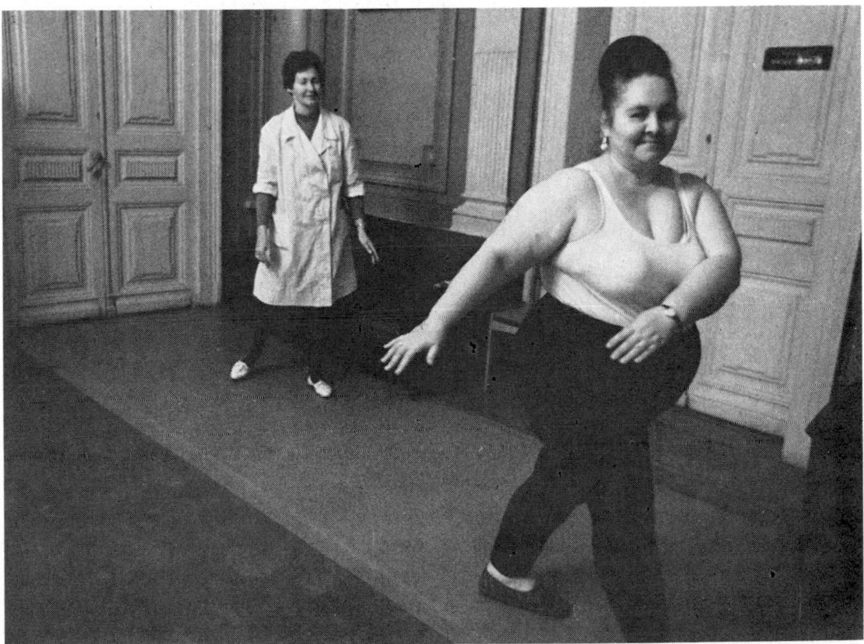

At a clinic in the nutritional institute in Moscow, patients are given instructions in physical exercise and special diets. (WHO photo by M. Jacot)

TABLE 5-6 **Energy Equivalents of Selected Foods and Beverages**

Food	Kilo-calories	Activity (minutes)				
		Walking[a]	*Riding Bicycle*[b]	*Swimming*[c]	*Running*[d]	*Reclining*[e]
Apple, large	101	19	12	9	5	78
Bacon, 2 strips	96	18	12	9	5	74
Banana, small	88	17	11	8	4	68
Beans, green, 1 c	27	5	3	2	1	21
Bread and butter	105	20	13	9	5	81
Cake, 1/12, 2-layer	356	68	43	32	18	274
Carbonated beverage, 1 glass, 8 oz	106	20	13	9	5	82
Carrot, raw	42	8	5	4	2	32
Cereal, dry, 1/2 c, with milk and sugar	200	38	24	18	10	154
Cheese, cottage, 1 tbsp	27	5	3	2	1	21
Cheese, cheddar, 1 oz	111	21	14	10	6	85
Chicken, fried, 1/2 breast	232	45	28	21	12	178
Cookie, chocolate chip	51	10	6	5	3	39
Doughnut	151	29	18	13	8	116
Egg, fried	110	21	13	10	6	85
Egg, boiled	77	15	9	7	4	59
French dressing, 1 tbsp	59	11	7	5	3	45
Halibut steak, 1/4 lb	205	39	25	18	11	158
Ham, 2 slices	167	32	20	15	9	128
Ice cream, 1/6 qt	193	37	24	17	10	148
Ice cream soda	255	49	31	23	13	196
Ice milk, 1/6 qt	144	28	18	13	7	111
Gelatin dessert, with cream	117	23	14	10	6	90
Mayonnaise, 1 tbsp	92	18	11	8	5	71
Milk, whole, 8 oz	166	32	20	15	9	128
Milk, skim, 8 oz	81	16	10	7	4	62
Orange, medium	68	13	8	6	4	52
Orange juice, 6 oz	92	18	11	8	5	71
Pancake with syrup, 1 tbsp	124	24	15	11	6	93
Peach, medium	46	9	6	4	2	35
Pie, apple, 1/6	377	73	46	34	19	290
Pizza, cheese, 1/8	180	35	22	16	9	138
Pork chop, loin, 2.7 oz, lean & fat	314	60	38	28	16	242
Potato chips, 1 serving (10 chips)	108	21	13	10	6	83
Sandwiches						
Club	590	113	72	53	30	454
Hamburger	350	67	43	31	18	269
Tuna fish salad	278	53	34	25	14	214
Sherbet, 1/6 qt	177	34	22	16	9	136
Steak, T-bone, 3 oz	235	45	29	21	12	181
Strawberry shortcake	400	77	49	36	21	308

TABLE 5-6 **Energy Equivalents of Selected Foods and Beverages (Continued)**

Alcoholic Beverages	Kilo-calories	Activity (minutes)				
		Walking[a]	*Riding Bicycle*[b]	*Swimming*[c]	*Running*[d]	*Reclining*[e]
Beer (regular), 8 oz	100	19	12	9	5	77
Beer (light), 8 oz	70	13	8	6	4	54
White wine, $3\frac{1}{2}$ oz	84	16	10	8	4	65
Dessert wine, 3 oz	124	24	15	11	6	95
Gin (80 proof), 1 oz	65	12	8	6	3	50
Rye (80 proof), 1 oz	65	12	8	6	3	50
Scotch (80 proof), 1 oz	65	12	8	6	3	50
Vodka (80 proof), 1 oz	65	12	8	6	3	50
Vermouth, dry, 1 oz	33	6	4	3	2	25
Vermouth, sweet, 1 oz	45	9	5	4	2	35
Bloody Mary, $1\frac{1}{2}$ oz liquor + 6 oz juice	130	25	16	12	7	100
Screwdriver, $1\frac{1}{2}$ oz liquor + 6 oz juice	175	34	21	16	9	135

Note: These values are based on the energy used by an adult male weighing approximately 154 pounds (70 kg) and should be adjusted for other individuals according to their weight and sex.

[a] Energy cost of walking for 70-kg individual = 5.2 kilocalories per minute at 3.5 m.p.h.

[b] Energy cost of riding bicycle = 8.2 kilocalories per minute.

[c] Energy cost of swimming = 11.2 kilocalories per minute.

[d] Energy cost of running, 180 steps/min. = 19.4 kilocalories per minute.

[e] Energy cost of reclining = 1.3 kilocalories per minute.

Source: Adapted from F. Konishi, Food energy equivalents of various activities, *Journal of the American Dietetic Association* 46:186, 1965.

Energy expenditure can be increased in other simple ways as well, with some advance planning. Dieters should be encouraged to park the car or get off the bus several blocks from their destination, and walk there quickly. Instead of waiting for the elevator, they should walk up a flight or two of stairs. In fact, walking at any time is an excellent exercise. It can be done virtually everywhere, requires no special equipment, and is especially suitable for people who, at least initially, find the more strenuous or competitive sports too taxing. A quick examination of daily activities can suggest many other creative ways to increase the amount of energy expended without spending a lot of time or money. This assumes, of course, that the dieter is young and healthy. Individuals who are extremely overweight, who have a history of illness, or who are middle-aged or older should consult their physician to establish an exercise program suited to their special needs.

Exercise often provides the "edge" for a dieter. Usually, dieting begins in a burst of determination, supported by quickly noticeable loss of weight and inches. But then many dieters get stuck on a plateau. Their bodies have adjusted to decreased energy intake. Physiologically, fat mobilization is still taking place, but some metabolic water is retained. This is when dieters typically get discouraged. But it is important not to give up; the weight will come off. At this point, increasing energy expenditure through exercise may speed weight loss without more rigid Calorie-counting on the part of the discouraged dieter. Then, too, exercise is something positive you can do to lose weight, as opposed to the negative aspect of giving up some favorite foods.

Role of Behavior Modification Techniques

We often eat in response not to biological cues of hunger and thirst, but to various social and psychological cues. Because eating habits are learned, they can be unlearned, and more appropriate eating behaviors substituted for those that produce and maintain obesity. In recent years, behavior modification techniques have been used with notable success in the treatment of obesity.

Before eating behaviors can be modified, however, it is necessary to identify them and, in particular, to locate those habits that are destructive and should be changed. Participants in behavior modification programs work closely, often in a group situation, with a group leader or therapist and keep extensive records of food intake and eating behavior. These records are regularly reviewed and analyzed. Clients keep a daily diary of the time and places of eating, of their physical position while eating, of the social aspects of the situation, of other activities associated with each eating experience, of the degree of hunger felt, of their mood at the time, of their choice of food, and of the amount of each food consumed, noting its energy value. Often, the client is also asked to note what events took place immediately before eating in order to identify conditions that lead to inappropriate food intake.

After this period of data collection, the client and therapist examine the data and identify problems, such as eating while watching television, eating too quickly at meal times, or snacking when bored or tense. The next step is to plan the strategy for changing, or modifying, a particular behavior that is associated with excessive food intake. Substitution of a new pattern has been found to be more likely to be successful than attempting to eliminate the negative habit altogether. A person who may find it impossible to stop eating snacks completely may still be able to change her or his snacking in some way—perhaps by substituting a low-calorie, high-nutrient food such as fruit for the usual potato chips and beer. It may not be possible to completely remove tension and boredom from anyone's life, but a client may be guided to pick up needlepoint or a crossword puzzle at such times instead of reaching for a soft drink or a cookie. A similar approach may be used to increase physical activity at the same time. If weight is lost, the modifications are continued. If weight is not lost, new modifications are tried.

The changes planned in behavior modification therapy are intended to decrease both the frequency and the quantity of food intake. Such changes are effective because obese individuals have eating habits that differ from those of normal-weight individuals. In one study, for example, it was found that obese subjects ate more rapidly, took larger bites of food, and chewed food less thoroughly than their nonobese tablemates (Drabman et al., 1977).

Changes will not become permanent unless they are reinforced in some way, thus motivating the client to persevere in the new eating pattern. A sequence of rewards is usually built into the modification program and formalized by a "contract" between client and therapist. For instance, when a

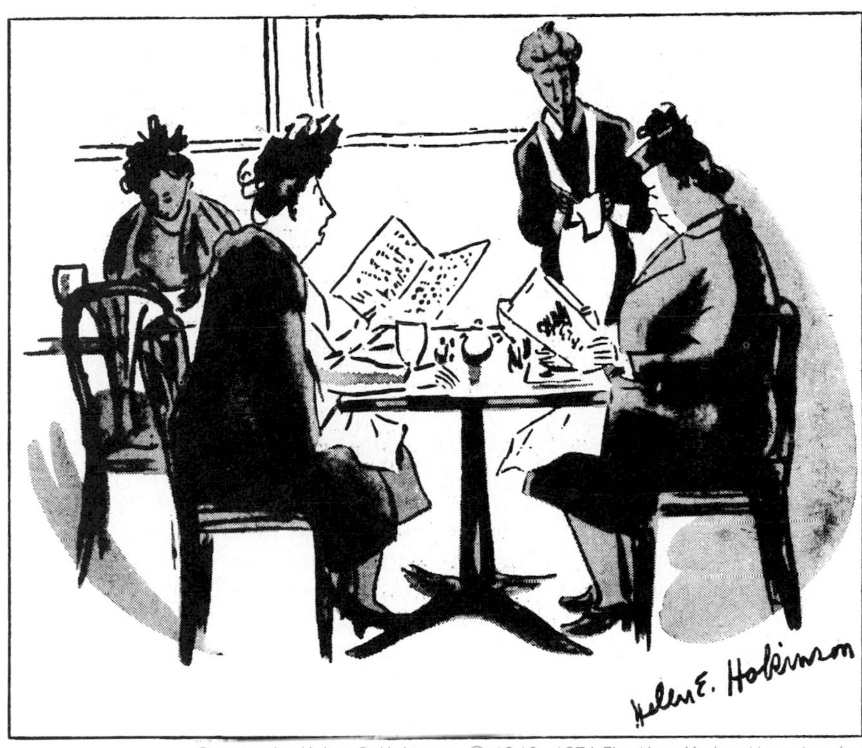

Drawing by Helen E. Hokinson; © 1948, 1976 The New Yorker Magazine, Inc.

"Sometimes I think Schrafft's doesn't *care* about calories."

certain weight loss is achieved, or when a certain negative behavior has not been resumed for a period of time, the client is entitled to buy a new outfit in a size that fits. The goal is permanent change and permanent normal weight; the adult individual must assume full responsibility for his or her own eating behavior.

Behavior modification for children is seldom successful unless the entire family becomes involved. Each family member is shown how to aid and encourage new eating habits in the overweight child and is thus given a share of responsibility for the outcome. Otherwise, the family is likely to subvert the child's efforts to change.

So far behavior modification, in conjunction with a balanced deficit diet to ensure nutritional adequacy, seems to be an effective addition to conventional methods of weight control. However, only long-term studies will indicate its effectiveness in achieving permanent weight loss.

Alternative Methods of Weight Reduction

Having decided to lose weight, most people want immediate results. They forget that the weight was gained slowly in the first place and must be lost the same way. So they succumb to a succession of diets and other treatments publicized in the popular press.

The media promises are indeed appealing. "Eat all you want and still lose weight" promises one advertisement. "Lose 30 pounds in 90 minutes!!!" touts another. (This extravagant claim, explained in small print at the bottom of the advertisement, actually referred to the 18 5-minute visits to a weight-loss clinic over a period of months!) There are diet guides directed at women, at drinking men and thinking men, at chubby children and at busy executives. Devices and treatments offer to banish pounds and inches, shape the legs, trim the tummy, and otherwise alter the user's shape. Numerous over-the-counter pharmaceutical preparations promise to decrease the appetite, fill the stomach, break down fat, and speed waste products out of the body.

The Food and Drug Administration does not have authority to interfere with the promotion of such programs and products *before* they reach the marketplace. The only recourse is legal action by consumers after purchase, based on injury or ineffectiveness. Obviously, the risk of complaints is insufficient to discourage the promoters of these diet "aids." As quickly as one plan disappears from the market, another rushes in to take its place.

Many dieters, recognizing obesity as a health problem, turn to their physicians. Because few physicians, however, have studied diet-management, all too often the result is a cursory examination and a printed diet sheet. Few of the millions of overweight Americans have ever been asked by their physicians for a diet history or instructed in any method of evaluating food intake patterns and determining energy requirements. Or the overweight turn to physicians who have developed reputations as "diet doctors," and who are just as ready as more commercial ventures to promise fast, effortless diet programs.

Weight-reduction "clinics," "medical centers," and "health spas" have also been springing up, competing aggressively for the money to be made by promising painless loss of poundage. Their fees are generally quite high and, too often, susceptible customers sign contracts before inquiring about the actual content of their programs.

KETOGENIC DIETS. Low-carbohydrate diets have been popular for a number of years. Some of these have such impressive-sounding names as the "Mayo Clinic Diet," (a title given to several different food regimens, all of which have been disavowed by that prestigious institution) or the "Air Force Diet" (similarly disclaimed by the U.S. Air Force). In this category too are Dr. Atkin's Diet Revolution, the Stillman Diet, and many other variants. These programs have in common a severe restriction of carbohydrate intake, while they allow large or even unlimited amounts of certain high-protein foods. They differ, however, in the amount of energy intake permitted and range from being calorie-restricted to "eat all the meat you want."

Promoters of these diets assert that fat people tend to convert carbohydrates into adipose tissue more rapidly than normal people. The fat and protein in the diets they recommend, however, are said to be burned in the metabolic process, and therefore cannot be stored as fat. But this is simply untrue: There is no consistent scientific evidence to indicate that energy provided from any one nutrient is utilized differently from energy from any other source.

In a low-carbohydrate diet, glycogen stores are rapidly depleted, an effect that is accelerated when calorie intake is also restricted. Fatty acids are metabolized at a rapid rate to provide energy in the form of ketone bodies for physiological functioning. Most body tissues can readily utilize the ketone bodies for energy needs, but the brain must first undergo a period of adaptation during which glucose is still required. Gluconeogenesis provides the glucose through an amino acid metabolic pathway. Meanwhile, acetyl CoA is being produced more rapidly than the Krebs cycle can metabolize it, and the number of ketone bodies in the blood increases to abnormal levels.

This physiological imbalance, known as *ketosis*, is decidedly unhealthy. Ketone bodies are acids. Their overproduction upsets the body's acid-base balance, a condition that cannot be tolerated by people with kidney disease—and that may precipitate kidney problems in previously normal individuals. Electrolyte loss, which may cause cardiovascular problems, also occurs in ketosis. In addition, ketone bodies compete with uric acid for kidney excretion, increasing the risk of gout in susceptible individuals. There is one small plus for ketosis: It acts as a mild appetite suppressant, which may be somewhat helpful to the dieter.

Proponents of ketogenic diets point to the rapid and often substantial initial weight losses as evidence that these diets work. "Lose 7 to 15 pounds in the first week," they promise—and indeed the scales often bear them out. But this initial loss is a depletion of water, not of fat. The exact mechanism of water loss on a low-carbohydrate diet is not known, but it may be related to the sodium loss induced by ketosis. In any event, the water and its weight will be regained when carbohydrate intake is resumed.

Contrary to claims, actual rate of fat loss is quite slow in ketogenic diets, because fats are not metabolized efficiently in the absence of carbohydrates. Without carbohydrates to regenerate oxaloacetate, the Krebs cycle is disrupted (see Figure 5-4), and ketone bodies accumulate. For this reason, a minimum of 50 grams (200 kcal) of carbohydrate per day should be included in any weight-loss diet. Furthermore, ketogenic diets often promote excessive cholesterol and saturated fat intakes.

Because of the strange food combinations advocated in low-carbohydrate diets, few people are able to adhere to them for very long. Because they do not alter the dieter's eating patterns, lost weight is often regained when regular eating is resumed. Thus, ketogenic diets often lead to the "yo-yo effect" of initial weight loss, followed by weight gain, followed by yet another unbalanced diet. This sequence may be even more dangerous for many individuals than being slightly overweight.

STARVATION. Ketosis results also from the most rigorous weight-loss program, starvation or prolonged fasting. Starvation regimens are not recommended for those who should lose 35 pounds or less and they are generally used only for the massively obese. Patients should be hospitalized for the duration, at least one and perhaps two or three months; only in that way can intake be controlled and medical supervision provided. Vitamin and mineral supplements and a minimum of two quarts of water a day must be taken. The metabolic processes are essentially the same as those in the low-carbohydrate diets, with ketone bodies providing the chief energy source for all tissues. Weight loss may be as high as one pound per day. There are, however, possible severe side effects, including nausea and loss of hair. The most serious consequence is the loss of muscle protein during the fasting period. Studies

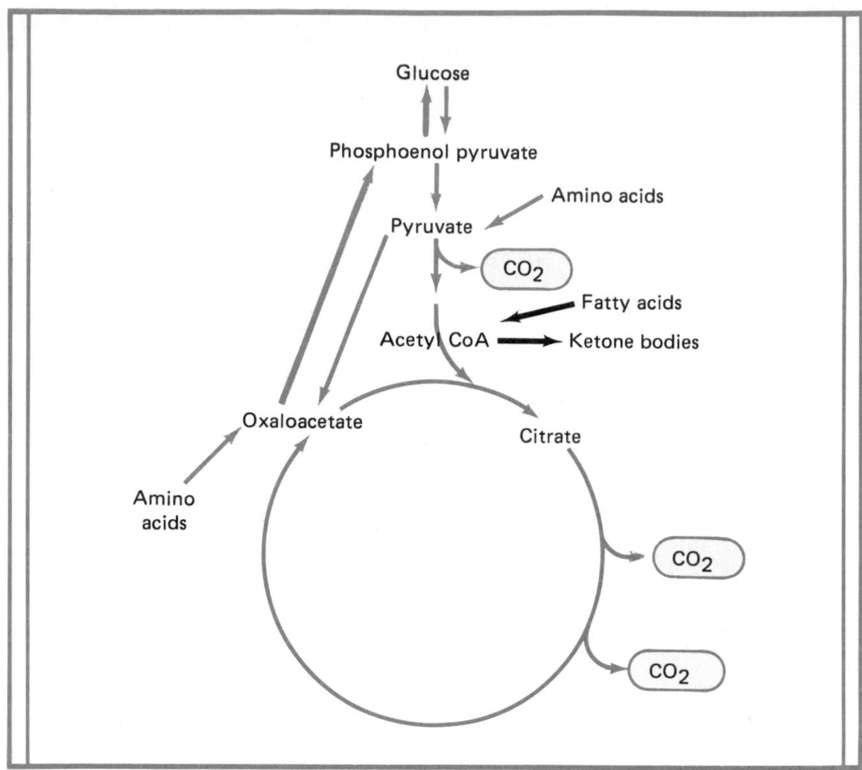

FIGURE 5-4

Disruption of the Krebs Cycle on a Low-Carbohydrate Diet

As carbohydrate intake is reduced, oxaloacetate, produced by the deamination of amino acids, is used for glucose synthesis via the intermediate PEP (phosphoenol pyruvate). Oxaloacetate is thus diverted from the reactions of the Krebs cycle. As fatty acids are metabolized to acetyl CoA, formation of citrate cannot occur. Instead, units of acetyl CoA are condensed to form ketone bodies.

have shown that 65 percent of the weight loss produced by fasting is traceable to a loss of lean body tissue and only 35 percent to loss of fat. This lean tissue loss can be avoided by administration of small amounts of protein to maintain tissue protein; on a *protein-sparing modified fast*, 3 to 6 ounces of dry milk, egg white, cottage cheese, or fish are added twice a day to the otherwise nonnutrient liquid and vitamin-supplemented intake.

Although part of the rationale for prolonged fasting is that it may break the chain of dietary habits that produce obesity and thus give obese patients a clean start, this does not seem to happen. In a recent study of 207 grossly obese patients (192 men and 16 women) who lost weight during prolonged fasting, near normal body weight was attained in approximately 50 percent of the cases. The longer the patient was able to fast, the greater was the observed weight loss. However, within two to three years, there was a steady return to prefasting weight level in all patients, regardless of length of fasting, extent of weight loss, or age of onset of obesity. Patients who had been obese since infancy tended to regain weight to levels *above* their prefasting point (Johnson and Drenick, 1977).

The presumed benefits of protein-sparing fasts have been questioned by some (VanItallie and Yang, 1977; Felig, 1978), and long-range studies of their effectiveness have yet to appear. However, approaches that gradually readjust the patient to the real world of eating following such a regimen have been tried and show promise. For example, the patient is weaned from the protein-sparing fast to an energy-restricted program in which regular foods are slowly introduced. Behavior modification therapy accompanies the next transition, to a normal weight-maintenance diet, with the aim of restructuring eating habits.

SURGERY, MEDICATION, AND OTHER APPROACHES. Perhaps the most drastic of all weight-loss procedures is intestinal bypass surgery. A loop of intestine 16 to 22 feet in length is surgically blocked off, leaving only a small length of functional intestine. Nutrient absorption is significantly decreased. Following bypass surgery (sometimes called jejuno-ilial bypass), most patients experience a steady weight loss for up to two years. Then, however, there is a leveling off, usually attributed to adaptation of the functioning intestinal segment to increase absorptive capacity. Because of the reduced absorption, key nutrients, including essential fatty acids, fat-soluble vitamins, and vitamin B_{12} must be exogenously supplied. In some cases amino acids and some minerals must also be supplemented.

This is major, and risky, surgery, with a 3 to 6 percent mortality rate. Serious side effects related to the lack of normal nutrient absorption include not only nutritional deficiencies but also fat deposits in the liver, other liver problems, nausea and/or diarrhea, and the development of renal stones. Positive benefits, on the other hand, have been reported, including improved self-esteem and general attitude and improvements in interpersonal relationships and career achievements (Solow et al., 1974). Other changes may include increased activity levels, changes in taste preferences, and decreased food intake. Because of the serious implications of this surgical procedure, patients must be carefully selected not only for degree of obesity but also for overall physical and psychological stability.

Reliance on drugs is another risky means of weight control. Americans have become so used to taking pills and potions for all sorts of major and minor problems that we expect pills to confer speedy slimness, too. Unfortunately, pills cannot do anything except suppress appetite and disrupt fluid balance and metabolism. Drugs can also be abused and become habit-forming.

Amphetamines have most often been prescribed for their appetite-depressing effects. However, these drugs are central nervous system stimulants and can lead to excitability, insomnia, constipation, and addiction. In addition, their appetite-depressing ability is short-lived, and ever-increasing amounts become necessary to maintain the same level.

Hope has been raised that a newer medication, fenfluramine, will be more useful in modifying food intake. This medication also suppresses appetite, but it depresses rather than excites the central nervous system, causing drowsiness instead of a high. It appears not to be addictive and thus has less potential for abuse.

Diuretics and laxatives have also been prescribed for the overweight person. Again, these substances do not attack the central problem and can lead to a temporary, and false, sense of security. Worse, they can lead to serious loss of water and electrolytes and interfere with nutrient absorption.

Excessive adiposity is often blamed on hormonal problems, and many obese individuals seek their physicians' agreement with this self-diagnosis. Actual hormonal contributions to obesity are rare; but thyroid, growth, and other hormones are often prescribed nonetheless, perhaps out of desperation on the part of physician as well as patient. Weight loss does sometimes occur when some of these preparations are taken; however, it is not permanent, and the potential for such serious complications as cardiovascular damage and interference with calcium and nitrogen balance is high.

A placental hormone, HCG (human chorionic gonadotropin), has been used as an adjunct to severely energy-restricted diets and seems to have appetite-depressing and mood-elevating effects. However, studies have not confirmed the effect of the hormone independently of the loss of weight due to the low-calorie (500 kcal, 2100 kJ) regimen.

Finally, there is a constantly increasing assortment of devices promising to rid the body of its fat by application to the body's external surface. There is a soap, for example, whose allegedly health-benefiting lather must be applied by special gloves; not only are the soap and gloves outrageously expensive, but they do not work (Yudkin, 1978). Or you might try "Love Legs," rubber stockings that supposedly trim heavy thighs by inducing perspiration. A similar claim has been made for "Instant Trim" as well as various gloves and girdles that promise to exercise parts of your body while you are doing something else. Perspiration, it must be emphasized, has no effect on fat cells; and any garment that is wrapped or worn tightly can dangerously impede circulation. None of these devices facilitates permanent weight loss in any way although they may produce temporary dehydration. One of the newest assertions of the gadget approach to weight reduction is that something called "cellulite" accumulates under our skin and must be removed by controlled exercise and massage with special lotions. This, too, is nonsense. But the public spends a fortune in a vain attempt to lose those extra pounds in an easy, painless way.

Many have found that the only regimen that works for them is a combination of controlled food intake and participation in a supportive group. The growing rosters of Weight Watchers, TOPS (Take Off Pounds Sensibly), Overeaters Anonymous, and similar groups attest to the success of such supportive approaches. Regular weigh-ins, shared experiences, and the genuine interest of others in the dieter's success seem to be effective. Such programs combine balanced deficit diets, behavior modification, and social and psychological support. They encourage exercise and provide the motivation of a periodic social event and group involvement along with hope for a positive outcome.

RECOMMENDATIONS. A number of approaches to weight loss have been examined briefly in this section. Table 5-7 shows the goals, advantages, and disadvantages of several currently popular weight-loss programs. In choosing a program, it is important to determine whether the prescriptions of the program make sense. Clearly, any program that does not call for restricting

TABLE 5-7 Comparison of Various Weight Reduction Methods

Method	Description	Promised Goals	Advantages	Disadvantages
1. Balanced Deficit	Reduction of energy intake Avoidance of concentrated sweets and foods of high fat content	Steady rate of weight loss	Nutritionally adequate No known medical risks Fosters development of appropriate eating behaviors (if not below 1,000 kcal/day)	Relatively slow weight loss
2. Weight Watchers	Weekly group meetings Reduction of energy intake by standardized meal plan	Steady rate of weight loss	Encouragement in group situation Nutritionally adequate Provides structured plan, beneficial for some	Relatively slow weight loss Does not provide for individual preferences in foods and life style
3. Behavior Modification	In conjunction with energy-restricted diet	Weight loss Changes in eating behaviors	Opportunity to learn new eating behaviors Allows for personal preferences in foods and lifestyles	Does not work for all individuals
4. Formula Diets	Liquid containing nutrients, usually in skim milk base Consumed to provide 900 kcal/day	"Easy" weight loss	Provides structured plan Nutritionally adequate (except lacking in fiber)	Monotonous Maintenance of weight loss usually not sustained Does not foster development of appropriate eating behaviors
5. "Liquid Protein"	High-protein/low-carbohydrate/low-fat diet Use of predigested protein	Rapid weight loss	Short-term rapid weight loss	Medically risky Nutritionally imbalanced Does not foster development of appropriate eating behavior Weight loss not maintained
6. Stillman's	High protein/high fat/low carbohydrate Meat, fish, eggs, vitamin supplement, fluid	Rapid weight loss	Short-term rapid weight loss	High-fat/high-cholesterol Medically risky for some individuals May become monotonous Weight loss not sustained

TABLE 5-7 **Comparison of Various Weight Reduction Methods (Continued)**

Method	Description	Promised Goals	Advantages	Disadvantages
7. Scarsdale	14-day diet with planned meals High-protein/ restricted-carbohydrate Combination of free and restricted portion sizes	Rapid weight loss	Short-term rapid weight loss Preplanned meals beneficial for some	Medically risky for cardiac patients Does not foster development of appropriate eating behavior Low in calcium
8. Starvation	Intake restricted to water and vitamin/mineral supplements for extended period of time	Rapid weight loss	Rapid weight loss for massively obese	Requires hospitalization Medically risky Loss of lean body mass Maintenance of weight loss usually not sustained
9. Drugs	(a) Amphetamines	Reduction in appetite leading to weight loss	"Easy and painless"	Weight loss not sustained Potentially serious side effects Does not foster appropriate eating behaviors
	(b) Laxatives/ diuretics: excretion of nutrients, water	Weight loss	"Easy"	Weight loss not sustained Risk of dehydration and electrolyte imbalance Does not foster appropriate eating behaviors
	(c) Thyroid hormones: induce hypermetabolic state	Weight loss	"Easy"	Medically risky Weight loss not sustained
10. Surgery	Decrease of intestinal absorption area	Weight loss	Effective for massively obese Steady weight loss for 1–2 years Positive psychological benefit	Surgical risk Serious medical side effects in many people

energy intake does not make sense! Any program that stresses a single food—grapefruit, perhaps—or eliminates an entire nutrient category—"no carbohydrate"—doesn't make sense because it is not nutritionally adequate. The only sure and safe way to lose weight is to reduce the total amount of energy intake by eliminating high-fat and highly-sugared foods, along with unnecessary snacks and alcoholic beverages; by eating smaller portions at scheduled meals; and by increasing physical exercise. Only a diverse diet provides all of the nutrients necessary for continued healthy living during weight loss. Nutritionists recommend a distribution of energy intake for weight-reduction diets in the proportions of 20 to 25 percent from protein, 30 percent from fat, and 45 to 50 percent from carbohydrate. Only readjustment of eating patterns will make lifelong weight maintenance possible.

Prevention remains the best tactic of all for weight control. Balancing intake with expenditure and making adjustments throughout life as metabolic needs change during different stages of the life cycle are the keys to preventing an overweight condition.

PERSPECTIVE ON The Liquid Protein Diet

A few years ago, the liquid protein diet was hailed as a new, easy, and safe way to lose weight. New and easy it was, but it was definitely not safe. By the end of 1977, the Food and Drug Administration had received notification of more than 40 deaths, and more than 100 cases of serious illness among people following this diet who had previously been apparently healthy, although fat (Glick, 1978).

Medically supervised "protein-sparing modified fasts" inspired the development of the over-the-counter liquid or powder protein preparations. The use of protein-supplemented fasting in a clinical setting, however, is quite different from consumer adaptations of nonsupervised programs. Prolonged fasting carries definite health risks, including anemia, impaired liver function, and mineral imbalances. Only severely obese patients, whose lives are at greater risk from the complications of their obesity and whose weight is resistant to more traditional methods of weight loss, are included in the supervised fasting programs. In the hospital, such patients are carefully monitored for complications and given, in addition to minimal amounts of high-quality protein, controlled quantities of water along with vitamin and mineral supplements.

Unlike the experimental diets, however, the commercially available liquid protein diets provide only low-quality amino acids with marginal nutritional value. This characteristic may not be fully perceived by dieters used to the concept of taking a liquid nutrient supplement as a diet aid. For many years now, various products have been available, usually in a milk and artificially flavored base, to substitute for one or more meals a day for the serious dieter. Although these products do nothing to revise inappropriate eating patterns, they do provide a substantial part of RDAs for most nutrients in a very calorie-restricted package. But the newer liquid protein preparations are almost totally lacking in nutrients. Their monetary value, however, was great; before the liquid protein craze faltered, it had become a $40 million market (*Consumer Reports*, 1978).

Why did some of the people using liquid protein die? Some showed abnormal cardiac function, perhaps due to mineral imbalance. Low blood and tissue levels of potassium, calcium, and magnesium were noted. Nevertheless, the definite cause of death has not been determined, even in the 12 patients who had been dieting under conventional medical supervision. In view of these problems liquid protein diets cannot be recommended as a weight-loss procedure. Indeed, because of the lack of definite information, it has been proposed that liquid protein supplements be considered as experimental treatment only, and that the procedures usually applied to experimentation with humans, such as getting informed, written consent of subjects, be required in addition to meticulous medical supervision (Felig, 1978).

THE UNDERWEIGHT CONDITION: NEGATIVE ENERGY BALANCE

Definition, Risks, and Treatment

Although obesity is classified as a major national nutrition problem, attention must also be paid to the relatively few individuals who exhibit varying degrees of underweight. By definition, an individual who is underweight weighs less than 90 percent of the ideal weight for his or her height, age, and body build.

In contrast to the risks associated with obesity, there are few medical risks attached to being underweight. There is, however, a somewhat increased susceptibility to infection, including tuberculosis, particularly during adolescence. Because underweight individuals have limited reserves of energy stored as adipose tissue, energy needs during periods of illness or stress, when appetite is diminished and food is not consumed, will be met by drawing from lean body mass.

Probably the greatest risk associated with the underweight condition affects young women who are pregnant; they have a higher risk of not completing pregnancy and of delivering low-birth-weight infants than do women of normal weight (see Chapter 12). In addition, women may have difficulty becoming pregnant because of low body weight and may also experience disturbances of their menstrual cycles. Recovery from severe illness, surgery, or other traumas may be more complicated and take longer for the underweight individual and require extensive medical treatment and nutritional therapy.

The degree of underweight common in Western society is subclinical and generally is not life threatening or even a significant medical risk. It is usually due to inadequate energy intake, excessive physical activity, or genetic predisposition. Of course, physical illnesses such as cancer, gastrointestinal disorders, chronic disease, or hyperthyroidism may produce serious weight loss. Illness may cause loss of appetite, leading to sharply reduced food intake, perhaps accompanied by malabsorption of energy-yielding nutrients and an increase in the rate of catabolism. In these cases, correction of the underlying condition should correct the weight problem as well. For most people who are chronically underweight, however, increased energy consumption is the key.

Increasing energy intake is not as easy as it may seem. Many underweight individuals simply do not like cakes, cookies, milkshakes, and other high-energy foods. Even for the underweight, empty calories are an unwise choice, except as supplements to a nutritionally adequate intake pattern. Nutritionists recommend instead a balanced diet of easily digested foods that are low in bulk (fiber). The goal is to increase energy without increasing the overall volume of food eaten. Raw fruit and salad will add bulk but not substantial energy and may satisfy the appetite before an adequate amount of energy-yielding food has been eaten. Fat-rich foods that increase energy without adding bulk are a good choice. Thus, it is possible to add cheese to egg dishes and sauces, cream or whole milk to soups, and butter, mayonnaise, or jams or jellies to sandwiches without significantly increasing the quantity of food to be eaten. Serving excessively fatty or sweet foods at meals can be counterproductive, however, since such foods are likely to depress appetite even further. Underweight individuals may respond more readily to the addition of snacks between their regular meals than to an addition of food at mealtimes. Thus, an afternoon snack of pie and milk, or a bedtime sandwich or muffin with butter and honey or jelly, would be good ways to add energy.

In some individuals, being underweight is associated with a rush-and-hurry lifestyle, or with a frantic, perhaps "nervous," approach to normal events and stresses. If there is a social-psychological component to an individual's lack of appetite, psychotherapy and/or behavior modification therapy may be desirable. In most cases, nutritionists find active and enthusiastic cooperation in their underweight patients, many of whom suffer serious psychological damage from their condition. Being teased about their "skinny" appearance is just as painful to underweight individuals as being teased about obesity is to many overweight individuals.

Anorexia nervosa

For some individuals, extreme thinness appears to be rewarding, not punishing. These people are likely to be uncooperative and resistant to any dietary changes that might reverse their extreme emaciation. For them, being thin assumes extraordinary importance, and maintaining their excessively underweight condition becomes the major preoccupation of their lives. In such individuals, thinness is a symptom of psychological disturbance and may even result in death.

This bizarre and often life-threatening condition is known as *anorexia nervosa*. It is most often seen in adolescent girls from middle-class and upper-class families. Adolescent males rarely suffer from this syndrome. Psychologists believe that these youngsters are struggling to establish a sense of control and a personal identity independent of authority figures such as parents (Bruch, 1978). Typically, they are perfectionists who cannot meet the goals they or their families have defined for them. They are dissatisfied with their achievements, unable to establish satisfactory social relationships, fearful of maturing, and inspired by the emphasis placed by our society on slenderness for women. Anorexic girls believe that by becoming thin they will gain respect and attention of others and achieve control over their lives. But their image of themselves is usually unrealistic and becomes even more distorted as they become enmeshed in the anorexic pattern. Even when they are as thin as the proverbial rail, these girls will look in a mirror and see themselves as being fat.

For an adolescent who has previously been overweight, the road to anorexia may begin as much needed and seemingly normal weight loss. As she grows thinner, she is indeed noticed and admired. Then panic sets in, as the newly thin girl fears that she will lose control of her food habits and once again gain weight. To avoid this, she begins to develop bizarre eating habits. She will plan her meals on a rigid schedule, often at unusual hours, and limit her intake to a small quantity of a particular food. A few decide not to eat at all. In an eating pattern adopted by anorexics, hunger does not disappear. It increases as the body's needs for nourishment increase and may prompt frantic eating binges during which huge quantities of food and fluid are devoured. This is predictably followed by extreme shame, remorse, and guilt, and the anorexic fights back with self-induced vomiting, laxatives, and an increased resolve to achieve domination over her body and its needs. The result is self-starvation, which produces weight loss, amenorrhea, constipation, abdominal pain, unusual growth of body hair, and severe metabolic defects. If anorexia nervosa is left untreated, death may result.

What can be done for a confused young anorexic, "a skeleton only clad with skin," weighing perhaps 65 pounds? The multidisciplinary approach recommended for other weight-control problems is equally applicable for anorexia nervosa, but first emergency medical and psychiatric treatments must be instituted (Bruch, 1978). After nutrient balance is restored, behavior modification may be used to change the anorexic patient's maladaptive eating patterns. Weight gain alone may represent a continuation of the patient's pathological desire to gain approval. The goal of therapy is a long-range change in attitude toward food and the development of a positive and secure self-image.

ON BALANCE

The principle of energy balance as applied to weight maintenance—energy taken in must be equal to energy expended—is simple enough in theory, but for many individuals this is an unattainable goal in practice. In only a minority of cases is marked energy imbalance caused by an underlying physiological or psychological disorder. The vast majority of energy imbalance problems are manifested as obesity and are due in part to inappropriate eating behaviors. These behaviors include a wide range of food intake patterns, including eating too often and eating too much. Foods eaten in excess, whether they have a high or low nutrient density, contribute to weight gain. Of course, foods that are of low nutrient density may cause additional nutritional problems as well. Physical activity also plays an important role in maintaining energy balance, and many observers believe that the increasingly sedentary American lifestyle is, at least in part, to blame for our national obesity problem.

SUMMARY

The human body requires energy for each of its functions. Normal growth and development, rehabilitation following illness or stress of any kind, normal cellular metabolic processes, and our daily activities all require energy. But all of these anabolic processes together consume only 30 to 40 percent of the energy our bodies derive from metabolizing food nutrients. The greatest portion of available energy is used to maintain body temperature.

Energy is defined as the capacity to do work, and food energy has traditionally been measured in kilocalories, (also called Calories), a unit of heat energy. However, the joule, a metric nonheat measure of energy is being increasingly used. One kilocalorie (kcal) is equivalent to 4.18 kilojoules (kJ). The energy content of foods is determined by use of a bomb calorimeter which literally burns (oxidizes) a measured sample of a particular food and determines the amount of heat generated.

Energy requirements of individuals are the total of a number of components, including the basal metabolic rate or energy needs at rest, the extent and kinds of physical activity, and the quantity of energy related to the ingestion of a meal. The last is known as the specific dynamic effect (SDE) of food. All energy needs are proportionate to the size (weight and height) of the individual. Standard tables have been derived from measurements of these factors in numerous individuals, and the Food and Nutrition Board has recommended that adult American males consume 2,700 kilocalories (11,340 kJ) per day, and adult females 2,000 kilocalories (8,400 kJ).

The energy-producing food nutrients are carbohydrates, fats, and protein, and the nonnutrient alcohol. Of these, fats provide the most concentrated source of energy. Energy supplied by food in excess of that required for body functions is stored as adipose tissue. A certain amount of subcutaneous fat and energy reserve is necessary, but a marked excess is unhealthy. Obesity is diagnosed in individuals who are 20 percent or more above their ideal weight for height, age, sex, and body build. More than 30 percent of the American adult population is estimated to be obese.

The causes of obesity are varied and complex, but in only a small minority of cases are they genetic or physiological. Our society places a premium on slenderness, and the millions of individuals trying to lose weight constitute a vast market for fad diets and other reducing aids. Most such methods are ineffective at best because they do not correct the underlying food habits that caused the problem, and they may be dangerous at worst. The best approach to weight control combines a balanced deficit diet (that is, balanced nutrient intake and a reduction in energy consumption) with behavior modification therapy to correct eating patterns; increasing physical activity also helps.

There is less medical risk attached to the underweight condition; however, anorexia nervosa, a self-induced state of virtual starvation affecting primarily adolescent girls, is caused by an underlying emotional disorder and can have severe consequences. Medical and psychological treatment is indicated to correct this disturbance.

BIBLIOGRAPHY

AMES, S. R. The joule—Unit of energy. *Journal of the American Dietetic Association* 357:415, 1970.

ASHWORTH, A. Metabolic rates of recovery from protein-calorie malnutrition: The need for a new concept of specific dynamic action. *Nature* 223:407, 1969.

BRAY, G. A., F. L. GREENWAY, M. E. MOLITCH, W. T. DAHMS, R. L. ATKINSON, AND K. HAMILTON. Use of anthropometric measures to assess weight loss. *American Journal of Clinical Nutrition* 31:769, 1978.

BRUCH, H. *Eating disorders.* New York: Basic Books, 1973.

BRUCH, H. *The golden cage: The enigma of anorexia nervosa.* Cambridge, Mass.: Harvard University Press, 1978.

Consumer Reports. After the last chance diet. Vol. 43:92, 1978.

DRABMAN, R. S., D. HAMMER, AND G. J. JARVIE. Eating rates of elementary school children. *Journal of Nutrition Education* 9(2):80, 1977.

FAO/WHO. *Energy and protein requirements.* FAO Nutrition Report Series No. 52; WHO Technical Report Series No. 522. Rome: Food and Agriculture Organization, 1973.

FELIG, P. Four questions about protein diets. *New England Journal of Medicine* 298:1025, 1978.

FINEBURG, S. K. The realities of obesity and fad diets. *Nutrition Today* 7(4):23, 1972.

FOOD AND NUTRITION BOARD, NATIONAL RESEARCH COUNCIL. *Recommended dietary allowances,* 8th ed. Washington, D.C.: National Academy of Sciences, 1974.

FRIEDMAN, M. I., AND E. M. STRICKER. The physiological psychology of hunger: A physiological perspective. *Psychological Review* 83(6):409, 1976.

GARN, S. M., S. M. BAILEY, P. E. COLE, AND T. T. HIGGINS. Level of education, level of income, and level of fatness in adults. *American Journal of Clinical Nutrition* 30:721, 1977.

GARN, S. M., AND D. C. CLARK. Trends in fatness and the origins of obesity. *Pediatrics* 57(4):443, 1976.

GLICK, N. Low-calorie protein diets. *FDA Consumer* 12(2):7, 1978.

HARPER, A. E. Remarks on the joule. *Journal of the American Dietetic Association* 57:416, 1970.

HEGSTED, D. M. Energy needs and energy utilization. *Nutrition Reviews* 32:33, 1974.

HIRSCH, J., AND J. L. KNITTLE. Cellularity of obese and nonobese human adipose tissue. *Federation Proceedings* 29:1516, 1970.

JAMES, W. P. T. *Research on obesity: A report of the DHSS/MRC group.* London: Her Majesty's Stationery Office, 1976.

JOHNSON, D., AND E. J. DRENICK. Therapeutic fasting in morbid obesity. Long term follow-up. *Archives of Internal Medicine* 137:1381, 1977.

JORDAN, H. A. In defense of body weight. *Journal of the American Dietetic Association* 62:17, 1973.

KONISHI, F. Food energy equivalents of various activities. *Journal of the American Dietetic Association* 46:186, 1965.

KONISHI, F., AND S. L. HARRISON. Body weight-gain equivalents of selected foods. *Journal of the American Dietetic Association* 70:365, 1977.

KREBS, H. A. The metabolic fate of amino acids. In *Mammalian protein metabolism,* ed. H. N. Munro and J. B. Allison, Vol. 1. New York: Academic Press, 1964.

LEVEILLE, G. A., AND D. R. ROMSOS. Meal eating and obesity. *Nutrition Today* 9(6):4, 1974.

MAYER, J. Why people get hungry. *Nutrition Today* 1(2):2, 1966.

New York Times. Fat is an energy issue. November 14, 1978, p. C2.

New York Times. Science watch: Obesity. December 12, 1978, p. C2.

PASSMORE, R., AND J. V. G. A. DURNIN. Human energy expenditure. *Physiologic Review* 35:801, 1955.

REISIN, E., R. ABEL, M. MODAN, D. S. SILVERBERG, H. E. ELIAHOU, AND B. MODAN. Effect of weight loss without salt restriction on the reduction of blood pressure in overweight hypertensive patients. *New England Journal of Medicine* 298:1, 1978.

SOLOW, C., P. M. SILBERFARB, AND K. SWIFT. Psychosocial effects of intestinal bypass surgery for severe obesity. *New England Journal of Medicine* 290:300, 1974.

STOFFERI, J. A study of social stereotype of body image of children. *Journal of Perspectives in Social Psychology* 7:101, 1967.

VANITALLIE, T. B., AND M. U. YANG. Current concepts in nutrition: Diet and weight loss. *New England Journal of Medicine* 297:1158, 1977.

Wall Street Journal. Fat people find slim pickings in job market. March 27, 1973, p. 1.

WINICK, M., ED. *Childhood obesity.* New York: John Wiley, 1975.

WINICK, M., J. A. BRASEL, AND P. ROSSO. Nutrition and cell growth. In *Current concepts in nutrition,* vol. 1: *Nutrition and development,* ed. M. Winick. New York: John Wiley, 1972.

YUDKIN, J. Obesity and society. *Bibliotheca Nutritio et Dieta* 26:146, 1978.

SUGGESTED ADDITIONAL READING

ASHER, P. Fat babies and fat children. *Archives of Disease in Childhood* 41:672, 1966.

CHARNEY, E., H. C. GOODMAN, M. MCBRIDE, B. LYON, AND R. PRATT. Childhood antecedents of adult obesity. Do chubby infants become obese adults? *New England Journal of Medicine* 295:6, 1976.

CROWLEY, A. The stigma and cost of obesity. *Dietetic Currents* 3(6):1976.

Dairy Council Digest. Current concepts of obesity. 46(4):19, 1975.

Dairy Council Digest. What's new in weight control? Vol. 49(2):7, 1978.

EID. E. E. Follow-up study of physical growth of children who had excessive weight gain in the first six months of life. *British Medical Journal* 2:74, 1970.

FERGUSON, J. M. *Habits, not diets: The real way to weight control.* Palo Alto, Calif.: Bull Publishing Co., 1976.

LLOYD, J. K., O. H. WOLF, AND W. S. WHELAN. Childhood obesity: A long-term study of height and weight. *British Medical Journal* 2:145, 1961.

MAHONEY, M. J., AND K. MAHONEY. *Permanent weight control: A total solution to the dieter's dilemma.* New York: W. W. Norton & Co., 1977.

MAYER, J. Liquid protein: The last word on the last chance diet. *Family Health/Today's Health* 10(1):40, 1978.

MAYER, J. *Overweight: Causes, costs, and control.* Englewood Cliffs, N.J.: Prentice-Hall, 1968.

Nutrition Reviews. Research on obesity. 35(9):249, 1977.

Nutrition Reviews. Morbid obesity: Long term results of therapeutic fasting. 36(1):6, 1978.

Nutrition Reviews. The nature of weight loss during short term dieting. 36(3):72, 1978.

RAVELLI, G. P., Z. A. STEIN, AND M. V. SUSSER. Obesity in young men after famine exposure in utero and early infancy. *New England Journal of Medicine* 295:349, 1976.

RITT, R. S., H. A. JORDAN, AND L. S. LEVITZ. Changes in nutrient intake during a behavioral weight control program. *Journal of the American Dietetic Association* 74:325, 1979.

Chapter 6

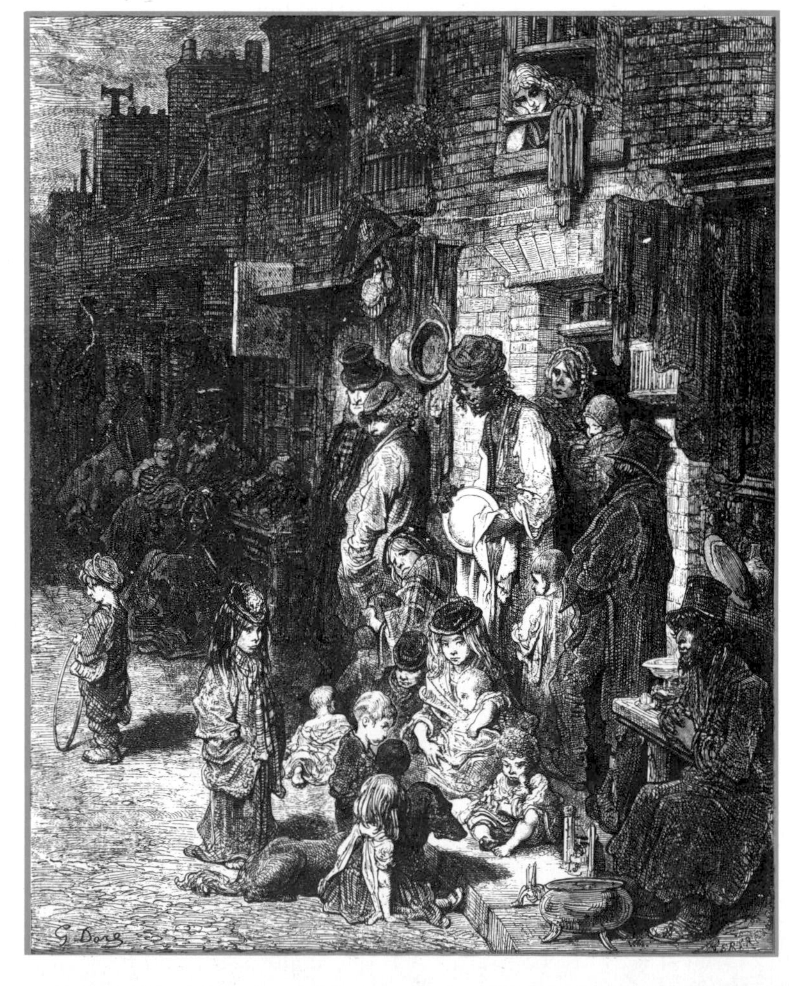

Wentworth Street, Whitechapel by Gustav Doré

Fat-Soluble Vitamins

When nineteenth-century researchers succeeded in establishing the dietary need for carbohydrates, fats, proteins, and the minerals calcium, iron, and phosphorus, they felt confident that all the nutrients essential to life had been identified. Despite the accumulation of evidence over the years that "protective substances" in citrus fruits could prevent scurvy and that brown rice diets cured beriberi, it had not occurred to researchers that there might be other organic substances in foods of which minute quantities were vital for good nutrition.

Then it was observed that purified diets which contained only the known essential nutrients could not support health and growth in laboratory animals, and that clear and consistent physical symptoms of disease appeared in animals maintained on such diets. What could be wrong? Were the diets causing infection? Were the ingredients poisonous? When further research showed that these diseases could not be transferred from one animal to another by inoculation, and that the same dietary ingredients did not poison animals fed natural diets, then the concept of "deficiency disease" was accepted as the only logical possibility remaining.

Not until 1912, however, did Casimir Funk, a Polish chemist, actually identify the mysterious, vital "food factor." It was neither a mineral-containing salt nor a protein but appeared to be a nitrogen-containing organic compound of rather small molecular weight. Funk called it a "vitamine," from the Latin word *vita* (life) and the biochemical term *amine* (an organic compound containing nitrogen). As researchers began to discover other essential "food factors," however, it became apparent that not all were amines. In 1920, to avoid confusion, the British biochemist J. C. Drummond introduced the term we use today—*vitamin.*

Vitamins are, by definition, organic compounds that (a) are required in trace amounts by the body, (b) perform specific metabolic functions, and (c) are not synthesized at all in the body, or are not synthesized in adequate quantities, and so must be provided by dietary sources. Unlike the nutrients discussed thus far, vitamins do not produce energy. Also, they differ widely from one another in chemical structure and thus in biochemical function. Because no one food contains all the vitamins required by the body, a diversified diet is necessary to ensure adequate intake of each of these substances.

Vitamins are involved in a wide range of metabolic processes and may serve structural functions as well. Over and over again, the absence rather than the presence of vitamins has demonstrated their importance and specific functions. From the time of Lind's attempts to alleviate scurvy in sailors (see Chapter 1), much of what we know about vitamins has come from studies of the so-called deficiency diseases such as xerophthalmia (vitamin A), beriberi (thiamin), pellagra (niacin), and rickets (vitamin D).

Vitamin deficiencies are reflected in decreased tissue and then serum levels of the vitamin, followed by a decrease in the related biochemical function, leading to the clinical symptoms of the corresponding deficiency state. A *primary deficiency* results simply from inadequate consumption of the nutrient in question relative to physiological need. In *secondary or indirect deficiency*, intake is adequate, but absorption may be inhibited, excretion may be accelerated, or function may be impaired.

Excess consumption of certain vitamins can also have adverse effects on the normal functioning of the body. This is because the two different kinds of vitamins—water-soluble and fat-soluble—are metabolized differently. Excessive amounts of water-soluble vitamins (such as vitamin C and the B-complex vitamins) are readily excreted from the body.

Vitamins A, D, E, and K, on the other hand, are fat-soluble. Because of this chemical property, they share a number of characteristics (although exceptions do occur), including: relative stability during processing, preservation, and preparation of foods; similar mechanisms of absorption and excretion; and storage in the liver and fatty deposits of the body. All consist solely of carbon, hydrogen, and oxygen. Because they can be stored, they do not have to be consumed on a daily basis. But for the same reason, excess consumption of vitamins A and D produces toxicity symptoms; under certain circumstances, vitamin E and some forms of vitamin K also may be toxic. These and other aspects of the fat-soluble vitamins are the subject of the present chapter.

VITAMIN A

Soon after Funk had proposed his vitamin theory, researchers at Yale University and the University of Wisconsin, working independently of each other, discovered another candidate for this new class of nutrients. They found that the source of fat in a diet fed to rats influenced growth and eye function. Removal of milkfat from a purified diet, or a diet whose only fats were lard or olive oil, produced stunted growth and eye lesions. However, with the addition of butterfat or egg yolk to the rats' diets, these symptoms were abated or even reversed.

The Wisconsin research team, Elmer V. McCollum and Marguerite Davis, named the chemically unidentified substance Fat Soluble A, based on the only chemical property they knew it to possess. Subsequently, the yellow pigment carotene was shown to have the same growth-promoting properties as

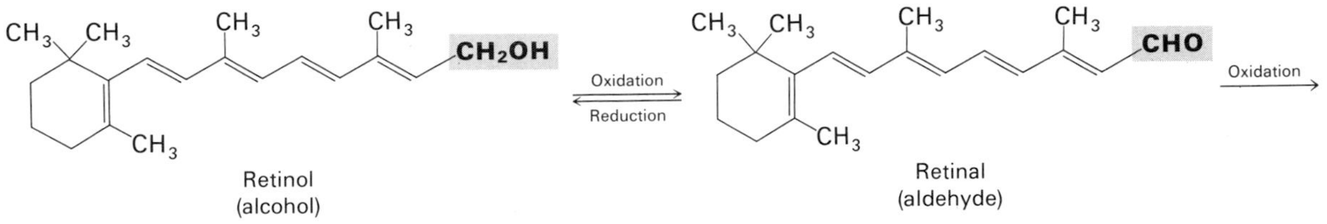

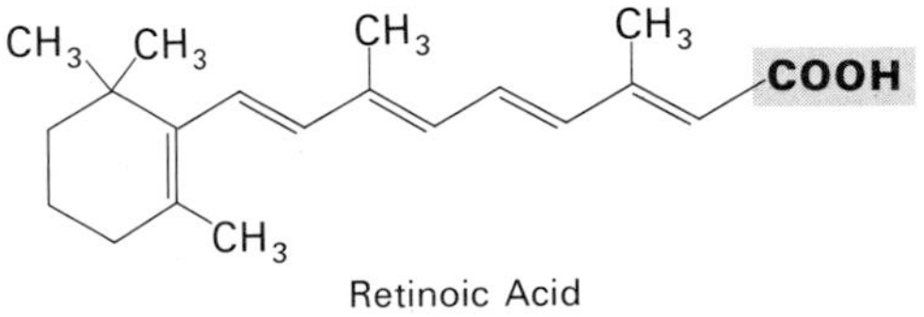

FIGURE 6-1

Chemical Structure of Preformed Vitamin A

A comparison of the structure of β-carotene (Figure 6-2) with the structure of vitamin A (Figure 6-1) makes clear that two molecules of retinal can be produced by cleaving the provitamin at the position marked by the dashed line in Figure 6-2. This reaction involves molecular oxygen.

vitamin A, and also to be a precursor of the newly identified substance found in animal products. In 1937 the vitamin was isolated from cod-liver oil, and in 1946 it was synthesized in the laboratory.

Chemistry and Properties

Retinol = Vitamin A alcohol

Retinyl ester = Vitamin A alcohol + fatty acid

Retinal = Vitamin A aldehyde

Retinoic acid = Vitamin A acid

(See Figure 6-1)

Vitamin A occurs both in a preformed state and in a precursor form that does not have activity until it is converted. Preformed vitamin A exists as three biologically active variants: retinol (an alcohol), retinal (an aldehyde), and retinoic acid. As Figure 6-1 shows, the three forms are chemically identical except for the single functional group that determines both how the compound is classified and its chemical behavior.

Figure 6-1 also demonstrates the chemical relationship of the three forms. Most of the preformed vitamin A in our food is the alcohol form, retinol. Retinol can be reversibly oxidized to the aldehyde form, retinal. This second form is the one involved in the visual response to dim light. Oxidation of retinal produces the acid form of the vitamin, retinoic acid. Although retinoic acid does not participate in the visual cycle and cannot be converted back to the aldehyde form, it does retain the same growth-promoting but not the reproduction-supporting properties of the other forms of the vitamin.

Biologically active vitamin A is found almost exclusively in foods of animal origin. But all three forms of vitamin A can be produced from a group of plant pigments known as *carotenes.* These yellow-orange pigments thus serve as precursors of the biologically active forms, or provitamins. Carotenes, which give carrots their characteristic color, are most commonly found in the leaves of green plants, where their color is masked by the darker green pigment chlorophyll. The most common provitamin form is β-carotene, a dark yellow-orange pigment whose chemical structure is shown in Figure 6-2.

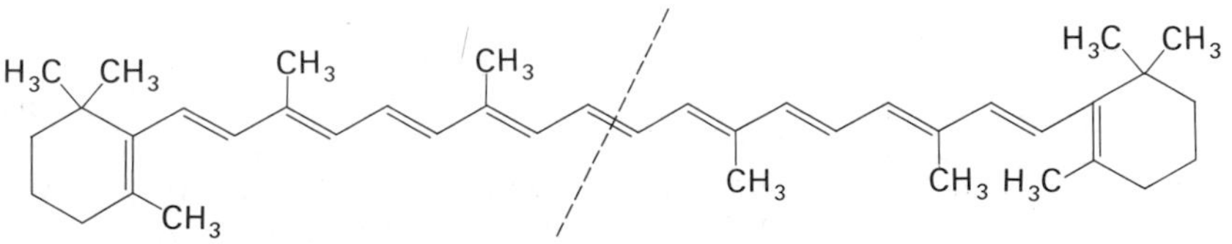

FIGURE 6-2

Chemical Structure of β-Carotene

Unlike its precursors, vitamin A is colorless. Both forms are soluble in fat and fat solvents, and are vulnerable to partial destruction by oxygen and ultraviolet light. They are relatively heat stable, although prolonged heat will reduce their activity.

Absorption and Metabolism

ABSORPTION. Preformed vitamin A in foods occurs primarily as a retinyl ester—that is, as a compound of retinol and a fatty acid. In the lumen of the small intestine, pancreatic and intestinal enzymes hydrolyze it to its components. Retinol is absorbed into the mucosal cells lining the intestine, where it is rapidly re-esterified (principally with palmitic acid) back to retinyl esters and "packaged" with extremely small lipid particles in the chylomicrons (see Chapter 3). In this form the retinyl esters enter the lymphatic system and then the general circulation which ultimately delivers them to the liver, the main storage site for vitamin A.

When the diet provides the carotene precursors, which are the major source of vitamin A for most animals, the path from ingestion to storage is almost the same. In the mucosal cells of the small intestine, the provitamins are converted to retinal, assisted by a cleavage enzyme. Further conversion to retinol (by reduction) is catalyzed by another intestinal enzyme. From this point on, the processes of esterification and transport are the same as those already described.

Theoretically, every molecule of β-carotene should yield two molecules of retinal, but the conversion mechanism is not completely efficient; the implications of this fact for dietary requirements will be discussed below. Molecules of the precursor forms that remain unhydrolyzed are also packaged in the chylomicrons along with the retinyl esters, and are transported to the liver as well. Some of the remaining β-carotene is apparently converted in the liver to retinal and then to retinyl esters, in which form it can be stored.

The absorption of vitamin A is affected by the same factors that influence fat absorption (Chapter 3). Thus, absence of bile or any generalized malfunction of the lipid absorption system will interfere with absorption of the vitamin. Absorption can also be adversely affected by the consumption of mineral oil or of drugs that bind bile salts (such as cholestyramine, a drug used to lower blood cholesterol).

METABOLISM. Although vitamin A is stored in the kidneys, the adipose tissue, and the adrenal glands, the primary site of storage is the liver. As noted previously, the vitamin is stored mainly in the form of retinyl esters. When vitamin A is needed by the body, esters are first hydrolyzed to retinol, which is then bound to a specific transport protein called retinol-binding protein (RBP). Bound to RBP, as retinol, vitamin A is quite stable and readily available to body tissues. But in other forms, such as retinal and particularly retinoic acid, it is quickly metabolized to products that are excreted in bile and urine.

Protein deficiency has a negative effect on vitamin A status, because the synthesis of RBP is slowed or halted, and thus the serum levels of vitamin A are diminished. Zinc deficiency has a similar effect, though the actual mechanism is not understood. Liver disease such as hepatitis will decrease serum levels of both vitamin A and RBP, but renal (kidney) disease actually increases the serum levels because efficiency of excretion is hampered. Among the drugs shown to affect vitamin A status are the oral contraceptives, which increase serum levels apparently by inducing RBP synthesis.

Physiological Functions

Vitamin A is known to affect almost every tissue in the body and to have a key role in a great variety of body functions and processes. Unfortunately, our knowledge of its biochemical activity is incomplete. There are gaps in our present understanding of vitamin A involvement in growth and tissue maintenance; its role in other metabolic processes is even less clear. The only function of vitamin A that is thoroughly understood is its role in the so-called visual cycle.

VISION. It had long been known that vitamin A deficiency caused night blindness, the inability of the eye to adjust to variations in light intensity. The mechanisms of the visual cycle were first described in detail by George Wald of Harvard University, who won a Nobel Prize in 1967 for his work.

Light intensity is perceived in the retina of the eye through two types of photoreceptors or light-sensitive cells. The *rods* are sensitive to low-intensity or dim light, while the *cones* respond to color and high-intensity or bright light. Both types of photoreceptor contain special pigments consisting of retinal and a protein molecule called *opsin*. The pigment in the rods is *rhodopsin* or visual purple; that in the cones is *iodopsin* or visual violet. Slight differences in the opsin component account for the different sensitivities of the two pigments. Although the visual cycle is virtually the same for both pigments, the effects of bright light on the eye are more dramatic at night than during the day (see Figure 6-3).

The ability to see in dim light after rhodopsin has been bleached by bright light is directly related to vitamin A status. The condition called "night blindness" often results from a diminished capacity for rhodopsin regeneration. A person with night blindness will require a longer time to recover from the blinding effects of, for example, the headlights of an oncoming car. It should be remembered, that only retinol and retinal can maintain the visual cycle. Retinoic acid cannot be reduced to retinol and, therefore, cannot cure night blindness. (Vitamin A, incidentally, cannot cure color blindness, which results from the absence of some color receptors in the cones.)

Vitamin A plays an additional important role in vision by maintaining the structure of the tissues of the eye. Prolonged vitamin A deficiency can result in permanent blindness.

MAINTENANCE OF EPITHELIAL TISSUES. Epithelial tissue constitutes the external surfaces of the body—the cells that form the outer layers of the skin and the mucous membranes that line the digestive, respiratory, and reproductive tracts. These tissues produce mucus and other secretions that help to lubricate and preserve the integrity of the tissue and to protect against invasion by bacteria and other microorganisms. Vitamin A is apparently

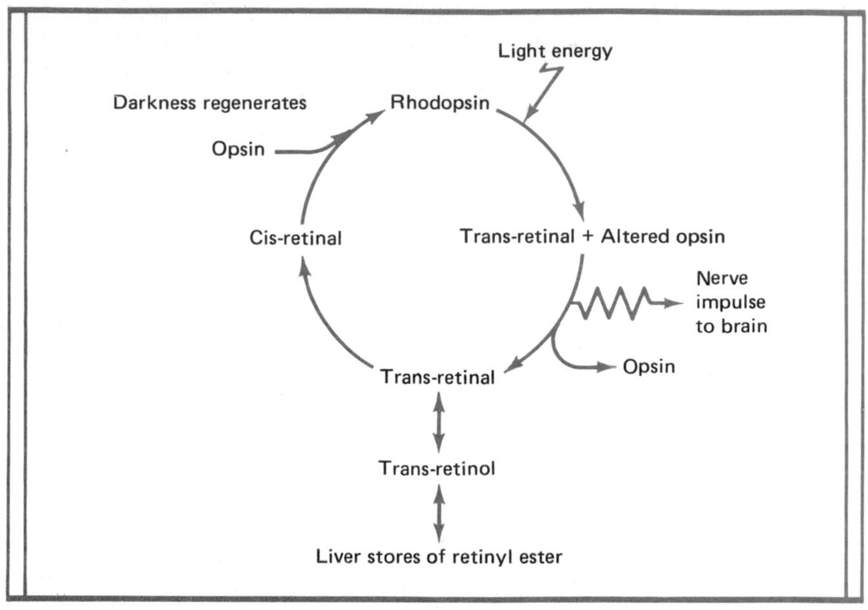

FIGURE 6-3
Role of Vitamin A in the Visual Cycle

The visual cycle begins when light enters the eye and strikes the rhodopsin molecule. As the pigment absorbs the light energy, changes take place in its retinal and opsin components, causing them to dissociate. In the process, a nerve impulse is generated and sent to the brain via the optic nerve. In effect, light energy has been transformed into a signal, a nerve impulse, which carries the "visual image" to the brain.

The effect of light causing the dissociation of rhodopsin into its component parts is known as bleaching. When rhodopsin is bleached, some of the released retinal is degraded. As it is degraded, more rhodopsin must be regenerated so that the visual process can continue. Retinol released from the liver is transported by RBPs to the photoreceptor cells of the retina. Here it is oxidized to retinal and combines with opsin to form rhodopsin. Thus, new rhodopsin is always being formed to replace the rhodopsin that is broken down when visual images are transmitted. If there is not enough stored vitamin A available to participate in the regeneration process, however, rhodopsin formation is slowed or interrupted, and dim-light perception is impaired.

Source: Adapted from R. Montgomery, R. L. Dryer, T. W. Conway, and A. A. Spector, *Biochemistry: A case-oriented approach* (St. Louis: C. V. Mosby Co., 1974), p. 31.

necessary for the synthesis of certain substances in mucus and other secretions.

In the absence of vitamin A, epithelial tissue does not produce mucus but becomes covered with keratin, a dry, water-insoluble protein that is the main constituent of hair and nails. With vitamin A deficiency, epithelial cells are gradually transformed from soft, moist tissue to hard and dry, or keratinized, areas. As more and more epithelial tissue is keratinized, there is less secretion of mucus and other protective substances. Consequently the incidence of infection is noticeably greater during vitamin A deficiency. (Intestinal lining does not actually become keratinized, but its secretion of mucus decreases.) Moreover, the loss of appetite noted in animals lacking vitamin A has been attributed in part to the keratinization and consequent loss of sensitivity of the taste buds.

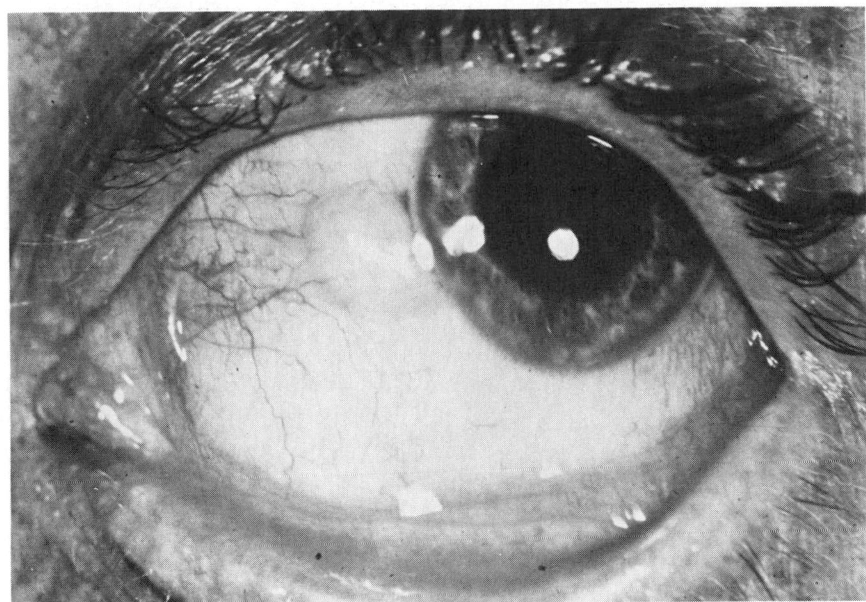

One of the early and typical signs of vitamin A deficiency is the development of a Bitot's spot, identified as a white patchy area on the epithelial tissue of the eyeball. (Lester V. Bergman & Associates, Inc.)

GROWTH. Vitamin A is required for the normal growth and development of bones and teeth. The precise mechanisms are not known but vitamin A is believed to be an essential factor in the metabolic activity of certain specialized cells involved in the formation of these tissues.

A growing long bone contains two growth areas, or "plates," one near each end of the bone. These plates consist of layers of rapidly growing cartilaginous tissue. New bone is formed by the mineralization of the tissue at the plate edge nearest the center of the bone. This process of bone formation and growth is the function of specialized cells known as *osteoblasts.* Although the mechanism is complex and little understood, it appears that vitamin A is necessary for development of healthy osteoblasts capable of mineralizing the cartilage growth plates of bones.

Bone formation does not stop with the end of normal bone growth, however. Bone tissue is broken down and reformed throughout the life of the individual. This continuous remodeling serves to keep the composition of bone constant. Again, osteoblasts perform the function of building new bone. The dissolution of bone is caused by enzymes released from specialized cells called *osteoclasts.* Research so far has indicated that vitamin A is apparently involved in transforming immature cells to osteoblasts and osteoclasts. Release of the enzymes that make possible the resorption of old bone also appears to require vitamin A.

Similarly, vitamin A is necessary for normal development and function of ameloblasts, specialized cells responsible for the formation of tooth enamel. In vitamin A deficiency, teeth develop imperfectly; tooth enamel is thin and tends to break or chip.

OTHER METABOLIC FUNCTIONS. Vitamin A also has important functions in the maintenance of membrane stability, in reproduction, and in the synthesis of a number of adrenal and thyroid hormones. What little is known about the effect of vitamin A on reproductive functions indicates this influence is related to its role in the synthesis of steroid hormones.

Our understanding of vitamin A function in other metabolic processes is even more limited. Research on how this important nutrient functions in the body has, however, produced some fascinating tentative results. For example, one group of researchers has found that experimentally induced cancer may be arrested in laboratory animals given vitamin A (Rogers et al., 1973). Similarly, large doses of a vitamin A-type compound have been reported to reverse tumor growth in some instances (Saffiotti et al., 1967). This interesting phenomenon is related to the vitamin's *pharmacological action*—that is, to large amounts used as medication. (A *nutritional* effect of a vitamin occurs with small, or trace amounts.) Clinical trials to determine its effectiveness continue to be conducted. Because public interest has been aroused by these preliminary reports, it cannot be emphasized too strongly that the observation is by no means proven. Consumption of large doses of vitamin A in the hope that it will prevent cancer is unwarranted and, as we shall see below, potentially harmful.

Dietary Requirements and Recommended Allowances

1 RE
= 1 μg retinol
= 6 μg β-carotene
= 12 μg other provitamin A carotenoids
= 3.33 IU retinol
= 10 IU β-carotene
= 20 IU other provitamin A carotenoids

UNITS OF MEASUREMENT. Until recently, vitamin A activity in foods, as well as recommended allowances, has been expressed in **International Units** (IU), originally defined as the amount needed to promote a specified growth rate in laboratory rats. One IU of vitamin A is equivalent to 0.3 micrograms (μg) retinol, 0.344 μg retinyl acetate, 0.6 μg β-carotene, or 1.2 micrograms of other provitamin A carotenoids. But this system, which reflects biological activity, does not take into consideration the body's absorption of the different dietary forms of vitamin A. In the form of retinol, vitamin A is completely absorbed into the body. By contrast, only one-third of dietary β-carotene (the most significant vitamin A food source) is utilized, and only half of that is converted to retinol. Thus the true effectiveness of β-carotene, weight for weight, is one-sixth that of retinol; and the effectiveness of other carotenoids is one-twelfth that of retinol. Accurate specification of the total dietary activity of the vitamin, then, requires specifying the percentage from each source.

To reflect utilization more accurately, the term "retinol equivalent," or RE, was introduced in 1967 by an FAO/WHO Expert Committee (FAO/WHO, 1967). By definition, one retinol equivalent is equal to one gram of retinol or equivalent amount of other compounds, corrected for efficiency of utilization. The Food and Nutrition Board of the National Research Council/National Academy of Sciences has recommended adoption of the new unit. Until the transition is complete, it has also recommended that both units be used and that food analyses provide separately the different sources of vitamin A.

RECOMMENDED DIETARY ALLOWANCES. The RDA for vitamin A is based on several factors, including the minimum amount required to eliminate clinical symptoms of deficiency, to maintain physiological function and adequate blood levels, and to promote storage. The RDA for adult American men is 1,000 RE (5,000 IU). The RDA for women has been set at 80 percent of that for men, on the basis of body weight (800 RE, or 4,000 IU). During pregnancy it is 1,000 RE (5,000 IU), and 1,200 RE (6,000 IU) is recommended for lactating mothers. For the first six months of life, the RDA is 420 RE (1,400 IU); for infants six months to one year of age, it is 400 RE (2,000 IU). The RDA for infants is based on the average content of retinol in human milk, and assumes this to be the sole source for the first half year.

Dietary Sources of Vitamin A

Considering the importance of vitamin A to health, it is fortunate that adequate amounts of this nutrient are easily obtained from a wide variety of plant and animal products (as carotenes in the former; as retinyl esters in the latter). In the United States, about half of dietary vitamin A comes from retinol, and half from provitamin A carotenoids. The most concentrated sources are liver and dark green and orange-yellow vegetables, but significant amounts are provided by whole milk, butter, cream cheese, and eggs. Skim milk and its products may be fortified with the vitamin, as may margarine and other dairy product substitutes. Though plant oils contain none, fish-liver oils are highly concentrated sources of vitamin A.

Because vitamin A can be stored by the body, daily intake is not necessary. For example, as Table 6-1 shows, a single (small) serving of liver provides enough vitamin A for nine days. However, many people do not like liver and will not eat it even though it is nutritious. Thus it is important to note the many types of common foods that contain vitamin A activity. Since food composition tables are still expressed in IUs, it is also important to remember that the usable carotene content of foods is variable. Dark green leafy vegetables contain carotenes, though their color is masked by the chlorophyll pigment. On the other hand, the pigments of many red or yellow-orange vegetables (kidney beans, turnips) have no significant carotene content.

In general, normal processing and cooking procedures cause little loss of vitamin A. In fact, mashing, cutting, or puréeing may increase the availability of provitamin A by rupturing plant cell walls. Because the vitamin is not soluble in water, there is little loss in most cooking methods. Vitamin A oxidizes readily under the influence of high heat, and drying accelerates this reaction. To retain vitamin A, vegetables should be steamed or simmered in a small amount of water. The diet should regularly include raw or slightly cooked vitamin A-rich foods, particularly carrots and green leafy vegetables.

Symptoms of Clinical Deficiency

Clinically significant symptoms of vitamin A deficiency are generally caused by a primary deficiency, that is, by insufficient dietary intake. Secondary deficiencies may be precipitated by absorptive disorders, including those caused by long-term use of mineral oil or prescribed drugs, or those caused by pancreatic or gall bladder disease, generally interfering with lipid metabolism. In laboratory animals, growth retardation, reproductive failure, and eye

TABLE 6-1
Vitamin A Content of Selected Foods
RDA for Adults
Men: 1000 RE
Women: 800 RE

Food	Serving Size	Vitamin A Content per Serving	
		IU	*RE*
Liver, beef, fried	3 oz	45,390	—[a]
Dandelion greens, cooked	½ c	10,530	—
Canteloupe, with rind (5″ diam.)	½ melon	9,240	—
Sweet potato, baked	1 large	9,230	—
Carrots, cooked, drained	½ c	8,140	—
Collards, cooked, drained	½ c	7,410	—
Spinach, cooked, drained	½ c	7,290	—
Spinach, raw, chopped	1 c	4,460	—
Winter squash, baked	½ c	4,305	—
Beet greens, cooked, drained	½ c	3,700	—
Broccoli, cooked, drained	⅔ c	3,205	—
Apricots, canned in syrup	½ c	2,245	—
Tomatoes, canned	1 c	2,170	—
Apricots, dried	5 halves	2,043	—
Tomato, raw	1 medium	1,640	—
Lettuce, romaine	1 c	1,050	—
Oysters	1 c	740	—
Green peas, canned	½ c	585	—
Milk, skim or low-fat, fortified	1 c	500	140
Margarine, fortified	1 tbsp	470	—
Butter	1 tbsp	460	114
Orange juice, from concentrate	6 oz	410	—
Cream cheese	1 oz	405	124
Lettuce, Boston type	¼ head	395	—
Cheese, pasteurized, processed American	1 oz	343	82
Egg, yolk	1 large	313	94

[a] Information not available.

lesions are common symptoms. In humans, eye lesions and increased susceptibility to infection are the classic signs of deficiency.

Night blindness, or nyctalopia, usually the first sign of vitamin A deficiency in humans, was described as early as 1500 B.C. in ancient Egypt, and primitive "cures" for the condition have been known and used for at least 3,500 years. Ancient Egyptian documents refer to the application of liver juice to the eye as a treatment for night blindness. The question that arises, of course, is how any vitamin A could enter the body, as it must, to be effective. It has been suggested that the tear ducts of the eye may have provided the necessary entryway. This suggestion is supported by the fact that xerophthalmia in rats can be cured by the direct application of retinol to the cornea of the eye (Wolf, 1978). In Java an almost identical treatment is still in use today. The one significant difference is that, following local application to the eyes, the liver itself is fed to the patient. But this consumption of liver is not considered by the Javanese to be part of the treatment! (Hussaini et al., 1978). It may well be that the Egyptian patients did in fact eat the liver from which the juice was derived but for some reason failed to record the fact. It is certainly

TABLE 6-1
(Continued)

Food	Serving Size	Vitamin A Content per Serving	
		IU	*RE*
Milk, whole	1 c	307	76
Cheddar cheese	1 oz	300	86
Yogurt, whole-milk	8 oz	280	68
Ice cream	½ c	272	66
Egg, whole	1 large	260	78
Lima beans, cooked	½ c	240	—
Banana	1 medium	237	—
Catsup	1 tbsp	210	—
Sardines, canned in oil	3 oz	190	—
Cottage cheese, creamed	½ c	170	50
Yogurt, low-fat, plain	8 oz	150	36
Apple	1 medium	120	—
Yogurt, low-fat, fruit	8 oz	104	25
Chicken, meat only	3 oz	80	—
Tuna fish	3 oz	70	—
Salmon, pink, canned	3 oz	60	—
Chickpeas	½ c	50	—
Hamburger, cooked	3 oz	30	—
Yogurt, non-fat	8 oz	16	5
Beets, canned, drained	½ c	15	—
White bread	1 slice	trace	trace

Sources: USDA, Agricultural Research Service, *Nutritive value of foods*, Home and Garden Bulletin No. 72, rev. ed. (Washington, D.C.: U.S. Government Printing Office, 1977); and C. F. Church and H. N. Church, *Food values of portions commonly used*, 12th ed. (Philadelphia: Lippincott, 1975). RE values are from Consumer and Food Economics Institute, *Composition of foods—dairy and egg products—raw, processed, prepared*, Agriculture Handbook No. 8-1 (Washington, D.C.: U.S. Government Printing Office, 1976).

known that Hippocrates, the Greek "father of medicine," prescribed eating liver as a cure for night blindness. This may also have significance for understanding the Egyptian practice, since Greek medicine was deeply indebted to the medical theory and practice of Egypt (Wolf, 1978).

Of greater concern than night blindness is the progressive hardening, or keratinization, of eye tissue which, if not corrected, can result in permanent blindness. We have already discussed the role of vitamin A in the maintenance of epithelial tissue, and nowhere is its absence so obviously destructive as in the eye. *Xerosis*, or drying out of the eye tissue, is the first in the sequence of lesions associated with xerophthalmia. Epithelial cells become dry and keratinized, particularly in the cornea. Gray-white patches called Bitot's spots may appear on the surface of the eye. Keratinization of the cornea continues with prolonged deficiency and may lead to permanent blindness. These symptoms of severe deficiency are found in India and in many of the developing countries of Southeast Asia, Africa, and Latin America.

Other signs of clinical deficiency include changes in bones and nerves. In children bone growth is stunted, thereby compressing the still-growing nerves of the central nervous system (brain and spinal cord). Changes in the epithelial tissue of the gastrointestinal tract lead to diarrhea, aggravating the victim's condition. Infections of eyes, ears, respiratory system, and reproductive tract are also common. Skin changes such as keratinization of the epithelial cells surrounding hair follicles (*follicular hyperkeratosis*) are often seen. The skin takes on a bumpy, dry appearance sometimes referred to as "toad skin."

PREVENTION AND TREATMENT. In many geographical areas vitamin A-containing foodstuffs, particularly carotene-containing plants, are available; but for cultural and other reasons, they are not consumed. The need for more effective use of these dietary sources is obvious. Fortification of skim milk has helped alleviate deficiency problems. Administration of large amounts of vitamin A in single doses reverses the clinical signs and symptoms, with the exception of blindness. Preventive administration of vitamin A has been effective in reducing the prevalence of xerophthalmia.

Deficiency is more prevalent in children, as might be expected, because their tissues have not had time to build up reserves of the vitamin. Most adults eating a diverse diet have reserves that are adequate for several months to a year.

Toxicity

Paradoxically, the mechanism that protects the body against vitamin A deficiency is also the cause of its potential toxicity. The fat-soluble nature of the nutrient permits its storage in liver and other tissues. Consequently, the potential for storage of excess amounts is always present. Excess carotene intake, however, does not result in vitamin A toxicity, although the skin may turn yellow due to the high level of carotene stored in the lipid layer under the skin. This could result from consumption of a 1-pound bag of carrots every day for several weeks. Normal skin color gradually returns as carotene intake is reduced.

Serious toxic effects result from excessive intake of preformed vitamin A. Studies of pregnant animals have established that large doses of vitamin A produce severe malformations in newborn offspring: abnormalities of the central nervous system, hydrocephalus ("water on the brain"), and encephalocoele (cranial hernia). Infants may also develop hydrocephalus if fed even ten times the appropriate RDA for several weeks. **Hypervitaminosis** A in older children and adults may produce a syndrome that resembles a brain tumor: headache, nausea, vomiting, ringing in the ears, and double vision. General symptoms observed at all ages include dryness of skin and mucous membranes, thinning hair, brittle nails, enlarged spleen, anemia, and pain in the muscles, bones, joints, and abdomen. Symptoms disappear when vitamin A is discontinued.

Not more than 2,000 RE (10,000 IU) of vitamin A per day should be taken without medical recommendation and supervision. Yet, in spite of the awareness of the dangers of excessive consumption of vitamin A, hypervitaminosis A has been on the increase in recent years, with numerous reports of intakes in the range of 25,000 to 100,000 IU per day. Such quantities present a real risk to health, especially to pregnant women and the fetus. Serious toxic effects are also caused by large doses of vitamin A sometimes used in the treatment of acne. Yet clinical trials have shown that even doses in the range of 50,000 to 150,000 IU per day have no consistent or long-lasting beneficial effect on this condition (American Academy of Pediatrics, 1971). Recently published results from clinical trials at the dermatology branch of the National Cancer Institute, however, suggest that a vitamin A derivative, a retinoid, might be temporarily useful in the treatment of *severe* acne. The mechanism appears to be that the retinoid interferes with the production of oil by sebacious glands. The drug is still classified as experimental; moreover, caution about its teratogenic effects is advised. The new drug could not, for example, safely be given to women who are pregnant or not using some method of contraception because it is one of a class of substances known to injure embryos (Peck et al., 1979).

Contributory causes of hypervitaminosis A appear to be the ease with which high-potency vitamin preparations can be obtained without a prescription, as well as parents who act on the mistaken notion that if vitamins are good, a lot of vitamins must be even better. The use of highly fortified "health" foods further complicates the problem.

The biochemical mechanism of vitamin A toxicity is not known. It has been suggested that sufficiently large amounts saturate the RBP system. The unbound vitamin A then circulates as retinal in association with plasma lipoproteins. In this form it may have direct toxic effects on cells (Smith and Goodman, 1976).

With public interest in the recent announcement that certain vitamin A-like compounds may prevent cancer, there has been concern that the incidence of vitamin A toxicity will increase. The tests performed so far have involved laboratory animals, in which cancer has been induced by powerful carcinogens; there is as yet no clear evidence for a similar effect on humans. The new form of the vitamin is *not* available to the public, and vitamin A supplements currently on the market are not known to have any cancer-preventing effect.

In summary, vitamin A is widely available in ordinary food sources, and for most people there is no need for supplementation, which may in fact be dangerous.

VITAMIN D

The identification of vitamin D and its role in human health is one of the most interesting discoveries in the history of medicine and nutritional science. The story of vitamin D, like that of vitamin A, begins in ancient times. Walking across a battlefield in 526 B.C., the Greek historian Herodotus observed a distinct difference in bone density between the Egyptian and Persian soldiers who had been opponents. The skulls of the slain Persians were fragile while those of the Egyptians were strong. The Egyptians' explanation of this difference was amazingly prophetic. They pointed out that while the

Persians wore turbans to protect themselves from the sun, Egyptians went bareheaded from childhood.

Undoubtedly the Persians suffered from what we now know to be the vitamin D deficiency condition called *rickets*, which is characterized by impaired bone formation and is especially damaging during the growth years. While it must have been a common condition from the time that people began to wear clothes and live in houses, rickets was not named or described in medical literature until about 1600. By 1900, according to some estimates, 90 percent of the young children in Europe were afflicted with this disease, which killed many of them. The condition was especially common among the poor. Children who lived in cities or were born in the fall or winter were those most often affected.

As late as 1917, the cause of rickets remained unknown. The first clue came in 1918 when Sir Edward Mellanby of the University of London found that cod-liver oil and butterfat prevented the disease. Because both contained Fat Soluble A, the vitamin recently discovered by McCollum and Davis, Mellanby erroneously concluded that rickets was due to a deficiency of Fat Soluble A.

The next clue was provided by McCollum and his colleagues at Johns Hopkins University. They demonstrated that cod-liver oil retained its anti-rickets effectiveness despite being heated and oxygenated until its vitamin A content had been destroyed. Moreover, they found that coconut oil, which contains no vitamin A, also prevented rickets. Apparently the "Fat Soluble A" discovered by McCollum and Davis consisted of more than one vitamin. By 1922, McCollum had demonstrated the existence of a new vitamin essential to the metabolism of bones. Because this vitamin was, by then, the fourth one discovered, it was called vitamin D.

One other puzzle remained. It was already known that sunlight, which provides ultraviolet light, could reduce and even cure rickets in rats and humans. That meant that there had to be some relationship between sunlight and the new vitamin. Indeed, shortly after McCollum's discovery, other

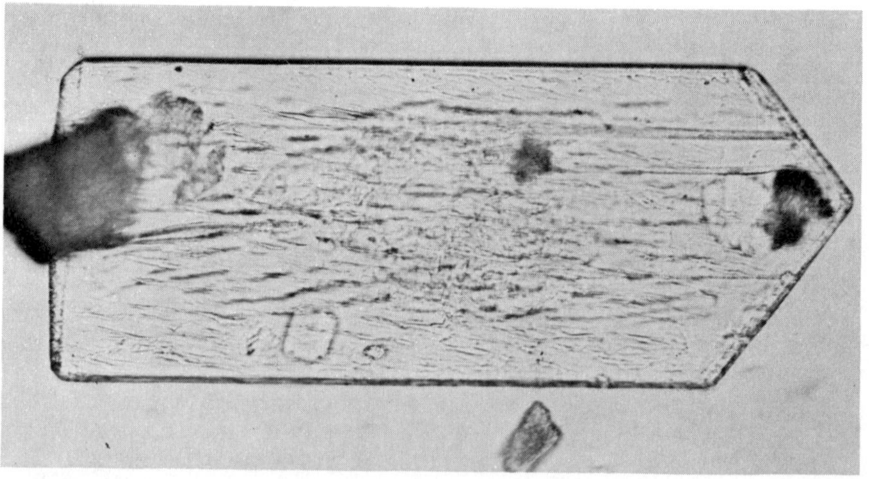

A crystal of ergosterol, the plant precursor of vitamin D_2. magnified 240 times. (Lester V. Bergman & Associates, Inc.)

researchers found that ultraviolet irradiation produced vitamin D in milk, yeasts, and certain other foods.

The connection between rickets as a nutritional deficiency disease, and lack of sunlight, city life, and autumn or winter birth as contributory factors, then became clear. Because their diets contained little meat or milk, the urban poor were more likely to be afflicted. Because they spent little time out of doors, and because city streets are more often shaded, city dwellers generally received less sunlight. And because of shorter days, weaker sunlight, and colder weather, infants born in the fall or winter were kept indoors and wore more clothing when out of doors during the most crucial early bone-developing period of life. We know now, too, that the rapid spread of rickets in northern European cities in the nineteenth century was one of the results of the industrial revolution, which removed people from the sunny open spaces of the countryside and put young children to work inside homes and factories. Even for those city dwellers who spent time outdoors, ultraviolet light was largely filtered out by the smoke from coal and wood fires.

Chemistry and Properties

Like vitamin A, vitamin D is an organic molecule composed of carbon, hydrogen, and oxygen arranged in a multi-ring structure; also, it can be formed from a provitamin. Plants, including yeast, contain a substance called ergosterol. Exposure to sunlight (ultraviolet light) converts this compound to *ergocalciferol,* or vitamin D_2. The skin and hair of animals, including humans, contain another sterol, 7-dehydrocholesterol, which is converted to *cholecalciferol,* or vitamin D_3, by ultraviolet light. "Calciferol" is a name descriptive of the function of vitamin D: calcium-bearing alcohol. Both forms are equally effective in humans (Hess et al., 1925). As a fat-soluble substance, vitamin D is, of course, insoluble in water. When crystallized it is colorless. It is also remarkably stable; exposure to heat, light, and oxygen does not readily affect its activity.

Figure 6-4 shows the similarities of the two forms of vitamin D and of their precursors. The origin of these compounds becomes even more evident if one compares their structure with that of cholesterol (see Figure 3-5).

Absorption and Metabolism

Because of its fat-soluble nature, the absorption of vitamin D into the body is similar to that of vitamin A described previously. Vitamin D is absorbed from the jejunum in the presence of bile. The vitamin enters the general circulation by means of chylomicrons transported via the lymph. The nutrient is removed from the circulation and is stored in the liver. The amounts stored, however, are very small, and storage does not play as important a role in vitamin D metabolism as it does in maintaining vitamin A status. As with vitamin A, factors that influence fat absorption also affect absorption of vitamin D. Thus disorders of fat absorption, ingestion of mineral oil, and drugs that bind bile acids (for instance, cholestyramine) will interfere with the absorption of vitamin D (as well as of other fat-soluble vitamins).

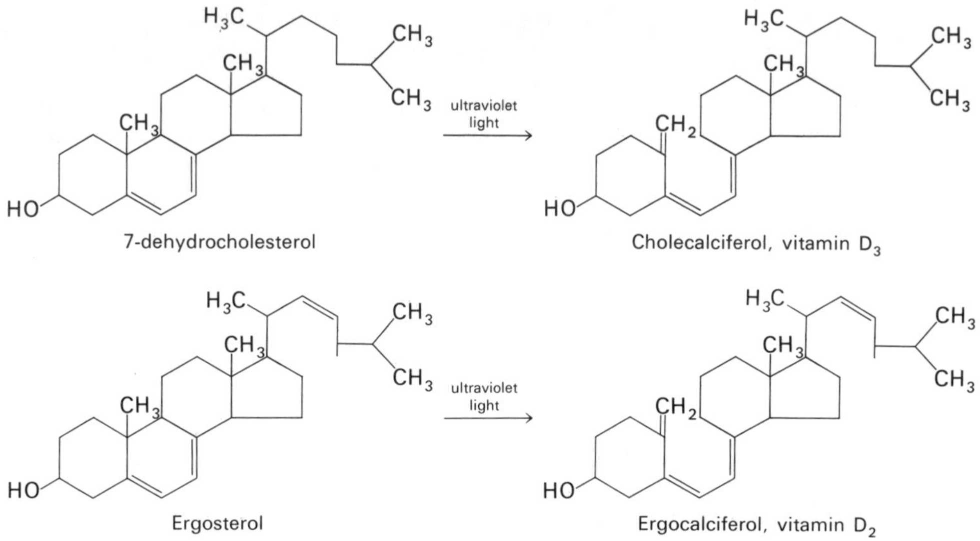

FIGURE 6-4

Structures of Two Forms of Vitamin D and Their Precursors

The opening of the second ring causes a shift in location of the double bonds.

HCC = 25-hydroxy-cholecalciferol

DHCC = 1,25-dihydroxy-cholecalciferol

Small reserves of vitamin D are found not only in the liver but also in the bone, brain, and skin. Some vitamin D metabolites are eliminated by excretion in the bile.

Recent research on the metabolism of vitamin D suggests that it should perhaps be classified as a prohormone because it can be totally synthesized in the body and because it exerts its metabolic effect only after being hydroxylated to two more active forms, HCC and DHCC. These substances fulfill the definition of hormones: synthesis in one tissue of the body, from which they are transported through the blood to another tissue where they exercise their specific effect. Synthesis of the prohormone form of vitamin D occurs in the skin and then the first hydroxylation takes place in the liver, where cholecalciferol (and ergocalciferol) is converted by a specific enzyme to HCC. It is then carried in the blood by a specific transport protein to the kidneys, where DHCC is produced by another enzymatic hydroxylation. In this form, vitamin D exerts its critical influence on the metabolism of calcium and phosphorus, and consequently on bone development. Parathyroid hormone (PTH), produced in the parathyroid glands, has a role in regulation of this process.

These and other recent discoveries concerning the biochemical activity of vitamin D continue its exciting history. They have been made possible only by the remarkable technological advances within the last two decades, including chemical synthesis of radioactive forms of the vitamin, chromatographic methods of bioassay, and high resolution mass spectroscopy (National Dairy Council, 1976).

Physiological Functions

A major function of vitamin D (that is, of DHCC) is to increase the absorption of dietary calcium and phosphorus, both of which are needed for bone mineralization. Vitamin D also acts directly on bone, aiding bone formation and also stimulating the release of reserve calcium into the blood. An intricate network of biochemical reactions, with vitamin D as a key factor at several points, carries out these functions.

Vitamin D initiates the synthesis of a specific calcium-binding protein (CaBP) that increases the absorption of calcium. The absorption of dietary phosphorus is similarly increased by vitamin D. These absorption processes take place by means of *active transport systems;* that is, the mineral is carried across cell membranes by specialized carrier molecules, and metabolic energy (ATP) fuels the process.

In bone itself, vitamin D enhances mineralization through a mechanism that is not yet completely understood. However, the mechanism by which this vitamin affects *release* of bone calcium to maintain serum calcium and phosphorus at the appropriate levels is more clear. Bone tissue functions as a calcium and phosphorus reserve in a regulatory system that tightly controls the levels of these minerals in the blood. When serum calcium or phosphorus levels fall, the parathyroid glands (four small glands embedded in the thyroid gland) respond by secreting PTH. This polypeptide hormone stimulates the kidney hydroxylase enzyme that converts HCC to DHCC. By this means, the most active form of vitamin D is produced in the required quantities to perform its metabolic functions on intestinal cells, bone, and (possibly) the kidney. In this way, vitamin D stimulates the release of calcium and phosphorus from the bone into the blood.

This seems paradoxical. Vitamin D is known to be necessary for the mineralization of bone, though the mechanism is not clear. Why then does it also promote the process of bone resorption? The answer, apparently, is that there are optimal serum levels of calcium and phosphorus that are required for bone mineralization. By maintaining these optimal levels, vitamin D in the form of DHCC and in the presence of PTH controls bone formation. These complex interactions are diagramed in Figure 6-5.

Vitamin D also appears to increase reabsorption of phosphorus and calcium by the kidney and prevents excretion of phosphorus in the urine. Thus, the overall effect of vitamin D is to provide the optimal amounts of calcium and phosphorus needed for bone mineralization by increasing their availability through increased absorption and preventing the loss of phosphorus in the urine. (Calcium and phosphorus will be discussed further in Chapter 8.)

Dietary Requirements and Recommended Allowances

UNITS OF MEASUREMENT. Vitamin D activity is expressed in International Units or as micrograms of cholecalciferol. One IU equals 0.025 micrograms (μg) of pure crystalline vitamin D_3. Vitamin D activity in a food is most often measured by means of the so-called line test. In this technique, rats with rickets are fed measured doses of a test material. Subsequent bone calcification can be determined through chemical staining of a longitudinal section of bone; the area of calcification is clearly visible as a line. The extent of calcification is proportional to the amount of vitamin D in the tested substance, and can be compared to standardized measurements of vitamin D_3 activity.

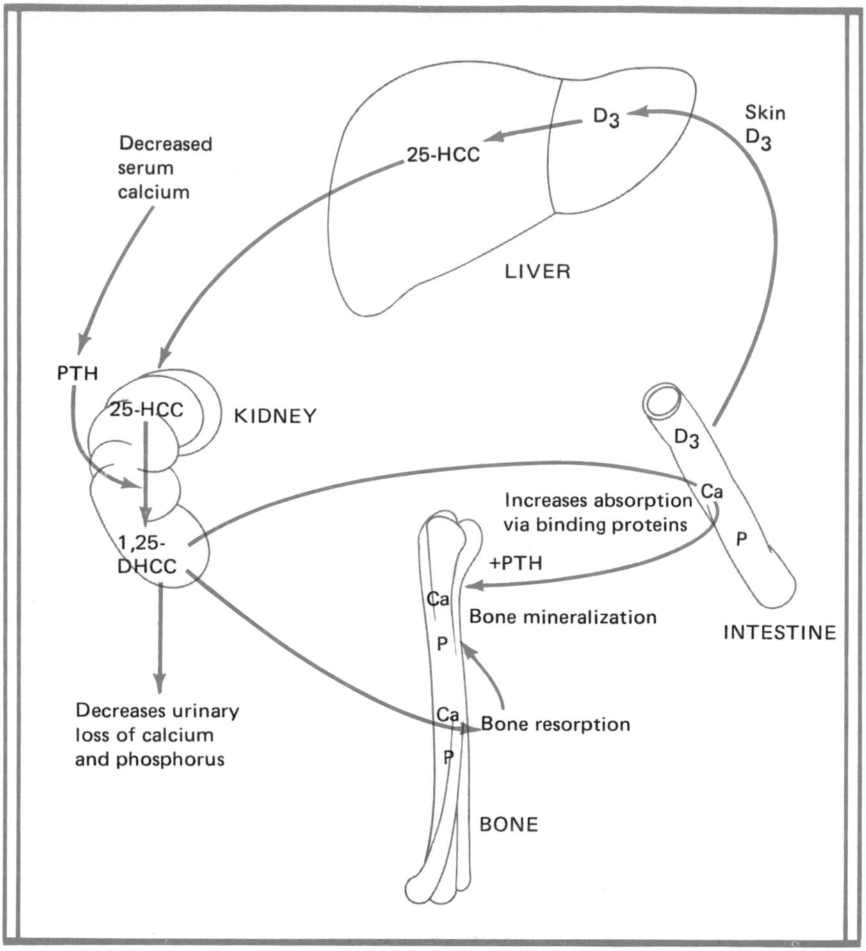

FIGURE 6-5

Metabolic Functions of Vitamin D

Activated vitamin D_3 increases absorption of calcium and phosphorus from the intestine, in conjunction with PTH promotes both bone resorption and mineralization, and prevents loss of urinary calcium and phosphorus. When serum calcium and phosphorus levels fall, there is an increase in production of PTH by the parathyroid glands, resulting in increased DHCC synthesis. When *both* calcium and phosphorus blood levels increase, the conversion of HCC to DHCC is diminished.

Because the line test is both time-consuming and expensive and only an indirect measure of vitamin D activity, researchers have sought to develop other techniques. Highly sensitive assay techniques have recently been developed to measure HCC and DHCC in human blood plasma.

RECOMMENDED DIETARY ALLOWANCES. A minimum dietary requirement for vitamin D is yet to be established. Sunlight, which may produce a substantial part of the amount required, is itself a variable. The amount of vitamin D formed by sunlight is dependent on various factors, including length and intensity of exposure and color of skin (the greater the pigmentation of the skin, the greater its screening effect against ultraviolet light).

The RDA for vitamin D is 10 μg (400 IU) per day from birth through 18 years of age. A daily intake of 2.5 μg (100 IU) is sufficient to prevent rickets, but the larger amount is associated with optimal calcium absorption and growth and includes a safety margin. During late adolescence and the adult years, the RDA is 7.5 μg (300 IU) and 5 μg (200 IU), respectively. An additional 5 μg is recommended during pregnancy and lactation.

Dietary Sources

Except for certain fish and fish-liver oils, the only *significant* natural source of vitamin D is that produced by sunlight. Fortified foods and commercial preparations are the only reliable common dietary sources. Table 6-2 lists the vitamin D values of various food products. In general, egg whites, vegetable oils, unfortified dairy products, cereals, beans, fruits, vegetables, and muscle meats are poor sources of vitamin D. Relatively good sources are egg yolk, butterfat, fortified dairy products, fish oils, and organ meats.

Human milk is an unreliable source of vitamin D, as is unfortified cow's milk. Because it contains both calcium and phosphorus and is an important food for children, milk is an appropriate vehicle for fortification with vitamin D. Today almost all milk is fortified by the direct addition of vitamin D_2 or D_3 concentrates. According to estimates made in 1973, approximately 98 percent of all homogenized milk sold commercially in the United States contained vitamin D in concentrations of 400 IU per quart (Fine, 1973). Thus, growing children who drink two cups of fortified milk every day are assured of half the recommended amount from this source alone. Breast-fed infants, however, should be given a vitamin D supplement, as should strict vegetarians (vegans).

Because vitamin D is highly resistant to heat, light, and oxidation, it is essentially unaffected by food processing and preparation procedures. Being fat soluble, vitamin D is stored in the body, though to a lesser extent than vitamin A. Daily intake, therefore, is not necessary, especially for adults. But those who have limited exposure to the sun—winter-born infants, city dwellers, the elderly—should have a dietary source of vitamin D.

Symptoms of Clinical Deficiency

The best known and most common deficiency condition resulting from lack of vitamin D is, of course, rickets. Metabolically, the visible symptoms of rickets are caused by inadequate absorption of calcium and phosphorus and, consequently, faulty mineralization of bones and teeth. In children lacking sufficient vitamin D, the bones remain too soft to withstand mechanical stress. The skeletal malformations characteristic of this condition include bow legs; enlargement of junctions between the ribs and their cartilaginous connection to the sternum or breast bone, forming a series of knobby protuberances sometimes called rachitic rosary; projection of the sternum ("pigeon breast"); narrow pelvis; and spinal curvature. Knock knees (enlarged knee joints), skull deformations, various muscle weaknesses, nervous irritability, and malformation of the teeth are additional symptoms of fully developed rickets.

Vitamin D deficiency in adults causes osteomalacia ("bone softening"), or adult rickets. The most common symptoms are weakening of the bone due to

TABLE 6-2
Vitamin D Content of Selected Foods
RDA for Adults
5μg cholecalciferol = 200 IU

Food	Serving Size	Vitamin D Content IU/Serving
Sardines	3½ oz	1,150–1,570[a]
Cod-liver oil	1 tbsp	1,275
Mackerel, raw	3½ oz	1,100
Salmon, fresh	3½ oz	154–550[a]
Oysters	3–4 medium	510
Salmon, canned	3½ oz	220–440[a]
Herring, canned	3½ oz	330
Herring, fresh	3½ oz	315
Tuna, canned in water	3½ oz	250
Shrimp	3½ oz	150
Milk, whole or skim, fortified	1 c	100
Liver, chicken, raw	3½ oz	50–67[a]
Liver, pork, raw	3½ oz	45
Halibut	3½ oz	44
Liver, beef, raw	3½ oz	9–42[a]
Egg, whole	1 large	25
Egg, yolk	1 large	25
Milk, human	1 c	0–24[a]
Liver, lamb, raw	3½ oz	20
Liver, calf, raw	3½ oz	0–15[a]
Cheese, cottage	½ c	10
Milk, cow, unfortified	1 c	0.7–10[a]
Cheese, cheddar	1 oz	3–8[a]
Cream, heavy	1 tbsp	8
Butter	1 tbsp	5
Ice cream	½ c	5
Clams	½ c	3
Bread, white enriched	1 slice	3
Butter	1 pat	2
Egg, white	1 large	0
Wheat germ	1 tbsp	0
Soybeans, cooked	½ c	0
Corn flakes	1 c	0
Oatmeal, cooked	¾ c	0
Margarine	1 tbsp	0
Vegetable oil	1 tbsp	0
Spinach	—	0
Apple	—	0
Ground beef	3 oz	0
Chicken	—	0
Beans	—	0
Yogurt	8 oz	—

[a] Ranges are given for food items in which a significant variability in vitamin D value is apparent. Values are influenced by season (amount of sunlight) in the case of dairy products. For liver, the older the animal the longer the time available to build up vitamin stores.

Sources: C. F. Church and H. N. Church, *Food values of portions commonly used,* 12th ed. (Philadelphia: Lippincott, 1975); J. A. Pennington, *Dietary nutrient guide* (Westport, Conn.: Avi Publishing Co., 1976); and E. Yendt, in *International encyclopedia of pharmacology and therapeutics,* vol. 1 (Elmsford, N.Y.: Pergamon Press, 1970), p. 139.

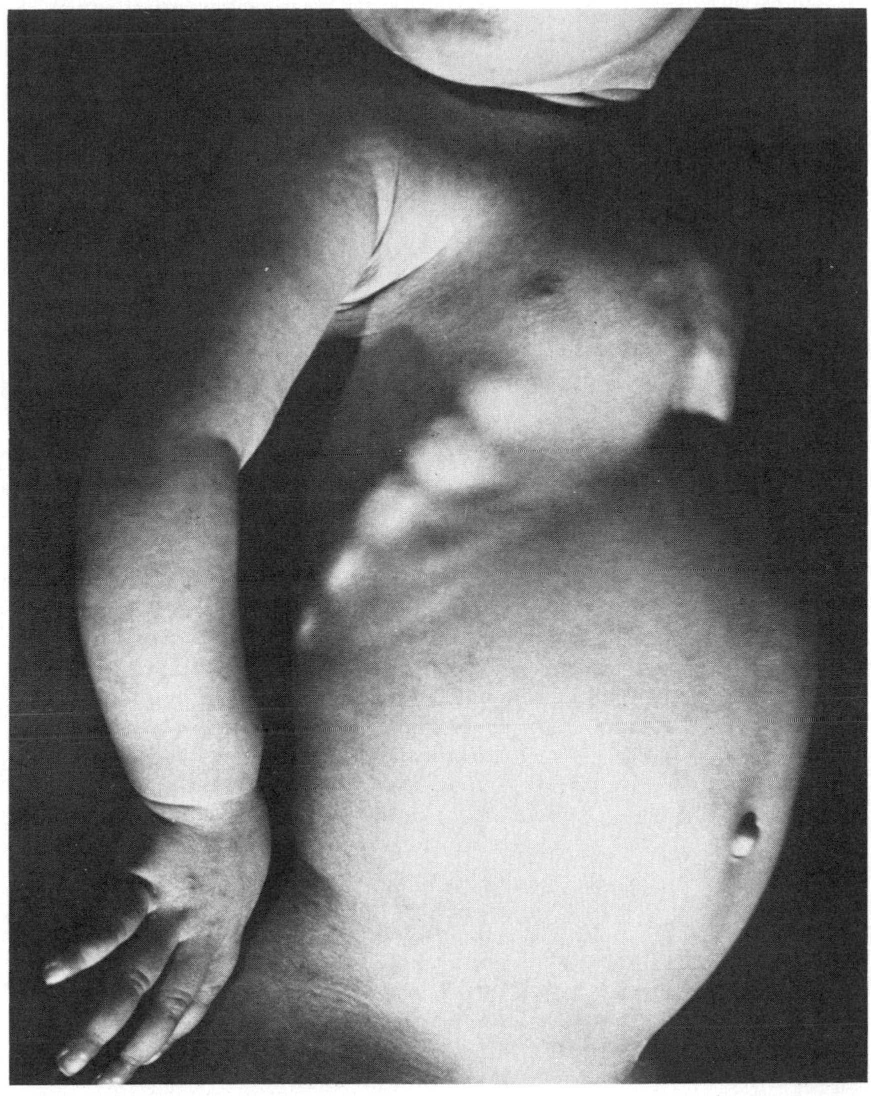

Rachitic rosary, an early symptom of rickets. (Children's Hospital Medical Center, Boston)

increased porosity and decreased density. This may result in various deformities, pain in the bones of the leg and lower back, general physical weakness including difficulty in walking, and spontaneous bone fractures.

Among adults, osteomalacia generally occurs in women, especially following repeated pregnancies, and among the elderly. Again, inadequate diet and/or insufficient sunlight are the major contributory factors. (Nutrition during pregnancy is discussed further in Chapter 12. Aspects of adult nutrition are treated in Chapter 14.)

The main cause of primary vitamin D deficiency is lack of sunlight. Absence of sunlight is more likely to be a significant contributory factor in premature infants and elderly people who spend very little time outdoors.

Other conditions may also prevent sufficient exposure. In parts of the Middle East, for example, clothing customs require almost complete covering of the body, especially for women. Also, ultraviolet light cannot penetrate smoke, soot, fog, or window glass, with implications for inhabitants of smog-bound cities.

Insufficient exposure to sunlight becomes increasingly important when the amount of dietary vitamin D decreases and may be a significant factor in the health of some infants. Human milk, although it is an excellent food for infants, is not a complete food, and cases of rickets in breast-fed infants continue to appear in the medical literature. It has recently been reported that human milk may contain a water-soluble form of vitamin D; however, this finding awaits confirmation. Since plant foods are a particularly poor source of vitamin D, the breast-fed child of a vegetarian mother is even more at risk (Fomon and Straus, 1978). Cases of rickets in vegetarian children have recently been reported in Boston (Dwyer et al., 1979). Vitamin D supplementation is especially important for such children, unless regular exposure to sunlight is assured.

Despite adequate sunlight and dietary intake, secondary vitamin D deficiency may develop under certain conditions. Some endocrine disorders and diseases of the liver or kidney apparently interfere with the synthesis of HCC and DHCC; as a result, there may develop what is known as vitamin D-resistant rickets. The same condition can arise from a particular genetic defect as well. Various drugs are also known to interfere with the metabolism of vitamin D. Cortisone therapy may produce osteoporosis or loss of bone tissue (as will Cushing's disease, in which there is excessive synthesis of hydrocortisone). Barbiturates and anticonvulsant drugs reduce the amount of available HCC and DHCC. As mentioned earlier, the bile necessary for absorption of vitamin D is decreased by cholestyramine, a drug used to reduce serum cholesterol in cardiovascular disease. Mineral oil also reduces absorption. (For a general discussion of the biochemistry and clinical applications of vitamin D, see Haussler and McCain, 1977).

Toxicity

Because individuals vary in their sensitivity to vitamin D, a minimal toxic dose has not been determined. But excessive amounts of dietary vitamin D are definitely hazardous. It is certainly possible to have too much of a good thing: The most common cause of hypervitaminosis D is dietary supplementation with cod-liver oil!

The symptoms of hypervitaminosis D are largely due to the resulting high levels of calcium in the blood (hypercalcemia). They include nausea, loss of appetite, weight loss, and calcification of bone and soft tissues. Particularly serious injury to the kidneys can result from calcification. In children, growth may be reduced.

Sensitive infants may develop hypercalcemia on an intake of 1,800 to 2,000 IU per day, since the toxicity threshold is only four to five times the RDA. Symptoms in adults with intakes exceeding 100,000 IU per day have been documented. Moreover, because the excess vitamin is contained in stored fat tissue, hypercalcemia may last for months after intake of the vitamin has ceased. Thus it is important to remember the hazards as well as the benefits of vitamin D and to control dietary intake. Except in the case of diseases that affect vitamin D absorption or metabolism, dietary intake should be limited to 400 IU (Food and Nutrition Board, 1979). A child (or adult) drinking a quart of milk a day should not receive vitamin D supplementation.

VITAMIN E

Vitamin E is one of the most controversial nutrients. Discovered in 1922 by H. M. Evans and K. S. Bishop at the University of California, Berkeley, it was first identified as a dietary factor essential for reproduction in rats. This function is reflected in the chemical name of the vitamin, *tocopherol*, which is derived from Greek words meaning "to bear offspring." It has since been promoted as a sex vitamin, as a cure for a number of nondeficiency diseases of the reproductive, circulatory, and nervous systems, and as a protective agent against aging and air pollution. These claims—and many similar ones—are based on inadequate evidence and are much disputed. But despite extensive research, mostly on experimental animals, the role of vitamin E in human nutrition is still not clear. Deficiency symptoms noted in animal studies have not been demonstrated in humans, although it has been established that small amounts are required by infants, especially those who are premature. Because vitamin E is found in a wide variety of foods common in the human diet, deficiencies are so unlikely in adults that none have yet been found. Nevertheless, research on the role of this vitamin continues. As one nutritionist has said, "There is the nagging suspicion that there is a very important use for the vitamin and we are just not smart enough to see it" (Tappel, 1973). Although the nutritional history of this substance has barely begun, a review of the findings thus far can be found in Mason (1977).

Chemistry and Properties

Vitamin E occurs naturally in four forms. When pure, all are oily yellow liquids and are completely soluble in fats and fat solvents. By far the most active and common form is α-tocopherol, whose structure is shown in Figure 6-6.

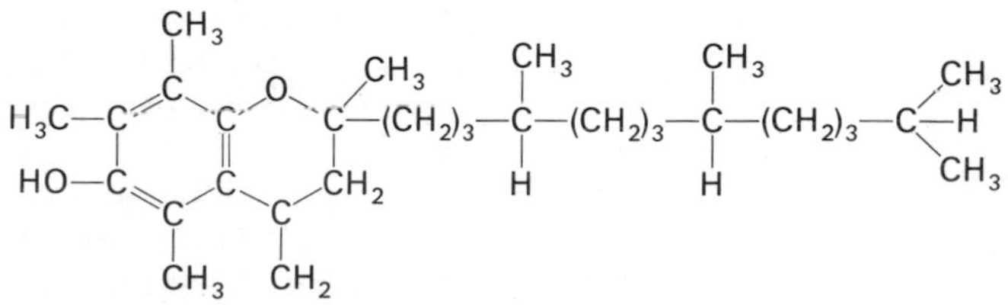

FIGURE 6-6
Chemical Structure of α-tocopherol

For the most part, vitamin E is highly stable. Neither boiling nor long periods of storage alone affect its activity. However, exposure to air or light, or contact with iron or copper, will cause the vitamin to decompose. The tocopherols oxidize readily—so readily, in fact, that they are oxidized before other substances in a mixture exposed to an oxidizing agent. For this reason, vitamin E is used as an antioxidant in foods to protect other substances, particularly vitamin A and polyunsaturated fatty acids (PUFA), from oxidation and, in the case of fatty foods, from becoming **rancid.**

Absorption and Metabolism

The process of absorption of vitamin E is much the same as that of other fats and fat-soluble substances. It requires bile, occurs in the mucosa of the small intestine, and its transport into the general circulation takes place via chylomicrons and lymph.

Vitamin E is carried in the blood by lipoproteins. It is stored primarily in adipose tissue, with smaller amounts found in liver and muscle tissue. The adrenal and pituitary glands contain significant concentrations of the vitamin. Vitamin E is released into the circulation whenever fat is mobilized. Its metabolites are excreted both in urine and in feces.

Absorption of vitamin E is less efficient than that of vitamin A; only 50 to 85 percent of the dietary intake of this vitamin actually enters the bloodstream. These figures are reduced by the presence of mineral oil or any of the other conditions that affect the absorption of fats generally. Efficiency of absorption is further impaired as intake increases. Tissue levels of vitamin E only double when intake is increased to ten times the RDA for the vitamin. For this reason, those who take megadoses of vitamin E are surely getting less than anticipated for their money (Tappel, 1973).

Physiological Functions

Few nutrients have generated as much public interest or clinical debate as has vitamin E. If all the claims made for its curative and health-promoting effects were true, it would indeed be a wonder nutrient. To put these claims in proper perspective, it is useful to note that they arose, at least in part, from a misinterpretation of research with laboratory animals, and in part from the nature of the earliest findings involving tocopherols.

Early research showed these substances to be essential for fertility in rats, and subsequent studies identified other deficiency conditions as well—for a number of laboratory animal species. But experimental animals can be fed a controlled diet and deliberately deprived of all vitamin E until a deficiency condition is produced. It would be extremely difficult, if not impossible, to produce a similar deficiency in humans. Vitamin E is widely available in a normal diet; it is stored throughout the body; and its release from storage ("turnover") is so gradual that depletion of body stores would take many months. No symptoms of vitamin E deficiency have been identified in humans without other medical disorders. Without deficiency symptoms, it is difficult to identify the function of a nutrient. Moreover, although vitamin E deficiency can produce certain conditions in animals, it has been shown that similar disorders in humans are unrelated to vitamin E status. For example, severe vitamin E deficiency causes a type of muscular dystrophy in animals; however, humans with this condition exhibit normal muscle tissue levels of the vitamin. Consequently, claims that vitamin E will prevent or cure muscular dystrophy in humans are simply not true. A deficiency disease induced in an animal cannot be compared with a genetic disease in humans.

Nonetheless, there is evidence to suggest that vitamin E plays an important role in a number of metabolic processes. Vitamin E may be required, although in minute amounts, for the synthesis of **heme** (a part of the hemoglobin molecule and of other metabolically essential body chemicals).

The best-understood activities of vitamin E, however, result from its antioxidant activity. Tocopherol reacts with compounds that have an unpaired electron and are therefore highly reactive as oxidizing agents. These compounds are known as *free radicals*. By reacting with them, vitamin E prevents the radicals from oxidizing polyunsaturated fats, vitamin A, various enzymes, and cell membrane constituents. In forestalling oxidative damage, vitamin E increases the stability of cellular and intracellular structures, particularly membranes.

In addition to their destructive potential as oxidizing agents, free radicals are believed to participate in the formation of "aging pigments," which may contribute to the aging process in various tissues. It has therefore been theorized that, by deactivating free radicals, vitamin E may be able to slow cell aging. So far, however, experimental tests on laboratory animals have not confirmed this hypothesis.

Additionally, vitamin E apparently works with certain other nutrients in complementary relationships that protect the integrity of numerous biochemical substances and cellular structures. For example, glutathione perioxidase is an enzyme that prevents oxidative destruction of PUFAs during a particular stage of cell development. Production of this enzyme requires specific proteins in association with the trace element selenium, and its function is enhanced by vitamin E as well (Tappel, 1973). Since the role of this enzyme is similar to one of the best-understood functions of vitamin E, this involvement is not surprising.

The antioxidant properties of vitamin E are those most extensively studied, but they do not explain all of its observed effects. Recent research, for example, has shown that administration of vitamin E in pharmacological doses interferes with the blood clotting process. The postulated mechanism involves a metabolite of the vitamin, tocopherylquinone, which is similar in structure to vitamin K. Vitamin K, as we shall see, promotes blood coagulation. According to the present hypothesis, tocopherylquinone acts as an antagonist to vitamin K. It is possible that, in its other roles as well, vitamin E acts through one or more metabolites, as vitamin D does through HCC and DHCC.

Dietary Requirements and Recommended Allowances

UNITS OF MEASUREMENT. One milligram of d-α-tocopherol has been designated as 1 α-tocopherol equivalent (αT.E.). Values for several forms of α-tocopherol are:

0.67 αT.E. = 1 mg dl-α-tocopheryl acetate (natural or synthetic)
0.74 αT.E. = 1 mg dl-α-tocopherol (synthetic)
0.91 αT.E. = 1 mg d-α-tocopheryl acetate
1.00 αT.E. = 1 mg d-α-tocopherol (naturally occurring)

Precise activity levels of the other tocopherols are not known at present.

BASIS OF REQUIREMENTS. The RDAs for vitamin E are based on studies of dietary intake, which are assumed to be adequate since no deficiencies have been identified. Studies have also indicated, however, that the vitamin E requirements increase directly as PUFA intake increases. In American diets, vitamin E intake varies directly with PUFA intake, since they are naturally found together in foods, for example in vegetable oils. Because the actual requirement for vitamin E is a function of PUFA intake, which is highly variable, precise requirements cannot be established. The Food and Nutrition Board has suggested an α-tocopherol:PUFA ratio of 0.6 milligrams of α-tocopherol per 1 gram of PUFA. Actual intakes in the United States seem to approximate a vitamin E:PUFA ratio of 0.4 milligrams per gram, but no adverse effects have been identified; the Food and Nutrition Board recommendation can, however, serve as a guide. The RDAs for adult men and women are 10 and 8 mg αT.E., respectively. RDAs for other age groups will be discussed later.

Dietary Sources

Since vitamin E is generally found with PUFAs, its main sources in the American diet are oils of vegetable origin. Animal fats are not useful sources nor are animal products in general, although liver and eggs contain fair amounts. Among other vegetable foods, cereals and legumes have moderate vitamin E content. In the processing of white rice and refined flour, however, much of their vitamin E content is removed. Fruits and leafy and root vegetables contain very little vitamin E, and most of that is in a less active form. Table 6-3 lists the tocopherol content of selected foods.

Because of its availability in the cooking oils (cottonseed, soybean, and corn) generally used in this country, it would be difficult not to consume the recommended dietary allowances of vitamin E. Moreover, since vegetable oils are the major dietary source, an increase of vitamin E intake in proportion to an increase in PUFA consumption is virtually automatic, unless the oil has become rancid. Further, there is little loss of vitamin activity in most cooking procedures. High heat, however, will oxidize tocopherols. In one study, oil used repeatedly for deep-frying doughnuts was tested at intervals for tocopherol content and went from 19.4 mg per 100 g to 10.7 mg in the course of a day's cooking. But much more dramatic was the combined effect of the used cooking oil and high temperature frying on the shortening used in the doughnut batter: As mixed into the batter, this shortening contained 92.8 mg of tocopherols per 100 g; in the last batch of cooked doughnuts, tocopherol content had been reduced to 6.8 mg per 100 g (Harris et al., 1950). Prolonged storage, especially of foods cooked in vegetable oils, will also result in loss of tocopherols by oxidation.

TABLE 6-3
Total Tocopherol Content of Selected Foods
RDA for Adults
Men: 10 mgαT.E.
Women: 8 mgαT.E.

Food	Serving Size	Tocopherol Content mg/serving
Wheat germ oil	1 tbsp	39.0
Baked blueberry pie, fresh	1/6 of 9″ pie	28.3
Corn oil, hydrogenated[a]	1 tbsp	15.8
Soybean oil, unhydrogenated[a]	1 tbsp	15.2
Corn oil, unhydrogenated[a]	1 tbsp	15.0
Soybean oil, hydrogenated[a]	1 tbsp	11.0
Safflower oil, stabilized	1 tbsp	8.8
Safflower oil, unstabilized	1 tbsp	5.4
Wheat germ	1 oz	3.8
Yellow corn meal	1/2 c	3.4
Margarine, corn oil	1 pat	2.3
Oatmeal, uncooked	1/4 c	1.9
Mayonnaise	1 tbsp	1.8
Salmon, broiled	3 oz	1.5
Navy beans, dry	1/2 c	1.5
Peas, fresh	1/2 c	1.5
Italian salad dressing	1 tbsp	1.4
Beef liver, broiled	3 oz	1.4
Tomato juice, canned	6 oz	1.3
Coconut oil	1 tbsp	1.2
Haddock, broiled	3 oz	1.0
Apple	1 medium	0.7
Bread, whole wheat	1 slice	0.6
Peas, frozen, cooked	1/2 c	0.6
Egg	1 medium	0.5
Ground beef, fried	3 oz	0.5
Chicken, breast with bones, broiled	3 oz	0.5
Banana	1 medium	0.5
Cream cheese	1 oz	0.3
Milk, whole	1 c	0.2
Celery	1 stalk	0.2
Ice cream	1/2 c	0.1
Potato, raw	1 large	0.1
Lettuce	1/8 head	0.1
Corn flakes	1 c	0.1
Potato, baked	1 large	0.08
Bread, white	1 slice	0.06
Butter	1 pat	0.05
Peas, canned	1/2 c	0.03

[a]Hydrogenation does not systematically alter the tocopherol content of vegetable oils. Note that the tocopherol content decreases when soybean oil is hydrogenated, whereas a slight increase occurs with the hydrogenation of corn oil.

Sources: R. H. Bunnel, J. Keating, A. Quaresimo, and G. K. Parman, Alpha-tocopherol content of foods, *American Journal of Clinical Nutrition* 17:1, 1965; P. L. Harris, M. L. Quaife, and W. J. Swanson, Vitamin E content of foods, *Journal of Nutrition* 40:367, 1950; and J. A. Pennington, *Dietary nutrient guide* (Westport, Conn.: Avi Publishing Co., 1976).

Symptoms of Clinical Deficiency

Because deficiency symptoms in humans have not been clearly identified, clinical deficiency can only be determined by measurement of serum levels of vitamin E or by red blood cell destruction by oxidation in premature infants. Low serum levels are found in newborns generally but rise within the first month of life, especially in breast-fed full-term infants. There are reports of deficiency symptoms—irritability, edema, and hemolytic anemia (caused by the destruction of red blood cells)—in premature infants fed a commercial formula with inadequate vitamin E content; these symptoms were reversed when vitamin E was administered. In adults, however, storage levels are apparently sufficient to ward off deficiencies for prolonged periods; adult male volunteers who received low-tocopherol diets for three years did not develop symptoms, although serum levels became quite low (Horwitt, 1960).

A few situations in which vitamin E supplementation is beneficial have been established. Several diseases, including cystic fibrosis and liver cirrhosis, as well as gastric surgery, result in malabsorption of lipids. The resulting deficiencies can be effectively treated with vitamin E and the other fat-soluble vitamins. Large (or pharmacologic) doses for several months can also relieve the condition known as intermittent claudication, or pain in the calf muscle during walking. In view of the large doses required for effectiveness in these conditions, and their specialized nature, the relief of symptoms should be considered a drug effect. Only the treatment of hemolytic anemia in premature infants can be considered to involve a *nutritional* effect of vitamin E in human deficiency disease.

Despite various claims, tests have failed to show that vitamin E has any positive effect on athletic performance or that it provides any protection against cancer or aging. There is some evidence that it may prevent lung damage from air pollution, though it does not reverse the symptoms. And there is no reliable evidence to give vitamin E a role in either human fertility or sexual performance, unless the person is subject to a placebo effect.

Toxicity

As we saw earlier, recent studies have shown an antagonistic relationship between very high vitamin E intake and blood coagulation, with large doses slowing the clotting rate. It has been suggested that this property of vitamin E could be beneficial to women taking oral contraceptives, since they are at greater risk of developing thrombosis (Horwitt, 1976). On the other hand, the anti-vitamin K activity of vitamin E increases the risk of hemorrhage in patients suffering from vitamin K deficiency and is a potentially toxic effect.

Daily intakes as high as 800 mg αT.E. have not been found to be toxic. Only in recent years, however, have large numbers of people been "prescribing" vitamin E for themselves; the long-term effect is not known at present. Certainly vitamin E does not produce toxic symptoms as severe and visible as those of vitamins A and D. However, one report has noted adverse symptoms associated with excess intake for as short a time as three months, and another has reported the occurrence of hemorrhage when excess vitamin E coincided with a vitamin K deficiency (Corrigan and Marcus, 1974). The potential for hypervitaminosis E definitely exists and should not be ignored.

VITAMIN K

Vitamin K was discovered by a Danish scientist, Henrik Dam, in 1929. He had earlier observed a hemorrhagic disease in newborn chicks. Blood analyses showed decreased levels of prothrombin, a factor involved in blood clotting. Although the chicks' diet had appeared to be entirely adequate, Dam found that hog-liver fat or alfalfa prevented the condition. He named the antihemorrhagic factor vitamin K, from the Danish word *koagulation*. In 1943 Dam received the Nobel Prize in physiology and medicine for his discovery.

Chemistry and Properties

Vitamin K is actually a group of yellowish **crystalline** (chemically pure) compounds belonging to a family of chemical substances called quinones. All forms are resistant to heat, air, and moisture but are vulnerable to destruction by strong acids, alkalis, and light. Only two major forms are found in nature, and vitamin K_1 (phylloquinone) is the only form synthesized by plants. Vitamin K_2 (menaquinone), itself a group of vitamins, is found in bacteria and in animals, in which it is a product of bacterial metabolism. The activity of K_2 is about 75 percent that of K_1. The most potent form of the vitamin, with more than twice the activity of K_2, is menadione, which is not present in nature but which can be synthesized in the laboratory. Animals convert menadione to menaquinone by adding the long side chain, which is needed for vitamin activity. Thus, it is the *ring* structure of vitamin K that cannot be synthesized by animals, who therefore need an exogenous source for optimal health. Both diet and synthesis by intestinal bacteria contribute to the supply needed. As you can see from Figure 6-7, the basic ring structure of these three forms is the same; they differ in the length and composition of their side chains.

Absorption and Metabolism

The absorption and initial metabolism of vitamin K are much the same as those of other fat-soluble vitamins, requiring bile and other factors which promote the absorption of fat-soluble materials. Any disorder of fat absorption will interfere with absorption of vitamin K. Chylomicrons transport the vitamin to the liver, where it is combined with β-lipoproteins before entering the general circulation. Although vitamin K is concentrated in the liver for a short time, storage in the body is minimal. Small amounts appear in skin, muscle, the kidneys, and the heart. Metabolites are excreted in bile and urine.

One notable difference between vitamin K and the other fat-soluble vitamins is that bacterial synthesis of vitamin K_2 in the intestine is an important source of vitamin K in humans.

Metabolic Function

Vitamin K has only one known function in humans and animals, and that is as a factor essential for blood clotting. The coagulation of blood is a complex

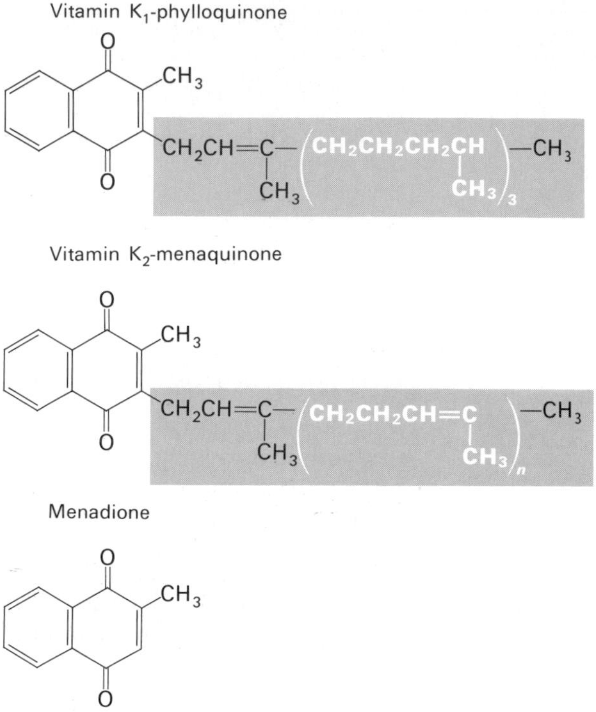

Vitamin K_1-phylloquinone

Vitamin K_2-menaquinone

Menadione

FIGURE 6-7
Chemical Structures of Three Forms of Vitamin K

series of reactions and, like so many other intricate biochemical mechanisms, is still only partly understood. Prothrombin, a protein factor necessary for clotting, forms only in the presence of adequate vitamin K in the liver. According to the most widely held theory, vitamin K functions as a cofactor of the enzyme that catalyzes one step in the synthesis of prothrombin.

Several other so-called clotting factors are also influenced by vitamin K. Thus a deficiency of the vitamin or the administration of an antagonist will interfere in several ways with synthesis of prothrombin and the other substances necessary for blood coagulation. Blood clotting time may be prolonged, which is normally undesirable but which may, in some circumstances, be preferred. (The mechanism of blood clotting is further discussed in Chapter 8 in conjunction with calcium metabolism.) Despite its great importance in blood clotting, administration of vitamin K has no therapeutic effect on hemophilia because this disease is caused by a genetic defect in another stage of the clotting mechanism.

Dietary Requirements and Recommended Allowances

UNITS OF MEASUREMENT. Vitamin K activity is often expressed as micrograms of menadione, a synthetic form of the vitamin. The most common bioassay technique for measuring the vitamin activity in foods makes use of chickens in which vitamin K deficiency has been produced. Measured amounts of the test food are fed to the chicks, and the resulting increased levels of blood prothrombin are determined. These levels are then compared to those produced by known quantities of vitamin K_1.

RECOMMENDED ALLOWANCES. The Food and Nutrition Board has set no RDA for vitamin K. Estimated safe and adequate daily dietary intakes have been established (Food and Nutrition Board, 1979). For adults, this estimate is 70-140 μg per day. From 50 to 60 percent of the vitamin K in the body is synthesized by the bacterial flora in the intestine, and the remainder is derived from food sources. Because vitamin K is found in a variety of foods and there is extensive synthesis by bacteria, there is little risk of inadequate vitamin status under normal conditions.

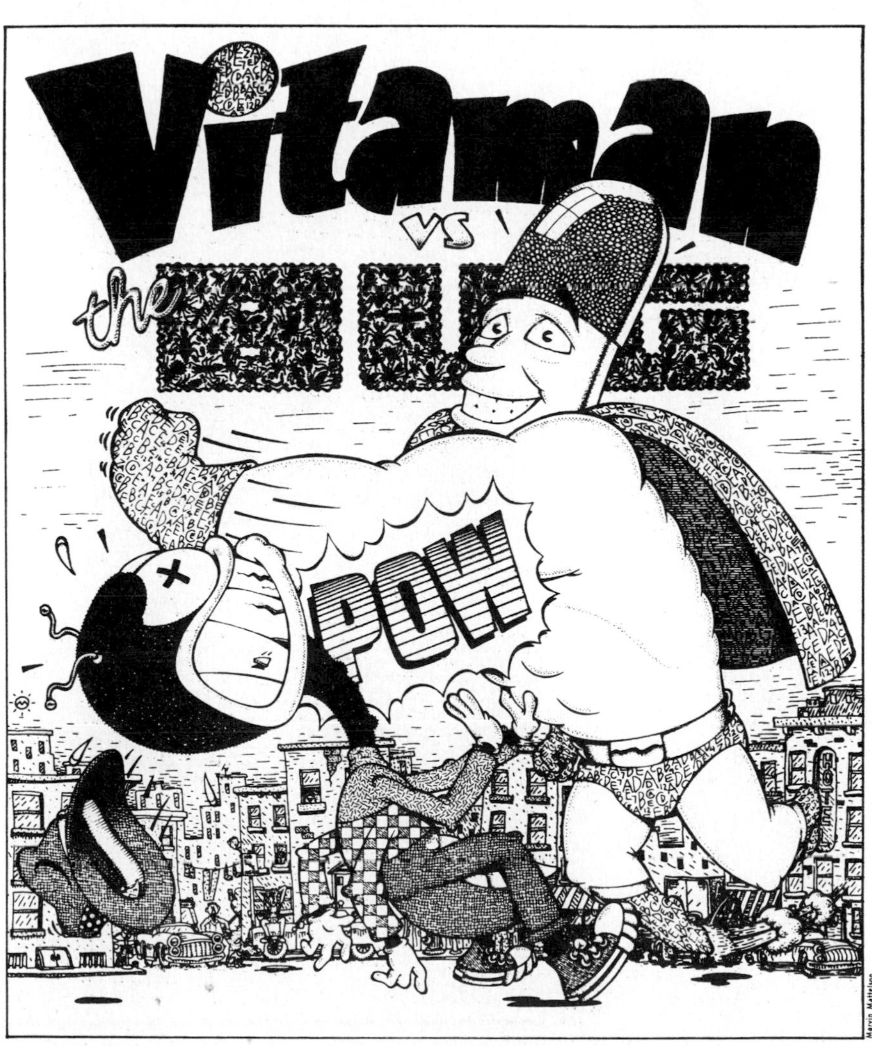

Vita Man vs The Bug. (Marvin Mattelson)

Dietary Sources

Since bacterial synthesis usually provides at least half of the required amount of vitamin K, there is little difficulty in completing the requirement from dietary sources. A selected list of foods and their vitamin K content appears in Table 6-4. In general, green leafy vegetables and members of the cabbage-cauliflower group are the best sources. These are followed by meats (especially liver) and dairy products, fruits, and cereals. Human milk, however, contains very little vitamin K.

It is a curious fact that one of the richest sources of vitamin K is non-dietary—tobacco! Unfortunately for cigarette smokers, only a small amount goes up in smoke from which (if inhaled) it is absorbed by the mucous membranes of the nasal passage and lungs. Baseball players and other users of chewing tobacco undoubtedly derive greater benefit.

TABLE 6-4
Average Vitamin K Content of Selected Foods
Estimated Safe and Adequate Daily Dietary Intake for Adults: 70–140 μg

Food	Serving Size	Vitamin K Content μg/serving
Turnip greens	½ c	195
Broccoli	½ c	160
Lettuce	⅛ head	90
Beef liver	3 oz	78
Cabbage	½ c	56
Asparagus	4 spears	34
Spinach	½ c	27
Pork liver	3 oz	21
Tea, green	1 tsp	19
Watercress	½ c	17
Peas, green	½ c	16
Bacon	4 strips	14
Ham	3 oz	13
Cheese	1 oz	10
Pork tenderloin	3 oz	9
Beans, green	½ c	8
Cow's milk	1 c	7
Tomato	1 med.	7
Ground beef	3 oz	6
Chicken liver	3 oz	6
Egg, whole	1 large	5.5
Potato	1 large	4.7
Applesauce	½ c	2.6
Banana	1 large	2.4
Corn oil	1 tbsp	1.5
Butter	1 pat	1.5
Orange	1 med.	1.3
Bread	1 slice	1.1
Tea, black	—	0.0

Source: Adapted from R. E. Olson, Vitamin K, in *Modern nutrition in health and disease*, 5th ed., ed. R. S. Goodhart and M. E. Shils (Philadelphia: Lea and Febiger, 1973).

Symptoms of Clinical Deficiency

Because of intestinal synthesis and widespread distribution of vitamin K in plant and animal foods, primary deficiency of this nutrient is highly unlikely. Newborn infants are an exception. Little vitamin K from the mother is received by the developing fetus (due to poor placental transfer), and the normal intestinal bacteria do not become established until about a week after birth. To raise low prothrombin levels and prevent hemorrhagic disease, injection of 1 milligram of vitamin K_1 immediately after birth has become standard procedure at many hospitals.

However, secondary deficiencies can result from a number of causes: sulfa drugs and antibiotics, which reduce bacterial synthesis; anticoagulants such as Dicumarol, which are antagonists of the vitamin; some anticonvulsant drugs, which increase the rate at which vitamin K is metabolized and eliminated; surgery involving the area of the intestine in which bacterial synthesis and absorption occur; and any condition that affects fat absorption. Secondary deficiency conditions should be compensated by supplying vitamin K, *except* where an anticoagulant effect is needed to prevent blood clot formation in certain heart and blood vessel conditions.

The only identifiable symptom of vitamin K deficiency is decreased efficiency of blood coagulation. In extreme form, as in chronic liver disease or therapy with some drugs, decreased coagulation efficiency may result in hemorrhage.

Toxicity

In pharmacological doses for prolonged periods, vitamin K can produce hemolytic anemia and jaundice in infants. Because of its toxic effect on red blood cell membranes, the synthetic form menadione (vitamin K_3) is no longer permitted in over-the-counter preparations. The water-soluble forms of vitamin K have a greater safety margin and should be used when vitamin K supplements are indicated.

PERSPECTIVE ON Drug–Nutrient Interactions

Throughout this chapter there have been references to medications that disrupt nutrient metabolism and consequently may induce secondary vitamin deficiencies. Recent research has increasingly demonstrated that these and additional interactions that occur between drugs and other nutrients in the body may have a negative impact on health.

Drugs may undermine nutritional status in a number of ways: through their effects on appetite, and through interference with the normal mechanisms of nutrient absorption, function, metabolism, and excretion. Conversely, the effectiveness of a drug for its prescribed purpose may be compromised by the action of various foods and nutrients on drug absorption, metabolism, and excretion. In this section we shall consider those interactions of particular importance to nutritional status and their clinical significance.

Drugs and Appetite. The suppression of appetite by amphetamines, sometimes prescribed in the treatment of depression as well as obesity, is a well-known drug–nutrient interaction. Some other drugs (the vitamin B-complex liquids, chloral hydrate) depress the appetite by causing nausea and gastrointestinal upset; some antibiotics decrease taste sensitivity. Other drugs are known to stimulate the appetite; among them are insulin, certain tranquilizers and antidepressants, oral contraceptives, and some antihistamines (Hartshorn, 1977). Whether appetite is depressed or stimulated, the balance of nutrient and energy intake is upset.

Drugs and Nutrient Absorption, Function, Metabolism, and Excretion. Nutrient absorption may be impaired by any of several mechanisms. Laxatives and cathartics increase intestinal motility, thereby reducing the time in which nutrients can be absorbed. Some of these pharmaceutical products interfere directly with nutrient absorption. We have already seen, for example, that mineral oil dissolves carotene, which is then eliminated in the feces. Drugs may also increase nutrient excretion by any of several mechanisms that effectively keep the nutrient from its binding sites on proteins or within tissues.

Any drug that binds bile salts or decreases their availability will greatly reduce the efficiency with which fats and fat-soluble vitamins can be absorbed. Some drugs can damage certain cells of the intestinal mucosa or directly interfere with transport mechanisms. Some cause excessive release and/or decreased synthesis of pancreatic enzymes, resulting in impaired digestion of fat, protein, and carbohydrate (National Dairy Council, 1977).

Nutrient synthesis can also be affected by drugs, as when antibiotics inhibit the manufacture of vitamin K in the intestinal tract or chloramphenicol decreases protein synthesis. Among the categories of medications that interfere with metabolism and absorption are anticholesterol drugs, such as cholestyramine; antibiotics, such as neomycin; anticonvulsants; and certain drugs used to treat diabetes and other conditions.

Drugs can also act as antivitamins by preventing either the synthesis of an active metabolite or conversion to a coenzyme form, by promoting retention of inactive forms, or by decreasing the natural body stores of a vitamin by increasing the activity of specific metabolic enzymes. There is considerable evidence that anticonvulsant drugs effectively counteract vitamin D by this last mechanism. Thus epileptics on long-term anticonvulsant therapy may develop osteomalacia.

Other important drug-nutrient interactions include the effect of antacids on mineral metabolism. For example, antacids containing aluminum inhibit absorption of phosphorus, ultimately increasing the excretion of both phosphorus and calcium; prolonged use may lead to significant demineralization of bone. The antacid property itself causes conversion of iron to insoluble and unabsorbable forms.

Clinical Significance of Drug–Nutrient Interactions. Individuals who already have borderline nutritional deficiencies, due to low nutrient intake and/or chronic diseases, are significantly at risk of developing clinically important effects of drug–nutrient interactions. Among the common reasons for lowered nutrient intake are alcoholism, psychological stress, chronic illness, and smoking. The latter specifically lowers vitamin C and vitamin E levels. As you may imagine, these conditions involve a large number of individuals in the population. The elderly, because of lowered energy and therefore food needs, are particularly vulnerable. Moreover, they often take several drugs simultaneously. The effects of any interaction, of course, depend on the dose and duration of drug treatment. Two or three days of medication are of no concern; neither are small doses, unless use is prolonged. Drug consumption for weeks or longer, however, is a potentially serious problem. Particularly at risk in such situations are the chronically ill who are likely to be long-term drug users, the elderly, growing children who have high nutrient requirements relative to total food intake, and women who are either pregnant or using oral contraceptives.

Effects of Food on Drugs. Conversely, some foods may interfere with drug utilization. For example, absorption of sulfanilamide and many other drugs is delayed and effectiveness decreased if they are taken simultaneously with food. But some medications, including lithium salts, enhance absorption when food and drug are ingested at the same time. Specific nutrients may also deter or promote absorption of individual drugs: Tetracyclines lose some effectiveness in the presence of foods containing iron, calcium, and other mineral salts.

We are already aware of many food–drug effects, but many more remain to be clarified. This is an area of inquiry for scientists in a variety of fields—toxicology, pharmacology, nutrition, and medicine. And the implications are important for everyone. March (1976) surveys scientific literature on nutrient–drug interactions.

In the meantime, the medical profession and the public should be made aware of the possibility of these interactions, and unnecessary drugtaking (whether prescription, over-the-counter, or illicit) should be discouraged. When drugs are prescribed, instructions for taking them before, during, after, or between meals, and any other instructions, should be carefully followed.

SUMMARY

Vitamins are organic compounds that are (1) required in trace amounts by the body, (2) perform one or more essential metabolic functions, and (3) must be provided at least in part from dietary sources. Much of our present understanding of these substances results from studies of the so-called deficiency diseases. Unlike other classes of nutrients, vitamins differ widely in chemical structure and, consequently, in metabolism and function.

It is useful to classify vitamins according to their solubility in water or in fats and fat solvents. Solubility affects a number of characteristics: distribution in foods, stability, absorption, metabolism, excretion, and potential toxicity. For example, the fat-soluble vitamins (A, D, E, and K) are all absorbed into the body in similar fashion from the intestine; efficient absorption requires bile and is affected by any factor or condition that affects bile or the absorption of fats. Compared to water-soluble vitamins, fat-soluble vitamins are more readily retained in the body, and their potential toxicity is therefore greater.

Vitamin A is relatively stable and occurs in three biologically active forms—retinol, retinal, and retinoic acid. Biologically active vitamin A is found almost exclusively in animal products (as retinyl esters). All three forms, however, can be derived from carotene precursors (provitamins), which are widely distributed plant pigments.

Vitamin A is known to affect almost all tissues and to function in a great number of processes, including vision, growth of bones and teeth, maintenance of epithelial tissue, and hormone synthesis. It is readily available from many dietary sources and significant amounts are stored in the body, especially the liver. Deficiency produces night blindness, xerophthalmia, and skin keratinization; administration of the vitamin can reverse many symptoms, especially in early stages. Conditions caused by vitamin A toxicity include birth defects, especially of the central nervous system; a syndrome that mimics brain tumor; anemia; and muscle and joint pain.

Vitamin D is chemically very stable and has two primary biologically active forms. Ergocalciferol, D_2, is derived from a plant precursor (ergosterol), and cholecalciferol, D_3, is derived from 7-dehydrocholesterol, found in the skin and hair of animals. Vitamin D serves chiefly to maintain optimum blood levels of calcium and phosphorus. This function is mediated by two metabolites of the vitamin—HCC and DHCC—produced in the skin and in plants and microorganisms by sunlight; commercial preparations and fortified foods are the only reliable *dietary* sources. It is stored in the body, but to a lesser extent than vitamin A. Clinical conditions resulting from deficiency are rickets in children and osteomalacia in adults. Symptoms of hypervitaminosis D include hypercalcemia, nausea, loss of weight and appetite, and calcification of bone and soft tissues.

Vitamin E is highly stable (though readily oxidized) and occurs in four natural forms, the most common and biologically active being α-tocopherol. Despite numerous claims for the curative and health-promoting powers of vitamin E, its role in human nutrition remains unclear. Evidence suggests that it may function mainly as a protective antioxidant agent. Vitamin E is very readily available from dietary sources. The only known deficiency condition is hemolytic anemia in premature infants. In pharmacological doses the vitamin can have certain beneficial effects but may carry some risks as well. Large doses also have an anticoagulant effect; thus excessive intake could lead to hemorrhaging in certain instances.

Vitamin K is a group of relatively stable compounds belonging to the chemical family of substances called quinones. Vitamin K_1 (phylloquinone) is the only form synthesized by plants. About half the amount of vitamin K in the body is a form of K_2 (menaquinone) synthesized by intestinal bacteria. Dietary sources supply the rest. The only known function of vitamin K is as a factor essential to blood clotting. The body stores minimal amounts of the vitamin, but it is found in many animal and plant products, and the metabolic need is for very small amounts. The only known deficiency symptom is prolonged blood coagulation time leading to hemorrhage. In pharmalogical doses over extended periods, vitamin K can cause hemolytic anemia and jaundice in infants.

BIBLIOGRAPHY

American Academy of Pediatrics, Committees on Drugs and on Nutrition. The use and abuse of vitamin A. *Pediatrics* 48:655, 1971.

Corrigan, J. J., Jr., and F. I. Marcus. Coagulopathy associated with vitamin E ingestion. *Journal of the American Medical Association* 230:1300, 1974.

Dwyer, J. T., W. H. Dietz, Jr., G. Hass, and R. Suskind. Risk of nutritional rickets among vegetarian children. *American Journal of Diseases of Children* 133:134, 1979.

FAO/WHO. *Requirements of vitamin A, thiamine, riboflavin, and niacin.* Report of a joint FAO/WHO Expert Committee. FAO Nutrition Meetings Report Series No. 41. WHO Technical Report Series No. 362. Geneva, 1967.

Fine, F. D. *Federal Register* 38:27924, 1973.

Fomon, S. J., and F. G. Strauss. Nutrient deficiencies in breast-fed infants. *New England Journal of Medicine* 299:355, 1978.

Food and Nutrition Board, National Research Council. *Recommended dietary allowances*, 9th ed. Washington, D.C.: National Academy of Sciences, 1979.

Harris, P. L., M. L. Quaife, and W. J. Swanson. Vitamin E content of foods. *Journal of Nutrition* 40:367, 1950.

Hartshorn, E. A. Food and drug interactions. *Journal of the American Dietetic Association* 70:15, 1977.

Haussler, M. R., and T. A. McCain. Basic and clinical concepts related to vitamin D metabolism and action. *New England Journal of Medicine* 297:974, 1977.

Hess, A. F., M. Weinstock, and F. D. Helman. The antirachitic value of irradiated phytosterol and cholesterol. *Journal of Biological Chemistry* 63:305, 1925.

Horwitt, M. K. Vitamin E and lipid metabolism in man. *American Journal of Clinical Nutrition* 8:451, 1960.

Horwitt, M. K. Vitamin E: A reexamination. *American Journal of Clinical Nutrition* 29:569, 1976.

Hussaini, G., I. Tarwotjo, and A. Summer. Cure for night blindness. *American Journal of Clinical Nutrition* 31(9):1489, 1978.

March, D. C. *Handbook: Interactions of selected drugs with nutritional status in man.* Chicago: American Dietetic Association, 1976.

Mason, K. E. The first two decades of vitamin E. *Federation Proceedings* 36:1906, 1977.

National Dairy Council. Recent developments in vitamin D. *Dairy Council Digest* 47(3):13, 1976.

National Dairy Council. Diet-drug interactions. *Dairy Council Digest* 48(2):7, 1977.

Peck, G. L., T. G. Olsen, F. W. Yoder, J. S. Strauss, D. T. Downing, M. Pandya, D. Butkus, and J. Arnaud-Battandier. Prolonged remission of cystic and conglobate acne with 13-cis-retinoic acid. *New England Journal of Medicine* 300:329, 1979.

ROGERS, A. E., B. J. HERNDON, AND P. M. NEWBERNE. Induction by dimethylhydrazine of intestinal carcinoma in normal rats and rats fed high or low levels of vitamin A. *Cancer Research* 33:1003, 1973.

SAFFIOTTI, U., R. MONTESANA, A. R. SELLAKUMAR, AND S. A. BORG. Experimental cancer of the lung. Inhibition by vitamin A of the induction of tracheobronchial squamous metaplasia and squamous cell tumors. *Cancer* 20:857, 1967.

SMITH, F. R., AND D. S. GOODMAN. Vitamin A transport in human vitamin A toxicity. *New England Journal of Medicine* 294:805, 1976.

TAPPEL, A. L. Vitamin E. *Nutrition Today* 8(4):4, 1973.

WOLF, G. A historical note on the mode of administration of vitamin A for the cure of night blindness. *American Journal of Clinical Nutrition* 31:290, 1978.

SUGGESTED ADDITIONAL READING

American Journal of Clinical Nutrition. Symposium on drug–nutrient relationships. Vol. 26:103, 1973.

BIERI, J. G., AND R. P. EVARTS. Vitamin E adequacy in vegetable oils. *Journal of the American Dietetic Association* 66:134, 1975.

BUNNELL, R. H., J. KEATING, A. QUARESIMO, AND G. K. PARMAN. Alpha-tocopherol content of foods. *American Journal of Clinical Nutrition* 17:1, 1965.

DALE, A. E., AND M. E. LOWENBERG. Consumption of vitamin D in fortified and natural foods and in vitamin preparations. *Journal of Pediatrics* 70:952, 1967.

DAM, H. The antihaemorrhagic vitamin of the chick. *Biochemical Journal* 29:1273, 1935.

DELUCA, H. F. A new look at an old vitamin. *Nutrition Reviews* 29:179, 1971.

DRUMMOND, J. C. LIX. The nomenclature of the so-called accessory food factors (Vitamins). *Biochemical Journal* 14:660, 1920.

FOOD AND NUTRITION BOARD, DIVISION OF BIOLOGY AND AGRICULTURE, NATIONAL RESEARCH COUNCIL COMMITTEE ON NUTRITIONAL MISINFORMATION. Supplementation of human diets with vitamin E. *Nutrition Reviews Supplement,* July 1974.

FOOD AND NUTRITION BOARD, NATIONAL ACADEMY OF SCIENCES, NATIONAL RESEARCH COUNCIL COMMITTEE ON NUTRITIONAL MISINFORMATION. Hazards of overuse of vitamin D. *Nutrition Reviews* 33:61, 1975.

HATHCOCK, J. N., AND J. COON. *Nutrition and drug interrelations.* New York: Academic Press, 1978.

HERBERT, V. Letter to the editor: Vitamin E report. *Nutrition Reviews* 35:158, 1977.

HORWITT, M. K. Status of human requirements for vitamin E. *American Journal of Clinical Nutrition* 27:1182, 1974.

INSTITUTE OF FOOD TECHNOLOGISTS' EXPERT PANEL ON FOOD SAFETY AND NUTRITION AND THE COMMITTEE ON PUBLIC INFORMATION. Vitamin E. *Nutrition Reviews* 35:57, 1977.

MCCOLLUM, E. V., AND M. DAVIS. The necessity of certain lipids in the diet during growth. *Journal of Biological Chemistry* 15:167, 1913.

OSKI, F. A., AND L. A. BARNESS. Vitamin E deficiency: A previously unrecognized cause of hemolytic anemia in the premature infant. *Journal of Pediatrics* 70:211, 1967.

ROE, D. Drug-induced vitamin deficiencies. *Drug Therapy* 4:23, 1973.

SMITH, J. E., AND D. S. GOODMAN. Vitamin A metabolism and transport. In *Present knowledge in nutrition,* 4th ed., ed. D. M. Hegsted. Washington, D.C.: Nutrition Foundation, 1976.

SUTTIE, J. W. Vitamin K and prothrombin synthesis. *Nutrition Reviews* 31:105, 1973.

WALD, G. Molecular basis of visual excitation. *Scientific American* 162:230, 1968.

WEICK, M. T., SR. A history of rickets in the United States. *American Journal of Clinical Nutrition* 20:1234, 1967.

Chapter 7

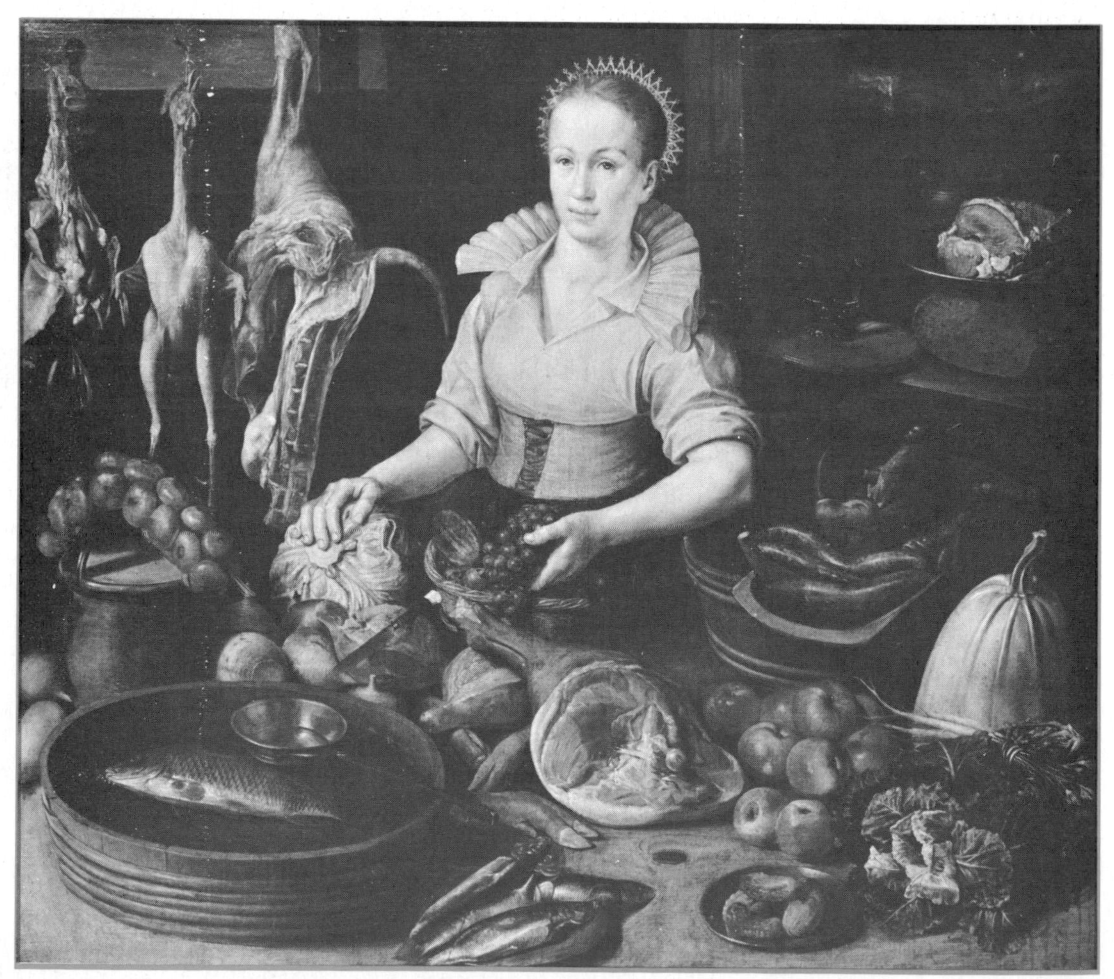

The Cook by Pieter Corneliszen Van Ryck

Water-Soluble Vitamins

In some respects, the water-soluble vitamins resemble their fat-soluble counterparts. They are organic molecules required in trace amounts by the body for specific metabolic functions, and they are classified as essential nutrients because the body cannot synthesize them in sufficient quantity and therefore must obtain them from other sources, usually dietary. But many characteristics common to the water-soluble vitamins are not shared by the fat-soluble group.

As we saw in the preceding chapter, the fat solubility of vitamins A, D, E, and K is the most important characteristic they have in common with one another. Not surprisingly, then, the water solubility of the vitamins to be discussed in this chapter is the characteristic that most clearly distinguishes them as a group. The solubility of these essential nutrients greatly influences their absorption into and storage in the body, their rate of excretion from the body, the frequency and amount of dietary intake required for nutritional health, the extent to which they are affected by food processing and preparation, and their potential toxicity.

TABLE 7-1
Classification of the Water-Soluble Vitamins

B-complex
Energy-releasing
Thiamin (B_1)
Riboflavin (B_2)
Niacin
Biotin
Pantothenic acid (B_3)
Hematopoietic
Folacin
Vitamin B_{12} (cobalamin)
Other
Vitamin B_6 (Pyridoxine)
Non-B-complex
Ascorbic Acid (C)

Another important difference between the two groups of vitamins involves their chemical composition. As we have seen, fat-soluble vitamins consist solely of carbon, hydrogen, and oxygen. Most of the water-soluble vitamins, however, contain nitrogen in addition; and several contain other elements such as sulfur, cobalt or, when changed to the physiologically active form, phosphorus. In chemical structure, however, the water-soluble vitamins differ as much from each other as they do from the fat-soluble group.

In terms of metabolic activity, the distinguishing characteristic of water-soluble vitamins (except for vitamin C) is their function as components of specific coenzymes. (Coenzymes themselves function as components of enzyme complexes essential for catalyzing many biochemical reactions.) Five of them—the so-called energy-releasing vitamins—are involved in producing energy from carbohydrate, fats, and protein. Two others—the hematopoietic vitamins—are necessary for red blood cell formation. As the classification scheme of the table at the left shows, these seven account for all but two of the water-soluble vitamins.

Vitamin B_6 has biological functions that are distinct from those specified above. In addition, all but one of the established water-soluble vitamins (vitamin C) belong to the B-complex vitamin group. This curious-looking but useful nomenclature resulted historically from the original system of naming vitamins alphabetically as they were discovered. A newly discovered vitamin was first assigned its own letter, unless it appeared to be similar in chemical structure and dietary source to one already discovered. In the latter case, the new vitamin was assigned the same letter along with a distinguishing number (e.g., B_6). When its chemical structure was determined, the vitamin was then given the appropriate chemical name. Although the chemical designation is the most acceptable identifying name, the use of letters and numbers has persisted, primarily because of their simplicity and convenience.

In the course of vitamin research, the status of some substances—the *vitaminlike factors*—has remained unclear. Moreover, certain substances, although sometimes popularly referred to as vitamins (for example, "B_{15}"), are not vitamins at all.

THIAMIN (VITAMIN B_1)

Like vitamins A and D, thiamin has an ancient medical history. Beriberi, the disease condition resulting from thiamin deficiency, was known to the Chinese as early as 2600 B.C. The name itself is a doubling of the word for

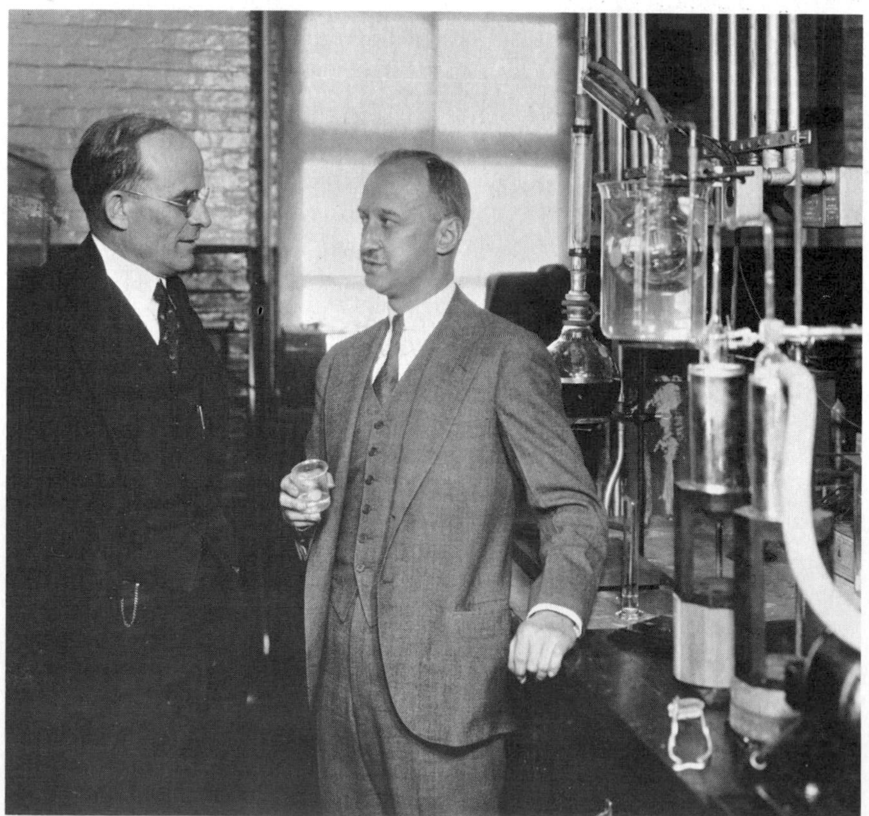

Robert R. Williams (left) and his colleague Robert E. Waterman, photographed in 1937 following the successful synthesis of thiamin. The beaker held by Waterman contains the synthesized vitamin. (Courtesy Research Corporation, New York)

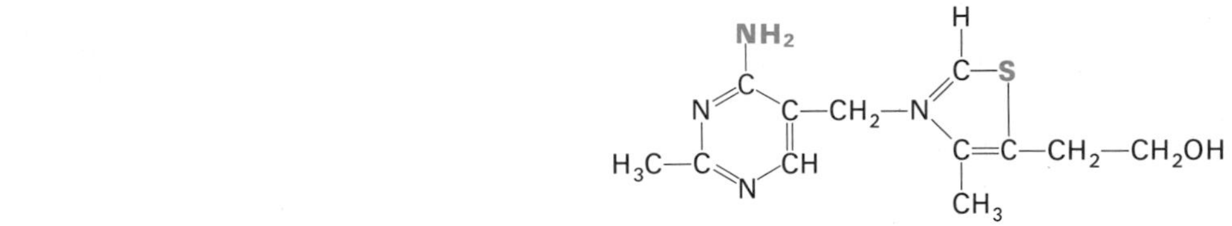

FIGURE 7-1
Structure of Thiamin

"weakness" in Sinhalese, the language of Ceylon, and aptly describes the major symptom of the disease. In 1855, a Japanese naval officer named Takaki effected one of the earliest known cures of beriberi by feeding his men a diet of milk and meat. Then, shortly before 1900, Christiaan Eijkman, a Dutch physician working in Java, recognized that chickens fed on polished rice developed the same symptoms as human victims of beriberi. (Polished rice has had the outer husk and bran removed in the process of milling.) Eijkman showed that the symptoms of chickens and humans both could be reversed by the addition of rice husks and bran to the diet. Eventually it was recognized that beriberi occurred widely among peoples whose diet consisted mainly of polished rice.

Casimir Funk was among the first to isolate the antiberiberi factor (from rice bran and yeast), and he was also the first to realize that this substance is an essential nutrient. The new factor received the designation "vitamin B," which it kept until subsequent research revealed that the substance actually consisted of several accessory food factors. Researchers therefore renamed the antiberiberi factor "vitamin B_1," as it is still commonly known. After the identification of its structure in 1926, vitamin B_1 received its modern chemical name, thiamin. (Although an "e" sometimes appears at the end of this name, the former spelling is preferred.) The first successful synthesis of the vitamin followed ten years later, in 1936.

Chemistry and Properties

It was because of the amine group in thiamin that Funk coined the term "vitamine" as a general name for accessory food factors. Thiamin also contains sulfur, hence the prefix "thi," from the Greek word for sulfur. Figure 7-1 shows the structure of thiamin. The addition of two phosphate groups produces the primary physiologically active form, thiamin pyrophosphate (TPP), as shown in Figure 7-2. This is the form in which thiamin acts as a

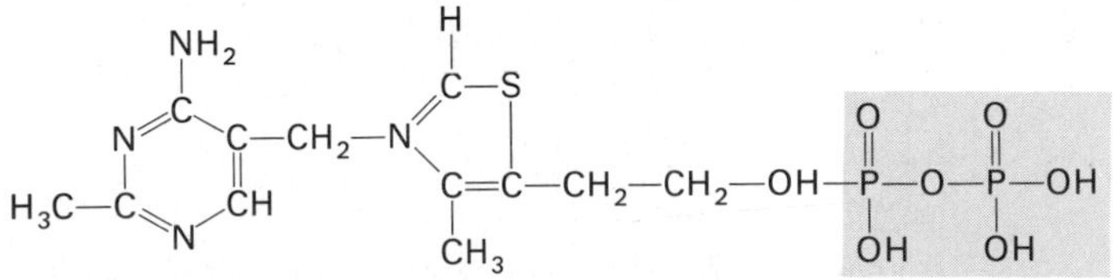

Thiamin Pyrophosphate (TPP) = Cocarboxylase

FIGURE 7-2
Structure of Thiamin Pyrophosphate

coenzyme in energy-producing reactions. Another form, thiamin triphosphate, possibly may be involved in nerve function and its absence related to certain symptoms of beriberi.

In its commercially available form, thiamin hydrocholoride, the vitamin is a pale yellow crystalline substance, resistant to oxidation and highly soluble in water. In dry form, thiamin is heat stable up to temperatures of 100°C, but in solution it becomes less stable. These properties are especially relevant to the preparation of foods containing thiamin; frying and broiling such foods or cooking them under pressure for too long will destroy the vitamin. Since water will dissolve and leach the vitamin from thiamin-containing foods, washing of such foods should be brief, and only small amounts of water should be used in cooking. Thiamin becomes somewhat more heat stable in an acidic solution, but is quite vulnerable to the presence of alkali. For this reason, baking soda (sodium bicarbonate), often added to cooking water to preserve vegetable color, will decrease thiamin activity and should not be used. Because of their alkaline content, antacids consumed in large quantities may also inactivate the vitamin. Finally, the sulfur dioxide used in processing dried fruits virtually destroys their thiamin content.

Absorption and Metabolism

Absorption of dietary thiamin takes place in the upper part of the small intestine. If present in very large amounts in the intestine, the vitamin is passively absorbed. Absorption of the usual small amounts, however, is by active transport and requires energy and sodium. Thiamin apparently is converted to its active form by the addition of phosphates in the mucosal cells of the intestine. From there, the vitamin enters the general circulation via the portal vein and the liver. Barbiturates and alcohol both decrease the absorption of thiamin from the intestine.

The body stores only small amounts of thiamin, mainly as thiamin pyrophosphate; the total reserve averages about 30 milligrams. Half of it is in muscle tissue, and the remainder is stored in the heart, liver, brain, and kidneys. Excess amounts are excreted in the urine. The use of diuretics containing mercury compounds increases urinary excretion of thiamin (as well as of other water-soluble nutrients).

Physiological Function

In its most important role, thiamin is crucial to the energy-generating reactions involving carbohydrates, fatty acids, and amino acids. It participates in these reactions in its coenzyme form, thiamin pyrophosphate (TPP), also known as cocarboxylase (see Figure 7-2). Specifically, it catalyzes the two decarboxylation reactions shown in general form here:

1. $\text{Pyruvate} \xrightarrow{\text{TPP}} \text{Acetyl CoA} + CO_2$

2. $\alpha\text{-Ketoglutarate} \xrightarrow{\text{TPP}} \text{Succinyl CoA} + CO_2$

The first reaction in effect "connects" the glycolytic to the Krebs cycle. The second reaction is part of the energy-releasing series of reactions in the Krebs cycle. Thiamin is also involved indirectly in metabolism of nucleic acids.

Altogether, thiamin participates in more than 20 different enzymatic reactions and is required for the metabolism of carbohydrates, proteins, and fats. Moreover, thiamin actually contributes to the body's supply of another B vitamin by assisting in the conversion of the amino acid tryptophan to niacin, as we shall see in our discussion of that vitamin.

It has been suggested that thiamin may play a role in nerve functioning as well, as a component of the nerve-cell membrane and in transmission of nerve impulses (Itokawa and Cooper, 1970). If true, this hypothesis could well account for the truly devastating effects that thiamin deficiency has on the nervous system. But thus far, experimental research has failed conclusively to support the hypothesis. How thiamin deficiency produces its neurological symptoms remains to be demonstrated.

Recommended Allowances and Dietary Sources

As noted above, the metabolism of carbohydrates, proteins, and fats requires thiamin. However, the actual requirements reflect the energy content of the diet and also the distribution of calories between carbohydrate, protein, and fat. A high dietary intake of carbohydrate increases the need for thiamin; protein and fat apparently require less, thus "sparing" the vitamin to some extent. The RDA for thiamin is based on several considerations, including the excretion of the vitamin and its metabolites and the effects of measured doses on clinical symptoms of deficiency.

The allowance is usually stated in proportion to energy allowance (0.5 mg/1,000 kcal). Thus, the RDAs for adult men and women are 1.4 and 1.0 milligrams per day, respectively. Additional thiamin is recommended during pregnancy and lactation. Because some evidence suggests that older people utilize thiamin less efficiently, it is recommended that they maintain an intake of not less than 1 milligram per day. Daily consumption is recommended for all ages, since excess thiamin is excreted, and the body will rapidly mobilize the small stores it has.

Thiamin occurs in a wide variety of plant and animal foods, but only a small number of these contain the vitamin in appreciable amounts (Table 7-1). Pork, legumes, wheat germ, and dried yeast are all excellent sources, but the latter two do not represent a significant part of most American diets. Because consumption of cereal grains and enriched grain products is generally substantial, these are probably the most practical daily sources. However, much of the thiamin content of cereal grains is concentrated in the outer coat of the seed (the bran) and is removed in the milling and refining process (compare, for example, the values for brown and for unenriched white rice as shown in Table 7-2). In enriched bread and similar products, the thiamin, riboflavin, niacin, and iron removed by processing are restored at a later stage of manufacture; these are good sources, because most individuals consume several slices of bread a day. Not all bread, however, is enriched. Enrichment is required only for bread intended for interstate transport. Milk and milk products contribute to daily thiamin intake too, but they are not particularly rich sources. With the exception of the citrus group, most fruits and vegetables are even less useful as major sources of this vitamin.

TABLE 7-1
Thiamin Content of Selected Foods
RDA for Adults
Men: 1.4 mg
Women: 1.0 mg

Food	Serving Size	Thiamin Content mg/serving
Yeast, dried brewer's	1 tbsp	1.25
Pork chop, lean, broiled	3 oz	0.92
Ham, baked, lean	3 oz	0.49
Bran flakes, 40%	1 c	0.41
Peanuts, roasted, salted	$\frac{1}{2}$ c	0.23
Peas, frozen, cooked	$\frac{1}{2}$ c	0.21
Liver, calf, cooked	3 oz	0.20
Asparagus, cooked	$\frac{2}{3}$ c	0.20
Soybeans, cooked	$\frac{1}{2}$ c	0.19
Oatmeal, cooked	1 c	0.19
Orange juice, frozen concentrate, diluted	6 oz	0.17
Orange	1 medium	0.13
Rice, white, enriched, cooked	$\frac{1}{2}$ c	0.12
Wheat germ, toasted	1 tbsp	0.11
Yogurt, nonfat milk	8 oz	0.11
Yogurt, low-fat, plain	8 oz	0.10
Milk, low fat, 2% solids	8 oz	0.10
Rice, brown, cooked	$\frac{1}{2}$ c	0.09
Bread, whole-wheat	1 slice	0.06–0.09
Yogurt, low-fat, flavored	8 oz	0.08
Hamburger, 21% fat, cooked	3 oz	0.07
Milk, whole	8 oz	0.07
Yogurt, whole-milk	8 oz	0.07
Banana	1 medium	0.06
Bread, white enriched	1 slice	0.06
Egg, whole	1 large	0.05
Apple	1 medium	0.05
Ice cream, 10% fat	1 c	0.05
Egg yolk	1 large	0.04
Fish (haddock, halibut)	3 oz	0.03
Chicken, light meat	3 oz	0.03
Cottage cheese, uncreamed	$\frac{1}{2}$ c	0.02
Peanut butter	1 tbsp	0.02
Rice, white, unenriched, cooked	$\frac{1}{2}$ c	0.02
Cheddar cheese	1 oz	0.01
Beer	8 oz	0.01
Cream cheese	1 tbsp	trace
Oils, butter, margarine	1 tbsp	0

Source: C. F. Adams, *Nutritive value of American foods in common units,* USDA Agriculture Handbook No. 456 (Washington, D.C.: U.S. Government Printing Office, 1975).

Clinical Symptoms of Deficiency

Beriberi, the disease caused by primary thiamin deficiency, is dangerous and, if untreated, lethal. The three known forms of beriberi—infantile, "wet," and "dry"—all involve impairment of the nervous, cardiovascular, and gastrointestinal systems. The chief biochemical feature of the disease is the accumulation of pyruvic and lactic acids, mainly in the blood and brain. There is a difference of opinion about whether thiamin deficiency alone causes neurologic damage, and some researchers believe that deficiencies of other B vitamins are involved as well. For this reason, supplementation with *all* B vitamins is advised as the best treatment of beriberi symptoms.

Infantile beriberi usually strikes nursing infants in the first six months of life. The cause is insufficient thiamin in the mother's milk, though she herself may show no clinical symptoms of beriberi. The disease has a rapid onset and a short course. Unless treatment begins promptly, the classic symptoms of labored breathing, bluish skin color (cyanosis), and rapid heartbeat are quickly followed by heart failure and death.

The major clinical symptoms of *wet beriberi* resemble those of congestive heart failure—edema, or swelling, of the legs and perhaps of the trunk and face as well, labored breathing, rapid heartbeat, and enlarged heart. Onset is gradual but the victim of wet beriberi runs the real danger of rapid deterioration and a fatal circulatory collapse.

In *dry beriberi* the edema of wet beriberi is absent, hence the name. Dry beriberi is a progressive, wasting disease in which the victim tires easily, the limbs feel heavy and weak, and the legs may develop areas of numbness and tingling sensations. There is difficulty in walking or in rising from a squatting position. If untreated, the disease will progress until the victim becomes bedridden and frequently dies of a chronic infection.

In areas of the world where people subsist on polished rice, and where enrichment is not a standard food-processing procedure, beriberi remains a problem. In the United States and Europe, however, it has been almost completely eliminated, although secondary deficiencies caused by drugs or malabsorptive disease sometimes occur. The most frequently seen form of secondary beriberi in Western countries is due to chronic alcoholism. The contributing factors include reduced intake of thiamin resulting from an inadequate diet, impaired intestinal absorption, and defective phosphorylation of thiamin after absorption. The extreme deficiency condition caused by alcoholism is known as the Wernicke-Korsakoff syndrome; unless diagnosed early and treated promptly, irreversible brain damage, usually requiring institutionalization, can occur. It is not clear to what extent the excess alcohol intake causes the symptoms and to what extent the resulting thiamin deficiency is responsible. A recent proposal suggests fortifying alcoholic beverages with thiamin as a preventive measure (Centerwall and Criqui, 1978). Such a solution raises a number of difficult and controversial questions: How much thiamin would be necessary to be effective? What form of thiamin should be used and how stable would it be in alcohol? Should alcohol be fortified with other nutrients as well? And if the proposal were implemented, would alcoholic beverages then qualify as a food? Further study is understandably required before such a suggestion is put into practice.

Toxicity

Because of thiamin's high solubility in water, large doses of the vitamin are readily excreted. Thus, there is a large margin of safety between even supplemented consumption and the amounts needed to produce toxicity. But intravenous injections of large amounts have caused sensitization reactions in some individuals.

RIBOFLAVIN (VITAMIN B_2)

During the 1920s researchers discovered that laboratory animals continued to grow, although not optimally, on diets of foods in which the antiberiberi factor had been destroyed by heat. Biochemists hypothesized the existence of a heat-stable vitamin B_2 and began to look for it. In 1933 Richard Kuhn and his colleagues finally succeeded in extracting 1 gram of a yellow crystalline substance from 5,400 liters of milk. Even earlier, in the nineteenth century, yellowish fluorescent pigments had been discovered in milk, eggs, yeast, and liver. The name *flavin*, from the Latin word for "yellow," was given to these substances. In 1932 Otto Warburg and W. Christian had found a "yellow enzyme" in yeast. It soon became apparent that the distinctively colored crystals found by Kuhn were the same as Warburg's yellow enzyme. The vitamin, which consists of a pigment, the flavin, attached to a chemical group similar to the pentose ribose, was synthesized in 1935 and named riboflavin.

Chemistry and Properties

Riboflavin (Figure 7-3) is a yellow-orange crystalline compound, slightly soluble in water. In solution it exhibits a yellow-green fluorescence. It is heat stable, acid resistant, and slow to oxidize. Because of its lower solubility in water and greater heat stability, riboflavin is less affected than thiamin by most normal cooking procedures. However, some losses do occur when vegetables are cooked for long periods of time in a large volume of water.

Riboflavin becomes unstable in alkaline solutions (caused, for example, by the addition of baking soda). Apparently vitamin B_2 in solution is destroyed by light. For this reason, foods cooked in uncovered vessels and exposed to light will lose some of their riboflavin content. Milk has a relatively high content of riboflavin, and opaque containers, such as waxed cardboard cartons, are generally used today to protect the vitamin from decomposition.

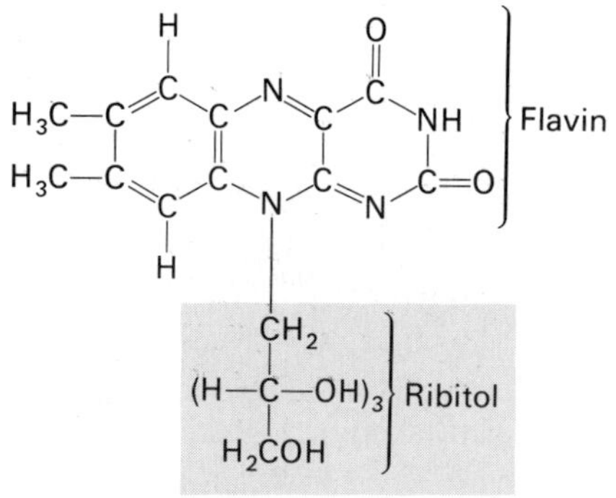

FIGURE 7-3
Structure of Riboflavin

Absorption and Metabolism

Like thiamin, riboflavin is absorbed from the small intestine, phosphorylated, and then transported to the liver via the portal vein. Absorption appears to involve a specific transport system, with albumin serving as the carrier by which riboflavin reaches the liver. Further phosphorylation of the vitamin takes place in the liver and other tissues of the body. One quite curious feature of riboflavin absorption is that, for reasons unknown, it increases with age. Ingesting a source of the vitamin as part of a meal also appears to improve absorption.

The liver, kidneys, and heart retain small reserves of riboflavin, but the total is quite small indeed, necessitating regular intake. When intake is low, however, the body's capacity for storing riboflavin appears to be greater than that for storing thiamin.

Excess riboflavin is excreted in the urine, but an even greater amount is found in the feces. Fecal riboflavin originates not from metabolized food but from bacterial synthesis of the vitamin in the intestine. Whether riboflavin of intestinal origin is absorbed and metabolized for use by the body (as is the case with vitamin K) and, if so, to what extent, is not known at present.

Riboflavin metabolism can be affected by certain drugs. For example, the antibiotic tetracycline increases urinary excretion of the vitamin. Certain types of diuretics have the same effect, as does probenecid, used in the treatment of gout. The latter drug decreases riboflavin absorption as well. Some oral contraceptives appear to lower serum levels of the vitamin but without causing any observable symptoms of deficiency. The antimicrobial sulfonamides (sulfa drugs) decrease bacterial synthesis of riboflavin, but the nutritional significance of this effect is not clear.

Physiological Function

Riboflavin, in its coenzyme form, plays a vital role in the release of energy from carbohydrates, fats, and proteins. In association with components of ATP, it enters these reactions as a component of two closely related coenzymes, *flavin mononucleotide* (FMN) (also known as riboflavin monophosphate) and *flavin adenine dinucleotide* (FAD). The structure of FAD is shown in Figure 7-4.

These coenzymes combine with various proteins to form active enzymes commonly known as flavoproteins. It is in the form of flavoproteins that riboflavin participates in the energy-producing reactions of the cell. We saw in previous chapters that the hydrogen generated (as 2H) in glycolysis and the Krebs cycle is transmitted through the electron transport system located in mitochondria, releasing H_2O and energy in the concentrated form of ATP. The flavoproteins are one of the carrier molecules to which hydrogen becomes attached as it moves through the electron transport system.

FAD has the ability to act as a carrier because it readily accepts hydrogen electrons and as readily gives them up. Thus, it exists in both reduced form ($FADH_2$) and in oxidized form (FAD). In this reaction,

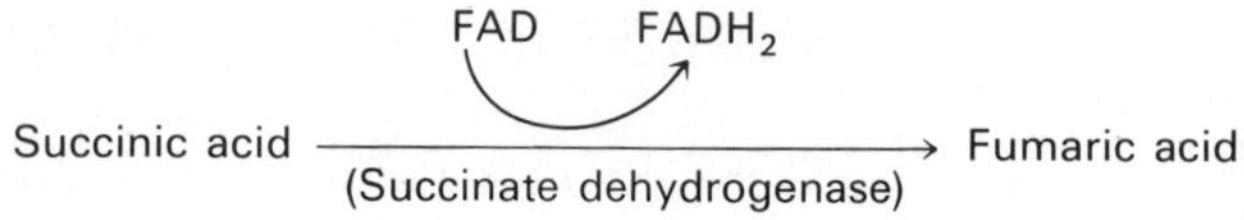

$$\text{Succinic acid} \xrightarrow[\text{(Succinate dehydrogenase)}]{\text{FAD} \curvearrowright \text{FADH}_2} \text{Fumaric acid}$$

FAD is transformed into $FADH_2$ when it accepts hydrogen atoms from succinic acid, leaving fumaric acid to serve as substrate for the next reaction.

FAD also plays a role in the complex series of reactions in which pyruvate and α-ketoglutarate are decarboxylated. In addition, this coenzyme is important for the oxidation of fatty acids and amino acids.

In the form of FMN, riboflavin is necessary for the activity of other enzymes associated with the electron transport system, cytochrome reductase and some of the amino acid oxidases. (The cytochromes, a group of iron-containing enzymes, are another important component of the electron transport system.) Thus, the flavoproteins catalyze hydrogen-transfer reactions. Riboflavin, moreover, may play a part in the synthesis of corticosteroids and in production of red blood cells.

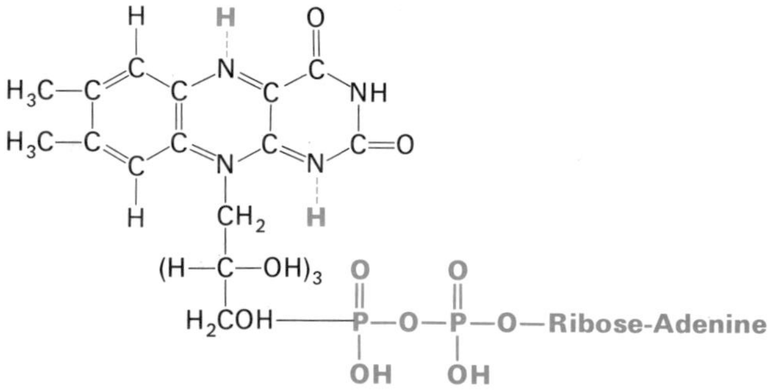

FIGURE 7-4
Structure of Flavin Adenine Dinucleotide (FAD).

Recommended Allowances and Dietary Sources

Recommended allowances for riboflavin are set at 0.6 milligrams of the vitamin per 1,000 kilocalories (4,200 kJ). Assuming an average daily intake of 2,700 kcal (11,340 kJ) for adult men and 2,000 kcal (8,400 kJ) for adult women, the recommended daily allowances are 1.6 mg and 1.2 mg respectively. Women should increase their intake to 1.5 mg/day during pregnancy and 1.7 mg/day during lactation.

Riboflavin, like thiamin, is found in many foods, but usually in relatively small amounts. A substantial part of daily intake is most likely to come from milk, milk products, organ meats, and green leafy vegetables. Consequently, vegetarians, especially those who exclude milk and milk products from their diet, can ensure adequate intake through regular use of baked products containing yeast and of green leafy vegetables and winter squash eaten in quantity. Whole grains and enriched flours and bread will increase intake also. Table 7-2 shows the riboflavin content of selected foods.

TABLE 7-2
Riboflavin Content of Selected Foods
RDA for Adults
Men: 1.6 mg
Women: 1.2 mg

Food	Serving Size	Riboflavin Content mg/serving
Liver, calf, cooked	3 oz	3.54
Yogurt, nonfat milk	8 oz	0.53
Milk, low-fat, 2% solids	8 oz	0.52
Yogurt, low-fat, plain	8 oz	0.49
Bran flakes, 40%	1 c	0.49
Milk, whole	1 c (8 oz)	0.41
Yogurt, low-fat, flavored	8 oz	0.40
Yeast, dried brewer's	1 tbsp	0.34
Yogurt, whole-milk	8 oz	0.32
Ice cream, 10% fat	1 c	0.28
Pork chop, lean, broiled	3 oz	0.27
Spinach, cooked	1 c	0.25
Asparagus, fresh, cooked	⅔ c	0.22
Ham, lean, baked	3 oz	0.20
Cottage cheese, uncreamed	½ c	0.20
Winter squash, baked	⅔ c	0.18
Hamburger, 21% fat, cooked	3 oz	0.17
Egg, whole	1 large	0.15
Broccoli, cooked	⅔ c	0.15
Cheddar cheese	1 oz	0.13
Peanuts, roasted, salted	½ c	0.10
Soybeans, cooked	½ c	0.08
Chicken, light meat	3 oz	0.08
Peas, frozen, cooked	½ c	0.07
Banana	1 medium	0.07
Egg yolk	1 large	0.07
Fish (haddock, halibut)	3 oz	0.06
Oatmeal, cooked	1 c	0.05
Wheat germ, toasted	1 tbsp	0.05
Orange	1 medium	0.05
Bread, white, enriched	1 slice	0.05
Apple, raw	1 medium	0.03
Bread, whole-wheat	1 slice	0.03
Cream cheese	1 tbsp	0.03
Rice, brown, cooked	½ c	0.02
Peanut butter	1 tbsp	0.02
Rice, white, cooked	½ c	0.01
Oils, butter, margarine	1 tbsp	0

Sources: C. F. Adams, *Nutritive value of American foods in common units*, USDA Agriculture Handbook No. 456 (Washington, D.C.: U.S. Government Printing Office, 1975); L. P. Posati and M. L. Orr, *Composition of foods—Dairy and egg products—Raw, processed, prepared*, USDA Agriculture Handbook No. 8-1 (Washington, D.C.: U.S. Government Printing Office, 1976).

Because riboflavin is only slightly soluble in water, losses of vitamin activity from cooking tend to be less than for other vitamins such as B_1, and C. But baking soda, because of its alkalinity, will destroy the vitamin. Foods with significant riboflavin content, such as milk, should be kept in opaque containers to protect against the rapid destruction of riboflavin caused by light.

Symptoms of Clinical Deficiency ("Ariboflavinosis")

Because B vitamins tend to occur as a group in foods, B vitamin deficiencies also tend to appear in association with one another. The clinical symptoms of riboflavin deficiency are much less dramatic than those of beriberi or niacin deficiency, and most of what we know about human ariboflavinosis comes from studies in which a riboflavin antagonist was administered to people. Observed symptoms include growth retardation and certain abnormalities of the eyes and mouth, particularly cracks at the corners of the mouth (cheilosis), a smooth and purplish tongue (glossitis), inflamed mouth, and dry, scaly facial skin.

Some of these symptoms may result from other deficiences of the B-complex group or even from other causes. For example, an allergy or a cold can cause cracks at the corner of the mouth. Therefore the particular symptom or condition will respond to riboflavin therapy *only if it is due to a deficiency of this vitamin.*

Toxicity

Riboflavin has no known toxic effects at any likely consumption levels.

NIACIN (NICOTINIC ACID, NICOTINAMIDE)

In 1867 a compound was obtained by chemical oxidation of nicotine and named nicotinic acid. In 1912 the same substance was identified in the antiberiberi materials extracted from rice polishings. Although Funk and others ascribed to it vitaminlike effects, the evidence to prove this ascription was not found until 1937, when Conrad Elvehjem and his colleagues found that nicotinic acid cured a condition called "blacktongue" in dogs.

The symptoms of blacktongue are similar to those of pellagra, a human disease which was widespread in Europe and the United States. It was first described in 1735 by Gaspar Casal, physician to Philip V of Spain, and one of the visible symptoms of deficiency bears Casal's name. Its appearance in Europe coincided with the introduction of corn (maize) from the New World to the countries bordering the Mediterranean where, in the form of cornmeal, it supplanted wheat as a staple foodstuff. The name *pellagra* comes from the Italian words meaning "rough skin"; dermatitis is one of the "four D's" that are characteristic of the disease. Diarrhea, dementia, and death are the others.

Until the early part of this century, pellagra was little known in the United States. But from 1910 to 1935, more than 150,000 cases were reported *annually*, mostly among the poor of the South. It was the worst nutritional disease outbreak in U.S. history. In 1914 Joseph Goldberger began a series of epidemiologic studies to determine its cause; these were to become a classic example of excellent epidemiological and clinical investigations of a nutritional disorder. By the end of 1917 he had succeeded in establishing the

Niacin (C_5H_4N—COOH) $\xrightarrow{\text{Glutamine} \rightarrow \text{Glutamic acid}}$ Nicotinamide (C_5H_4N—$CONH_2$)

FIGURE 7-5
Niacin and Its Conversion to Nicotinamide

connection between pellagra and the poor diet. About the same time, blacktongue in dogs came to be recognized as the canine form of the disease. This second discovery led to the eventual identification of nicotinic acid, or niacin, as the antipellagra (pellagra-preventive) factor.

Chemistry and Properties

Niacin is a water-soluble, white, crystalline powder with a sour taste. The vitamin is very stable under a wide variety of conditions, being resistant to the degradative effects of light, heat, oxygen, acid, and alkali. Consequently, losses that occur in cooking are due largely to its solubility in water. Niacin is readily converted to nicotinamide, the physiologically active form of the vitamin which becomes part of the coenzyme synthesized from it (see Figure 7-5).

Crystals of nicotinic acid (niacin) magnified 200 times. (Lester V. Bergman & Associates, Inc.)

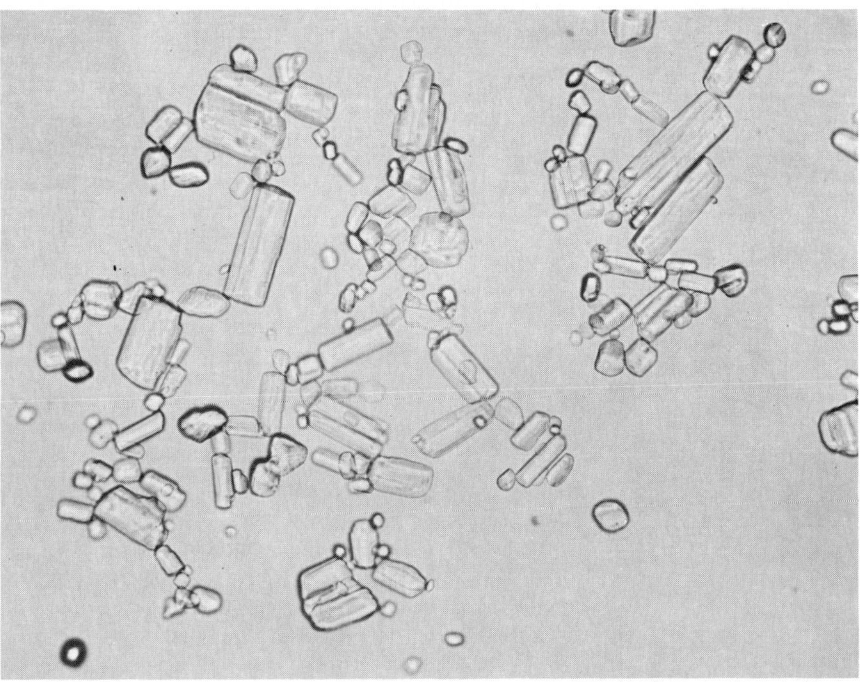

Absorption and Metabolism

Absorption of niacin into the body takes place, probably by passive diffusion, in the upper part of the small intestine. The process is both rapid and efficient. The body stores only limited amounts and excretes any excess in the urine.

Niacin is distinguished from all the other water-soluble vitamins by having a dietary precursor—the amino acid tryptophan. The oxidative conversion of tryptophan to niacin requires three other B-complex vitamins—thiamin, riboflavin, and pyridoxine (B_6). On the basis of some experimental evidence, it has been estimated that 1 milligram of niacin can by synthesized from approximately 60 milligrams of dietary trypotophan. As low as this conversion rate is (compared, for example, to that of carotene to vitamin A), the tryptophan content of foods should be considered in estimating the dietary requirement for niacin. But the estimated rate of conversion may not always be the same. For example, conversion is probably less efficient in people who consume diets low in niacin or low in tryptophan. More than a dozen metabolites of niacin have been identified.

Physiological Function

In its role in various metabolic reactions, niacin very much resembles riboflavin. First, it functions mainly as a component of two closely related coenzymes, *nicotinamide adenine dinucleotide* (NAD) and *nicotinamide adenine dinucleotide phosphate* (NADP). The structure of NADP differs from that of NAD (shown in Figure 7-6) by addition of a single phosphate group (represented in the diagram by an asterisk). As the illustration shows, NAD contains nicotinamide, adenine, ribose, and two phosphate groups. The adenine and phosphates come from ATP.

Second, NAD and NADP combine with various proteins to form a third important group of carrier enzymes involved in the energy-producing reactions of the cell. Third, like the riboflavin coenzymes, NAD and NADP exist in both oxidized and reduced forms, enabling them to act as hydrogen carriers:

$$\text{NAD(P)} \rightleftharpoons \text{NAD(P)H}$$

As such, the two coenzymes take part in many of the hydrogen-transfer reactions necessary for the oxidation of glucose, amino acids, and fats. NAD

FIGURE 7-6
Structure of NAD and NADH
* Additional phosphate group attached to ribose in NADP (see text).

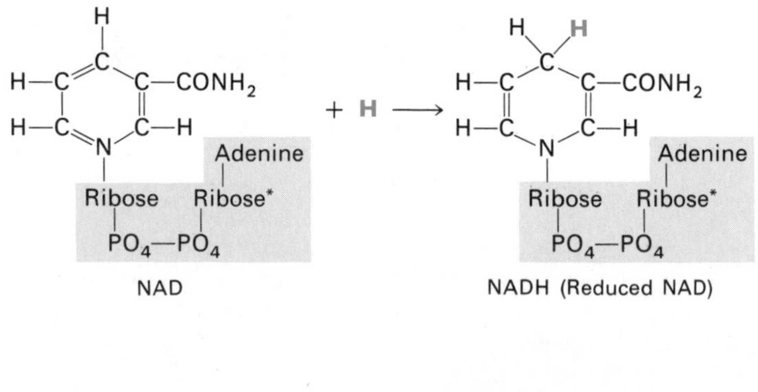

NAD + H ⟶ NADH (Reduced NAD)

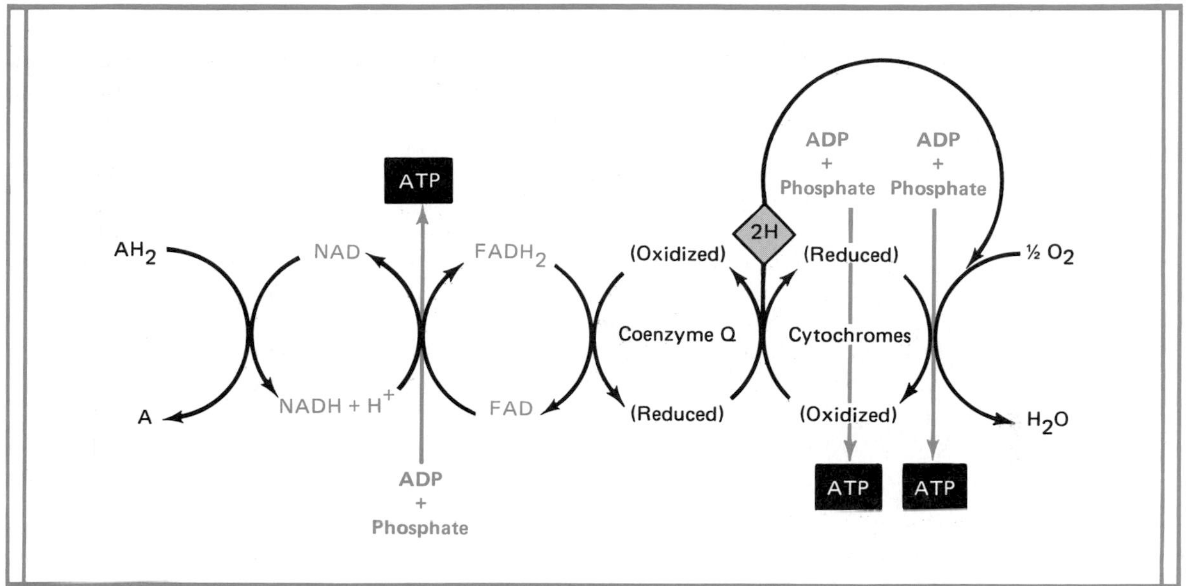

FIGURE 7-7
The Electron Transport System
Water and ATP are produced through a series of reactions located in the mitochondrial membrane. Reduced substances (AH_2) such as malate and lactate are oxidized (A), and the hydrogen atoms are transferred to NAD and/or FAD and then to Coenzyme Q (ubiquinone). Electrons are transported through a series of iron-containing proteins, the cytochromes. Finally, hydrogen ions, electrons, and oxygen combine to form water. The high-energy compound ATP is generated at three places along the electron transport chain.

appears in both glycolysis and the Krebs cycle and is important in the functioning of the electron transport system (see Figure 7-7). NADP, which is produced in the pentose pathway of carbohydrate metabolism, plays an essential role in the synthesis of fatty acids and of cholesterol. (The roles of vitamins as coenzymes in energy metabolism are diagrammed and summarized in Figure 7-18.)

Recommended Allowances and Dietary Sources

The Food and Nutrition Board has set RDAs for niacin in relation to energy intake and recommends an allowance of 6.6 milligrams of niacin per 1,000 kilocalories (4,200 kJ); the niacin RDA for adult men is, therefore, 18 mg, and for adult women 13 mg. The Food and Nutrition Board recommends also the consumption of at least 13 mg total niacin per day as a minimum, even for energy intakes below 2,000 kcal (8,400 kJ) per day. These allowances are intended to allow a substantial margin of safety. Because physiolgical requirements for niacin are increased during pregnancy and lactation, the RDAs have also been increased by 2 mg and 5 mg respectively for those situations.

The RDA is expressed as niacin equivalents because the effective niacin value of food is dependent upon its tryptophan content as well. For this reason, niacin equivalents have been defined. One niacin equivalent is equal to 1 mg of preformed niacin or 60 mg of tryptophan. Both sources should be considered when estimating niacin intake.

Meat, poultry, and fish contain more niacin than do fruits, vegetables, and grains, which in turn contain more than dairy products and eggs. It should be noted that, although niacin was first identified as a product of the oxidation of nicotine, this component of tobacco has no vitamin activity. Cooking

TABLE 7-3 Niacin Content of Selected Foods
RDA for Adults Men: 18 mg Women: 13 mg

Food	Serving Size	Tryptophan[a] Content mg	Niacin Equivalents mg	Niacin[b] Content mg	Total Niacin Content mg
Round steak	3 oz	194	3.2	5.1	8.3
Chicken	2 pieces	125	2.1	5.8	7.9
Beans, pinto	½ c	181	3.0	2.1	5.1
Milk, whole	1 c	113	1.9	0.2	2.1
Corn meal	½ c	34	0.6	1.2	1.8
Egg, whole	1 large	97	1.6	0.03	1.63
Banana	1 medium	31	0.5	0.8	1.3
Bread, white, enriched	1 slice	23	0.4	0.6	1.0
Ice cream	½ c	34	0.6	0.07	0.67
Orange	1 medium	5	0.1	0.5	0.6
Carrot, raw	1 medium	8	0.1	0.4	0.5
Green beans, canned	½ c	17	0.3	0.2	0.5

[a]From M. L. Orr and B. K. Watt, *Amino acid content of foods*, USDA Home Economics Research Report No. 4 (Washington, D.C.: U.S. Government Printing Office, 1968).
[b]From C. F. Adams *Nutritive value of American foods in common units*, USDA Agriculture Handbook No. 456 (Washington, D.C.: U.S. Government Printing Office, 1975).

methods have little effect on the content of niacin, which is quite stable, unless cooking water is drained off. Table 7-3 lists the amounts of preformed niacin available in various food products and some niacin equivalents as well. Approximately 1.4 percent of animal protein is tryptophan; vegetable protein is approximately 1.0 percent tryptophan (Orr and Watt, 1957). Thus, one cup of milk, which contains 120 mg of tryptophan, can provide 2 mg of the vitamin to the body in addition to 0.25 mg of preformed niacin. Thus, milk is a better source than its low niacin content alone would indicate. So, for the same reason, are eggs.

Many foods, particularly grains, contain niacin in chemically bound forms that the body cannot metabolize. This fact explains why even some cereal-based diets may lead to niacin deficiency and pellagra. But it does not answer the fascinating question of why pellagra has never been a serious problem in Central and South America, where corn is the staple. The answer is that the treatment of corn with lime salts (a common procedure in those areas) releases the bound forms of niacin, thereby making it available for absorption. In addition, the beans that usually constitute a large part of every meal in Latin America have significant tryptophan content.

Symptoms of Clinical Deficiency

Pellagra is the primary clinical manifestation of niacin deficiency. Specifically, it results from a prolonged diet low in both niacin and protein. Since the body can synthesize niacin from tryptophan, a pellagra-producing diet must generally be deficient or marginal in the latter as well. Goldberger noted that the diet characteristic of pellagra victims in the United States in his day consisted largely of cornmeal, fatback, and molasses (Darby et al., 1975). The disease appeared most frequently in the spring, following a lengthy period in which the diet was likely to be particularly deficient.

Because of the key role of nicotinamide in energy metabolism, niacin deficiency affects many body systems, most dramatically the skin, gastrointestinal tract, and nervous system. The symptoms are numerous, but pellagra is best known by three of the "four D's"—dermatitis, diarrhea, and dementia. Although the onset is gradual, unless the disease is treated the fourth "D"—death—will follow. The dermatitis takes the form of a symmetrical rash on exposed areas of the body. (The phrase *Casal's necklace* is often used to refer to such a collar of dermatitis around the neck.) The mouth, tongue, and intestines become inflamed. Disturbances of the nervous system can be severe, causing mental confusion, anxiety, and psychosis. Numerous mental institutions primarily for pellagra victims were established when this disease was rampant, before it was realized that the mental symptoms were due to a nutritional deficiency disease (Darby et al., 1975).

Many symptoms of pellagra resemble those resulting from thiamin and riboflavin deficiencies. In fact, recent research suggests that pellagra is a "mixed deficiency" disease, and that thiamin, riboflavin, and possibly vitamin B_6 deficiencies may contribute to its development. These three vitamins are necessary for the synthesis of niacin from tryptophan, so the lack of any of them could deprive the body of a potentially significant amount of niacin.

Diets based on millet or sorghum may produce pellagra in some instances, even though these grains contain high concentrations of available niacin as

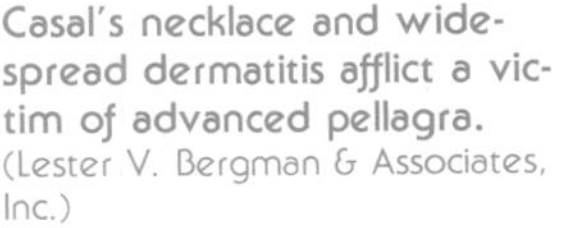

Casal's necklace and widespread dermatitis afflict a victim of advanced pellagra. (Lester V. Bergman & Associates, Inc.)

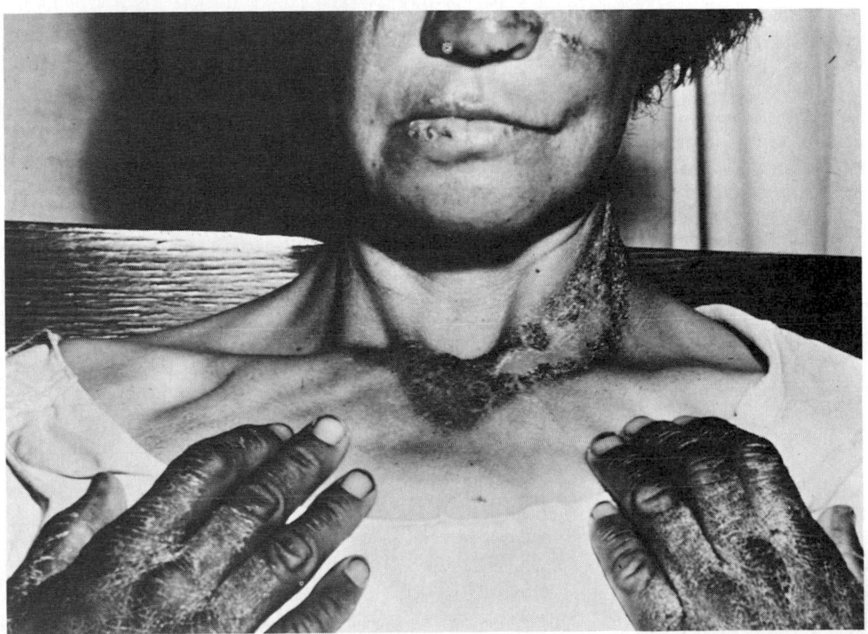

well as reasonable amounts of tryptophan. But they also contain considerable amounts of leucine, an amino acid that either interferes with the synthesis of niacin from tryptophan or alters niacin metabolism in some other, as yet unidentified way.

Secondary niacin deficiencies, due to diseases affecting ingestion, absorption, or metabolism of the vitamin, may accompany amebic dysentery, hookworm, and malaria. Cirrhosis of the liver, and therefore chronic alcoholism, can also cause secondary pellagra.

The recommended treatment for pellagra is 50 to 250 milligrams per day of nicotinamide and the other B-complex vitamins, in addition to an adequate diet. Though it still occurs in the corn-eating countries of Europe, pellagra has all but disappeared in the United States. Its disappearance was largely due to two factors: first, changes in people's economic status, and therefore diet, as the country began to recover from the agricultural and economic depression of the early 1930s; and second, a greater understanding of the vitamin and its preventive effects. For example, Figure 7-8 shows that bread enrichment, which began in 1938, further accelerated the decline in pellagra mortality.

It has only recently been pointed out that, in the period from 1920 to 1960, more than twice as many women as men succumbed to pellagra, a ratio that remained fairly constant in every year throughout this period (Miller, 1978). Is the differential due to different food habits of men and women? Do women have greater requirements for niacin? Are women more vulnerable to niacin and/or tryptophan deficiency? These questions suggest further areas for research.

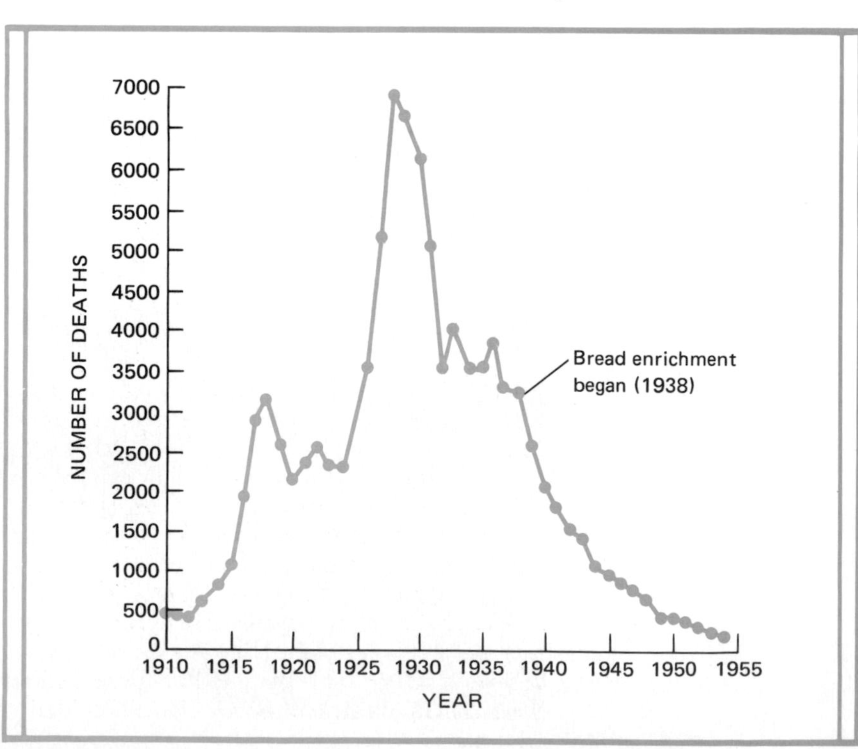

FIGURE 7-8

Deaths from Pellagra in the United States

Fatalities from pellagra began climbing during World War I, briefly stabilized in the prosperity of the early twenties, and climbed sharply as economic conditions worsened toward the end of that decade. A partial decline in fatalities followed, but not until a nationwide program of enriching bread was initiated in 1938 did mortality from pellagra begin its sharp downward plunge.

Source: National Center for Health Statistics

Toxicity

In large amounts, niacin (not nicotinamide) produces vasodilation; tingling sensations; flushed skin, especially on the face; and liver damage. For a time, pharmalogical doses of niacin (3 grams or more per day) were prescribed to lower serum cholesterol and lipoprotein levels; however, the Coronary Drug Project Research Group has stated that there is no evidence that niacin will improve the survival chances of anyone who has had a heart attack (1975). It was found that niacin may contribute slightly to preventing the recurrence of minor heart attack but that the side effects were serious enough to require great caution in its use. Among those side effects were increased likelihood of heartbeat irregularity and various gastrointestinal disorders (Coronary Project Drug Research Group, 1975).

Massive doses of niacin can cause liver toxicity and, if continued for a long period of time, may cause diabetes and activate peptic ulcers. In pharmacological amounts, then, niacin is by no means a completely harmless water-soluble vitamin.

Pharmacologic doses of niacin have also been advocated for the treatment of schizophrenia; this application will be discussed later in this chapter. However, the magnitude of the doses recommended in this context are dangerous and should not be administered without a physician's supervision.

BIOTIN

Biotin is one of the most widely available and most scientifically elusive vitamins. Before its final identification, biotin was independently "discovered" at least three times and acquired half a dozen different names! It was originally discovered in 1901 and named "Bios" for its growth-promoting properties in microorganisms. Subsequent research showed Bios to be one component of a complex of water-soluble B vitamins, from which it could be separated. In the early 1930s, Fritz Kögl began to look for a source of this growth factor, by this time called Bios II*b*. In 1936, a 16-stage extraction procedure and 550 pounds of dried duck-egg yolks yielded 1 milligram of a highly active growth factor which was given the name of biotin.

At about the same time, other researchers found a substance they called coenzyme R, which stimulated growth in some bacteria, and eventually the similarity between coenzyme R and biotin was noted. In the meantime, Margaret Boas (in 1927) and others had observed that when rats were given raw egg white as their only source of dietary protein, they developed dermatitis and bleeding skin, paralysis, weight loss, and "spectacle eye," a characteristic loss of hair around the eyes. Cooking the egg whites prevented such symptoms, but so did the addition of other foods, which were presumed to contain, variously, "protective factor X" and "vitamin H."

Eventually these lines of research converged in 1940 when Paul György demonstrated that Kögl's biotin was related to his own "vitamin H." With the identification of the vitamin's chemical structure in 1942, and its synthesis the following year, biotin was officially added to the roster of water-soluble vitamins.

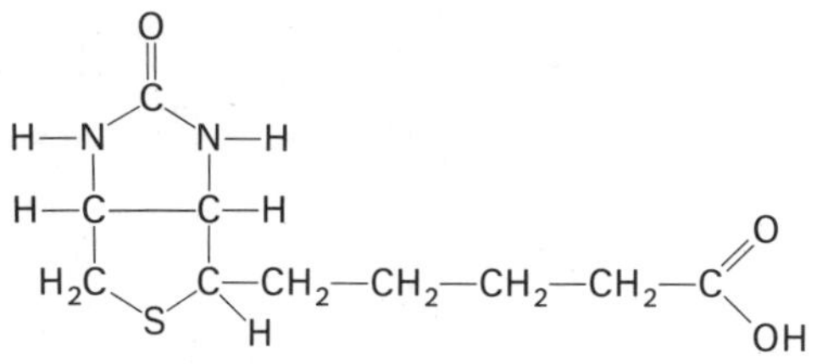

FIGURE 7-9
Structure of Biotin
* Active site, which picks up CO_2 for transfer.

Chemistry and Properties

Biotin is a white crystalline substance somewhat soluble in water but quite heat-stable. The former property leads to some loss of the vitamin during cooking, while the latter protects it during cooking, processing, and storage. The vitamin is also alcohol-soluble and vulnerable to oxidizing substances, alkalis, and strong acids. Biotin, like thiamin, contains sulfur (see Figure 7-9).

Absorption and Metabolism

As far as is known, only one substance—the protein avidin, found in raw egg whites—will interfere specifically with biotin absorption from the intestine. Avidin combines with biotin and prevents it from being absorbed. Significant amounts of biotin are synthesized by bacteria in the body, and in this form the vitamin is very likely available for absorption and use.

Biotin occurs in all the cells of the body, although in minute amounts. The liver and kidneys contain the highest concentrations. In plant and animal foods and in body tissues, the vitamin is protein-bound, in which form it serves its conenzymatic functions.

Excess biotin is excreted in the urine. Excretion of three to six times the amount of biotin ingested has been demonstrated, emphasizing that bacterial synthesis contributes large quantities to the body's available supply.

Physiological Function

One of the most active biological substances known, biotin functions as a coenzyme in a large number of important metabolic reactions. In particular, the vitamin acts as a carbon dioxide carrier in CO_2-fixation reactions (carboxylation), which lengthen carbon chains. Note, in Figure 7-9, the HN group in the biotin molecule to which CO_2 becomes temporarily attached in these reactions. Three important examples are:

1. Pyruvate $\xrightarrow{CO_2}$ Oxaloacetate
2. Acetyl CoA $\xrightarrow{CO_2}$ Malonyl CoA $\longrightarrow$ Fatty acids
3. Proprionyl CoA $\xrightarrow{CO_2}$ Methylmalonyl CoA $\longrightarrow$ Succinate

The third reaction is particularly important in the oxidation of odd-number carbon chains (such as the odd-number fatty acids). Again, look ahead to Figure 7-18 to see how these three reactions fit into the overall pattern of energy metabolism.

In addition to its established role in fatty-acid synthesis, biotin has a part in several transcarboxylation reactions of amino acid metabolism and may be involved in protein and carbohydrate metabolism. Other processes that may require biotin include antibody formation and the synthesis of pancreatic amylase.

Recommended Allowances and Dietary Sources

The Food and Nutrition Board has established no dietary allowance for biotin because there is insufficient evidence on which to base an RDA. It did, however, recommend in 1979 that the daily intake be 100–200 micrograms for adults.

Normal dietary intake is estimated to be 100 to 300 micrograms per day. This amount, plus that from bacterial synthesis, makes the possibility of deficiency so improbable that it seems not to occur, except when large quantities of raw eggs are eaten for long periods.

Milk and various milk products are among the best sources of the vitamin since one or more appear fairly frequently in most diets. See Table 7-4 for a more extensive list. The biotin content of many foods, however, has not been determined.

Symptoms of Clinical Deficiency

Natural biotin deficiency is not known to occur in humans except with excessive consumption of raw eggs. However, because major amounts of biotin are synthesized by intestinal bacteria, the use of antibiotics could affect the amounts of the vitamin available for absorption from the intestine. Oxytetracycline and the sulfonamides are both known to reduce bacterial populations that synthesize biotin. Thus some of the symptoms that appear with long-term use of these drugs may in fact be symptoms of secondary deficiency of biotin or other vitamins.

Some evidence suggests that biotin deficiency may be the actual cause of two types of dermatitis—seborrheic dermatitis and Leiner's disease. Biotin is highly effective in the treatment of both conditions in infants. In adults, however, neither condition responds to vitamin therapy. Experimentally induced deficiency in humans produces a grayish, dry, scaly skin; loss of appetite; lassitude; muscle pain; and nausea. Eating an occasional raw egg will not produce deficiency symptoms. According to one estimate, the avidin content of more than 20 raw eggs per day for several weeks would be required to create a biotin deficiency.

TABLE 7-4
Biotin Content of Selected Foods
Estimated Safe and Adequate Daily Dietary Intake 100–200 μg

Food	Serving Size	Biotin Content μg/serving
Liver, beef, fried	3 oz	82
Oatmeal, cooked	1 c	58
Soybeans, cooked	½ c	22
Clams, canned, drained	½ c	20
Egg, whole, cooked[a]	1 medium	13
Salmon, broiled or baked	3 oz	10
Milk, whole	8 oz	10
Rice, brown, cooked	½ c	9
Shrimp, cooked	3 oz	9
Chicken, fried	3 oz	9
Ice cream, 10% fat	1 c	8
Sardines, canned	2 medium	7
Milk, low-fat + 2% solids	8 oz	7
Mushrooms, canned	½ c	7
Halibut, cooked	3 oz	7
Avocado	½ medium	6
Banana	1 medium	6
Beans, white, cooked	½ c	6
Peanut butter	1 tbsp	6
Cashews	6–8	5
Milk, skim	8 oz	5
Frankfurter, cooked	2	4
Rice, white, enriched, cooked	½ c	4
Hamburger, 21% fat, cooked	3 oz	3
Cantaloupe	¼ melon	3
Orange	1 medium	3
Apple, raw	1 medium	2
Carrots, cooked	½ c	2
Cottage cheese, creamed	½ c	2
Wheat germ	1 tbsp	1.3
Cheddar cheese	1 oz	1.0
Butter	1 tsp	1
Bread, whole wheat	1 slice	0
Bread, white	1 slice	0
Oils, fats, margarine	1 tbsp	0

[a]But raw egg white consumed in quantity inhibits absorption of biotin; see text.
Source: J. A. Pennington, *Dietary nutrient guide* (Westport, Conn.: Avi Publishing Co., 1976).

Toxicity

Biotin has no known toxic effects. Animals have tolerated large doses for extended periods with no signs of toxicity.

PANTOTHENIC ACID

Like biotin, pantothenic acid first appeared in the Bios complex of vitamins and was accordingly designated vitamin B_3. Roger J. Williams, who discovered the vitamin, gave it its chemical name in 1938, from *pantos*, the Greek word meaning "everywhere." The name reflects its widespread distribution in plants and animals. Pantothenic acid was synthesized in 1940.

Chemistry and Properties

Pantothenic acid (see Figure 7-10) is a yellow oily liquid. However, calcium pantothenate, the calcium salt of pantothenic acid, is crystalline. This commercially available form is a white, alcohol- and water-soluble substance that is quite stable in neutral solution but decomposes easily in both alkaline and acid solutions. Dry heat also destroys the vitamin.

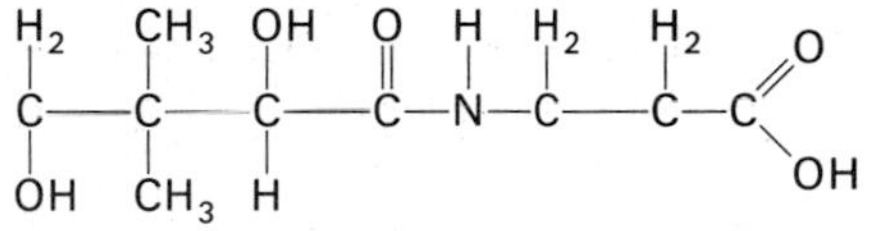

$$HO{-}CH_2{-}C(CH_3)_2{-}CH(OH){-}C(=O){-}NH{-}CH_2{-}CH_2{-}COOH$$

FIGURE 7-10

Structure of Pantothenic Acid

Absorption and Metabolism

Little is known about the absorption of pantothenic acid. Salts of the acid are probably absorbed from the intestines by passive diffusion. In the body tissues, the vitamin is converted to its important coenzyme form coenzyme A (see Figure 7-11). Pantothenic acid is also a component of acyl-carrier protein (ACP), important in fatty acid metabolism.

Limited reserves of pantothenic acid are stored in the liver, adrenal glands, brain, kidneys, and heart. Little is known about excretion of this vitamin except that it is found in urine.

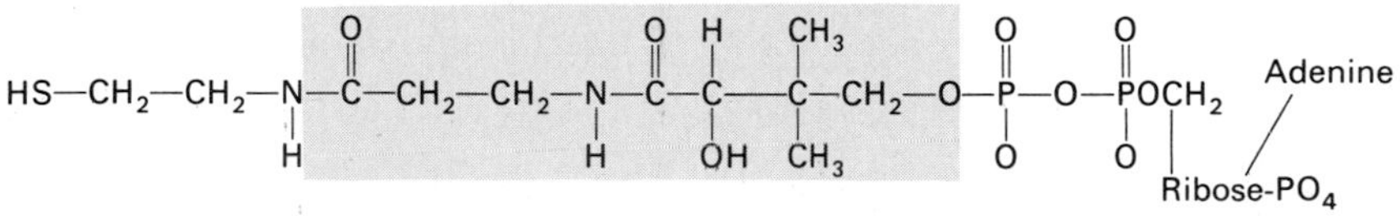

$$HS{-}CH_2{-}CH_2{-}NH{-}C(=O){-}CH_2{-}CH_2{-}NH{-}C(=O){-}CH(OH){-}C(CH_3)_2{-}CH_2{-}O{-}P(=O)(O){-}O{-}P(=O)(O){-}OCH_2{-}\text{Ribose-PO}_4{-}\text{Adenine}$$

FIGURE 7-11

Structure of Coenzyme A

Physiological Function

The great importance of pantothenic acid results from its function as a component of coenzyme A and acyl-carrier protein (ACP). The extensive functions of acetyl CoA are summarized diagrammatically in Figure 7-12. ACP transports acetyl CoA from the mitochondria to the cytoplasm and participates in all the subsequent reactions of fatty acid synthesis.

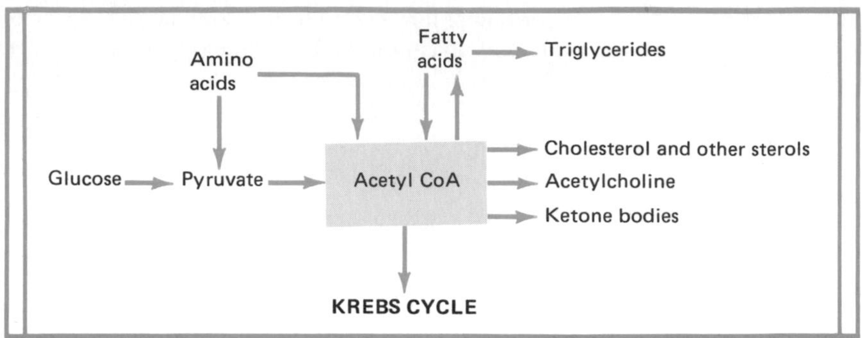

FIGURE 7-12

Sources and Functions of Acetyl CoA

Acetyl CoA, which derives from the oxidative breakdown of carbohydrate, protein, and fat, initiates the Krebs cycle by combining with oxaloacetate to form citric acid. Acetyl CoA also functions in the synthesis of fatty acids, sterols (including cholesterol), and poryphyrin, the pigment component of hemoglobin. And in the synthesis of acetylcholine, a very important neurotransmitter, the acetyl group is provided by acetyl CoA.

Recommended Allowances and Dietary Sources

Because of insufficient evidence concerning requirements for pantothenic acid, the Food and Nutrition Board simply suggests a dietary intake of 4 to 7 milligrams per day. Estimates place the average dietary intake of Americans at between 10 and 20 milligrams per day. Deficiency is most unlikely.

All foods contain pantothenic acid, although fruits contain only negligible amounts. Liver, eggs, yeast, salmon, and heart contain some of the highest concentrations; but other good sources include mushrooms, cauliflower, molasses, and peanuts (see Table 7-5). Although grains represent an important source of the vitamin, about 50 percent of their content is lost in milling.

Little pantothenic acid activity is lost in most cooking methods, but temperatures above the boiling point, as in a pressure cooker, will cause significant loss. Frozen vegetables and meats lose considerable pantothenic acid during processing and storage.

Clinical Symptoms of Deficiency

The difficulty of establishing an RDA for pantothenic acid arises chiefly from the difficulty of identifying a clinical deficiency of the vitamin in humans. No dietary deficiency is known, and artificially induced deficiencies appear to require extended consumption of a purified diet in combination with metabolic antagonists of the vitamin. The resulting symptoms include insomnia, fatigue, irritability, numbness and tingling of the hands and feet, muscle cramps, and impaired production of antibodies. Administration of the vitamin eliminates all symptoms. Because food processing can result in vitamin losses, and because clinicians generally are not looking for pantothenic acid deficiency, concern has recently arisen that "borderline" deficiencies may occur in people who do not consume diversified diets. More study is needed. Deficiency symptoms can be produced in other species; rats, for example, develop gray hair, which may account for the false claim by some vitamin advocates that pantothenic acid will prevent graying of hair in humans. Humans, however, are very different from rats in this respect, and contrary to all claims, the vitamin has not been shown to prevent gray hair in humans.

Pantothenic acid has been used successfully in some instances to treat the

TABLE 7-5
Pantothenic Acid Content of Selected Foods
Estimated Safe and Adequate Daily Dietary Intake 4–7 mg

Food	Serving Size	Pantothenic Acid Content μg/serving
Liver, beef, fried	3 oz	6,035
Egg, whole	1 medium	1,100
Avocado	½ medium	1,100
Mushrooms, canned	½ c	1,000
Milk, skim	8 oz	984
Ice cream, 10% fat	1 c	900
Chicken, fried	3 oz	765
Milk, whole	8 oz	732
Soybeans, cooked	½ c	525
Lamb leg, roasted	3 oz	510
Banana	1 medium	450
Orange, raw	1 medium	450
Pork, roasted	3 oz	425
Collard greens, cooked	½ c	425
Potato, baked	1 medium	400
Frankfurter, cooked	2 links	360
Beer, 4.5% alcohol	12 oz	360
Hamburger, 21% fat, cooked	3 oz	340
Corn, cooked	½ c	340
Broccoli, cooked	½ c	315
Cantaloupe	¼ melon	300
Rice, brown, cooked	½ c	300
Halibut, broiled	3 oz	255
Peanut butter	1 tbsp	238
Cottage cheese, creamed	½ c	228
Bread, whole wheat	1 slice	184
Tuna, canned	2 oz	180
Rice, white enriched, cooked	½ c	150
Apple	1 medium	150
Cheddar cheese	1 oz	140
Wheat germ	1 tbsp	132
Bread, white enriched	1 slice	92
Oils, butter, margarine	1 tbsp	0
Sugar	1 tbsp	0

Note: The vitamin contents in the table are given in micrograms (μg), whereas the suggested intake is 4 to 7 mg. One mg is equivalent to 1,000 μg. But note also the many different kinds of foods which contain significant amounts of pantothenic acid.
Source: J. A. Pennington, *Dietary nutrient guide* (Westport, Conn.: Avi Publishing Co., 1976).

neurologic symptoms of patients who have received streptomycin. More commonly, the vitamin is used to stimulate the gastrointestinal tract following surgery. However, doses of 10 to 20 grams will cause diarrhea.

Toxicity

No toxic effects, except for diarrhea after doses of 10 to 20 grams, are known to result from consumption of pantothenic acid in large quantities.

VITAMIN B_6 (PYRIDOXINE)

The history of vitamin B_6 has been less eventful than that of most of the vitamins. Although studies of its metabolism and interaction with regulatory systems continue, the vitamin has no classic deficiency disease, such as beriberi and pellagra, associated with it. Researchers began looking for a new vitamin when they found that none of the known B-vitamins was effective against acrodynia, a type of dermatitis in rats. In 1934 György reported that the "vitamin B_2 complex" contained a distinct chemical substance in addition to riboflavin. This substance, isolated by several laboratories in 1938 and synthesized in 1939, was a crystalline compound which was given the name pyridoxine. It also proved effective against acrodynia when added to the diets of deficient rats.

Chemistry and Properties

Vitamin B_6 is not a single substance but rather a complex of three closely related compounds (Figure 7-13). Structurally the vitamin molecule has a pyridine ring with an alcohol (pyridoxine, or pyridoxol), an aldehyde (pyridoxal), or an amine (pyridoxamine) group attached. All three forms are nutritionally active and can be converted to the active coenzyme form. Although "pyridoxine" is still used to refer to all three, the preferred designation is "vitamin B_6."

Vitamin B_6 is an odorless, white, crystalline compound, soluble in both water and alcohol. Although heat stable in acid solution, the vitamin becomes heat labile in alkaline solution. It is also relatively vulnerable to destruction by light.

FIGURE 7-13

Structure of the Three Forms of Vitamin B_6

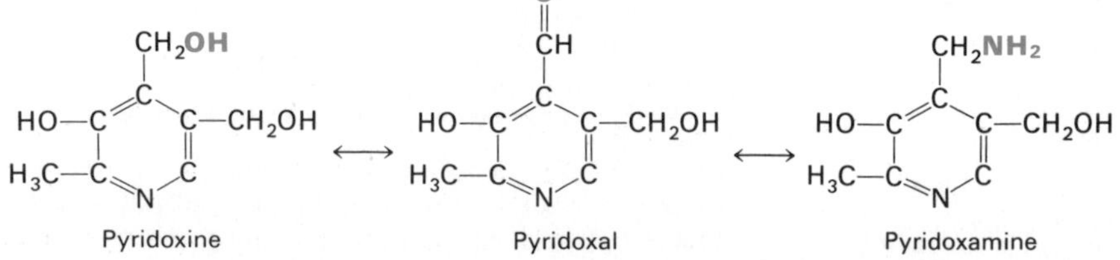

Pyridoxine ⟷ Pyridoxal ⟷ Pyridoxamine

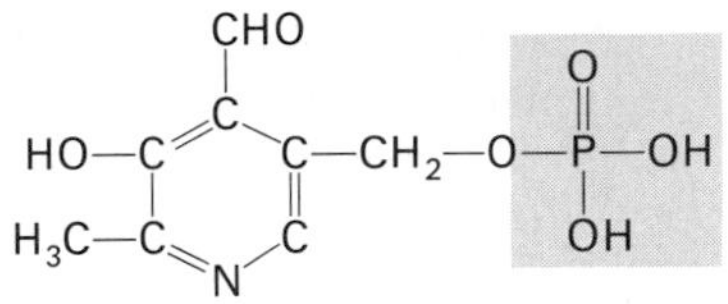

FIGURE 7-14
Structure of Pyridoxal Phosphate (PLP)

Absorption and Metabolism

Like other water-soluble vitamins, vitamin B_6 enters the body from the upper part of the small intestine. Absorption is rapid except in cases of acute infantile celiac disease (a malabsorption syndrome), chronic alcoholism (in which synthetic preparations of the vitamin appear to be more easily absorbed), and intestinal bypass operations (sometimes used as a treatment for extreme obesity).

After absorption, all three forms are converted to pyridoxal phosphate, the active coenzyme form (see Figure 7-14). Although pyridoxal phosphate is found in all the tissues of the body, there is no real storage. The vitamin is excreted in the urine, mainly as pyridoxic acid, along with small amounts of pyridoxal and pyridoxamine.

Physiological Function

Unlike the water-soluble vitamins discussed so far, vitamin B_6 has no direct role in energy metabolism. Rather it functions chiefly as a coenzyme in the synthesis and breakdown of amino acids, a role that makes it of great importance in protein metabolism. In these reactions, the coenzyme is usually pyridoxal phosphate (PLP), although pyridoxamine phosphate catalyzes certain reactions. PLP is required as a coenzyme in four amino acid-metabolizing reactions:

1. Transamination in amino acid metabolism, such as the conversion of alanine to pyruvate, the end product of glycolysis.
2. Decarboxylation, in the synthesis of neurotransmitters (such as serotonin and norepinephrine) and of histamine, which acts as a vasodilator. The latter results from the decarboxylation of the amino acid histidine.
3. Transsulfuration, of which the conversion of one amino acid, serine, to another, cysteine, is an example.
4. Side-chain transfers as in conversion of methionine to cysteine.

PLP also plays an important part in other reactions. In the release of glucose-1-phosphate from glycogen in liver and muscle tissue, PLP apparently does not act as a coenzyme; instead, PLP maintains the enzyme phosphorylase in its active form so the reaction can proceed. Here a deficiency of vitamin B_6 could result in lowered blood glucose levels. As a coenzyme, PLP also affects a reaction in which a heme precursor, necessary to the formation of hemoglobin, is produced. In addition, PLP may play a part in converting linoleic acid to arachidonic acid, although the evidence for this role is, thus far, less convincing than for other functions of the vitamin.

Another important function of PLP is to aid in the conversion of tryptophan to niacin, discussed previously (p. 268), which may explain why some of the symptoms of B_6 deficiency are similar to those of pellagra.

Recommended Allowances and Dietary Sources

Because of the association between protein metabolism and vitamin B_6, requirements for the vitamin are proportionate to protein intake. Since vitamin B_6 deficiency is not a critical health problem anywhere in the world, estimates of dietary requirements are based on data from studies of experimentally induced deficiency symptoms and from measurements of several clinical parameters. Moreover, although the vitamin occurs in a great variety of foodstuffs, albeit in small quantities, tissue levels are easily depleted by a number of physiological and pathological factors.

At present the RDA for vitamin B_6 is 2.2 milligrams per day for men and 2 milligrams per day for women. Pregnancy and lactation increase the allowances by 0.6 milligrams and 0.5 milligrams respectively. Women using oral contraceptives show abnormalities in tryptophan metabolism, a condition eliminated by large doses of the vitamin. The significance of this clinical finding, however, is controversial and unclear. Therapeutic doses have also alleviated depression in some women, probably as a result of the vitamin's role in the synthesis of the neurotransmitter serotonin. But there is no reason for women generally to supplement vitamin B_6 intake.

The RDA for infants is 0.3 to 0.6 milligrams per day. These figures are derived from studies initiated about two decades ago, when the vitamin B_6 content of a commercial infant formula was accidentally destroyed by overprocessing. The deficiency in infants fed this formula resulted in irritability and convulsions. When vitamin B_6 was administered to the affected babies, recovery was prompt.

There is evidence to suggest that the need for vitamin B_6 increases with age, but the data are insufficient to establish a firm RDA for the older age groups.

Various medical conditions and drug therapies affect vitamin B_6 metabolism and thus the requirements for the vitamin. Certain antitubercular drugs (INH) and the antibiotic chloramphenicol will bind vitamin B_6, resulting in neurological symptoms unless the vitamin is pharmacologically supplemented. Since several diuretics and hydralazine, an antihypertensive drug, increase excretion of the vitamin, supplementation may be needed in these cases as well.

Table 7-6 lists the vitamin B_6 content of selected foods. Note that the content is expressed in micrograms, although the RDA is stated in milligrams. The best dietary sources include yeast, organ and muscle meats, whole grain cereals, legumes, and bananas.

Symptoms of Clinical Deficiency

The only known disease condition attributable to vitamin B_6 deficiency is microcytic anemia, characterized by smaller than average red blood cells.

TABLE 7-6
Vitamin B_6 Content of Selected Food Items
RDA for Adults
Men 2.2 mg
Women 2.0 mg

Food	Serving Size	B_6 Content μg/serving
Liver, beef, fried	3 oz	569
Banana	1 medium	480
Avocado	½ medium	420
Hamburger, 21% fat, cooked	3 oz	391
Chicken, fried	3 oz	340
Halibut, broiled	3 oz	289
Lamb leg, roasted	3 oz	272
Corn, cooked	½ c	246
Beer, 4.5% alcohol	12 oz	216
Potato, white, baked in skin	1 medium	200
Collard greens, cooked	½ c	170
Spinach, cooked	½ c	161
Haddock, fried	3½ oz	140
Rice, brown, cooked	½ c	127
Peas, green, cooked	½ c	110
Walnuts	8-10 halves	109
Broccoli, cooked	½ c	107
Milk, whole	8 oz	98
Milk, skim + 2% solids	8 oz	98
Frankfurter	2	98
Orange, raw	1 medium	90
Cantaloupe, raw	¼ melon	90
Tomato, raw	½ medium	74
Wheat germ	1 tbsp	55
Ice cream, 10% fat	1 c	54
Egg, whole	1 medium	49
Peanut butter	1 tbsp	46
Cottage cheese, creamed	½ c	46
Apple	1 medium	45
Bread, whole wheat	1 slice	41
Grapefruit	½ medium	30
Rice, white, enriched, cooked	½ c	30
Soybeans, cooked	½ c	30
Cheddar cheese	1 oz	22
Bread, white, enriched	1 slice	9
Oils, fats, margarine, butter	1 tbsp	0

Note: Vitamin content is expressed in micrograms; recommended intakes are in milligrams.
Source: J. A. Pennington, *Dietary nutrient guide* (Westport, Conn.: Avi Publishing Co., 1976).

Associated symptoms include muscle weakness, irritability, and difficulty in walking. Because vitamin B_6 is so widely available in food sources, deficiency cannot be produced experimentally unless an antagonist such as deoxypyridoxine is administered. Induced symptoms include nausea, neuritis, dermatitis, and mouth and tongue lesions different from those caused by riboflavin or niacin deficiency. The most extreme symptoms were observed after use of the overprocessed infant formula referred to above. These involved severe convulsions, clearly demonstrating the importance of this vitamin in the functioning of the central nervous system.

There is increasing concern based on recent evidence that present-day normal American diets may be somewhat low in vitamin B_6. Although no clinical signs have been documented, biochemical evidence of borderline "deficiency" has been obtained in some studies. This points up the need for further study, appropriate food choices, and perhaps supplementation in some cases.

Because the conversion of tryptophan to niacin cannot proceed in the absence of PLP, a relative lack of vitamin B_6 may make a small contribution to a niacin deficiency and, consequently, to the development of pellagra.

Toxicity

The possibility of toxic effects from normal dietary amounts of vitamin B_6 is considered to be extremely remote. Therapeutic doses of up to 150 milligrams per day may produce slight side effects including sleepiness. At intakes of 200 mg per day, human subjects have become metabolically dependent on large intakes of the vitamin, which can result in deficiency when the large intakes are discontinued. Intakes of 300 mg or more per day do have definite toxic effects.

FOLACIN

In 1931, Dr. Lucy Wills reported finding a characteristic type of anemia in pregnant women in India. She induced the same disease in monkeys fed a diet based on polished rice and white bread and found that no known vitamin cured it. Neither did the purified liver extract used to treat pernicious anemia (see page 289). Yeast, however, which was ineffective against pernicious anemia, caused an improvement in the condition. The yeast apparently contained an antianemia factor ("Wills' Factor") that differed from the effective component of liver extract.

In 1941 a substance that promoted bacterial growth was isolated from spinach leaves and named folic acid from the Latin *folium,* "leaf." Folic acid was found to be an effective treatment for dietary anemias in laboratory animals and, in 1945, a cure for the megaloblastic anemia of pregnancy. It was synthesized in 1948.

Chemistry and Properties

Like vitamin B_6, folacin (a term that comprises folic acid and related compounds) is actually a complex of several biologically active forms. The technical name—pteroylglutamic acid (PGA)—indicates its chemical composition: pteroic acid plus one, three, or up to seven glutamate molecules. Figure 7-15 shows the monoglutamate form, which is used in food supplements and therapy. The para-aminobenzoic acid (PABA) portion of pteroic acid was formerly thought to be a vitamin for humans, but we now recognize that PABA cannot be utilized by humans.

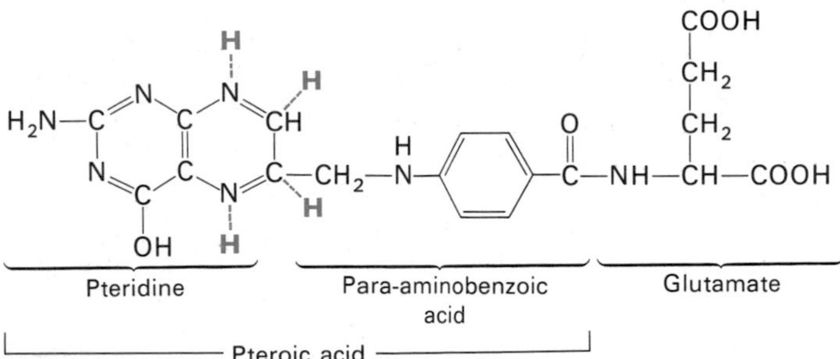

FIGURE 7-15
Structure of Folic Acid, Monoglutamate Form
In tetrahydrofolic acid (THFA), hydrogen ions are added as indicated.

Folacin compounds are water-soluble, yellow, and crystalline. The monoglutamate form is very heat stable, but the vitamin becomes heat labile in acid solution. When dry, folacin is easily destroyed by sunlight. Storage and high-temperature processing cause considerable loss of vitamin activity.

Absorption and Metabolism

Folacin is absorbed by mucosal cells in the upper part of the small intestine. But the vitamin must first be prepared for absorption by removal, with the aid of the hydrolytic enzyme folate conjugase, of most of its glutamate molecules. For this reason, the rate of absorption may vary inversely with the number of glutamates attached; studies are being conducted to determine the extent to which glutamate chain length affects the digestion and therefore the availability of the vitamin.

Once absorbed, folacin is bound to a protein for transport and storage. This form, probably methylated, occurs in all cells, but the liver contains approximately half the body's stores. Small amounts of at least one metabolite are excreted in the urine.

Several pharmaceutical compounds affect the metabolism of folacin. The antitubercular drugs aminosalicylic acid and cycloserine, certain anticonvulsants, and alcohol reduce absorption. (Chronic alcoholics, in fact, cannot absorb the common dietary forms; synthetic preparations, however, are better absorbed.) Trimethoprim and pyrimethamine, both antimalarial drugs, inactivate the vitamin, as does methotrexate, a strong folic acid antagonist used in cancer chemotherapy. Also, oral contraceptives and the hormonal changes of pregnancy produce significant decreases in serum levels of folic acid.

Physiological Function

In its principal role, folic acid is a coenzyme necessary for transferring single carbon units (such as formyl and methyl) during various reactions involved in metabolism of certain amino acids and in the synthesis of the nucleotide bases of nucleic acids (see Chapter 4). Folic acid is, first, reduced to tetrahydrofolic acid (THFA) in a reaction that requires the presence of the niacin-containing coenzyme NADPH. A 1-carbon fragment is then added to one or two of the nitrogen molecules of pteroic acid, and in this methylated form folacin participates in metabolic reactions.

While THFA is needed for synthesis of all the nucleotides, it is particularly important in the formation of thymine which is, as we saw in Chapter 4, a distinctive component of DNA. Without THFA, thymine cannot be synthesized; and without thymine, DNA synthesis and red blood cell formation is impaired. This appears to be the ultimate cause of the megaloblastic anemia observed in folic acid deficiency.

THFA also plays a part in several interconversions of histidine to glutamic acid. This reaction forms the basis of a widely used bioassay of serum levels of folic acid.

Recommended Allowances and Dietary Sources

The RDA for folacin is 400 micrograms (μg) per day for adults. During pregnancy and lactation the allowance should be increased to 800 μg and 500 μg, respectively, in view of the importance of folic acid to nucleic acid synthesis, and therefore cell division. The allowance for infants, 30–45 μg per day, is easily supplied in most cases from human or cow's milk. (Goat's milk, however, is not a good source.)

Folacin occurs in most green vegetables and in a wide variety of foods, including liver, fish, poultry, most meats, and legumes. Unfortunately, there are discrepancies in the published values of the folacin content of foods, due to the different assay methods used. Ideally, data for content of both the free (monoglutamate form) and the total or polyglutamate forms should be reported, because the extent to which the body utilizes polyglutamate forms remains unknown. Perloff and Butrum (1977) have recently published both free and total folacin values for several hundred food items; some of their data appears in Table 7-7.

In its monoglutamate form, folic acid is very stable to heat. The heat stability of other forms varies considerably, however. Moreover, all forms appear to be somewhat more vulnerable to degradation by microwave cooking than by conventional methods.

Symptoms of Clinical Deficiency

Megaloblastic anemia represents the chief disease condition caused by folacin deficiency. Other symptoms include disturbances of the gastrointestinal tract, lesions of the tongue, and retarded growth.

It is interesting to compare the types of anemia produced by deficiencies of vitamin B_6 and folic acid, as diagrammed in Figure 7-16. A lack of folic acid, of course, interferes with DNA synthesis and therefore cell division, resulting in enlarged but undivided red blood cell precursors. Hence the term *hematopoeitic*, or "blood-forming," for this vitamin. By contrast, deficiency of vitamin B_6 (and/or iron; see Chapter 8) tends to inhibit the maturation of cells and may result in *microcytic* (small-cell) anemia.

Because folic acid metabolism occurs in close association with vitamin B_{12} (see below), some of the same symptoms appear in the absence of either of

TABLE 7-7

Folacin Content of Selected Foods

RDA for Adults 400 μg

Food	Serving Size	Folacin Content μg/serving	
		Free Folacin	*Total Folacin*
Yeast, brewer's	1 tbsp	14	313
Liver, beef, cooked	3 oz	—[a]	123
Spinach, raw	1 c	65	106
Orange juice, fresh or frozen, reconstituted	6 oz	63	102
Lettuce, romaine	1 c	33	98
Spinach, cooked	½ c	54	82
Beets, cooked	½ c	32	66
Orange, raw	1 medium	45	65
Avocado, raw	½ medium	36	59
Broccoli, cooked	½ c	21	44
Beans, red, cooked	½ c	—	34
Banana	1 medium	26	33
Egg, whole, raw	1 medium	20	29
Cottage cheese	1 c	—	29
Brussels sprouts	½ c	4	28
Yogurt	1 c	—	27
Tomato, raw	½ medium	14	26
Egg yolk, raw	1 medium	18	23
Wheat germ	1 tbsp	15	20
Lettuce, head or leaf	1 c	19	20
Bread, whole-wheat	1 slice	8	16
Shredded wheat	1 oz	3	14
Almonds, shelled	approx. 11	5	13
Peanut butter	1 tbsp	3	13
Apple	1 medium	5	13
Tuna fish, canned	3 oz	7	13
Milk, whole	1 c	12	12
Bread, white	1 slice	3	10
Cucumber, pared	½ small	8	10
Ham, smoked	3 oz	—	9
Mushrooms, raw	½ c	7	8
Sesame seeds	1 tbsp	4	8
Haddock, frozen	3 oz	3	8
Chicken, without skin, dark meat, cooked	3 oz	—	6
Egg white, raw	1 medium	1	5
Cheddar cheese	1 oz	<0.5	5
Pork, cooked	3 oz	—	4
Beef, ground, cooked	3 oz	—	3
Chicken, without skin, light meat, cooked	3 oz	—	3
Cornflakes	1 oz	3	3
Apricots, dried	5 halves	2	2.5
Butter or margarine	1 tbsp	<0.5	<0.5

[a]Dash indicates value not available.

Source: Adapted from B. P. Perloff and R. R. Butrum, Folacin in selected foods, *Journal of the American Dietetic Association* 70:161, 1977.

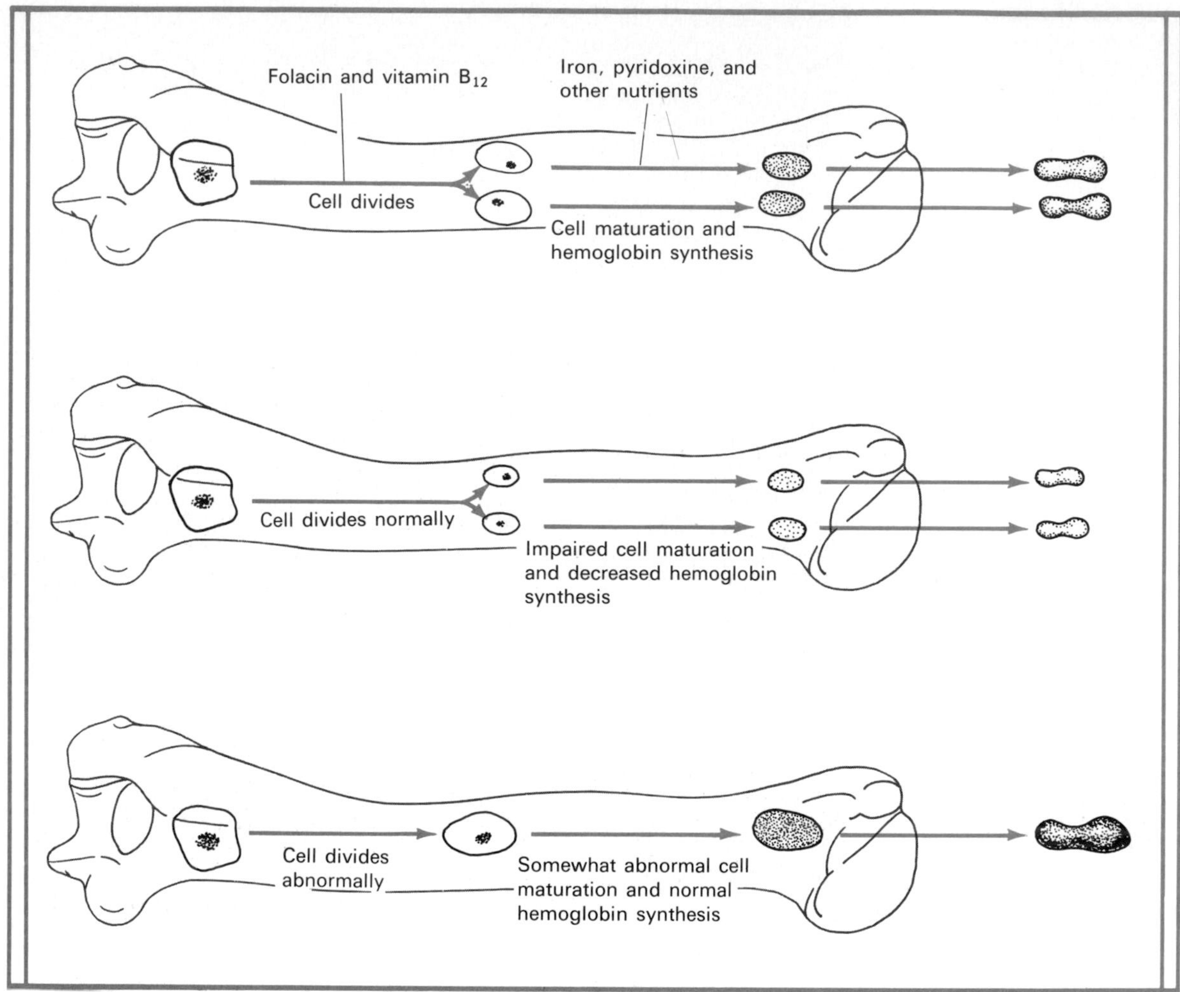

FIGURE 7-16
Normal and Abnormal Red Blood Cell Development
Top: Production of normal red blood cells. Center: Production of abnormally small and lightly colored red blood cells in iron and pyridoxine deficiency. Bottom: Production of abnormally large red blood cells in folacin or vitamin B_{12} deficiency, resulting from defective cell division.

these vitamins. Folacin will cure the symptoms of anemia resulting from vitamin B_{12} deficiency, but it is ineffective against the more serious neurological symptoms. Thus a potentially lethal B_{12} deficiency could be temporarily masked by folic acid supplementation, and therefore large supplements of folacin should not be used unless the possibility of vitamin B_{12} deficiency has been ruled out.

Toxicity

To date, no toxic effects are known. However, folacin excess may interfere with the effectiveness of anticonvulsant drugs.

VITAMIN B_{12} (COBALAMIN)

A form of anemia whose victims, usually older adults, invariably died within two to five years after becoming ill was identified in London in the middle of the nineteenth century and called pernicious anemia for its inexorable and ultimately fatal progress. In 1926 in Boston, G. R. Minot and W. P. Murphy showed that ingestion of one pound of raw liver daily cured pernicious anemia, and William B. Castle observed that anemia patients had abnormal gastric secretions. Postulating that an *intrinsic factor* (in gastric secretions) was needed for absorption of an unknown *extrinsic factor* (from food), Castle theorized that the pernicious anemia victims lacked intrinsic factor, and that a combination of extrinsic and intrinsic factors prevented the disease. When it was found that the common microorganism *Lactobacillus lactis* needed the antianemia (extrinsic) factor as much as humans did, the search for the unknown substance was greatly facilitated. A protein-free liver extract proved to be even more active in preventing the disease than liver itself, and in 1948 vitamin B_{12} was isolated (independently in both England and the United States) from liver extract. Dorothy Hodgkin determined the structure in 1956. The vitamin was not synthesized until 1973.

Chemistry and Properties

Vitamin B_{12} is a large, complex molecule that contains cobalt. Figure 7-17 shows the chemical structure of one of the naturally occurring forms, hydroxycobalamin. The vitamin takes several other forms in serum and tissues. One of the most potent biological compounds to be found in the body, cobalamin is a water- and alcohol-soluble, reddish crystalline substance. Vitamin B_{12} is stable to heat but vulnerable to strong acids, alkalis, and light.

Absorption and Metabolism

The absorption of vitamin B_{12} requires both calcium and Castle's intrinsic factor, which turned out to be a large glycoprotein secreted by the stomach wall. Intrinsic factor first combines with dietary B_{12} in the stomach and then apparently helps to attach the vitamin to receptors in the lower ileum.

Once absorbed into the mucosal lining, B_{12} is carried by a transport protein (transcobalamin) through the general circulation to the tissues. It is stored in the liver in amounts that are substantial by comparison to the quantities actually needed by the body, and in this respect differs from all other water-soluble vitamins. Cobalamin that exceeds the storage capacity is excreted in the urine.

In large concentrated doses, small but significant amounts of vitamin B_{12} are absorbed by passive diffusion (which does not require intrinsic factor). Even such small amounts—1 to 3 percent—of a large dose of such a potent compound would account for the success of Minot's and Murphy's raw liver treatment for pernicious anemia.

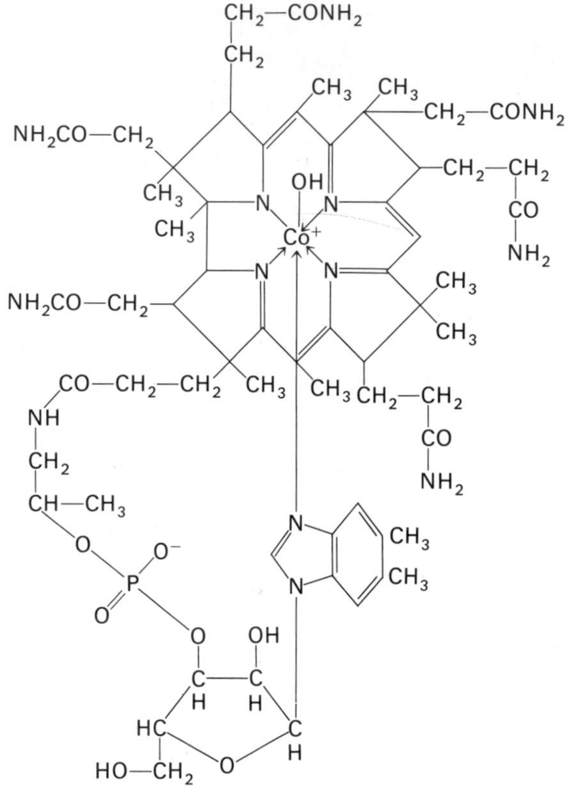

FIGURE 7-17
Structure of Vitamin B_{12} (Hydroxycobalamin)
The arrows indicate electrical force.

Iron and vitamin B_6 deficiencies, inherited deficiency of intrinsic factor, gastritis, and, apparently, age, all decrease the absorption of B_{12}. Pregnancy increases absorption but also increases the need for the vitamin.

Physiological Function

In its adenosyl or methyl forms, vitamin B_{12} is an essential coenzyme involved in reactions in all cells of the body. Along with folic acid, it is necessary for the formation of the thymine nucleotides of DNA. A lack of either of these vitamins results in megaloblastosis, or the development of red blood cells that are enlarged because normal cell division has not taken place.

Vitamin B_{12} also affects nervous system functioning, in part because it stabilizes glutathione, a component of several enzymes needed for carbohydrate metabolism. An absence of vitamin B_{12} would, therefore, interfere with the energy supply that fuels nerve cells. But this vitamin is also necessary for the formation and maintenance of myelin, the protective sheathing around the axons of nerve cells. In its adenosyl coenzyme form, vitamin B_{12} functions in the metabolism of odd-numbered fatty acids, which are important in myelin formation. This reaction also requires biotin. And the metabolism of single-carbon units (as in the conversion of homocysteine to methionine) is likewise dependent on a coenzyme of vitamin B_{12}.

Recommended Allowances and Dietary Sources

Although vitamin B_{12} is needed for such major reactions, human requirements are very small. The RDA of 3 μg (micrograms) for adults, and 4 μg for pregnant or lactating women, is more than adequately met by most diets in the United States, which contain anywhere from 7 to 30 μg. A dietary intake of 15 μg per day is recommended for those whose liver stores are depleted by illness (fever or hyperthyroidism, for example).

The best sources of vitamin B_{12} include beef and other liver, seafood, meat, eggs, and milk (see Table 7-8). Vitamin B_{12} is not synthesized by plants or animals. It is therefore available primarily in foods of animal origin because these have accumulated it from the microorganisms that make it. This raises

TABLE 7-8
Vitamin B_{12} Content of Selected Foods
RDA for Adults
3 μg

Food	Serving Size	B_{12} Content μg/serving
Liver, beef, fried	3 oz	68
Clams, canned	½ c	19.1
Oysters, canned	3½ oz	18.0
Sauerkraut, canned	½ c	16
Peas, frozen, cooked	½ c	11
Pineapple, canned	½ c	9
Peach, raw	1 medium	7
Carrots, cooked	½ c	5
Cucumber, raw, pared	¼ small	4
Celery, raw	1 stalk	4
Lamb leg, roasted	3 oz	2.63
Tuna, canned	2 oz	1.32
Frankfurter	2	1.16
Yogurt, fruit-flavored, low-fat	8 oz	1.060
Milk, skim + milk solids	8 oz	0.946
Milk, whole	8 oz	0.871
Egg, whole	1 large	0.773
Cottage cheese, creamed	½ c	0.704
Halibut, broiled	3 oz	0.85
Hamburger, 21% fat, cooked	3 oz	0.76
Pork, roasted	3 oz	0.42
Chicken, fried	3 oz	0.36
Ice cream, 10% fat	½ c	0.31
Cheddar cheese	1 oz	0.234
Bacon	2 slices	0.11
Butter	1 tbsp	0.01
Fruits	—	0
Vegetables	—	0
Grains, cereals	—	0
Nuts, legumes, seeds	—	0
Oils, margarine	—	0

Sources: J. A. Pennington, *Dietary nutrient guide* (Westport, Conn.: Avi Publishing Co., 1976), and L. P. Posati, and M. L. Orr, *Composition of foods—Dairy and egg products—Raw, processed, prepared,* USDA Agriculture Handbook No. 8-1 (Washington, D.C.: U.S. Government Printing Office, 1976).

some interesting and controversial questions pertaining to vegetarian diets.

Vegetarian diets that include milk and eggs provide an adequate source of vitamin B_{12}. But vegans, vegetarians who exclude all animal products from their diet, are ultimately at considerable risk. In several studies of vegans, serum levels of B_{12} in about half the cases measured were in the low range characteristic of pernicious anemia. Some illness and at least two deaths have been attributed to B_{12} deficiency (Smith, 1965). Yet a number of subjects tested appeared to be quite healthy despite having eaten plant foods exclusively for years. Extensive previous storage in the liver probably accounts for this; furthermore, over time the body may adapt to the miniscule amounts that might be present in plant foods due to bacterial content of soils and water.

It has been proposed that in some foods, such as groundnuts (peanuts) and perhaps other nuts and legumes, bacterial fermentation may produce the vitamin (Smith, 1965). *Trace* amounts may be present in plants grown in very rich soil: The presence of large amounts of bacteria in the soil may enable some plants to absorb small amounts of vitamin B_{12}. Another explanation for the lack of deficiency in many vegans has been refuted; although bacteria in the human intestine can indeed synthesize B_{12}, the vitamin is not absorbed that far down the intestine.

Interestingly, most vegetarians in India do use some animal products, particularly yogurt, and may in that way receive adequate amounts of B_{12}. Tofu (soybean curd), a fermented legume product, may serve the same function for vegetarians in China and Japan.

A different controversy has arisen over a report claiming that high intake of vitamin C destroys B_{12} (Herbert and Jacob, 1974). A report refuting this claim has also appeared (Newmark et al., 1976). Differences in methods of measuring B_{12} content may account for these discrepancies.

Symptoms of Clinical Deficiency

Blood and nervous system disorders are the primary symptoms of B_{12} deficiency. The characteristic blood defect is megaloblastic anemia, or presence of large (but fewer) red blood cells. This symptom can also result from folic acid deficiency. The nervous disorders associated with vitamin B_{12} deficiency are due both to defective synthesis of myelin and disrupted metabolism of fatty acids.

Pernicious anemia, on the other hand, is due not to a primary vitamin B_{12} deficiency, but to a lack of intrinsic factor necessary for absorption of the vitamin. It can be cured, however, by massive doses of vitamin B_{12} without intrinsic factor. This disease may be caused by an inborn error of metabolism and also is often a result of aging. Various malabsorptive conditions (Carmel, 1978) and surgical removal of the ileum will also prevent normal vitamin B_{12} absorption. In some areas of the world, a particular species of tapeworm found in fish has the ability to break down the B_{12}-intrinsic factor complex, thereby creating a deficiency. Daily injections of small doses (1 μg) or monthly injections of larger doses of vitamin B_{12} are often used to prevent the onset of pernicious anemia in these cases.

In recent years nutritionists have become increasingly concerned about the

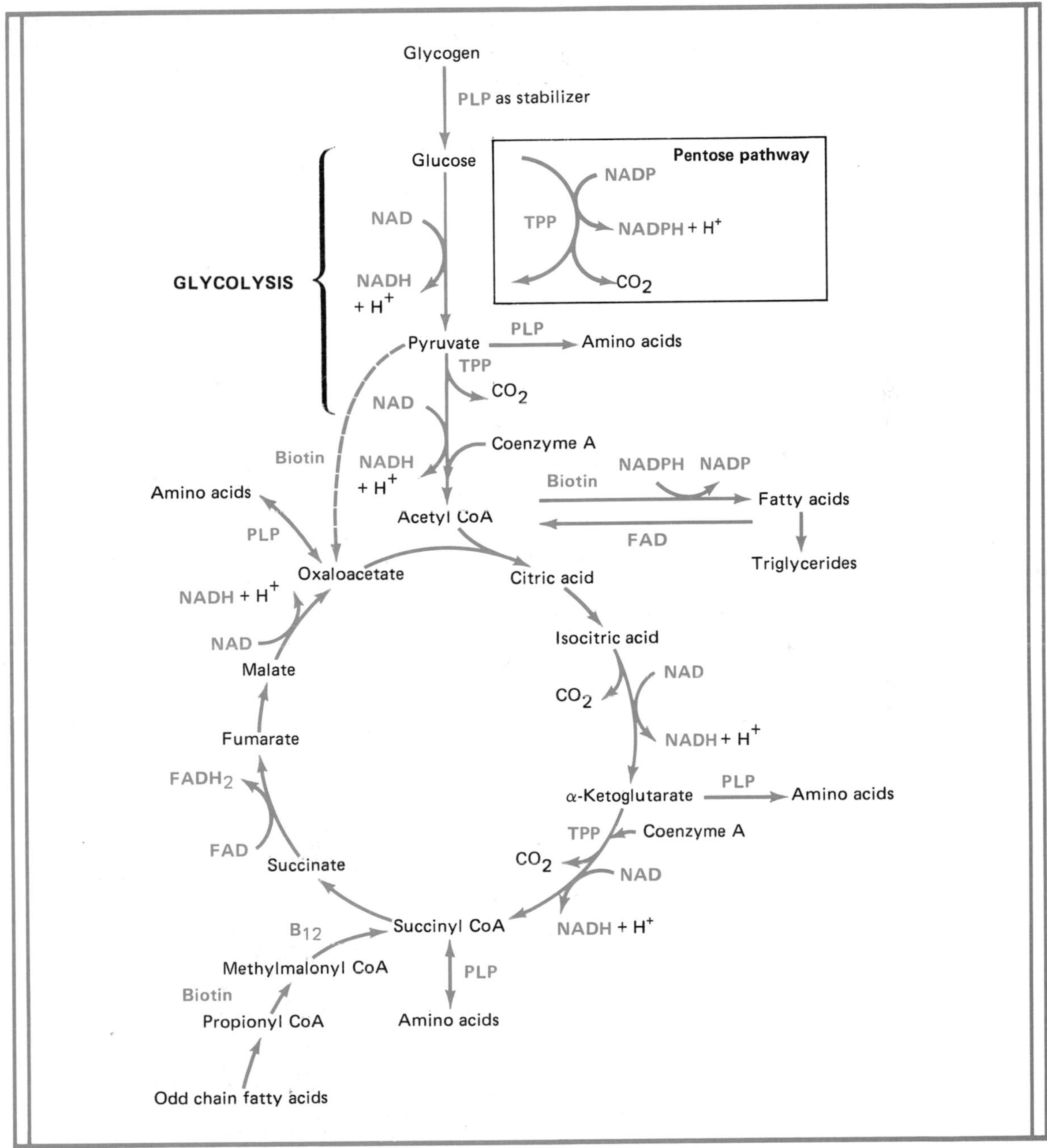

FIGURE 7-18
Summary of Coenzyme Functions of the B Vitamins

Key:
NAD contains Niacin
FAD contains Riboflavin
PLP contains Pyridoxine
TPP contains Thiamin
CoA contains Pantothenic acid

effects on B_{12} status of strict vegetarian diets. The average adult has a five-to-six-year supply stored in the liver, but children eating vegetarian diets and not having accumulated such stores run a greater risk of deficiency. Even more disturbing is the potential risk to infants who are nursed by strict vegetarian mothers. The mother's milk may contain very little vitamin B_{12}, and the infant will have little stored in the liver. At least two cases of severe B_{12} deficiency in infants have recently been reported in the United States, and more are anticipated (Higginbottom et al., 1978; Frader et al., 1978). Typically, the mother has been a vegan for several years before becoming pregnant. Her child, fed exclusively on breast milk, seems normal for several months, but then begins to lose control of head and body movements and becomes lethargic. By six months of age, weight is lost, the infant can no longer sit up unaided, and clinical symptoms include megaloblastic anemia and even coma. Fortunately, response to vitamin B_{12} therapy is rapid.

Strangely, the mothers in these cases showed only marginal deficiency of the vitamin, emphasizing the role of body storage in adults, and therefore the greater need of infants and young children eating vegetarian foods. Vegetarian diets for children should include milk and/or eggs; otherwise, supplementation with a vitamin preparation containing cobalamin is essential. Pregnant and lactating women who are vegetarians should also receive supplementary vitamin B_{12}.

Toxicity

Vitamin B_{12}, like folic acid, is not known to have any toxic effects at any reasonable intake levels.

SUMMARY OF B VITAMINS

These water-soluble vitamins play important roles in the metabolism of carbohydrates, proteins, and lipids and cannot be studied apart from the macronutrients. Because of their coenzyme functions, it is possible to identify the precise reactions in metabolic pathways in which the B vitamins participate. These are shown in Figure 7-18.

ASCORBIC ACID (VITAMIN C)

Scurvy, described as early as 1500 B.C. and much later identified as ascorbic acid deficiency, is one of the oldest known vitamin deficiency diseases. In our own day, ascorbic acid is probably the most familiar and the most controversial of the vitamins.

The story of how Lind, a surgeon with the British navy, first demonstrated a cure for scurvy—and whose prescribed treatment was responsible for British

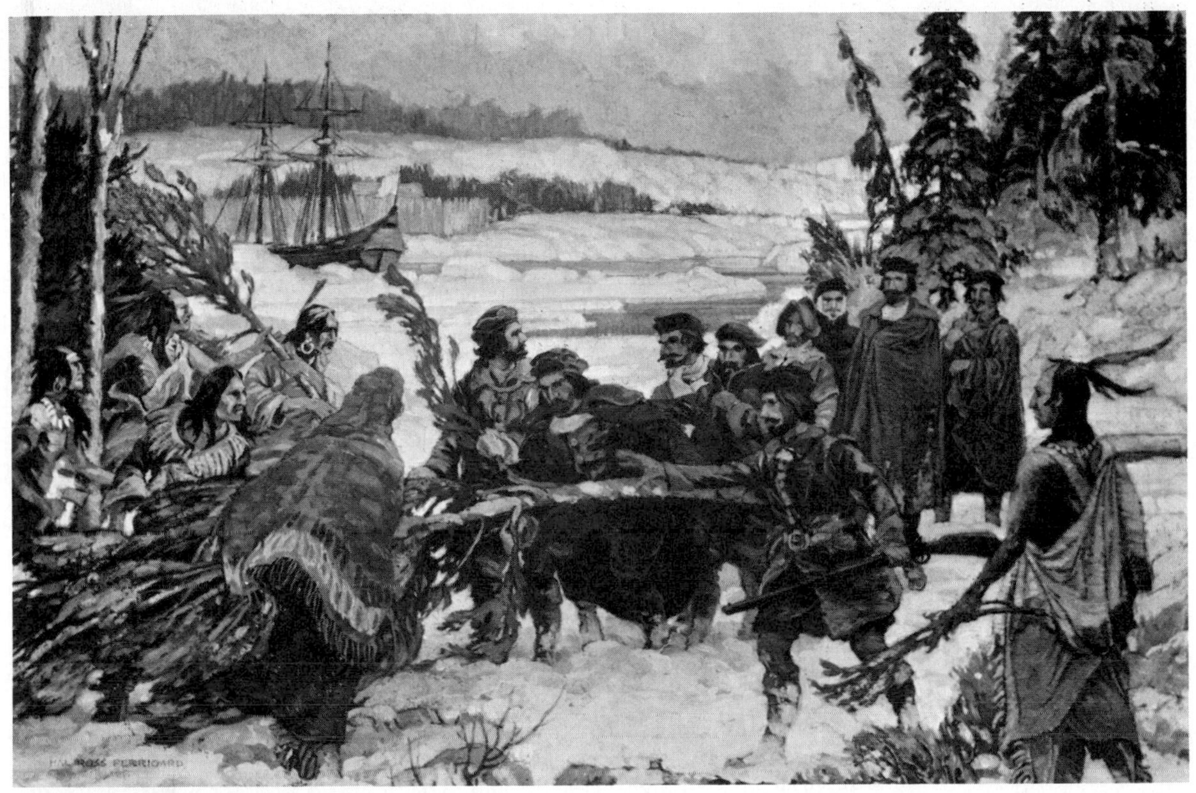

Indians showing explorer Jacques Cartier and his followers the source of their cure for scurvy, made from branches of the juniper tree, depicted in an oil painting by H. R. Perrigard. (Public Archives Canada)

sailors being familiarly known as "limeys"—has been told in Chapter 1. In *A Treatise on Scurvy,* Lind tells not only of his own experiments, but cites the experiences of the French explorer Cartier and his party of 110 men. Stranded along the iced-in St. Lawrence River in the winter of 1535, the explorers became afflicted with the gruesome symptoms of an unfamiliar and fatal disease—swollen limbs, blotched and hemorrhaging gums and skin, loss of teeth, and severe weakness. Soon eight had died, and more than fifty others were in critical condition, until local Indians recognized the disease and told them the cure: ingestion of a solution containing pine needles and bark.

In 1907, Axel Holst and Theodor Fröhlich induced scurvy in guinea pigs, a species that, along with all primates and a few other animal species as well, cannot synthesize the antiscurvy factor. In 1928 Albert Szent-Györgyi isolated a highly active hydrogen carrier from the adrenal gland, cabbages, and oranges. Because Szent-Györgyi was then concerned with hydrogen reactions in cell respiration, he failed to recognize the vitamin properties of the substance and named it hexuronic acid. Several years later, an active crystalline substance was isolated from lemon juice and named for its antiscurvy properties (from the Latin, *scorbutus,* "scurvy"; *ascorbic* means "without scurvy"). Almost immediately, Szent-Györgyi and a colleague determined that ascorbic acid was identical with hexuronic acid. The new vitamin was synthesized in 1933.

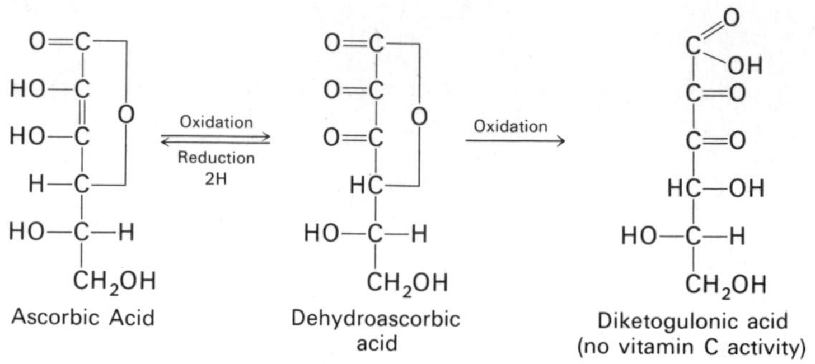

Oxidation ⇌ Reduction 2H; Oxidation →

Ascorbic Acid — Dehydroascorbic acid — Diketogulonic acid (no vitamin C activity)

FIGURE 7-19
Structure of Ascorbic Acid and Related Oxidation/Reduction Reactions

Chemistry and Properties

Ascorbic acid is a white, water-soluble, crystalline substance, stable when dry. However, in solution it becomes the least stable of all vitamins and oxidizes readily in light, air, and especially when heated or in alkaline solution. Oxidation is further accelerated in the presence of copper or iron. All of these oxidation-enhancing factors imply potential loss of vitamin activity during certain food preparation and storage conditions.

The 6-carbon structure of vitamin C makes it chemically similar to glucose (see Figure 7-19). The biologically active forms are L-ascorbic acid and its oxidation product L-dehydroascorbic acid, which has about 80 percent of the activity of the unoxidized form. Further oxidation converts the dehydroascorbic acid to diketogulonic acid, which has no antiscorbutic activity at all (see Figure 7-19); this latter reaction is irreversible.

Absorption and Metabolism

Vitamin C is readily absorbed through the mucosa of the small intestine. From there it passes through the portal vein to the liver and is then distributed to tissues throughout the body. The transport mechanism may differ from species to species, according to whether or not a species can synthesize ascorbic acid.

In humans, body stores total about 1,500 milligrams, with moderate reserves in the liver and spleen, and high concentrations but small amounts in the adrenal glands. The high concentration in the adrenal glands suggests that ascorbic acid may be involved in synthesis of adrenal steroids. Serum and tissue levels appear to be in equilibrium. Thus, white blood cells, which take up vitamin C, provide a basis for evaluating vitamin C status in humans.

The body excretes vitamin C primarily as ascorbic acid and as the metabolite oxalic acid in the urine, with very small amounts expired as carbon dioxide. The amount excreted daily represents about 3 percent of the total body reserves. Excretion increases with the administration of adrenal steroids, salicylates, sulfonamides, and tetracycline. Though the finding has been disputed, cigarette smoking appears to decrease plasma levels of vitamin C. Findings suggesting that oral contraceptives adversely affect ascorbic acid metabolism are also in dispute.

Physiological Function

Ascorbic acid is apparently the only water-soluble vitamin that is not known to serve as a coenzyme in any metabolic pathway. While much is known about its physiological functions, the biochemical involvements of this vitamin remain unclear.

The most important role of vitamin C is in the formation of collagen, a major component of all connective tissues in the body—skin, bones, teeth, muscle, tendon, cornea, and so on. Ascorbic acid is necessary for transformation of the amino acids proline and lysine into hydroxyproline and hydroxylysine. These hydroxy forms provide the tertiary structure which gives stability to the collagen molecule (see Chapter 4). The major symptoms of scurvy, which result from the breakdown of connective tissue, demonstrate the importance of vitamin C. Vitamin C further contributes to the formation of collagen needed for healing wounds, and therapeutic doses are sometimes used in treatment of postsurgical patients and burn victims.

Vitamin C, furthermore, apparently functions in conversion of amino acids for neurotransmitter synthesis and also is important in enhancing absorption of iron (see Chapter 8). It has been suggested that vitamin C lowers serum cholesterol levels, although contrary evidence has also been presented (Peterson et al., 1975). There has been a report, too, that pharmacological doses may help to dissolve gallstones (Ginter, 1976).

But undoubtedly the most controversial issue concerning ascorbic acid function involves its alleged power in preventing and curing the common cold. Studies have presented a mixed picture, but some suggest that large doses of ascorbic acid have an antihistaminelike effect; others, however, suggest no effect at all.

Recommended Allowances and Dietary Sources

While 10 milligrams per day of ascorbic acid is all that is needed to prevent scurvy, optimal health requires more. The RDA is 60 mg for adults, with increases to 80 mg and 100 mg for pregnant and lactating women respectively.

PERSPECTIVE ON
Vitamin C and the Common Cold

The argument for vitamin C as an effective preventive agent was introduced by Nobel Prize winner Linus Pauling in *Vitamin C and the Common Cold* (1970). In this book he advocates daily consumption of 1 to 3 grams of ascorbic acid, asserting that 1,000 milligrams a day will result in 45 percent fewer colds and 60 percent fewer sick days. Subsequently there have been claims that megadoses of ascorbic acid are effective in preventing other and more serious illnesses, including heart disease and cancer. Public response was overwhelming, and vitamin C supplements of all sizes, shapes, and forms—tablets, timed capsules, powders, and liquids, from rose hips, acerola, and other sources, and in doses of from 100 to 1,000 milligrams—sold like the proverbial hotcakes. Controversy followed, as opponents pointed out that the body excretes excess amounts of the vitamin and that Pauling's theoretical arguments were not backed up by documented and controlled case studies.

To date, a number of studies have been conducted, but evidence is negative to inconclusive. When Chalmers (1975) analyzed 14 such studies, he found that only 8 had been validly designed and conducted; generally the differences in the numbers of colds per year and the durations of illness produced small and statistically insignificant results in favor of ascorbic acid supplementation, while the differences in severity of symptoms were larger and more significant. Anderson and colleagues found, for example, that vitamin-dosed subjects experienced 7 percent fewer episodes of illness and 12 percent fewer sick days (not statistically significant), but 30 percent fewer days of severe illness, which was significant (Anderson, 1977).

Some of the conflicting evidence produced by various studies has been fascinating and suggests avenues for further research. For instance, at least one study of school children has shown that girls experience fewer cold symptoms when receiving vitamin C supplementation than do boys, but a repeat test did not produce the same results (Coulehan et al., 1976). Again, a study of pairs of twins showed no overall significant differences in the effect of vitamin C on cold incidence or symptoms—but younger girls apparently did benefit more from increased intake than did older girls or boys of any age. The most interesting finding in this study, however, was that the youngest group of boys grew an average of 1.3 centimeters more than their untreated cotwins in the five months in which they were studied; it is suggested that there may be a stage of development in which young boys are particularly sensitive to increases in ascorbic acid intake (Miller et al., 1977). But the growth effect was apparent in only one of the six age and sex groups studied, and the numbers involved in this test were relatively small.

Anderson calls attention to the effect of prior nutritional status of test subjects, pointing out that subjects whose vitamin C intake is normally high will be less likely to have their tissue levels affected by increased intakes, and therefore may demonstrate less apparent benefit during a test (Anderson, 1977). He also raises the question of the role of saturation versus maintenance levels of ascorbic acid. Because animal species that synthesize vitamin C apparently maintain tissue saturation levels at all times, it has been theorized that human intakes should aim for this level too. Human tissues achieve ascorbic acid saturation with body stores of about 4,000 milligrams, and it is estimated that daily intakes of about 120 mg will maintain tissue saturation in most individuals. (The recommended daily allowance of 60 mg will maintain body stores at about 1,500 mg.) Proponents of this view hold that the traditional approach to requirements for a vitamin as being the amount needed to prevent its deficiency symptoms are outmoded. In the case of ascorbic acid, it is pointed out that, while as little as 10 mg per day are adequate to avoid symptoms, optimum health probably requires much more. Anderson and others have suggested that saturation levels are probably desirable in aiding the body's resistance to stress (including attack by cold viruses and other stresses as well), and that the presence of the vitamin in every body cell argues that it has a widespread and positive role in maintaining tissue health, rather than simply the traditional preventive role of merely protecting against scurvy.

In view of the provocative but conflicting evidence, what can be recommended? First, researchers generally agree that any effect of ascorbic acid on the common cold is pharmacological rather than due to its nutritional activity (at least, in terms of what we know at this time about how it acts biochemically). Many of those most antagonistic to Pauling's strong claim do admit that, although the vitamin may not prevent onset, it does appear to reduce the severity of cold symptoms. However, a strong psychological component was suggested when it was found that in one study a large number of volunteers were able to determine by taste and appearance of the dose whether they were in the placebo or vitamin C group; when results from those who had correctly guessed their status and may have responded accordingly were eliminated, no significant differences in severity or duration remained (Chalmers, 1975).

There is probably no reason for most people to avoid moderate increases in intake, especially at times of physical illness or other stress. The best way to do this would be to increase consumption of fresh fruits and vegetables, which will provide additional nutrients as well. It should be borne in mind, however, that toxic effects have been reported on daily intakes greater than 1 gram, and there is reason for concern about the effect of long-term high ascorbic acid dosage on calcium status (Chalmers, 1975) and kidney function. Some proponents of vitamin C are reportedly taking from 6 to 10 *grams* per day, and this is definitely not advisable. The possibility of toxicity for some individuals from even 1-gram amounts over a period of time precludes recommending intakes over 500 milligrams per day for the general public, especially in the absence of definitive evidence of any major benefit.

Because body stores are limited, daily intake is necessary. Individuals with chronic illness and those recovering from surgery should receive additional amounts.

In addition to citrus fruits and their juices, which are well known as sources of vitamin C, tomatoes, green vegetables, and other fruits such as most melons and berries also contain significant quantities. Potatoes, not generally thought to provide exceptional amounts of this vitamin, may nonetheless be an important source for population groups consuming large quantities; one medium baked potato will provide about one-half of the recommended allowance for an adult. With the exception of liver, foods of animal origin generally have little or no ascorbic acid content (see Table 7-9).

Because vitamin C is so vulnerable to light, air, and heat, care must be taken in food preparation to preserve its activity. Cut foods should not be left exposed for long periods; there should be as little cutting and chopping before cooking as possible; baking soda should never be added to cooking water; minimal quantities of water should be used in cooking; vegetables should be put into water that has already come to a boil and should not be overcooked. Vegetable cooking liquids should be reused in soups; and foods should be covered and stored in opaque containers.

Symptoms of Clinical Deficiency

The numerous symptoms of ascorbic acid deficiency include lassitude and general weakness, swollen joints and aching bones, spongy and bleeding gums, delayed wound healing, muscle cramps, and dry scaly skin. Infants with scurvy assume a characteristic "frog's leg" position, are generally irritable, have particularly sensitive lips and limbs, and have little appetite. Unless the mother is deficient, breast-fed infants rarely get scurvy. But bottle-fed infants on some formulas should be given supplements.

In the United States, scurvy has almost completely disappeared, although alcoholics and the elderly, as well as some of those with bizarre eating habits, may show deficiency, usually due to decreased consumption of fresh fruits and juices. Interestingly two sources of vitamin C have fallen victim to "progress," and sporadic outbreaks of scurvy have been the result. In the southern states, it was the custom, particularly among rural people, to drink the liquid in which green vegetables had been cooked; this "pot likker" was a good source of the vitamin C that long cooking and a large volume of water had leached out of greens. But a rising standard of living eliminated this dietary custom in many families, and children developed scurvy. Children also became "victims" of pasteurization, which destroys the ascorbic acid content of milk along with microorganisms.

For somewhat different reasons, it might be expected that Eskimos, especially in the Arctic, would have a relatively high incidence of scurvy, since their diet contains almost no foods of plant origin (unlike the sub-Arctic Eskimo, who do get some fruits, berries, and vegetables). Apparently the fact that the Eskimos eat much of their animal food frozen, raw, or only partially cooked preserves what little vitamin C is in their diet. Table 7-10 lists the vitamin C content of some Eskimo foods; it is interesting to compare these figures with those of the typical American diet in Table 7-9.

TABLE 7-9
Ascorbic Acid Content of Selected Foods
RDA for Adults
60 mg

Food	Serving Size	Ascorbic Acid Content mg/serving
Orange juice, frozen concentrate, diluted as directed	6 oz	90
Strawberries, fresh	1 c	88
Broccoli, fresh, cooked	3 spears	81
Broccoli, frozen, cooked	3 spears	66
Orange	1 medium	66
Grapefruit juice, canned	6 oz	63
Cantaloupe	1/4 melon	45
Grapefruit	1/2 medium	37
Liver, calf, cooked	3 oz	31
Asparagus, cooked	2/3 c	31
Potato, white, baked	1 medium	31
Cranberry juice cocktail	6 oz	30
Tomato juice, canned	6 oz	29
Spinach, frozen, cooked	1/2 c	27
Winter squash, mashed	1 c	27
Sweet potato, baked	1 medium	25
Liver, beef, cooked	3 oz	23
Avocado, raw	1/2 medium	16
Vegetable juice cocktail	6 oz	16
Tomato, raw	1/2 medium	14
Lemonade, frozen concentrate, diluted as directed	6 oz	13
Soybeans, cooked	1/2 c	13
Tomato soup, prepared with water	1 c	12
Banana	1 medium	12
Apricots, raw	3	11
Green beans, fresh, cooked	2/3 c	10
Clams, raw, meat only	3 oz	8
Apple	1 medium	6
Yogurt, plain	8 oz	2
Milk, whole	8 oz	2
Milk, low-fat	8 oz	2
Yogurt, fruit-flavored	8 oz	1
Bread, white, enriched	1 slice	trace
Cheddar cheese	1 oz	0
Fish	3 oz	0
Hamburger, 21% fat, cooked	3 oz	0
Poultry	3 oz	0
Oils, butter, margarine	—	0
Egg, whole	1 medium	0

Source: C. F. Adams, *Nutritive value of American foods in common units*, USDA Agriculture Handbook No. 456 (Washington, D.C.: U.S. Government Printing Office, 1975).

Toxicity

Because it is water-soluble and readily excreted, and because the body's capacity for storage of ascorbic acid is limited, toxic effects have long been thought unlikely. Indeed, even in doses as high as several hundred milligrams per day, little toxicity has been demonstrated. But ingestion of very large doses, in the range of one to several grams per day, does have potentially serious effects for some people. There is, for example, evidence that high intakes can cause kidney stones and gout in susceptible individuals. Other evidence has suggested that vitamin C may act as a vitamin B_{12} antagonist, but this has been challenged. The ability of ascorbic acid to enhance absorption of dietary iron may pose the threat of iron overload to sensitive individuals. A more serious problem, potentially affecting larger numbers of individuals, is that urine tests to determine desirable insulin requirements for diabetics are falsified by consumption of large doses of ascorbic acid. Very large doses may acidify the urine and produce a burning sensation during urination.

A single case study related to megadosage of vitamin C for migraine headaches has suggested the possibility that prolonged intake of such quantities may lead to nutritional dependency (Ball and Calloway, 1978). Additional fragmentary evidence suggests that individuals who have been consuming significant amounts of ascorbic acid should wean themselves slowly until moderate levels of intake are achieved (Anderson, 1977).

Some physicians have warned that ingestion of megadoses of ascorbic acid during pregnancy may produce a vitamin C-dependent infant. In such a case, a condition known as "rebound scurvy" could develop when the infant receives only normal amounts of the vitamin after birth. Once the fetal metabolic system has adapted to the higher amounts by removing the excess vitamin C more rapidly than normal, even the normal amounts ingested by the newborn are removed at the faster-than-normal rate, depressing serum and tissue levels (Anderson, 1977).

TABLE 7-10
Ascorbic Acid Content of Foods in Eskimo Diet

Food	Ascorbic Acid Content mg/100g (3½ oz)
Arctic char (a fish): frozen, raw	0.48
Caribou, 2-year-old, male: muscle	
frozen, raw	0.76
roasted, medium rare	0.43
Seal	
pup	
muscle, in soup	0.66
liver, boiled	30.49 (only significant source)
3-year-old female, muscle	
frozen, raw	0.43
cooked in soup	0.47
4-year-old male, muscle: frozen raw	0.62

Source: K. Hoppner, J. M. McLaughlan, B. G. Shah, J. N. Thompson, J. Beare-Rogers, J. Ellestad-Sayed, and O. Shaefer, Nutrient levels of some foods of Eskimos from Arctic Bay, N.W.T., Canada, *Journal of the American Dietetic Association* 73:257, 1978.

VITAMINLIKE FACTORS

At different times in the history of vitamin research a number of substances have been candidates for classification as vitamins. Some—like those discussed thus far in this chapter and those discussed in Chapter 6—have been "elected," so to speak. Some have been "defeated," and some elected only to be recalled later. As our knowledge of nutritional metabolism grows, one or more of these substances may yet receive recognition as vitamins. The compounds with the best qualifications are choline, inositol, ubiquinone, lipoic acid, para-aminobenzoic acid, and the bioflavinoids. At present, however, each is considered to lack one or more of the three essential criteria that characterize this nutrient class.

Choline

Choline is apparently synthesized in all plant and animal species. Its greatest importance is as a precursor of the neurotransmitter acetylcholine; dietary choline directly affects acetylcholine levels as well as the density of acetylcholine receptors in the brain. For this reason, pharmacological doses of choline have been used to treat brain disorders that are apparently related to deficiency of choline functioning, such as tardive dyskinesia and Huntington's disease. Choline is also a component of phospholipids and lecithins, which form an essential part of cell membranes and lipoproteins; deficiency produces structural and functional abnormalities in cells. And choline is needed, along with methionine, to prevent the development of fatty liver. Food sources include wheat germ, egg yolk, organ meats, and legumes; the average American diet provides about 800 milligrams, an ample supply, per day. (For a recent review of what is known about this substance, see Kuksis and Mookerjea, 1978a.)

Inositol

This colorless, water-soluble substance whose structure resembles that of glucose is widely found in plants, especially in grains, nuts, fruits, and vegetables, as well as in yeast and milk. Because the body, it has been learned, apparently synthesizes enough for all metabolic requirements, inositol is no longer considered to be a vitamin. Its main function in humans is as a component of muscle phospholipids. Phytic acid, an inositol-phosphate compound found in some plants and seeds, binds zinc, iron, and calcium in the human gastrointestinal tract and therefore may significantly decrease absorption of those minerals. (For a review of present knowledge about inositol, see Kuksis and Mookerjea, 1978b.)

Ubiquinone

Also known as Coenzyme Q, and chemically related both to vitamins E and K, this compound derives its name from its ubiquitous distribution in animals and plants. Because adequate amounts are synthesized in body cells, food sources are not necessary. Ubiquinone is a component of the phospholipids that form the mitochondrial membranes, and in this way it plays a very important part as an electron carrier in the electron transport system (see Figure 7-7).

Lipoic acid

Lipoic acid is a sulfur-containing fat-soluble molecule for which no human dietary requirement is known. Acting as a coenzyme in conjunction with thiamin, niacin, riboflavin, and pantothenic acid, lipoic acid participates in the conversion of (1) pyruvate to acetyl CoA, and (2) α-ketoglutarate to succinyl CoA. Thus, it plays an important role in the metabolism of carbohydrate, protein, and fat. It is not classified as a vitamin, however, because it can be synthesized in the body in physiologically effective amounts.

Para-aminobenzoic acid

Para-aminobenzoic acid (PABA) functions as a growth factor for bacteria and lower animals. It is a component of folic acid and can completely satisfy the need in rats and mice for dietary folic acid. For these reasons, it was accorded vitamin status at one time. But it is not clear whether PABA has any metabolic role other than as a component of folic acid, and it is no longer considered a vitamin for humans or other animals.

Bioflavinoids

The bioflavinoids were discovered by Szent-Györgyi, in 1936, as a mixture of compounds in lemon peel and red peppers that he named citrin (a designation later dropped). The active component in citrin was briefly called vitamin P for its role in maintaining permeability of capillary membranes. Experimentally induced bioflavinoid deficiency in animals results in a syndrome marked by increased capillary permeability and fragility. This deficiency effect has some relationship to the role of vitamin C. Apparently the bioflavinoids have an antioxidant effect that protects ascorbic acid from oxidative destruction. But this is an indirect and nonessential effect. At present there is not enough evidence to include these substances among the vitamins.

NONVITAMINS

Laetrile

In 1952, the biochemist Ernst T. Krebs, Jr. (not related to Sir Hans Krebs) announced the development of a drug he called Laetrile, which was asserted to be a cure for cancer and safe when injected. Subsequently, he claimed that Laetrile was a vitamin (B_{17}). Krebs, his father, and others produced and promoted Laetrile as a cancer preventive and cure and have charged that the medical establishment and the Food and Drug Administration are in collusion to keep it from the public.

Laetrile is found in apricot and peach pits and almond kernels; it is a glucose-related compound that contains cyanide and is known chemically as amygdalin. Although it has been promoted for a quarter of a century, the anticancer effectiveness of Laetrile remains to be demonstrated. Contrary to the contentions of the Krebs's and their associates, this substance has been the subject of numerous tests. The National Cancer Institute sought a widespread analysis of Laetrile treatment and solicited case histories showing improvement from 385,000 physicians, 70,000 other health professionals, and all pro-Laetrile organizations. The progress of 68 patient cases, along with an equal number of controls who had received conventional treatment, were presented to a panel of 12 cancer specialists who did not know the treatment used for each patient. Evaluation of patient progress attributed only two completely favorable responses and four partially favorable responses to Laetrile (Ellison et al., 1978).

Laetrile does not meet the essential criteria for being a vitamin. It has no known metabolic function essential to nutritional health, and its absence from the diet produces no deficiency symptoms. (The only criterion that it does meet is that it is not synthesized in the human body!) More important, it

PERSPECTIVE ON Megavitamin Therapy

A vitamin, by definition, is a substance required by the body in very small amounts. As the discussion of the common cold (above) made clear, even the amounts needed to "saturate" body tissues are quite small as well. Up to and including saturation, vitamins in the body function as coenzymes or hormonelike compounds. Once saturation is reached (and in some cases total saturation of the body with a nutrient may be neither beneficial nor desirable), any additional amount of vitamin becomes just another chemical. This is because, at saturation levels, the metabolic system is already working at full capacity. From a nutritional point of view, then, there is no need for vitamin doses that exceed the saturation level. Many people mistakenly consume large amounts of vitamins in the belief that if some is good, more is better. What they are actually getting are small amounts of vitamin (the portion that can be utilized metabolically) and large amounts of what may act essentially as a chemical or drug.

The use of vitamins in dosages of at least ten times the RDA is popularly known as **megavitamin therapy,** although it is certainly not a *vitamin* therapy. Another term, **orthomolecular medicine,** was coined by Pauling some ten years ago (from the Greek *ortho,* "right") to describe treatment based on substances that naturally occur in or are used by the body, such as insulin or vitamins. Orthomolecular treatment with niacin has been used to lower lipid serum levels, and niacin, ascorbic acid, and other water-soluble vitamins have been used in the treatment of schizophrenia.

The use of vitamin megadoses for schizophrenia actually began in the 1950s, when Abram Hoffer and Humphrey Osmond noted similarities between schizophrenia symptoms and the disoriented mental states of pellagra patients. They treated newly admitted schizophrenics with massive doses of niacin with what appeared to be success. In recent years, proponents of orthomolecular therapy have claimed that this approach is useful in the treatment of autism, hyperactivity in children, alcoholism, arthritis, allergies, cancer, and a number of other conditions. However, these claims have failed to gain acceptance from the medical or psychiatric communities.

Schizophrenia is believed to be several different conditions sharing a number of symptoms of mental derangement, with multiple causes including both genetic and environmental factors. There is some evidence that biochemical disturbances are in-is not a harmless substance. Its cyanide content is potentially lethal, and symptoms of toxicity have been reported. Some observers, however, do believe that it is harmless.

Laetrile has become a political issue as well as a medical question. Because it is not an approved drug, it cannot be legally sold as such in most of the United States and has been banned from interstate commerce. Some people feel that these restrictions interfere with their freedom to choose their own medical treatment. In June 1979 the Supreme Court unanimously upheld the right of the Federal Government to prohibit interstate transport of laetrile, to seize the substance, and to prosecute distributors. However, as of that date, laetrile could legally be distributed in 17 states (Greenhouse, 1979).

The claims made for Laetrile present a number of dilemmas. Since present evidence does not support its alleged benefits, should sales be allowed? Do individuals have the right to choose their own treatment—and possibly to choose a treatment that is not only not therapeutic but that may even be harmful? Again, if a seriously ill patient fully believes that this substance, and nothing else, will help, is there a danger in allowing its use? Might it not have, in fact, a placebo effect that may well help to relieve suffering?

volved, but it is not clear what the particular chemical substances may be, how they act, or indeed whether they are a cause or result of the problem. Most of the successes attributed to orthomolecular treatment of schizophrenia are anecdotal testimonials. The role of vitamin megadoses remains unclear for several reasons: This psychosis is characterized by alternating periods of severe breakdown and remission; orthomolecular treatment has usually been an adjunct to other therapies; and no double-blind studies have been conducted in recent years.

On the other hand, large doses of vitamins are helpful when used for a known therapeutic purpose. For example, where certain inborn errors of metabolism are involved, a vitamin megadose will "stimulate" an enzyme that does not appear to be fully functional, or will result in adequate absorption of the nutrient when the absorptive process is defective. Large amounts of vitamin D, in the active form of DHCC, are given to stimulate the production of calcium-binding protein in the intestine. Large doses can also compensate for the effects of prescribed medications that antagonize vitamins and interfere with absorption, such as anticonvulsants, the antitubercular drug INH, oral contraceptives, and others. Here, however, the vitamin is being administered, albeit in massive amounts, for a *nutritional* purpose. In such cases, it is important to achieve equilibrium between the medication and the vitamin megadose, because an excess of the vitamin may also neutralize the effects of the drug.

Reports to date of the successful use of vitamins in megadosages are tantalizing, but unbiased evidence is as yet scanty. Nevertheless, many people take various high-dose vitamin preparations for their alleged benefits, ranging from increased energy and enhanced sexual performance to prevention of heart disease and cancer. All such reports should be viewed with caution, because they are frequently not based on *scientific evidence.*

Because many vitamins, especially the fat-soluble ones, do have toxic effects, especially in massive amounts, self-dosing is definitely not advisable. As more and more people have been routinely taking more vitamins in large quantities, more side effects are becoming apparent. Thus, concentrated ascorbic acid, previously thought to be totally innocuous, causes gastrointestinal discomfort and diarrhea for many people and may have more serious consequences. However, moderate supplementation of some vitamins, at levels no greater than the allowance set by the Food and Nutrition Board, may be useful for some individuals. But remember that a vitamin pill contains only one or a few vitamins; it cannot supply any of the other nutrients the body needs. It is always best to obtain necessary vitamins from foods, not from pills.

The answers to these questions are still not clear, even to many who believe the substance to have no healing powers (Ingelfinger, 1977). But it is clear that, in tragically too many cases, Laetrile therapy prevented use of effective traditional therapies until it was too late (Holden, 1976). (One such case is described in Nolen, 1974.) In summary, then, there is no known nutritional need or proven therapeutic use for Laetrile.

Pangamic acid

Pangamic acid, also known as pangamate and recently promoted as vitamin B_{15}, was patented in 1949 by the same people who developed Laetrile. Claims are made that it is a wonder drug that provides "extra" energy and cures a host of physical ailments besides (Nobile, 1978). Pangamate's developers, however, have never furnished any proof (other than testimonials) of its vitamin properties and curative powers. Nevertheless, it is widely used in the Soviet Union and in a number of European and other countries. Claims made for it by the Soviets include maintenance of tissue levels of oxygen, and this would seem to accord with claims made for its energy-giving property; however, it apparently does not increase body intake of oxygen but, rather, removes greater amounts of oxygen from blood into tissues, which may, in fact, be hazardous rather than beneficial (Mayer and Dwyer, 1978).

Like Laetrile, pangamate is found in apricot pits and all other seeds, hence the name given to it by Krebs, from *pan,* "all," and *gamete,* "seed." Also as with Laetrile, it does not meet the criteria for a vitamin. Lacking evidence for its effectiveness as a drug or for its safety, and with the chemical makeup of various preparations in dispute, the Food and Drug Adminstration has refused to approve its sale as a drug or dietary supplement (Herbert, 1979).

SUMMARY

The water-soluble vitamins are distinguished from their fat-soluble counterparts in three major ways:

1. Solubility—their water solubility substantially determines such properties as limited body storage and excretion in urine.
2. Chemical composition—in addition to carbon, hydrogen, and oxygen, most water-soluble vitamins also contain nitrogen, and several contain sulfur, cobalt, or phosphorus.
3. Metabolic function—except for ascorbic acid, all the water-soluble vitamins are known to function as components of one or more coenzymes.

Thiamin (B_1) participates in more than 20 enzyme reactions necessary for the metabolism of carbohydrates, fats, and proteins. Its active form is a sulfur-containing molecule, thiamin pyrophosphate (TPP or cocarboxylase). Many foods, especially whole grains, contain thiamin in varied amounts. Thiamin deficiency, or beriberi, was described as early as 2600 B.C. and takes several forms, all involving impairment of the nervous, cardiovascular, and gastrointestinal systems.

Riboflavin (B_2) is a component of the coenzymes flavin mononucleotide (FMN) and flavin adenine dinucleotide (FAD). It combines with various proteins to form flavoprotein enzymes, which function as hydrogen carriers. A wide variety of food provides small amounts of riboflavin, usually in association with other B vitamins. Deficiency symptoms, which are probably associated with deficiencies of other vitamins as well, include growth retardation and various abnormalities or lesions of the eyes, mouth, tongue, and skin.

Niacin, also known as nicotinic acid and nicotinamide, resembles riboflavin in metabolic function. Niacin forms two related coenzymes, nicotine adenine dinucleotide (NAD) and nicotine adenine dinucleotide phosphate (NADP). These combine with various proteins to form enzymes that act as hydrogen carriers. Niacin is found in many foods and also is synthesized in the body from the amino acid tryptophan in a reaction that requires thiamin, riboflavin, and vitamin B_6. The serious niacin-deficiency condition pellagra is characterized by "the four D's"—dermatitis, diarrhea, dementia, and death. Pharmacological doses may be toxic to the liver and may cause diabetes or peptic ulcer.

Biotin, a widespread and potent vitamin, was not identified chemically until 1942. It is a sulfur-containing, heat-stable growth factor which functions chiefly as a coenzyme in fatty acid synthesis (CO_2-fixation reactions) and amino acid metabolism (transcarboxylation reactions). No RDA for biotin has been established, nor have any deficiency or toxic effects been identified.

Pantothenic acid, named for its extremely wide distribution, functions mainly as a component of coenzyme A (CoA), the compound that combines with oxaloacetate to initiate the Krebs cycle and in acyl carrier protein. No RDA for pantothenic acid has been established, nor has any natural deficiency been identified in humans.

Vitamin B_6 (pyridoxine) has three forms, all of which are active as the coenzyme pyridoxal phosphate (PLP). Among other functions, PLP participates in reactions essential to amino acid metabolism. The only known natural clinical deficiency is microcytic anemia in infants. Therapeutic doses may cause mild toxicity, and dependency and severe toxicity may result from larger intakes.

Folacin was identified ten years after the discovery of a deficiency anemia that did not respond to any of the known B-complex factors. Its primary function is as a coenzyme involved in the synthesis of thymine, a nucleotide in DNA. Folacin deficiency produces megaloblastic anemia (immature, enlarged red blood cells).

Vitamin B_{12} (cobalamin), identified in 1948 as the anti-pernicious anemia factor, is a large, complex, cobalt-containing molecule. Like folic acid, vitamin B_{12} is essential for DNA synthesis, and it is essential also for nervous system function. Since it is found only in foods of animal origin, individuals on strict vegetarian diets, especially pregnant and lactating women, breast-fed infants, and children, should receive supplementation.

Ascorbic acid (vitamin C) was identified as the antiscurvy factor in 1932. It functions chiefly in maintaining the structure of collagen, the major component of all connective tissue. It also enhances iron absorption. The role of ascorbic acid in prevention of the common cold is disputed. Vitamin C is found in many fruits and vegetables. Possible toxic effects may result from long-term high doses and include gout, kidney stones, lessened calcium retention, and vitamin dependence.

Vitaminlike factors are important biological substances that have been classified or may yet be classified as vitamins but at present lack one or more of three defining characteristics. On the other hand, Laetrile ("B_{17}") and pangamic acid ("B_{15}") are actually nonvitamins since they satisfy none of the important criteria for vitamins.

BIBLIOGRAPHY

ANDERSON, T. W. New horizons for vitamin C. *Nutrition Today* 12(1):6, 1977.

BALL, L., AND E. CALLOWAY. Vitamin C and migraine: A case report. *New England Journal of Medicine* 299:364, 1978.

CARMEL, R. Nutritional vitamin B_{12} deficiency. Possible contributory role of subtle vitamin B_{12} malabsorption. *Annals of Internal Medicine* 88:647, 1978.

CENTERWALL, B. S., AND M. H. CRIQUI. Prevention of the Wernicke-Korsakoff syndrome. A cost-benefit analysis. *New England Journal of Medicine* 299:285, 1978.

CHALMERS, T. C. Effects of ascorbic acid on the common cold: An evaluation of the evidence. *American Journal of Medicine* 58:532, 1975.

CORONARY DRUG PROJECT RESEARCH GROUP. Clofibrate and niacin in coronary heart disease. *Journal of the American Medical Association* 321:360, 1975.

COULEHAN, J. L., S. EBERHARD, L. KAPNER, F. TAYLOR, K. ROGERS, AND P. GARVY. Vitamin C and acute illness in Navajo school children. *New England Journal of Medicine* 295:973, 1976.

DARBY, W. J., K. W. MCNUTT, AND E. N. TODHUNTER. Niacin. *Nutrition Reviews* 33:289, 1975.

ELLISON, N. M., D. P. BYAR, AND G. R. NEWELL. Special report on Laetrile: The NCI Laetrile review. Results of the National Cancer Institute's retrospective Laetrile analysis. *New England Journal of Medicine* 299:549, 1978.

FRADER, J., B. REIBMEN, AND D. TURKOWITZ. Vitamin B_{12} deficiency in strict vegetarians. *New England Journal of Medicine* 299:1319, 1978.

GINTER, E. Chenodeoxycholic acid, gallstones, and vitamin C. *New England Journal of Medicine* 295:1260, 1976.

GREENHOUSE, L. High court upholds Laetrile ban. *The New York Times*, June 19, 1979, p. 1.

HERBERT, V. Pangamic acid ("vitamin B_{15}"). *American Journal of Clinical Nutrition* 32:1534, 1979.

HERBERT, V., AND E. JACOB. Destruction of vitamin B_{12} by ascorbic acid. *Journal of the American Medical Association* 230:241, 1974.

HIGGINBOTTOM, M. C., L. SWEETMAN, AND W. L. NYHAN. A syndrome of methylmalonic aciduria, homocystinuria, megaloblastic anemia, and neurologic abnormalities in a vitamin B_{12}-deficient breast-fed infant of a strict vegetarian. *New England Journal of Medicine* 299:317, 1978.

HOLDEN, C. Laetrile: Quack cancer remedy still brings hope to sufferers. *Science* 193:982, 1976.

INGELFINGER, F. J. Laetrilomania. *New England Journal of Medicine* 296:1167, 1977.

ITOKAWA, Y., AND J. R. COOPER. Ion movements and thiamin. II. The release of the vitamin from membrane fragments. *Biochimica et Biophysica Acta* 196:274, 1970.

KUKSIS, A., AND S. MOOKERJEA. Choline. *Nutrition Reviews* 36:201, 1978a.

KUKSIS, A., AND S. MOOKERJEA. Inositol. *Nutrition Reviews* 36:233, 1978b.

MAYER, J., AND J. DWYER. Calcium pangamate isn't a vitamin. *Boston Globe,* August 16, 1978, p. 50.

MILLER, D. F. Pellagra deaths in the United States. *American Journal of Clinical Nutrition* 31:558, 1978.

MILLER, J. Z., W. N. NANCE, J. A. NORTON, R. W. WOLAN, R. S. GRIFFITH, AND R. J. ROSE. Therapeutic effect of vitamin C. A co-twin study. *Journal of the American Medical Association* 237:248, 1977.

NEWMARK, H. L., J. SCHEINER, M. MARCUS, AND M. PRABHUDESAI. Stability of vitamin B_{12} in presence of ascorbic acid. *American Journal of Clinical Nutrition* 29:645, 1976.

NOBILE, P. Will vitamin B_{15} cure what ails you? *New York Magazine,* March 13, 1978, pp. 39–41.

NOLEN, W. A. *A doctor in search of a miracle.* New York: Random House, 1974.

ORR, M. L., AND B. K. WATT. *Amino acid content of foods.* USDA Home Economics Research Report No. 4. Washington, D.C.: U.S. Government Printing Office, 1957.

PAULING, L. *Vitamin C and the common cold.* San Francisco: W. H. Freeman & Co., 1970.

PERLOFF, B. P., AND R. R. BUTRUM. Folacin in selected foods. *Journal of the American Dietetic Association* 70:157, 1977.

PETERSON, V. E., P. A. CRAPO, J. WEININGER, H. GINSBERG, AND J. OLETSKY. Quantification of plasma cholesterol and triglyceride levels in hypercholesterolemic subjects receiving ascorbic acid supplements. *American Journal of Clinical Nutrition* 28:584, 1975.

SMITH, E. L. *Vitamin B_{12}.* New York: John Wiley, 1965.

SUGGESTED ADDITIONAL READING

ANDERSON, T. W., B. W. REID, AND G. H. BEATON. Vitamin C and the common cold: A double blind trial. *Canadian Medical Association Journal* 107:503, 1971.

ANDERSON, T. W., C. F. ENLOE, JR., H. L. HARTLEY, R. PASSMORE, L. C. PAULING, AND A. SZENT-GYÖRGYI. To dose or megadose: A debate about vitamin C. *Nutrition Today* 13(2):6, 1978.

COURSIN, D. B. Convulsive seizures in infants with pyridoxine-deficient diets. *Journal of the American Medical Association* 154:406, 1954.

FOMON, S. J., AND R. G. STRAUSS. Nutrient deficiencies in breast-fed infants. *New England Journal of Medicine* 299:355, 1978.

FOOD AND NUTRITION BOARD, NATIONAL RESEARCH COUNCIL. *Folic acid, biochemistry and physiology in relation to the human nutrition requirement.* Washington, D.C.: National Academy of Sciences, 1977.

FOOD AND NUTRITION BOARD, NATIONAL RESEARCH COUNCIL. *Human vitamin B_6 requirement.* Washington, D.C.: National Academy of Sciences, 1978.

GOLDBERGER, J. The prevention of pellagra. A test diet among institutional inmates. *Public Health Reports* 30:3117, 1938.

GOLDSMITH, G. A., O. N. MILLER, AND W. G. UNGLAUB. Efficiency of tryptophan as a niacin precursor in man. *Journal of Nutrition* 73:172, 1961.

HERBERT, V. Megavitamin therapy. *Contemporary Nutrition,* October 1977.

HUDIBURGH, N. K., AND A. N. MILNER. Influence of oral contraceptives on ascorbic acid and triglyceride status. *Journal of the American Dietetic Association,* 75:19, 1979.

MINOT, G. R., AND W. P. MURPHY. Treatment of pernicious anemia by a special diet. *Journal of the American Medical Association* 87:470, 1926.

NUTRITION TODAY. Report: Discovery and synthesis of vitamin B_{12} celebrated. Vol. 8(1):24, 1973.

RIVLIN, R. S., ED. *Riboflavin.* New York: Plenum Press, 1975.

SEBRELL, W. H., AND R. E. BUTLER. Riboflavin deficiency in man. *Public Health Reports* 54:1212, 1939.

SYDENSTRICKER, V. P., S. A. SINGAL, A. P. BRIGGS, N. M. DEVAUGHN, AND H. ISBELL. Preliminary observations on "egg white injury" in man and its cure with a biotin concentrate. *Science* 95:176, 1942.

WILLIAMS, R. R. *Toward the conquest of beriberi.* Cambridge, Mass.: Harvard University Press, 1961.

Chapter 8

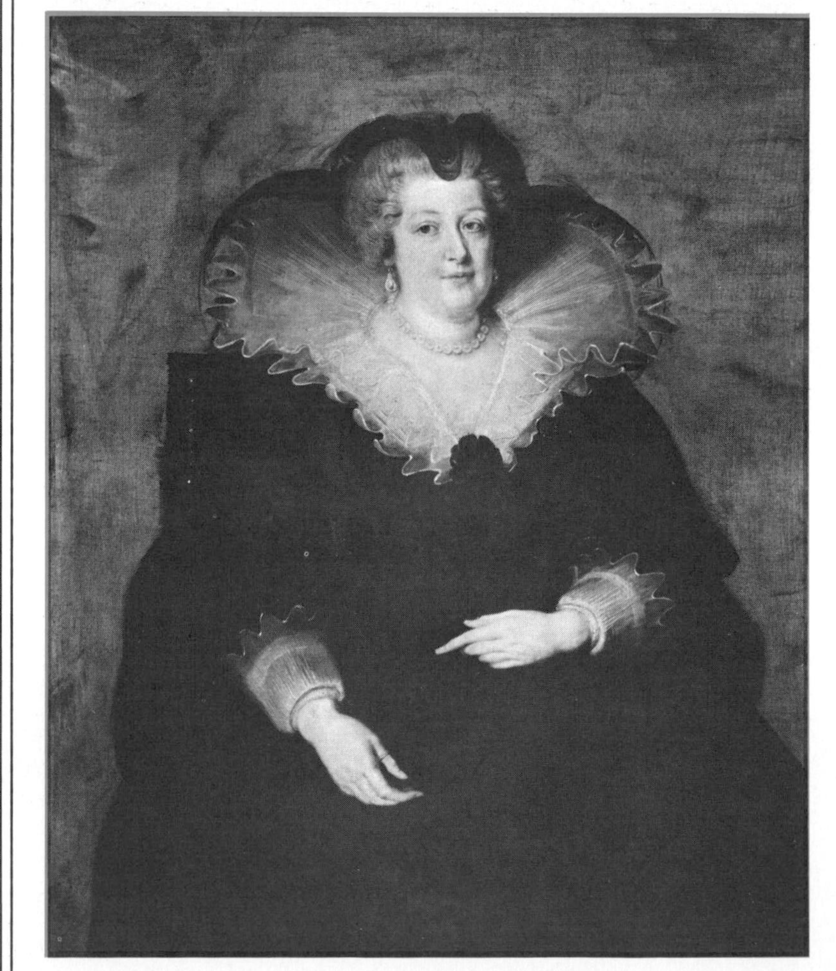

Maria de'Medici by Peter Paul Rubens

Minerals

About 50 of the more than 100 known elements are found in body tissues and fluids, and four of these 50—carbon, hydrogen, oxygen, and nitrogen—make up 96 percent of our body weight. In varying combinations, these four elements are fundamental components of one or more of the five nutrient classes: carbohydrate, protein, lipids, vitamins, and water. Twenty-one additional elements have been classified as essential nutrients; they account for most of the remaining 4 percent of body weight. Their chemical nature and similarities of function justify classifying them together as a single nutrient category, the *minerals.* This class of nutrients consists of those chemical elements that (1) are known (or strongly suspected) to be essential for nutritional health in humans and (2) are required in milligram quantities in the daily diet. (See Table 1-2 for the percentage amounts of different elements in the body.)

The additional two dozen or more elements found in the body have no known essential function and are classified as *contaminants.* These enter the body via air, food, and water and, for the most part, pose no health problem. Under certain circumstances and in sufficient quantity, however, they can be toxic and even lethal. Three well-known examples are lead, mercury, and strontium-90.

The essential minerals can be divided into two subgroups on the basis of dietary requirement: The so-called *macro* or **major minerals** are required in amounts of 100 milligrams or more per day; **trace minerals** are required in amounts no greater than a few milligrams per day. In contrast to the much larger requirements established for carbohydrate, protein, and lipids, the small requirements for minerals resemble those for vitamins.

The essential minerals have wide distribution in the tissues and fluids of the body. They occur chiefly (1) as components of various important organic molecules such as metalloenzymes (the iron-containing cytochromes), amino acids (sulfur in cysteine and methionine), and others (iron in hemoglobin, iodine in thyroid hormones); (2) as structural components of certain tissues (calcium, phosphorus, and fluorine in dental tissue); and (3) as free ions (sodium, calcium, and potassium) in blood and other body fluids. As free ions, minerals play an important part in water and acid-base balance, nerve impulse transmission, and muscle contraction, and as catalysts for enzymatic reactions.

Major Minerals
Calcium
Phosphorus
Magnesium
Sodium
Potassium
Chlorine
Sulfur
Trace Minerals
Iron
Copper
Zinc
Iodine
Fluorine
Chromium
Cobalt
Manganese
Molybdenum
Selenium
Silicon
Tin
Vanadium
Nickel

In terms of quantitative distribution most minerals function primarily as structural components of body tissues.

The essential minerals resemble water-soluble vitamins in another respect: Most are not stored by the body in significant amounts, and so must be supplied in the daily diet. When dietary intake is adequate, the quantities of nearly all essential minerals found in the body and the various body compartments are closely regulated. If the body is viewed as a system with an input and an output, it becomes clear that absorption and excretion can serve to control mineral balance. In fact, tissue levels of some minerals are controlled by the efficiency of absorption. For minerals whose absorption is almost completely efficient, the amounts excreted in urine are modified according to the needs of the organism. These controls protect the body against both deficiency and potentially toxic accumulations, and can be described as "gatekeeper" regulatory mechanisms. In addition there exist other internal control mechanisms that regulate the distribution of minerals throughout body tissues.

Chemically, the essential minerals are the simplest nutrients found in the body. Nonetheless, nutritional scientists still have a great deal to learn about these elements. Until recently, research has been greatly hampered by the difficulty of measuring the minute quantities in which minerals exist in the body and in foods. In the past decade, however, technological advances have led to the development of new analytical techniques. With the resulting increase in knowledge has come the discovery that the functions of some minerals are interrelated. The absorption, metabolism, mode of action, and, indeed, the dietary requirements for many minerals may be modified by the presence or absence of other minerals.

THE MAJOR MINERALS

Of the essential minerals, seven are required in amounts greater than 100 milligrams per day, are present in the body in quantities representing at least 0.05 percent of body weight, or both. These seven major minerals are calcium, phosphorus, magnesium, sodium, potassium, chlorine, and sulfur.

Calcium

Calcium is, after carbon, hydrogen, oxygen, and nitrogen, the most abundant element in the human body. In the form of the doubly positive ion Ca^{++}, calcium is also the most abundant cation in the body. Though it is best known for its role in bone development, this mineral has other very important functions.

DISTRIBUTION IN THE BODY. The calcium content of the average healthy adult is a little less than 2 percent of body weight and represents half of the total mineral content of the body. Thus for a body weight of 70 kilograms (154 lb), the calcium content is 1,200 to 1,250 grams. Of this amount, almost all (99 percent) is deposited in bone and dental tissue. The remaining 1 percent is located in extracellular fluid, including blood.

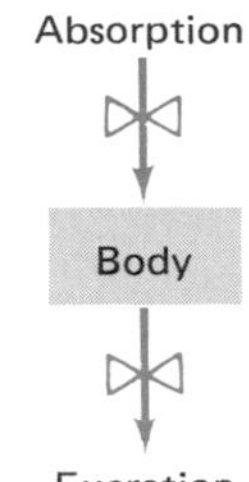

Symbol for the "gatekeeper" mechanism that regulates intake and output.

METABOLISM AND PHYSIOLOGICAL FUNCTIONS: I. ABSORPTION. Calcium is absorbed into the body from the small intestine primarily by active transport, which requires the assistance of vitamin D. Some passive diffusion also occurs. The body normally absorbs between 30 and 40 percent of ingested calcium. Active absorption appears to be controlled by a "gatekeeper" mechanism of the kind described above. The rate of absorption increases with decreased dietary intake of calcium, and with the increased physiological need for the mineral that occurs during growth, pregnancy, and lactation.

A number of other factors affect calcium absorption as well. Parathyroid hormone (PTH) increases calcium absorption by increasing the conversion of vitamin D to its active form (see Chapter 6). Amino acids appear to increase the solubility of calcium and therefore enhance its absorption. Lactose also increases the solubility of calcium. Since lactose is the primary sugar in milk and since milk is commercially fortified with vitamin D, this beverage is an excellent source of the mineral.

Factors that decrease calcium absorption include vitamin D deficiency; decreased intestinal acidity (high pH), more common in later age; diarrhea; and any condition that generally results in malabsorption. Oxalic acid, which is found in chocolate, spinach, beet tops, collard greens, and several other vegetables, combines with dietary calcium to form an insoluble compound, thereby binding calcium and making it unavailable for absorption. But normally this is not a concern because the total amount of dietary calcium greatly exceeds the amount of dietary oxalate, so that the effect of the latter is insignificant. Phytic acid, which is found in relatively large amounts in the outer layers of cereal grains and therefore in cereal products containing unrefined grain, also binds dietary calcium to form an insoluble complex known as **phytate.** Here again the effect is not significant unless extensive consumption of phytic acid-containing foods is accompanied by low calcium intake. This may be a concern to strict vegetarians (vegans), although a well-varied vegetarian diet should compensate for any imbalance. Free fatty acids, particularly the saturated variety, may also combine with calcium to form the type of insoluble complexes known as soaps.

Further, it has long been believed that the absorption of calcium is maximized when dietary calcium and phosphorus are present in approximately equal amounts. There is evidence that diets with a low calcium: phosphorus ratio produce bone resorption in rats and dogs due to decreased calcium absorption (*Nutrition Reviews*, 1973). This finding has generated some concern because in most American diets phosphorus intake is greater than that of calcium, resulting in a calcium:phosphorus ratio of 1:2 (National Center for Health Statistics, 1977). Studies with monkeys who were fed diets with low calcium:phosphorus ratios, however, showed no evidence of bone disease during a seven-year observation period (Anderson et al., 1977). Extension of these experiments to humans has demonstrated that at a wide range of calcium intakes calcium absorption was unaffected when dietary phosphorus was increased (Spencer et al., 1978). These and other studies have produced no evidence to date that diets with a low calcium:phosphorus ratio are detrimental to healthy humans. Future studies will undoubtedly attempt to confirm these findings and to clarify the significance of the dietary calcium:phosphorus ratio.

METABOLISM AND PHYSIOLOGICAL FUNCTIONS: II. FUNCTIONS. Following absorption, calcium enters the blood stream and is transported to body tissues. The major site of deposition is bone. In the process of bone mineralization, an inorganic calcium-containing complex interacts with an organic substance, cartilage. The inorganic complex, known as *hydroxyapatite*, consists of phosphorus and hydroxide ions in addition to calcium. The organic components of cartilage are collagen and mucopolysaccharides. Bone, then, constitutes the major reservoir of body calcium, accounting for about 99 percent of the total. Readily available stores of the mineral are located particularly in the ends of long bones, known as trabeculae. When the trabecular stores become exhausted (which might happen as a result of a prolonged dietary calcium deficiency) and dietary intake continues to be insufficient, calcium is withdrawn from the shafts of the bones to meet physiological needs. As calcium is removed, the bone becomes weakened.

Bone formation or **ossification** begins during fetal development, proceeds rapidly during the growth years, and continues throughout life as a dynamic metabolic process. As we saw in Chapter 6, bone mineralization is mediated by bone-synthesizing osteoblasts, and bone resorption by bone-destroying osteoclasts. Together these two types of specialized cells are responsible for the continuous remodeling of bone.

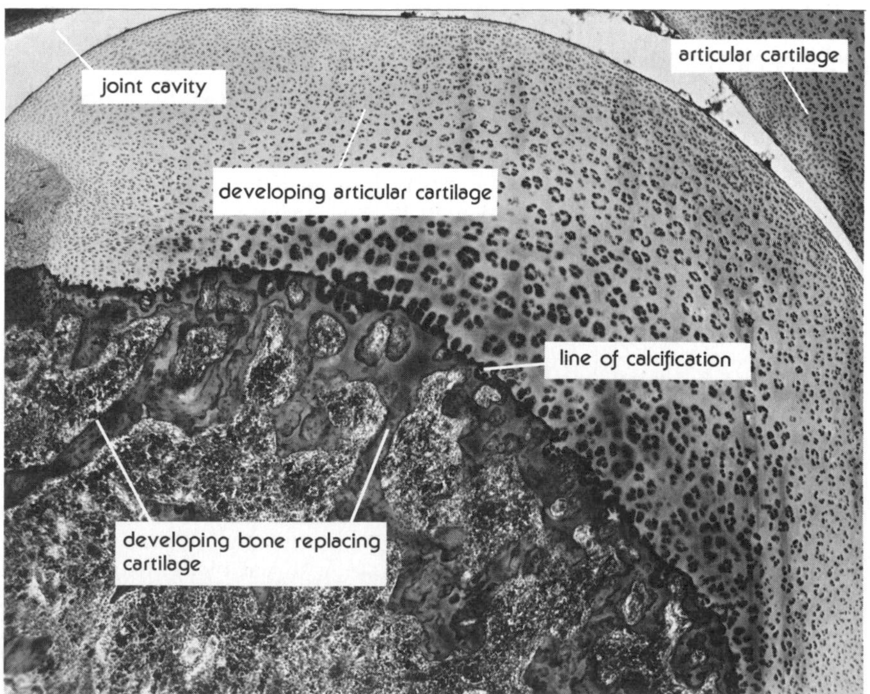

Developing bone and cartilage in the finger of a human fetus.
articular cartilage
joint cavity
developing articular cartilage
line of calcification
developing bone replacing cartilage
(Lester V. Bergman & Associates, Inc.)

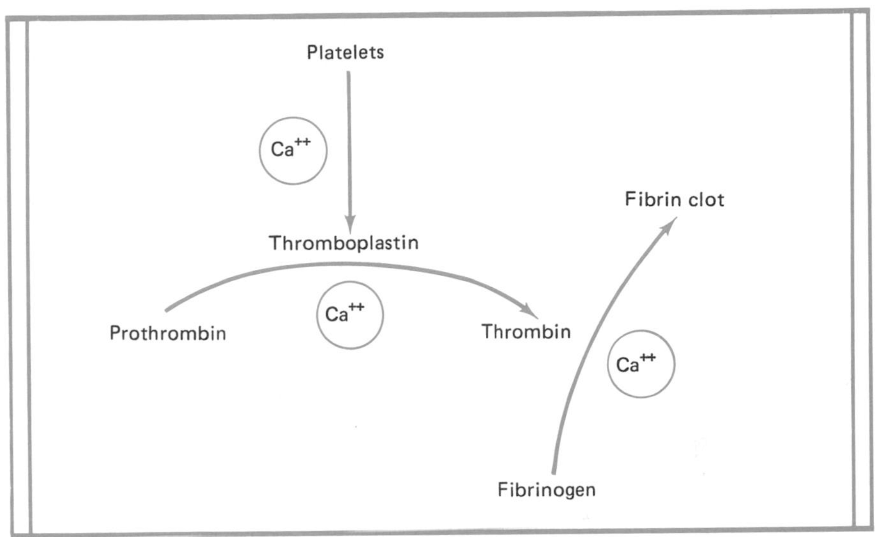

FIGURE 8-1
The Role of Calcium in the Blood Clotting Process
Calcium is a factor at three key points in the clotting process. This process begins with the exposure of collagen in the walls of the broken blood vessels, causing platelets to gather in the vicinity of the wound. In the presence of Ca^{++}, (1) platelets release thromboplastin, which, in the presence of Ca^{++}, (2) activates prothrombin and causes it to change to thrombin, which, again in the presence of Ca^{++}, (3) converts soluble fibrinogen to insoluble fibrin, thus forming the hardened, protective blood clot which seals off the outside of the wound. This is a "cascade" reaction, in which each successive step is initiated by the step that immediately precedes it.

Thus calcium enters and leaves the skeleton continuously. The relative rates of mineralization and resorption are key factors in determining the structural integrity of bone. Estimates indicate that between 600 and 700 milligrams of calcium are removed from, and added to, the bones of a normal adult *every day*. At that rate, the total calcium content of the skeleton is replaced once every five years.

Tooth formation, which also begins during fetal development, requires calcium. This process resembles bone formation in several respects: Calcium and phosphorus (as well as magnesium and fluorine) mineralize an organic (protein) matrix to give teeth their rigidity. (The importance of nutrients to dental health during the growth years will be discussed in Chapter 13.) Unlike bone calcium, tooth calcium cannot be replaced once it has been lost.

Calcium plays an important part in other body processes as well. In particular, blood clotting requires calcium at several steps in a series of interconnected reactions (see Figure 8-1). Calcium is required for the absorption of dietary vitamin B_{12} (Chapter 7); for the synthesis of the neurotransmitter acetylcholine; for activation of several important enzymes, such as pancreatic lipase; and for the regulation of muscle relaxation and contraction.

The great importance of calcium is emphasized by the fact that serum levels of the mineral are maintained within very narrow limits. The normal range of serum calcium is 9 to 11 mg/dl. *Hypocalcemia* results in tetany, a condition characterized by stiff, contracted muscles and increased nerve activation. *Hypercalcemia,* on the other hand, produces calcium deposition in soft tissues, such as the heart and kidneys. But these conditions result from abnormalities in the regulating mechanisms rather than from dietary deficiency or excess of calcium. Hypercalcemia also results from excessive vitamin D intake.

The maintenance of serum calcium within strict limits is so important that several mechanisms exist to regulate it. (There is a similarity between this multiple regulatory system and that of blood glucose described in Chapter 2.) Serum calcium can be raised by increasing the activation rate of vitamin D and thereby increasing absorption of dietary calcium; the peptide hormone secreted by the parathyroid glands, PTH, serves this function. And vitamin D and PTH both act to release calcium from storage sites in bone and to reduce urinary excretion of the mineral. But if serum calcium exceeds optimal levels, an antagonist of PTH is produced by the thyroid gland. This antagonist, the peptide hormone calcitonin, indirectly counteracts the effects of PTH by decreasing the conversion of vitamin D to its active form, thus diminishing the absorption of dietary calcium. At the same time, calcitonin directly slows the rate of release of calcium from bone. The mechanism by which the hormone acts on the kidney to modify urinary excretion remains unclear. These controls act in combination as a "gatekeeper," letting calcium "in" and "out" as needed.

METABOLISM AND PHYSIOLOGICAL FUNCTIONS: III. EXCRETION. Perspiration, feces, and urine all provide routes for loss of body calcium. Under normal circumstances perspiration losses amount to 15 to 20 milligrams per day. Profuse sweating may lead to greater losses. Fecal calcium consists both of unabsorbed dietary calcium and of calcium secreted into the gut from endogenous sources such as digestive juices. Fecal loss of endogenous calcium ranges from 125 to 180 milligrams per day; variable amounts of dietary calcium are lost in the feces, depending on dietary intake.

Calcium loss through urinary excretion, usually 100 to 200 milligrams per day, appears to be fairly constant for any one individual but varies widely from individual to individual. However, recent research has demonstrated that urinary loss is greatly influenced by the amount of protein consumed in the diet—the higher the intake of protein, the greater the loss of urinary calcium. Moreover, increased consumption of calcium does not compensate for the losses resulting from high protein intake, since the additional calcium is not absorbed in proportion to urinary excretion. A recent study has confirmed that a high-protein diet (approximately 150 grams per day) increases urinary calcium excretion. Moreover, dietary phosphorus also modifies the loss of urinary calcium: A high phosphorus intake (2,525 mg/day) reduced urinary calcium excretion and improved calcium balance. However, the demonstrated effect of phosphorus did not completely eliminate the effect of the high-protein diet on either urinary calcium excretion or calcium balance in the experimental subjects (Hegsted et al., 1979). Consequently, a diet rich in protein, especially if it is low in calcium, carries with it the potential risk of calcium deficiency. Because the average American diet contains a large amount of protein, additional protein intake may have an adverse effect on calcium status. High protein intake probably explains, at least in part, why

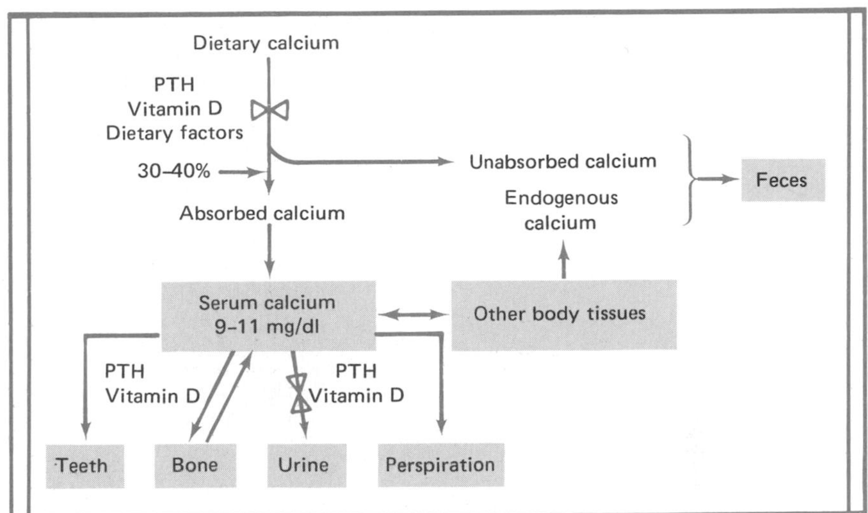

FIGURE 8-2
Summary of Calcium Metabolism

Eskimos, who commonly ingest as much as 200 grams of protein per day, have a high incidence of osteoporosis, a condition characterized by bone resorption and weakening.

A summary of calcium metabolism is presented in Figure 8-2.

DIETARY ALLOWANCES. The present RDA for adults is 800 milligrams. This value was established by adding the average daily losses and correcting for the average absorption rate:

$$\left.\begin{array}{r}175 \text{ mg (urine)} \\ +125 \text{ mg (feces)} \\ +\ \ 20 \text{ mg (perspiration)}\end{array}\right\} = 320 \text{ mg/day} \div 40\% = 800 \text{ mg/day}$$

Some nutritionists consider the RDA to be unrealistically high since many people appear to be in good health although consuming lesser amounts of calcium. Moreover, the Food and Agricultural Organization recommends a daily intake of only 400 to 500 milligrams for adults.

But others consider the present RDA to be too low, especially for women. There is some evidence that a daily intake of 1,200 milligrams is necessary to maintain calcium balance in this group, and a recent report suggests that calcium supplementation can minimize and even reverse osteoporosis in older women (Albanese et al., 1978). Although it has been postulated that adaptation to low intakes occurs, it may be that such adaptation is not ideal and that effects of long-term suboptimal intake begin to appear in later life. Related to these considerations, and in view of the high protein intakes in the American diet, there have been suggestions that the calcium RDA should be increased.

DIETARY SOURCES. The primary sources of dietary calcium are dairy products (with the exception of butter), which provide 75 percent of the calcium in the American diet (Marston and Friend, 1976). Milk, cheese, ice cream, and yogurt are significant sources.

TABLE 8-1 **Calcium Content of Selected Foods**
RDA for Adults 800 mg

Food	Serving Size	Calcium Content mg/serving
Yogurt, plain, low-fat	8 oz	415
Sardines, Atlantic, in oil	1 can = $3\frac{1}{4}$ oz	402
Milk, low-fat + protein fortified	1 c	352
Yogurt, fruit-flavored, low-fat + milk solids	8 oz	345
Milk, skim	1 c	302
Milk, whole	1 c	291
Salmon, red, canned	$3\frac{1}{2}$ oz	285
Yogurt, whole-milk, plain	8 oz	274
Cheddar cheese	1 oz	204
American cheese, pasteurized, processed	1 oz	174
Tofu (soybean curd)	1 cake ($2\frac{1}{2}'' \times 2\frac{3}{4}'' \times 1''$)	154
Oysters, raw	½ c	113
Collard greens, cooked	½ c	110
Spinach, frozen, cooked	½ c	100
Ice cream, 10% fat	½ c	88
Beet greens, cooked	½ c	72
Soybeans, cooked	½ c	66
Molasses, medium	1 tbsp	58
Orange	1 medium	54
Beans, navy type, cooked	½ c	48
Clams, raw, meat only	4 or 5	48
Beans, green, cooked	⅔ c	42
Beans, red kidney, cooked	½ c	35
Egg	1 large	28
Egg yolk	1 large	26
Bread, whole-wheat	1 slice	25
Lentils, cooked	½ c	25
Cottage cheese, uncreamed	½ c	23
Bread, white, enriched	1 slice	21
Bran flakes, 40%	1 c	19
Yeast, dried brewers	1 tbsp	17
Halibut, broiled	3 oz	15
Apple, 3″ diameter	1	12
Apricots, dried	5 medium halves	12
Broccoli, frozen, cooked	3 spears	12
Liver, calf, cooked	3 oz	11
Hamburger, 21% fat, cooked	3 oz	9
Peanut butter	1 tbsp	9
Chicken, white meat, cooked	2 pieces	6
Egg white	1 large	4
Sugar, brown	1 tsp	3
Butter or margarine	1 pat = 1 tsp	1
Vegetable oil	1 tsp	0
Sugar, white	1 tsp	0

Sources: C. F. Adams, *Nutritive value of American foods in common units,* USDA Agriculture Handbook No. 456 (Washington, D.C.: U.S. Government Printing Office, 1975); L. P. Posati, and M. L. Orr, *Composition of foods—Dairy and egg products—Raw, processed, prepared,* USDA Agriculture Handbook No. 8-1 (Washington, D.C.: U.S. Government Printing Office, 1976).

Other foods of high protein content provide variable amounts of this mineral. Clams, oysters, shrimp, and canned salmon (including the soft bones) are moderately good sources, although they are not eaten frequently or in large amounts by most people. Red meats, poultry, and most fish are not considered good sources. Liver, many readers will be pleased to learn, is *not* a good source. By contrast, tofu, or soybean curd, contains significant amounts of calcium. Nuts, seeds, and legumes are good sources, and with vegetables constitute the primary source of calcium for vegetarians. Spinach, collard greens, beet greens, and other leafy dark green varieties provide the largest amounts of calcium among vegetables. Fruits contain smaller quantities. Bread and grain products contribute some calcium, especially if the mold-preventive calcium propionate and dry milk solids have been added.

Table 8-1 indicates the calcium content of selected food items. In contrast to some sources of vitamins, no one food can provide the RDA for calcium in a single serving. This table does not indicate, however, a number of nondietary sources, such as water supply, rocks used for grinding and cooking (for example, in Mexico, South America, and Japan), and contaminants in many of the foods available in traditional societies.

DISTURBANCES IN CALCIUM METABOLISM. Hypocalcemia and hypercalcemia may result from disturbances in the calcium regulating system. It is a matter of considerable controversy whether osteoporosis is due to a dietary deficiency of calcium. This disorder, which can be defined as reduction of total bone mass and must be distinguished from osteomalacia (adult rickets; see Chapter 6), is particularly common among the elderly in all parts of the world, including the United States. At present, while the evidence does not support classifying osteoporosis as a calcium deficiency disease, it does suggest a role for the mineral in prevention and treatment. Apparently a number of factors are involved, and additional research is needed to clarify this role.

The role of calcium in periodontal disease is even less clear. This condition involves the progressive breakdown of gum tissue and supporting bone and is by far the main cause of tooth loss in adults. Calcium status may be one of several factors related to this disorder.

Phosphorus

The presence of phosphorus in the activated forms of various energy-releasing vitamins and ATP gives some indication of just how important this mineral is in the physiology and biochemistry of the body. But phosphorus has not received as much attention as other nutrients. This neglect may be due to the fact that phosphorus occurs in all plant and animal cells, and therefore in all cell-containing foods, as well as in noncellular foods such as milk. As a result, deficiency is almost unknown in humans except under certain unusual circumstances.

DISTRIBUTION IN THE BODY. Phosphorus is the second most common mineral in the body and resembles calcium in its distribution in body tissues. Phosphorus represents 0.8 to 1.2 percent of human body weight, approximately 650 grams, or about half the amount of body calcium. Bones and teeth contain 80 to 90 percent of body phosphorus, the remainder being found in body cells and the blood.

METABOLISM AND PHYSIOLOGICAL FUNCTIONS: I. ABSORPTION. Dietary phosphorus is absorbed into the body as soluble phosphate ions (PO_4^-). Combination of phosphorus with iron and magnesium will decrease its absorption. Similarly, the phosphorus-containing phytic acid found in whole-grain cereals combines with calcium to form phytate, which, because it is insoluble, prevents both the calcium and phosphorus from being absorbed. Altogether, as much as 30 percent of dietary phosphorus passes through the gastrointestinal tract without being absorbed. As it does with calcium, vitamin D increases absorption of phosphorus from the intestine.

METABOLISM AND PHYSIOLOGICAL FUNCTIONS: II. FUNCTIONS. The 70 percent or more of dietary phosphorus that enters the body functions in a variety of roles:

1. In the mineralization of bones and teeth (as a major component, along with calcium, of hydroxyapatite). Decreased mineralization of bone results as much from phosphorus deficiency as it does from calcium deficiency.
2. As a component of various compounds essential for energy metabolism including the phosphorylated vitamins (thiamin, niacin, riboflavin, pyridoxine), and ATP, the production of which also requires phosphorus-containing intermediates.
3. In absorption and transport of nutrients. Glucose must be phosphorylated in order to be absorbed from the intestine and to enter the cells of the body. Phospholipids represent the chief means of transporting lipids throughout the body fluids.
4. As components of the nucleic acids (DNA and RNA), which are vital to heredity and protein synthesis.
5. In the regulation of acid-base balance. Phosphate compounds are effective buffers.

Serum levels of phosphorus range from 35 to 45 mg/dl. Like calcium, body phosphorus remains in dynamic equilibrium between cells and fluids and is continuously released from and incorporated into bone.

METABOLISM AND PHYSIOLOGICAL FUNCTIONS: III. EXCRETION. In contrast to calcium, for which absorption is controlled, urinary excretion provides the gatekeeper mechanism for regulating the amount of phosphorus in the body. Relatively small amounts, representing nonabsorbed and endogenous phosphorus, are excreted in the feces. As Figure 8-3 indicates, both vitamin D and PTH affect the rate at which the kidneys reabsorb phosphorus to increase serum levels of the mineral. Vitamin D increases reabsorption from the kidney, while PTH increases urinary excretion of phosphorus.

DIETARY ALLOWANCES. Except for infants, the recommended allowances are the same as those for calcium—that is, 800 milligrams for adults. For newborn infants, the allowances for calcium and phosphorus are 360 and 240 milligrams, respectively. Infants are at risk of developing hypocalcemia and possibly tetany not only because of the depressing effect of phosphorus on calcium absorption, but also because in the first months of life PTH is not produced quickly enough or in adequate quantity in response to lowered

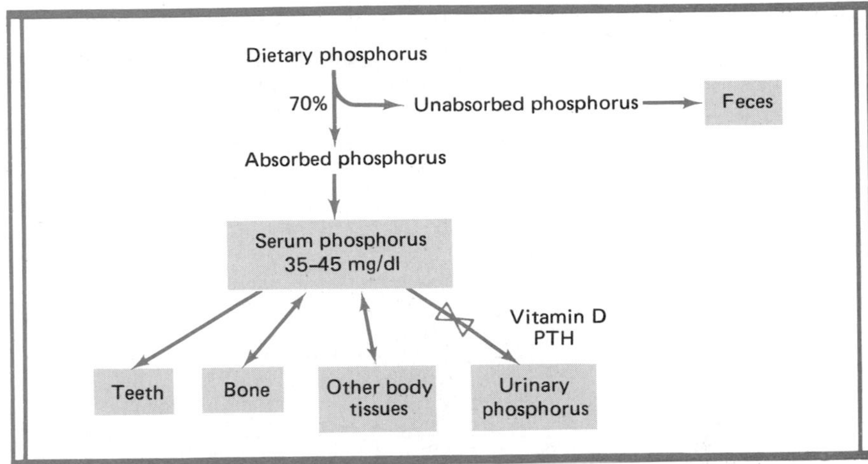

FIGURE 8-3
Summary of Phosphorus Metabolism

serum calcium levels. Therefore, to prevent neonatal tetany (or neonatal hypocalcemia), the recommended allowance provides for a relative reduction of phosphorus to give a calcium:phosphorus ratio of 1.5:1.0 in newborns.

DIETARY SOURCES. Because of the widespread distribution of phosphorus in foods, primary deficiency is highly unlikely. The milk and meat groups provide the most important sources of the mineral. High-protein foods in general are good sources, and carbonated beverages contain significant amounts of phosphorus, up to 500 milligrams in 12 ounces. Table 8-2 lists the phosphorus content of a variety of foods. It should be noted that the phosphorus values given in food composition tables include the amounts present in phytic acid, and therefore may not all be biologically available. However, during the leavening and baking of whole-wheat bread, phosphorus is released from phytic acid, minimizing calcium and phosphorus malabsorption. Habitual consumption of unleavened bread, in which the phytic acid remains intact, may contribute to the development of bone disease, particularly when vitamin D and calcium intakes are low.

DISTURBANCES IN PHOSPHORUS METABOLISM. Although primary deficiency of phosphorus is rare, excessive and long-term use of antacids that contain aluminum hydroxide can produce symptoms of hypophosphatemia—weakness, anorexia (loss of appetite), and bone demineralization. Other factors and conditions, including use of anticonvulsants (e.g., phenobarbital), vitamin D deficiency, certain metabolic abnormalities, and inadequate reabsorption by the kidneys, can produce symptoms of phosphorus deficiency. Hyperphosphatemia can result from renal disease.

Magnesium

The characteristic purgative effects of magnesium became known, almost two centuries before the element itself was identified, with the accidental discovery of a pool of bitter-tasting water in the village of Epsom, England, in

TABLE 8-2
Phosphorus Content of Selected Foods
RDA for Adults
800 mg

Food	Serving Size	Phosphorus Content mg/serving
Liver, beef, cooked	3 oz	405
Yogurt, low-fat + milk solids	8 oz	326
Yogurt, fruit-flavored + milk solids	8 oz	271
Chicken, cooked	3½ oz	266
Milk, skim	1 c	247
Milk, 2% fat	1 c	232
Milk, whole	1 c	228
Yogurt, plain, whole-milk	8 oz	215
American cheese, pasteurized, processed	1 oz	211
Haddock, fried	3 oz	210
Tuna, canned	3½ oz	188
Swiss cheese	1 oz	171
Soybeans, cooked	½ c	161
Hamburger, 21% fat, cooked	3 oz	159
Cheddar cheese	1 oz	145
Bran flakes, 40%	1 c	125
Potato, baked in skin	1 medium	101
Egg	1 large	90
Egg yolk	1 large	86
Peas, green, cooked	½ c	79
Frankfurter	1	76
Cottage cheese, uncreamed	½ c	75
Ice cream, 10% fat	½ c	67
Peanut butter	1 tbsp	61
Bread, whole-wheat	1 slice	57
Collard greens, cooked	½ c	50
Broccoli, cooked	½ c	48
Avocado	1 half	47
Raisins	small box = 1½ oz	43
Spinach, cooked	½ c	34
Orange	1 medium	33
Rice, cooked	½ c	28
Bread, white, enriched	1 slice	28
Banana	1 medium	27
Tomato	1 medium	25
Carrots, cooked	½ c	24
Green beans, cooked	½ c	23
Egg white	1 large	4
Butter	1 pat = 1 tsp	1
Margarine	1 pat = 1 tsp	0.7

Sources: C. F. Adams, *Nutritive value of American foods in common units,* USDA Agriculture Handbook No. 456 (Washington, D.C.: U.S. Government Printing Office, 1975); L. P. Posati, and M. L. Orr, *Composition of foods—Dairy and egg products—Raw, processed, prepared,* USDA Agriculture Handbook No. 8-1 (Washington, D.C.: U.S. Government Printing Office, 1976).

1618. People who drank the water felt healthfully purified, and later in the century its salts were crystallized and marketed, to great acclaim. Sir Humphrey Davy isolated magnesium, the key component of Epsom salts, in 1808, and since then this element has become well known for its use in photographic flashes, flares, and incendiary bombs, and as a metal greatly valued for its lightness in space-age technology.

Magnesium is to plants what iron is—as we shall see below—to animals. Just as iron is the "core" atom of hemoglobin, magnesium is the "core" atom of chlorophyll, the green pigment that enables plants, in the presence of light, to transform carbon dioxide and water into carbohydrates. It thus has some claim to being, after carbon, the element most important to life.

DISTRIBUTION IN THE BODY. The human body contains considerably less magnesium than it does either calcium or phosphorus. The total magnesium content of an adult weighing 70 kilograms (154 lb) averages between 20 and 28 grams. Of this total, a little over half (55 percent) occurs in bone; slightly more than one quarter (27 percent) in muscle; and the remainder in other soft tissues, serum, and red blood cells.

METABOLISM AND PHYSIOLOGICAL FUNCTIONS. The body absorbs about 35–40 percent of dietary magnesium by active transport from the intestine. However, the percent absorbed varies inversely with dietary intake. That is, as dietary magnesium increases in quantity, the efficiency of absorption decreases. In this respect magnesium resembles calcium and may even share the same transport system. Many of the factors that influence calcium absorption also affect the absorption of magnesium, though to a lesser degree; the intestine apparently is not a major control point in magnesium metabolism. Also, there is little fecal excretion of endogenous magnesium.

The physiological importance of magnesium is clearly reflected in the number and variety of its functions in the body. Many of these functions depend on the mineral's ability to interact with calcium, phosphate, and carbonate ions. In a complicated relationship, magnesium plays an important role in bone metabolism. Equally important, this mineral catalyzes many essential enzymatic reactions, playing a crucial role in glucose and fatty acid metabolism, amino acid activation, and synthesis of ATP. Protein synthesis also requires magnesium, directly or indirectly, at several different stages. Magnesium is also important (along with calcium, sodium, potassium, and phosphorus) in nervous activity and muscle contraction. At certain stages of neuromuscular activity the interaction between magnesium and calcium is antagonistic; at others, synergistic (enhancing). Such interactions are particularly significant because the metabolism of calcium, sodium, and potassium are all affected by any deficiency of magnesium.

Serum levels of this essential mineral are controlled by urinary excretion, which is influenced by the adrenal hormone **aldosterone** (see Chapter 9). When usual amounts of magnesium are ingested, urinary excretion normally amounts to 100 to 200 milligrams of the mineral per day. This amount, however, is rapidly diminished if intake decreases, and as quickly increases in response to more ample supplies.

DIETARY ALLOWANCES. Because the magnesium content of foods is

TABLE 8-3
Magnesium Content of Selected Foods
RDA for Adults
Men: 350 mg
Women: 300 mg

Food	Serving Size	Magnesium Content mg/serving
Peanuts, roasted	¼ c	63
Banana	1 medium	58
Beet greens, raw	1 c	58
Avocado	1 half	56
Molasses, blackstrap	1 tbsp	52
Cashew nuts	9 medium	52
Milk, 2% fat, protein fortified	1 c	40
Swiss chard, raw	1 c	37
Milk, whole	1 c	33
Yogurt, fruit-flavored, + milk solids	8 oz	33
Collard greens, raw	1 c	31
Milk, skim	1 c	28
Peanut butter	1 tbsp	28
Spinach, raw	1 c	28
Oysters, raw	6 medium	27
Yogurt, plain	8 oz	26
Macaroni, cooked	1 c	26
Pork, fresh, roasted	3 oz	25
Turkey, light meat, roasted	3 oz	24
Wheat bran	1 tbsp	20
Wheat germ	1 tbsp	20
Hamburger, lean, cooked	3 oz	20
Haddock, fried	3 oz	20
Bread, whole-wheat	1 slice	19
Carrots, raw	1 medium	19
Yeast, brewer's	1 tbsp	18
Chicken, broiled w/o skin	3 oz	16
Orange, peeled	1 medium	15
Apple, 3″ diameter	1	14
Beans, green, frozen	½ c	14
Ice cream, 10% fat	½ c	9
Cheddar cheese	1 oz	8
American cheese	1 oz	6
Bacon, cooked	3 strips	6
Egg, whole	1 large	6
Bread, white	1 slice	5.5
Cornflakes	1 c	4
Egg yolk	1 large	3
Egg white	1 large	3
Mushrooms, raw	¼ c	2
Butter	1 pat = 1 tsp	trace
Vegetable oil	1 tbsp	0

Sources: C. F. Adams, *Nutritive value of American foods in common units,* USDA Agriculture Handbook No. 456 (Washington, D.C.: U.S. Government Printing Office, 1975); L. P. Posati, and M. L. Orr, *Composition of foods—Dairy and egg products—Raw, processed, prepared,* USDA Agriculture Handbook No. 8-1 (Washington, D.C.: U.S. Government Printing Office, 1976); Consumer and Food Economics Institute, *Composition of foods, raw, processed, prepared,* USDA Handbook No. 8, rev. ed. (Washington, D.C.: U.S. Government Printing Office, 1963).

highly variable, dietary intakes of the mineral are also variable. According to current estimates, typical American diets provide from 180 to 480 mg of magnesium per day, or 120 mg per 1,000 kcal. Various studies have led to the establishment of RDAs of 350 mg for adult males, and 300 mg for adult females (Food and Nutrition Board, 1979). Thus, intake of 300 mg of magnesium would require a 2,500 kcal intake. Many individuals, therefore, especially women, may not consume the recommended amounts of magnesium. It appears that women lose less of the mineral and are able to maintain equilibrium levels on lower intake than men (Krehl, 1967). Symptoms of magnesium deficiency are not prevalent, and the body may well adjust to less than optimal intakes.

DIETARY SOURCES. Of commonly eaten foods, in the portions usually consumed, dairy products are the best sources of magnesium, followed (in order of decreasing content) by breads and cereals, vegetables, meats and poultry, and fruits. Of the vegetables, green leafy types are best, owing to their chlorophyll content. Legumes and whole grains also contain significant amounts of magnesium. Some loss of the mineral results from food processing and preparation, including loss when cooking water is discarded. Table 8-3 gives the magnesium content of selected foods.

Milk of magnesia should not be considered a dietary source of magnesium. Commonly used as a laxative, it acts osmotically by drawing water from cells into the intestine and by increasing intestinal motility. Consequently the use of milk of magnesia as an antacid (to neutralize stomach acidity) may produce diarrhea as a side effect. Because of its effect on water balance, overuse of this substance represents a potential hazard to those with kidney problems.

DISTURBANCES IN MAGNESIUM METABOLISM. Because of the mineral's wide availability in foods and because of the body's reserve in bone, depletion of body stores proceeds slowly. This may mask a borderline deficiency, and magnesium deficiency may be more common than is generally recognized.

Primary deficiency can result from dietary insufficiency, malabsorption, and prolonged, severe diarrhea and vomiting. Secondary deficiency can be caused by diuretics, overconsumption of alcohol, kidney disease, acute pancreatitis, and cirrhosis of the liver, among other disease conditions.

Regardless of cause, magnesium deficiency produces clinical symptoms indistinguishable from hypocalcemic tetany—mainly muscle contraction and nervous irritability. Other common symptoms include tremor, disorientation, and confusion.

Sodium

Although sodium can be obtained from a variety of foods, by far the best-known source is common table salt, or sodium chloride (NaCl). This compound is unique in that its historical importance has been much greater than its undeniable value as a source of nutrients would seem to justify. Wars have been fought over salt deposits. Women and children have been traded for salt. Long before similar methods were known in Europe, the Chinese had developed sophisticated techniques for obtaining salt from underground

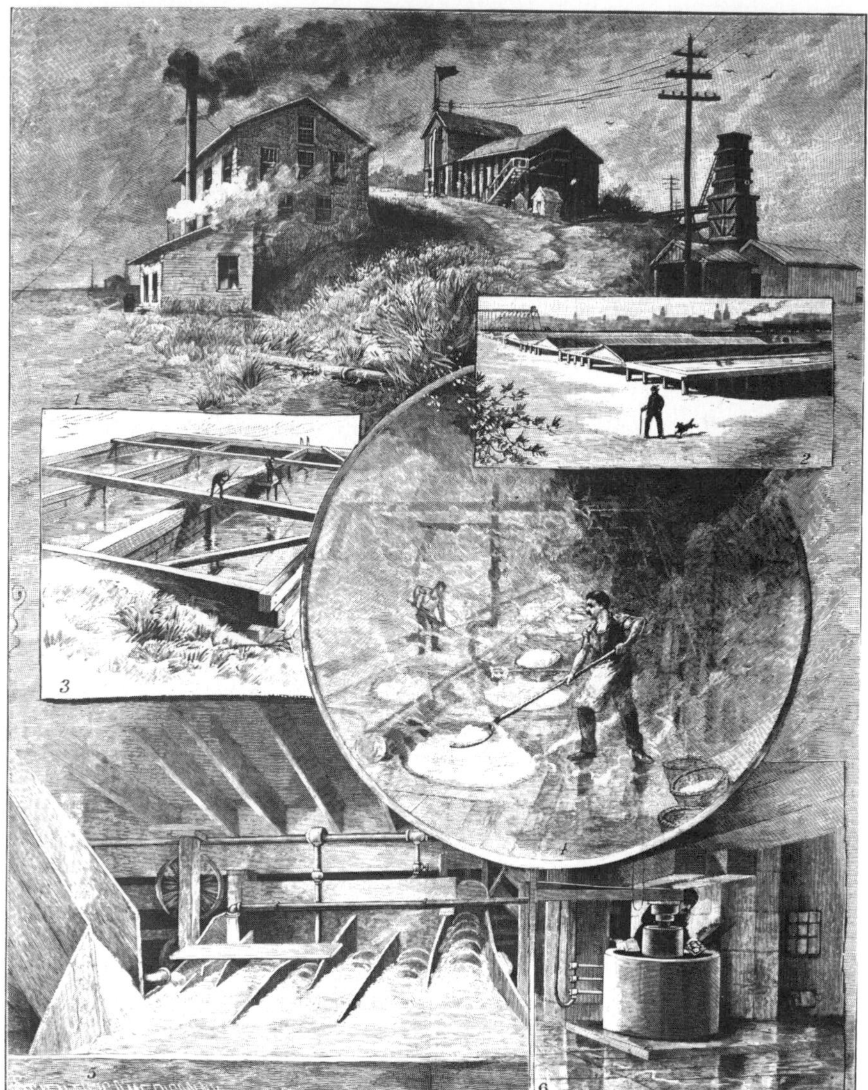

Manufacture of commercial salt in New York State, late 19th century. (The Bettmann Archive)

1. New York State pumping station and reservoir.
2. Solar evaporation.
3. Settling vats.
4. Salt boiling in kettles.
5. Washing salt.
6. Centrifugal drier.

deposits that were too deep to be mined directly. And today salt is the one mineral source for which the demand is so great that the production of dietary salt constitutes a significant industry in itself.

Herbivorous animals (cattle, deer, horses) are attracted to salt licks, but carnivores are not. Exclusively meat-eating animals apparently ingest adequate amounts of sodium with the flesh they consume. The early human diet, consisting of nondomesticated, largely carnivorous animals, provided an adequate sodium supply. But when agriculture developed, dietary intake of grains, vegetables, and domesticated herbivorous animals increased. Additional sources of salt became important during the early agricultural period, from 5,000 to 10,000 years ago in different parts of the world (Krehl, 1967).

Human sodium intakes can vary tremendously. Some people consume none other than that occurring naturally in the foods they eat. Others put salt "on everything," while the majority steer a course somewhere between these two extremes.

DISTRIBUTION IN THE BODY. The adult body contains about 120 grams of sodium. Approximately half of the total body sodium is found in body fluids outside the cells, with an additional third bound to the skeletal surface. Intracellular sodium represents only about 10 percent of that contained in the body.

METABOLISM AND PHYSIOLOGICAL FUNCTIONS. Dietary sodium is absorbed rapidly and with almost perfect efficiency, very little being lost in the feces. Absorption, therefore, does not regulate sodium metabolism.

The concentration of sodium (and other ions) in the different body fluids affects the direction of fluid movement between body compartments. In turn, the control of fluid volume is directly related to blood pressure.

Sodium also functions in the control of acid-base balance, plays a part in both carbohydrate and protein metabolism, and has a major role in the generation of nerve impulses. (A nerve impulse arises, in part, from the electrical change produced by the sudden flow of sodium ions across the nerve-cell membrane—from the outside to the inside of the nerve cell.)

As noted above, the feces normally contain very little sodium. The kidneys represent the main regulatory means for controlling the sodium content of the body. Except for losses through perspiration, the amount excreted in the urine usually balances dietary intake. Since the gatekeeper mechanism in this case is reabsorption in the tubules of the kidneys, the kidneys are able to maintain sodium balance over a wide range of dietary intakes. As Figure 8-4 indicates, however, ultimate control lies in the adrenal glands, which produce aldosterone. This hormone increases reabsorption of sodium by the kidney.

FIGURE 8-4
Summary of Sodium Metabolism

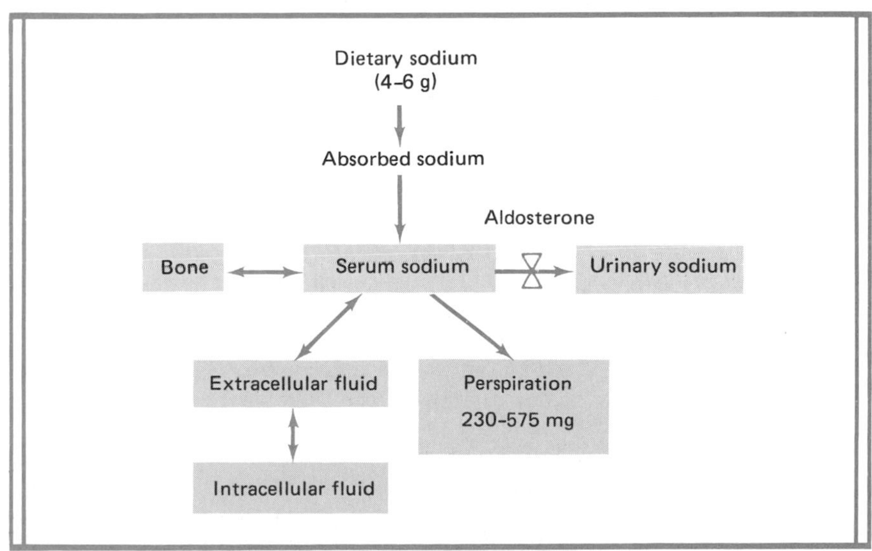

PERSPECTIVE ON
Sodium and Hypertension

The relationship between sodium and hypertension is based on the capacity of this mineral to "attract" water. When the serum level of sodium increases, the body retains water, thereby decreasing the serum sodium concentration. Blood pressure, which depends in part on blood volume, increases as retained water increases. In this way, serum levels of sodium can affect blood pressure. But sodium is not the sole cause of hypertension. If it were, all individuals would be affected in proportion to the sodium content of their diets. This is definitely not the case. Hypertension appears to be multifactorial in origin.

Among factors, other than sodium intake, that may cause elevated blood pressure are genetic predisposition, obesity, smoking, a "high-strung" or "Type A" personality, a pressured lifestyle, and general life stresses. Nonetheless, epidemiological evidence shows a clear association between sodium intake and hypertension. In populations where the daily intake is normally less than 0.5 grams of sodium per day, hypertension is almost unknown and blood pressure remains stable throughout life. In the United States blood pressure increases with age, and an estimated 20 percent of the population has hypertension; some estimates, in fact, are even higher. A diet of salty foods, as found in northern Japan, is accompanied by a frequency of hypertension several times that seen in the United States.

Patients with heart or kidney ailments have a greatly diminished capacity for excretion of sodium, with the result that sodium and fluid are retained. Because of its association with heart disease, stroke, and kidney failure, hypertension is a widespread health problem.

Some medications also modify urinary excretion. Diuretics, for example, increase sodium loss.

Loss of sodium through perspiration depends on the volume of sweat. Normal losses range from 230 to 575 milligrams per day, but heavy sweating can result in losses as great as 8 grams per day! Cystic fibrosis, a disease that affects the sweat glands, also leads to large losses of the mineral.

DIETARY ALLOWANCES AND SOURCES. The Food and Nutrition Board has not established an RDA for sodium. The average daily intake of salt, which is the chief source of dietary sodium, ranges from 6 to 24 grams. Since sodium constitutes 40 percent (by weight) of salt, this intake is equivalent to 2.4 to 9.6 grams of the mineral per day. (A pinch of salt contains 267 mg of sodium; 1 teaspoon contains 2,132 mg.) Studies have indicated that the average individual *requires* only 0.5 to 1.0 grams for nutritional health. However, this is a minimal amount and the Food and Nutrition Board (1979) recommends a daily intake of 1100–3300 mg for adults (or 1.1 to 3.3 g).

Most dietary sodium comes from table salt, but it is found also in other inorganic salts used during some food processing procedures. But sodium is found in a wide variety of foods as well (see Table 8-4)—so readily found, in fact, that it is quite difficult to eliminate this mineral from the diet. Meats and many dairy products are naturally rich in the mineral, and most processed foods contain sodium either as salt added to enhance flavor, or in a variety of preservative compounds. Moreover, salt is commonly added to food during cooking and also at the table. Drinking water contains variable amounts of salt, possibly including "road salt" used to melt snow and ice in winter. Many

Hypertension is generally treated with drugs that increase sodium excretion (diuretics) or that modify the tone and flexibility of blood vessels; dietary restriction of sodium intake; and weight loss. The loss of excess weight lowers moderately elevated blood pressure even without a reduction of sodium intake. Unfortunately, most people find taking a pill easier than eating less food or modifying their customary eating habits in any way. (Their physicians may find it more convenient as well!) For this reason, and because most Americans have become accustomed to the taste of highly salted foods, low-sodium diets are difficult for many patients to maintain.

Salt substitutes are often recommended for the hypertensive patient but should be used with caution. Most are not really substitutes, since only 50 percent of the sodium of ordinary table salt is replaced. Moreover, the replacement is usually potassium chloride, which may lead to excessive serum levels of potassium and place an additional burden on the kidneys. For persons with kidney disease, potassium-containing salt substitutes can be quite dangerous. For similar reasons, individuals with liver disease should not use ammonium-containing compounds. Patients should read content labels carefully before using, and use these substances only with a physician's approval. Those who must decrease their salt intake can find helpful and flavorful ideas in the many good cookbooks dealing with this dietary problem. The use of other seasonings, such as lemon juice, garlic, ginger, and many herbs and spices, will add flavor and variety to meals.

Can hypertension be prevented by decreasing sodium intake? Because the disorder is multifactorial in origin and its precise cause is literally unknown in the majority of cases, there are no definitive answers. Prudence, however, suggests that persons who are predisposed to hypertension would be well advised to use the salt shaker less often and to limit their intake of highly salted foods.

drugs contain sodium as well. Considering this multiplicity of sources, sodium deficiency resulting from dietary insufficiency is a rather remote possibility.

DISTURBANCES IN SODIUM METABOLISM. Lowered serum levels of sodium can result from insufficient production of adrenocortical hormones and from prolonged, excessive sweating. Prolonged diarrhea and vomiting can also produce sodium depletion. Addition of salt to drinking water (1 g $NaCl$/1 liter H_2O) or to food quickly relieves deficiency symptoms, which include nausea, giddiness, muscle cramps, and vomiting. In extreme cases, the result of sodium deficiency is circulatory failure.

Potassium

DISTRIBUTION IN THE BODY. Functionally, potassium is closely associated with sodium. But in contrast to sodium, potassium is concentrated within the cells. Nerve and muscle cells are especially rich in potassium. Fluid outside the cells contains less than 5 percent of the total body amount (approximately 250 g).

METABOLISM AND PHYSIOLOGICAL FUNCTIONS. The body absorbs potassium efficiently, and very little potassium appears in the feces.

The main functions of potassium are the same as those of sodium: maintenance of fluid balance and volume. Other functions include a role in carbohydrate metabolism, enhancement of protein synthesis, and muscle contraction and nerve impulse conduction.

TABLE 8-4
Sodium Content of Selected Foods
Estimated Safe and Adequate Daily Dietary Intake for Adults
1100–3300 mg

Food	Serving Size	Sodium Content mg/serving
Soy sauce	1 tbsp	1,319
Bouillon	1 cube	960
Olives, green, large	10	926
Ham	3 oz	770
Frankfurter	1	627
Cottage cheese, creamed	½ c	425
American cheese, pasteurized, processed	1 oz	406
Rice, cooked in salted water	½ c	383
Tomato juice, canned	6 fl. oz	364
Salad dressing, Italian	1 tbsp	314
Table salt	1 pinch	267
Bran flakes, 40%	1 c	207
Peas, canned, cooked	½ c	200
Beets, canned, cooked	½ c	200
Cheddar cheese	1 oz	176
Liver, beef, cooked	3 oz	156
Bacon, cooked	3 slices	153
Haddock, cooked	3 oz	150
Milk, 2% fat, protein fortified	1 c	145
Bread, white, enriched	1 slice	134
Bread, whole-wheat	1 slice	132
Milk, skim	1 c	126
Milk, whole	1 c	120
Peanut butter	1 tbsp	97
Egg, whole	1 large	69
Chicken, meat only	3½ oz	64
Ice cream, 10% fat	½ c	58
Celery	1 stalk	50
Egg, white	1 large	50
Hamburger, 21% fat, cooked	3 oz	49
Spinach, cooked	½ c	45
Margarine, salted	1 pat	41
Butter, salted	1 pat	41
Tuna fish	3½ oz	41
Beets, fresh, cooked	½ c	36
Carrots, cooked	½ c	26
Raisins	small box = 1½ oz	12
Egg yolk	1 large	8
Broccoli, cooked	½ c	8
Potato, baked	1 large	6
Avocado	1 half	5
Soybeans, cooked	½ c	2
Orange	1 medium	2
Peas, fresh, cooked	½ c	1
Banana	1 medium	1

Sources: C. F. Adams, *Nutritive value of American foods in common units,* USDA Agriculture Handbook No. 456 (Washington, D.C.: U.S. Government Printing Office, 1975); L. P. Posati, and M. L. Orr, *Composition of foods—Dairy and egg products—Raw, processed, prepared,* USDA Agriculture Handbook No. 8-1 (Washington, D.C.: U.S. Government Printing Office, 1976).

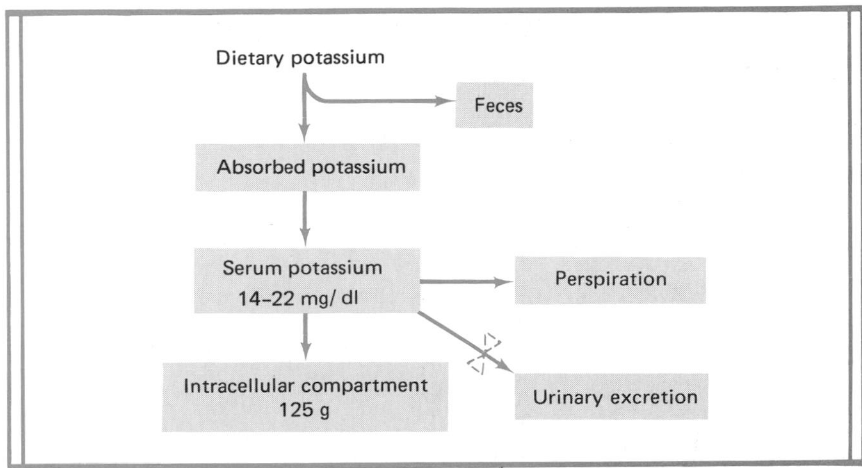

FIGURE 8-5
Summary of Potassium Metabolism

The gatekeeper mechanism for regulating body potassium is urinary excretion, which removes excess amounts of the mineral. Aldosterone increases excretion of potassium, just the opposite of its effect on sodium. The body cannot conserve potassium as efficiently as sodium, and the potential for deficiency is thus greater. Potassium is also lost through perspiration; heavy exercise in hot conditions can cause potassium losses that exceed 6 grams per day. For a summary of potassium metabolism, see Figure 8-5.

DIETARY ALLOWANCES AND SOURCES. Although the Food and Nutrition Board has not yet established an RDA for potassium it recommends a daily intake of 1875–5625 mg for adults. It is estimated that the typical American diet provides 2 to 6 grams per day.

Because the mineral is widely distributed in foods (see Table 8-5), obtaining sufficient dietary potassium presents no difficulty. Meat and dairy products (other than cheese, from which potassium is lost in the whey) are good sources. Fruits, vegetables, and whole-grain products are also good sources of potassium; these foods have the added advantage of being low in sodium.

Preparation and cooking cause some potassium loss. Water leaches out the mineral, and the loss increases with the amount of surface area exposed. To conserve potassium, food should not be finely cut, cooked in a large amount of water, or cooked in water for an extended period of time. On the other hand, these methods provide a way to reduce the potassium content of foods for those on restricted diets, as in the case of kidney disease; potatoes, for example, are cut into small cubes, soaked in water which is discarded, and finally cooked in additional water.

DISTURBANCES IN POTASSIUM METABOLISM. Potassium deficiency is rare but may result from starvation, drugs that increase its urinary excretion (such as diuretics used in the treatment of hypertension), diarrhea, and adrenal tumors (which increase the production of aldosterone). Aldosterone production is also increased when physiological or emotional stress stimulates the anterior pituitary gland to release **ACTH** (the "stress hormone"), with

TABLE 8 5
Potassium Content of Selected Foods
Estimated Safe and Adequate Daily Dietary Intake for Adults
1875–5625 mg

Food	Serving Size	Potassium Content mg/serving
Potato, baked in skin	1 medium	782
Avocado	1 half	680
Yogurt, plain, low-fat + milk solids	8 oz	531
Soybeans, cooked	½ c	486
Yogurt, fruit-flavored + milk solids	8 oz	442
Banana	1 medium	440
Chicken, meat only	3½ oz	412
Milk, skim	1 c	406
Milk, 2% fat + milk solids	1 c	397
Milk, 2% fat	1 c	377
Milk, whole	1 c	370
Yogurt, plain	8 oz	351
Raisins	small box = 1½ oz	328
Liver, beef, cooked	3 oz	323
Haddock, fried	3 oz	300
Spinach, cooked	½ c	291
Orange	1 medium	291
Tuna, canned	3½ oz	276
Collard greens, cooked	½ c	249
Tomato	1 medium	222
Hamburger, 21% fat, cooked	3 oz	221
Broccoli, cooked	½ c	207
Apple	1 medium	165
Carrots, cooked	½ c	162
Peas, green, fresh, cooked	½ c	157
Bran flakes, 40%	1 c	137
Celery	1 stalk	136
Ice cream, 10% fat	½ c	128
Frankfurter	1	125
Peanut butter	1 tbsp	100
Green beans, cooked	½ c	95
Bread, whole-wheat	1 slice	68
Coffee, prepared	1 c = 6 oz	65
Egg, whole	1 large	65
American cheese, pasteurized, processed	1 oz	46
Egg, white	1 large	45
Bacon, cooked	2 slices	35
Bread, white, enriched	1 slice	33
Rice, cooked	½ c	28
Cheddar cheese	1 oz	28
Cottage cheese, uncreamed	½ c	24
Cranberry juice	6 oz	19
Egg yolk	1 large	15
Butter or margarine	1 pat = 1 tsp	1

Sources: C. F. Adams, *Nutritive value of American foods in common units*, USDA Agriculture Handbook No. 456 (Washington, D.C.: U.S. Government Printing Office, 1975); L. P. Posati, and M. L. Orr, *Composition of foods—Dairy and egg products—Raw, processed, prepared*, USDA Agriculture Handbook No. 8-1 (Washington, D.C.: U.S. Government Printing Office, 1976).

consequent potassium loss. Clinical symptoms of deficiency include nausea, vomiting (which itself can result in potassium loss), muscle weakness, tachycardia (rapid heart beat), and—in extreme cases—cardiac failure.

Hyperkalemia, or excess potassium in the blood, occurs in cases of renal failure because the kidneys lose the ability to excrete the mineral. Severe dehydration will also produce hyperkalemia. The consequences of this condition are muscle weakness and cardiac arhythmias that lead to heart failure.

Chlorine

DISTRIBUTION IN THE BODY. As the chloride ion (Cl^-), chlorine is the primary anion found in fluid outside the cells and particularly in cerebrospinal fluid. Less than 15 percent of the body's total of 74 grams (for adults) is in intracellular fluid. Chlorine is mostly associated with sodium but also occurs in protein-bound forms.

METABOLISM AND PHYSIOLOGICAL FUNCTIONS. The body absorbs almost all dietary chlorine. The most usual source of dietary chlorine is as a component of common table salt.

Chlorine has a number of important functions in the maintenance of nutritional health. It helps maintain the acid-base balance of the blood. Chlorine is also a component of the hydrochloric acid in gastric juice and is therefore involved in the digestion of dietary protein and vitamin B_{12}. Other functions include the mineral's role in maintaining the flow and composition of body fluids and the activation of amylase enzymes that accelerate the hydrolysis of starch.

The regulatory control of chlorine levels involves the same mechanism that regulates sodium—reabsorption in the tubules of the kidneys. Excess chlorine appears in the urine. Variable amounts are lost via the feces and sweat. Because of its presence in hydrochloric acid, significant amounts of the mineral may be lost through vomiting.

DIETARY ALLOWANCES AND SOURCES. No RDAs have been established for chlorine, but the Food and Nutrition Board has recommended an intake of 1700–5100 mg per day for adults. Intake is usually adequate as long as sodium intake is sufficient. The amount of salt in the average diet assures a more than adequate dietary supply.

DISTURBANCES IN CHLORINE METABOLISM. Abnormal chlorine metabolism commonly occurs in association with disturbances in sodium metabolism. Vomiting and diarrhea can produce chloride loss, resulting in hypochloremic alkalosis. The latter may also accompany hypokalemia.

Because the kidneys excrete excess chloride, *dietary* chlorine has no known toxicity. (Note the emphasis on "dietary"—chlorine gas is deadly!)

Sulfur

DISTRIBUTION IN THE BODY. All body cells contain sulfur, chiefly as a component of the amino acids methionine and cysteine found in some proteins. Sulfur also occurs in a number of important metabolic compounds,

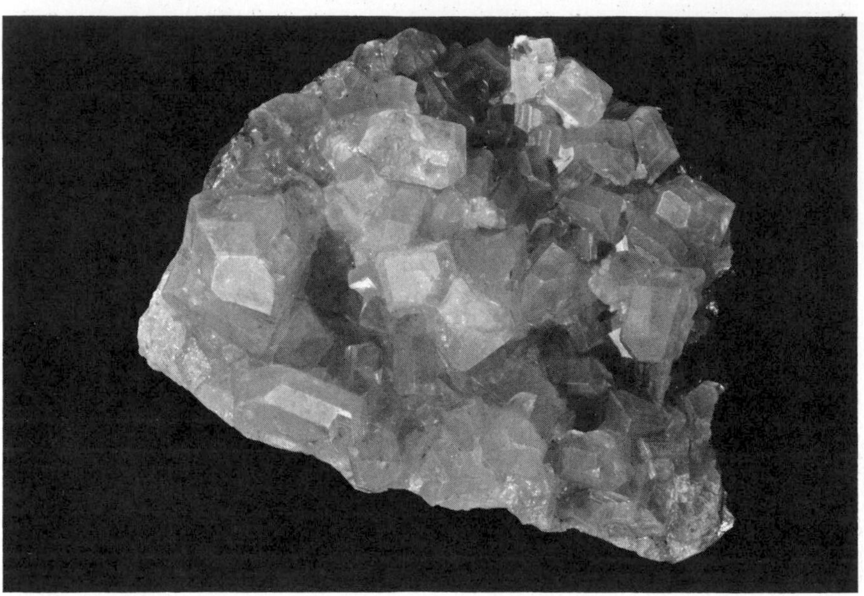

Sulphur crystals. (Courtesy of the American Museum of Natural History)

including acetyl CoA and the water-soluble vitamins thiamin and biotin. Because of the specific structural amino acids they contain, hair, skin, and nails are especially high in sulfur content.

METABOLISM AND PHYSIOLOGICAL FUNCTIONS. The body absorbs sulfur mainly in the form of sulfur-containing amino acids and absorbs the remainder as inorganic sulfate.

The important functions of sulfur include its roles as a component (1) of sulfur-containing amino acids; (2) of the sulfur groups of various compounds essential to certain oxidation-reduction reactions: coenzyme A, thiamin, biotin, glutathione; (3) in the structure of insulin and other hormones, and of the anticoagulant heparin; (4) of such compounds as the mucopolysaccharides and sulfated lipids that are components of the structural tissues of the body; and (5) of taurocholic acid, a bile acid derived in part from the amino acid cystine.

Sulfur is excreted in the urine as inorganic sulfate. Urinary output averages 2 grams per day and is proportional to nitrogen excretion (because most of the sulfate is derived from amino acid metabolism). Small amounts are excreted in the feces.

DIETARY ALLOWANCES AND SOURCES. No RDA has been established for this mineral. The sulfur content of foods parallels that of methionine and cystine. Adequate intakes are not a problem in the average American diet, with large protein intake from varied sources. Approximately 1 percent of dietary protein is sulfur. However, the amino acid composition of protein must be considered by strict vegetarians, since grains are low in the sulfur-containing essential amino acids (see Chapter 4). Vegetarians who consume a variety of foods in addition to grains are not likely to be at risk of developing a sulfur deficiency.

TRACE MINERALS

Although essential trace elements differ chemically from vitamins, they resemble the latter in several important respects: they are required by the body in very small amounts; they influence biochemical reactions, functioning either as components or activators of enzymes, vitamins, or hormones; and their nutritional function is influenced by other members of the same nutrient class.

At present the main problem facing researchers who study these micronutrients is the accurate determination of optimal nutritional requirements. The problem is important because many trace elements, although essential in very small quantities, can be toxic in larger amounts. (Copper and fluorine are two well-known examples.) The difficulty of determining requirements is aggravated because trace minerals are effective in such tiny amounts in the body, and because absorption of trace minerals is affected dramatically by the composition of the diet (fiber, phytates, and other nutrients). Only in recent years have new techniques of biochemical assay begun to analyze and accurately measure these elusive substances. In addition, the widespread use of processed foods from which trace minerals have been removed is of concern to nutritionists because inadequate intakes may be a result.

Each micronutrient can be classified in one of three groups, depending on what is known about its dietary requirement: (1) those for which a well-defined allowance has been established (iron, zinc, and iodine); (2) those for which "provisional" allowances have been suggested (copper, chromium, manganese, molybdenum, fluorine and selenium); and (3) the "newer" trace elements, which occur in such minute amounts that present analytical techniques do not permit even an estimate of dietary requirement (cobalt, silicon, tin, vanadium, and nickel). Our discussion will generally follow this grouping.

Iron

The importance of iron to the synthesis of hemoglobin in red blood cells is well known, but it is not generally appreciated that iron has other functions as well. Iron-deficiency anemia is a widespread health problem in the United States, particularly among children and women of childbearing age regardless of socioeconomic status. Iron deficiency anemia is rightly a major nutritional concern.

DISTRIBUTION IN THE BODY. Despite its great importance, the total body content of iron averages no more than several grams (0.004 percent of body weight). All body cells contain some iron, but the mineral is concentrated in red blood cells. For men, the average total body concentration ranges from 40 to 50 milligrams per kilogram of body weight. Of this amount, 60 to 70 percent is present in hemoglobin, 30 percent is stored, and the remainder functions as a component of various substances, in particular of the cytochrome enzymes of the electron-transport system (see Chapter 7). Hemoglobin and storage levels of iron are generally lower for women than for men, with the total storage iron for women ranging from 35 to 50 milligrams per kilogram of body weight.

METABOLISM AND PHYSIOLOGICAL FUNCTIONS: I. ABSORPTION. Absorption provides the gatekeeper mechanism for regulating iron metabolism. Since the body has no effective means of eliminating iron, and excess amounts are toxic, the body strictly regulates the quantities permitted to enter. Indeed, absorption of iron—which may vary from 2 to 40 percent of intake, with an average in the 5 to 15 percent range—is a complex process which is not completely understood.

Many factors influence the amount of iron absorbed. Of major importance are (1) metabolic need, which increases when iron stores are low following hemorrhage or blood donation, and during pregnancy, lactation, and growth; (2) the nature of the dietary iron; and (3) the presence or absence of other dietary nutrients that influence the absorption of iron. But to understand just how these factors affect absorption requires some understanding of the general regulatory mechanism involved.

There are two types of dietary iron, *heme* and *nonheme*. Heme iron is found in hemoglobin (hence its name) and muscle myoglobin, and is obtained exclusively from meats. The one factor that appears to determine absorption of organically bound or heme iron is iron status. If body stores are adequate, approximately 25 percent of ingested heme iron will be absorbed. Absorption can be as high as 35 percent if stores are depleted. Thus, absorption of dietary heme iron is inversely proportional to iron status (Monsen et al. 1978).

Absorption of nonheme iron, found in both animal and vegetable foods, is a much more complex process than that of heme iron. Inorganic iron occurs in foods primarily in oxidized form as the ferric ion (Fe^{+++}). The reduced form, ferrous iron (Fe^{++}), is more readily absorbed, however, because it is more soluble in digestive juices. Thus factors that affect the reduction of iron also affect its absorption. Particularly important in this respect is the pH or acidity of the stomach and the upper part of the small intestine. The presence of both ascorbic acid and fructose increases absorption by enhancing the conversion of ferric to ferrous ion.

Another absorption-enhancing factor for nonheme iron is present in meat, poultry and fish, as an otherwise unidentified "meat factor." Protein per se does not enhance absorption of nonheme iron, but beef, lamb, liver, pork, chicken, and fish do, and are therefore considered to contain the "meat factor" (in addition to the heme iron that is absorbed). Milk, cheese, eggs, and some other substances may actually decrease absorption: Specific factors known to decrease the availability of nonheme iron include antacids, tannic acid (in tea), phytates, phosvitin (in egg yolk), and calcium and phosphate salts.

Both heme and nonheme iron enter the mucosal cells lining the upper intestine. (Heme iron is first absorbed as part of the porphyrin component of hemoglobin. Then it is released to join the "pool" of inorganic iron in the mucosa on which the body draws as necessary.) The iron binds with a specific protein to form a compound known as ferritin. This molecule acts as a "holding bin" of sorts and never actually leaves the mucosal cell. Ferritin is

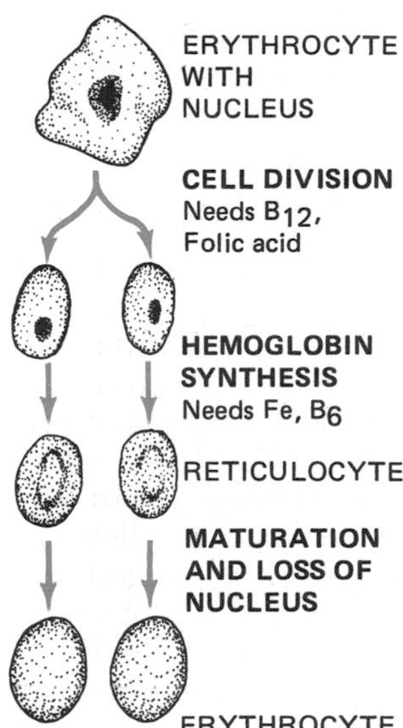

Normal Production of Red Blood Cells

lost when the mucosal cells are sloughed off into the intestinal lumen. Iron is transported by the protein transferrin, which circulates in the blood. When body stores are adequate, the transferrin molecules are "fully booked" with iron and will not accept any more iron "passengers" from the mucosal cells. When body stores are low, however, the transferrin molecules contain less iron and will more readily pick up "new" iron atoms from ferritin molecules in the mucosal cells. Thus, only a small portion of absorbed iron actually enters the circulation. That portion varies according to the amount being carried by the circulating transferrin molecules, which in turn depends on the iron stores. Clearly, iron absorption is a tightly regulated process.

Transferrin delivers iron to the bone marrow, where red blood cells (erythrocytes) are synthesized, and to such storage sites as the spleen and liver, where iron is stored as the proteins ferritin and hemosiderin. Transferrin also shuttles iron to other tissues, as well as between tissues, of the body. The synthesis of erythrocytes was diagrammatically shown in Figure 7-16.

Unlike other cells, erythrocytes lose their nuclei in the course of maturation. Because they are, therefore, lacking any DNA, cell replication and protein synthesis cannot occur. This is why they become "old" and "die" and must be replaced by new red blood cells synthesized "from scratch." This process begins in the bone marrow, where stem cells are produced. These in turn give rise to white blood cells, platelets, and erythroblasts, the nucleus-containing cells. Each erythroblast divides, in the presence of vitamin B_{12} and folic acid, to form two new cells which, in the presence of vitamin B_6, incorporate iron to synthesize hemoglobin. It is estimated that 2.5 million erythrocytes, 20,000 white blood cells, and 5 million platelets are sent into the circulation every *second* (Bessis, 1961).

Amino acid pool
Amino acids
Globin
Hemoglobin
Heme
Fe
Released to circulation
Bile pigments
Bilirubin
Bile

Recycling of Hemoglobin Components

METABOLISM AND PHYSIOLOGICAL FUNCTIONS: II. FUNCTIONS. The major function of iron is oxygen transport. It accomplishes this as a component of two different transport molecules, hemoglobin in red blood cells and myoblobin in muscle. Four heme groups combine with the protein globin to form a single molecule of hemoglobin. Each red blood cell contains over 250 million hemoglobin molecules, which means that a single cell can transport to the body more than a billion molecules of oxygen from their entry point in the lungs. The oxygen is required by the body for energy production by aerobic metabolism. Hemoglobin also transports CO_2, a byproduct of cellular metabolism, back to the lungs for excretion.

The amount of iron in myoglobin is only one quarter that in hemoglobin, or one atom of iron per molecule of myoglobin. This protein functions as a temporary oxygen reserve in muscle metabolism.

As a component of cytochromes in the electron transport system, iron has an important role in cell respiration. Other essential iron-containing compounds include such enzymes as catalase and xanthine oxidase. The latter is involved in the catabolism of purines, one of the components of nucleic acids, thereby giving iron a part in cell division and protein synthesis. Finally, iron is a cofactor of various enzymes, such as aconitase, which catalyzes the conversion of citric acid to isocitric acid in the Krebs cycle.

METABOLISM AND PHYSIOLOGICAL FUNCTIONS: III. EXCRETION. Red blood cells have an average life span of 120 days. As they die, their iron is recycled very efficiently by the body. The regeneration process begins with the removal of the red blood cells by the liver, bone marrow, and spleen, where breakdown of the hemoglobin molecule into heme and globin occurs. Globin is then broken down into its constituent amino acids, which are recycled into the body's available pool of amino acids. The iron in heme may be stored in the spleen and liver, or released into the circulation, to be picked up by transferrin and transported back to the bone marrow for incorporation into new red blood cells. The noniron portion of heme is converted to bile pigments, primarily bilirubin, which can be reutilized in the synthesis of new erythrocytes, or is excreted in the bile.

So efficient is this recycling process that very little iron is excreted on a daily basis—less than 0.1 milligram in the urine, 0.5 milligram from the intestine, and even smaller amounts in perspiration and sloughed skin. Most of the iron present in feces represents *unabsorbed* dietary mineral, though a small part of fecal iron comes from sloughed mucosal cells and digestive juices. A summary of iron metabolism is presented in Figure 8-6.

Iron Availability in Three Types of Meals

Low Availability
Less than 1 oz meat, poultry, or fish *Or* Less than 25 mg ascorbic acid
Medium Availability
1–3 oz meat, poultry, or fish *Or* 25–75 mg ascorbic acid
High Availability
More than 3 oz meat, poultry, or fish *Or* More than 75 mg ascorbic acid *Or* 1–3 oz meat, poultry or fish, plus 25–75 mg ascorbic acid

Source: E. R. Monsen et al., Estimation of available dietary iron, *American Journal of Clinical Nutrition* 31:134, 1978.

DIETARY ALLOWANCES. Although the body requires relatively little iron to replace daily losses, it absorbs only a small portion of the dietary amount. For this reason, and because of the complex interactions involved in absorption, dietary allowances for iron have been based on measurements of the amounts excreted. For adult men, body losses of iron normally amount to 1 mg per day. Women, however, because of their additional losses in menstruation, have an average iron loss of 1.8 mg per day. Correcting these figures for an average absorption rate of 10 percent, allowances have been established at 10 and 18 mg per day for men and women respectively. (Iron allowances at other stages of the life cycle are discussed in Chapters 12, 13, and 14.)

Estimates indicate that the average American diet supplies 6 mg of iron for every 1,000 kcal of food (Monsen et al., 1967). Thus, men should be able to meet the RDA for iron by consuming 1,700 kcal per day, well below the amount of food eaten by the average man. Women, on the other hand, would have to consume food totaling 3,000 kcal per day, much more than most women can, should, or want to eat. Not surprisingly, a very high proportion of American women do indeed have iron deficiencies of varying degrees.

Determination of actual iron needs and provision of adequate iron for women are difficult because the actual amount of dietary iron that is absorbed depends on a number of factors, including the amount of stored iron in the individual and the kinds of foods served at a given meal. (Absorption of nonheme iron, it will be remembered, is in direct proportion to the ascorbic acid and "meat factor" present in the same meal, while both nonheme and heme iron are absorbed in inverse proportion to body stores.)

A working estimate of absorbable iron can be calculated from the amounts of five components in a given meal: total iron, heme iron, nonheme iron, ascorbic acid, and amount of meat, poultry, or fish. On the basis of these determinations, a meal can be classified as one of high, medium, or low availability of iron (Monsen et al., 1978).

The average individual cannot, of course, be expected to work out these calculations. A realistic guideline for obtaining adequate absorbable iron is based on estimates that a minimum of 25 milligrams of ascorbic acid in a meal will double the amount of iron absorbed, and 1 gram of meat tissue has the approximate effect of 1 milligram of ascorbic acid.

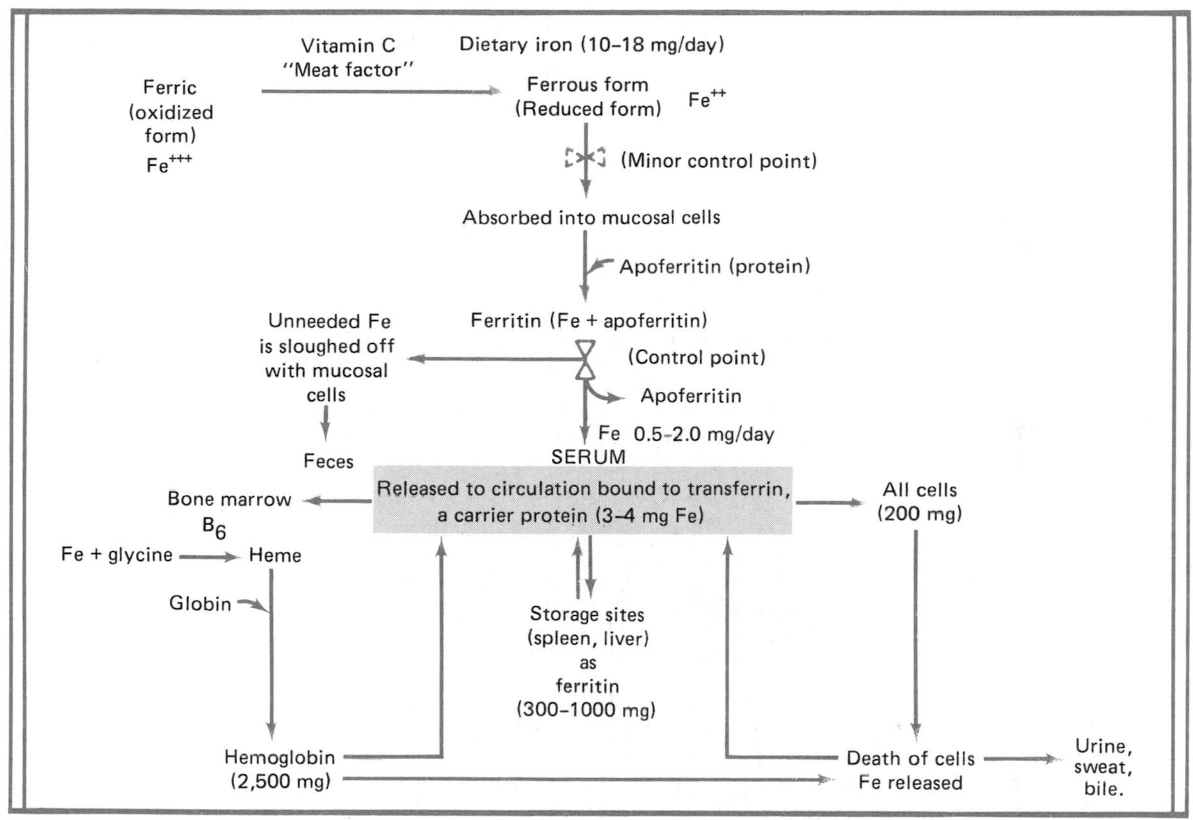

FIGURE 8-6
Summary of Iron Metabolism

For most people, then, the simple addition of a source of ascorbic acid—tomato juice, green pepper, a piece of melon—to every meal, and/or consumption of 3 ounces of meat, poultry, or fish, will significantly enhance the availability of iron in their diet. Vegetarians, however, cannot enhance availability with "meat factor" foods and must depend on larger quantities of ascorbic acid-containing foods to compensate. A high-available-iron vegetarian meal might include kidney beans with tomato sauce, broccoli, and pineapple. (And the factors that may hinder absorption—such as egg and tea—should be considered as well; drinking tea with a high-availability meal will transform it into a poorer source of absorbable iron.) In order to meet their needs, women should try to consume two "high-availability" meals per day.

DIETARY SOURCES. Food composition tables reflect *total* iron content and do not distinguish between heme and nonheme iron or otherwise indicate the amount of absorbable iron. Meat, poultry, and fish contain anywhere from 30 to 60 percent of their iron in the heme form. Fruits, vegetables, milk, eggs, and dairy products contain nonheme iron only. Dried fruits, legumes, and meats (especially liver!) and seafood are generally good sources of iron; eggs and milk are poor sources. Table 8-6 indicates the iron content of a variety of foods.

Certain dietary factors, such as phytate and fiber, decrease the absorption

Cast iron cooking vessels sold by Sears, Roebuck & Company in the late 19th century. When these were the everyday cookwares of everybody, iron deficiency was rare. (New York Public Library Picture Collection)

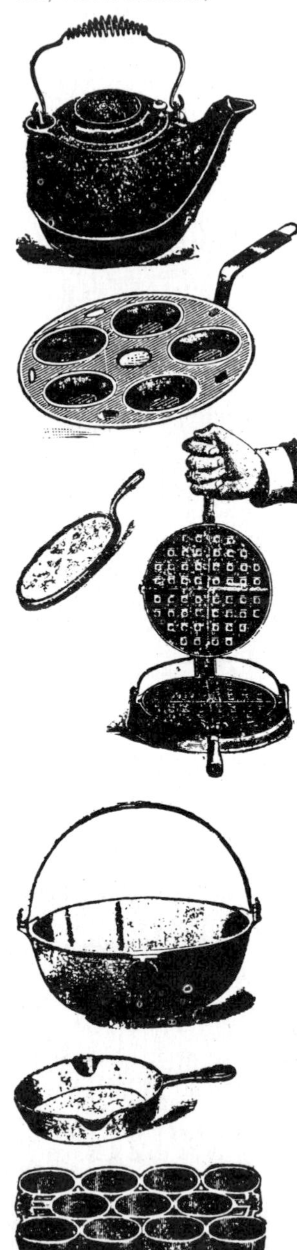

of iron. The method of preparing iron-containing foods can also affect iron availability. Boiling in water, for example, will leach significant amounts of the mineral, which is then lost if the water is discarded. Cast iron cooking vessels, on the other hand, can be an important supplementary source of the mineral. Iron cooking vessels have been used for centuries throughout the world, and the Chinese wok and Mexican *comal* or tortilla griddle have certainly added to the dietary supply of this mineral in their native lands. In North America and Europe, the mid-twentieth century shift to aluminum, stainless steel, and enamel vessels may well have increased the risk of iron-deficiency anemia.

IRON DEFICIENCY. In iron deficiency, body stores are depleted, and consequently the ability to synthesize hemoglobin is drastically reduced. Clinical anemia is the result of a long-term deficiency, since the elimination of all iron stores is a slow process.

Clinically, decreased serum iron, which follows tissue depletion, is reflected in decreased saturation of transferrin, and less than 10 to 12 grams of hemoglobin per 100 milliliters of serum. Symptoms include chronic fatigue, headache, and pallor. There are also indications that iron deficiency increases susceptibility to infection (Strauss, 1978). The characteristic symptoms of iron-deficiency anemia are also symptomatic of numerous other conditions, including depression. Therefore, clinical iron-deficiency anemia can only be determined by a variety of blood tests to evaluate iron status.

Iron deficiency can arise from several different causes: decreased intake, decreased absorption, hemorrhage or abnormal bleeding (including bleeding due to hookworm infestation), and excessive blood donations (1 pint of blood contains 250 mg of iron). Iron deficiency, however, is not the only cause of anemia, which by definition represents a decreased number of red blood cells. Folate and vitamin B_{12} deficiencies cause anemia of a different kind (as we saw in Chapter 7) resulting from changes in the shape and development of red blood cells. Severe pyridoxine and protein deficiencies also cause anemia.

Infants, young children, adolescents, and women of childbearing age are especially susceptible to iron deficiency anemia. Iron supplements, usually in the form of ferrous salts with ascorbic acid added to increase absorption, can be used to build up iron stores. For many women, this is indeed advisable. However, because of individual variation, not all women need iron supplementation, even if their dietary intake falls below the recommended allowance of 18 milligrams per day. Unfortunately, by the time a clinical deficiency can be identified, iron stores have been depleted. A special effort should be made, therefore, to include iron-rich foods in the diet on a daily basis.

IRON TOXICITY. For a small percent of the population, iron accumulation and not deficiency is a problem. Because the body lacks a mechanism for excreting excess iron, the mineral accumulates in the body, particularly in soft tissues such as liver, lungs, and pancreas. Iron accumulation causes necrosis, or cell destruction and death, as it distorts the structure of the cells of these tissues.

The resulting condition, known as *hemosiderosis,* appears to involve aggregates of ferritin molecules (hemosiderin), formed when large amounts of iron are complexed to ferritin. Hemosiderosis occurs frequently among Bantu

PERSPECTIVE ON
Iron Enrichment of Foods

In 1970 the American Bakers Association and the Millers' National Federation petitioned the Food and Drug Administration to allow an increase in the amount of iron they were permitted to add to bread and flour. The proposed enrichment levels were 40 mg/lb for flour and 25 mg/lb for bread, compared to the present levels of 16.5 mg/lb for flour and 12.5 mg/lb for bread. The FDA announced its intention to approve the petition. What followed was one of the longest and hottest nutrition controversies in FDA history.

The petition owed its origin to evidence that a significant segment of the population had subnormal levels of hemoglobin. Iron-deficiency anemia had been found to be one of the most common nutritional problems in the United States, with an incidence of more than 25 percent among infants, adolescent girls, and pregnant women who are not given a supplement. Women generally and people at the lowest socioeconomic level are the two population groups in which deficiency is most widespread. Proponents of the enrichment proposal cited the loss of iron from extradietary sources that had formerly been a significant factor, such as cast iron cooking vessels and various iron-containing contaminants. Because the average diet supplies significantly less than the RDA for women, they argued, there was every reason to further fortify two common food items like bread and flour.

The FDA was persuaded, and published in the *Federal Register* its intention to increase iron fortification levels threefold. The announcement was seen by a physician who had for years been treating a patient with hemochromatosis. She and two other hematologists protested to the FDA. The FDA first postponed, then reconsidered, and ultimately withdrew approval of superenrichment (*Nutrition Today*, 1978).

In the years between the initial proposal and the final decision, the issues were debated by physicians, nutritionists, hematologists, and consumers. The organizations supporting "superenrichment" included the American Medical Association, the American Dietetic Association, and the Food and Nutrition Board of the National Research Council, among others. But their influence with the FDA weakened when it was pointed out that many individuals who were avid supporters of the proposal were in key positions in more than one of the organizations lobbying for approval. Further, in a period of several years none of these groups had presented new evidence to indicate that the potential benefits outweighed potential risks. A group of medical and research experts met to analyze evidence for and against the proposal in February of 1972. This group recommended to the Food and Drug Commissioner that the superenrichment proposal be rejected. This was a particular surprise because several of those recommending proposal rejection had previously supported the plan (*Nutrition Today*, 1972).

Among the points that gave the experts pause were the following: The need for increasing fortification levels was not sufficiently established; the proposed amounts of supplementation were not based on laboratory determinations of real need; and significant numbers of individuals would be at risk if the proposed enrichment levels were implemented.

Extensive new research findings are still not available to counter these and other points. However, some suggestive evidence has come from Sweden, where for some 30 years flours have contained 22 milligrams of iron per pound, providing an increased intake of 42 percent. A study, initiated because of an unusual incidence of hemachromatosis in one area of that country, showed that a number of men did have elevated serum iron values, although women did not (Crosby, 1977). This evidence is not sufficient to implicate fortification in these findings, but it certainly does suggest that the risk of danger due to increased iron intake may well be greater than the potential benefit. Nutritionists will continue to emphasize the importance, especially for women and young children, of a varied diet to meet iron requirements, and, if necessary to prevent and/or correct iron deficiency, the use of supplements.

TABLE 8-6
Iron Content of Selected Foods
RDA for Adults
Men: 10 mg
Women: 18 mg

Food	Serving Size	Iron Content mg/serving
Bran flakes, 40%	1 c	12.4
Liver, beef, cooked	3 oz	7.5
Oysters	½ c, raw	6.6
Clams	4–5 raw	5.3
Molasses, blackstrap	1 tbsp	3.2
Hamburger, 21% fat, cooked	3 oz	2.6
Beans, navy, cooked	½ c	2.6
Soybeans, cooked	½ c	2.5
Beans, red kidney, cooked	½ c	2.2
Split peas, cooked	½ c	2.1
Shrimp, canned	½ c	2.0
Spinach, cooked	½ c	2.0
Tuna fish, canned	3½ oz	1.6
Raisins	small box = 1½ oz	1.5
Chicken, meat only	3½ oz	1.4
Molasses, medium	1 tbsp	1.2
Potato, baked in skin	1 medium	1.1
Frankfurter	1	1.1
Egg, whole	1 large	1.04
Apricots, dried	5 medium halves	1.0
Egg yolk	1 large	0.95
Rice, cooked, enriched	½ c	0.9
Haddock, cooked	3 oz	0.9
Collard greens, cooked	½ c	0.8
Bread, whole-wheat	1 slice	0.8
Banana	1 medium	0.8
Avocado	½ fruit	0.7
Bread, white, enriched	1 slice	0.6
Cranberry juice	6 oz	0.6
Lobster, cooked	½ c	0.6
Orange	1 medium	0.6

men of South Africa as a result of the high iron content of their beer, which is fermented in iron pots. Absorption is facilitated by the acid content of the beer, as well as of other dietary items. This demonstrates that the regulation of iron absorption is not absolute, and in fact fails at very high levels of iron intake.

Hemosiderosis also results from types of anemia characterized by excessive breakdown of red blood cells. Because the iron and amino acids of hemoglobin are reutilized, transferrin can become completely saturated in the case of excessive erythrocyte turnover, with the result that iron unable to attach to transferrin will be deposited in soft tissues. Hemosiderosis may also occur following excessive blood transfusion.

Hemochromatosis, an abnormal increase in tissue iron deposition, is an advanced state of hemosiderosis. It is associated with pathological changes in tissue structure and function and may lead to liver damage, diabetes, and heart failure if untreated. Hemochromatosis is caused by a disturbance in the

TABLE 8-6
(Continued)

Food	Serving Size	Iron Content mg/serving
Broccoli, cooked	½ c	0.6
Tomato	1 medium	0.5
Crabmeat, canned	½ c	0.5
Carrots, cooked	½ c	0.5
Bacon, cooked	3 slices	0.5
Green beans, cooked	½ c	0.4
Apple	1 medium	0.4
Cottage cheese, uncreamed	½ c	0.3
Salami	1 slice = 1 oz	0.3
Peanut butter	1 tbsp	0.3
Bread, white, unenriched	1 slice	0.2
Coffee, prepared	1 c = 6 oz	0.2
Cheddar cheese	1 oz	0.19
Yogurt, low-fat, fruit-flavored	8 oz	0.16
Milk, 2% fat + protein	1 c	0.15
Milk, whole	1 c	0.12
Milk, 2% fat	1 c	0.12
American cheese, pasteurized, processed	1 oz	0.11
Yogurt, plain	8 oz	0.11
Milk, skim	1 c	0.10
Celery	1 stalk	0.10
Ice cream, 10% fat	½ c	0.06
Swiss cheese	1 oz	0.05
Butter	1 pat = 1 tsp	0.01
Egg white	1 whole	0.01

Sources: C. F. Adams, *Nutritive value of American foods in common units,* USDA Agriculture Handbook No. 456 (Washington, D.C.: U.S. Government Printing Office, 1975); L. P. Posati, and M. L. Orr, *Composition of foods—Dairy and egg products—Raw, processed, prepared,* USDA Agriculture Handbook No. 8-1 (Washington, D.C.: U.S. Government Printing Office, 1976).

control of iron absorption. Termed "idiopathic hemochromatosis," this unexplained increase in absorption of iron from a normal diet is of genetic origin.

Treatment for both of these rare but dangerous conditions includes administration of an iron-binding agent to solubilize the iron so that it can be excreted in the urine, or phlebotomy (medically supervised bleeding).

Copper

This mineral is of increasing interest to nutritionists for its importance in iron metabolism, contributing to iron absorption and the formation of hemoglobin. The recognition that bottle-fed infants may under certain circumstances develop anemia that is more responsive to copper treatment than to iron therapy has spurred research on this essential nutrient.

DISTRIBUTION IN THE BODY. The human body contains 75 to 150 milligrams of copper. All body tissues contain some copper, but the greatest concentrations are found in the liver, brain, heart, and kidneys. Blood copper is apportioned in roughly equal amounts between red blood cells and plasma. In plasma, copper occurs as the copper-protein complex called ceruloplasmin.

METABOLISM AND PHYSIOLOGICAL FUNCTIONS. Absorption takes place in the duodenum of the intestine, but relatively little is known about regulatory control of the process. Approximately 30 percent of dietary copper is absorbed. Molybdenum, zinc, cadmium, and other trace minerals interfere with absorption. Following uptake of absorbed copper from the intestine, the liver stores the mineral or releases it as ceruloplasmin, which accounts for 95 percent of the copper found in serum. Albumin binds the remaining 5 percent.

Ceruloplasmin is involved in various stages of iron metabolism. In particular, it is necessary for the conversion of ferrous to ferric iron, important during various stages of iron metabolism. Copper enhances iron absorption and stimulates the mobilization of iron from stores in the liver and other tissues. Copper-containing enzymes play a part in various oxidation reactions in energy metabolism and in the metabolism of fatty acids. The mineral itself activates certain enzymes. The major route of copper excretion is via the bile.

DIETARY ALLOWANCES AND SOURCES. The Food and Nutrition Board has established provisional recommended ranges for dietary intake of copper, but not RDAs. From copper balance studies in adults, it has been determined that the body needs from 1.5 to 2.0 mg/day. The provisional recommendations by the Food and Nutrition Board are 2 to 3 mg/day for adults. The interactions of copper with other trace minerals, and the lack of sufficient data, compound the difficulty of setting a reliable RDA for copper.

The average diet contains 2 milligrams or more copper per day. Drinking water may be a source of variable amounts as well. The richest sources of the mineral include nuts, shellfish, liver, kidney, raisins, and legumes. Just as it is a poor source of iron, milk is a poor source of copper.

A number of factors influence the copper content of foods. Environmental factors include copper content of soil, geographic location (such as nearness to industrial complexes that may release copper-containing wastes), use and kind of fertilizers, origin of water supply, and the season. Handling and processing also affect copper content. Water, equipment, and various contaminants may introduce copper, while milling, grinding, and cooking in water tend to remove it.

It should be noted that laboratory analyses of foods have produced a wide range of copper values, and consequently the copper contents of foods reported in the literature vary widely. The values listed in food composition tables are approximations only. Table 8-7 gives the copper content of selected foods. Consumption of a diversified diet should ensure sufficient intake of the mineral.

COPPER DEFICIENCY AND TOXICITY. The broad scope of copper's functions can be judged by the range of symptoms that result from deficiency: anemia, cardiovascular lesions, degeneration of the nervous system, skeletal

TABLE 8-7
Copper Content of Selected Foods
Estimated Safe and Adequate Daily Dietary Intake for Adults
2.0–3.0 mg

Food	Serving Size	Copper Content mg/serving
Oysters	6 medium	14.2
Lobster	1 c	2.45
Liver, beef, cooked	3 oz	2.38
Bran flakes, 40%	1 c	0.51
Avocado	1 half	0.49
Potato, baked in skin	1 medium	0.36
Soybeans, cooked	½ c	0.30
Banana	1 medium	0.26
Haddock, cooked	3 oz	0.16
Apple	1 medium	0.14
Chicken, meat only	3½ oz	0.14
Spinach, cooked	½ c	0.13
Peas, green, cooked	½ c	0.12
Tuna, canned	3½ oz	0.12
Raisins	small box = 1½ oz	0.11
Tomato	1 medium	0.11
Green beans, cooked	½ c	0.09
Peanut butter	1 tbsp	0.09
Milk, whole	1 c	0.09
Broccoli, cooked	½ c	0.08
Bacon, cooked	3 slices	0.08
Bread, whole-wheat	1 slice	0.06
Bread, white, enriched	1 slice	0.06
Carrots, cooked	½c	0.06
Egg, whole	1 large	0.05
Egg yolk	1 large	0.05
Milk, skim	1 c	0.05
Frankfurter	1	0.05
Beef, ground	3 oz	0.05
Coffee, prepared	6 oz	0.04
Swiss cheese	1 oz	0.03
Cheddar cheese	1 oz	0.03
Celery	1 stalk	0.03
Ice cream, 10% fat	½ c	0.03
Rice, cooked	½ c	0.02
American cheese	1 oz	0.02
Cottage cheese	½ c	0.01
Egg white	1 large	0.01
Margarine	1 pat = 1 tsp	trace
Butter	1 pat = 1 tsp	0

Source: J. T. Pennington, and D. H. Calloway, Copper content of foods, *Journal of the American Dietetic Association* 63:143, 1973.

defects, various hair abnormalities, and loss of taste acuity. Copper deficient infants exhibit low serum copper levels, anemia, and bone demineralization. Copper imbalances usually result from genetic defects in control mechanisms. One such inherited defect produces a fatal condition called Menke's syndrome (or kinky-hair disease), caused by defective absorption of copper from the intestine. Symptoms include rapid degeneration of nerve tissue, skeletal abnormalities, a "steely" texture of the hair, vascular lesions, and subnormal body temperature. Copper deficiency can also arise from malnutrition, diarrhea, malabsorption, and kidney disease.

Toxicity due to an excess of dietary copper is rare. Daily intakes of more than 20 milligrams of copper, however, produce nausea and vomiting.

An inherited condition, Wilson's disease, produces chronic copper toxicity due to defective excretion. Ceruloplasmin levels decrease and copper gradually accumulates in the tissues. The symptoms of this progressive disease include tissue necrosis (especially in the liver), mental deterioration, tremor, and loss of coordination.

Zinc

Although long known to be essential for animals, the importance of zinc in human nutrition began to be appreciated about 20 years ago. The impetus for the revised view of zinc's relevance to human nutrition came with evidence of zinc deficiency in Iran and Egypt in the early 1960s.

DISTRIBUTION IN THE BODY. The human body contains 2 to 3 grams of zinc. It occurs in all tissues, with highest concentrations in the choroid membrane of the eye and the male reproductive organs. The liver, skeletal muscle, and bone contain somewhat lower concentrations. Zinc also occurs in blood (most of it in erythrocytes) and in the pancreas as a component of insulin.

METABOLISM AND PHYSIOLOGICAL FUNCTIONS. Absorption of zinc from the upper part of the small intestine is about 30 percent efficient. Although the mechanism of absorption remains to be identified, it is thought that the process is energy dependent and increases with body size, physiological need, and dietary zinc content. Calcium, phytate, and dietary fiber interfere with absorption.

As a component of insulin, a hormone that regulates carbohydrate metabolism, zinc is extremely important to nutritional health. It is also a component of at least 20 metalloenzymes—including carbonic anhydrase (necessary for CO_2 transport from red blood cells to the lungs), carboxypeptidase (needed for peptide digestion), and alcohol dehydrogenase as well as other dehydrogenase enzymes. It plays an essential part in the synthesis of DNA, RNA, and proteins. Mobilization of vitamin A from the liver requires zinc, and the mineral also plays a part in wound healing, perhaps in the synthesis of collagen.

According to a recent study, zinc appears to be a necessary activator of the conjugase enzyme associated with absorption of the polyglutamate forms of folic acid. Polyglutamate absorption was decreased by approximately half when zinc depletion was experimentally induced (Tamura et al., 1978). Further research is needed to clarify the role of zinc in other physiological systems.

In addition to fecal excretion of unabsorbed zinc, the daily loss of endogenous zinc amounts to 2 to 3 milligrams. Urine and perspiration account for

TABLE 8-8
Zinc Content of Selected Foods
RDA for Adults
15 mg

Food	Serving Size	Zinc Content mg/serving
Oysters, fresh	6 medium	124.9
Turkey, dark meat, cooked	3 oz	3.7
Liver, beef	3 oz	3.31
Lima beans, canned, cooked	½ c	2.72
Pork, lean, cooked	3 oz	2.6
Beef, ground, cooked	3 oz	2.12
Turkey, light meat, cooked	3 oz	1.8
Yogurt, fruit-flavored	8 oz	1.68
Yogurt, plain	8 oz	1.34
Bran flakes, 40%	1 c	1.3
Almonds	¼ c	1.24
Peanuts, roasted	¼ c	1.17
Swiss cheese	1 oz	1.11
Milk, skim	1 c	0.98
Milk, whole	1 c	0.93
Wheat germ	1 tbsp	0.9
Cheddar cheese	1 oz	0.88
Whole egg	1 large	0.72
Ice cream, 10% fat	½ c	0.71
Egg yolk	1 large	0.58
Potato, baked	1 medium	0.44
Cottage cheese, uncreamed	½ c	0.34
Lentils, cooked	½ c	0.18
Spinach, cooked	½ c	0.17
Cream cheese	1 oz	0.15
Orange juice	6 oz	0.13
Lettuce, chunks	1 c	0.12
Banana	1 medium	0.04
Egg white	1 large	0.01
Butter or margarine	1 pat = 1 tsp	trace

Sources: L. P. Posati, and M. L. Orr, *Composition of foods—Dairy and egg products—Raw, processed, prepared,* USDA Agriculture Handbook No. 8-1 (Washington, D.C.: U.S. Government Printing Office, 1976); H. H. Sandstead, Zinc nutrition in the United States, *American Journal of Clinical Nutrition* 26:1257, 1973.

about 0.5 milligrams per day each, and the remainder is lost in pancreatic and intestinal secretions. The control points of zinc metabolism remain to be identified.

DIETARY ALLOWANCES AND SOURCES. Metabolic studies indicate that a dietary intake of 8 to 10 milligrams per day suffices to produce zinc equilibrium in adults. Allowing a substantial margin, and correcting for absorption, the adult RDA has been set at 15 milligrams. It should be remembered, however, that this figure is supported by limited research.

Data on dietary sources also are limited. As Table 8-8 shows, oysters are by far the richest source of zinc. High protein foods, such as meats and egg yolks, contain valuable amounts. Fruits, vegetables, and egg whites are poor sources of zinc. Milling of cereals reduces their zinc content, and the zinc found in whole-grain products may be largely unavailable due to the presence of phytic acid. The interrelationships between dietary zinc, copper, calcium, and protein are only beginning to emerge.

ZINC DEFICIENCY AND TOXICITY. The major symptoms of zinc deficiency are delayed growth and maturation, including sexual maturation. Other symptoms include delayed wound healing and impaired taste acuity (hypogeusia). These symptoms reflect the importance of zinc in nucleic acid and protein synthesis. Most studies of zinc deficiency have been of boys. Girls suffer growth retardation, but no studies have been done on the effect of zinc deficiency on sexual maturation in girls. Concern has recently been expressed that suboptimal intake may be more common than previously thought.

Zinc apparently has no significant toxic effects, although vomiting, diarrhea, and abdominal cramping have been reported following consumption of beverages stored in galvanized containers. However, because long-term effects of prolonged high consumption are not known, zinc supplements should be taken only when prescribed for therapeutic reasons.

Iodine

As a nutrient, iodine is well known for its association with iodized salt and the unsightly iodine deficiency condition called goiter. Although the causal connection between iodine and goiter was established only about a century ago, iodine-containing substances were used long before that by the Chinese, Egyptians, and Incas to treat the goitrous condition.

DISTRIBUTION IN THE BODY. The total amount of body iodine averages between 20 and 30 milligrams, of which 75 percent is found in the thyroid gland. The thyroid gland is a two-lobed structure that lies across the trachea. Its major function is the synthesis and storage of thyroid hormones. The remaining 25 percent of body iodine is found in all body tissues, and especially in skeletal muscle, blood, and the ovaries.

METABOLISM AND PHYSIOLOGICAL FUNCTIONS. The body absorbs dietary iodine (primarily as iodides) with nearly 100 percent efficiency. After entry into the blood and distribution throughout the extracellular fluid, about 30 percent of the absorbed iodine is trapped by the thyroid. Since there is no mechanism for the conservation of additional iodide, the remainder of the absorbed iodine is excreted in the urine.

Iodide functions in the synthesis of two thyroid hormones—thyroxine (T_4) and triiodothyronine (T_3)—which are essential for normal metabolism. Synthesis of these hormones begins with the formation of a large iodine-containing protein called thyroglobulin, which contains many tyrosine molecules. Enzymatic hydrolysis of thyroglobulin releases the hormones into the blood, which distributes them to all tissues.

The two thyroid hormones accelerate biochemical reactions in all cells of the body, causing greater utilization of oxygen and an increased metabolic rate. Consequently these hormones have a profound and far-reaching influence on growth and development, protein synthesis, and energy metabolism. The mechanisms by which thyroid hormones produce these effects have yet to be clearly identified. The hormones also play a part in the conversion of carotene to vitamin A and in the synthesis of cholesterol.

The thyroid gland is able to compensate for low dietary iodine intake by expanding its activity (and size), thereby maximizing the use of the limited supply. The most important regulator of thyroid activity is a pituitary product called thyroid-stimulating or thyrotropic hormone (TSH). The regulation of thyroid hormone synthesis and release by TSH involves a number of feedback mechanisms.

Although several disturbances of thyroid hormone metabolism exist, anything more than the briefest description is beyond the scope of this book. The condition known as *hypothyroidism* (or underactive thyroid) results in subnormal levels of thyroid hormones in the blood, a consequence of insufficient synthesis. The form of hypothyroidism known as myxedema produces a clinical picture of coarse hair, yellowish skin, decreased tolerance to cold, and a tendency to be overweight. Although rare, this condition is the basis for the claim that obesity results from an undcractivc thyroid. Myxcdcma, howcvcr, does not stem from iodine deficiency but rather from a metabolic error in hormone synthesis.

On the other hand *hyperthyroidism*, or overactive thyroid, occurs when the regulatory mechanisms that control thyroid hormone synthesis do not function. A person with Graves' disease, as one type of hyperthyroidism is called, is nervous, has a voracious appetite but loses weight, demonstrates an increased metabolic rate, and cannot tolerate heat. A frequent symptom, known as exophthalmia ("popeye"), is a visible protrusion of the eyeballs.

Thyroid hormones are sometimes suggested as a part of weight-loss regimens because of their effect in increasing the metabolic rate. But this method of treating obesity is potentially dangerous and can cause cardiac failure. Moreover, the hormones are not permanently effective against weight gain.

DIETARY ALLOWANCES AND SOURCES. The RDA for iodine for both adult men and women has been set at 150 micrograms per day, with increases recommended during pregnancy and lactation.

In the United States important sources of the mineral are iodized salt and bread to which iodine-containing dough conditioners have been added. In recent years, the dietary intake of iodine appears to have increased, although the sources of the additional amounts remain to be determined. Present iodization of table salt adds 100 milligrams of potassium iodide for each kilogram of sodium chloride. Thus 1 teaspoon of table salt contains 420 micrograms of iodine, far more than the RDA.

Drinking water supplies variable amounts of the mineral and tends to reflect the amount present in the soil. Iodine content of foods varies considerably according to the type of soil, animal feed, fertilizers, and processing methods used. Seafood, although an excellent source of iodine, provides a very small proportion of dietary intake because of its infrequent appearance in the average diet. Because of the variability of iodine content in foods, and because it is present in such small amounts, accurate determinations are not available for most food items. Fish, seafoods, and seaweeds are usually good sources. Bread and dairy products may be good sources as well, as will any

Tyrosine

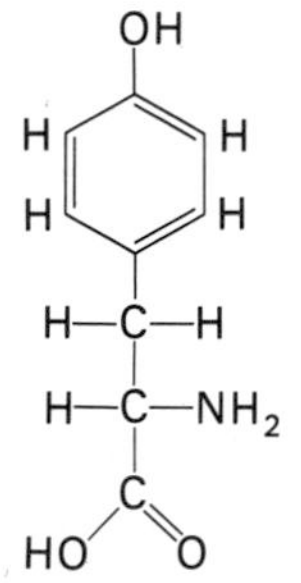

T_3 (Triiodothyronine)

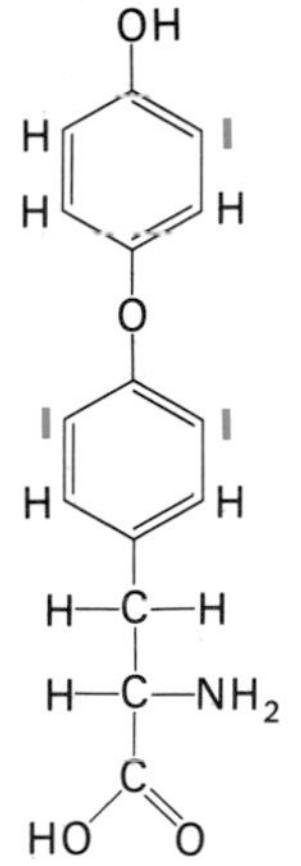

T_4 (Thyroxine)

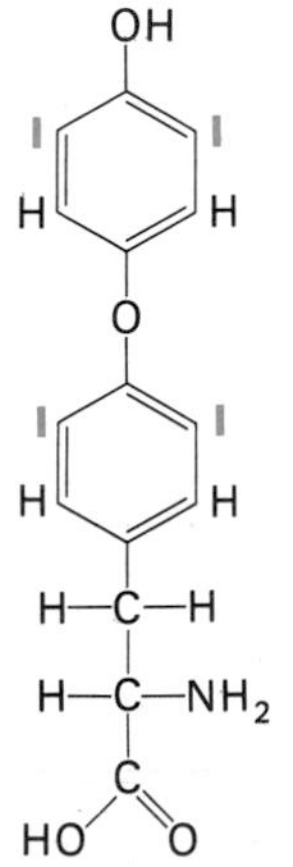

Substitution of iodine for 3 or 4 hydrogen atoms on two linked tyrosine molecules produces T_3 or T_4 respectively.

prepared foods using iodized salt. A single pinch of iodized salt contains about 50 micrograms of iodine, as does an 8-ounce glass of milk—fully one-third the RDA. Most vegetables contain little iodine: Spinach, broccoli, and potatoes all contain less than 10 micrograms per serving (Kidd et al., 1974).

IODINE DEFICIENCY. The most common consequence of iodine deficiency is simple goiter, or swelling of the thyroid gland. In response to decreased serum levels of thyroid hormones caused by a lack of dietary iodine, TSH is released. TSH controls thyroid metabolism in part by increasing the number and size of thyroid cells. This in turn increases the efficiency of the gland's iodine-trapping mechanism and enables it to accelerate synthesis and release of its key hormones. Thus, simple goiter is a useful compensatory mechanism and generally does not pose any serious medical problem. Development of goiter was for centuries a sign of puberty in girls and considered normal and desirable. In fact, goiter was so common that many Renaissance paintings depict the beautiful women of the day showing enlarged thyroids among their other physical endowments (see page 312). Today we know that estrogen alters thyroid hormone metabolism, and thus may result in goiter if iodine intake is marginal. In extreme cases a goiter may become so enlarged as to interfere with breathing.

Goiter may also develop from ingestion of "goitrogens"—compounds that compete with iodine for thyroid uptake or that interfere with thyroid hormone synthesis. Such goitrogens are to be found in cabbages and brussels sprouts. Another goitrogen, thiocyanate, occurs in cassava, which is a dietary staple in areas in Africa that have a high incidence both of goiter and of *cretinism*. Cretinism is a much more serious form of thyroid hormone deficiency. This condition is present at birth in infants who were deprived of iodine during fetal development because their mothers had a profound deficiency of thyroid hormone due to severe and prolonged iodine deficiency. The symptoms of cretinism include lethargy (as a result of very low basal metabolism), mental retardation, stunted growth, enlarged tongue, and dry skin.

Congenital hypothyroidism also produces the same symptoms but is the result of a genetic defect rather than of iodine deficiency. In both of these conditions, mental and physical retardation can be prevented if thyroid hormones are administered soon after birth. Since early diagnosis is essential, mandatory screening of all newborn infants for hypothyroidism has been suggested.

Recently concern has developed that dietary intake of iodine may be excessive. Over a long period of time, ingestion of large amounts of iodine (25 to 50 times the recommended levels) can suppress the synthesis of thyroid hormones, resulting in a hyperactive and enlarged thyroid, a condition known as "iodide goiter." Indeed, the sensitivity of the thyroid gland makes iodine one of the very few nutrients of which both excess and deficiency can produce the same effect.

Fluorine

The body contains less than 1 gram of fluorine, which has an interesting history in relation to dental health. The presence of fluoride in bones and teeth was discovered early in the last century. Dentists in Colorado Springs had observed that people living in the area had unusual teeth: Their teeth had dark brown stains (so-called mottled enamel) and the incidence of dental caries was exceptionally low. The stains, although esthetically unappealing, had no adverse effects on health. By 1931 investigators established that naturally occurring fluorides in the water supply were responsible for both of the observed effects.

METABOLISM AND PHYSIOLOGICAL FUNCTIONS. Passive absorption of fluorine is rapid and takes place primarily in the stomach, but some may be absorbed from the intestine as well. Efficiency of absorption ranges from 75 to 90 percent of the amount ingested, with approximately half retained in the teeth and bones.

The function of fluoride appears to be the protection of bone and—especially—dental tissue, an influence that it exercises primarily during prenatal life, infancy, and childhood. Fluoridated water, however, is of some benefit to adults as well as to children. There is also some evidence that an adequate dietary intake of the mineral throughout life protects against osteoporosis in the elderly.

Fragmentary evidence suggests that fluorine may also enhance wound healing and, by enhancing iron absorption, protect against the anemias that accompany pregnancy and lactation.

The body excretes fluoride mainly in the urine, although small amounts are lost in sweat and feces. Urinary loss is very rapid, the excess amount being excreted within 24 hours.

Range of Fluoride in Selected Foods

Food	Fluoride Content μg/g
Spinach	0.1 -20.3
Cheese	0.16- 1.71
Potatoes	0.4 - 5.20
Fish	1.0 - 8.0

DIETARY ALLOWANCES AND SOURCES. Although RDAs for fluorine have not been established, the Food and Nutrition Board provisionally recommends that water supplies be fluoridated at a level of 1 ppm (or 1 mg/liter) to provide 1.5 to 4 milligrams per day for adults.

The amounts of fluoride from dietary sources other than fluoridated water are unreliable. Most plant and animal foods reflect the variable contents of soil, water supply, and other factors and contain only minor amounts of the mineral. Fish products and seaweed (important components of Japanese diets) are exceptions, and tea provides 0.3 milligrams per cup. Grains and vegetables are sometimes good sources, as are bone meal, meats, fish, and dairy products. As an example of the variability of fluoride content of food, nuts usually have anywhere from 0.3 to 1.45 micrograms per gram, but values as high as 7.8 micrograms per gram have been recorded. Fluoridated water used during processing and preparation increases the fluoride content of food, as does cooking with Teflon vessels. Boiling water in aluminum ware, on the other hand, greatly reduces fluoride content.

Because the mineral occurs in such small amounts in foods and is so rapidly excreted, fluorine toxicity is rare. In areas where fluoride is naturally present in the water supply at levels approximating 6–8 ppm, tooth enamel becomes mottled, but no adverse effects on health have been documented. In rare instances in which fluoride has been ingested, usually accidentally, in amounts greater than 2,500 times recommended levels, fatal poisoning has resulted. Chronic ingestion of more than 50 milligrams per day, which may result from environmental pollution, can produce bone and tooth malformations. However, it has been thoroughly documented that the levels provided by artificially fluoridated water pose no health hazard and in fact are beneficial.

PERSPECTIVE ON
The Politics of Fluoridation

Despite the undeniable role of fluoride in the prevention of tooth decay, the history of attempts to fluoridate municipal water supplies has been rocky indeed. The persistent opposition to fluoridation would perhaps be more understandable if dental caries were not a major health problem. In 1942, almost 200,000 potential draftees were rejected because they had fewer than 12 sound teeth (in proper position)—out of a total of 32! And by that time, ten years of Public Health Service research had already demonstrated conclusively that fluoride significantly reduced the number of cavities.

In the 1940s there was, in fact, a good reason to hesitate before adding a little-studied mineral to public drinking water: Virtually nothing was known about possible side effects. In 1954 a ten-year study of children in two New York towns, one of which had a fluoridated water supply, was concluded. The study identified only one medically significant difference between the two groups: 60 percent fewer cavities developed in children who drank the fluoridated water. In subsequent years, many other studies have essentially led to the same conclusion. Information concerning water fluoridation was gathered from all over the world and was analyzed by the World Health Organization, which published its report in 1970. Only one sign of physiological or pathological change was associated with the presence or absence of fluoride in the water supply: In study after study, those who drank fluoridated water had significantly fewer cavities than those who did not. A representative of the American Dental Association testified at a 1978 Congressional hearing that "Fluoridation may well be the most thoroughly studied community health measure of recent history."

The recommended concentration of fluorine is only 1 ppm. Nonetheless, opposition has been long and persistent. Since 1973, when it seemed as though fluoridation might at last be gaining acceptance, hundreds of communities in the United States have voted against it. (Fluoridation is perhaps the only public health measure subject to popular vote, a fact that makes it vulnerable to politics.) Cost is not the problem, amounting to no more than about $0.40 per person per year. But the politics of fluoridation is not restricted to the United States. In 1976 Holland dropped its plans to fluoridate public water supplies. And Great Britain undertook a reevaluation before going ahead with fluoridation.

Fluoridation has been attacked on a number of grounds, political and medical. Early opponents characterized the measure as a "communist conspiracy" to poison the population. More recently objection has been taken on the grounds that such measures limit the citizens's freedom of choice of medical treatment. Other accusations charge fluoridation with causing birth defects, cancer, heart disease, mutations, and allergic reactions. Every such charge has been the subject of at least several scientific studies which have all exonerated fluoride. For example, separate studies by the National Cancer Institute, the U.S. Center for Disease Control, and the National Heart, Lung, and Blood Institute in 1976 and 1977 could find no evidence to connect cancer with fluoridation.

Although many people who oppose fluoridation are honestly motivated, the obviously well-financed and skillfully organized opposition groups often raise doubts about their real goal. An official of the American Dental Association has been quoted as saying that the real aim of these groups "is to create the illusion of a scientific controversy" (*Consumer Reports*, 1978). There is in fact no *scientific* controversy; on the contrary, scientific evidence has proven the values of fluoridation and has not identified any medical risk.

Other Trace Elements

Until quite recently, little has been known about the functions in the body of a number of trace elements, but in the last few years evidence has accumulated to show that minute amounts of a number of minerals are essential to human health and must be provided in the diet. As a result, provisional allowances have been set for manganese, molybdenum, selenium, and chromium. These elements, along with cobalt, are now known to be integral constituents of essential body compounds. Silicon, tin, vanadium, and nickel are being carefully studied, because their essentiality for humans is increasingly suspected.

CHROMIUM. Because chromium was implicated as a participant in glucose metabolism in 1959, it has been more actively studied than most of the other trace elements and evidence for its essentiality, although scattered, has continued to accumulate. The total amount of this mineral to be found in the human body averages less than 6 milligrams but is highly variable. The hair, spleen, kidney, and testes contain the highest concentrations; heart, pancreas, lungs, and brain have lower concentrations. The amount of chromium in the body declines with age, possibly as a result of depletion of body stores, but most likely due to decreased dietary intake.

Absorption—in the organically bound form known as *glucose tolerance factor* (GTF)—is 10 to 25 percent efficient. However, the body absorbs only about 1 percent of inorganic chromium from the diet. Daily loss, mainly via urinary excretion, averages between 7 and 10 micrograms.

The major function of chromium is to enhance the activity of insulin in the metabolism of glucose and particularly in maintaining the rate at which glucose is removed from blood for uptake into cells. Chromium also activates several enzymes and may play a role in protein and lipid metabolism.

A scattering of studies shows a wide range of values for dietary intake, from 50 to 400 micrograms per day. In the absence of specific information about need and utilization, the Food and Nutrition Board offers provisional allowances of 0.05 to 2.0 milligrams (50 to 200 μg) per day for adults. Good sources include yeast, beer, liver, cheese, bread, and beef. Black pepper contains chromium but is seldom consumed in amounts sufficient to make this a useful dietary source. Refining of sugar and flour removes most of the chromium contained in these sources. Even good sources contain varying amounts of the mineral in different samples tested, due to variations in water and soil content and methods of processing and preparation.

Impaired glucose tolerance appears to result from chromium deficiency. Symptoms shown by laboratory animals have included growth retardation, hyperglycemia, glycosuria, and elevated serum cholesterol, along with a generally reduced ability to cope with psychological stress. Severely malnourished children have shown improved glucose removal following chromium therapy. Some researchers feel that many Americans may have a chronic deficiency (Levander, 1975). However, evidence is far from sufficient to offer a clear-cut theory of how chromium exerts its effects or, indeed, precisely what those effects are. Although no evidence exists of toxicity from dietary sources, until more is learned about this trace mineral, supplements are not advised.

COBALT. The first evidence for a nutritional role for cobalt came about 45 years ago when an anemia-like disease of cattle in Australia and New Zealand was cured by administration of iron compounds. It was subsequently demonstrated that the effective portion of the compound was a cobalt salt and, eventually, that it functioned as part of vitamin B_{12}. This is still the only known role for cobalt, although there is some evidence that it has an effect on thyroid function.

Dietary cobalt can be utilized only in its physiologically active form, cobalamin, or vitamin B_{12}; inorganic cobalt is excreted and has no known function. (Inorganic cobalt is needed in diets of cattle, however, because vitamin B_{12} is produced by gastrointestinal microorganisms during the ruminant digestive process. But because intestinal synthesis of vitamin B_{12} is limited or nonexistent in humans, cobalt must be obtained in the active form.) Thus it is the vitamin B_{12} content of foods, and not their cobalt content, that supplies human needs for this element. Although cobalt is present in a variety of foodstuffs (meats and dairy products and, to a lesser extent, in cereals, grains, and vegetables), the physiologically active form (as described in Chapter 7) must be consumed.

The body of the average human male contains only 1.1 milligrams of cobalt. Small amounts are lost in feces, sweat, and hair, while urine is the main excretory route. Cobalt shares the same transport route as iron and is absorbed in proportion to iron need. Although at times cobalt absorption may, for this reason, be relatively great in proportion to human need for cobalamin, toxicity is rare. Excessive intakes may have a thyroid-stimulating effect and cause stimulation of the bone marrow, resulting in excessive production of erythrocytes (polycythemia). Cobalt is often used as an antifoaming agent in beer; consumption of large amounts of this beverage have been associated with polycythemia and cardiovascular effects. For most persons however, cobalt toxicity is not likely to occur.

MANGANESE. The total body content of this mineral is about 10 to 20 milligrams, which is distributed throughout all tissues but with the highest concentrations occurring in the pancreas, liver, kidneys, and intestines. Manganese absorption tends to be inefficient (less than 20 percent) and varies inversely with the amount of dietary calcium and iron. Little is excreted in the urine, with the major excretory route being the bile.

Studies of laboratory animals have shown that manganese is required for normal growth, nervous function, and lipid and carbohydrate metabolism. Although the mineral appears to function much the same way in humans, further study is needed. For example, animal research data has clearly established that manganese has a role in glucose metabolism and is a cofactor or component of many enzymes in the body. Many metabolic pathways require manganese, although its mechanism of action remains unclear.

Dietary intake of manganese averages between 2.5 and 7 milligrams per day. Because manganese deficiency is almost unknown in humans, the Food and Nutrition Board has established a provisional requirement of only 2.5–5 milligrams per day for adults.

As Table 8-9 shows, a wide range of foodstuffs contain generous amounts of manganese. Whole grains and tea are especially rich in the mineral, but nuts, vegetables, and fruits are also good sources. As with other trace minerals, the manganese content of foods depends in large part on agricultural and processing conditions.

To date, manganese deficiency has been demonstrated only in animals, whose requirements are far greater than those of humans. Deficiency in animals affects bone, brain tissue, and reproductive function. Because substantial amounts of manganese are found in many common foods, intakes for most people probably far exceed need. But the possibility of manganese

TABLE 8-9
Manganese Content of Selected Foods
Estimated Safe and Adequate Daily Dietary Intake for Adults
2.5–5 mg

Food	Serving Size	Manganese Content µg/serving
Tea	1 c (1 tsp tea)	400–2,700
Raisins	small box = 1½ oz	201
Rice, cooked	½ c	146
Spinach, cooked	½ c	128
Carrots, cooked	½ c	120
Broccoli, cooked	½ c	119
Orange	1 medium	52
Peas, green	½ c	51
Bran flakes, 40%	1 c	48
Apple	1 medium	46
Milk, whole	1 c	46
Milk, skim	1 c	46
Swiss cheese	1 oz	37
Bread, white	1 slice	36
Eggs	1 large	30
Tomato	1 medium	30
Chicken, meat only	3½ oz	21
Green beans, cooked	½ c	15
Liver, beef, cooked	3 oz	14
Butter	1 pat = 1 tsp	5
Beef, ground, cooked	3 oz	4

Note: The mineral contents in the table are given in micrograms (µg), whereas the provisional requirement is 2.5–5 milligrams (mg). One milligram is equivalent to 1,000 µg.

Source: Adapted from H. Q. Schroeder, J. J. Balassa, and I. H. Tiptin, Essential trace metals in man: Manganese. *Journal of Chronic Diseases* 19:545, 1966.

deficiency should be considered in certain cases. In particular, pregnant women consuming diets high in calcium and low in manganese may risk deficiency because of the requirements of the developing fetus. Growing children, who may require more of this mineral, and adults on weight-reduction diets may also develop deficiencies. (Deficiencies of other minerals are known to occur in such cases as well.)

Toxicity from dietary intake appears to be highly unlikely. However, miners of manganese ores may develop a syndrome from inhaling ore dust. The symptoms resemble those of viral encephalitis. Tremor and loss of coordination characterize severe cases. But this is not associated with an excess of dietary manganese (Schroeder et al., 1966).

MOLYBDENUM. Total body content of this mineral is very small, as is the provisional daily allowance of 150 to 500 micrograms. As a component of xanthine oxidase, molybdenum plays an essential role in the metabolism of the purine components of nucleic acids and the formation of uric acid. It is also a cofactor for various flavoprotein enzymes. High sulfate intakes decrease absorption and increase urinary excretion of the mineral.

The estimated dietary intake of 45 to 500 micrograms per day probably more than meets human requirements. Although present in small amounts, molybdenum is widely distributed in foodstuffs. Whole-grain cereals, legumes, and organ meats are good sources of the mineral.

No deficiency of molybdenum is known in humans. Since the mineral competes with copper, excess molybdenum produces symptoms of copper deficiency in animals. Increasing the sulfate content of the diet prevents copper deficiency by increasing excretion of molybdenum. These interrelationships between minerals are fascinating and have spurred much research.

SELENIUM. The body content of this mineral, totaling only a few micrograms, is distributed throughout the body tissues, with highest concentrations in the kidney, liver, spleen, pancreas, and testes. It is readily absorbed and is excreted in urine and feces.

Because selenium and vitamin E were known to spare each other, it was long thought that the mineral must function as an antioxidant. This has been confirmed by the finding that selenium specifically functions as a component of glutathione peroxidase, a powerful antioxidant that protects cell membranes from destruction.

Little is known about the dietary requirement for selenium—estimated to be 75 micrograms—and no RDA has been set. Provisional allowances of 50 to 200 micrograms per day have been recommended. In general, the selenium content of foods varies with their protein content. Meats, seafoods, egg yolk, and milk are good sources. Cereals are not reliable sources since their selenium content depends on the amount of this mineral in the soil. Milling of grains causes little loss, but the addition of sugar in processing appears to produce significant loss of selenium. Cooking has little effect on selenium content, but boiling the few vegetables that do have high selenium content, such as mushrooms and asparagus, will leach the mineral. Generally, though, fruits and vegetables are poor sources.

Despite numerous studies, no specific disease condition has been associated with selenium deficiency in humans, although a variety of symptoms is exhibited in animal species (Levander, 1975). However, children recovering from kwashiorkor have shown improved additional weight gain with selenium supplementation (Schwarz, 1961).

Selenium is toxic. Cattle that graze on selenium-rich land develop a condition with the descriptive name "blind staggers." Increased dental caries have been reported among schoolchildren living in areas of selenium-rich soil. Selenium also produces chronic fatigue, irritability, and damage to such tissues as nails and hair. However, long-term ingestion of 2,400 micrograms or more daily would be required to produce these effects (Food and Nutrition Board, 1977).

SILICON, TIN, VANADIUM, AND NICKEL. All of these minerals, originally believed to be mineral contaminants (like lead), have been reappraised since the inducement of deficiency conditions in experimental animals. If a nutrient is essential to one or more species of mammals, there is a good chance that humans require it also.

Silicon, after oxygen the most common element on earth, is nevertheless found only in trace amounts in the body. The highest concentrations are found in the connective tissues generally and in the collagen of skin and bone.

Deficiency studies of animals suggest that silicon may have an essential role in bone calcification and the synthesis of mucopolysaccharides. Confirmation of the latter role would mean that silicon participates in other processes involving growth and maintenance of connective tissue, embryonic development, and wound healing. Silicon may play a part in aging—the silicon content of skin, aorta, and thymus decreases with age, while that of other tissues remain constant throughout life (Carlisle, 1976). Silicon may also contribute to the structure and resilience of all connective tissue (Schwarz, 1973). The human requirement for silicon is unknown.

Tin has been found to be an essential mineral for rats. Induced tin deficiency in rats resulted in poor growth, loss of hair, and other symptoms (Mertz, 1974). At present, where and how tin functions in the human body remain to be determined. It occurs in water and some foods and especially in canned foods.

Vanadium deficiency has been induced in rats and chickens. Symptoms include impaired growth and abnormal bone development. Research data indicate that vanadium functions in iron and lipid metabolism and perhaps in development of bones and teeth (Hurley, 1976). Its site and mode of function in humans remain to be determined. Vanadium is found in root vegetables, nuts, seafood, some grains, and vegetable oils.

Nickel deficiency has been induced in several different species of laboratory animals, variously affecting growth, serum cholesterol levels, and red blood cell count, and having other manifestations as well. The organ most usually affected is the liver. Nickel, like vanadium, appears to be involved in lipid metabolism, but its function in humans has not been established. It occurs in legumes, tea, pepper, cocoa, grains, and a variety of fruits and vegetables.

Knowledge of these trace elements is still evolving. The bioassay techniques to measure the involvement of the minute quantities in which these elements occur in the human body are themselves still evolving as well. The need for these elements is already clear, however, and emphasizes the importance of consuming a diversified diet. Foods fortified with vitamins and iron do not contain trace minerals, nor do the vitamin supplements available at health food or drug stores. We cannot, therefore, meet our requirements for them through artificial sources. Our food supply contains *all* of the many nutrients we need—including those for which the need cannot yet be measured.

SUMMARY

In addition to carbohydrate, lipid, protein, and vitamins, the body requires a group of some 20 elements called *minerals*. Each of the *macro* minerals is required in amounts of 100 milligrams or more per day, represents 0.05 percent of body weight, or both; each *trace* element is required in amounts of no more than a few milligrams per day.

The minerals commonly occur as components of important organic molecules such as hemoglobin, thyroid hormone, and metalloenzymes. They also form inorganic compounds (as in bone) and function as free ions in the blood and other body fluids. The minerals help to maintain acid-base and fluid balance; act as catalysts of reactions in hormonal and metabolic processes; are involved in muscle contraction and nerve-impulse transmission; and are components of essential body compounds, both structural and functional.

The seven major minerals are calcium, phosphorus, magnesium, sodium, potassium, chlorine, and sulfur.

Calcium functions chiefly as a component (with phosphorus) of hydroxapatite, the main structural component of bone and dental tissue, and plays an important part in blood coagulation, synthesis of the neurotransmitter acetylcholine, activation of certain enzymes (e.g., pancreatic lipase), regulation of muscle contraction, and nerve impulse transmission.

Phosphorus, like calcium, functions in the mineralization of bones and teeth. Energy metabolism requires phosphate-containing compounds (for example, ATP and certain phosphorylated vitamins), as does the absorption of glucose. Phosphorus is an essential component of phospholipids in membranes and of nucleic acids; phosphates are also effective buffers.

Magnesium interacts with calcium and with phosphate and carbonate ions in many of its functions, which include bone metabolism, catalysis of many enzyme reactions (including glucose, fatty acid and amino acid metabolism, and protein synthesis), muscle contraction, and nerve activity.

Sodium maintains osmolarity and acid base balance, and affects extracellular fluid volume (and thus blood pressure) and nerve-impulse transmission. Because of the very widespread distribution of sodium chloride in natural and processed foods, and its extensive use as table salt, sodium deficiency is rare. Excessive intake, however, is associated with high blood pressure.

Potassium, like sodium, functions in maintaining fluid balance and osmolarity, muscle contraction, and nerve activity. It also plays a role in carbohydrate metabolism (particularly glycogen synthesis and glucose oxidation) and, indirectly, in protein synthesis.

Chlorine also helps to maintain acid base balance and osmolarity. As a component of hydrochloric acid in gastric juice, chlorine has an important part in digestion. The mineral also activates amylase (which hydrolyzes starch and glycogen) and functions in nerve activity.

Sulfur has a variety of functions as a component of sulfur-containing amino acids, compounds associated with oxidation-reduction reactions (e.g., CoA, thiamin, biotin), insulin and other hormones, and structural compounds (mucopolysaccharides and sulfated lipids).

The trace minerals about which most is known are iron, copper, zinc, iodine, and fluorine. Much less is known about chromium, cobalt, manganese, molybdenum, selenium, and even less about silicon, tin, vanadium, and nickel.

Iron functions chiefly as a component of oxygen-transporting hemoglobin found in red blood cells. It is also a component of myoglobin (for oxygen reserve in muscle), and such enzymes as catalase, xanthine oxidase, and the cytochrome enzymes of electron transport, and as a cofactor of aconitase in the citric acid cycle.

The classic disease condition resulting from deficiency is iron deficiency anemia (although anemia can have a number of causes). Excess iron produces hemosiderosis, characterized by necrosis of the liver and other soft tissues.

Copper, as a component of ceruloplasmin, is essential for incorporation of iron in hemoglobin. It also increases iron absorption and stimulates iron mobilization from tissue stores. Copper-containing enzymes function in energy metabolism and the metabolism of fatty acids and connective tissues.

Zinc is a component of at least 20 metalloenzymes; its more important functions include CO_2 transport and peptide digestion. Zinc also has a part in protein and nucleic acid metabolism, mobilization of vitamin A from the liver, and wound healing. Deficiency of the mineral retards growth and sexual maturation and delays wound healing.

Iodine functions in the synthesis of two thyroid hormones (thyroxine and triiodothyronine), which are "metabolic accelerators" and which are essential to normal metabolism. Iodine deficiency results in the classic symptom of goiter. Hypothyroidism (underactive thyroid), of which myxedema is a form, and hyperthyroidism (Grave's disease) are not related to dietary intake but represent metabolic errors.

Fluorine protects bone and especially dental tissue. An increased number of dental caries results from inadequate fluorine intake.

Little is known about the other trace minerals. *Chromium*—as GTF—enhances the activity of insulin and several other enzymes. *Cobalt's* only known function is as a component of vitamin B_{12}, the only form of this mineral the body can utilize. *Manganese* appears to be essential for growth, nervous function, and metabolism of lipids and carbohydrates. *Molybdenum* functions in purine metabolism. *Selenium* has antioxidant properties and functions as a component of glutathione oxidase, which destroys lipid peroxides. No deficiency condition has been identified, but the mineral is toxic, causing the "blind staggers" in animals and a variety of chronic symptoms in humans who live in areas where selenium-rich soils transfer large amounts of the mineral to plant foods.

Silicon, tin, vanadium, and *nickel* have yet to be established as essential nutrients, although there is some evidence that they have roles in maintenance of nutritional health. Silicon appears to be needed for structure and maintenance of connective tissue; and tin, vanadium, and nickel also appear to be involved in growth, with the latter two elements possibly involved in lipid metabolism.

BIBLIOGRAPHY

Albanese, A. A., E. J. Lorenze, Jr., and E. H. Wein. Osteoporosis: Effects of calcium. *American Family Physician,* October 1978.

Anderson, M. P., R. D. Hunt, H. J. Griffiths, K. W. McIntyre, and R. E. Zimmerman. Long-term effect of low dietary calcium: phosphate ratio on the skeleton of *Cebus albifrons* monkeys. *Journal of Nutrition* 107:834, 1977.

Bessis, M. The blood cells and their formation. In *The cell,* Vol. 5, ed. J. Brachet and A. E. Mirsky. New York: Academic Press, 1961.

Carlisle, E. M. Silicon. In *Present knowledge in nutrition,* 4th ed., ed. D. M. Hegsted. Washington, D. C.: Nutrition Foundation, Inc., 1976.

Consumer Reports. Fluoridation: The cancer scare. 43:392, 1978.

Crosby, W. H. Current concepts in nutrition: Who needs iron? *New England Journal of Medicine* 297:543, 1977.

Food and Nutrition Board. Selenium and human health. *Nutrition Reviews* 11(34):347, 1977.

Food and Nutrition Board, National Research Council. *Recommended dietary allowances,* 9th ed. Washington, D. C.: National Academy of Sciences, 1979.

HEGSTED, D. M., S. SCHUETTE, M. ZEMEL, AND H. M. LINKSWILER. The effect of level of protein and phosphorus intake on calcium balance in young adult men. *Federation Proceedings* 38:765, 1979 (Abstract No. 2839).

HURLEY, L. S. Manganese and other trace elements. In *Present knowledge in nutrition,* ed. D. M. Hegsted. 4th ed, Washington, D.C.: Nutrition Foundation, Inc., 1976.

KIDD, P. S., F. L. TROWBRIDGE, J. B. GOLDSBY, AND M. Z. NICHAMAN. Sources of dietary iodine. *Journal of the American Dietetic Association* 65:420, 1974.

KREHL, W. A. Magnesium. *Nutrition Today* 2(3):16, 1967.

LEVANDER, O. A. Selenium and chromium in human nutrition. *Journal of the American Dietetic Association* 66:338, 1975.

MARSTON, R., AND B. FRIEND. *National food situation.* Economic Research Service, Bulletin No. NFS-158. Washington, D.C.: U.S. Government Printing Office, November 1976.

MERTZ, W. The newer essential trace elements, chromium, tin, vanadium, nickel and silicon. *Proceedings of the Nutrition Society* 33:307, 1974.

MONSEN, E. R., I. N. KUHN, AND L. FINCH. Iron status of menstruating women. *American Journal of Clinical Nutrition* 20:842, 1967.

MONSEN, E. R., L. HALLBERG, M. LAYRISSE, D. M. HEGSTED, J. D. COOK, W. MERTZ, AND C. A. FINCH. Estimation of available dietary iron. *American Journal of Clinical Nutrition* 31:134, 1978.

NATIONAL CENTER FOR HEALTH STATISTICS. Dietary intake findings United States, 1971–74. Vital and Health Statistics, Series 11, No. 202, DHEW Pub. No. (HRH) 77-1647, Hyattsville, Md., July 1977.

Nutrition Reviews. Dietary phosphorus, PTH, and bone resorption. Vol. 31:124, 1973.

Nutrition Today. The dietary iron controversy. Vol. 7(2):2, 1972.

Nutrition Today. Anatomy of a decision. Vol. 13(1):6, 1978.

SCHROEDER, H. A., J. J. BALASSA, AND I. H. TIPTON. Essential trace metals in man: Manganese. *Journal of Chronic Diseases* 19:545, 1966.

SCHWARZ, K. Development and status of experimental work on factor 3-Selenium. *Federation Proceedings* 20:666, 1961.

SCHWARZ, K. A bound form of silicon in glycosaminoglycans and polyuronides. *Proceedings of the National Academy of Sciences* USA 70:1608, 1973.

SPENCER, H., L. KRAMER, D. OSIS, AND C. NORRIS. Effect of phosphorus on absorption of calcium in man. *Journal of Nutrition* 108:447, 1978.

STRAUSS, R. G. Iron deficiency, infections, and immune function: A reassessment. *American Journal of Clinical Nutrition* 31:660, 1978.

TAMURA, T., B. SHANE, M. T. BAER, J. C. KING, S. MARGEN, AND E. L. R. STOKSTAD. Absorption of mono- and polyglutamyl folates in zinc-depleted man. *American Journal of Clinical Nutrition* 31:1984, 1978.

SUGGESTED ADDITIONAL READING

BOWERING, J., A. M. SANCHEZ, AND M. I. IRWIN. A conspectus of research on iron requirements of man. *Journal of Nutrition* 106:985, 1976.

Consumer Reports. Attack on fluoridation: Six ways to mislead the public. 43:392, 1978.

CULLEN, R. W., A. PAULBITSKI, AND S. M. OACE. Sodium, hypertension, and the U.S. dietary goals. *Journal of Nutrition Education* 10:59, 1978.

ELWOOD, P. E. The enrichment debate. *Nutrition Today* 12(4):18, 1977.

FINCH, C. A. Iron metabolism. *Nutrition Today* 4(2):2, 1969.

GRAHAM, D. M., AND A. A. HERTZLER. Why enrich or fortify foods? *Journal of Nutrition Education* 9(4):166, 1977.

HARRISON, H. E. Phosphorus. In *Present knowledge in nutrition,* 4th ed., ed. D. M. Hegsted. Washington, D.C.: Nutrition Foundation, Inc, 1976.

HEANEY, R. P., R. R. BECKER, AND P. D. SAVILLE. Calcium balance and calcium requirements in middle-aged women. *American Journal of Clinical Nutrition* 30:1603, 1977.

HOLDEN, J. M., W. R. WOLF, AND W. MERTZ. Zinc and copper self-selected diets. *Journal of the American Dietetic Association* 75:23, 1979.

KREHL, W. A. Sodium: A most extraordinary dietary essential. *Nutrition Today* 1(4):16, 1966.

KREHL, W. A. The potassium depletion syndrome. *Nutrition Today* 1(2):20, 1966.

KREHL, W. A. Selenium, the maddening mineral. *Nutrition Today* 5(4):26, 1970.

LANE, H. W., AND J. J. CERDA. Potassium requirements and exercise. *Journal of the American Dietetic Association* 73:64, 1978.

LEIBEL, R. L. Behavioral and biochemical correlates of iron deficiency. *Journal of the American Dietetic Association* 71:398, 1977.

LINKSWILER, H. M. Calcium. In *Present knowledge in nutrition,* 4th ed., ed. D. M. Hegsted. Washington, D.C.: Nutrition Foundation, Inc., 1976.

MENEELY, G. R., AND H. D. BATTARBEE. Sodium and potassium. *Nutrition Reviews* 34:225, 1976.

MERTZ, W. Trace elements. *Contemporary Nutrition* 3(2):1, 1978.

MESSER, H. H., AND L. SINGER. Fluoride. In *Present knowledge in nutrition,* 4th ed., ed. D. M. Hegsted. Washington, D.C.: Nutrition Foundation, Inc., 1976.

PENNINGTON, J. T., AND D. H. CALLOWAY. Copper content of foods: Factors affecting reported values. *Journal of the American Dietetic Association* 63:143, 1973.

REISIN, E., R. ABEL, M. MODAN, D. S. SILVERBERG, H. E. ELIAHOU, AND B. MODAN. Effect of weight loss without salt restriction on the reduction of blood pressure in overweight hypertensive patients. *New England Journal of Medicine* 298:1, 1978.

SANDSTEAD, H. H. Zinc, a metal to grow on. *Nutrition Today* 3(1):12, 1968.

SHILS, M. E. Magnesium. In *Present knowledge in nutrition,* 4th ed., ed. D. M. Hegsted. Washington, D.C.: Nutrition Foundation, Inc., 1976.

STADTMAN, T. C. Biological function of selenium. *Nutrition Reviews* 35:161, 1977.

ULMER, D. D. Current concepts: Trace elements. *New England Journal of Medicine* 297:318, 1977.

UNDERWOOD, E. J. Cobalt. In *Present knowledge in nutrition,* 4th ed., ed. D. M. Hegsted. Washington, D.C.: Nutrition Foundation, Inc., 1976.

Chapter 9

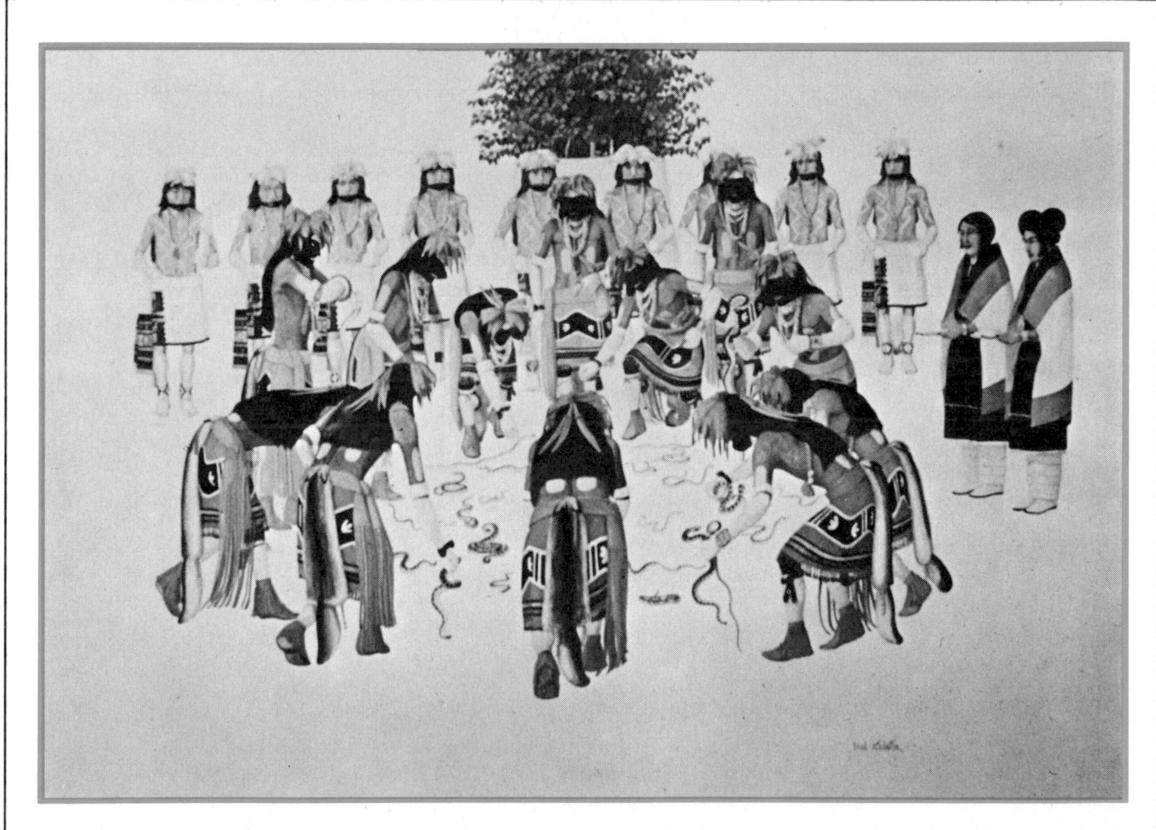

The Snake Dance by Fred Kabotie

Water Balance

Water . . . is the image of the ungraspable phantom of life; and this is the key to it all.

—Herman Melville,
MOBY DICK

From the beginning of recorded history, water has been exalted in all cultures as the source of life, the healer of illness, the secret of immortality. The horned water serpent of the Pueblo Indians; the river Lethe whose waters, according to Greek mythology, brought forgetfulness; the Christian ritual of baptism—these are only a few examples of the universal recognition given to water throughout human existence.

It is, in fact, generally believed that water was the primordial environment in which living cells, which would give rise to all subsequent life forms, first appeared. Biologically speaking, we haven't strayed too far from those origins. The millions of minute cells that make up our bodies may be viewed as tiny fluid-filled aquatic organisms, moving in a sea of flowing body fluids. Body fluids—*water*—normally comprise from 45 to 60 percent of the weight of healthy adults—and a similar proportion of the weight of every kind of living organism. Body fluids are never static but always in motion. Water enters the body with ingested foods and beverages and is excreted in perspiration, respiration, feces, and urine. As it travels through the various body systems, it is constantly assisting or participating in biochemical reactions or otherwise facilitating essential body processes.

Water intake and output are normally in equilibrium, and about 2,400 milliliters (2.5 quarts) are ingested and excreted by the average adult every day (Strand, 1978). Interrelated regulatory systems in the brain, kidneys, and endocrine glands maintain water balance between intake and output and control the distribution of water within the body as well. Normally there are no significant fluctuations in body water levels. Although the body can tolerate a loss of most of its fat and carbohydrate content, and of about 50 percent of its protein, a loss of only 10 percent of body water is life threatening, and deficits greater than 20 percent are invariably fatal. Tales of survival after weeks of starvation are common, but more than a few days' survival without water is rare.

WATER AS A CHEMICAL

Water is a vital nutrient, and yet its role is quite different from that of the other nutrients previously studied. It is not digested before being absorbed from the intestine. It does not supply energy for growth, maintenance, or physical work. But as a substance with unique chemical and physical properties, it provides a suitable **medium** for the chemical reactions that occur in the body. In addition, water participates in biological reactions and plays an important role in the regulation of body temperature.

Model of Four Water Molecules Joined by Hydrogen Bonds

A single water molecule is triangular in shape, with one oxygen atom attracting the electrons from the two hydrogen atoms, which then become relatively positive in charge. The electronegative oxygen atom can attract other positive ions (cations), while the hydrogen atoms attract negative ions (anions). This chemical property decreases the strength of attraction between cations and anions and permits them to dissolve in a water solution. Since most biological compounds have areas of positive and negative charge, water is an excellent **solvent.**

Another fascinating property of water is that it remains liquid at room— and body—temperatures, although its component elements are gases at these same temperatures. If it were not for the strong attraction water molecules have for *one another,* a result of hydrogen bonds, water would be a volatile substance under normal living conditions. Large amounts of heat are needed to break the hydrogen bonds that allow water to "stick" to itself, accounting for the observation that water has a high *heat capacity;* that is, it takes a relatively large amount of heat to increase the temperature of water. As a result, this liquid is a relatively poor conductor of heat. This property is important in the economy of the body: Although water helps to distribute heat evenly throughout the body, it absorbs the heat produced without becoming "hot" itself.

Compared to other molecules of the same size, water has a high *latent heat of vaporization,* the amount of heat necessary to produce a vapor from a liquid. Only at 212°F (100°C) are all the hydrogen bonds between water molecules broken, allowing water to boil up to form water vapor. In contrast, vaporization of other common liquid chemicals occurs at much lower temperatures. This special property of water is important, because one of the ways the body dissipates excess heat is through evaporation of water from the skin. If water were vaporized at lower levels of energy (heat), humans could not survive the external heat of tropical climates or the internal heat of high fevers. Rather, the body's fluid supply would quickly sizzle away.

FUNCTIONS OF WATER

The chemical properties of water are responsible for its functions in the body.

Regulation of Body Temperature

Metabolic reactions produce energy, some of which is trapped as ATP and some of which is released as heat. A portion of this heat is used for the maintenance of body temperature. But the body must dispose of excess heat, which would otherwise inactivate enzymes necessary for vital metabolic processes. The major routes for loss of excess heat at low environmental temperature and humidity are radiation and conduction. Smaller amounts of heat are dissipated as "insensible perspiration." Six hundred kilocalories are used in the evaporation of every liter of fluid from the surface of the body. As a result, loss of water by insensible perspiration is estimated to be 20 to 30 milliliters per hour, and loss of heat to be about 12 to 18 kilocalories per hour (Guyton, 1976). The amount of heat lost by insensible evaporation is in direct proportion to body surface area and in inverse proportion to the amount of subcutaneous fat. This layer of fat acts as an insulator, preventing effective heat transfer—a bonus in winter and a detriment in summer.

When environmental temperature or humidity rise, body heat cannot be effectively lost by radiation and conduction. If the ambient temperature is greater than that of the skin, the body actually gains heat. Under this condition, the only way for the body to cool itself is by sweating (sensible perspiration). When environmental temperature and humidity become so high that perspiration cannot evaporate and exert its cooling effect, heat stroke may result, with body temperatures soaring as high as 107° to 110°F (42° to 43°C). Ambient temperatures higher than 90°F (32°C) and relative humidity greater than 80 percent may produce this condition, particularly during exertion. Heat stroke is life threatening, not only because of water loss due to continued sweat production, but also because elevated body temperatures inactivate cellular enzyme systems. Irreversible cell damage may follow.

The temperature-regulating capacity of water is also apparent when a fever "breaks," which is signalled by heavy perspiration. As water evaporates from the skin, it has a cooling effect and elevated body temperatures start to subside. Prolonged fevers are dangerous because the body's heat cannot be released to the external environment. As in heat stroke, irreversible cell damage occurs when the body temperature exceeds 106°F (41°C).

Solvent for Biochemicals

The solvent properties of water underlie some of its other body functions and are nutritionally important in several ways. Enzymes, hormones, and coenzymes are dissolved in watery body fluids and act on metabolites (amino acids, carbohydrates, vitamins, minerals) that are similarly dissolved. Water also serves as a solvent for waste products—urea, carbon dioxide, and various electrolytes—destined for excretion. As a solvent containing these substances, water assists in their transport to and from all cells of the body.

Lubrication

Water serves as a lubricant in digestion and other body processes. The water in saliva facilitates chewing and swallowing, ensuring that foods will slide easily down the esophagus. Water contained in other digestive fluids sustains movement throughout the gastrointestinal system. The watery fluid surrounding joints, eyeballs, and other body parts helps them to move smoothly. And water is a component of various mucous secretions that help maintain tissue tone and condition.

Hydrolysis and Other Biological Reactions

Water is an active participant in hydrolysis, a major chemical process of digestion. During this process water molecules are ionized into hydrogen (H^+) and hydroxyl (OH^-) groups, each of which reacts with other substances. Sucrose, for example, is hydrolyzed into fructose and glucose, forms in which it can be utilized by body cells (see Chapter 2). In addition, water serves as a reactant in intracellular reactions and plays an important role in the maintenance of electrolyte balance.

DISTRIBUTION OF BODY WATER

The amount of water contained in the body varies with age, tissue composition, and sex. It is highest in earliest life—a human embryo is an average 97 percent fluid, and the body of a newborn baby is about 77 percent water (Wolf, 1958). Dehydration proceeds slowly but steadily throughout life. In an adult male of normal weight, water represents about 60 percent of body weight. Loss of water in all tissues continues and is probably involved in many of the physical alterations associated with aging.

Although water is present in all tissues, its relative proportion varies. Bone is 10 percent water, teeth only 5 percent, while adipose tissue contains from 25 to 35 percent. In comparison, muscle tissue is 72 percent water. Thus, as body fat increases, the relative percentage of body water decreases. In lean, muscular adults, water accounts for 70 percent of total body weight, but in obese adults, only 50 percent. Because women of normal weight have a higher percentage of adipose tissue than men, they have a lower percentage of body water.

Compartmentalization

Approximately 60 percent of the body's total water content is contained inside the cells and is said to make up the **intracellular compartment.** The remaining 40 percent, located in the many areas outside the cells, makes up the **extracellular compartment,** which has two major subdivisions (see Figure 9-1): **Intravascular fluid,** representing 20 percent of the extracellular fluid in the body, is the liquid component of blood, and is present in the heart, arteries, veins, and capillaries. **Interstitial and transcellular fluid,** accounting for 80 percent of the extracellular fluid in the body, includes the fluids bathing all the cells, as well as such diverse substances as cerebrospinal fluid, the ocular fluid lubricating the eyes, the synovial fluid that lubricates joints, various secretions (saliva, bile, gastric juice, mucus), and lymph.

The locations of body fluid are considered as separate compartments, but they do not exist in isolation from one another. Rather, compartmentalization is dynamic, with a constant exchange of fluid and other substances between compartments (see Figure 9-2). A variety of forces operates to maintain the equilibrium of fluids and body chemicals in all compartments.

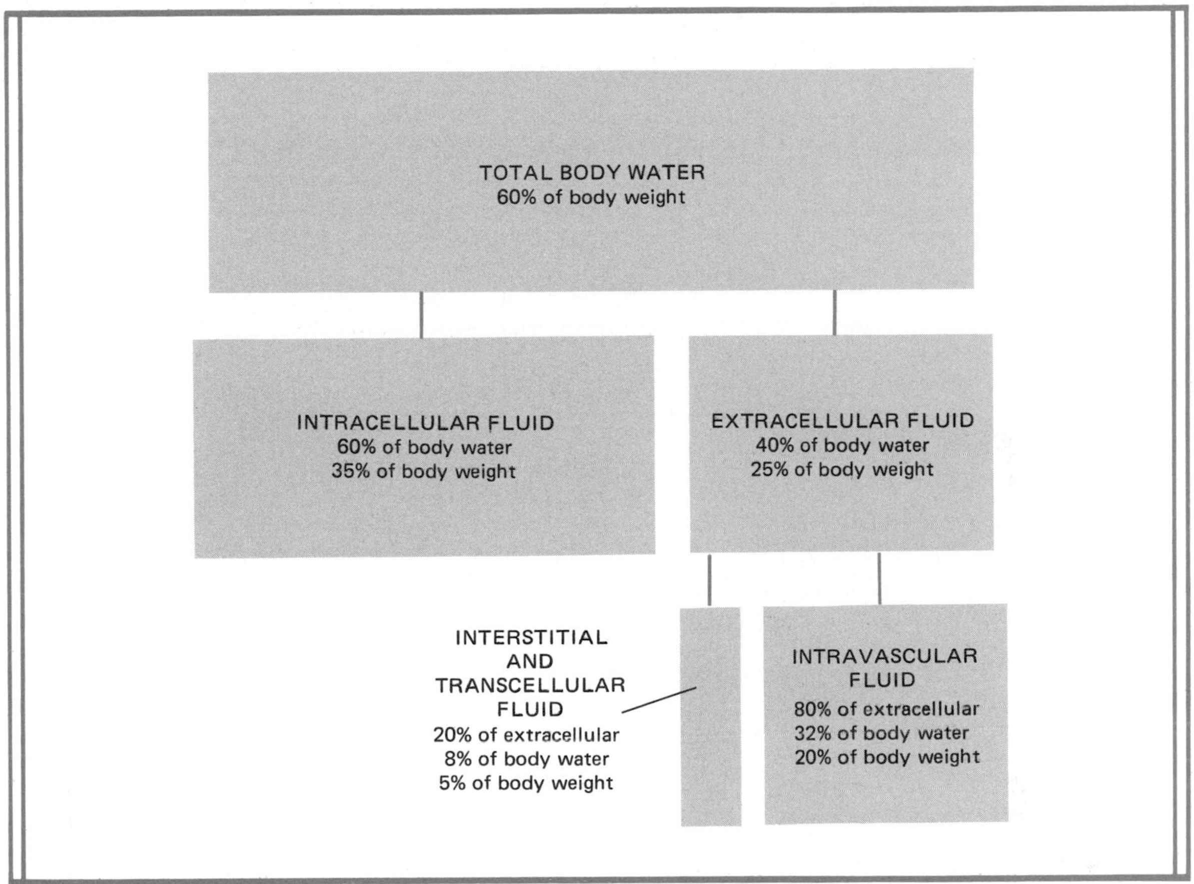

FIGURE 9-1
Fluid Compartments of the Body

Operation of these forces depends to a large extent on the content of the different body fluids.

CONTENT OF BODY FLUIDS. In addition to fluid, every cell in the body contains the various nutrients required for all metabolic processes. Substances dissolved in the body fluids are termed **solutes.** Three categories of solute affect movement of body fluids: electrolytes, large molecules such as the plasma proteins, and smaller molecules such as glucose and urea.

Electrolytes are molecules that dissociate in a water solution into anions (negatively charged particles) and cations (positively charged particles). Chloride, bicarbonate, phosphate, and sulfate are the major anions; sodium, potassium, calcium, and magnesium are the most important cations contained in body fluids.

Within each compartment the total concentration of cations equals the total concentration of anions, making the solutions electrically neutral. By far the most common cation in extracellular fluid is sodium, while chloride is the most common anion. In intracellular fluid, however, potassium is the most

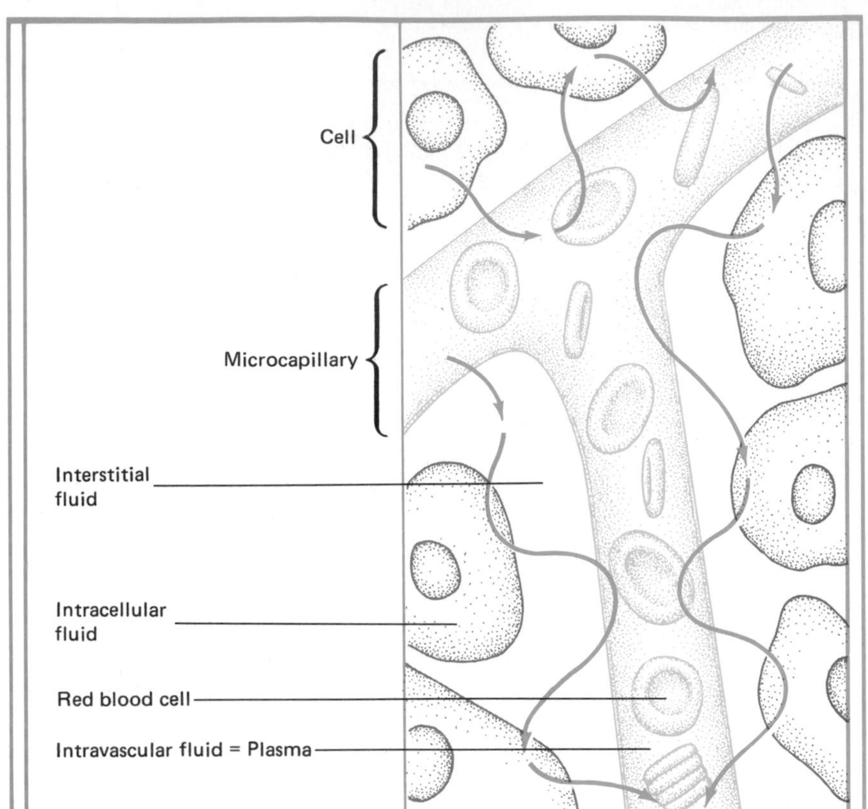

FIGURE 9-2

Relationship of Body Fluid Compartments

Interstitial fluid is the vehicle for the exchange of nutrients, oxygen, and metabolic waste products between the microcapillaries and the cells.

Source: Adapted from J. R. Robinson, Water, the indispensable nutrient, *Nutrition Today* 5(1):16, 1970.

TABLE 9-1 **Ionic Concentration of Body Fluids**

Cation	Anion	Extracellular Fluid		Intracellular Fluid	
		Cation mEq/l	*Anion mEq/l*	*Cation, mEq intracellular water*	*Anion, mEq intracellular water*
Na^+		142		11	
K^+		5		164	
Ca^{++}		5		2	
Mg^{++}		3		28	
	Cl^-		103		
	HCO_3^-		27		10
	HPO_4^{--}		2		105
	SO_4^{--}		1		20
	Protein		16		65
	Organic acids		6		5
Total		155	155	205	205

$$\text{mEq} = \frac{\text{Weight of Substance (mg)}}{\text{Molecular weight} \div \text{Valence (charge)}}$$

Source: Adapted from D. A. Black, *Essentials of fluid balance*, 4th ed. (Philadelphia: Lippincott, 1968), p. 9.

Major Cations	
Sodium	Na^+
Potassium	K^+
Calcium	Ca^{++}
Magnesium	Mg^{++}
Major Anions	
Chloride	Cl^-
Bicarbonate	HCO_3^-
Phosphate	HPO_4^{--}
Sulfate	SO_4^{--}

common cation, and phosphate the most common anion. Extracellular fluid has a high sodium:potassium ratio, about 28:1, while intracellular fluid has a potassium:sodium ratio of approximately 15:1. Body fluids, then, differ in electrolyte content and concentration according to their location and function (see Table 9-1 and Figure 9-3).

Maintenance of Fluid and Electrolyte Balance

Cell membranes are selectively permeable, allowing water and some solutes to pass through. Several mechanisms control the flow of these substances within and among body tissues. Water is constantly flowing across—entering and leaving—every cell membrane; as much as 100 times the cell volume passes through the membrane every second, and yet total cell volume remains unchanged (Strand, 1978). The movement of water molecules through a membrane is known as **osmosis.** The specific electrolyte content and concentration in the fluids on either side of the membrane control the flow of water; fluid moves from the area of low to high electrolyte concentration in order to equalize the concentrations on both sides of the membrane.

The primary mechanisms underlying water transport through cell membranes are osmosis and **filtration pressure.** The greatest part of fluid exchange in the body takes part through the capillaries, whose walls are so thin that fluid and small solute particles pass through easily. Thus water, urea, and glucose move readily across capillary membranes, while hemoglobin and serum albumin, being large molecules, are retained within the capillaries. These large plasma protein molecules within the capillaries create *colloidal osmotic pressure* that tends to retain water in the capillaries and prevent its transfer into the interstitial spaces. Meanwhile, water and small particles are "pushed" out of the capillaries by the hydrostatic or filtration pressure exerted

FIGURE 9-3

Electrolyte Composition of Various Body Fluids

(a) Sweat, normal; (b) Bile fistula; (c) Gastric juice, total fasting; (d) Saliva.

Source: N. M. Methany and W. D. Snively, Jr., *Nurses handbook of fluid balance*, 2nd ed. (Philadelphia: Lippincott, 1974).

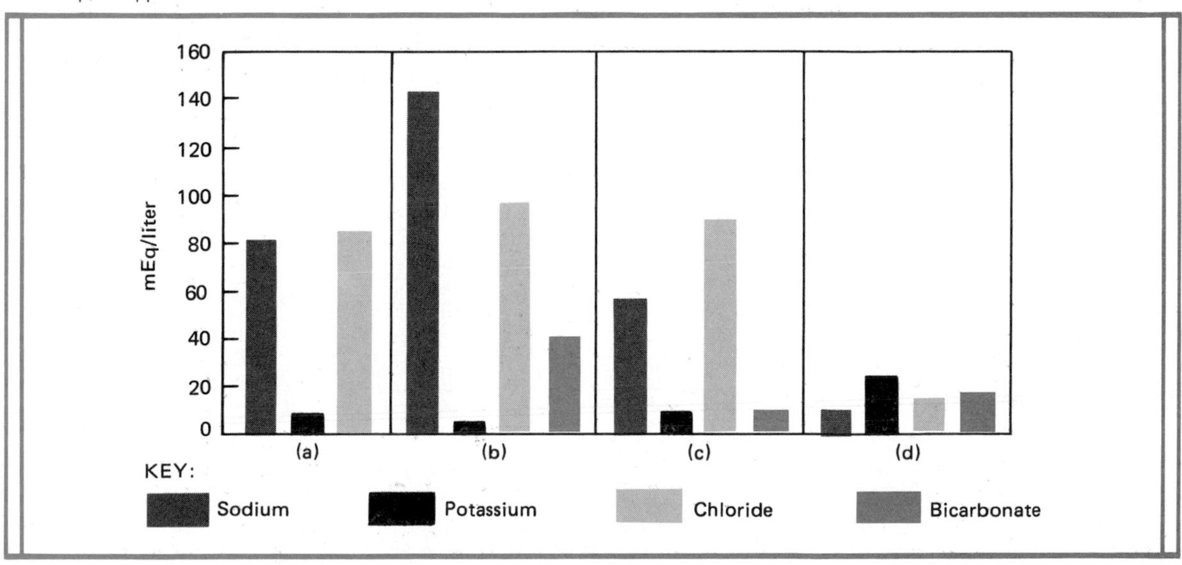

TABLE 9-2
Permeability of Capillary Membranes to Molecules of Different Molecular Weights

Substance	Molecular Weight	Membrane Permeability cm^3/sec/100 g tissue
Water	18	3.7
Urea	60	1.83
Glucose	180	0.64
Sucrose	342	0.35
Myoglobin	17,000	0.005
Hemoglobin	68,000	0.001
Serum albumin	69,000	0.000

Source: Adapted from F. L. Strand, *Physiology: A regulatory systems approach* (New York: Macmillan, 1978), p. 51, Table 4-3.

by the beating heart. This exchange is constantly occurring. Table 9-2 shows the size of protein and other solute molecules and the relative ease with which they pass through capillary membranes.

Under normal circumstances, despite the constant flow of body fluids, the electrolyte balance characteristic of each compartment and kind of cellular or extracellular location is maintained. Cell membranes, being selectively permeable, keep specific proportions of different ions or other solutes in their respective places at a great expense of energy. Water balance, then, is maintained by the varied distribution of osmotically active solutes in the different compartments and cells. Overall volumes of blood and intracellular fluids are stabilized, even, if necessary, at the expense of interstitial fluid, which in effect serves as a "resource" for the maintenance of blood and cell fluid volumes.

Changes in permeability of membranes also affect water movements. The physiological state of an individual can alter membrane permeability, largely through the effects of hormones.

Under normal circumstances, the lymphatic circulation serves as an additional control mechanism, draining moderate amounts of excess fluid from the tissues and eventually returning them to the blood circulation. Under some pathological circumstances, however, this balance is thrown off, and excess fluid is retained in the interstitial space, resulting in **edema.** A sharp increase in blood pressure is one of several reasons why this might occur. Other causes are infections of the lymph vessels and severe protein malnutrition. In this last instance, the concentration of the plasma proteins becomes so low that fluid is not drawn back into the capillaries and instead accumulates in interstitial fluid, leading to the characteristic bloated appearance of victims of kwashiorkor.

WATER BALANCE

Water, like the nutrients previously discussed, is at the center of a metabolic system that comprises sources of intake, body uses, and routes of output (see Figure 9-4).

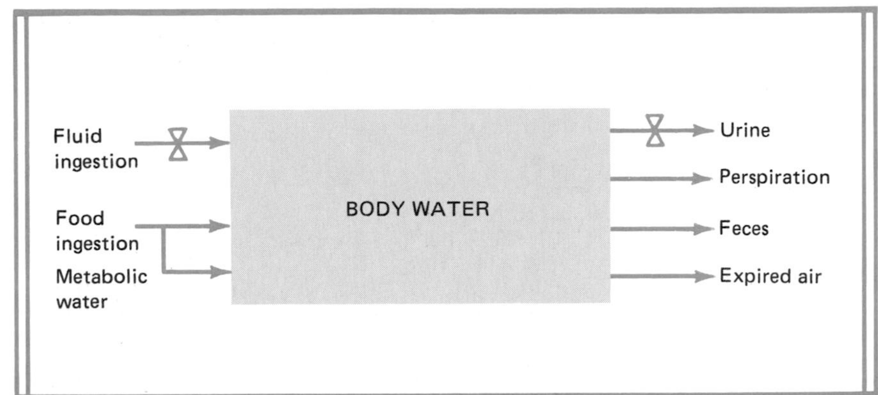

FIGURE 9-4
Normal Routes of Water Intake and Output
Major regulatory controls are indicated. Thirst sensations increase fluid ingestion, and several mechanisms influence urine volume.

Sources of Intake

Dietary fluids and foods constitute the primary sources of water. Consumption of soda, coffee, tea, juice, alcoholic beverages, milk, and just plain tap water typically tallies up to about 1,100 to 1,200 milliliters per day (1 to $1\frac{1}{4}$ quarts). Solid foods contribute another 500 to 800 milliliters of water each day. All foods, except pure fats such as vegetable oil, contain water, with some foods having higher water content than others. Table 9-3 presents the water content of a variety of common foods. Note that vegetables, fruits, and fluid milk products contain more than 75 percent water, whereas meats and fish provide from 50 to 65 percent. Breads (approximately 35 percent water) and dry cereal products (less than 5 percent) do not contribute significant amounts of water.

Metabolism itself provides an additional 300 to 400 milliliters of water each day; when protein, carbohydrate, and fat are oxidized they yield approximately 0.4, 0.6, and 1.1 milliliters of water per gram, respectively. Catabolism of fat stored in the body is yet another potential source of water, producing approximately 1 liter of water for 1 kilogram of adipose tissue.

Mechanisms of Loss

Urine production in the kidneys accounts for most of the body's water output. The lungs, skin, and feces also provide routes for water loss.

THE KIDNEYS. Although a detailed description of kidney function is beyond the scope of this text, several of the vital processes that take place in these organs will be discussed.

The body's total volume of blood passes through the kidneys many times each day, at a rate of about $1\frac{1}{4}$ quarts (1,200 ml) per minute. In this short time a specific part of the kidney's functional units known as *nephrons* (each kidney contains 1 million nephrons!) acts as a filter, producing a protein-free filtrate containing water, glucose, amino acids, minerals, and metabolic waste products.

TABLE 9-3
Water Content of Selected Foods

Food	Serving Size	Water Content ml/serving	ml/100 g
Milk, skim	1 c	222.6	90.6
Cantaloupe	$\frac{1}{4}$ 5″-diam. melon	217.0	91.2
Milk, low-fat, 2% solids	1 c	214.0	87.0
Milk, whole	1 c	213.3	87.4
Yogurt, plain	1 c	193.0	85
Yogurt, fruit-flavored	1 c	170.2	75
Orange	1 medium	129.0	86
Apple	1 medium	126.6	84.4
Banana	1 medium	113.5	75.7
Spinach, frozen, cooked	$\frac{1}{2}$ c	87.2	91.8
Beans, green, cooked, drained	$\frac{1}{2}$ c	59.7	91.8
Fish, haddock, cooked	3 oz	56.1	66.0
Soybeans, cooked	$\frac{1}{2}$ c	55.3	73.7
Rice, cooked	$\frac{1}{2}$ c	54.4	72.5
Chicken, light meat, cooked	3 oz	54.2	63.8
Hamburger, 21% fat, cooked	3 oz	46.1	54.2
Carrots, raw	$\frac{1}{2}$ large	44.1	88.2
Egg	1 large	42.0	73.7
Ice cream	$\frac{1}{2}$ c	41.7	63.2
Lettuce	$\frac{1}{2}$ c chunks	35.3	95.4
Cream cheese	1 oz	14.3	51.1
Cheddar cheese	1 oz	10.4	37.1
Bread, whole-wheat	1 slice	8.4	35.0
Bread, white, enriched	1 slice	8.2	35.6
Apricots, dried	5 halves	4.5	25.0
Corn flakes, dry	1 c	1.0	3.6
Butter	1 tsp	0.8	16.0
Margarine	1 tsp	0.8	15.5
Popcorn	1.5 c	0.8	3.8
Peanut butter	1 oz = 2 tbsp	0.5	1.8
Margarine, whipped	1 tsp	0.5	15.5
Saltine crackers	2	0.3	4.3
Oils	1 tsp	0.0	0.0

Source: C. F. Adams, *Nutritive value of American foods in common units*, USDA Handbook No. 456 (Washington, D.C.: U.S. Government Printing Office, 1975).

The filtrate then passes into long tubules whose cells selectively reabsorb most of the glucose, amino acids, and electrolytes in the filtrate, along with 80 percent of the water. This complex separation and reabsorption process produces urine containing primarily sodium, urea, and other waste products of metabolism dissolved in water. Ordinarily, there is no glucose in the urine. The kidneys have a highly efficient active transport system that passes glucose back into the blood. Only when blood glucose exceeds approximately 160 mg/dl does it surpass its renal threshold and spill into the urine.

Active transport mechanisms also move additional quantities of potassium, hydrogen, and other ions from the blood capillaries across the cells of the kidney tubules, where they are secreted into the urine. This secretion process serves the important function of adjusting acid-base balance in the body. The kidneys' combined filtration, reabsorption, and secretion systems help to regulate the osmotic pressure of body fluids, to control fluid and electrolyte balance, and to maintain acid-base equilibrium.

Under normal circumstances, urine production in the kidneys ranges from 900 to 1,400 milliliters per day, depending on fluid intake. However, metabolic disturbances and altered dietary intake are quickly detected by the kidneys. If there is a decrease in extracellular fluid volume (as in hemorrhage), the kidneys respond by decreasing urine volume. If water consumption is excessive, urine volume is increased. High-protein, high-salt, and low-carbohydrate diets all tend to increase urine volume, because they present the kidneys with a large solute load of urea, sodium, and ketone bodies, respectively. Increasing water intake with these diets will dilute solute concentrations but increase urinary output. Conversely, low-protein, low-salt, and high-carbohydrate diets are useful in situations where water intake and output must be minimized. Before and during space flights, for example, astronauts consume controlled diets to limit water requirements and waste production.

FECAL WATER LOSSES. Of the approximately 8 liters of water secreted into the gastrointestinal tract as part of digestive juices per day, only about 200 milliliters is excreted in the feces. Much of the water of digestive fluids is normally reabsorbed in the colon. Diarrhea and high-fiber diets decrease reabsorption and thus increase fecal water loss.

THE LUNGS. Another 300 milliliters of water vapor is exhaled through the lungs each day. High altitudes and strenuous exercise increase the respiration rate to meet the body's oxygen needs. Under these conditions, respiratory water loss also increases. Dehydration and physical debilitation are often experienced by mountain climbers at high altitudes, when several liters of water may be expired in the course of a day.

THE SKIN. Each day from 400 to 500 milliliters of water is lost through the skin as "insensible" perspiration, the nonvisible sweating that occurs even when the body is at rest. Insensible perspiration increases in dry climates. In the pressurized cabins of airplanes, for example, very dry air and rapid air circulation combine to cause large insensible losses of water, contributing to the feelings of lethargy and fatigue known as "jet lag." Although beverages are usually served to passengers, fluid intake may not be sufficient to replace the quart or more of water lost through insensible perspiration even on short flights. The heavy perspiration that we experience in hot, humid weather contributes to water losses through the skin in addition to normal loss.

Taken together, normal water losses through the urine, feces, insensible perspiration, and respiration total about 1,900 to 2,400 milliliters per day for an adult living in the temperate zones, closely matching the average daily fluid input. Under normal conditions, the water intakes and outputs are balanced.

REQUIREMENTS

There is no RDA for water. Needs vary from individual to individual in response to changes in both the external and internal environments. Age, activity level, health status, air temperature, and even the time of day influence water requirements. The Food and Nutrition Board (1974) indi-

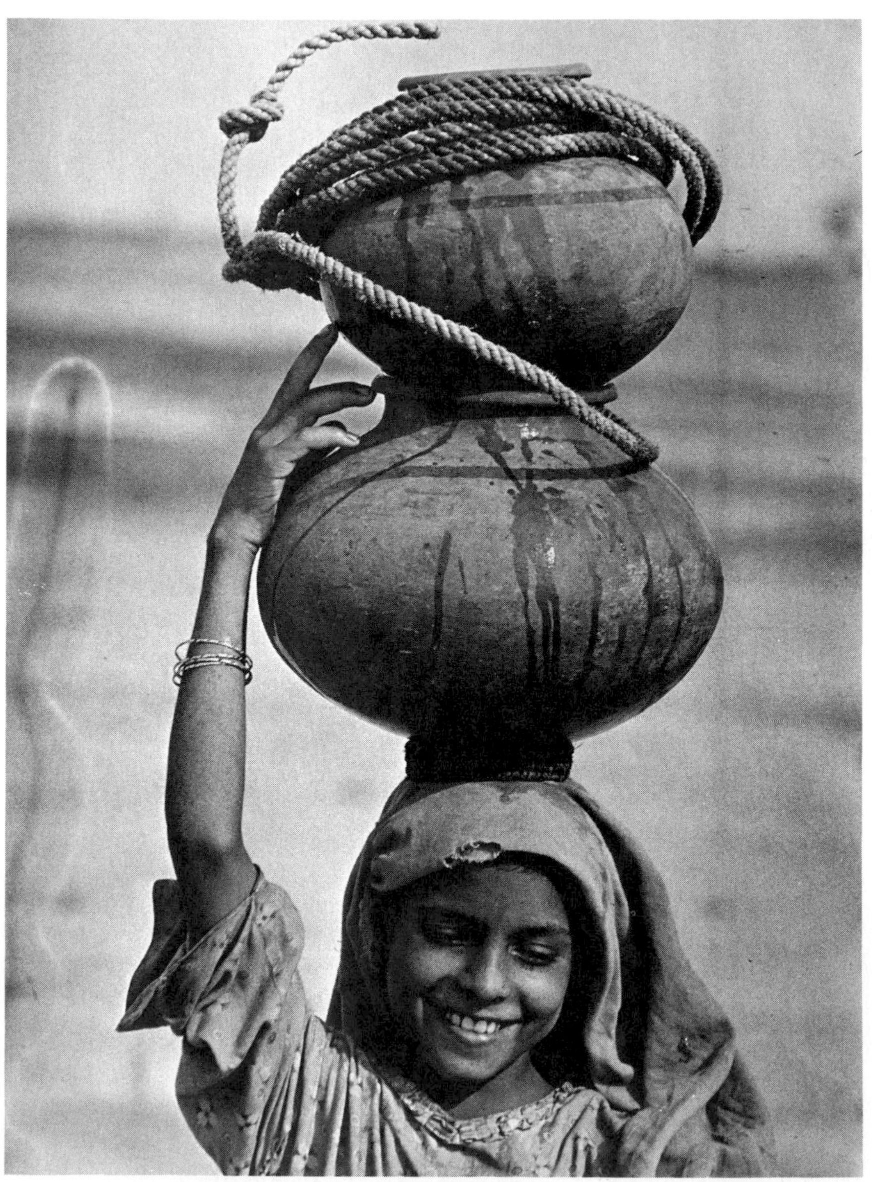

A girl returning from a well with a *gadhas* full of water, in Uttar Pradesh, near New Delhi, India. In most of the developing nations, water must be drawn by hand and carried to the home, often from a distance. (Lynn McLaren, Rapho/Photo Researchers, Inc.)

cates that, "under ordinary circumstances," a reasonable daily water allowance for adults would be 1 milliliter per kilocalorie, providing about 2.5 to 3 quarts, including that contained in foods. The daily allowance for infants is 1.5 milliliters per kilocalorie (0.5 to 1.5 quarts in the first year), an approximate reflection of the higher water content of the body at younger ages, the increased surface area in relation to body weight, and the high basal metabolic rate of infants.

REGULATION OF WATER BALANCE

Water is unique among nutrients because the body has a set of intricate warning mechanisms that detect negative water balance. Of course, the body also has hunger warning systems, but they do not indicate specific nutrient deficits. When people feel hungry, they know that the body is calling for food, but they usually don't know which specific carbohydrates, proteins, fats, vitamins, or minerals are lacking. Thirst, on the other hand, means just one thing: Take a drink. Whether one chooses milk, tea, coffee, or any other fluid, the basic nutrient supplied is still water, just what the body ordered.

Regulation of Water Intake

The thirst warning system involves a complex network of signals and responses. Dehydration and decreased blood volume increase electrolyte concentration in extracellular fluids, thus raising the osmotic pressure of the blood. A decrease of normal body fluids by as little as 1 percent causes thirst. Three interrelated sensing systems become activated, making the individual aware of the need for water intake.

The most familiar sensing system consists of the nerve endings in the mouth and pharynx. As body fluid levels decrease, secretion of saliva decreases as well, and these nerve endings perceive the increasing dryness of the mouth.

Another sensing system consists of thirst receptors in the hypothalamic portion of the brain. Decreases in fluid in the extracellular compartment result in higher electrolyte levels and greater osmotic pressure. As the osmotic pressure draws fluid from the intracellular compartment, cells become dehydrated. This signals the thirst center of the hypothalamus, which also triggers drinking behavior.

A third network is activated when sodium content of extracellular fluid is depleted. As water leaves that compartment to raise the sodium concentration, blood volume diminishes, and fluid levels in the intracellular compartment are increased. The fluid-filled cells do not, however, send nonthirst signals. Rather, the decrease in blood volume stimulates volume receptors in the heart, which in turn signal the hypothalamic thirst center. This might happen, for example, on a low-sodium diet, or as a result of hemorrhage, prolonged diarrhea, or vomiting.

As ingested water enters the system, it is rapidly dispersed into the blood stream. As the extracellular compartment regains its fluid volume, osmotic balance between compartments is achieved. The various thirst receptors are no longer stimulated, and the sensations of thirst vanish—until the cycle begins again.

Regulation of Water Output

The kidneys are the primary control mechanism for regulating water output, and they function chiefly by adjusting urine volume. As decreased extracellular fluid volume results in an increase in osmotic pressure, cells of the posterior pituitary gland are stimulated to secrete antidiuretic hormone (ADH). This polypeptide, also known as vasopressin, acts on the tubules of the kidneys causing increased reabsorption of water, resulting in the production of more concentrated urine. As reabsorption causes fluid volume levels of extracellular fluid to rise, osmotic pressure becomes equalized, cells regain their full fluid volume levels, and ADH secretion is halted.

Another hormone, aldosterone, also acts in the kidneys to help maintain water balance. A steroid hormone produced in the adrenal gland, aldosterone is released in response to sodium depletion, reduced blood volume, or

FIGURE 9-5

How Water Balance Is Maintained

The maintenance of water balance is shown in this diagram devised by E. P. Adolph of the University of Rochester. When the body is dehydrated (left of zero water load), gain by drinking (hatched area) exceeds water loss via urine excretion and evaporation from lungs and skin. When there is an excess of water in the body (right of zero water load), urine output increases and drinking stops so that water loss exceeds the small gain from the oxidation of the hydrogen of foodstuff (indicated by broken line). These regulatory processes compensate for deficits or excesses of water and tend to bring the body to a zero water load, where the curves of total gain and loss cross.

Source: A. V. Wolf, Body water, *Scientific American* 199(5): 125, 1958.

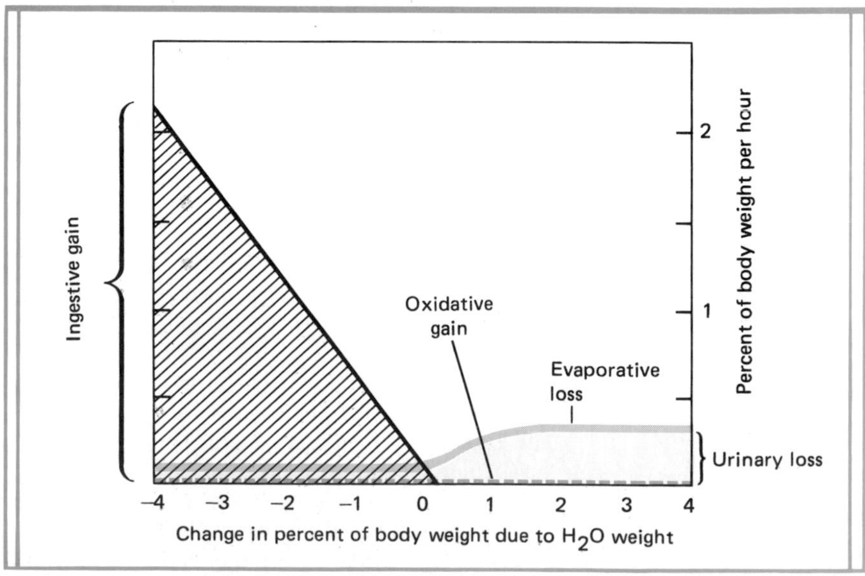

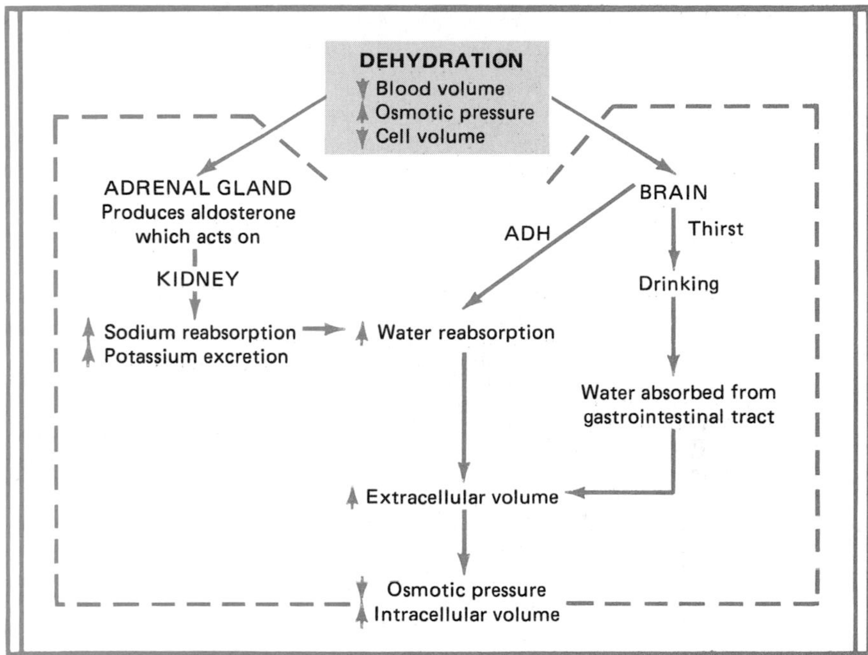

FIGURE 9-6
Summary of Water Balance
Dehydration results in water conservation, mediated by behavioral (thirst) and hormonal (aldosterone and ADH) mechanisms. Restoration of water balance turns off the signals to the brain and adrenal gland.

increased extracellular potassium concentration. In the kidney, aldosterone increases reabsorption of sodium, thus leading to greater sodium concentration inside kidney cells. As a result, the cells of the tubules reabsorb additional water. These increased quantities of sodium and water move from the kidney into the plasma, thus increasing plasma volume and sodium content.

Recall that the sodium:potassium ratios characteristic of the intracellular and the extracellular compartments must be maintained. When the decrease of sodium or increase of potassium in the blood results in an increase in aldosterone production, potassium is drawn from the blood into the kidneys, where it enters the urine for excretion. Release of aldosterone, then, results in retention of sodium and water and excretion of potassium. (See Figure 9-5.)

DISTURBANCES IN WATER BALANCE

Regulatory systems in the kidneys, the hypothalamus, and several other glands ordinarily function in remarkable harmony, finely tuning water and electrolyte balances throughout the body and within its numerous parts (see Figure 9-6). But there are a number of external and internal conditions that overtax these mechanisms. Because maintenance of water balance is critical, any condition resulting in significant depletion or excess is dangerous unless corrected promptly.

Dehydration

Dehydration may result from unusual fluid loss as well as from decreased fluid intake. Hemorrhage, diarrhea, vomiting, or ADH insufficiency directly diminish blood volume. Abnormal sweating, or seepage from extensive burns or other severe wounds, represent loss of interstitial fluid.

Fluid loss consists not only of water, but of electrolytes as well. Because the body's fluid compartments are contiguous and interdependent, water and electrolyte losses in any compartment have an impact throughout. Vomiting, for example, causes losses of hydrochloric acid as well as water from the stomach, and results not only in dehydration but also in electrolyte imbalance. The loss of acid directly causes an excessive concentration of sodium and potassium ions in the remaining body fluids.

In diarrhea the fluid loss from the intestines includes sodium-containing bile, pancreatic, and intestinal secretions. The result is dehydration. The changed osmotic pressure due to this electrolyte imbalance causes more water and sodium to move from the intravascular and interstitial areas into the gastrointestinal tract. Blood volume and cell volume decrease, and too little water is available for the kidneys. These organs respond by increasing sodium retention by the aldosterone mechanism we examined above, so that water will also be reabsorbed. Meanwhile, to maintain the potassium:sodium ratios, potassium ions move out of cells into interstitial spaces. At the same time, the kidneys are recycling the retained sodium back into the blood to increase the *volume* of blood. Potassium must move out of the blood, to be lost in the urine. This deprives muscles of the potassium ions needed for contraction, producing weakness and diminished reflex responsiveness. Severe potassium depletion will affect the functioning of heart muscle and may result in cardiac failure.

For most adults, the mild diarrhea that accompanies occasional stomach upsets or viral infections does not cause significant risk. Even mild diarrhea, however, may have severe consequences for the very young and the elderly, as may any other dehydrating condition. Although the bodies of infants and children contain a higher percentage of water than adults' bodies do, their total water content is, of course, quite small. Because of their high metabolic rate and increased surface area, their water requirements are relatively high. This makes infants quite vulnerable to sudden water losses. Because the elderly have a low percentage of body water, and renal mechanisms for water reabsorption may be impaired, they also are at risk. Metabolic losses of nutrients may be significant as well. When any dehydrating condition exists, at any age, care should be taken to restore fluid and electrolyte balance by ingestion of fluids—water, weak tea, bouillon, orange juice, gelatin dessert, or soft drinks. With the very young or the elderly, fluids may have to be forced or administered intravenously. Even in mature adults, if the condition is severe or prolonged, it may be necessary to administer fluid and electrolyte intravenously.

CHOLERA. An extreme dehydrating condition is cholera, a gastrointestinal disturbance caused by toxin-producing microorganisms. The rapid and voluminous watery diarrhea of cholera creates a sudden and significant loss of both fluid and electrolytes. Therapy limited to antimicrobial agents may kill the

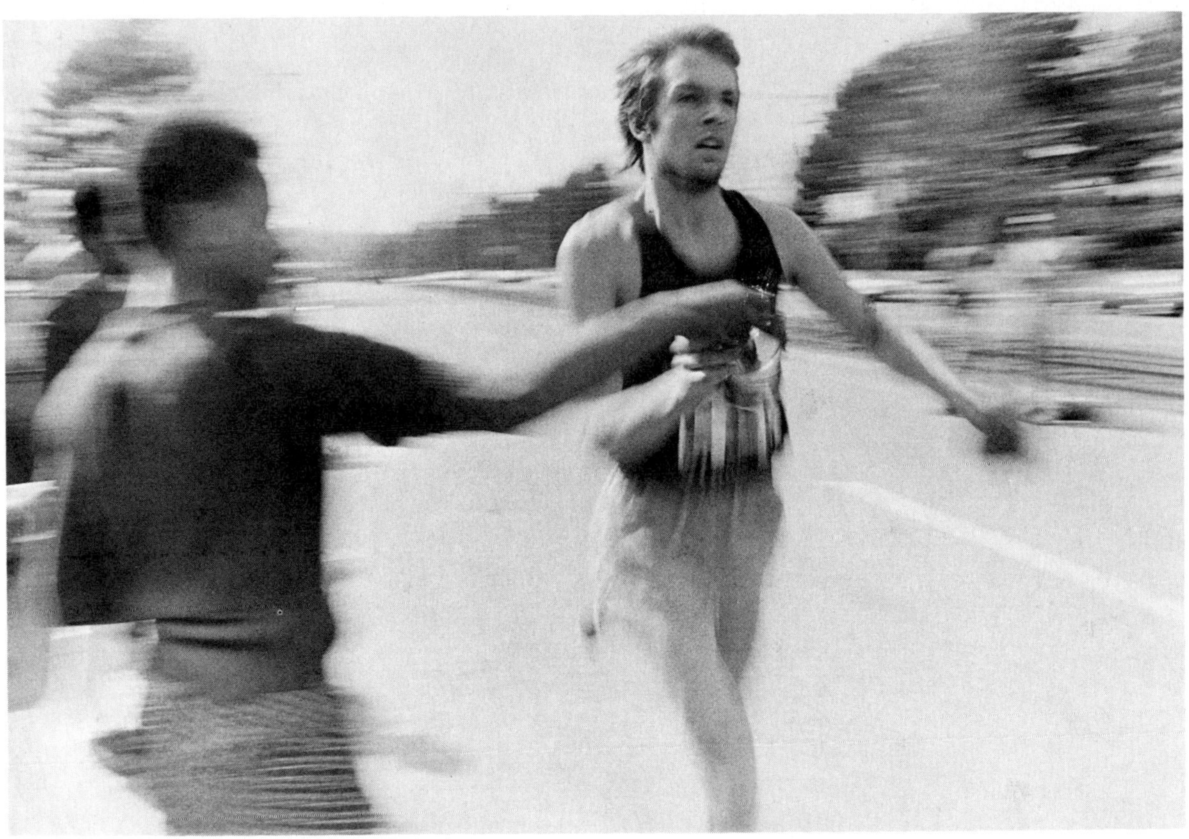

A runner in the Boston Marathon of 1973 receives a drink while racing. (Rocky Weldon/De Wys)

infecting organism but does not combat the severe dehydration that is the primary cause of fatalities from cholera. Immediate and constant therapy with a solution of water and electrolytes is essential.

PROFUSE SWEATING. Profuse sweating represents water loss from the interstitial spaces; sodium and chloride, the major electrolytes of interstitial fluid, are lost as well. Although intense thirst may be perceived, it is not advisable to drink more than 2 quarts of tap water in this situation. Rapid ingestion of plain water further dilutes the depleted salts in the extracellular compartment. In order to equalize electrolyte concentrations, water enters the cells. Cellular overhydration leads to painful muscle contractions ("heat cramps"), weakness, and a decrease in blood pressure. The Food and Nutrition Board recommends that when more than 4 quarts (approximately 4 liters) of water have been consumed to replace sweat losses, additional water intake should be accompanied by 2 grams of sodium chloride for each quart. It is not generally realized that the need for salt is related to water replacement, not to the amount of perspiration. Individuals not adapted to heavy work or exercise in a hot environment may experience salt depletion heat exhaustion due to inadequate replacement of *salt* following heavy perspiration. This is a hazard of which many vacationers are not sufficiently aware, as they spend hours on the tennis courts or otherwise overexert on the first day at a semitropical resort. This condition may also occur in individuals who attempt to carry on a normal activity load during a heat wave, or in athletes, such as football players, who train during the summer.

Water Intoxication

Several years ago there appeared reports about a woman who died after drinking too much water in a misguided attempt to "cleanse" her body of impurities. At about the same time, a young victim of child abuse also died after her father forced her to consume excessive quantities of water. Both deaths were due to **water intoxication**, an intake of fluid that exceeds the maximal rate of urinary flow. As hard as the kidneys work, they cannot keep up with tremendous influxes of water. Fluid volume of cells increases, and cellular constituent substances become diluted. Cells in all parts of the body, including the brain, are affected. The light-headedness, confusion, and poor coordination that result resemble inebriety and give the condition its name. More severe symptoms follow: throbbing headache, nausea and vomiting, weakness, tremors, convulsions, coma, and finally, death. These symptoms are due primarily to the relative lack of salt in the body. Administration of salt in early stages of water intoxication can halt or prevent muscular and other symptoms. Cessation of fluid intake is, of course, essential.

Other Influences on Water Balance

The body is a remarkable machine, but there are limits to its ability to sustain external or internal insults. Under normal conditions the interacting water regulatory mechanisms keep in fine balance with one another. But any of several normal, disease, and accidental conditions can cause fluid imbalance. In each case the regulatory systems are upset, but in different ways.

WATER RETENTION AND FEMALE HORMONES. We have seen that maintenance of water balance involves the hormones ADH and aldosterone. However, other hormones as well act in concert with these. The thyroid hormones, for example, increase reabsorption of sodium in the kidney tubules; other hormones modify the action of ADH. Estrogen and progesterone, the two primary female hormones, are of particular interest in relation to their effects on fluid regulation.

Many women are aware of greater body fluid retention immediately prior to and at the start of their menstrual periods and during the last trimester of pregnancy. It used to be thought that premenstrual edema was due to high progesterone levels at these times. However, it now appears that progesterone is an aldosterone antagonist, increasing sodium and water excretion and causing retention of potassium (Williams, 1974). Sodium loss, and therefore water loss, caused by progesterone production in physiological amounts are transient effects.

Estrogen, on the other hand, has a slight resemblance to aldosterone and initially causes water loss followed by a period of sodium and, therefore fluid retention. Premenstrual edema is a complex phenomenon, with variable effects in different women, and even in an individual woman at different times of life. It is clear that changes in water balance during the menstrual cycle, pregnancy, and the use of oral contraceptives are caused by changing relationships of estrogen and progesterone, but the mechanism causing these effects is not fully understood. Other hormones may be involved as well.

DIABETES. The dynamics of water and electrolyte balance have particular significance for individuals with diabetes, heart disease, and, of course, kidney failure. Diabetes mellitus, characterized by spillage of glucose into the urine, was discussed in Chapter 2. Another type of diabetes is known as diabetes insipidus, because of the bland, diluted quality of the urine, as opposed to the honeylike urine of the condition associated with lack of insulin. Diabetes insipidus is caused by abnormalities in ADH production or response, and results in the production of enormous quantities of urine (5 to 15 liters per day) and feelings of extreme thirst. When the condition is caused by deficient production of ADH by the pituitary, it can be treated with ADH replacement. Patients with diabetes insipidus caused by kidney cells that are unresponsive to the action of ADH are less fortunate and must rely on drinking large amounts of water to compensate for the extreme urinary loss.

DIURETICS. Edema, or fluid accumulation within the tissue spaces, accompanies various conditions, including congestive heart failure. Diuretic drugs are used to help correct this imbalance. Many diuretics inhibit the action of aldosterone, increasing sodium loss in the urine and drawing water away as well. As water is lost, accumulated interstitial fluid moves out of the tissues and into the vascular compartment on the way to the kidneys. Some diuretics also cause potassium depletion, an unwanted side effect. To counteract this, patients taking these drugs are advised to ingest potassium, either in the form of supplements or in foods, such as bananas and citrus fruits, that are rich in this mineral (see Chapter 8).

Some people use diuretics to promote weight loss. It should be apparent that diuretics rid the body of electrolytes and water, not of fat. Any weight loss that might follow indiscriminate use of diuretics may fool the mind of the dieter but not the body. Dehydration, potassium deficits, and other undesirable situations may follow. Meanwhile, the fat is unaffected.

Ethanol, the alcohol found in beverages, acts as a diuretic and inhibits the secretion of ADH by the pituitary gland. The increased volume of urine observed following a cocktail party is due not only to the fluid volume of the beverages consumed, but to their inhibition of ADH secretion. Instead of being reabsorbed in the kidneys, fluid goes directly into the urine. The persistent thirst felt several hours later, and the headachy "hangover" characteristic of "the morning after," signal the need to replenish the fluids lost the night before. The effect depends on the amount of alcohol in the blood, which in turn is directly related to the amount consumed and inversely related to the length of time over which the alcohol is imbibed.

DROWNING. Drowning frequently results from drastic electrolyte imbalances and concomitant rapid shifts in water between the body's fluid compartments. The mechanisms of death by drowning in sea water and in fresh water are quite different. Body fluids contain 0.9 percent salt. Because sea water is 3.5 percent salt, its accumulation in the lungs causes a rush of water from the blood and across the alveolar membranes of the lungs in a vain attempt to dilute the sodium concentration. Death follows due to accumulation of water in the lungs (pulmonary edema) and hemoconcentration (decreased fluid in the blood). On the other hand, drowning in fresh water fills the lungs with relatively unsalted water, which rushes through the alveolar membranes into the bloodstream and then into red blood cells. The influx of water causes the erythrocytes to fill to the bursting (hemolysis) point. The large quantities of potassium released by hemolysis damage the heart muscle, and death due to cardiac arrest follows.

CURRENT ISSUES

According to Sir Edmund Hillary, his expedition succeeded in conquering Mt. Everest where others had failed because care had been taken to provide plentiful supplies of water for the last, highest stages of the climb (Mitchell et al., 1976). Hillary knew well that water lost by the combination of extreme exertion and high altitudes could rapidly lead to dehydration and debilitation since, at high altitudes, the amount of water lost in respiration increases, as it does during exercise at any altitude. In addition, the temperature-regulating capacity of body fluids is reduced, because 600 kilocalories of body heat are lost with every liter of water expired or evaporated. Climbers become chilled easily, especially at night when there is no production of body heat by exercise. Chilling may interfere with sleep, thus impairing the next day's performance (Robinson, 1970).

Most of us will never climb mountains or sleep out at altitudes of 20,000 feet, but water is just as vital for performance of our daily activities. In recent years, people of industrialized nations have been learning that their water supply cannot be taken for granted. The problem of ensuring adequate supplies of potable water has beome an important medical and social concern.

The water flowing out of the tap in our homes has a long history. As part of the great water cycle, the molecules in tap water, in one form or another, rained on or flowed across the earth billions of years ago. It has been used and reused all over the globe, by countless beings of every species, in all the eons past. Although recurrent water shortages make it seem that water is disappearing from the planet, what is really happening is that those molecules of water have shifted to inaccessible phases of the water cycle.

One significant change in water supplies, however, makes water recycled in our lifetimes quite different from the water of a billion years ago. Detergents, pesticides, industrial byproducts, nuclear wastes, and newly created chemicals have placed the mark of modern technology upon the world's waters. This has occurred because water, both inside and outside of the body, is such an excellent solvent. The rain washing over lawns, houses, and parking lots will carry with it chemical fertilizer, paint flakes, particles of asbestos roofing, puddles of gasoline, oil, and brake fluid, and soot and industrial waste particles from the air. All join the stream of water seeping through the ground on its way back into reservoirs and wells. Unless the water passes through an extensive natural filtration system or a sophisticated one of human construction, many of these pollutants will eventually appear in the water supply.

In the United States, responsibility for regulating the safety of the water supply long rested with the Food and Drug Administration, and water was classified as a food. In 1974, with the passage of the Safe Water Drinking Act, responsibility shifted to the Environmental Protection Agency, which evaluates water not only as a food, but also as a medium for transportation, waste disposal, and other processes. The EPA sets standards for water quality, and conducts tests to detect contamination as well. It is active in developing legislation to control water pollution and to discover new methods for ensuring safe water levels of naturally occurring elements.

Despite safeguards, well-known pollutants and previously unsuspected contaminants continue to enter our water supplies. Contaminants may come from the aging pipes, perhaps made of lead, iron, or copper, that transport water from reservoir to home. Even presumably safe chemicals, such as chlorine, which is purposely added to drinking water to reduce bacterial contamination, may be suspect. Chlorine in drinking water may combine with organic substances to produce chloroform, in high amounts a known carcinogen, but no safer disinfectant substitute has been found (Safe Drinking Water Committee, 1977). The Safe Drinking Water Committee, in an 18-month study undertaken for the EPA, cited asbestos particles in water as the greatest potential health hazard. But the committee found that in Duluth, Minnesota, where mineral particle contamination of water supply lasted for 20 years, the cancer rate was not significantly high (Safe Drinking Water Committee, 1977).

Some scientists claim that, at low levels, such carcinogens may not be especially harmful. A recent Louisiana study, however, suggested a definite relationship between pollutants in the Mississippi River water supply and incidence of all cancers, of cancer of the urinary organs, and of cancer of the gastrointestinal tract (Page et al., 1976). This association, however, remains to be proved.

Cancer is not the only concern. Seepage into drinking water of salt used for snow removal has been associated with findings of unusually high blood pressure in high school students in Boston (*New York Times*, 9/18/78). The Massachusetts Department of Public Health advocates sanding of roads instead of salting to avoid this problem.

Many people have turned off their water faucets and turned on to bottled water. Spring water comes from streams deep underground. Some spring waters pass through naturally occurring mineral deposits, picking up small quantities of these minerals and, consequently, taking on a distinctive taste or smell. Some are naturally carbonated. Many mineral waters have been touted as natural health remedies, and their trace elements may, in fact, have some value. But increasing numbers of people are using bottled waters, not for what they do contain, but for what they don't. No chlorine, no known carcinogens, no detergents, no lead particles leached from decaying water pipes can be detected.

Not all bottled waters come from underground springs. Distilled water, which accounts for about 75 percent of the bottled water sold in the United States, is produced by recondensing the vapor of regular tap water that has

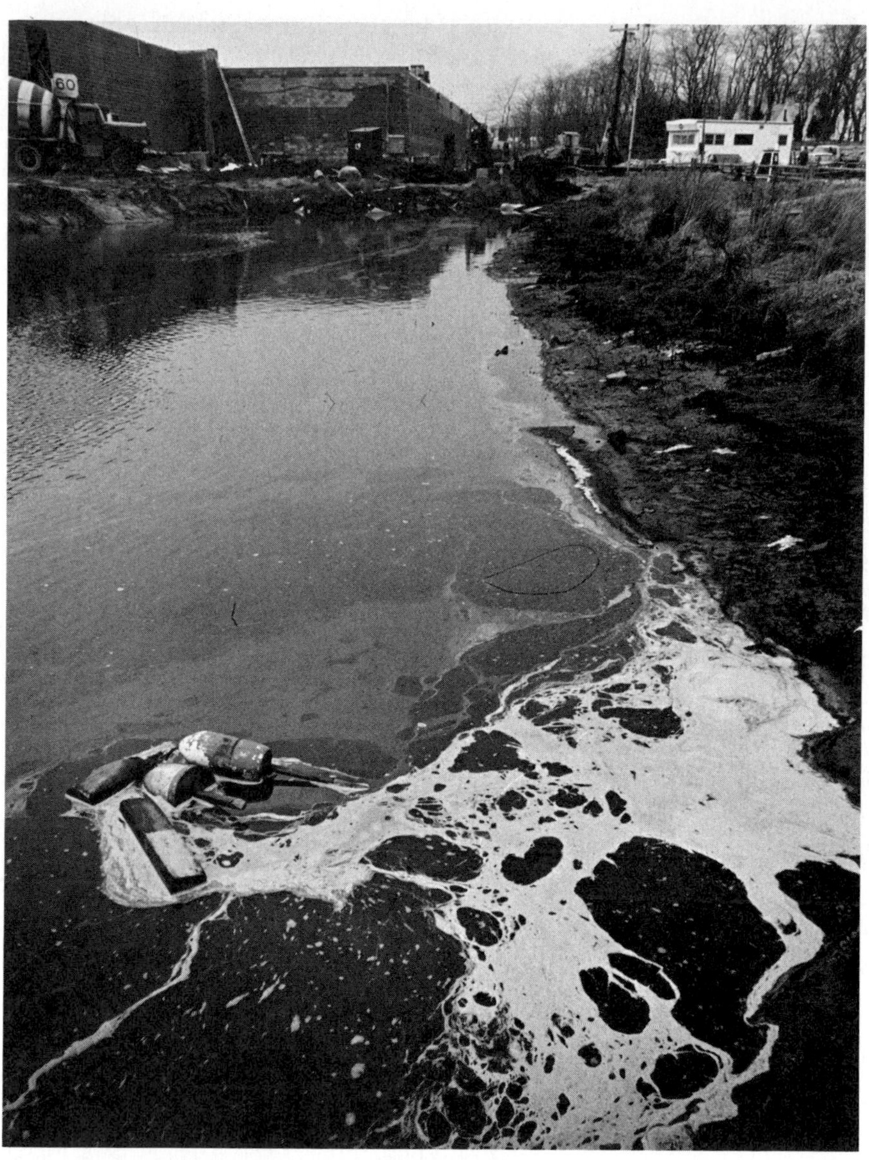

A polluted stream . . . (Gordon S. Smith/Photo Researchers, Inc.)

been boiled. Dissolved minerals as well as contaminants are left behind. Therefore, distilled water does not provide the beneficial mineral content found in spring and even tap waters. And it is often sold in plastic containers which may themselves be, as some critics believe, a possible source of contamination.

The consumer, as usual, faces a choice—and cost becomes a factor in that choice. The cost of bottled water is higher than the cost of any local water supply, ranging from about 50 cents per *gallon* for purified water, to over one dollar per *quart* for some high-status (generally imported) mineral waters. But until they are assured of uncontaminated tap water, many people feel this is

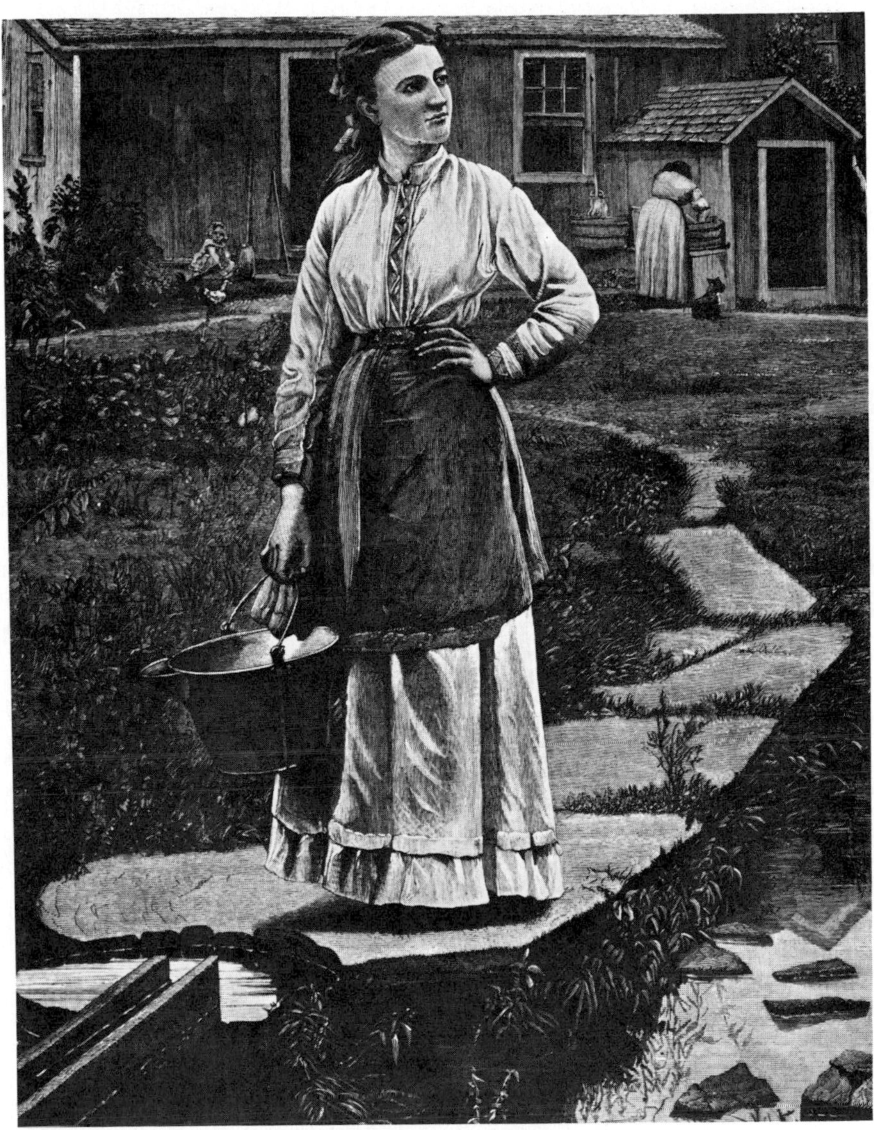

. . . and how it used to be: an early 19th century painting, Going to The Spring, by J. G. Brown. (The Bettmann Archive)

a small price to pay for peace of mind for themselves, for their families, and even for their water-loving plants.

SUMMARY

Water is the most vital of all the nutrients, and yet it functions differently from them.

Water absorbs heat, thus helping to regulate body temperature. Evaporation of water from the skin in the form of sweat also serves this function. As a major component of the fluids involved in digestion, absorption, and metabolism, water serves as a solvent for metabolites and other substances, and is an ion donor and recipient in several biochemical reactions. In addition, it is the transport medium in which digestive products and wastes move through the body. It is essential for the maintenance of electrolyte balance. Finally, water serves as a lubricant for body tissues.

The amount of water in the body varies with age, tissue composition, and sex. A newborn baby's body is 77 percent water, and that of a normal adult male, about 60 percent. Adipose tissue is 25 to 35 percent water, while muscle tissue is 72 percent water. Therefore lean muscular individuals have proportionately more fluid than do the obese, whose bodies are only about 50 percent water. Women's bodies have less water than men's, and the percentage of body water is lowest in old age.

About 60 percent of the body's water is contained inside cells in the *intracellular compartment*. The *extracellular compartment* contains the remainder, of which some 20 percent is *intravascular fluid*, the liquid component of blood, and 80 percent is *interstitial and transcellular fluid*. Although these locations of body fluid are considered separate for conceptual purposes, in reality compartmentalization is dynamic, with fluids and their contents constantly flowing between the compartments.

Various organic molecules and the inorganic electrolytes are contained in body fluids. Electrolytes are minerals that ionize in water solution; anions are negatively charged and cations are positively charged.

Chloride, bicarbonate, phosphate, and sulfate are the primary anions; sodium, potassium, calcium, and magnesium are the most important cations.

In each compartment, body fluids have distinctive electrolyte composition. Water tends to flow from one compartment to the other until electrolyte concentration is equalized. Sodium and potassium, in particular, tend to draw water from areas of low salt concentration to areas of higher concentration; this principle is commonly expressed as "water follows salt." Cell membranes are selectively permeable, and water and various solutes enter and leave. The major influence on movement of water molecules through cell membranes is *osmotic pressure*, which increases when concentration of electrolytes and other solutes increases.

The amount of water in the body is kept at a relatively constant level. Water intake from beverages, foods, and metabolic oxidative processes is balanced by water outflow through the urine, the feces, insensible perspiration, and respiration. Although there is no RDA for water, the Food and Nutrition Board recommends an intake of 1 milliliter per kilocalorie.

When the body needs more water, saliva production decreases, and thirst warning centers sense resultant mouth dryness, increased extracellular electrolyte concentration, and decreased blood volume. These effects trigger drinking and the release of antidiuretic hormone (ADH). The kidneys respond by increasing reabsorption of water and producing more concentrated urine. Aldosterone and other hormones also participate in the control process.

Rapid water losses due to hemorrhage, diarrhea, vomiting, ADH insufficiency, extensive burns, or excessive perspiration may overwhelm regulatory mechanisms and lead to impaired cellular function due to electrolyte losses. Water intoxication due to excessive drinking is also damaging. Diuretic drugs may help to reverse fluid accumulation and its consequences in some cases.

Maintenance of adequate supplies of pure water is an important medical and social concern. Proven and suspected pollutants have been found in the water supply in many areas. Prevention of contamination of water supplies is a major concern of the Environmental Protection Agency and of civic and consumer organizations as well.

BIBLIOGRAPHY

FOOD AND NUTRITION BOARD, NATIONAL RESEARCH COUNCIL. *Recommended dietary allowances,* 8th ed. Washington, D.C.: National Academy of Sciences, 1974.

GUYTON, A. C. *Textbook of medical physiology,* 5th ed. Philadelphia: Saunders, 1976.

MITCHELL, H. S., H. J. RYNBERGEN, L. ANDERSON, AND M. V. DEBBLE. *Nutrition in health and disease,* 16th ed. Philadelphia: Lippincott, 1976.

New York Times. Salt in drinking water linked to blood pressure. September 18, 1978.

PAGE, T., R. H. HARRIS, AND S. S. EPSTEIN. Drinking water and cancer mortality in Louisiana. *Science* 193:55, 1976.

ROBINSON, J. R. Water, the indispensable nutrient. *Nutrition Today* 5(1):16, 1970.

SAFE DRINKING WATER COMMITTEE, NATIONAL RESEARCH COUNCIL. *Summary report: Drinking water and health.* Washington D.C.: National Academy of Sciences, 1977.

STRAND, F. L. *Physiology: A regulatory systems approach.* New York: Macmillan, 1978.

WILLIAMS, R. H., ED. *Textbook of endocrinology,* 5th ed. Philadelphia: Saunders, 1974.

WOLF, A. V. Body water. *Scientific American* 199(5):125, 1958.

SUGGESTED ADDITIONAL READING

ANDERSON, B. Thirst and brain control of water balance. *American Scientist* 59:408, 1971.

CHEN, L. C. Control of diarrheal disease morbidity and mortality. *American Journal of Clinical Nutrition* 32:2284, 1978.

JOHNSON, R. E. Water and osmotic economy on survival rations. *Journal of the American Dietetic Association* 45:124, 1964.

KELLER, E. What is happening to our drinking water? *Chemistry* 48(2): 16, 1975.

MOHLMAN, H. T., B. J. KATCHMAN, AND A. R. SLONIM. Human water consumption and excretion data for aerospace systems. *Aerospace Medicine* 39:396, 1968.

SMITH, N. J. *Food for sport.* Palo Alto: Bull Publishing Co., 1976.

In Retrospect II

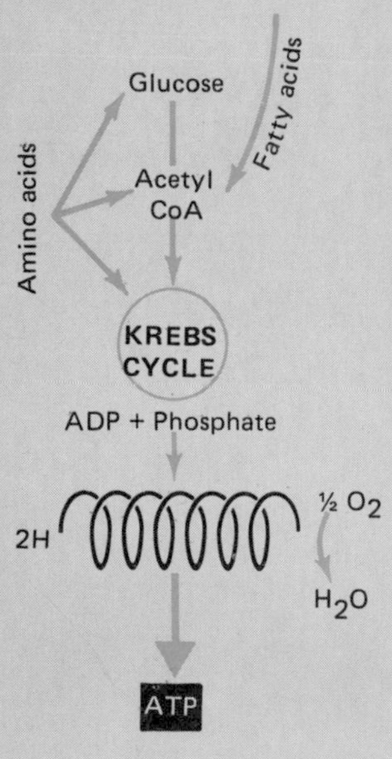

In Part One of this text, nutrition has been presented as both a science and a process. Concepts of biology and chemistry as they relate to nutritional science were introduced and explained, and the processes by which the nutrients present in foods are transformed metabolically into the substances of which our bodies are composed were described. The interconversions between the energy-yielding nutrients (carbohydrates, lipids, and proteins) were presented in In Retrospect I (see pages 163 to 167). The final products of metabolism of these nutrients are CO_2 and H_2O and, in the case of amino acids, urea (see Figures I-1 and I-2).

We ingest food, not nutrients. Immediately following ingestion, however, with the start of digestion in the mouth, we can begin to speak of nutrients and chemicals. In the time between ingestion and excretion, many metabolites are produced. Some, as we have seen, are incorporated into the structure of the human organism. Some are essential for normal functioning of that organism. And some are part of the various interconnected cycles that maintain homeostasis or balance of systems, structures, and substances. The metabolism of carbohydrate, fat, and protein also produces chemical energy, necessary to fuel body processes, which is trapped in the cells as ATP.

Although vitamins, minerals, and water are not energy-producing nutrients, they participate in the chemical reactions of the energy-producing nutrients and are also necessary to maintain structure, function, and regulation. In particular, the water-soluble vitamins function as coenzymes in metabolic reactions, facilitating the metabolism of carbohydrate, protein, and fat (as we saw in Chapter 7), and assisting in the synthesis of such important body compounds as nucleic acids. Each of the fat-soluble vitamins (Chapter 6), in its own specific way, also helps to maintain the function of the body. Similarly, minerals are essential to many metabolic reactions and promote structural and functional integrity of the organism as well (Chapter 8). And water, often labeled "the forgotten nutrient," is on a day-to-day basis the most essential of all (Chapter 9).

Each of these categories of nutrient has been presented separately, as a discrete entity. But in the total economy of the body, it is the interaction of all these nutrients that makes the organism the intricately detailed but marvelously integrated machine that it is.

The body creates its own regulators, in the form of hormones, special transport proteins, enzymes, coenzymes, and other substances, from the nutrients provided in food. The endocrine system, in which hormones are produced, is the primary regulator of body processes. Several hormone systems, and their roles in controlling enzyme activity, modulating transport processes, and thus influencing both the direction and rate of the various metabolic pathways, have been described in the preceding chapters. Absorption and excretion are regulated by these substances as well. The regulatory mechanisms maintain constancy in the internal environment, regardless of variations in the external environment. These homeostatic processes cushion body systems against fluctuations in the supply of nutrients. Homeostatic regulators are at work constantly, on a daily and even minute-to-minute basis, compensating for the ever-changing biological and environmental demands on the system and ensuring that the human body functions to its fullest potential.

The body is wonderfully adaptable to continual shifts in supply and demand. Adaptation, however, can only go so far. When poor nutrition, disease, or exceptionally harsh demands deplete the substrates necessary for growth, energy, and maintenance, the regulatory mechanisms can no longer function at optimal levels. Under prolonged assault, some body systems stop functioning altogether, and eventually all come to a halt. Illness, and ultimately death, are the result. The integrity of particularly vital systems—levels of glucose and calcium in the blood, water and electrolyte balance, and others—are protected by several regulatory mechanisms, each of which compensates for fluctuations in nutrient supplies.

A great deal of what we now know about the integration of body substances and systems has been learned in a relatively brief time. Nutrition is indeed a twentieth-century science, and the research techniques that have made present knowledge possible have largely been developed and used within the last few decades. Today's knowledge goes only so far, and we have repeatedly seen that the precise mechanism by which one or another body chemical interacts to produce a specific result is not completely clear. Much remains to be learned about all of the nutrients—about their presence and availability (not necessarily, as we have seen, the same thing) in the food supply, and about how they function individually and as part of the "team" of chemicals present in our bodies. In Part Two of this text the roles of the individual nutrients and the basic concepts of nutritional science will be shown in terms of their integration into everyday living at all of the stages of the human life cycle, and as they reflect external influences, such as lifestyle, food supply, and even politics and international relations.

PERSPECTIVE ON
Nutrition for Athletes

Athletes, whether amateur or professional, pursue an unending search for that tantalizing "edge" in competition, the reserve and endurance that will put them out front, surging ahead of their opponents. In pursuit of that extra something, many have turned to **supernutrition** or even to drugs. Careful attention to nutrition can indeed help athletes achieve their bodies' full potential, while undernutrition will surely hinder athletic ability. But whether "supernutrition" can create super performance is debatable. And drug-taking for purposes of extending endurance in athletic competition is physiologically dangerous as well as unethical.

Nevertheless, many athletes, coaches, and trainers advocate certain nutritional supplements and dietary regimens to increase strength and endurance. Although there may be a factual basis for some recommendations, most perceived benefits are more psychological than physiological in origin. Research has shown, for example, that beyond a particular high level of athletic performance, additional physiological manipulations rarely have an influence (Darden, 1977). Subjectively, however, athletes seldom know why they perform well one day and poorly the next and may well attribute success or failure to a food eaten prior to the event. The strength of such a belief may aid performance, or deprivation of a favored food or regimen may impair performance because an athlete is insecure without it (Van Itallie, 1968). Many sports superstitions focus on one particular nutrient category as the key to improved performance.

Individual nutrient and energy requirements are largely determined by individual growth rates and activity levels. Athletes, because of their great activity levels, require quantities of nutrients and, especially, energy, that are extraordinary by comparison with the nutrient intake of the average individual. This has created an aura of mystery about the nutritional requirements for athletes.

Protein. A popular training practice is consumption of great quantities of meat, intended to replace protein losses presumably incurred during strenuous muscular exertion. This long-lived belief is at least as old as the Olympic games. Because wrestlers were not classified by weight in ancient Greece, heavyweights had a distinct advantage. Trainers who introduced weight-increasing meat diets (which would be high in kilocalories) had observable success (Mayer, 1972). Their method has had long-lasting repercussions: Vasily Alexeev, the 345-pound Russian Olympic gold-medal winner in weight-lifting, reportedly consumes 1,500 grams of protein each day, more than ten times the RDA, even for a man of his height, massive build, and high activity level. Nutritionists speculate that this diet has produced tremendous hypertrophy of Alexeev's liver and kidneys (Darden, 1977).

The truth is that protein is not used as fuel in well-nourished individuals performing strenuous physical activities (Astrand and Rodahl, 1977). When the protein metabolism of cross-country skiiers racing 20 to 50 miles in one day was compared with that of comparable athletes on a rest day, no significant differences were observed (Astrand, 1968). Only when carbohydrate and fat supplies are depleted (hardly likely to happen to a well-fed athlete) does protein become a source of metabolic energy.

Further, very little protein is needed to produce muscle tissue, 70 percent of which is water (Darden, 1977). Excessive protein can deprive the body of more useful fuel and is expensive as well. Metabolism of excess protein produces excess body heat, which is detrimental to athletes. And water loss will be increased as well, as the increased urea production must be excreted in urine—at best a nuisance in athletic performance, and possibly dangerous as a potential source of severe water imbalance and increased likelihood of cramping.

Like all individuals, athletes require essential amino acids in the proper proportions, as found in proteins from animal products and plant food combinations. Nutritionists recommend that athletes consume 1 gram of protein per kilogram of body weight per day. This requirement is easily met in the high-energy diet (as much as 4,000 kcals per day) necessary for active individuals, and it is more than the RDA. Protein intake above this level is not only unnecessary, but may actually be detrimental (Serfass, 1977). A carefully planned vegetarian diet can also meet these requirements (Smith, 1976).

Fat. Fat-containing foods are concentrated sources of energy and are usually consumed in relatively large amounts to meet the unusual energy needs of athletes. Because they delay gastric emptying, however, there is good reason to avoid consuming fatty foods immediately before strenuous activity.

Dietary fat should not be confused with *body* fat. Body fat is a reserve source of energy and may contribute as much as 70 percent of the energy required during prolonged aerobic work. But even the leanest athletes have adequate body fat to meet this sporadic metabolic demand (Serfass, 1977). Adding to body fat, by consuming too many kilocalories as protein, carbohydrate, or fat, would not improve the body's functioning during strenuous exercise. Excessive fat stores actually decrease strength and power, simply because the body must work harder to move its increased bulk.

Carbodydrate. Carbohydrate is the most efficent fuel for energy production during maximum exertion. The body ordinarily contains limited stores of carbohydrate in the form of liver and muscle glycogen. These glycogen stores are essential for the repeated muscular contractions athletes perform.

Some "single-effort" sports, such as diving, broad jumping, and pole vaulting, and short-duration sports, such as sprinting and skiing, do not tax the usual stores of glycogen. However, the sustained effort required by sports, such as long-distance running, that involve endurance or extreme or prolonged stress may eventually deplete glycogen stores. Once depleted, muscles fail to contract. The result is exhaustion, a form of fatigue familiar to marathon runners, wrestlers, and rowers.

Research has shown that, over a period of time, decreased carbohydrate intake accompanied by exercise greatly reduces glycogen stores in the body. After several days on a low-carbohydrate regimen, an abrupt increase in carbohydrate intake dramatically increases glycogen stores and, consequently, physical stamina. This intake sequence is known as **carbohydrate loading.** Studies have shown that, following a period of low carbohydrate intake, a diet consisting of 75 to 90 percent carbohydrate maintained for three to four days before competition will maximally increase muscle glycogen storage (Costill, 1978). Forgac (1979) has recently outlined the specific phases of this diet.

In Sweden, where the carbohydrate-loading concept was developed, long-distance runners on this regimen significantly improved in running time, most notably in the final stretches of a long race. While nonloaders slowed markedly in the course of an event, carbohydrate loaders were able to maintain a fast pace (Slovic, 1975).

Word of the advantages of this diet soon reached athletes and the general public. A survey of runners in the 1974 Trail's End Marathon in Oregon found that 50 percent of the early finishers had used the carbohydrate-loading regimen during training (Slovic, 1975). Today the figure would be much higher. Diets emphasizing starches such as pasta and bread are particularly popular, with good nutritional reason. The polysaccharides in these foods are absorbed relatively slowly and stimulate production of insulin over a longer period, unlike simple sugars. This is the crucial factor in promoting glycogen storage (Costill, 1978) because insulin increases deposition of glycogen in the liver and muscles. Epinephrine (adrenalin), the adrenal hormone released into the circulation during times of stress, releases glycogen from storage. The stress of competition and physical exertion rushes epinephrine to the muscles, sending glycogen-derived glucose throughout the body and bringing peak efficiency to muscular performance.

Increased glycogen stores, however, also increase body water. The added weight may make the body work harder, thus decreasing its efficiency (Astrand and Rodahl, 1977). In addition, there have been reports of cardiac abnormalities and angina in older athletes who have tried the carbohydrate-loading regimen (Serfass, 1977). Because of these risks, carbohydrate loading should only be attempted under supervision.

Vitamins and Minerals. There is no evidence that vitamin intake in excess of body requirements confers any physiological benefit. In fact (as we saw in Chapter 6), high intake of some vitamins (fat-soluble A and D) carries a danger of toxicity. Athletes who take megadoses of various vitamin and mineral preparations are not receiving any significant benefit.

The ample diet required to provide high energy content ensures adequate intake even of those vitamins and minerals that are depleted during strenuous activity. Consumption of whole-grain or enriched bread products, for example, supplies adequate quantities of the B-complex vitamins necessary for metabolism of carbohydrate, protein, and fat. Supplements are unnecessary.

Reports of special benefits from particular vitamins are not scientifically valid. Vitamin E, for example, has been called a "supernutrient" by some trainers. But despite some early, promising reports, no consistent effect of this vitamin on physical endurance has been demonstrated (Lawrence et al., 1975).

Mineral supplementation is also commonly found in the athletic regimen. This practice, unlike vitamin supplementation, does have some physiological basis. Heavy exercise causes sweating, which depletes the body's stores of sodium, potassium, and other minerals. Potassium deficiency is particularly damaging in athletes, since it interferes with glycogen formation in muscle tissue (Knochel, 1978) and results in cramping. This can be avoided by inclusion of potassium-rich foods such as oranges and bananas in the diet. Ingestion of salt tablets is seldom necessary and may be dangerous. Because excessive salt intake traps water in the extracellular compartments of the body and depletes intracellular fluid, water imbalance with potentially serious effects may result.

Some female athletes (approximately 5 percent) experience excessive menstrual flow during strenuous exercise and may therefore lose more iron than other women. Supplements are often recommended during menstrual periods as well as careful attention to consumption of iron-rich meals at all times. This is not a universal problem, however; a significant number of female athletes fail to menstruate at all during times of heavy physical exertion (Drinkwater, 1973). Some of these women have high levels of androgen, but whether these hormonal abnormalities are the cause or the result of their highly developed musculature is a topic of debate (Darden, 1976). More likely, the reduction of body fat as a percentage of total body weight in well-trained female athletes results in the observed amenorrhea.

Fluids. Exercise-induced sweating produces significant loss of water and minerals, particularly in hot, humid environments. That dehydration is a serious threat is apparent in many reports of death due to heat stroke after athletic matches (Serfass, 1977).

Because athletes have a larger than normal percentage of muscle tissue which contains a high percentage of water, water constitutes a larger percentage of their body weight. For this reason, they may find their after-exercise thirst is slaked by drinking fluids in amounts that do not fully replace lost fluid. Athletes should, therefore, drink according to a schedule to maintain adequate hydration and optimum performance and not merely enough to satisfy thirst (Smith, 1976).

To meet the particular fluid and mineral needs of athletes, special drinks have been developed containing sugar, water, and electrolytes, such as the popular "Gatorade," and these are commonly used during athletic training. The same benefits, however, can be obtained if knowledgeable attention is paid to ordinary food and water intake.

Drugs. If we define as food that which is ingested to supply nutrients used in the body, then drugs could not properly be considered in our discussion of food and sports (Darden 1976). However, many foods contain pharmacologically active substances that may affect the body's use of the nutrients in foods. For these reasons, and because drugs are a major concern in sports, it is appropriate to discuss the categories of several drugs frequently used, and abused, by athletes.

Stimulants are particularly popular, both in "natural" and prescription form. Alcohol is often thought to be a stimulant, but it is not. Although alcohol temporarily decreases fatigue, the actual depressant effect of even moderate doses seriously impairs coordination.

Coffee, tea, and cola drinks contain caffeine, a potent stimulant known to increase motor activity, speed reaction time, and avert feelings of fatigue. These effects, however, are relatively short-lived.

Amphetamines are frequently used stimulants that act on the respiratory and arousal centers of the brain and in the peripheral nervous system, stimulating neurons that cause muscles to contract. In the form of popular brand name "pep pills" such as Dexedrine, Benzedrine, and Ritalin, amphetamines are often used. Their actual effects vary from athlete to athlete, depending upon the individual's personality, motivation, and fatigability, and some find that these impair their performance (Darden, 1977). Sedatives, barbiturates, tranquilizers, and other relaxant drugs are also often used, an indication that many players believe they perform better when excitement and tension are reduced, not stimulated.

Pain killers are often used in the sports world. Such drugs as Novocain (procaine HCl) and Xylocaine (lidocaine) have local anesthetic action, numbing nerve endings in injured sections of the body and permitting an athlete to perform before healing has occurred. But there is danger of seriously aggravating an unhealed injury. Antiinflammation agents are usually injected into painful joints, tendons, and muscles. Cortisone, the best known of these, is a synthetic form of a powerful adrenal hormone. Although it produces temporary pain relief, cortisone actually impedes healing; it may also weaken resistance to microbial infection and has significant effects on the metabolism of carbohydrate and proteins.

Perhaps the most controversial drugs currently taken by athletes are oral anabolic-androgenic steroids. These drugs are synthetic analogues of testosterone and other male hormones. Research has shown that androgens are involved in the anabolic processes of protein building and nitrogen retention. It is believed that the greater presence of androgens in males is responsible for their greater strength and muscle mass (Darden, 1976). Anecdotal reports from both male and female athletes claim significant gains in endurance and muscle power with the use of this class of drug. Controlled scientific testing, however, has failed to substantiate these positive effects (American College of Sports Medicine, 1977). Research studies do show a substantial risk of side effects ranging from inconvenient to serious. These include, in male athletes, decreased testicular size and function and decreased sperm production, and, in female athletes, delayed puberty, masculinization, voice changes, hirsutism (excess body hair), and menstrual disorders. Abnormal liver function, with various complications, has also been noted. Although many of these side effects may be benign and reversible, long-range effects are unknown, and several drug-related deaths have been reported.

Acknowledging these maximal risks and minimal benefits, the American College of Sports Medicine (1977) recently issued a position statement on the use and abuse of anabolic-androgenic steroids: In the absence of conclusive scientific evidence that these drugs either aid or hinder athletic performance, the reported benefits were classified as "placebo effects" generated by positive expectations on the part of trainers and athletes. Nevertheless, reliance on "magic" drugs remains an epidemic problem in sports today. A major dilemma for athletes and coaches is that "the other team" may well be using them. Recognizing this, the International Olympics Committee, standing strongly against such drug use, allocated $1.4 million for drug testing at the 1980 Winter Olympics in Lake Placid, New York. In previous competitions, drug testing has indeed disclosed numerous abuses of the international sports ban on stimulants and steroids. The 1977 women's shot-put gold medalist from East Germany and the men's discus thrower from Finland, along with other athletes, lost their European Cup medals and were barred from participation in international competition for 18 months, because of steroid violations. Other recent drug disqualifications have been reported in Olympic qualifying matches held in France, West Berlin, and Canada (*Amdur*, 1978).

Increasing concern over drug use makes it likely that testing programs will be increasingly extended to non Olympic competition. Horses are now routinely tested by urinalysis for drug detection before races. Will college athletes be next?

For sound nutritional recommendations for devising balanced diets suited to individual athletic programs, see Smith (1976) and Darden (1977).

BIBLIOGRAPHY

AMDUR, N. Mounting drug use afflicts world sports. *New York Times*, November 20, 1978, p. C-1

AMERICAN COLLEGE OF SPORTS MEDICINE. Position statement on the use and abuse of anabolic-androgenic steroids in sports. *Medicine and Science in Sports* 9(4):xi, 1977.

ASTRAND, P.-O. Something old and something new . . . very new. *Nutrition Today* 3(2):9, 1968.

ASTRAND, P.-O., AND K. RODAHL. *Textbook of work physiology*, 2nd ed. New York: McGraw-Hill, 1977.

COSTILL, D. L. Sports nutrition: The role of carbohydrates. *Nutrition News* 41(1):1, 1978.

DARDEN, E. *Nutrition and athletic performance*. Pasadena, Calif.: Athletic Press, 1976.

DARDEN E. The nutrition of Olympic athletes. *Journal of Home Economics*, March 1977, pp. 40–43.

DRINKWATER, B. L. Physiological responses of women to exercise. In *Exercise and sport sciences reviews*, Vol. 1, ed. J. H. Wilmore. New York: Academic Press, 1973.

FORGAC, M. T. Carbohydrate loading—A review. *Journal of the American Dietetic Association* 75:42, 1979.

KNOCHEL, J. P. Nutrition for athletes. American Dietetic Association, *Abstracts of 1978 meetings*, September 27, 1978.

LAWRENCE, J. D., R. C. BOWER, W. P. RIEHL, AND J. L. SMITH. Effects of alphatocopherol acetate on the swimming endurance of trained swimmers. *American Journal of Clinical Nutrition* 28:205, 1975.

MAYER, J. *Human nutrition.* Springfield, Ill.: Chas. C Thomas, 1972.

SERFASS, R. C. Nutrition for the athlete. *Contemporary Nutrition* 2(5):1, 1977.

SLOVIC, P. What helps the long distance runner run? *Nutrition Today* 10(3):18, 1975.

SMITH, N. J. *Food for sport.* Palo Alto, Calif.: Bull Publishing Co., 1976.

VAN ITALLIE, T. If we only knew. *Nutrition Today* 3(2):3, 1968.

SUGGESTED ADDITIONAL READING

LANE, H. W., AND J. J. CERDA. Potassium requirements and exercise. *Journal of the American Dietetic Association* 73:64, 1978.

NELSON, R. A. What should athletes eat? Unmixing folly and facts. *The Physician and Sportsmedicine* 3:67, 1975.

WERBLOW, J. A., H. M. FOX, AND A. HENNEMAN. Nutritional knowledge, attitudes, and food patterns of women athletes. *Journal of the American Dietetic Association* 73:242, 1978.

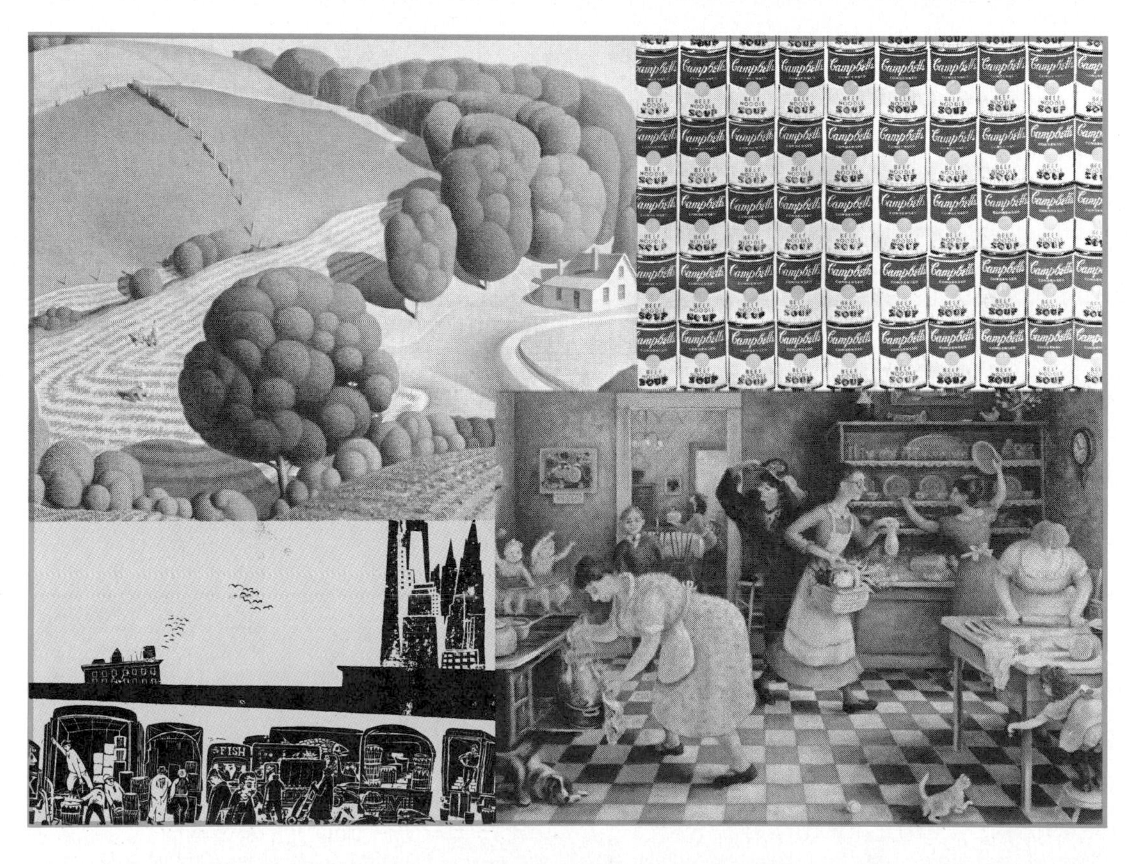

PART TWO NUTRITION FOR EVERYDAY LIVING

Chapter 10

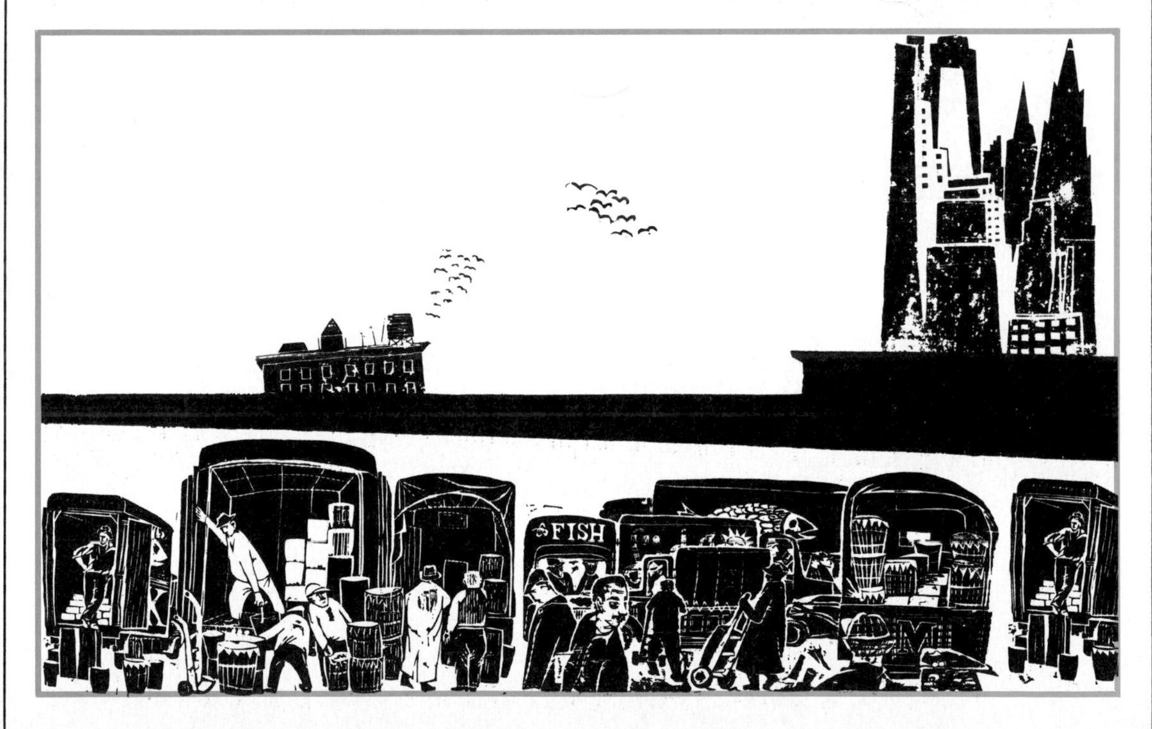

Fulton Fish Market by Antonio Frasconi

Assessing Nutritional Status and Planning an Adequate Diet

We are all food *consumers.* As economic consumers, we select and purchase food. As biological consumers, we ingest, digest, absorb, and metabolize it. Both consumption processes have become centers of attention for today's public. Books, magazines, newspaper articles, radio and television programs all provide a constant flow of information about food budgeting, "healthful eating," wise marketing, menu planning, and gourmet cookery. But despite our preoccupation with food and demand for information about it, and despite the fact that we have an abundance of food in this country, many people, either through ignorance or neglect, choose foods that do not provide adequate supplies of key nutrients.

Nutrition has become an increasing concern to professionals involved with preventive as well as curative health care, as evidence mounts to implicate dietary factors in the incidence of heart disease, cancer, diabetes, and other illnesses. Poor nutritional status is associated with prolonged recovery periods following illness or injury, adding to the duration and cost of hospitalization (Butterworth, 1974).

Since good nutrition is consonant with good health, it is important to identify existing nutritional shortcomings and disorders and to identify nutrient-related problems, not only in patient populations but in the presumably healthy general public as well. Four major methods—anthropometric, clinical, biochemical, and dietary—are used to assess nutritional status. Because a particular finding may be due to any of several causes, no one of these methods is sufficient to diagnose a nutritional deficiency state. A child's failure to achieve an adequate rate of growth, for example, could be *documented* by anthropometric measurements, but might be *caused* by heredity, disease, nutrition, or other factors. Only biochemical, clinical, and dietary data could confirm that the growth failure was caused by inadequate nutrient intake.

These assessment tools are also used to identify individuals or populations who are "at risk" of developing nutritional deficiencies, as well as to evaluate the effectiveness of nutrition education or supplementary feeding programs; they can also determine relationships between nutrient intake and the onset or prevention of chronic nutrition-related disease, such as coronary heart disease, diabetes, and some forms of cancer. No association between a disease condition and nutritional factors can be determined if food intake patterns are not known. These methods can also help to identify nutrients that may be inadequately provided by the available food supply; once nutrient deficiencies or excesses are determined, necessary changes can be instituted.

In this chapter we shall examine not only the different means by which professionals assess nutritional status but also some of the aids to nutritional choice that have been designed to assist the general public. Educated consumers are the key to improving nutritional status on a broad scale.

TOOLS FOR ASSESSING NUTRITIONAL STATUS

In a particular individual, clinical symptoms of nutrient deficiency and abnormalities of growth, development, or physiological function are the ultimate results of long-standing deprivations. Visible signs of nutritional deficiency do not appear until the body's stores of nutrients have been depleted. For most nutrients this will not happen until daily intake has fallen far short of need for a prolonged period of time. Examination of an individual's food behaviors may suggest the existence of a nutritional deficiency, and laboratory tests may confirm the tentative diagnosis. On the other hand, biochemical data indicate tissue depletion of nutrients before clinical signs become apparent, and a study of food intake patterns may strengthen the argument. A variety of standardized anthropometric, clinical, biochemical, and dietary assessment techniques are used to determine nutritional status of individuals and groups. Each of these methods has advantages and disadvantages. Taken together they can confirm suspicions and provide the factual data on which corrective measures must be based.

Anthropometric Assessment

Anthropometric (human measurement) assessments, such as height, weight, skinfold thickness, wrist circumference, and similar indices of physical dimension provide a gross indication of over- or undernutrition. Measurements of numerous individuals, representative of the total population, provide standards against which data for an individual can be compared. Individual anthropometric measurements that vary significantly from standards may indicate a nutrition-related problem, although they are not definitive.

HEIGHT AND WEIGHT. A person's potential for overall growth and body build is determined by heredity, but nutritional and other environmental factors can modify this potential considerably. Especially for young children, measurements of height are reliable indicators of normal growth and development, and imply adequate nutritional status. Similarly, height measurements also indicate abnormal growth that may be due to dietary deficiency.

There are several standards for height and weight, many of which often appear in popular publications. Some of the familiar charts and tables, however, are based on information obtained thirty or more years ago, when they were derived from measurements of relatively few children from selected geographical and cultural backgrounds. While these data were at one time useful, the figures are generally not applicable to today's population. Much has been learned in the intervening years about the importance of representative sampling for establishing valid baseline data. In addition, control of infectious disease and improved nutrition have allowed children to more nearly achieve their growth potential. For these reasons, newer data have been obtained, using more accurate sampling and measurement techniques, and have been published by the National Center for Health Statistics (NCHS, 1976).

These new standards are based on measurements of large numbers of boys and girls from birth through age 18, who were selected from diverse geographical areas and cultural backgrounds, and who more nearly represent the national population as it currently exists. Growth charts based on data of this type provide guidelines against which individual growth rates and patterns can be compared. These standardized measurements for appraising juvenile growth and development are presented in Chapter 13.

Published tables of normal adult weight, categorized by sex and height, also exist. Many of these are based on insurance company surveys of policyholders. Although such surveys have been criticized for ignoring the substantial segment of the population that does not buy insurance, other criticisms are of greater significance. Until very recently these tables showed "suggested average weights" increasing with age until the latest years of life, when weights decreased slightly. Although many adults do indeed tend to gain weight as they grow older, this weight gain is neither "normal" nor beneficial. Newer, revised actuarial tables (see Appendix D) now list "desirable" rather than "average" weights. An adult's desirable weight is that which is normal at age 25. Unlike earlier tables, these take body build (small, medium, or large frame) into account, although there are not at present any objective guides for accurately determining body build.

Despite the limitations mentioned, height-weight tables are useful in defining extremes and are particularly useful to monitor an individual over a period of time. Marked changes in an individual's weight (or in the case of children, changes in the *pattern* of growth and development) may indicate a nutritional problem. A child whose height and weight were at the median level (at the 50th percentile) at birth and during the preschool years, but whose growth rate decreases to the 25th percentile at age 10, should be examined for the presence of disease or other factors, including malnutrition, that produce growth retardation.

Measuring skinfold thickness with calipers. (Cambridge Scientific Industries)

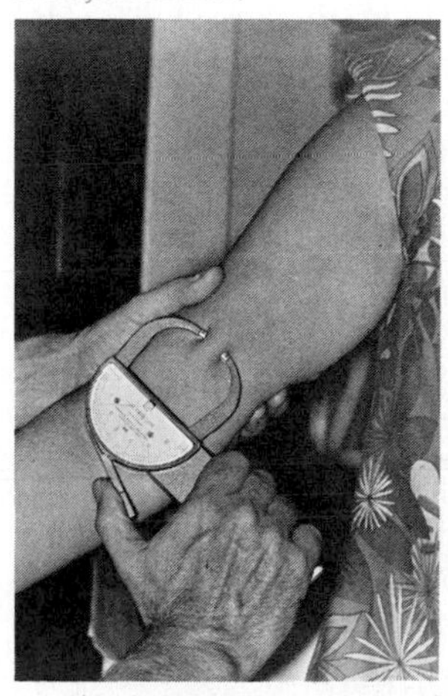

OTHER ANTHROPOMETRIC INDICES. Measurement of skinfold thickness, midarm muscle circumference, chest and head circumferences, and the use of X-rays to determine wrist bone development are also helpful in identifying abnormal growth. In certain situations, they can provide significant additional data about an individual's condition. Their disadvantage, in comparison to more easily and inexpensively obtained height and weight measures, is that they require specialized equipment and technicians trained in their use.

The increased precision of these techniques does not guarantee better diagnosis of nutritional problems, however. The most complex and sophisticated anthropometric measurements are nonspecific. That is, while they may indicate signs of general undernutrition, they cannot pinpoint specific nutrient deficiencies or metabolic disorders. With obesity, for example, overweight reflects excess energy intake but does not indicate the nature of the underlying causes. And unplanned weight loss can be due to many factors. Outside of a research laboratory, these indices generally add little to what can be learned by simple height and weight determinations, which have the additional advantages of not discomforting the patient and which can be performed by any individual with little difficulty and fair accuracy, using equipment that is readily available in clinics, physicians' offices, or other health care facilities.

Clinical Assessment

Anthropometric data collected during routine physical examinations reflect general health status. The physician uses this information as a guide and supplement in the clinical examination, a more thorough search for visible signs that reflect long-term disease processes. Severe nutritional deficiencies cause characteristic signs, directly related to the biochemical function of the nutrient involved, which can be observed during the physical examination. The most important of these have been mentioned in Part One of this text. Among the most apparent deficiency conditions are bone abnormalities due to lack of vitamin D or calcium, changes in eye appearance and function due to lack of vitamin A, and goiter resulting from lack of iodine. Such dramatic physical effects reflect long-term dietary deficits: Consumption of a nutritionally inadequate diet for a few days or even a few weeks will not produce marked clinical symptoms. And in developed nations, frank nutritional deficiencies such as kwashiorkor, beriberi, and pellagra are rarely seen at this time, although they may have existed in the past and isolated cases are occasionally reported. Some clinical observations and their nutritional causes are listed in Table 10-1.

Although such symptoms would seem easy to identify, many are puzzling when they do appear. There is a large area of subjectivity in all clinical observation. What looks like emaciation to some physicians may be "thinness" to others. This is a significant problem in clinical surveys of large populations, which depend on diagnostic reports from many physicians. Too, many physicians are not alert to signs of nutritional deficiency primarily because such deficiencies are so rare in this country. Careful training and exact specification of clinical criteria are required if intra- and interexaminer errors are to be avoided. Nevertheless, clinical observation is the most useful assessment method for screening large groups for signs of overt nutritional deficiency, and is often used for studies of experimental subject groups. Clinical assessment is quick and easy to perform and causes relatively little discomfort or inconvenience to the subjects being studied, but it does require the presence of a physician or a highly trained technician.

A number of extensive clinical studies have been designed to provide information about nutritional status and to identify populations at risk for nutritional deficiency. Documentation of clinical signs associated with malnutrition requires immediate intervention, but it is important to remember that by the time a clinical sign of deficiency is apparent, underlying tissue depletion and metabolic disruption have already occurred.

TABLE 10-1 **Some Clinical Observations Used in Nutritional Assessment**

Part of Body	Observation	Deficiency/(Excess)
Hair	Dry, brittle	Protein
	Can be plucked easily	Protein
	"Flag sign"	Protein
Eyes	Dryness of conjunctiva and cornea	Vitamin A
	Increase in blood vessels in cornea	Riboflavin
Lips and mouth	Cheilosis (cracking)	Niacin, riboflavin
	Smooth dark tongue	Niacin
	Magenta (purple) tongue	Riboflavin, folacin
	Bleeding gums	Vitamin C
	Dental caries	Fluoride/(sucrose) Protein Calcium
	Mottled enamel	(Fluoride)
Neck	Goiter	Iodine/(iodine)
Skin	Roughness at base of hair follicle	Vitamin A, essential fatty acid
	Dermatitis with sun sensitivity	Niacin
	Masolabial dermatitis	Pyridoxine, riboflavin
	Pinpoint hemorrhages	Vitamin C
	Paleness	Iron
Nails	"Spoon-shape"	Iron
Extremities or torso	Edema	Protein, niacin
	Rachitic rosary	Vitamin D, calcium
	Scorbutic rosary	Vitamin C
	Frog legs	Vitamin C
	Bowed legs	Vitamin D
	Emaciation, muscle wasting	Energy, protein
	Obesity	(Energy)
	Abnormal reflexes	Thiamin, vitamin B_{12}

Such studies can also be of value in conjunction with other assessment data, particularly in the identification of populations at risk of developing nutritional deficiencies. A particular symptom or set of symptoms may be noted with unusual frequency in the group being examined. This indicates the need to seek out other members of that population who are not yet affected, or who may have less obvious **subclinical signs** of deficiency that would be overlooked in an ordinary physical examination.

Clinical assessment, by itself, cannot confirm a diagnosis of a specific nutritional deficiency or risk of deficiency. Some clinical signs are *nonspecific*. For example, dermatitis may be related to deficiency of B vitamins, vitamin A, protein, or essential fatty acids or to factors totally unrelated to nutrient deficiency, including colds and allergies. The list of observations in Table 10-1 may include some that are personally familiar to you, but that does not necessarily mean that your diet is inadequate. Dry hair or pale complexion, for example, may reflect genetic or environmental factors. On the other hand, if these signs coincide with anthropometric indicators and with the biochemical signs we shall present next, dietary inadequacies may indeed be the causative factor.

Biochemical Assessment

Biochemical tests, which are based on an understanding of the metabolism and function of nutrients, are a useful adjunct to anthropometric and clinical assessment. They can confirm suspicions of existing long-term deficiencies and can also provide an early warning of clinical deficiency symptoms. Body measurements and clinical assessments reflect long-term and previous nutritional status, but biochemical analyses reflect the most recent situation.

Inadequate intake, inefficient digestion, disturbances in metabolism, or altered excretion of nutrients show up quickly in the chemical composition of body fluids. Blood and urine, in particular, provide an accessible window on current nutritional status. Most nutrients and/or their metabolites can be detected in either or both of these fluids. A sample of blood, for instance, contains all the substances that are currently circulating to every cell in the body. A urine sample contains wastes and byproducts that indicate how those substances have been used in the cells. For example, a low urinary level of a particular substance may reflect inadequate intake, abnormal metabolism, or malabsorption from the digestive tract (in which case, the fecal content of that substance will be abnormally high, a situation that can be detected by different biochemical tests). A high urinary level, on the other hand, may suggest an excessive supply of certain nutrients or physiological abnormalities.

Generally, decreased levels of nutrients or their metabolites in blood and urine reflect depleted tissue reserves of the nutrient in question. However, this is not always the case: Under certain conditions, vitamin A stores in the liver may not be released into the blood, and blood levels of the vitamin will be abnormally low even though tissues are not depleted.

Analysis of nutrient levels in various body tissues would also provide this information, but that would involve the discomfort of obtaining a tissue sample, as well as a certain amount of risk. For this reason, routine biochemical assessments utilize less invasive techniques, with biopsies requested only as a last resort or to confirm other findings implicating particular organs.

BLOOD ANALYSES. Measurements of the constituents in the blood provide clues about the level and function of nutrients in the body. Levels of some nutrients—vitamins, protein, lipids, and some minerals and other substances—can be measured directly. Fasting blood samples (usually taken in the morning before breakfast) are preferred, since they more accurately reflect the body's long-term stores of nutrients rather than those recently ingested.

In addition to direct measurements of nutrients in the blood, indirect analyses have been developed, particularly for the vitamins with cofactor activity; these tests are based on the metabolic function of the nutrient in question. For example, thiamin status may be determined by measuring blood pyruvate levels. As a result of thiamin deficiency, the cofactor necessary for the conversion of pyruvate to acetyl coenzyme A cannot be synthesized, and this reaction cannot occur at a normal rate. Thus, excess pyruvate accumulates in the blood.

Pyruvate
↓ Thiamin pyrophosphate
Acetyl CoA

Another kind of indirect test measures enzyme activity with and without the addition of cofactors necessary to the assay system. For example, glutamic-oxaloacetate transaminase, an enzyme contained in red blood cells, requires pyridoxine, thiamin, and riboflavin as cofactors in its catalytic function. If the activity of this enzyme increases markedly after the addition of vitamin B_6 to a blood sample, a pyridoxine deficiency is suspected. Other examples of functional tests used in nutritional assessment include red blood cell hemolysis to determine vitamin E status, and prothrombin (clotting) time as an indicator of vitamin K status (see Chapter 6).

A knowledge of the regulatory mechanisms controlling each nutrient is important for accurate interpretation of biochemical results. For example, abnormal serum calcium levels do not usually result from a dietary deficiency of this mineral; rather, they are more likely to reflect a disturbance in one or more of the interconnected mechanisms that maintain calcium homeostasis, or they may be secondary to protein status.

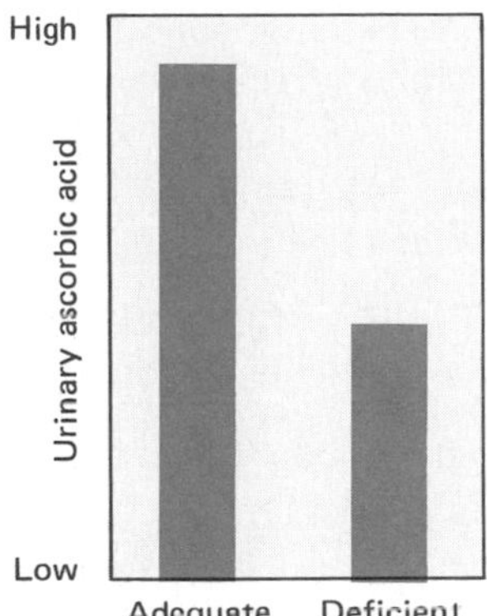

Urinary Ascorbic Acid Excretion after Load Dose of Vitamin C

URINE ANALYSES. Analysis of urine can detect normal or abnormal amounts of some nutrients or of their metabolites. Direct analysis can be done for a number of substances; glucose and albumin are among the most common. In addition, tissue reserves of water-soluble nutrients can be estimated by means of a "load" or "saturation" test: For example, administration of a large dose of ascorbic acid is followed by measuring the urinary excretion of vitamin C. With adequate tissue reserves of the vitamin, a large percentage of the administered dose will be excreted. Conversely, if the body's tissue reserves are low, a high percentage of the loading dose will be retained in the body, and less will appear in the urine.

Indirect, functional measures are also employed in urinalysis. For example, a "loading" dose of tryptophan, which is converted to nicotinic acid, may be administered before urine is collected for evaluation of vitamin B_6 status. Vitamin B_6 is required in the conversion of xanthurenic acid to nicotinic acid (niacin), a step in the normal metabolism of tryptophan. Therefore, in B_6 deficiency, a load dose of tryptophan will create an accumulation of xanthurenic acid, which will be excreted in the urine because there is insufficient vitamin B_6 available to further convert it to nicotinic acid.

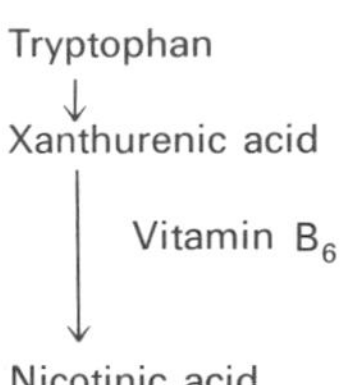

Collection of urine samples is somewhat more difficult than collection of blood samples. Although the momentary discomfort of drawing blood is avoided, the inconvenience factor is substantially increased. Ideally, biochemical tests are performed on a 24-hour sample of urine, which reflects the quantitative daily output of many substances rather than the relative output at any one time of day. Few subjects are willing to take the time and care required to collect 24-hour, or even 12- or 6-hour, urine samples. In most cases, a single specimen must suffice, from which quantitative estimates of daily excretion are calculated.

OTHER BIOCHEMICAL ANALYSES. Stool specimens and even hair specimens also may be collected and studied to complement the biochemical data obtained from blood and urine analyses. Although stool examination for parasites, blood, and fats is useful, stool sampling is unpleasant and not generally used for routine nutritional assessments. It is, however, essential for detection of a number of gastrointestinal disorders.

Collecting hair samples is no problem, but analyses of hair for protein, copper, zinc, and other trace metals are seldom performed except in a research setting. The ease of sampling promises to make them more useful in the future, but as yet standardized data of mineral levels in hair are not available.

Major disadvantages of many biochemical tests are the specialized equipment and carefully trained technicians needed to administer them. For these reasons, too, such tests are often expensive to conduct. As a result, many cannot be routinely used in field studies. Another drawback is that people often object to collecting urine samples, or being "stuck" to give a blood sample. And finally, many biochemical analyses can show only what's *in* the body—not how it got there or why. Unless specifically designed for a particular purpose, they cannot distinguish between primary and secondary nutrient deficiencies or otherwise indicate causal factors such as the effects of illness, anxiety, environmental pollutants, or heredity.

Biochemical studies do provide more specific information about nutrient status than the other methods described previously. Whereas anthropometric and clinical measures can only describe an individual's external appearance, biochemical tests are a "window" on the inner workings of the body.

Dietary Assessment

The three assessment techniques described thus far—anthropometric, clinical, and biochemical—can provide a great deal of data about an individual's physiological status and may give some indications of dietary deficiencies. But they do not answer the most important question posed by nutritionists: What is the food and nutrient intake? Dietary surveys do just that.

Conducting a dietary survey is more than a matter of asking a large number of people what they ate for dinner the night before. Some subjects will not remember at all, and many will omit one or more food items, either intentionally or unintentionally. The problems involved in learning about all the food eaten the previous day or week are even greater.

Dietary surveys are the only method by which actual intake can be assessed, and they can confirm or deny suspicions raised by other methods of assessment. If clinical and biochemical data suggest thiamin deficiency, for example, only an evaluation of actual food consumption will indicate whether the vitamin deficiency is likely to exist or whether the cause of the symptoms must be found elsewhere. Dietary assessment can also suggest that biochemical tests should be performed.

Dietary assessments also enable health care professionals to compare the food patterns of an individual or group with a desirable standard, usually the RDAs. This might be important, for example, in analyzing the nutritional status of a particular ethnic or socioeconomic group or of an individual. Also, diet surveys make it possible to note trends in consumption patterns of specific population subgroups, as in the study of growth patterns and diets of children consuming vegetarian diets.

Several techniques of dietary evaluation are used. Despite some disadvantages, **dietary recall** is a simple, rapid assessment method that is particularly useful for surveying large population groups. Typically, subjects are asked what foods, in what portion sizes, were consumed in the previous 24-hour period. A particular advantage of the recall method is that respondents will not have had the opportunity to deliberately modify their usual food behaviors, something that frequently happens when people realize that someone is interested in what they eat. Even though an individual's responses may be somewhat inaccurate or unrepresentative of typical intakes (the previous day may have been a birthday or a sick-day), the responses of the group as a whole provide a good qualitative estimate of general dietary behaviors in that particular population.

Because asking about yesterday's meals does not really provide very accurate information, specific kinds of diet surveys have been developed for specific purposes. When it is important to obtain accurate dietary information about long-term patterns of consumption, *household or population assessment* methods are used. In **household surveys** a trained interviewer typically visits the home to record all the foods on hand at the start of the study and instructs family members on how to record all food purchases made during the study. At the end of the study, the amounts and kinds of foods remaining in the house are also noted. Adjustments for food wasted within the home, that used for animal food, and that contributed by meals eaten outside the home must be made as well. Calculations estimate the nutrients available to the household during the study period. Adjustments are made for the number, age, and sex of people in the household, but they may not always correct for possible uneven distribution among family members. In addition, there is no guarantee that the food purchaser has not altered usual food buying habits during the study.

On a larger scale, the same type of survey could be used to record the quantities of foods produced in a particular region, city, or country, the amounts imported or exported, and the amounts lost in processing or allocation to animal feed. This information can serve to identify general patterns or trends of consumption, or ethnic or socioeconomic food habits, to predict food shortages and surpluses, and to diagnose inadequacies in a population's available diet.

When it is important to obtain accurate dietary information about a specific individual, as might be necessary for diagnostic purposes, other methods are used. *Food intake records* are written reports of foods eaten during a specified length of time, typically three to seven days. Although this reporting method minimizes the problem of atypical days, it introduces the problem of long-term diligence. Record keeping is boring, and boredom increases with time. Not surprisingly, accuracy decreases as the duration of record keeping increases. One recent study (Gersovitz et al., 1978) found, for example, that few subjects kept accurate records for more than four days. Only well-educated, highly literate subjects maintained accuracy for a longer period. Thus, the need for diligence and literacy is a distinct disadvantage of diet records; however, some way of motivating the subjects (visits or phone calls from a trained interviewer or a reward of some kind) often helps.

In both the recall and record methods, respondents must be advised about portion sizes. Use of plastic food models, or description of portions in common household measures, increases the accuracy of the data obtained.

Weighed diets are carefully quantified records of the weights of all foods served to an individual or family, with the weight of uneaten food subtracted. Thus, the amount consumed can be calculated. Proponents of the weighed diet technique argue that the weighing process ensures accuracy, even with bored or poorly educated subjects. However, weighing foods and keeping records is tedious and time-consuming, and, unless highly motivated, the average person will not do it for a long period. When precise weighing techniques are necessary for metabolic studies, trained observers are required. The disadvantage of this, however, is that the presence of observers may put

PERSPECTIVE ON
Nutrition Surveys in the United States

Information about national agricultural production and industrial processing and sale of food products has been gathered for decades. These statistics are known as disappearance data, reflecting the amounts of each kind of food absorbed into the economy. This information is used to plan farm production, imports, exports, and food assistance programs, but it does not describe the actual diets of real people. That would require a nationwide dietary survey.

Collecting intake data from the entire population of more than 200 million Americans, however, would not be feasible. Instead, sophisticated sampling methods, such as those used by polling and research organizations, select a random sample of individuals and/or families whose food consumption patterns are then intensively studied. From the resulting data, it is possible to project statistics that are accurate, with a small margin of error, for a larger population segment.

The Ten-State Nutrition Survey (TSNS) of 1968–1970, conducted by the Nutrition Program of the U.S. Department of Health, Education, and Welfare, was the largest nutrition survey ever performed in the United States until that time. The impetus for the TSNS came from an outpouring of public concern after congressional hearings in 1967 disclosed an unexpectedly high incidence of hunger and malnutrition in the United States, and numerous reports of starving children and emaciated older people appeared in the press and on television. Because the focal point of the survey was the extent of malnutrition in low-income populations, the sample was composed primarily of families with annual incomes of less than $3,000 and was drawn from low-income communities in states in which average family incomes were higher (California; Massachusetts; Michigan; New York, including New York City; and Washington) or lower (Kentucky, Louisiana, South Carolina, Texas, and West Virginia) than the national average. In this survey the population studied was therefore *not* a representative sample of the entire population within a county or state. The sampling technique used identified 30,000 families; 24,000, comprising more than 86,000 individuals, were finally studied (Center for Disease Control, 1972). Each examination included a complete medical history, anthropometric measurements (height and weight; knee and wrist diameters; calf, arm, shoulder, and head circumferences), dental evaluation, and serum hemoglobin and hematocrit determinations. Evaluation of dietary intake was based on information gained from a 24-hour die-

Dietary Intakes as Determined by the HANES Survey of 1971–1972

Age	Caloric intake						Actual mean amounts of dietary intake: Protein (grams)		Calcium (milligrams)	
	Above poverty level			Below poverty level			Above poverty level	Below poverty level	Above poverty level	Below poverty level
	Total	White	Black	Total	White	Black				
Under 5 years	1,598	1,607	1,507	1,511	1,592	1,387	59.01	55.81	927	803
6 to 11 years	2,103	2,118	1,943	1,933	2,059	1,690	77.64	71.66	1,127	911
12 to 17 years	2,401	2,423	2,164	1,990	2,076	1,877	91.61	75.96	1,144	888
18 to 44 years:										
Male	2,806	2,834	2,607	2,529	2,573	2,502	111.22	101.10	1,028	934
Female	1,680	1,690	1,546	1,602	1,651	1,510	68.53	62.17	642	598
45 to 59 years	1,961	1,973	1,724	1,560	1,633	1,461	83.36	63.52	727	583
60 to 74 years	1,679	1,686	1,559	1,434	1,455	1,365	69.40	57.72	666	583

Note: These intakes should of course be compared with the recommended standards of intake for these nutrients.

Source: U.S.D.H.E.W., Public Health Service, National Center for Health Statistics, *Health and Nutrition Examination Survey, 1971–72.*

tary recall. High-risk subgroups of infants, young children, adolescents, pregnant and lactating women, and elderly people received more detailed biochemical, physical, dental, and anthropometric assessment. Because of the particular concerns that had given rise to the TSNS, income status and racial and ethnic characteristics were also noted.

The TSNS confirmed dramatically that a significant percentage of the low-income population was malnourished. It also showed that specific nutritional problems varied in different population subgroups: Overall, malnutrition was most often found in low-income groups, highest among the migrant farm workers of Texas and low-income blacks. Generally, the incidence of malnutrition increased as income levels decreased. Low-income pregnant black women had significantly lower energy and protein intakes than did pregnant white women from higher-income families. Iron deficiencies were found in all racial, age, and income groups. Vitamin A deficiencies were noted in Mexican-Americans and in children of all cultural backgrounds. Adult black women were most likely to be obese although obesity was also prevalent in adolescent white males. Adolescents generally had the highest incidence of dental caries, as well as the greatest number of indicators of malnutrition.

The study concluded that these and other observed nutritional deficiencies were due not simply to lack of food availability, but to poor food choices and inequitable distribution of food to family members. The surprising incidence of nutritional problems in the population studied in the TSNS suggested the need for nutrition surveys that would be more representative of the United States population as a whole. In 1971, the first Health and Nutrition Examination Survey (HANES) was directed to include nutrition in the usual health examination survey. The HANES Survey used probability sampling methods to select a random sample of subjects aged 1 to 74 years, from all sections of the country. Subjects underwent complete clinical examinations, anthropometric assessments, and biochemical (blood and urine) determinations. To provide further details, a smaller sample of participants completed a 24-hour food recall and a food history questionnaire focusing on the three-month interval prior to the study (Dresser et al., 1978). A second HANES program, the U.S. Health and Nutrition Survey of 1976–1979, was undertaken. The mass of data collected by both HANES programs is still being analyzed. (Some of the findings of the 1971–1972 HANES Survey are presented in the table.) Preliminary findings indicate that:

- Iron deficiency, documented by both dietary and biochemical data, is prevalent in all segments and all age groups of the U.S. population, and biochemical deficiency is found particularly in children aged 1 to 5 years. Males aged 18 to 44 were the only subgroup showing mean iron intake above the recommended dietary allowances (Abraham et al., 1974).
- Blacks of all ages and income groups show a higher prevalence of nutrient deficiencies for vitamins A, C, and D, thiamin, calcium, phosphorus, and iodine than do whites.
- Black women aged 45 to 74, and white women in general, have a higher incidence of obesity than all men, regardless of income level. However, white men have a higher incidence of obesity than do black men.

Comparison of recent HANES findings with older nutrition surveys is also yielding interesting data. For example, an unexpected, and as yet unexplained, beneficial decrease in serum cholesterol levels of middle-aged women over the last decade has become apparent (Habicht et al., 1978). This kind of change illustrates the need for ongoing surveillance of national nutritional status.

Actual mean amounts of dietary intake

Iron (milligrams)		Vitamin A (international units)		Vitamin C (milligrams)	
Above poverty level	Below poverty level	Above poverty level	Below poverty level	Above poverty level	Below poverty level
8.35	7.90	3,217	3,413	74.88	58.78
10.43	10.40	4,042	4,174	79.77	61.11
12.72	11.55	4,340	3,688	79.54	72.51
16.60	15.63	5,169	5,265	94.85	70.95
10.58	9.68	4,038	3,765	81.02	64.16
12.91	10.26	5,489	7,006	91.62	66.32
11.41	9.57	6,914	4,216	99.15	70.63

RELATIVE IMPORTANCE OF NUTRITIONAL PROBLEMS IN THE TEN-STATE NUTRITION SURVEY 1968-1970

LOW-INCOME-RATIO STATES KENTUCKY, LOUISIANA, SOUTH CAROLINA, TEXAS, WEST VIRGINIA

ETHNIC GROUP	AGE	SEX	iron	protein	vitamin A	vitamin C	riboflavin	thiamine	iodine	growth & development	obesity
BLACK	0–5 years	both	High	O	High	O	High	O	O	High	–
	6–9 years	both	High	Low	Low	O	Medium	O	O	Low	–
	10–16 years	females	High	Low	Low	O	Medium	Low	O	Low	Medium
		males	High	O	Low	O	Medium	Low	O	Low	Medium
	17–59 years	females	High	Low	O	Low	Medium	O	O	–	High
		males	High	O	O	Medium	Medium	O	O	–	O
	over 60 years	females	High	Low	O	O	Medium	O	O	–	Medium
		males	Medium	Low	O	Medium	Medium	O	O	–	O
WHITE	0–5 years	both	Medium	O	Low	O	Low	O	O	Medium	–
	6–9 years	both	Medium	O	Low	O	Low	O	O	Medium	–
	10–16 years	females	Medium	O	Low	O	Low	Low	O	Low	Low
		males	Medium	O	Low	O	Low	Low	O	Low	Medium
	17–59 years	females	Medium	O	O	O	O	O	O	–	Medium
		males	Medium	O	O	Medium	O	O	O	–	Low
	over 60 years	females	Medium	O	O	O	O	O	O	–	Medium
		males	Medium	O	O	Medium	O	O	O	–	O
SPANISH-AMERICAN	0–5 years	both	Medium	O	High	O	Medium	O	O	Medium	–
	6–9 years	both	Medium	O	High	O	Medium	O	O	Medium	–
	10–16 years	females	Medium	Low	High	O	Medium	O	O	Low	–
		males	Medium	O	High	O	Medium	O	O	Low	–
	17–59 years	females	Medium	Low	High	O	Low	O	O	–	–
		males	Medium	Low	High	O	Low	O	O	–	–
	over 60 years	females	Medium	Low	High	O	Low	O	O	–	–
		males	Medium	Low	High	Medium	Low	O	O	–	–
Pregnant and lactating women			High	Medium	–	–	–	–	–	–	–

HIGH-INCOME-RATIO STATES CALIFORNIA, MASSACHUSETTS, MICHIGAN, NEW YORK (and NEW YORK CITY), WASHINGTON

iron	protein	vitamin A	vitamin C	riboflavin	thiamine	iodine	growth & development	obesity	SEX	AGE	ETHNIC GROUP
High	O	Medium	O	Low	O	O	Medium	–	both	0–5 years	BLACK
Medium	O	Low	O	Low	O	O	Medium	–	both	6–9 years	
Medium	O	Medium	O	Low	Low	O	Low	Low	females	10–16 years	
Medium	O	Low	O	Low	Low	O	Low	O	males		
Medium	O	O	O	Low	O	O	–	Medium	females	17–59 years	
Medium	O	O	O	Low	O	O	–	O	males		
Medium	O	O	O	Low	O	O	–	Medium	females	over 60 years	
Medium	O	O	Low	Low	O	O	–	O	males		
Low	O	Low	O	Low	O	O	Medium	–	both	0–5 years	WHITE
Low	O	Low	O	O	O	O	Medium	–	both	6–9 years	
Low	O	Low	O	O	O	O	Low	Low	females	10–16 years	
Low	O	Low	O	O	O	O	Low	Low	males		
Low	O	O	O	O	O	O	–	Medium	females	17–59 years	
Low	O	O	O	O	O	O	–	Low	males		
Low	O	O	O	O	O	O	–	Medium	females	over 60 years	
Low	O	O	Low	O	O	O	–	O	males		
Medium	O	O	O	O	O	O	Medium	–	both	0–5 years	SPANISH AMERICAN
Medium	O	O	O	O	O	O	Medium	–	both	6–9 years	
Medium	O	O	O	O	O	O	Low	–	females	10–16 years	
Medium	O	O	O	O	O	O	Low	–	males		
Medium	O	O	O	O	O	O	–	–	females	17–59 years	
Medium	O	O	O	O	O	O	–	–	males		
Medium	O	O	O	O	O	O	–	–	females	over 60 years	
Medium	O	O	O	O	O	O	–	–	males		
High	Medium	–	–	–	–	–	–	–	Pregnant and lactating women		

LEGEND: HIGH; MEDIUM; LOW; O MINIMAL; – NOT AVAIL

Ten-State Nutrition Survey, 1968–1970: Relative Importance of Nutritional Problems
Source: Center for Disease Control, *Ten-state nutrition survey in the United States, 1968–1970*, Highlights, DHEW Publication No. (HSM) 72-8134 (Atlanta, Ga.: Health Services and Mental Health Administration, 1972).

Some moderation is also needed, however. If all surveys were to collect the enormous amount of data generated by the TSNS or HANES, it might take years before important nutritional problems were detected. Researchers have suggested that new surveys limit themselves to proven, significant variables and to limited target populations. Among the nutrients considered most important in public health programs are protein, iron, iodine, niacin, thiamin, ascorbic acid, and vitamins A and D. Sodium, cholesterol, saturated and unsaturated fatty acids are also important because of their possible significance in cardiovascular disease. And energy intake must be given major consideration as well because of the high incidence of obesity. But priorities change and research plans must change accordingly. The National Center for Health Statistics in July 1977 awarded a contract to the National Academy of Public Administration to identify the principal nutritional concerns for further investigation.

the observees on "good behavior," changing their typical eating patterns. Weighed diets are more feasible in an institutional setting, and studies in hospitals, prisons, and the Armed Forces have used this method.

Diet histories are interview or questionnaire surveys of subjects' usual dietary pattern. A diet history does not determine the precise foods eaten on a given day or week. Rather, it describes the kinds and amounts of foods typically eaten and the frequency of their consumption in a specified period of days, weeks, or months. Subjects frequently receive a check-off list of many different foods and drinks and a set of food models to be used in estimating portion sizes. They simply search the list for foods they have eaten during the particular time period and then estimate the number and sizes of portions consumed. An interviewer can also elicit information about food likes and dislikes, usual number of meals consumed per day, and other pertinent information. Although this recall approach may appear to offer the same disadvantages as other recall techniques and often results in overestimates of consumption, Morgan et al. (1978) reported that it is more accurate than 24-hour recall or diet records. Comparison of subjects' current diet histories with earlier patterns of consumption can provide an important measure of dietary changes that may relate to diseases or environmental variables. In addition, a dietary history can also be used to substantiate information obtained from a 24-hour recall and food intake record.

After individual, family, or group intakes have been determined, the quantity of food consumed must be translated into the quantity of nutrient intake. Then these levels can be compared with a standard, usually the RDAs.

Generally, consistent intake of less than two-thirds of the RDA for one or more nutrients has been shown to be associated with risk of nutritional deficiency in an individual or population group. Anthropometric, clinical, and biochemical data would be sought to confirm suspicions. Figure 10-1 diagrams the interactions of the primary assessment techniques.

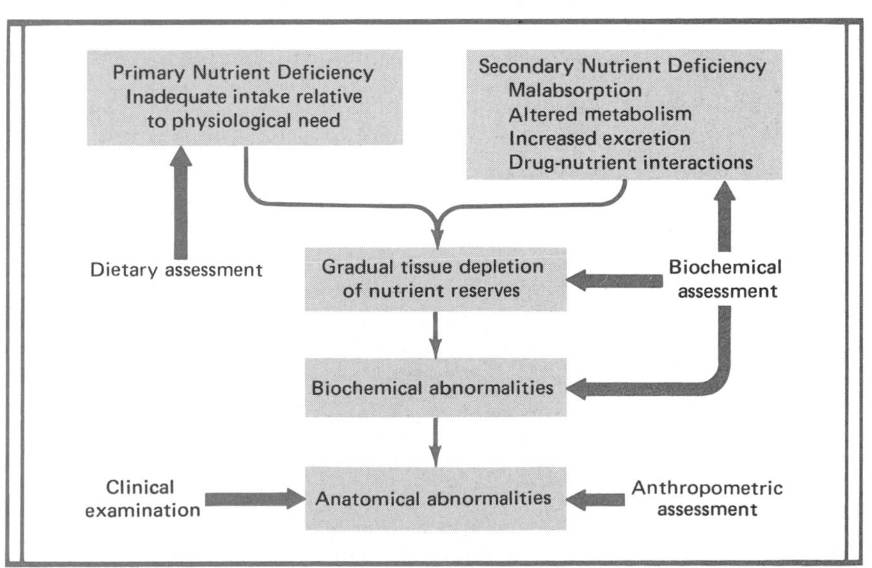

FIGURE 10-1
Development of Nutrient Deficiency and Tools for Assessment

Source: Adapted from W. A. Krehl, *Med. Clin. N. Am.* 48:1129, 1964.

Of course, mere identification of current or changing consumption patterns does not benefit health. Intervention must follow identification of a problem. In cases of severe deficiency, immediate refeeding and medical care is, of course, urgent. Planning, redistribution of food supplies, and nutrition education programs are required for individuals and groups at nutritional risk. And some attention must be paid to those not known to be at risk as well. Education programs and maintenance of food supplies will help to ensure that their currently adequate nutritional status will continue in the future.

TOOLS FOR PLANNING AN ADEQUATE DIET

Our discussion of dietary assessment indicated the need for estimates of adequate and suboptimal nutrient intake based on standardized information. To obtain these measurements, nutritionists first had to determine average levels of the nutrients contained in various foods, since, after all, nutrients are almost never ingested in pure form. To complicate matters further, both naturally grown and manufactured foods tend to vary in their nutrient content. In metabolic nutrition research this natural variability is neutralized by laboratory analysis of samples of any food to be eaten by the subject being studied. But this procedure is inconvenient and impractical for large-scale research or field studies. Food composition tables provide average nutrient values, based on quantitative analysis of many samples of each food item.

Food composition tables are widely used by professional nutritionists. With the RDAs, they provide a means by which diets and menus can be planned to meet the needs of individuals of all ages under normal conditions and under some special conditions as well. Because these guides are too complex for everyday use by most people, meal-planning aids for the general public and for particular purposes have also been devised.

Food Composition Tables

In 1869, Wilbur Atwater chemically analyzed Indian corn, which was the first American food to be studied for its nutrient content. By 1880 tables of food composition had been issued for numerous European products. In 1892 Atwater and Woods published the results of their investigations of about 900 foods, most of them meats. In the same year the USDA issued its Bulletin No. 11 summarizing the composition of more than 3,000 food items, mostly animal feeds, which had been analyzed before 1890. *The Chemical Composition of American Food Materials*, USDA Bulletin No. 28 by Atwater and Woods in 1896, is considered the classic American food table. This first comprehensive list of more than 600 edible items included their content of protein, carbohydrate, fat, ash, and water, as well as energy density.

Tables in use at present are compiled not only by the government, but by educational and industrial research groups as well. Most include data for a

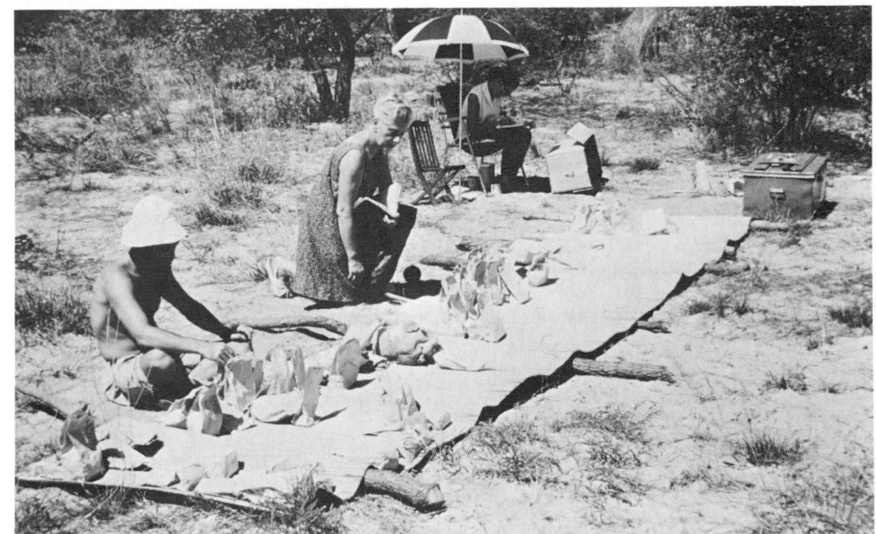

Samples of foods in the diets of peoples around the world are analyzed to determine their nutrient content. Here anthropologist Marjorie Whiting supervises the preparation of plant samples, which must be dried, packaged, and labeled, for analysis. (For more information about nutritional anthropology, see Chapter 15.) (Nancy DeVore)

minimum of five vitamins and five or more minerals now known to be essential nutrients, as well as food energy, protein, and lipid content. The new tables reflect the increasing variety of foods available in this country, and they also provide data on the different forms in which they are consumed. Although early tables gave data only for food in its raw form, tables issued by the USDA since 1940 have included values for fresh, canned, dried, and cooked forms of foods. More recently, values for frozen and commercially prepared foods have been added.

As new nutrients have been discovered and new assay methods developed to identify them in foods, tables have been issued focusing on one nutrient or a group of related nutrients; excerpts from some of these have appeared in previous chapters. In 1968, for example, when enough data had been accumulated to publish recommended dietary allowances for seven new nutrients (vitamins E, B_6, B_{12}, and folacin and the minerals phosphorus, iodine, and magnesium) there was a demand for information on their occurrence in foods (Watt and Murphy, 1970).

Changing commercial and home cooking or processing methods also affects the nutrient content of foods. Cooking by moist or dry heat, freeze drying as opposed to flash freezing, fast microwave roasting as compared with slow oven baking—all present the need for re-evaluation of nutrient content. In addition, yesterday's carrot may not be the same as today's. Vitamin content of a food can vary with the season, geographical area where it was produced, growing conditions, and genetic factors; mineral content is affected by soils, weather, and water supply. Garden-to-table time, storage facilities, and cooking methods also affect nutrient content (Erdman, 1978). As scientific breeding practices produce new strains, nutrient composition is altered. It has been estimated, for example, that young frying chickens sold during the 1960s contained about one-tenth more water, about half as much fat, and about 30 percent fewer calories than young chickens sold 20 to 40 years earlier. Differences in breeding, feeding, and processing account for much of this change.

Another familiar product, commercial white bread, has also changed significantly. Unlike the bread of the 1920s, which was made with water, white bread today is mixed with milk and has added calcium-rich mold inhibitors. Today's bread has nearly three times the calcium content of the bread Grandma used to eat (Watt, 1962).

Then too, new foods must be analyzed. "Health" foods and foods of ethnic groups—Chinese, Italians, Mexicans, Cubans, Native Americans, black Americans, and others—have become increasingly popular today in all segments of the population. Many of the foods characteristic of these groups remain to be evaluated for nutrient content. In addition, recent discoveries concerning inborn errors of metabolism and other metabolic disorders have led to a demand for information about the distribution and amount of specific amino acids in foods (Watt and Murphy, 1970).

In recent years, methods of laboratory analysis have increased in accuracy and reliability. Food chemists are repeating tests to obtain specific or more useful data, as well as testing newly developed or currently popular items. But some of the nutrient content in foods may not actually be used by the body. Many of the factors affecting this nutrient **bioavailability** are still unknown. It is known, however, that certain gastrointestinal disorders and ingested drugs reduce absorption from the intestine and thus limit nutrient bioavailability. The factors affecting utilization of micronutrients can be complex, as in the case of iron. As knowledge increases about the ways in which nutrients and other chemicals present in foods (phytates, for example) interact, new research must identify these substances in foods and food tables must make the new data available.

Health care professionals, and many consumers, too, are acquainted with a printed format that can be kept for frequent reference. Since publication of Atwater's USDA Bulletin No. 28, and its revisions in 1899 and 1906, the USDA has issued many food composition tables. The most recent major revision is Handbook No. 8, *Composition of Foods—Raw, processed, prepared* (Watt and Merrill, 1963). To make available the information that has become known since 1963, a revised Handbook No. 8 is now being prepared. Sections are released as they are ready: 8-1, *Dairy and egg products,* including more than twice as many food items as in the earlier edition; 8-2, *Herbs and spices,* containing information for 43 items of which only two had appeared in the earlier edition; 8-3, *Baby foods;* and 8-4, *Fats and oils,* were issued by late 1979. (Table 10-2 presents the data for an egg as shown in Handbook 8-1). The Food Composition Table in this textbook (Appendix, Table H) includes data from the 1963 Handbook, supplemented by information from these newly issued additions and from USDA Handbook No. 456 (Adams, 1975) as well. This last was based on Handbook No. 8 and presents values for 1,500 foods in terms of common household measures and market units instead of the 100-gram portions used in the 1963 volume, thus making the information more accessible for wider use. The complete revision of Handbook No. 8 is scheduled to contain information on more than 4,000 food items. In addition to previous sections, information on the following categories is being included: soups, sauces, and gravies; poultry; pork; sausages and luncheon meats; nuts and seeds; legumes; fish and shellfish; fruits; vegetables; beef; lamb and game; cereal grains; bakery products; sugars and sweets; beverages; and mixed dishes. The data tabulated are for water, energy, protein, fat, total carbohydrate, fiber and ash, mineral elements (calcium, iron, magnesium, phosphorus,

TABLE 10-2 Nutrient Composition of an Egg as Adapted from Handbook 8-1

EGG, CHICKEN, WHOLE, fresh and frozen, raw

Nutrients and Units		Amount in Edible Portion of Common Measures of Food: *Approximate measure and weight* *1 egg = 50 g*[a]	*1 c = 243 g*
PROXIMATE:			
Water	g	37.28	181.20
Food energy	kcal	79	384
	kJ	330	1,606
Protein (N × 6.25)	g	6.07	29.50
Total lipid (fat)	g	5.58	27.09
Carbohydrate, total	g	.60	2.92
Fiber	g	0	0
Ash	g	.47	2.28
MINERALS:			
Calcium	mg	28	136
Iron	mg	1.04	5.08
Magnesium	mg	6	30
Phosphorus	mg	90	438
Potassium	mg	65	316
Sodium	mg	69	336
Zinc	mg	.72	3.50
VITAMINS:			
Ascorbic acid	mg	0	0
Thiamin	mg	.044	.211
Riboflavin	mg	.150	.731
Niacin	mg	.031	.151
Pantothenic acid	mg	.864	4.197
Vitamin B_6	mg	.060	.292
Folacin	mcg	32	158
Vitamin B_{12}	mcg	.773	3.759
Vitamin A	RE	78	379
	IU	260	1,264
LIPIDS:			
Fatty acids:			
Saturated, total	g	1.67	8.14
4:0	g		
6:0	g		
8:0	g		
10:0	g		
12:0	g		
14:0	g	.02	.07

Nutrients and Units		Amount in Edible Portion of Common Measures of Food: *Approximate measure and weight* *1 egg = 50 g*[a]	*1 c = 243 g*
16:0	g	1.23	5.98
18:0	g	.43	2.08
Monounsaturated, total	g	2.23	10.83
16:1	g	.19	.90
18:1	g	2.04	9.93
20:1	g		
22:1	g		
Polyunsaturated, total	g	.72	3.52
18:2	g	.62	3.01
18:3	g	.02	.08
18:4	g		
20:4	g	.05	.23
20:5	g		
22:5	g		
22:6	g		
Cholesterol	mg	274	1,331
Phytosterols	mg		
AMINO ACIDS:			
Tryptophan	g	.097	.472
Threonine	g	.298	1.449
Isoleucine	g	.380	1.846
Leucine	g	.533	2.591
Lysine	g	.410	1.992
Methionine	g	.196	.953
Cystine	g	.145	.703
Phenylalanine	g	.343	1.666
Tyrosine	g	.253	1.227
Valine	g	.437	2.124
Arginine	g	.388	1.888
Histidine	g	.147	.713
Alanine	g	.354	1.723
Aspartic acid	g	.602	2.926
Glutamic acid	g	.773	3.757
Glycine	g	.202	.982
Proline	g	.241	1.171
Serine	g	.461	2.242

[a]Weight applies to large egg.

Source: L. P. Posati and M. L. Orr, *Composition of foods—Dairy and egg products—Raw, processed, prepared,* Agriculture Handbook No. 8-1 (Washington, D.C.: U.S. Government Printing Office, 1976), p. 123.

potassium, sodium, and zinc), nine vitamins (ascorbic acid, thiamin, riboflavin, niacin, pantothenic acid, vitamin B_6, folacin, vitamin B_{12}, and vitamin A), individual fatty acids, total fatty acids, cholesterol, total phytosterols, and 18 amino acids. Nutrient values will be expressed as the amount present in the edible portion of 100 grams, common household measures, and 1 pound of food as purchased.

So much data have accumulated that the most sophisticated tables are maintained and updated by computer. Two well-known computer-stored "nutrient data bases" are the Extended Table of Nutrient Values (ETNV) of the International Dietary Information Foundation, Inc., and the Nutrient Data Bank (NDB) of the Nutrient Data Research Center of the United States Department of Agriculture.

The ETNV, when it was first published in 1969, included data on 79 nutrients and other dietary factors for approximately 600 single foods and 1,500 commercially or domestically compounded foods containing several ingredients. New data are constantly being added; use of the ETNV is restricted to nonindustrial researchers.

The NDB contains data for approximately 100 nutrients and related factors and 215 food constituents with nutritional value. Nutrient information provided by food industry sources will contribute to the NDB, which will serve as a resource for continual updating of Handbook No. 8 (Hertzler and Hoover, 1977).

Dietary Standards

The RDAs, Recommended Dietary Allowances, which we introduced in Chapter 1 and have referred to throughout Part One, are issued in the form of a table (see Appendix, Table A) showing desirable amounts for daily intakes of energy and many nutrients. The energy levels have been estimated to meet the average needs of population groups of healthy individuals; the nutrient levels should meet or exceed the needs of practically all healthy persons.

The RDAs are not intended for use by consumers nor are they goals for individual dietary intakes. Rather, they are standards against which nutrient intakes can be compared. They are used to evaluate the nutrient content of population food supplies, of foods provided in government-sponsored or other feeding programs, and for related purposes (Hegsted, 1975).

Many observers have in recent years called attention to shortcomings of the RDAs. It has been suggested that this standard should be more applicable and understandable to consumers; that requirements should also be expressed in terms of nutrient density (that is, per 100 kcal) (Hansen et al., 1978); and that additional nutrients now known to be essential should be included. It has been suggested, furthermore, that consumers should be represented on the Food and Nutrition Board, which determines the RDAs. Presently, the Board is composed of nutritional biochemists—that is, scientists. Still others complain that the RDAs do not consider the role of such nutrient-related factors as fiber and cholesterol, and therefore do not define "acceptable" levels of intake. (The proposed U.S. Dietary Goals, which do suggest guidelines for cholesterol, fat, and sugar intake, are discussed in Chapter 16.)

Perhaps a more important concern is that the RDAs by definition encourage a tendency to think in terms of getting "enough" of a nutrient, even though for some nutrients (energy and protein for example) a majority of Americans are apparently consuming a "nutrient excess." Nevertheless, the RDAs represent the best estimate we have at present to evaluate nutritional status and to plan food supplies for population groups. Continued research and reinterpretation of data can be expected to further refine the nutrient allowances and to clarify the appropriate uses of the RDAs.

Figures derived from the RDAs, the U.S. Recommended Daily Allowances (U.S. RDA), are used by the Food and Drug Administration as the basis for nutritional labeling. Their derivation and use are discussed in the following section.

Tools for the Consumer

Although the RDAs were designed for professional use, a person does not have to be a professional nutritionist to learn to use them. As a nutrition student, you have an advantage. You will probably use the RDAs in conjunction with food composition tables to estimate your own nutrient intake. Although you may find it somewhat tedious to calculate nutrient levels for a variety of foods, and then to relate these calculations to RDA standards, you will probably have little difficulty doing it. But most consumers need a more accessible and easy-to-use guide to menu planning. Several consumer-oriented assessment systems have been designed to fill specific needs.

BASIC FOOD GROUPS. Most students are aware of the "Basic Four." This food guide was developed in consideration of the nutrient content of foods in different broad groups; key nutrients were identified as those which should be monitored. It has been assumed that if a few "index" nutrients were considered, the other 40-odd nutrients necessary for health would naturally accompany them when a variety of foods was consumed. It has also been assumed that the simpler the system, the more likely it is to be accepted and used, especially by children and poorly educated segments of the population. For this reason, the food guide promoted by the USDA is based on five groups: milk, meat, vegetables and fruits, breads and cereals, and other foods.

The *milk group*, providing high-quality protein, riboflavin, calcium, and, when fortified, vitamin D, includes all types of milk used in beverages, in natural and processed cheese, yogurt, ice cream and ice milk, in commercial soups, and in puddings. Products from the milk group supply about 75 percent of the calcium, over 35 percent of the riboflavin (vitamin B_2), and more than 20 percent of the protein available in the average American diet. Two servings are recommended for adults.

The *meat group*, noted for its high-quality protein, B vitamins, iron, and other trace elements, includes meats (beef, veal, pork, lamb, wild game), fish, poultry, eggs, meat alternatives (dry beans, peas, lentils, peanut butter), and nuts. Two servings from this group per day are recommended for most adults and children; pregnant women should choose three. Foods in the meat group supply over 50 percent of the protein, over 40 percent of the iron, and over 50 percent of the niacin in our diet. Since different foods from this group provide different percentages of these nutrients (see Table 10-3), choices must be made carefully. Legumes contain no vitamin B_{12}, but they are fairly rich sources of folacin. Meats, on the other hand, are good sources of B_{12} but only poor sources of folacin. Food guides often recommend certain choice combinations, because protein bioavailability depends upon the presence of complementary amino acids that are not found together in a single nonmeat

TABLE 10-3 Percentage Contribution of Food Groups to Nutrients Available for Consumption in the Average U.S. Diet

Food Group	Energy	Protein	Fat	Carbo-hydrate	Calcium	Phosphorus	Iron	Magnesium
Milk	11.1	22.0	12.5	6.7	74.6	35.0	2.5	21.7
Meat	24.9	52.8	40.6	2.3	9.1	39.6	41.9	27.2
Meat, poultry, fish	20.0	42.6	34.1	0.1	4.0	28.5	30.9	14.1
Eggs	1.8	4.8	2.7	0.1	2.2	5.0	4.7	1.2
Legumes and nuts	3.1	5.4	3.8	2.1	2.9	6.1	6.3	11.9
Fruit and Vegetable	8.6	7.0	0.9	17.3	9.6	10.9	18.8	25.9
Citrus fruits	0.9	0.5	0.1	2.0	1.0	0.7	0.8	2.3
Other fruits	2.1	0.6	0.3	4.6	1.2	1.1	3.3	3.9
Dark green/dark yellow vegetables	0.2	0.4	trace	0.5	1.5	0.6	1.5	2.0
Other vegetables[a]	5.4	5.5	0.5	10.2	5.9	8.5	13.2	17.7
Grain	19.2	17.6	1.3	34.7	3.4	12.2	27.9	17.9
Other[b]	36.1	0.6	44.5	39.0	3.4	2.3	9.0	7.3

[a] Includes potatoes and tomatoes.
[b] Includes fats, oils, sugars.
Source: Adapted from *National Food Review*, USDA, Washington, D.C., 1978.

"meat group" food, and other considerations (for example vitamin B_{12} content) must be made as well. Again, diversity is the watchword.

The *vegetable and fruit group* includes fresh, canned, frozen, and dried fruits and vegetables (except for dried beans and peas which are considered legumes; see meat group). Although corn is listed as a vegetable, it is also found in the grain group (corn grits and cornmeal). Fruits and vegetables supply over 90 percent of the vitamin C and almost 50 percent of the vitamin A in our diet, as well as significant amounts of other vitamins and minerals. Four fruit or vegetable servings are recommended each day.

The *bread and cereals group*, also called the grain group, includes breads, breakfast cereals, grits, noodles, pastas, barley, buckwheat, corn, oats, rice, rye, wheat, and all other related products. These foods supply about 40 percent of the thiamin and 30 percent of the iron and niacin in a typical American diet. Four daily servings are recommended.

Some common food items are missing from these groups: fats, such as butter, oil and margarine, and honey, sugar, jam, jelly, and candy. An *other* category has been established for these items, as well as for desserts, condiments, and beverages. Intakes should be adjusted to energy needs.

Another shortcoming of the Basic Four plan is that food portions may not necessarily coincide with standard "servings." Few home-prepared hamburgers, for example, are a uniform 3-ounce size, the quantity defined as one serving. In addition, some foods clearly belonging to basic food groups actually have minimal nutritional value. Beets and applesauce are often cited as examples. Finally, only a few nutrients—the key or index nutrients—from the approximately 45 essential nutrients are specifically identified in this grouping system. Although different combinations of a variety of foods within each group can provide all the other nutrients, there is no guarantee that people will know which combinations to choose (Pennington, 1976).

Vitamin A	Thiamin	Riboflavin	Niacin	Vitamin B_6	Vitamin B_{12}	Ascorbic acid
13.0	8.6	39.0	1.4	10.6	20.1	3.9
27.9	33.2	30.6	52.1	53.5	78.4	1.1
22.4	25.9	24.3	45.2	47.4	70.5	1.1
5.5	2.0	4.5	0.1	1.8	0	0
trace	5.3	1.8	6.8	4.3	0	trace
48.3	16.4	8.7	15.0	26.7	0	91.4
1.6	2.7	0.5	0.8	1.2	0	27.4
5.5	1.7	1.5	1.6	5.6	0	11.6
20.2	0.8	1.0	0.6	1.7	0	8.8
21.0	11.2	5.7	12.0	18.2	0	43.6
	41.6	21.0	27.9	8.9	1.5	0
10.5	0.1	1.6	3.5	0.1	0	3.6

Recently, computer evaluation of 20 menus derived from the Basic Four demonstrated that daily intakes met or surpassed current RDAs for only 8 of the 17 nutrients tested, and provided 60 percent or less of the RDA levels for vitamin E, vitamin B_6, magnesium, zinc, and iron. Adding foods from an "others" category primarily to increase vitamin E content with intake of fats and oils helped somewhat, but still failed to meet many RDAs. This is not necessarily a problem, because RDAs are overestimates of nutrient needs for most people. But modification of the Basic Four has been suggested to emphasize those nutrients most underrepresented. One proposed method will simply increase portion sizes of foods from the meat and fruit and vegetable groups, as well as add fats and oils (King et al., 1978). (For a further analysis of the shortcomings of the Basic Four and a more elaborate alternative, see Pennington, 1976.) Despite shortcomings, however, the basic food groups are the easiest tool developed to date for use by the general public, and it is particularly useful in demonstrating desirable food intakes to children, the elderly, and population groups at high risk of nutritional deficiency—those sectors which it is most important to reach.

Early 20th century advertisement for commercially-baked bread. (The Bettmann Archive)

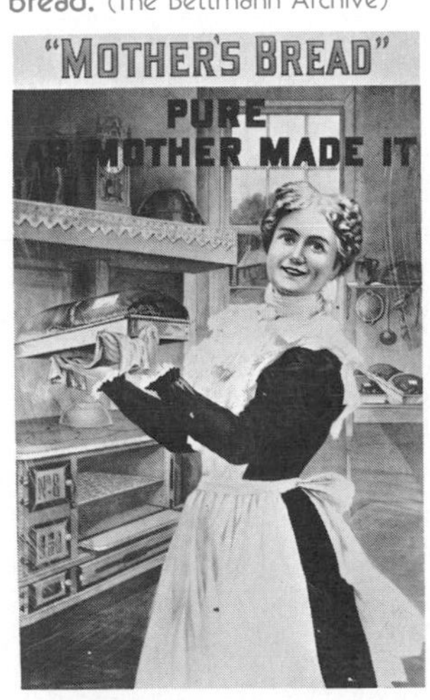

EXCHANGE LISTS. Exchange lists, introduced in 1950 for use by persons with diabetes mellitus, also present foods in various groups. These lists have become popular for use in planning fat-restricted, low-cholesterol, and weight-reduction diets as well. They contain food suggestions in specified portions in six different categories: milk, vegetables, fruit, bread (including cereals and starchy vegetables), meat, and fat. Sugar-rich foods (soft drinks, candies, cakes, and so on) are not included in any of the exchange groups, since they should not be included in the diets of people with diabetes.

The exchange lists were revised in 1976 to reflect changes in knowledge and philosophy, stressing foods of low-cholesterol and low fat content with lower energy values. The milk exchange group became based on nonfat milk; the meat group was subdivided into high-, medium-, and low-fat meats and their equivalents. Thus, the exchange lists emphasize kilocalories, nutrients, and low-fat foods.

Each of the six exchange lists contains foods of similar energy and nutrient content with emphasis on carbohydrate, fat, protein, and energy values. (See Appendix, Table G.) A good deal of flexibility in meal planning can be built in. Depending on the needs of an individual, diets can be worked out providing for daily consumption of, for example, two milk exchanges, two vegetable exchanges, three fruit exchanges, five bread/cereal exchanges, six medium-fat meat exchanges, and three fat exchanges. Such a plan will provide approximately 1,250 kilocalories. An individual who prefers to drink 1 cup of whole milk instead of skim milk must eliminate two fat exchanges from the daily meal plan under this system.

Exchange lists were designed for use by patients in consultation with a dietitian or other health professional. Without guidance as to how to use them for individual needs, they are not particularly useful. Further, because they focus on energy, fat, protein, and carbohydrate, meals based on these lists may not provide adequate amounts of other essential nutrients. In nutrition education programs using the exchange lists, the vitamin A and vitamin C content of fruits and vegetables is stressed, and food sources of other vitamins and minerals are pointed out as well. The importance of making diversified choices within each group is also explained.

Another drawback is that exchange lists do not include many foods that are popular with particular ethnic groups or "combination" or commercially available foods that are difficult to assign correctly to a single exchange list. Some food companies, however, publish information about the "exchange list" value of their products. Another aspect of this system of which consumers must be aware is that the amount listed for an "exchange" is not always equivalent to what is commonly considered a "serving"; meats are listed in 1-ounce amounts, for instance. These shortcomings, however, can be overcome by professional consultation and client education. The exchange list system is particularly useful for its intended purposes of planning diets for individuals with special needs, and it has been found generally easier to live with on a long-term basis than other diet plans.

NUTRITION LABELING. Food manufacturers have striven for years to produce easy-to-follow directions for preparation of their products that can be understood even by children and uneducated adults. Usually, they have been successful. If manufacturers can do this for their directions, why can't they do it for nutritional value? The answer, of course, is that they can. Nutrition labels on many food packages represent the government's and the food industry's current efforts to assist consumers in planning nutritious meals. But, as many consumer groups have indicated, nutritional labels are not as easily understood as manufacturers' package directions. During the summer and fall of 1978, the FDA held hearings throughout the country to find out from consumers where nutritional labels were falling short. The preliminary results of these hearings are discussed more fully in Chapter 16.

One area of consumer confusion is a misunderstanding of the United States Recommended Daily Allowances (U.S. RDAs), which form the standard for a part of nutritional labeling policy. U.S. RDAs are dietary standards that are derived from tables of the RDAs (Recommended Dietary Allowances) published by the Food and Nutrition Board in 1968. The U.S. RDAs replace the "minimum daily requirements" that were formerly used on the labels of mineral and vitamin preparations, breakfast cereals, and some other products. Because they are derived from the RDAs, they too provide a margin of safety for the typical consumer. In order to simplify nutritional labeling as much as possible, four tables of U.S. RDAs were developed. The most familiar is that which is used for adults and children over 4 years of age (Table 10-4). The U.S. RDA for a given nutrient is the highest RDA of that nutrient for children and adults, excluding pregnant and lactating women; thus, with a few exceptions, the RDA for 18-year-old males became the U.S. RDA. Examination of these standards will make it obvious that, for most individuals, allowances are even higher than the RDAs; this fact should be considered when comparing dietary intake to the U.S. RDAs.

Other U.S. RDA tables are for infants, children under 4 years of age, and for pregnant and lactating women (Appendix, Table C.); these figures appear on the labels of foods for these special groups.

Figure 10-2 shows examples of food labels, giving both ingredient and nutrition information. Ingredient information is required on all manufactured food products, unless these products have a so-called standard of

TABLE 10-4
U.S. Recommended Daily Allowances for Adults and Children over 4 Years of Age

	Nutrients	U.S. RDA
Must be listed on label	Protein	65 g[a]
	Vitamin A	5000 IU
	Vitamin C (ascorbic acid)	60.0 mg
	Thiamin (vitamin B_1)	1.5 mg
	Riboflavin (vitamin B_2)	1.7 mg
	Niacin	20.0 mg
	Calcium	1.0 g
	Iron	18.0 mg
May be listed on label	Vitamin D	400 IU
	Vitamin E	30 IU
	Vitamin B_6	2.0 mg
	Folacin (folic acid)	0.4 mg
	Vitamin B_{12}	6.0 μg
	Phosphorus	1.0 g
	Iodine	150 μg
	Magnesium	400 mg
	Zinc	15 mg
	Copper	2.0 mg
	Biotin	0.3 mg
	Pantothenic acid	10.0 mg

[a]For proteins with a Protein Efficiency Ratio (PER) less than that of casein (<2.5), the U.S. RDA is 65 g. For foods providing high-quality protein such as meat, fish, poultry, eggs, and milk (PER ≥2.5), the U.S. RDA is 45 g. Proteins with a PER less than 20% that of casein may not be expressed on the label as a percent of U.S. RDA.

Source: *Federal Register* 38 (13), (January 19, 1973).

FIGURE 10-2
Nutritional Information on Food Labels

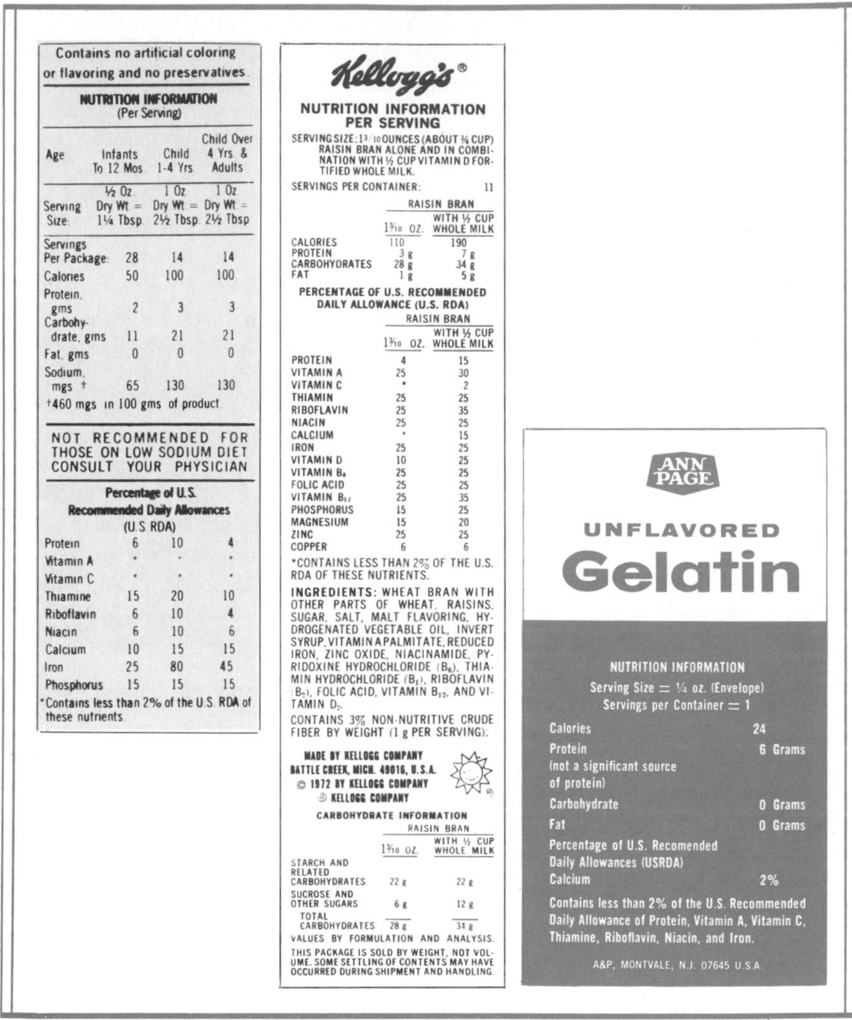

Contains no artificial coloring or flavoring and no preservatives.

NUTRITION INFORMATION
(Per Serving)

Age	Infants To 12 Mos.	Child 1-4 Yrs.	Child Over 4 Yrs. & Adults
Serving Size:	½ Oz. Dry Wt. = 1¼ Tbsp.	1 Oz. Dry Wt. = 2½ Tbsp.	1 Oz. Dry Wt. = 2½ Tbsp.
Servings Per Package:	28	14	14
Calories	50	100	100
Protein, gms	2	3	3
Carbohydrate, gms	11	21	21
Fat, gms	0	0	0
Sodium, mgs †	65	130	130

†460 mgs in 100 gms of product.

NOT RECOMMENDED FOR THOSE ON LOW SODIUM DIET CONSULT YOUR PHYSICIAN

Percentage of U.S. Recommended Daily Allowances
(U.S. RDA)

Protein	6	10	4
Vitamin A	*	*	*
Vitamin C	*	*	*
Thiamine	15	20	10
Riboflavin	6	10	4
Niacin	6	10	6
Calcium	10	15	15
Iron	25	80	45
Phosphorus	15	15	15

*Contains less than 2% of the U.S. RDA of these nutrients.

Kellogg's®

NUTRITION INFORMATION PER SERVING

SERVING SIZE: 1 3/10 OUNCES (ABOUT ¾ CUP) RAISIN BRAN ALONE AND IN COMBINATION WITH ½ CUP VITAMIN D FORTIFIED WHOLE MILK.

SERVINGS PER CONTAINER: 11

	RAISIN BRAN 1 3/10 OZ.	RAISIN BRAN WITH ½ CUP WHOLE MILK
CALORIES	110	190
PROTEIN	3 g	7 g
CARBOHYDRATES	28 g	34 g
FAT	1 g	5 g

PERCENTAGE OF U.S. RECOMMENDED DAILY ALLOWANCE (U.S. RDA)

	RAISIN BRAN 1 3/10 OZ.	RAISIN BRAN WITH ½ CUP WHOLE MILK
PROTEIN	4	15
VITAMIN A	25	30
VITAMIN C	*	2
THIAMIN	25	25
RIBOFLAVIN	25	35
NIACIN	25	25
CALCIUM	*	15
IRON	25	25
VITAMIN D	10	25
VITAMIN B_6	25	25
FOLIC ACID	25	25
VITAMIN B_{12}	25	35
PHOSPHORUS	15	25
MAGNESIUM	15	20
ZINC	25	25
COPPER	6	6

*CONTAINS LESS THAN 2% OF THE U.S. RDA OF THESE NUTRIENTS.

INGREDIENTS: WHEAT BRAN WITH OTHER PARTS OF WHEAT, RAISINS, SUGAR, SALT, MALT FLAVORING, HYDROGENATED VEGETABLE OIL, INVERT SYRUP, VITAMIN A PALMITATE, REDUCED IRON, ZINC OXIDE, NIACINAMIDE, PYRIDOXINE HYDROCHLORIDE (B_6), THIAMIN HYDROCHLORIDE (B_1), RIBOFLAVIN (B_2), FOLIC ACID, VITAMIN B_{12}, AND VITAMIN D_2.

CONTAINS 3% NON-NUTRITIVE CRUDE FIBER BY WEIGHT (1 g PER SERVING).

MADE BY KELLOGG COMPANY
BATTLE CREEK, MICH. 49016, U.S.A.
© 1972 BY KELLOGG COMPANY
® KELLOGG COMPANY

CARBOHYDRATE INFORMATION

	RAISIN BRAN 1 3/10 OZ.	RAISIN BRAN WITH ½ CUP WHOLE MILK
STARCH AND RELATED CARBOHYDRATES	22 g	22 g
SUCROSE AND OTHER SUGARS	6 g	12 g
TOTAL CARBOHYDRATES	28 g	34 g

VALUES BY FORMULATION AND ANALYSIS.

THIS PACKAGE IS SOLD BY WEIGHT, NOT VOLUME. SOME SETTLING OF CONTENTS MAY HAVE OCCURRED DURING SHIPMENT AND HANDLING.

ANN PAGE

UNFLAVORED
Gelatin

NUTRITION INFORMATION
Serving Size = ¼ oz. (Envelope)
Servings per Container = 1

Calories	24
Protein (not a significant source of protein)	6 Grams
Carbohydrate	0 Grams
Fat	0 Grams
Percentage of U.S. Recomended Daily Allowances (USRDA) Calcium	2%

Contains less than 2% of the U.S. Recommended Daily Allowance of Protein, Vitamin A, Vitamin C, Thiamine, Riboflavin, Niacin, and Iron.

A&P, MONTVALE, N.J. 07645 U.S.A.

identity (that is, they conform to standard "recipes" which indicate specific levels of mandatory ingredients), such as mayonnaise. Ingredients must be listed on the label in order of decreasing weight in the product. Nutritional labeling, on the other hand, is mandatory for (1) products for which a nutritional claim is made ("low-calorie," "low-salt," "vitamin-fortified," "nutritious"), (2) products that have been fortified (a nutrient not normally present in a food is added, such as vitamin D to milk), or (3) products that have been enriched (in which nutrients are added to replace those lost during processing, such as thiamin, riboflavin, niacin, and iron to wheat flour). Nutritional labeling is optional for other products.

At the present time, federal law requires that when nutritional labeling is used the following information must be provided in a specific order: serving size, servings per container, and energy, protein, carbohydrate, and fat content per serving. In addition, nutrient values for protein, vitamin A, vitamin C, thiamin, riboflavin, niacin, calcium, and iron expressed as percentages of the

High-quality Protein 2 eggs
13 g protein U.S. RDA = 45 g % U.S. RDA = 13 ÷ 45 = 29%
Lower-quality Protein 1 c lima beans
13 g protein U.S. RDA = 65 g % U.S. RDA = 13 ÷ 65 = 20%

U.S. RDA are required. Additional information for vitamin D, vitamin E, vitamin B_6, folacin, vitamin B_{12}, phosphorus, iodine, magnesium, zinc, copper, biotin, and pantothenic acid can also be provided, but it is not mandatory. Manufacturers may also include information about saturated and unsaturated fat content, and cholesterol and sodium contents as well.

An additional comment must be made about the U.S. RDA for protein. Because quantitative requirements for dietary protein are dependent on the quality of the protein (a reflection of its amino acid content), three different standards exist. The U.S. RDA for a high-quality protein such as provided by milk, meat, poultry, or eggs is 45 grams. However, for proteins (both singly and in a food combination) of lesser quality, the U.S. RDA is 65 grams. The effect of the difference is that *more* of a lesser-quality protein must be consumed to achieve the same "level" of the standard as a high-quality protein. An example should serve to clarify this point: Although two eggs and 1 cup of lima beans both have 13 grams of protein, consumption of these foods by themselves will provide 29 percent and 20 percent of the U.S. RDA for protein, respectively. It should also be noted that unflavored gelatin (two envelopes contain 12 grams of protein) is of such low-protein quality that the package label states parenthetically "not a significant source of protein." A nutrient which is present at less than 2 percent of the U.S. RDA per serving is so identified either by an asterisk or a statement to that effect.

Nutrition information panels can provide a relatively easy way for consumers to learn which foods are good sources of particular nutrients, which foods provide the most nutrients for the money spent, and also which provide the most nutrients in relation to the energy content. They can serve as guidelines for selection of a nutritionally balanced diet. Because current regulations do not address all the scientific and consumer issues involved, the FDA is considering changes that will increase consumer knowledge about the nutritional value of foods available in the marketplace (see Chapter 16).

INDEX OF NUTRITIONAL QUALITY. In an attempt to provide a definition of a "nutritious food" that would be of value to both consumers and professionals alike, nutritionists at Utah State University developed the Index of Nutritional Quality (INQ) (Sorenson et al., 1976).

Intuitively, we know that the nutritional quality of a food or combination of foods is a function of its nutrient content; what is perhaps not as obvious is that a value judgment of whether a food is nutritious should also consider the nutrient needs of an individual and the food's contribution to total energy intake as well. The INQ attempts to qualitate and relate these important variables.

When individual food choices are limited either in quantity or variety, perhaps for health or economic reasons, it becomes increasingly important to select foods that provide an adequate intake of essential nutrients. The INQ was developed to identify foods that have a beneficial nutrient:energy ratio, relative to a standard. When originally introduced, the standard used was the U.S. RDA, but refinement of the INQ concept has led the research group to prefer a standard energy level (1,000 or 2,000 kcal) as the energy reference point. The INQ is defined as follows:

$$\text{INQ} = \frac{\text{Amount of nutrient in food/kcal of food}}{\text{Allowance for nutrient /kcal allowance}}$$

Standards Used for INQ Determination

2,000 kcal
50 g protein
4,000 IU vitamin A
60 mg vitamin C
1.2 mg riboflavin
900 mg calcium
16 mg iron
3,000 mg sodium
5,000 mg potassium
350 mg cholesterol
78 g total fat

Source: R. G. Hansen and B. W. Wyse, Using the INQ to evaluate foods, *Nutrition News*, 42(1):2, 1979.

The reference values for adults currently used for some nutrients are listed in the margin.

The INQ for *each* nutrient in a food or food combination can be determined. For example, the calcium INQ for whole milk can be calculated from the formula given above. Although the figures in the numerator are those for 1 cup of milk, it is important to recognize (and will become apparent) that the calcium INQ will remain constant regardless of the amount of milk consumed.

$$\text{INQ}_{\text{calcium}} = \frac{290 \text{ mg calcium}/160 \text{ kcal}}{900 \text{ mg calcium}/2{,}000 \text{ kcal}} = 4.0$$

Rearrangement of the INQ formula results in a simplified equation:

$$\text{INQ} = \frac{\%\text{ standard of nutrient in food}}{\%\text{ standard of energy in food}}$$

$$\text{INQ}_{\text{calcium}} = \frac{290 \text{ mg calcium}/900 \text{ mg calcium}}{160 \text{ kcal}/2{,}000 \text{ kcal}} = \frac{0.32}{0.08} = 4.0$$

Stated in this way, it becomes apparent that 1 cup of milk provides 32 percent of the calcium allowance and 8 percent of the energy allowance; based on total adult requirements, therefore, milk supplies four times as much calcium as energy. Indeed, an INQ equal to 1.0 or more for any nutrient indicates that the food has a beneficial nutrient:energy ratio for that particular nutrient. The previous example shows that milk is a good source of calcium relative to energy. An examination of Table 10-5 reveals that milk has several nutrient INQs greater than 1.0 and also provides more than 30 percent of the dietary standard for two nutrients. In comparison, a chocolate candy bar, because it is energy dense, is less nutritious, both in terms of its nutrient:energy ratio (INQ) and its contribution to nutrient requirements (% standard).

INQs for all nutrients in a single food, meal, or total diet can be determined. The nutritional quality of foods can also be shown in a type of bar graph (see Table 10-6). In this example, protein, vitamin C, riboflavin, calcium, and iron are present in a favorable ratio to the energy content of the meal. Other meals consumed during the day should include foods to increase nutrient intakes to 100 percent of the standard and compare favorably with the energy standard, as shown by the length of the energy bar. Meals in which

TABLE 10-5
INQ: Comparison of Milk and Chocolate Candy Bar

	Milk		Chocolate Candy Bar	
	INQ	*% Standard*	*INQ*	*% Standard*
Energy	1.0	8.0	1.0	7.4
Protein	2.0	16.0	0.6	4.4
Calcium	4.0	32.0	0.9	7.2
Iron	0.09	0.75	0.26	1.9
Vitamin A	0.95	7.6	0.3	2.0
Thiamin	1.16	9.3	0.003	0.02
Riboflavin	4.1	32.9	1.12	8.3
Vitamin C	0.48	3.8	0.0	0.0

TABLE 10-6 **INQs for Meal of Bread (B), Cheese (C), and Strawberries (S)[a]**

Nutrient	Amount	INQ	%Std	0 — 25% — 50%
Energy[b]	295.0 kcal	1.00	14	BBBBBCCCCSS
Protein	12.8 g	1.74	26	BBBBBBBBCC*CCCCCCCCSS
Vitamin A	456.2 IU	0.77	12	CCCCCCCSS *
Vitamin C	87.9 mg	11.93	176	SSSSSSSSSSS*SSSSSSSSSSSSSSSSSSSSSSS ⟶ (176%)
Riboflavin	0.3 mg	1.78	27	BBBBBCCCCC *CCCSSSSSSS
Calcium	287.0 mg	2.16	32	BBBBCCCCCC *CCCCCCCCCCCCCSSS
Iron	3.0 mg	1.12	17	BBBBBCSSSS*SS
Sodium	456.0 mg	0.77	11	BBBBBCCCC *
Potassium	362.0 mg	0.61	8	BBSSSSS *
Cholesterol	29.0 mg	0.66	8	CCCCCCC *
Fat	11.3 g	0.98	14	BBCCCCCCCC*

*Indicates the 1.0 INQ point on each nutrient bar.
[a] 1 slice white enriched bread, 1 slice whole wheat bread, 1 ounce cheddar cheese, and ⅔ cup strawberries. Each letter represents the relative contribution of that food to the nutrient bar.
[b] Energy bar: Nutrient bars should meet or exceed this in length. The bars for cholesterol and fat, however, should not exceed the length of the energy bar.
Source: Adapted from R. G. Hansen and B. W. Wyse, Using the INQ to evaluate foods, *Nutrition News,* 42(1):2, 1979.

the energy bar is longer than the nutrient bars are less nutritious than those in which the reverse is true.

The two parameters—INQ and the percent standard—provide useful information in selecting nutritious foods. Individuals who wish to reduce their energy intake while maintaining an adequate nutrient intake should plan their meals to meet their desired level of energy consumption *and* choose foods with most or all of the nutrient INQs equal to or greater than 1.0.

This new concept of quantifying a "nutritious food" has been used to assess the nutritional quality of household diets (Abdel-Ghany, 1978) and as a nutrition education tool in elementary schools (Brown et al., 1979). Nutrient-density bar graphs are potentially useful as the basis for nutritional labeling of food products, and thus they might become a more visible tool for the consumer.

NUTRITION SCORECARD. The nutrition scorecard, perhaps familiar to some students, was developed by a consumer-oriented group, Center for Science in the Public Interest (CSPI). The scorecard assigns points to each food, based on its nutrient content. The more nutrients, the higher the point score. Points are subtracted for sugar, corn syrup, or saturated fat content. Protein, vitamins (A, thiamin, riboflavin, niacin, and C), iron, calcium, trace minerals, starch, fiber, naturally occurring sugars (carbohydrates), and unsaturated fats all add to a food's total score (Jacobson and Wilson, 1974).

In the nutrition scorecards shown on this page the winner is the hamburger. Although it loses points for its fat content, contributions of protein and vitamins boost its score. The chocolate bar, on the other hand, cannot overcome the burden of all that refined sugar.

It should be noted that in the final scorecard, only the total scores are given. Thus two foods with equally high or low scores may have quite different nutritional compositions. Milk has a rating of 39 because of its high protein, calcium, and riboflavin levels. In comparison, tomato juice, rated 37,

Nutrition Scorecard

Hamburger	
Protein	20
Carbohydrate	0
Fat	−13
Vitamins	19
Minerals	8
	34

Chocolate Bar	
Protein	3
Carbohydrate	
Natural	3
Sugar, syrup	−48
Fat	− 4
Vitamins	7
Minerals	6
	−33

Source: M. F. Jacobson and W. Wilson, *Food scorecard* (Washington, D.C.: Center for Science in the Public Interest, 1974).

receives most of its points for vitamins A and C. These similar scores might lead consumers to conclude that milk or tomato juice could be used interchangeably. Only if they knew the individual nutrient scores for these products could consumers understand that both foods have a place in their diets, but for quite different reasons.

The scorecard listings also do not include ratings for all the nutrients known to be important. Many vitamins and trace minerals are not considered when the score is calculated. Nevertheless, the scorecard approach does provide an easily understood measure of relative nutritional value—something lacking in many other systems. Youngsters in particular enjoy making food comparisons and picking the "winners." At the same time, they are learning to make informed dietary choices, as long as the limitations of the system are made apparent.

Consumer Responsibility

Tools exist to aid professionals in evaluating the nutritional status of individuals and population subgroups. But there is a great deal of nutritional ignorance and misinformation in the general public. Nutritionists in government and private agencies must begin to communicate the scientific principles of nutrition to consumers, and consumers must take a more active role in seeking the tools that can help them. The best protection for any consumer, until nutrition education and labeling catch up with public need, is selection of a varied diet, rich in foods such as fruits, vegetables, grains, fish, meats or meat substitutes, and milk. Because no one food provides *all* the nutrients needed by the human body, selections of diverse foods from each of the major categories will help to meet daily needs for even the least-known nutrients. It should also be apparent that "good" and "bad" foods cannot be absolutely defined. It is the *combination* of foods, in appropriate amounts, that make the difference.

SUMMARY

Improper nutrition has been implicated in the etiology of chronic, debilitating diseases and in common subclinical symptoms of impaired mental and physical performance. In our society today, the problem is most often not lack of food, but improper balance of energy and key nutrients in the diet.

Standardized assessment methods are used to identify nutritional deficiencies in individuals and in population groups. The four major categories of testing are: *anthropometric* assessment, human measurements of body size and body composition which include height, weight, and skinfold thickness; *clinical* assessment, a survey of visible, physical signs that relate to long-term disease processes; *biochemical* assessment, analysis of the chemical composition of body fluids and tissues, commonly emphasizing blood and urine testing; and *dietary* assessment, records of the foods consumed over a particular period of time.

Although each of these assessment tools can be used alone, they provide the most useful data when used together, as has been done in nutrition surveys such as the Ten-State Nutrition Survey. *Food composition tables* provide a great deal of information about individual foods, and they are widely used by professionals for meal planning and other purposes. The *Recommended Dietary Allowance* (RDA) tables are also used by professionals for meal planning and for evaluation of nutrient intakes.

Because food composition tables and RDAs are too complex for the average consumer, several simplified tools have been developed. Among these are the five basic food groupings, exchange lists, and the Index of Nutritional Quality (INQ).

More useful information for consumers is provided by nutrition labeling on many food packages; present federal regulations require that manufacturers indicate the number of kilocalories, grams of carbohydrate, protein, and fat in a single serving, and also list the content of selected nutrients as a percentage of the U.S. RDA when they make a nutritional claim for their product. Food labels have been criticized for their complexity, and consumer education groups are working to simplify labels and to increase the public's use and understanding of the information they do contain. Until nutrition education and labeling catch up with public needs, the consumer's best protection against nutritional deficiencies and excess is selection of a varied diet, in amounts appropriate to achieve or maintain optimal body weight.

BIBLIOGRAPHY

Abdel-Ghany, M. Evaluation of household diets by the Index of Nutritional Quality. *Journal of Nutrition Education* 10(2):79, 1978.

Abraham, S., F. W. Lowenstein, and C. L. Johnson. Preliminary findings of the first health and nutrition survey, United States, 1971–1972: Dietary intake and biochemical findings. DHEW Publication No. (HRA) 74-1219-1, January 1974.

Adams, C. F. *Nutritive value of American foods in common units.* USDA Agriculture Handbook No. 456. Washington, D.C.: U.S. Government Printing Office, 1975.

Brown, G., B. W. Wyse, and R. G. Hansen. A nutrient density nutrition education program for elementary schools. *Journal of Nutrition Education* 11(1):31, 1979.

Butterworth, C. E. The skeleton in the hospital closet. *Nutrition Today* 9(2):4, 1979.

Center for Disease Control. *Ten-state nutrition survey in the United States, 1968–1970.* Highlights, DHEW Publication No. (HSM) 72-8134. Atlanta, Ga.: Health Services and Mental Health Administration, 1972.

Dresser, C. M., S. Abraham, and M. D. Carroll. Eating styles today. *Abstacts of the Annual Meeting of the American Dietetic Association,* September 1978, p. 13.

Erdman, J. W. Bioavailability of nutrients from foods. *Contemporary Nutrition* 3(11):1, 1978.

Gersovitz, M., J. P. Madden, and H. S. Wright. Validity of the 24-hr. dietary recall and seven-day record for group comparisons. *Journal of the American Dietetic Association* 73:48, 1978.

Habicht, J.-P., J. M. Lane, and A. J. McDowell. National nutrition surveillance. *Federation Proceedings* 37:1181, 1978.

Hansen, R. G., B. W. Wyse, and G. Brown. Nutrient needs and their expression. *Food Technology* 32:44, 1978.

Hegsted, D. M. Dietary standards. *New England Journal of Medicine* 292:915, 1975.

Hertzler, A. A., and L. W. Hoover. Development of food tables and use with computers. *Journal of the American Dietetic Association* 70:20, 1977.
Jacobson, M. F., and W. Wilson. *Food scorecard.* Washington, D.C.: Center for Science in the Public Interest, 1974.
King, J. C., S. H. Cohenour, C. G. Corruccini, and P. Schneeman. Evaluation and modification of the Basic Four food group. *Journal of Nutrition Education* 10(1):27, 1978.
Morgan, R. W., M. Jain, A. B. Miller, N. W. Choi, V. Matthews, L. Munan, J. D. Burch, J. Feather, G. R. Howe, and A. Kelly. A comparison of dietary methods in epidemiologic studies. *American Journal of Epidemiology* 107(6):488, 1978.
National Center for Health Statistics. NCHS growth charts, 1976. *Monthly Vital Statistics Report*, Vol. 25, No. 3, Supplement (HRA) 76-1120. Rockville, Md.: Health Resources Administration, 1976.
Pennington, J. A. *Dietary nutrient guide.* Westport, Conn.: Avi Publishing Co., 1976.
Sorenson, A. W., B. W. Wyse, A. J. Wittwer, and R. G. Hansen. An index of nutritional quality for a balanced diet. *Journal of the American Dietetic Association* 68:236, 1976.
Watt, B. K. Concepts in developing a food composition table. *Journal of the American Dietetic Association* 40:297, 1962.
Watt, B. K., and A. L. Merrill. *Composition of foods—Raw, processed, prepared.* USDA Agriculture Handbook No. 8. Washington, D.C.: U.S. Government Printing Office, 1963.
Watt, B. K., and E. W. Murphy. Tables of food composition; Scope and needed research. *Food Technology* 24:674, 1970.

SUGGESTED ADDITIONAL READING

Ahlstrom, A., and L. Rasanen. Review of food grouping systems in nutrition education. *Journal of Nutrition Education* 5(1):13, 1973.
Arroyave, G. Biochemical evaluation of nutritional status in man. *Federation Proceedings* 20:39, 1961.
Elvehjem, C. A. The significance and limitations of food composition tables. *Federation Proceedings* 5:280, 1946.
Frank, G. C., G. S. Berenson, P. E. Shilling, and M. C. Moore. Adapting the 24-hr. recall for epidemiologic studies of school children. *Journal of the American Dietetic Association* 71:26, 1977.
Garn, S. M., F. A. Larkin, and P. E. Cole. The real problem with 1-day diet records. *American Journal of Clinical Nutrition* 31:1114, 1978.
Gebhardt, S. E., R. Cutrufelli, and R. H. Matthews. *Composition of foods—Baby foods—Raw, processed, prepared.* USDA Agriculture Handbook No. 8-3. Washington, D.C.: U.S. Government Printing Office, 1978.
Hansen, R. G., B. W. Wyse, and A. W. Sorenson. *Nutritional quality index of foods.* Westport, Conn.: Avi Publishing Co., 1979.
Hertzler, A. A., and H. L. Anderson. Food guides in the United States. *Journal of the American Dietetic Association* 64:19, 1974.
Hollingsworth, D. F. Dietary determination of nutritional status. *Federation Proceedings* 20:50, 1961.
Huenemann, R. L. Interpretation of nutritional status. *Journal of the American Dietetic Association* 63:123, 1973.
Journal of the American Dietetic Association. What is an exchange? 69:609, 1976.
Lowenstein, F. W. Preliminary clinical and anthropometric findings from the first Health and Nutrition Examination Survey, USA, 1971–1972. *American Journal of Clinical Nutrition* 29:918, 1976.

MADDEN, J. P., S. J. GOODMAN, AND H. A. GUTHRIE. Validity of the 24-hour recall: Analysis of data obtained from elderly subjects. *Journal of the American Dietetic Association* 68:143, 1976.

MARSH, A. C., M. K. MOSS, AND E. W. MURPHY. *Composition of foods—Spices and herbs—Raw, processed, prepared.* USDA Agriculture Handbook No. 8-2. Washington, D.C.: U.S. Government Printing Office, 1977.

MCMASTERS, V. History of food composition tables of the world. *Journal of the American Dietetic Association* 43:442, 1963.

MURPHY, E. W., B. K. WATT, AND R. L. RIZEK. Tables of food composition: Availability, uses, and limitations. *Food Technology,* January 1973, p. 41.

NATIONAL NUTRITION CONSORTIUM, INC., WITH R. M. DEUTSCH. *Nutritional labeling—How it can work for you.* Bethesda, Md.: The National Nutrition Consortium, Inc., 1975.

PETERKIN, B. The RDA or U.S. RDA? *Journal of Nutrition Education* 9(1):10, 1977.

POSATI, L. P., AND M. L. ORR. *Composition of foods—Dairy and egg products—Raw, processed, prepared.* USDA Agriculture Handbook No. 8-1. Washington, D.C.: U.S. Government Printing Office, 1976.

SCHAEFER, A. E. The national nutrition survey. *Journal of the American Dietetic Association* 54:371, 1969.

SHENKIN, A., AND L. W. STEELE. Clinical and laboratory assessment of nutritional status. *Proceedings of the Nutrition Society* 37:95, 1978.

Chapter 11

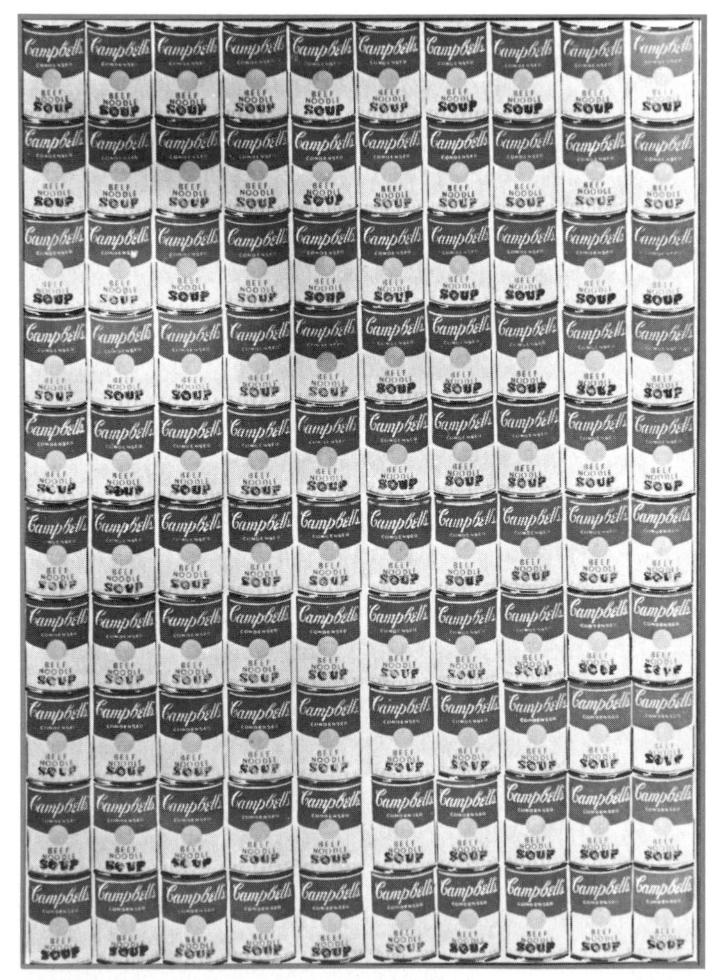

One Hundred Campbell's Soup Cans by Andy Warhol

Food and Contemporary Society

How do we decide what, where, when, and why to eat? Chapter 1 presented some of the universal factors that influence eating habits of people everywhere; the focus of this chapter will be on the United States.

In the United States at present, public interest in food and nutrition is high and visible, perhaps more so than ever before. One reason is the American consumer's new-found preoccupation with health. This, joined with concern about the increasing impact of government and industry in our lives, has led to the rise of consumerism. Economic factors have also begun to cause changes in our food behaviors and even in the way we think about food. American lifestyles not only reflect these concerns but also actively influence the types of food we eat and where we eat them.

This chapter explores the ways in which social changes and public attitudes affect today's patterns of food consumption. In the next three chapters the special nutritional needs and problems at different stages of life are discussed; these too can be related to contemporary lifestyles. In Chapter 15 we shall examine problems of food supply and nutrition in other parts of the world. And the final chapter examines some of the policy issues currently being debated and discusses the responsibility shared by all Americans to provide, and expect, food that is healthful, nutritious, and tasty.

A CHANGING SOCIETY

America has proven to be a land of plenty beyond the wildest dreams of pilgrim and pioneer. Though malnutrition remains a pressing concern, widespread undernutrition is not a public health issue. This is not to say, however, that things are so perfect that every American gets enough to eat. But we are not a nation of hungry people—and this very fact has implications for what and why we eat.

Our eating behaviors satisfy more than our physiological needs. Maslow has defined a hierarchy of needs, the most basic being physiological, with safety, belongingness-love, esteem, and self-actualization added in stepwise fashion.

Until the most basic needs have been satisfied, the higher needs must be ignored (Maslow, 1970). We all eat because we are hungry, but most of us eat to satisfy social and emotional needs as well. People buy caviar to impress their friends or because they like the taste of it, not because it's the only food available. Many overweight individuals turn to food for solace, perhaps in response to the need to be loved. But all of us eat for emotional reasons at times. We eat out of habit, or because it's that time of day. No one needs five meals a day, but few would give up a morning and afternoon coffee break because they really weren't hungry. We sit down at a table, over food, to talk things over or exchange views with family, friends, or associates. At lunch, business deals are transacted and job interviews conducted.

For most of human existence, food supplies consisted solely of what nature provided: fish, birds, wild plants, and animals. Available food resources varied with the geographical location of the human community. Much later in human history, plants were cultivated, and animals were captured and domesticated; this resulted in a food supply that was both more dependable and more varied.

Locating food is no longer the problem that it was for our prehistoric ancestors. A greater variety of food items is available today than could have been imagined barely a generation ago. There are some 10,000 different products in supermarkets, and the food industry is constantly creating new ones to tempt consumer tastes. This wide selection of foods presents a new kind of problem: *choice*. Behind every supermarket purchase lies a complex decision-making process in which convenience, economy, nutritional knowledge, individual tastes, cookery know-how, home storage capabilities, and several other factors are balanced. Shoppers are aware of these considerations, but they may be less aware of the other factors that determine what they eat—factors that they take for granted.

Social and Technological Factors

From the early years of our country's history, right up through a good part of the last century, most people grew their own food. In 1976, a mere 7 percent of the U.S. population produced not only enough food for the nation's needs, but millions of tons for export as well (Lowenberg and Lucas, 1976). Mechanization, fertilizers, improvements in plant strains and in food processing techniques and transportation—all these developments have allowed agricultural productivity to increase geometrically. American farms are the most productive in the world.

URBANIZATION AND SUBURBANIZATION. As fewer people have been needed on the farm to produce our food, millions have moved to towns and cities to find work. Largely because of the increased complexity of most jobs, and the increasing number of technologically demanding jobs, we have become a nation of specialists: hematologists, computer programmers, market researchers, educational administrators—and hundreds of other kinds of workers that did not exist a century ago. But recent demographic movements away from cities represent new growth for "bedroom communities" and subdivisions, not a return to the land. The rural or farm population of the United States continues to decline significantly every year.

With increased urbanization, simply prepared home-grown foods have been replaced by the store-bought variety, grown months before, hundreds or thousands of miles away, often preseasoned and precooked. "Suburbanization" has, if anything, confirmed and exacerbated this trend. Consumers now load up their station wagons at the supermarket once a week and bring everything home to the pantry and freezer, further lengthening the time as well as the physical distance between field and table.

FAMILY STRUCTURE. Some of these same economic and social forces have led to radical changes in the organization of American families. The traditional extended family—several generations living together under one roof—has never been the norm in the United States. The American family has always tended to be nuclear. This country was founded and continually populated by young persons and couples who left home and crossed the ocean. In later generations, young couples struck out for the West; now they leave the country and move to the city, or leave the city for the suburbs.

But, even if they did not live with their children, it was traditionally customary for grandparents to live nearby and to help in raising the grandchildren. Today it is uncommon to find grandparents living in the same neighborhood, or even in the same state, as their offspring. In this age of the car and airplane, succeeding generations tend to live farther apart.

Today, families are being started later, and are smaller, than in any previous generation. Increasing numbers of young men and women are electing to stay single, or are postponing marriage until they are in their twenties or even thirties. The number of one- and two-member households has increased dramatically during the past decade, and the trend shows no signs of reversing. Although the majority of families (53 percent) still include at least one parent with a child under 18, well over a third (38 percent) of all families consist of *only* two persons (Bureau of the Census, 1977). Some of these are single-parent families, some are young married couples who have postponed or decided against child-rearing, and some are older couples whose adult children have moved elsewhere, even before they marry—another recent social phenomenon.

The postwar baby boom is over. As we are reminded almost daily, the number of 18-year-olds will decrease steadily throughout the 1980s. Today women are postponing their child-bearing until their education is completed and their careers are launched. Not only are women having their children later, but they are having fewer of them. Movements such as ZPG—zero population growth—have won many converts to the idea of having no more than two children. The birth rate (number of live births per thousand population) reached its lowest level a few years ago. The total fertility rate (births per thousand women of childbearing age) in the United States rose from 1,768 in 1976 to 1,815 in 1977—1.8 children per woman, even lower than the ZPG goal of 2.1 children per woman.

At the other end of the human lifespan, people are living longer. This means that more older people are living *alone*, since grandparents typically make their homes away from their children. Approximately 15.5 million Americans live by themselves, with 6.5 million of these age 65 or over (Shaw and Pinto, 1978).

The trend toward smaller, isolated families directly affects the housing, energy, manufacturing, and food industries. Because of the greater number of families, more houses and apartment buildings are needed, which in turn consume more gas and fuel oil for heating. More beds and sofas, carpets and dinnerware, dishwashers and automobiles are produced and purchased. But smaller families also mean fewer people at the table, which normally means less elaborate meals with food requiring less preparation time. Mealtimes become less personal and more routine as the nightly family get-together gives way to the TV dinner.

WORKING WOMEN. In 1960, 40 percent of women aged 25 to 54 were in the work force, whereas today 60 percent are employed outside the home (Shapiro and Bohmbach, 1978). This remarkable shift, which has really been a social revolution taking place generally, is itself due to a number of economic and social factors. Increasing numbers of single and divorced women must support themselves and their families. The constant inflation of the 1970s left many middle-income couples unable to live in the style to which they had become accustomed on only one income. The women's movement not only motivated more women to seek career satisfaction but also opened up more job opportunities for them.

Women who work obviously have less time to devote to food shopping, preparation, and serving. Sales of convenience foods and appliances to save food preparation time (food processors, slow cookers, microwave ovens, freezers) have been steadily increasing for years. Families also eat out more—over one-third of all money spent on food in the United States is spent for meals consumed away from home (Burros, 1978; Shapiro and Bohmbach, 1978).

While women are still the primary "gatekeepers" to family food patterns (Gifft et al., 1972), increasingly the entire family has become involved in the meal preparation process. It is no longer remarkable to find husbands and children shopping and cooking.

ECONOMICS. Many American families own their own homes and most have cars, television sets, washers, driers, and an almost endless array of other consumer goods. Despite inflation, ours remains an affluent society. But the steadily increasing costs of necessities—housing, fuel, food—is causing most people to make changes in their way of life and in their plans for the future. Prices of all basic food items—milk, meat, produce, bread, and coffee—as well as luxuries—sugar, chocolate, and imported foods—have risen dramatically in relatively few years.

As a result of advanced product technology and marketing techniques, the percentage of personal income spent on food in the United States is the lowest of almost any country in the world. But the percentage has been increasing at a rapid rate. Consumers have been fighting back by instituting boycotts (refusing, for example, to buy high-priced coffee, or observing "meatless Wednesday"); by growing their own vegetables, even in apartment and penthouse gardens; and by choosing lower-cost sources of protein. Meat-stretching extenders such as beans, pasta, and texturized vegetable protein (TVP) figure prominently in cookbooks. Stories bearing headlines such as "How I Feed My Family of Four on $38.98 a Month" are featured in magazines. Newspapers devote their food pages to exotic recipes using low-cost foods (mussels, kidneys, eggplant, turnips) and to "wise shopping tips."

But it is hard to beat the law of supply and demand. A consumer boycott may help bring down the price of coffee, but the prices of margarine, pork, and white wine have gone up as people turn to them as substitutes for butter, beef, and distilled liquors. Ironically, a boycott of beef can lead to long-term shortages and even higher prices as cattle raisers cut back on production.

CULTURAL INFLUENCES. Many factors influence food preferences, but cultural influences usually are the decisive ones. The Ifugao people of the Philippines, for example, eat dragonflies; we do not (Lee, 1957). In most places of the world, sour foods are unpopular; yet in a part of India such foods are the most prized.

Cultural preferences extend to texture, viscosity, and color as well as flavor. Perhaps because they usually serve it as a side dish, Americans prefer their rice light and fluffy. Where rice is the staple, however, it is heavy and gummy. The American staple, bread, has also been turned into fluff. The stuff that laborers used to pull out of their pockets at lunchtime was much more substantial than that which most of us consume today.

Although the great American cultural "melting pot" does its best to blend the hallmarks of traditional cuisines, pride encourages us to perpetuate all the aspects of our own ethnic culture, including its distinctive foods. Regional variations can be distinguished—the ethnic mix is different in Baltimore and New Orleans, in Chicago and Los Angeles. Ethnic foods are becoming widely popular, as education and travel create new awareness of the foods of other cultures. We have long been familiar with Chinese, Mexican, French, and Italian cuisine. In recent years restaurants devoted to Greek, Cuban, Japanese, and Indian cookery have opened in many cities and adventurous home cooks are exploring new culinary territory with enthusiasm.

Food and Nutrition Are "In"

Wednesday is Food Day in the *New York Times*, the Boston *Globe*, and newspapers across the country. Television takes us into the kitchen with Julia Child or the Romanovs and brings us information affecting our food choices on the evening news (for example, in features on the rising cost of feeding a family or new research relating certain foods to heart disease) and in commercials. Even the introduction of a new product may be given air time—a recent news item presented nitrite-free bacon.

Food has become a status symbol. Gourmet club members exchange recipes and invite one another for dinners. "Adventures in eating" clubs go on restaurant expeditions. There are gourmet magazines, cooking schools, and lavishly illustrated "coffee-table" cookbooks. A recent traveler to China may remind guests of that fact by serving a Chinese meal complete with chopsticks. A recent newspaper article giving recipes on how to make chocolate pudding from scratch received an unprecedented response, and an entire cookbook devoted to making your own "prepared" foods—from catsup to ice cream—is aimed at the same audience (Witty and Colchie, 1979). Where food was once only a necessity of life, it has become for today's affluent society a visible sign of one's education and status, and food preparation and consumption have become for many people a source of entertainment as well as sustenance.

Where Will the Next Meal Come From?

A changing country and changing lifestyles affect not only the kinds of foods we eat, but also where we get them and how we prefer to cook them. Dinner tonight in many an American home will be broiled chicken taken out of the home freezer last night to defrost; frozen green beans, bought three weeks ago; spinach, prewashed, tossed in a commercial Italian dressing; cherry pie made from canned cherries and a crust mix, or selected from the frozen dessert section in the supermarket two days ago; ground coffee from a vacuum-packed can; milk from a paper carton, use-dated; sugar bought a month ago.

In the year 1850 foodstuffs were supplied by home gardens, local orchards and farms, general stores, and, on the frontier, perhaps by a peddler. Bought goods were sold loose by weight or the piece. Home canning and preserving (jelly-making, salting, and smoking) and storage in a root cellar were the only means by which food could be stored for any length of time. Otherwise, the variety of foods on the table was closely related to the local agricultural season. Milk, which Americans today consume in quantities startling to foreigners, was notoriously unreliable. Cider was one substitute, drunk especially in New England. By 1900, gas ranges had been invented and iceboxes provided storage for perishables. The general store gave way, in cities and towns at least, to the grocery store, the butcher, the fishmonger, the fruit-and-vegetable store, the bakery, and the milk delivery van. In the 1920s the electric refrigerator was beginning to replace the icebox and the pantry shelf; increasing ownership of automobiles allowed shoppers to travel greater distances to stores and to carry home much more than a single day's food needs. Today we get our foods preeminently from supermarkets, which in 1976 sold 75 percent of all groceries in the United States (Lowenberg et al., 1979). Like its forerunner, the general store, the supermarket still provides a means of socializing, a place to exchange opinions on brands, prices, and personal food choices.

But we also get our meals (particularly lunch) in restaurants of many kinds and price ranges, both near and far from home, during our working days, our weekend golfing or museum-going, and our vacations. And institutional cafeterias at schools, factories, and corporate offices provide 2 percent of all meals eaten per week (Shaw and Pinto, 1978).

SUPERMARKETS. The consumer walking into a supermarket today has a seemingly huge choice. But are those products responses to demand, to what the consumer "really" wants, as manufacturers claim and some consumers believe? Or does the food industry in fact create demand, telling consumers what they want by supplying particular food products, as some nutritionists and consumer advocates argue? One fact is incontrovertible: No consumer can buy a product that is not on the shelf.

It has been suggested (Wheeler, 1978) that shoppers' choices are made primarily on the basis of four concerns: knowledge (do I think this is nutritious?); attitudes (do I feel like eating it?); practicality (can I afford it?); and timing (should I buy it now?). The response to each of these depends on a complex interaction of individual and social history and experience; actions and statements by government experts and by food manufacturers and suppliers also influence the choice.

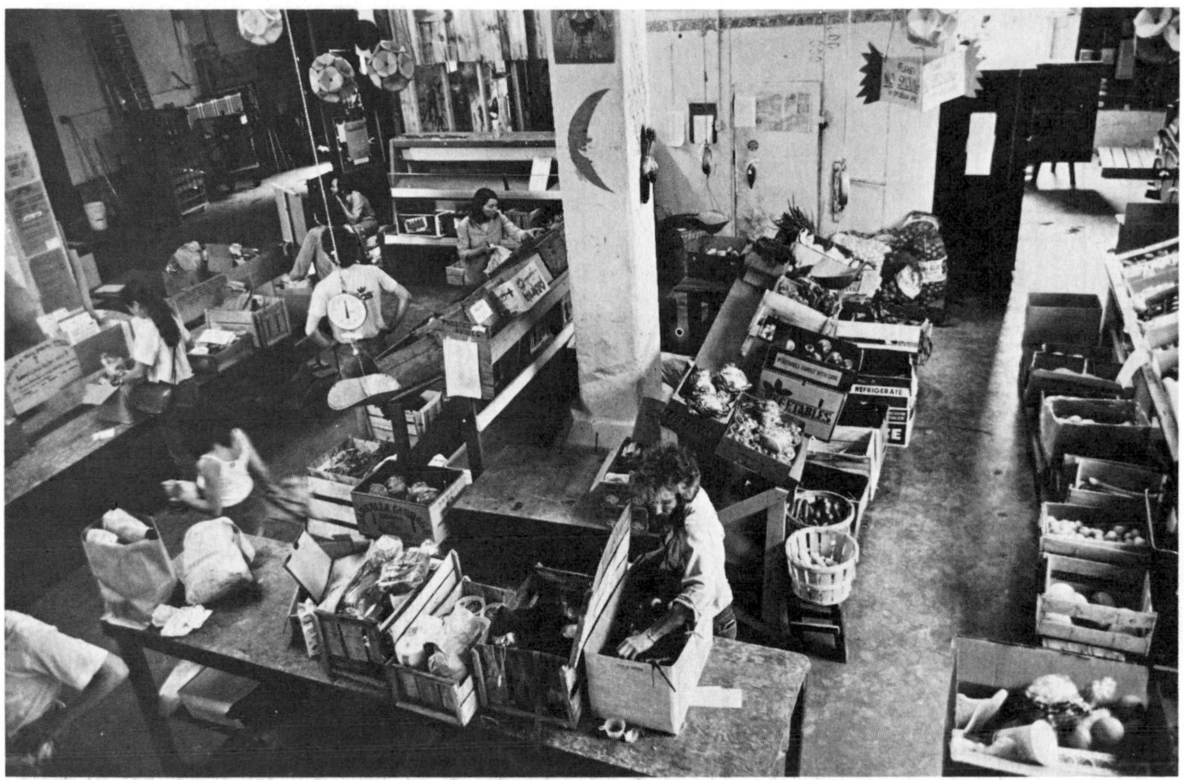

The Boston Food Coop, a no-frills supermarket. (Jim Harrison, Stock, Boston)

All food marketing tactics—package design, advertising, and even shelf position—are designed to urge the consumer to answer "Yes" to these four questions. Several studies of consumer ratings of supermarkets reveal that price is the most important consideration (Lowenberg et al., 1979). Supermarkets have an inherent advantage over smaller stores in their ability to buy in bulk and therefore to sell at lower cost. They also enhance their price advantage in a variety of ways, traditionally by offering house brands. These are items manufactured to specifications by nationally known producers but given a private label and priced lower than the national brand. The supermarket chain sustains no economic loss because the private label is not advertised.

A recent extension of the house brand idea is the "no frills" or generic item, manufactured to low-cost specifications and simply packaged. A pared-down label in stark black and white gives only the name of the food product, weight of contents, and FDA-mandated ingredients list (see Figure 11-1). These products sell for about 35 percent less than national brands and about 10 percent less than house brands; they sell best among upper and lower socioeconomic groups, and less well to middle-income shoppers (Pope, 1978).

Two major factors contribute to the reduced cost of these generic products. First, the quality of the product (defined by such parameters as texture, color, and uniformity of size and shape) is usually less than that of the more

**INFORMATION ON FAT AND CHOLESTEROL CONTENT IS PROVIDED FOR INDIVIDUALS WHO, ON THE ADVICE OF A PHYSICIAN, ARE MODIFYING THEIR TOTAL DIETARY INTAKE OF FAT AND/OR CHOLESTEROL.
*CONTAINS LESS THAN 2% OF THE U.S. RDA OF THESE NUTRIENTS.
INGREDIENTS: ROASTED PEANUTS, SALT, MODIFIED STARCH, PAPRIKA, AND DEXTRIN.
DISTRIBUTED BY COMPASS FOODS, INC.
MONTVALE, N.J. 07645 U.S.A.
0 11141 59430 3
Dry Roasted
PEANUTS
NO OILS USED IN PROCESSING
THESE PEANUTS ARE NOT AS LARGE AND HAVE FEWER WHOLE NUTS THAN NORMAL. FRESHNESS AND FLAVOR ARE NOT AFFECTED.
NET WT. 12 OZ.
340 g
Dry Roasted PEANUTS
NUTRITION INFORMATION PER SERVING
SERVING SIZE 1 OZ (28.35 grams)
SERVINGS PER CONTAINER 12
CALORIES 180
PROTEIN 7 grams
CARBOHYDRATE 6 grams
FAT** (70% OF CALORIES FROM FAT) 14 grams
POLYUNSATURATED 3 grams
SATURATED 2 grams
CHOLESTEROL** (0 mg. per 100 gm.) 0 milligrams
PERCENTAGE OF U.S. RECOMMENDED DAILY ALLOWANCES (U.S. RDA)
PROTEIN 10
VITAMIN A *
VITAMIN C *
THIAMINE 4
RIBOFLAVIN 2
NIACIN 20
CALCIUM *
IRON 2

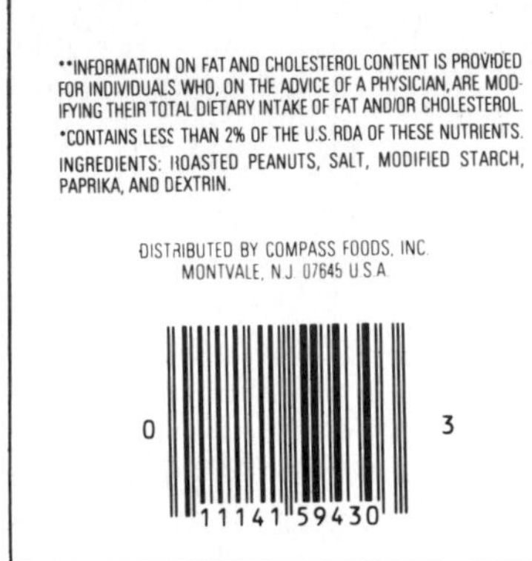

FIGURE 11-1
Example of a Label from a "No Frills" or Generic Item

expensive items. These "imperfect" food products are less costly for the manufacturer, who then passes the savings on to the consumer. Although lower quality may affect palatability, it does not affect the wholesomeness or safety of the final product; in addition, nutritional values of similar items are comparable. Second, minimal advertising campaigns and simple packaging methods save money for the manufacturer, the supermarket, and ultimately the consumer.

Another marketing device used by supermarkets and by individual food manufacturers to appeal to the consumer's interest in prices is the "special." This is a less-certain road to consumer savings because the psychological enticement to save may persuade the shopper to buy products that are not really needed, not really liked, or not really nutritious. "Cents-off" coupons offer the same advantages and disadvantages.

The vast array of foods that attracts the consumer to a supermarket can obscure an absence of real choice. The ten varieties of white bread on the shelf do not satisfy a consumer who wants whole-wheat bread but cannot find it. Not one additive-free sausage may be stocked, even though five national brands are available. Prepackaging can prevent the shopper from checking quality; a recent study has shown that 78 percent of consumers wanted packaged carrots, but only 14 percent wanted to buy prepacked fresh peaches (Lowenberg et al., 1979). Prepacking may also force the shopper into either taking home more food than can be used before spoilage or simply going without.

Modern supermarkets are based on self-service, and marketing plans make use of the shopper's self-propelled routing through the aisles to encourage sales. Foods are carefully placed: Items with the highest profit margin are habitually stocked at adult eye level; items attractive to children are placed just high enough for the toddler to see and grab. The largest cans and packages, usually less expensive by unit cost, are stacked on the easy-to-overlook bottom shelf or the difficult-to-reach upper one. The most profitable products are often displayed on the outer walls, to which shoppers gravitate naturally.

The modern technologies of preservation make many previously seasonal foods available year-round. Frequently, processed foods are less expensive than the unprocessed products, and are generally of comparable nutritional value. Delays in transportation, sitting in the sun without refrigeration, bruising during shipping and handling, and other causes of damage may reduce nutrient content of freshly picked produce—unless it is purchased at or near the original source. Frozen and canned products often preserve the original nutrient content with high efficiency, because the processing is done at or near the point of origin of the produce.

Prices of processed foods reflect the addition of sauces, spices, and other foods to the basic product, as well as labor and overhead. Consumers may educate themselves by comparing, for example, the price of raw potatoes with those of the many canned, frozen, boxed, and bagged potato products available in their supermarkets. But for the shopper to whom time saved in food preparation is a paramount consideration, the prepared food even at a higher price will be preferable. Moreover, any one consumer wants different things at different times, sometimes opting for convenience, sometimes for nutrition, sometimes for taste, and sometimes for price. The supermarket is large enough to satisfy a variety of decisions.

In the debate over whether the consumer is really queen—and king—in the domain of food supply and demand, the reliance of the food industry on marketing research suggests that demand does create supply. Only one of every ten manufacturers' product ideas survives to be test-marketed by consumer panels. Only one of every ten of these test-marketed products survives for general distribution (Rice, 1978). All told, 4,000 to 5,000 food products are introduced each year; scarcely a handful are truly innovative. Those that survive a rigorous marketing trial do so because they satisfy one or another desire; many recently introduced foods, for example, have appealed to consumer desires for no-preservative, no-artificial-color foods, for fewer calories, or for nutritious and cheaper alternatives to meat.

Gaps do exist in what is available. One table sauce manufacturer found that some consumers are dissatisfied with the prevailingly sweet, bland ketchups on the market and hired a marketing research company to conduct a computer analysis of psychophysics, or human sensory perceptions, to formulate the precise recipe—how much sugar, how much thickener—to satisfy buyers (Rice, 1978). Because 97 percent of American households routinely use ketchup, and 44 percent buy it once a month (Rice, 1978), a new spicier ketchup would widen choice and also fulfill the primary aim of every manufacturer: to make a profit. The "computer-assisted" sauce has been test-marketed in several cities.

Manufacturers capitalize on the consumer desire for "natural" or "old-fashioned" flavor in their advertising. What the public perceives as "natural," however, is partly what it is accustomed to. An egg fresh from the chicken has a startlingly heavy tang compared to a supermarket egg; a whole generation has grown up on frozen orange juice and learned to prefer its taste to that of fresh-squeezed juice. Flavor preference in general has moved to the "light" end of the spectrum; light liquor mixes, wines, and beer are taking over large shares of the market as they are introduced (*Food Product Development*, August 1978).

Supermarkets are becoming more responsive to consumer needs and wants, offering advice from nutritionists, recipes for dieting and other special needs, and "best buys" labels. One chain offers bilingual information on nutrition; another has nutrition information leaflets to be picked up in every aisle. The best time to alter eating habits is while the shopping basket is being filled, and efforts to do so, however rare, must be welcomed.

New kinds of supermarkets are making their appearance. Conscious of growing consumer resentment at rising prices and increased skepticism about the nutritional quality of food industry products, retailers are seeking a more positive image. Handsome graphic design, striking colors, piped-in music, and streamlined fixtures enhance appeal and tempt customers to linger longer. Special services—custom-cut meats in freezer portions, telephone orders and delivery service, appetizer and bakery departments—build customer loyalty.

New ways to merchandise food are being tested. In a Washington, D.C., suburb, customers phone in their orders from a computerized catalogue, and later in the day they can pick up the completed order at a warehouse—at savings of 5 to 15 percent over prices in local traditional supermarkets. Delivery is available for an additional charge. Other stores that offer a telephone and pick-up service do not offer discounts, appealing instead to the customer's desire to save time. "No frills" markets carry limited brand selections of basic items; customers help themselves to merchandise still in half-opened shipping cartons and pack their own groceries, saving up to 30 percent of food costs. These and similar new approaches are already found in many parts of the country.

Supermarkets are a necessary part of contemporary life. We may grow our own herbs in window boxes or back yards and raise tomatoes or a favorite lettuce for the unusual pleasure of eating a variety rarely available in the shops. But the year-round variety of foods, safely transported, preserved, and packaged, which supermarkets make available, cannot be duplicated.

RESTAURANTS. Whether at an elegant "tablecloth" restaurant, a truck stop, or a vending machine, Americans spend about 35 percent of their food dollars eating away from home—$57 billion in 1977. Three out of four respondents to a recent survey said that at least one member of their family eats out once a week or more (Shaw and Pinto, 1978). Although eating at home is still the norm, eating out is clearly a most popular recreation; more than that, it is part of the way we live now. For our parents and grandparents it was a much rarer event: part of courtship, or to celebrate a wedding, a graduation, a raise, a birth, a new job, or a new home.

In 1976, fast-food chains were patronized by 73 percent of all American households and accounted for 25 percent of U.S. restaurant sales. More traditional eating establishments—ranging from diners and cafeterias to fancy "tablecloth" restaurants—accounted for 60 percent.

Lunch is the meal most likely to be eaten out, breakfast the least likely; dinner falls in-between (see Figure 11-2). Almost one in three Americans eats lunch away from home—one in twelve at a fast-food restaurant. Put another way, Americans average two lunches and one dinner a week and about one breakfast every two weeks away from home (Shaw and Pinto, 1978).

Men eat out more frequently than women, as they have always done, but no longer by a decisive margin; men now consume 56 percent of all meals eaten away from home. The increasing number of working women, who eat out more often than do nonworking women, has narrowed the gap. Men in

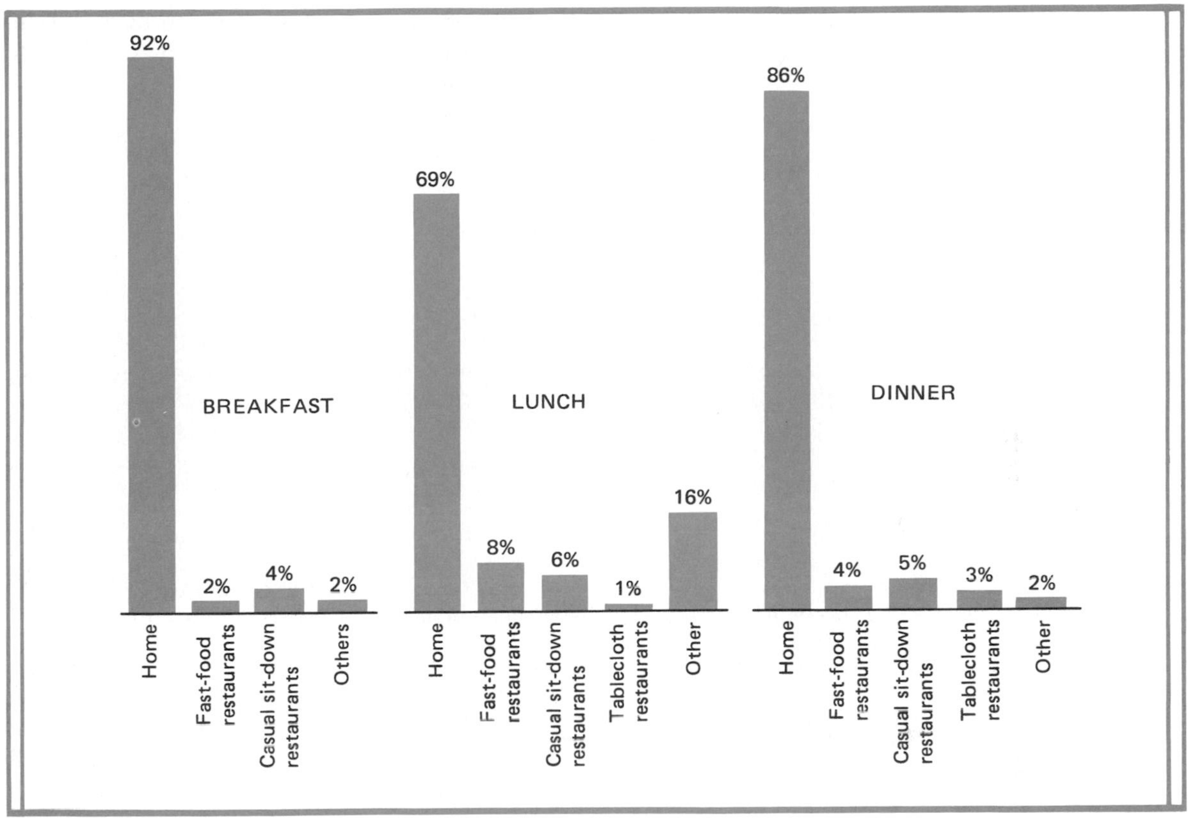

FIGURE 11-2
Where Meals Are Eaten

Source: Adapted from R. E. Shaw and D. Pinto, Where's your next meal coming from?, *The Nielsen Researcher*, No. 1, 1978, pp. 5, 6.

the 22 to 34 age group eat nearly half of their lunches away from home, and women in that age group, close to a third (Telser, 1978). But no segment of the population is excluded from the phenomenon—all ages, all incomes, all ethnic groups, and all social strata take part.

This democratization of dining out is paralleled by the variety of foods available in restaurants. Affluence, travel, education, and the opportunities given by our mobile society to mix with people of different ethnic backgrounds have broadened American tastes for new and "foreign" foods. New immigrant groups such as the Bengali and Vietnamese begin to open restaurants in neighborhoods where they settle, widening the food experience of all diners. The rapid spread of pizza throughout the nation following World War II, and the more recent proliferation of taco and souvlaki stands and Szechwan-style Chinese restaurants, attest to our appetite for new taste experiences.

Both men and women do business over the "three-martini" lunch. And use of the company credit card removes economic constraints, so these tend to be substantial meals, although the imbibing may be of Perrier water or wine instead of martinis. Among a small sample of Boston sales and marketing executives, a majority reported eating out at a tablecloth restaurant at least once a week. Interestingly, they did not eat chicken—perhaps because it was

PERSPECTIVE ON
Fast Foods

Fast-food outlets fit comfortably into our way of life. Teenagers grab a snack on the way home from school; working mothers can bring home Colonel Sanders instead of a bag of groceries. Some restaurants offer birthday parties for children, special gimmicks for holidays, and even lotteries. And the chains have begun bringing their food to us, accepting contracts to service cafeterias in schools, factories, and even aircraft carriers. A generation of adults has already grown up on burgers and fries. Fast-food outlets will soon account for a quarter of all meals consumed in this country, at a price tag of $25 billion annually.

Speed and economy remain the mainstays of the fast-food business. Limited menus offer economies in purchasing, distribution, preparation, equipment, and training of personnel—economies that do make it possible to serve millions of meals at moderate cost. Bulk purchasing, assembly-line operation, centralized design and advertising, and management expertise all make the expansion of food chains possible.

As tastes become more sophisticated, though, the fast-food industry is attempting to keep up. First it was hot dogs, pizza, and "submarines" (or hoagies, grinders, or heroes, depending on locality). Then hamburgers (our way or your way), fried chicken, and fried fish became the fast foods of choice. Now ethnic foods are making their appearance, along with breakfast choices, salad bars, and soft frozen yogurt.

But how well are we eating at these places? Only recently has information about the nutritional content of fast foods been available. (Examination of Appendix Table H will allow you to compare the nutritional values of different fast-food meals.) The nutrient composition of additional items is also available in other publications (Appledorf, 1974; Donovan and Appledorf, 1972, 1973; Appledorf and Kelly, 1979) and often from the food chains themselves.

A typical meal at a fast-food restaurant is relatively high in energy content, with substantial contributions made by the fat in fried foods and meats and by the sweeteners in beverages commonly purchased, such as soft drinks and shakes. The most frequently eaten meal—cheeseburger, fries, chocolate shake, and apple pie—contributes 1,180 kcal, with 39 percent of those kilocalories provided by fat, 50 percent by carbohydrate, and 11 percent by protein. This is obviously not a small contribution to the day's energy intake, and it may in fact be more than half of the total daily energy requirement.

Usual meals at fast food restaurants are adequate, even generous, in protein content, primarily derived from animal sources. Intakes of niacin, thiamin, ascorbic acid, vitamin B_{12}, and vitamin D compare favorably with the RDAs, depending of course on the particular food items selected. Vitamin A content tends to be low in most fast-food meals.

Consideration of the types of foods served at most fast-food restaurants will indicate that the crude fiber content is minimal. Although measures of crude fiber content underestimate total dietary fiber (Chapter 2), the amount of undigestible material in most fast foods is undeniably low.

Data provided in the Appendix demonstrate that fast-food restaurants are not suitable choices for people who must adhere to a sodium-restricted diet. Even the mildest restriction, 2 grams of sodium per day, would be difficult to achieve at a fast-food outlet, especially when other meals eaten during the day must be considered.

Other concerns related to the popularity of fast-food establishments focus on the limited number of food selections available. Moreover, people tend to order the same meal each time they go to a given restaurant, further reducing the variety of food consumed. The introduction of "fast-food lunches" into school systems has increased the opportunity of children to consume fast foods. Because of the importance of consuming a variety of foods to provide a nutritionally balanced and adequate diet, it becomes even more necessary to incorporate additional food varieties into the total dietary plan.

Frequent consumption of fast-food meals will not aid someone with a weight problem; and the appropriate strategy in this case is not to skip other meals. Adequate diets must provide enough of the essential nutrients needed for health and well-being, and not be planned only on the basis of calories. Lower-calorie foods can be selected at a fast-food restaurant by choosing an unsweetened beverage, milk or plain water, passing up dessert (or bringing an apple along), and eating single portions. Foods eaten during the rest of the day

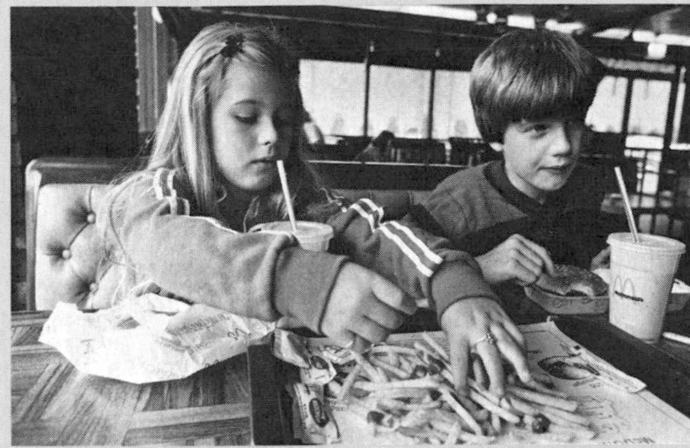

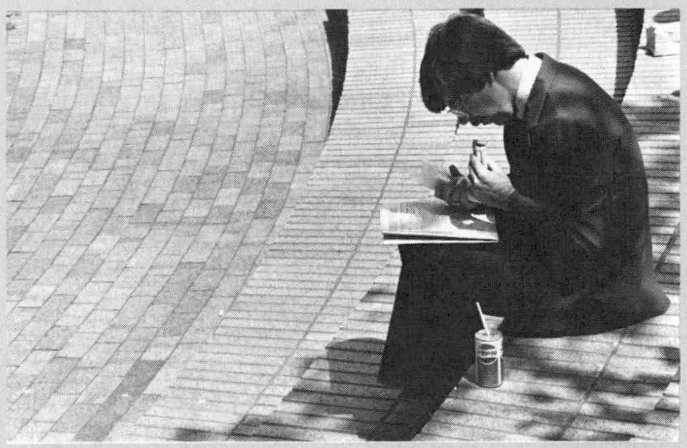

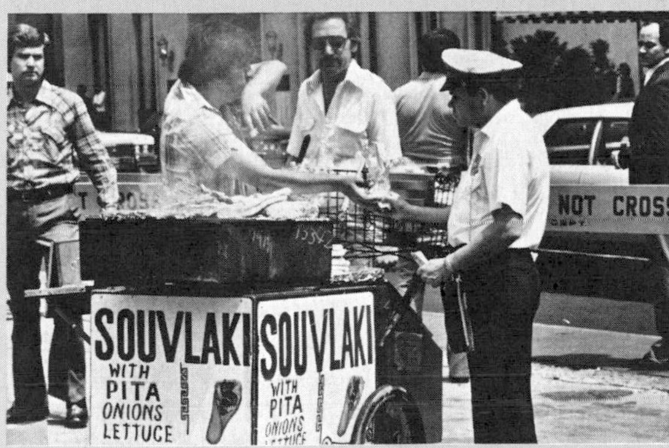

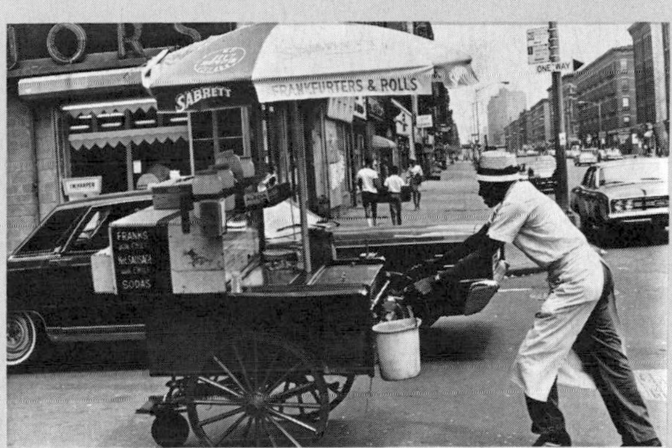

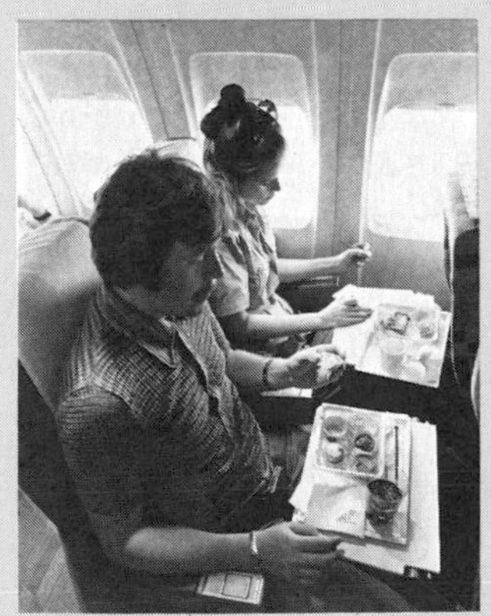

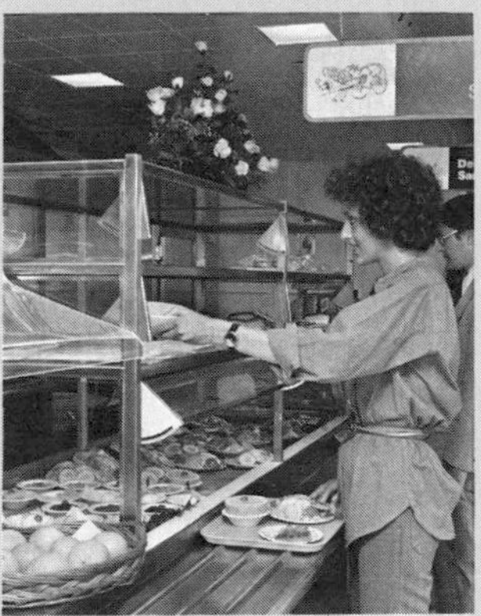

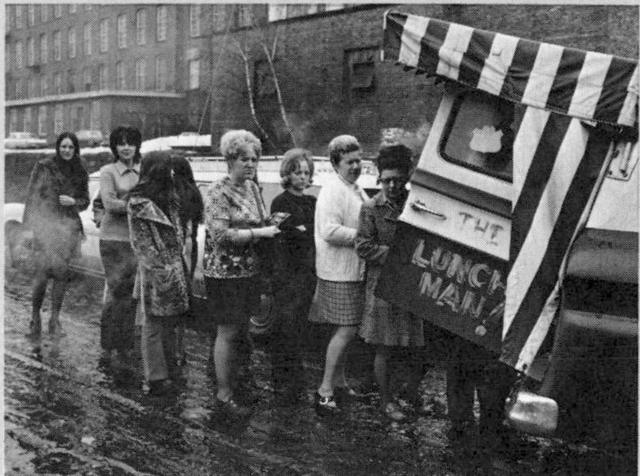

The American way of lunch. (top left Andy Levin, Black star; top right Susan Berkowitz; middle left Enrico Natali, Rapho/Photo Researchers, Inc.; middle right John Veltri, Rapho/Photo Researchers, Inc.; bottom left Chester Higgins, Jr., Rapho/Photo Researchers, Inc.; bottom middle Peter Menzel, Stock, Boston; bottom right Susan S. Perry, Woodfin Camp & Associates)

should include milk, a serving of dark green or yellow vegetables, and fruit or fruit juice.

Choices would be more informed if the nutrient composition of fast foods were more widely available for consumers to add to their own basic nutrition knowledge. Policies concerning the display of nutrition information to customers have been proposed (*Federal Register*, 11/19/76). The response of the industry to these policies may influence whether they become mandatory or remain on a voluntary basis (see Chapter 16).

served frequently at home. Their attitudes about food were also interesting; even in the younger age group, both men and women considered Scotch and martinis to be men's drinks, and wine, women's.

Neither price, nor nutrition, nor taste push consumers into restaurants. A typical fast-food meal is twice as expensive as the equivalent meal eaten at home (Isom, 1976). But in one national survey, 63 percent of the consumer sample thought of fast-food restaurants as cheaper than or about the same price as a home-cooked meal (Shaw and Pinto, 1978). While consumers may not believe that restaurant food is more nutritious than home cooking, 95 percent of a husband-and-wife sample believed that restaurant meals are "nutritionally balanced" (*Food Product Development*, March 1978). Consumers do not even prefer the taste of the food they get at restaurants. Most prefer home cooking—especially for steaks, fried chicken, meats other than steaks, and vegetables. Seafood, ethnic foods, hamburgers, and hot dogs taste better to a majority of respondents when eaten away from home (Telser, 1978).

INSTITUTIONS. Food is eaten away from home, not only at restaurants and fast-food chains, but also in cafeterias at school and work, at museums and other tourist locations, on airplanes, in trains, and in camps. Children particularly have become accustomed to institutional meals. Today school lunches are a $4-billion-a-year industry, the fourth largest food sector in the country (Young et al., 1978). Suburban sprawl, regional school systems, and integration programs require bus rides, so that children can no longer return home for lunch. Furthermore, lunch periods are short: Even children who live nearby cannot return home for the 20-minute lunch break allotted in some schools. Although some children still bring their lunch, most eat the food provided at school, because working mothers have less time to pack lunches.

Working people generally do not go home for lunch. Some bring a bag lunch, which is money-saving but time-consuming to prepare; others buy lunch. Many company cafeterias provide excellent food at low cost to cultivate employee goodwill, save workers travel time, cut down desk time lost after lunch, and provide fringe benefits for employees with both the lowest and the highest salaries. Large, prosperous corporations have established their own eating places at their headquarters and larger branches. Many provide both executive dining rooms and employee cafeterias.

Employee cafeterias range from beverage and sandwich machines to meals complete with tablecloth, wine, flowers, and soft music. Some cafeterias offer one or two different hot meals every day, several sandwich choices, a salad bar, and high-quality pastries. Others cater to special tastes and concerns with such items as diet plates, ethnic foods, and vegetarian menus. A captive audience need not mean unpalatable food.

Some school and camp cafeterias also cater to the special requirements of today's young people; they may offer a diet menu, a vegetarian selection, or some ethnic specialties. Variety and imagination of both school and camp menus is by no means universal, however, and many children do not enjoy meals in these settings. Foodservice managers may have to use great ingenuity to adapt meals to the conservative tastes of some children.

Because they must cater to people with a wide range of tastes and food preferences, foodservice operations on trains and airplanes and at museums and other tourist attractions tend more and more to provide bland, precooked foods, often pleasing no one. Elaborate dining cars with formally dressed waiters and long printed menus exist only in railroad history. In Europe the premium-priced Trans Euro Express trains still provide elegant, high-priced menus in their dining cars. But in Europe, as in America, most trains that do serve food offer only limp sandwiches and coffee in disposable cups. Carousels with infrared heat lamps are growing in popularity; they are established at many museums of the Smithsonian Institution in Washington, D.C., for example. Microwave ovens, which allow precooked main courses to be reheated en masse, are a necessity on airplanes where time and space are at a premium, and they have now spread to hospitals and even restaurants.

The limited-menu snack bars at many museums and other tourist attractions are little better than vending machines, but they keep preparation and service costs low. Increasingly, more of our meals as a nation will come from mass-feeding situations—as we spend more years in school, work for larger corporations, and have more time to travel.

CONTEMPORARY CONCERNS

Our national preoccupation with food has two facets. One focus is on the sociable and status aspects. The other reflects a growing concern over controversial issues relating to food and nutrition. This concern takes many forms and has resulted in some new trends in eating patterns.

Substantial numbers of individuals and groups have chosen to abandon the "traditional American diet" for a variety of reasons. Some advocate new methods of food production or distribution to achieve certain public benefits. The vegetarian movement has many converts. Other people are concerned with removing from their diets—and from supermarket shelves—an item or ingredient believed to be dangerous or unhealthy. Still others are looking for "miracle" foods or nutrients, and they patronize health food stores exclusively. For these and other reasons, countless people are consuming meals that would have seemed somewhat strange even to them only a few years ago—and assuring themselves and others that they never felt better in their lives.

Are these new foodways sound, or are they simply "quirky"? Not all nontraditional eating patterns can be dismissed as food faddism, which has been defined as "an unusual pattern of food behavior enthusiastically adopted by its adherents" (Schafer and Yetley, 1975). The growth of vegetarianism, an eating pattern considered weird not too many years ago, is perhaps the most obvious of today's new eating trends. It has been, in one or another form, so widely adopted that it is now accepted as a healthful way of eating, as long as a wide range of food items is consumed (see Chapter 4).

Many of the concerns that motivate new eating patterns are real and valid. Some individuals may, however, be led into harmful eating habits because of a lack of factual information, or because they are persuaded by visible and articulate adherents of a particular position. In the following pages we shall examine some of the issues that have encouraged alternative eating behaviors in recent years.

Ecology

Pesticides and fertilizers are used to protect or increase crop yield, which is both profitable to farmers and has made possible a plentiful supply of food at reasonable prices for consumers. Pesticides retard losses due to insects, rodents, and other wildlife. Fertilizers replace or add nutrients to the soil. Concern over environmental pollution from synthetic chemicals as suspected danger to life forms, however, has led many people to avoid foods grown with the aid of factory-produced pesticides and fertilizers.

Instead, people have turned to foods grown without fertilizers or pesticides, given minimal or no food processing, and not preserved with "additives." Those who are extremely concerned over this issue have turned to so-called **organic foods.** This term generally refers to foods grown by methods that use plant-and-animal-derived (instead of factory-produced) fertilizers and plant rotation or mechanical rather than chemical means of averting insects and other predators. Organically raised livestock are fed only with organically raised feed and receive no dietary supplements or chemicals to accelerate growth.

Virtually all our food is "organic" in the strictest sense of the word—because it is derived from plants and animals which contain the element carbon. Only water and salt, of substances commonly consumed, are *not* organic. The same chemicals are present in inorganic or commercial fertilizers as in the "natural" ones, but they may have already been broken down into simpler, more readily absorbed forms, and do not always include carbon. It really doesn't matter—just as the human body metabolizes ingested nutrients into the forms needed for cell processes, plants use the chemicals taken up from the soil as the raw materials for their cellular activities and growth.

Soil conditions markedly affect crop yields; in depleted soil, plants will not grow. Within limits, the mineral content of plants tends to parallel the mineral content of the soil. However, a far more significant factor in the nutrient composition of a plant is genetics. Whether fertilized or not, corn will never contain as much calcium as spinach. But as long as crops are grown in nutrient-rich soils, it matters little whether the nutrients are produced in a factory or a compost heap or manure pile. And as long as livestock receive a diet of nutrient-rich grasses, grains, and other plant products, they will not lack essential nutrients. But soils do become depleted, and nutrients must be returned to the earth, in one form or another.

Are commercial fertilizers harmful? Only if they contain a component that is harmful. But generally speaking, fertilizers contain only chemicals normally found in soils and needed by plants.

Pesticides may, however, be another story. These substances may be carried into the water supply, to be consumed by fish, animals, and ultimately humans. Concern over their ill effects began with the publication of *Silent Spring* by Rachel Carson in 1962. A number of these chemicals has been recently withdrawn from the market following reports of damage to other than their intended victims. Unfortunately, even "organic" growing methods are no guarantee that a food is free from pesticides. Chemicals persist in soils from year to year: pesticides sprayed on one field blow onto another. The result is that organically grown foods and feeds may contain significant amounts of pesticide residues (Leverton, 1974). Alternate methods of pest control are presented in Chapter 16.

The alleged benefits of organic production usually come at a higher price than comparable meats and produce purchased in standard supermarkets. Also, because production and distribution of organically produced foods is usually on a small scale, deliveries may be infrequent or irregular. To avoid purchasing merchandise that is less than fresh, wise shoppers can find out on what day delivery of desired items takes place and plan their purchases accordingly. The additional cost seems to many people well worth the peace of mind that they achieve when they know they are not consuming a chemically assisted, repellent-sprayed piece of fruit (Stephenson, 1978). As in most aspects of life, choices are made on the basis of striving for an optimum balance of perceived risks and benefits.

Health

Searching for wholesome foods that have not been tampered with, consumers have eagerly greeted "health" and "natural" foods. The word "natural" has been applied to cereal, bread, cheese, ice cream, and even beer, while soft drinks, snacks, and dozens of other products have the word "health" on their labels. In 1978, the Federal Trade Commission (FTC), the regulatory agency concerned with advertising claims, recommended restrictions on the use of the words "organic" and "natural" in advertising and a ban on claims for "health" foods altogether. The FTC defined a **natural food** as one that is minimally processed and contains no artificial ingredients. The FTC would not, however, permit advertising claims that such items are nutritionally superior to more highly processed food items (MacDougall, 1978).

The FDA, concerned over accuracy of package labeling, also prohibits claims of improved benefits and can intervene if false information about ingredients or health benefits is given or if a product is found to be dangerous. Thus, sassafras tea, which contains a substance shown to cause liver cancer in rats, was removed from sale in 1976. But other herb teas contain substances not yet tested, which may also be harmful (Stephenson, 1978).

Some items sold in "health food stores" may even be *unhealthy*. Arsenic may be found in kelp tablets; potassium chloride may cause hyperkalemia, and in fact recently caused the death of an infant in Florida. Many people use sea salt, believing that it is chemically different from ordinary salt. Only minute amounts of trace elements—and its higher price—distinguish it from its ordinary cousin. Those on sodium-restricted diets should be aware that tamari (fermented soy sauce), also sold in health food stores, can make a substantial contribution to sodium intake; 1 tablespoon of tamari contains 3 *grams* of salt (Hausman, 1978).

Cholesterol and saturated fat are also "health" issues. But "organic" cheese and milk from organically raised and fed cows contain as much fat as any other kind. Purchase of a product labeled "organic" or "natural" or of anything on the shelves in a "health food" store is not any guarantee that one is buying a nutritionally different, or better, product. Consider the popular granola-type cereals made of several different varieties of grains and nuts. Most of these are not only presweetened, but oil—usually highly saturated coconut oil—is added when the cereal grains are toasted. These products, widely advertised as "health" or "natural" foods, are not as good nutritional buys as are old-fashioned unsweetened cereals. Eating them would not contribute to the health of anyone seeking to reduce saturated fat—or energy—intakes (Hausman, 1978).

Excess energy intake is a nationwide health problem as discussed in Chapter 5. FDA surveys in 1974 and again in 1975 found that in 55 to 57 percent of all households at least one member was on a weight-loss diet (Food and Drug Administration, 1974, 1975). The concern with weight loss is pervasive, and the food industry has responded: new food—and nonfood—products have been developed for this large market, and dieters are the target of such advice and advertising. Some of the products aimed at scale-watchers may help them to lose weight, but many are frauds that take advantage of consumer gullibility. Further, many people confuse "health foods" with "diet foods," and erroneously believe that consumption of organic or natural foods will aid in weight loss.

Preservatives are substances added to foods to prolong shelf life and to maintain or enhance nutritional quality. They may appear as wax or powder on fruits and vegetables, or they may be invisible (additives will be discussed in Chapter 16). It is claimed that all foods sold in health food stores are free of preservatives. But unless the store takes great care in handling, repackaging, and storing its products, contamination will set in and the food quality will deteriorate in a very short time. Precisely because they do not contain preservatives, organic foods often appear shriveled, deteriorating, and even insect-infested (Leverton, 1974).

Consumerism

For many people, a major issue is distrust of the government, of the food industry, of advertising, and of big business in general. Often this is perceived as a problem of individualism, of the need to assert the human against the mass. People do not want to be supervised, red-taped, spindled, or mutilated—or told what to eat or what foods must contain and package labels must say. They believe that advertising claims, as well as government regulation, are an unnecessary interference with their lives and rights.

One reflection of these concerns has been the substantial numbers of people, especially young individuals and families, who have chosen to live simply on small farms and to produce their own food supply. The back-to-nature, living-on-the-earth movement is as much a revolt against the "establishment" as it is a positive statement about how to lead healthful lives.

Another reflection has been the development of the consumer movement. Books and magazines discuss the pitfalls of corporate production and the undesirable consequences of the "bigness" of the food industry. Groups of people monitor products (not only foods and food-related products such as cookwares, but all consumer goods) for safety and reliability. Lobbyists present findings and advocate positions, backed by organized and vocal consumer activists, to state and federal policy makers. Newsletters, radio talk shows, special television programming, and news features keep consumers concerned and aware of each other's activities.

Consumers can directly affect the cost and quality of their food supply. Cooperative purchasing groups—sometimes even health food coops—have lowered costs to consumers. Members take turns purchasing and delivering food and staffing the store. Profits are returned to members in the form of purchase bonuses, vouchers, or discounts keyed to the relative number of hours each member has contributed. Also, as some health food stores are growing into chains, they are able to offer extended service and lower costs to consumers. Aware consumers will be able to judge which products sold in these stores are honestly advantageous; conscientious owners and managers will provide guidance and purchase only the best quality and avoid those products that trade under false slogans.

CHANGING CONSUMPTION PATTERNS

So far in this chapter we have looked at some of the socioeconomic developments that have resulted in alterations in our eating habits in this century and at some of the personal concerns that have led to great public interest in and awareness of issues relating to food. The results of these concerns have varied enormously, from an increase in different kinds of "food fads" to reorientation of personal food preferences. Apparently, the wide publicity given to the cholesterol issue, for example, led many people to change their eating patterns, and the results seem to be encouraging. A decrease in mortality due to coronary heart disease has been documented in recent years (Keen, 1978), although it is clear that dietary changes are not the sole cause of these statistics. Some of these concerns have led to the spread of much misinformation, and an almost pathological overconcern has developed in psychologically susceptible individuals. There are people who won't buy any item with chemical names in the list of ingredients, for example. The remainder of this chapter examines some of the food intake patterns resulting from these developments and concerns and the ways in which changing food patterns become translated into new nutritional patterns.

Food Consumption Trends

In *The Changing American Diet*, Brewster and Jacobson (1978) compiled data produced by the USDA, making information about our food and nutrient supply in the United States more widely available to consumers. Several points should be made, however, about the nature of the data used: It is based on what is known as "disappearance data"—that is, how much of a food enters the marketplace. It is derived by several estimates: The USDA determines the quantity of food production in a certain year, using farm reports and processing industry data; this production figure is then adjusted for imports and exports, nonfood use, and stocks available at the beginning and end of the time period being investigated; and the weights of some products are further adjusted for some waste between the farm and retail store.

Per capita figures of food consumption are calculated on the basis of the current U.S. population, obtained from census data. It should be noted that after 1941, the amount of food used in the feeding of the military was deducted, and the "available food" was simply divided by the number of people in the civilian population.

The final figures do not account for waste at home or at the retail store, do not distinguish between different population groups, and do not reflect difference in actual consumption among different age groups. They are truly national averages and indicate what is available for consumption, not what is actually eaten by each individual.

Nonetheless, these data are truly informative despite these limitations, because the *relative patterns* of food consumption can be monitored over a period of time. With this in mind, let us examine some of the changes in our food consumption patterns over the years. Overall changes in the broad categories of food items can be seen in Table 11-1.

Per Capita Protein Consumption in the United States, 1978

Product	Protein g per day
Red meat	24
Flour	17
Milk and milk products	14
Poultry	9
Eggs	6
Cheese	5
Potatoes	5
Fish	4
Vegetables	3
Peanuts	2
Other	3
Total	92

Source: USDA, Economics, Statistics and Cooperatives Service, *National Food Review*, No. 5, December 1978.

MEAT, POULTRY, AND FISH. Pork was the most frequently consumed meat in the nineteenth century—"bringing home the bacon" and "pork-barrel politicians" have been permanent additions to our language. For the last few decades, however, beef has been king. We ate almost twice as much beef in 1976 as we did in 1950—a development that may be explained both by our growing national affluence and by our increased patronage of fast-food (hamburger and roast beef sandwich) restaurants. Now that beef consumption is decreasing due to inflation, pork consumption is rising.

Fish consumption has remained relatively stable throughout this century, but poultry consumption has increased dramatically. Improved production and marketing methods are the primary reasons for the upward trend in chicken and turkey availability.

FRUITS AND VEGETABLES. Per capita consumption of most fruits and vegetables reached high levels during the war years of the 1940s, declined sharply in the affluent 1950s, and began a steady increase in the 1970s. Data for homegrown produce are not included in the available figures, and so it is quite possible that actual fruit and vegetable consumption is higher than these statistics indicate. The recent increases in these categories reflect growing nutritional interest and knowledge as well as new concern about food prices.

Sales of fresh produce have not increased, however. In fact, sales in these categories have decreased and are only recently inching upward again. The increase in total consumption is due to the steady increase in the use of canned and frozen fruits and vegetables, which know no season and are of reliable quality. They are, furthermore, convenient to purchase, store, and prepare. The price differential between fresh and processed vegetables has also narrowed, and in many instances it may be more economical to purchase the frozen variety.

SNACKS. The $7.6 billion worth of snack foods sold in 1977 includes only bagged potato chips, corn chips, nuts, and the like. It does not include the more than $10 billion worth of soft drinks sold—great quantities of which are downed while munching—or the tons of billions of dollars worth of ice cream and beer. Still, nearly a quarter of all shoppers pick up snack foods before they leave the store, whether they intended to or not (*Food Product Development*, October 1978).

TABLE 11-1 Food Consumption in the United States (per capita per year)

Year	Meat, poultry, fish: Meat	Poultry	Fish	Total[a]	Eggs	Dairy products, excluding butter (milk equivalent)[b]	Fats and oils, including butter: Butter	Total[a]	Fruits, including melons: Citrus Fresh	Citrus Processed	Other Fresh	Other Processed	Total[a]
1900–1913	141	18	13	172	37	177	18	41	17	0	151	8	176
1925–1929	129	17	14	159	40	191	18	48	31	f	139	18	188
1935–1939	120	16	13	149	36	202	17	49	47	2	127	23	199
1947–1949	141	22	13	176	47	236	11	46	52	14	112	30	208
1957–1959	144	34	13	192	45	239	8	49	33	25	87	37	182
1965	148	41	14	203	40	235	6	51	28	23	77	38	166
1970	165	49	15	228	40	226	5	56	28	35	77	39	178
1975	158	49	15	222	35	216	5	57	28	46	74	34	181
1976[e]	165	53	15	233	35	222	4	59	29	47	78	34	188

NOTE: All quantities are in pounds except dairy products, which are in quarts.

Year	Vegetables, excluding potatoes and sweet potatoes: Dark green & deep yellow Fresh	Dark green & deep yellow Processed	Other, Including tomatoes Fresh	Other, Including tomatoes Processed	Total[a]	Potatoes, sweet potatoes: White[c] Fresh	White[c] Processed	Sweet potatoes Fresh	Sweet potatoes Processed	Total[a]	Dry beans, peas, nuts, soya products	Flour & cereal products	Sugar & other sweeteners	Miscellaneous[d]
1909–1913	14	f	172	17	203	182	f	23	f	205	16	291	89	10
1925–1929	24	1	166	25	217	142	f	20	f	162	17	237	119	13
1935–1939	27	2	171	31	231	128	f	19	f	147	19	204	110	16
1947–1949	27	4	157	43	232	111	f	12	f	123	17	171	110	19
1957–1959	19	6	130	54	209	88	6	7	1	101	17	148	106	15
1965	17	6	124	60	206	68	12	5	1	86	16	144	112	15
1970	17	7	124	64	212	59	19	4	1	83	16	141	120	14
1975	18	7	125	66	217	58	22	4	2	84	18	139	114	12
1976[e]	18	7	127	62	213	54	22	4	2	80	18	140	119	12

[a] Components may not add to total due to rounding.
[b] Milk equivalent based on calcium content.
[c] Includes revised estimates for processed potatoes, beginning 1957–1959.
[d] Includes coffee, tea, and chocolate liquor equivalent of cocoa and chocolate products.
[e] Preliminary.
[f] Less than 0.5 lb.

Source: L. Page and B. Friend, The changing United States diet, *BioScience* 28(3):192, 1978. Yearly data, except for 1976, based on USDA Agricultural Economics Report No. 138 (Washington, D.C.: U.S. Government Printing Office, 1978).

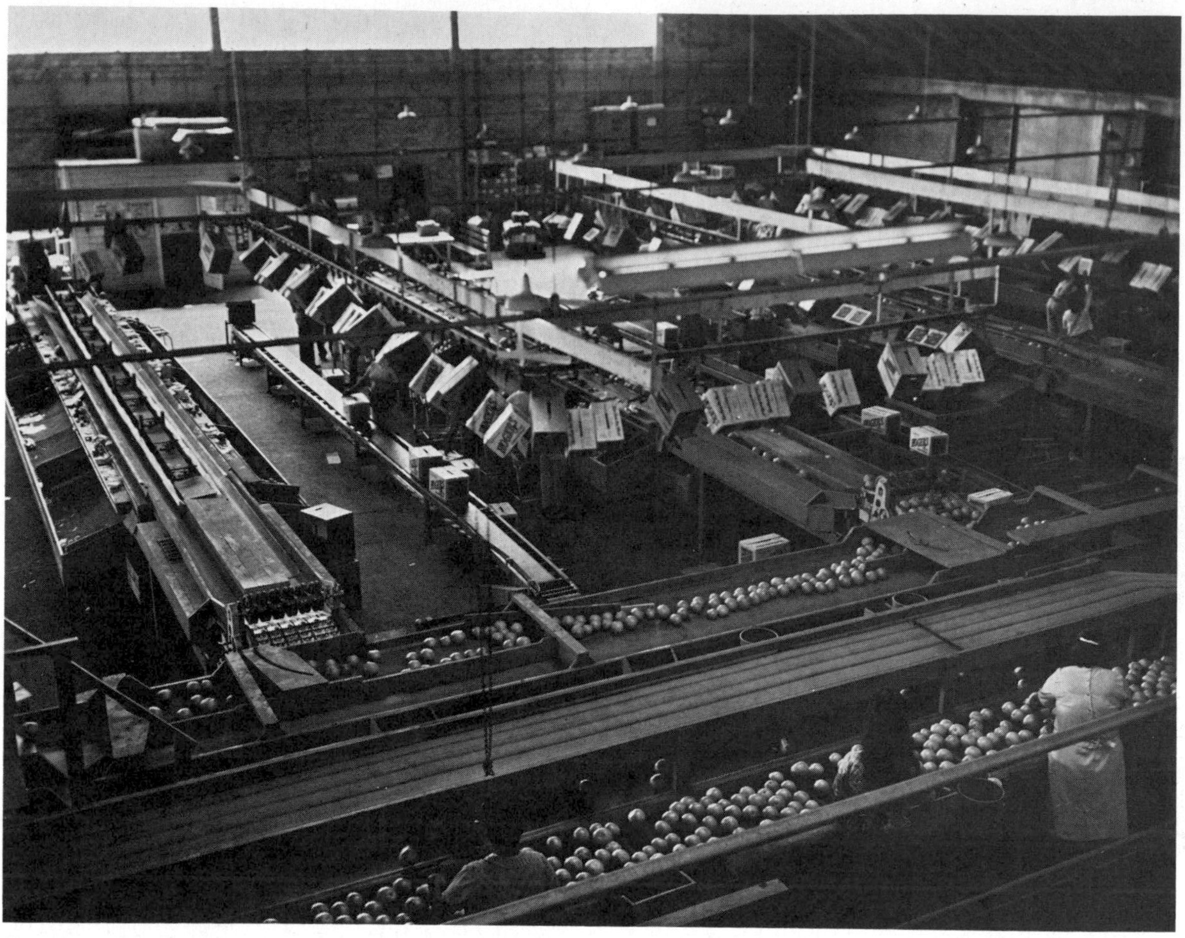

Oranges move on a conveyer belt for sorting and crating at a citrus packing house. (Grant Heilman, Lititz, Pa.)

And soft drinks are sliding down our throats at an incredible rate: 500 8-ounce servings per person annually. Consumption has more than doubled during the past ten years, even in the face of concern over the sugar content of soft drinks. In fact, diet soft drinks captured 11 percent of the market in 1976 (Brewster and Jacobson, 1978), and despite concern over the possible carcinogenicity of artificial sweeteners, the percentage is rising.

Regular soft drinks are most popular with 18- to 24-year-olds and consumption decreases progressively at later ages. Diet soft drinks, on the other hand, achieve their greatest popularity with 35- to 44-year-olds (Christon, 1977). Most soft drinks are sold at food stores (55 percent) or by vending machines (21 percent), not at fast-food restaurants where they have to compete with shakes.

Ice cream consumption has been increasing over the past 30 years, even after a boom during the first half of the twentieth century. Consumption of ice milk and other varieties of frozen dairy products has also increased: Ice milk, lower in fat than ice cream, is used in "shakes." Frozen yogurt is becoming increasingly popular.

The "natural" trend has extended to snack foods, too. Even soft drinks and potato chips have gone "natural." But when the artificial green coloring agent was removed from a popular frozen limeade, the drink looked more like lemonade and lost consumer acceptance (MacDougall, 1978). Natural potato chips are made from unpeeled potatoes rather than peeled ones and contain no preservatives.

Soon the average adult American will be absorbing 3 gallons of alcohol per year, a figure that has been steadily on the rise since the end of Prohibition in 1933. But in this area of consumption perhaps more than in any other, relatively few of us are average. There are millions of alcoholics and tens of millions of teetotalers. Beer consumption has risen every year for a quarter of a century. And just when the weight-conscious started to avoid it, light beers with somewhat lower calorie content were developed. Approximately 157 million barrels of beer were shipped in 1977—22.4 gallons per person (*Food Product Development*, April 1978). Depending on how hot the summers are, analysts expect even larger shipments in the future, with light beers accounting for an ever greater share of the market.

There is one snack item of which less is being consumed than previously. Candy consumption in this country has declined by almost a quarter during the past ten years, from 20.3 to 15.4 pounds per person (*Business Week*, 8/14/78).

OTHER CHANGES. It is difficult to escape the conclusion that Americans are simply eating more—of almost everything. But there are some foods which we are eating less: apples, down 70 percent from 1910 to 1976; butter and fresh cabbage, down 76 and 65 percent, in the same period. Coffee consumption has decreased 44 percent from 1946 to 1976. And there was a 48 percent decrease in consumption of wheat flour (used in bread, pastry, macaroni, and so on) from 1910 to 1976. In fact, consumption of all grain and cereal products has decreased dramatically from 300 pounds per person per year in 1910 to 140 in 1976. Further, we are consuming a smaller variety of these products. Rye, barley, buckwheat, and corn meal were common items in the diets of our forebears, but are seldom found in our pantries today.

Overall consumption of whole milk has declined, largely due to concern about fat content. But consumption of skim milk, cheese, and yogurt has increased in the last decade—each for different reasons. Skim milk is a low-fat alternative to whole milk; cheese is a meat alternate and reflects the growing interest in gourmet cookery; and yogurt is perceived as a health and diet food item. Although starting from a low base, the increase in yogurt consumption is indeed phenomenal—up 400 percent from 1967 to 1978, now at 2 pounds per person per year (Brewster and Jacobson, 1978).

Nutrient Content of Today's Foods

Contrary to popular belief, energy and carbohydrate intake is lower than at the turn of the century, and we consume about as much protein as ever (Scala, 1978). (Figure 11-3 compares the relative proportion of total calories provided by each of the three macronutrients in 1909–1913 and 1976.) But our energy is being provided more by fats, sugars, and meats, and our protein

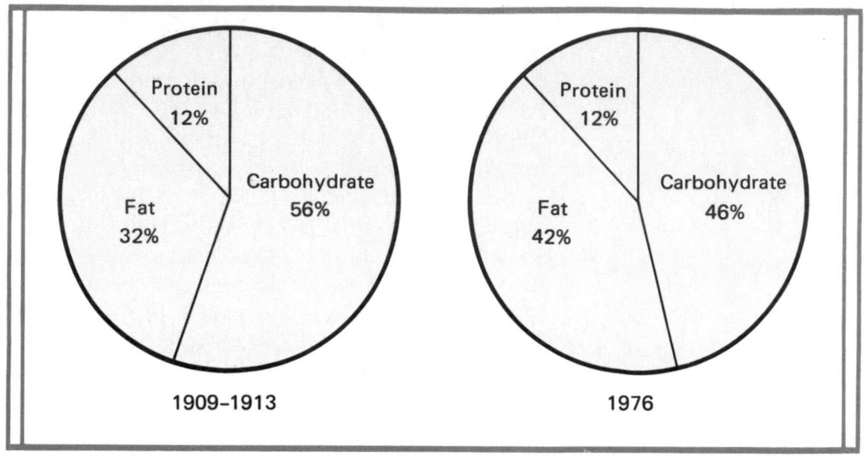

FIGURE 11-3

Calories from Energy-Yielding Nutrients

Per capita civilian consumption.

Source: L. Page and B. Friend, The changing United States diet, *BioScience* 28(3):196, 1978.

more by meat, instead of by the traditional cereals and grains. In 1910, fat and sweeteners supplied 44 percent of our calories; by 1976, they were providing 60 percent. The percentage of energy intake from complex carbohydrates fell from 37 to 21 during the same period. Flour and cereal products supplied 36 percent of protein at the beginning of the century, but now they supply only 17 percent; meat, poultry, and fish once provided 30 percent but now account for 42 percent (Brewster and Jacobson, 1978).

ENERGY. Our overall caloric intake from all foods (excluding liquors) declined steadily until the early 1960s, but it has risen since then and is now almost as high (3,300 kcal per day) as it was 70 years ago (3,480 kcal per person per day). Remember that these figures reflect disappearance data and, while undesirably high, do not reflect *real* individual intakes. In part they may indicate only that we are more wasteful of our foods; it has been shown that smaller households throw out more food than larger ones do, and the typical American household is shrinking, accounting for proportionally more waste.

Most of the recent increase in energy intake has come from fat, which furnishes over twice as much kilocalories per gram as protein or carbohydrates. In the 1909–1913 period, only 16 percent of the fat consumed came from vegetable sources; in 1976 the figure was 43 percent (Brewster and Jacobson, 1978). Fat and oil consumption increased by 1 gram per day in 1978, provided mostly from vegetable products (Marston and Page, 1978). Foods of animal origin, in the form of meat, eggs, milk, butter, and cheese supply the rest.

VITAMINS AND MINERALS. Less vitamin A is derived from sweet potatoes than formerly, but more comes from meat and other vegetables. Overall, then, vitamin A consumption has stayed about the same over the years, although a slight decrease has been noted in recent years (Marston and Page, 1978).

Intakes of thiamin, riboflavin, niacin, and iron tend to change in parallel fashion since they are usually found in the same foods. Consumption of these nutrients slowly declined until the late 1930s and increased when bread enrichment began in the 1940s. Meat provides proportionally more of these nutrients than it did fifty years ago and vegetables proportionally less.

Vitamin B_6 is another nutrient of which less was consumed during the Depression years. We now eat as much as in 1909 but about 15 percent more than in 1935. The flour-refining process removes much of the B_6 from grains, but today the vitamin is being added to several foods, including breakfast cereals and baby formulas. Throughout this century the disappearance data figures have hovered around the adult RDA of 2 milligrams of vitamin B_6 per adult per day.

Because we're eating more meat, we're getting about 14 percent more vitamin B_{12} than 70 years ago. Animal-origin foods are the only natural source of the vitamin, but other foods such as breakfast cereals are fortified with it, so that now 1.5 percent of our intake of B_{12} comes from flour and cereals (Brewster and Jacobson, 1978). A slight decrease in the availability of vitamin B_{12} was noted in 1978, due to a reduction in beef production (Marston and Page, 1978). Adequate consumption of vitamin B_{12} is a concern for those on strict vegetarian eating patterns.

Everybody knows that citrus fruits are rich in vitamin C, but so are vegetables, especially potatoes and tomatoes. Since improved transportation and the development of frozen juices have multiplied our consumption of citrus products, and Vitamin C–fortified drinks have also increased in number and use, it's little wonder that we're getting more vitamin C than ever.

Calcium intake parallels the consumption of milk. All the pregnant mothers and babies of the post–World War II baby boom pushed milk and calcium consumption to record levels. Calcium availability has decreased somewhat since then and tends to be unevenly distributed among the population.

Magnesium is one nutrient of which substantially less is being consumed, perhaps because it is not normally added to fortified foods. Daily personal consumption fell from 408 milligrams in 1909–1913 to 339 milligrams in 1965, but it has stayed almost exactly the same since then. Since these figures reflect disappearance data only, it is very likely that most people are getting less magnesium than the adult RDAs of 350 milligrams for men and 300 for women. The decrease in magnesium consumption parallels the decreased consumption of breads and cereals. These products provided 38 percent of the nutrient in 1909–1913 but only 18 percent in 1976 (Brewster and Jacobson, 1978). Dairy products, processed potatoes, and poultry however, are providing a greater proportion of dietary magnesium than formerly (Marston and Page, 1978).

Accurate figures for phosphorus intakes are not available. This mineral is a component of some food but exact quantities are not known. One producer of phosphates states that about 0.4 grams per person per day are derived from additives; the National Academy of Sciences has estimated the figure at 1.8 grams (Brewster and Jacobson, 1978). This latter figure is even higher than the total amount—just over 1.5 grams—derived from meats, vegetables, and dairy products. Total phosphorus intake has remained almost static during this century, although in earlier years a larger proportion of the mineral was provided by grains and cereals.

Consumption trends for some major vitamins and minerals, as well as for the three macronutrients, are summarized in Table 11-2.

TABLE 11-2 **Nutrient Content of the United States Diet (per capita per day)**

Year	Food Energy Calories	Protein g	Fat g	Carbo-hydrate g	Calcium g	Phos-phorus g	Iron mg	Magne-sium mg
1909–1913	3,480	102	125	492	.82	1.56	15.2	408
1925–1929	3,460	95	134	476	.86	1.51	14.4	388
1935–1939	3,260	90	132	436	.90	1.47	13.8	379
1947–1949	3,230	95	140	403	1.00	1.55	16.8	369
1957–1959	3,140	95	143	375	.98	1.53	16.3	347
1965	3,150	96	144	372	.96	1.52	16.7	339
1970	3,300	100	156	380	.94	1.55	18.0	342
1975	3,220	99	152	370	.91	1.52	18.3	341
1976[a]	3,300	101	157	376	.93	1.55	18.6	344

Note: Quantities of nutrients based on per capita food consumption estimates (retail weight), including home gardens, prepared by Economic Research Service, USDA. Data include iron, thiamin, riboflavin, and niacin added to flour and cereal products; other nutrients added primarily as follows: Vitamin A value to margarine, milk of all types, milk extenders; vitamin B_6 to cereals, meal replacements, infant formulas; vitamin B_{12} to cereals; ascorbic acid to fruit juices and drinks, flavored beverages and dessert

GAZING INTO THE CRYSTAL BALL

Where do we go from here? What will our foodways be in the near—and not so near—future? What new fads, new concerns, new products, new food technologies, new information about diet and health, and new lifestyle developments will come along to alter our menus and meals?

It is clear that events on international and national scales affect us in the kitchen and at the table. The Depression of the 1930s is only a memory to half of the population. Even World War II was not experienced by today's young adults. And yet our national food intake patterns changed most dramatically during the 1930s and 1940s.

Today's world event with the greatest impact on our food consumption patterns is undoubtedly the energy crisis. As prices rise and supplies diminish, costs of food increase at every point in the production-to-market chain. Even the cost and convenience of getting to the market are being affected, as drivers try to eliminate excessive car travel and plan shopping excursions more carefully than ever before. Energy costs for food preparation are rising as well.

Will consumers try to economize by eating at home more, buying less expensive products, and growing their own? It seems unlikely, because of our educational and occupational systems, that there will be a decline in the number of meals eaten away from home. Many people, however, are already choosing to substitute less-expensive foods and are experimenting with new items. Home-grown produce may be fresher and may taste better, but it may not prove to be more economical in terms of time and productivity. Large home crops mean that time must be found to can foods or prepare them for freezing; and space in freezers and pantries must be available for storage. Few homes built in this century were equipped with root cellars, in which the home-grown produce of earlier centuries was kept through the winter. And,

Year	Thiamin mg	Ribo-flavin mg	Niacin mg	Vitamin B_6 mg	Vitamin B_{12} μg	Vitamin A Value IU	Ascorbic Acid mg
1909–1913	1.64	1.86	19.2	2.26	8.4	7,600	104
1925–1929	1.55	1.87	18.0	2.05	8.1	8,000	106
1935–1939	1.43	1.84	17.3	1.96	7.7	8,300	112
1947–1949	1.91	2.30	21.4	1.99	9.0	8,800	114
1957–1959	1.84	2.30	21.1	1.99	8.9	8,100	104
1965	1.81	2.30	21.9	2.02	9.1	7,700	97
1970	1.92	2.37	23.6	2.22	9.9	8,200	110
1975	1.95	2.36	24.0	2.20	9.5	8,000	118
1976[a]	2.04	2.46	25.2	2.26	9.6	8,100	118

powders, milk extenders and cereals. Includes revised potato series in Supplement for 1975 to *Food Consumption, Prices, Expenditures*, Agriculture Economic Report 138, Table 26.

[a] Preliminary.

Source: L. Page and B. Friend, The changing United States diet, *BioScience* 28(3):192, 1978.

too, tastes have not yet changed back to the kinds of foods that were easily and economically grown and stored in those years—whole grains and root vegetables.

Predictions for the future can foresee only the continuation of trends already in progress. They cannot anticipate new and dramatic developments. Thus we can prophesy that concerns about diet and health will continue to motivate increasing numbers of people; that production and distribution of all manner of foods will increasingly depend on new technologies, research, and computers; that concern over increasing costs will lead to the expansion of cooperative markets; and that interest in international foods will lead to greater availability of food products of other cultures.

Expensive food specialty shops—"Bakery Boutique," "International Cheese"—continue to open; people are not willing to forego all luxuries even in the face of inflation. But more and more people are combining their economic and health concerns with their creative impulses and discovering ways to prepare *healthy* gourmet foods *cheaply*, guided by an increased production of cook books devoted to these aspects of food preparation.

Today's work force will continue to grow, both in absolute numbers and as a percentage of the working-age population. Women will contribute substantially to the increase (and the male component of the work force may even decrease as men exercise options for household and child care for longer periods of time). The work force will get progressively older. There will be more single-parent families, more households without children, and more retired people. However, after a decline in births, a "mini" baby boom is taking place, as women who postponed childbearing are establishing families. But sales of infant foods and formulas will again level off.

Consumer pressure will probably moderate television food advertising directed to children to some extent. But what will today's children, brought up on Big Macs and Whoppers, pizzas and shakes, eat when they set up homes of their own?

In the long run, probably, the most important factor in our food future is economics, both for the food industry and for the consumer. Technologies that can result in greater productivity and efficiency for the food industry, and greater purchasing power for the consumer, will be readily accepted. New product development will be with us for years to come. We already are eating "reformed" ham and potato chips and "extruded" snacks that pop out of machines in the shape of stars or squiggles. "Space sticks" or "astronaut foods" have been available for some time. Technology has given us instant breakfasts and even dehydrated martinis are now possible (you *do* have to add ice, water, and the olive) (Wells, 1979). Dehydrated foods are relatively less expensive than other varieties because they are lighter in weight (for both supplier and consumer) and can be stored and transported at lower energy cost (*Food Product Development*, October 1978). More foods will be processed and packaged at the factory rather than at individual grocery stores. Computers will increasingly be silent partners at every stage of the distance from producer to consumer. They give suppliers, supermarkets, and restaurants—especially fast-food chains—more efficient control over inventories, which means money savings that can be passed on to consumers.

"Aquaculture"—the raising of fish in a controlled environment—is already practiced in Israel and parts of Asia; as concern over pollution of natural water increases, this will become an increasingly attractive possibility. Chickens and turkeys will be bred larger in the future and will contain less fat.

TVP—textured vegetable protein—is here already. Meat substitutes made from spun strands of soy flour look and (almost) taste like the real thing and have comparable amounts of protein. Unlike meat, TVP has no cholesterol; but it also lacks vitamin B_{12} and some of the essential amino acids found in meat (Mayer, 1976). It is also high in sodium.

Optimistically, as the population becomes better educated and as the media respond to increased public concern about food and nutrition, more information will be available to more people. There is no question that Americans are concerned about what goes into their bodies, its possible effects on their health and appearance, and how much it costs. As additional research provides more answers, more accurate information will be available on which to base our food choices.

SUMMARY

For most of human existence, people's food supplies consisted only of what nature placed before them. But in today's technological society, a greater variety of food items is available than could ever before have been imagined. The twentieth century has been characterized by a sharp reversal of the producer-to-consumer ratio until, in 1976, only 7 percent of the U.S. population was producing enough food not only to satisfy the needs of the national population but for export as well. Among developments making this plenty possible have been genetic research, the chemical fertilization industry, new means of transportation and refrigeration, marketing techniques, and more.

Our food behaviors are shaped not only by productivity and availability, but also by social and cultural influences. These include: urbanization and suburbanization; changes in the family structure and the growing number of smaller household units; postponement of childbearing; increase in the number and proportion of working women of all ages; increase in mobility; inflation; energy shortages; and ethnic diversity. There is also a growing interest in food and cookery as well as a heightened awareness of health and nutrition.

Most food purchases are made in supermarkets—75 percent of all groceries sold in 1976 came from this source. At the same time, more meals are being consumed outside the home, at restaurants ranging from "fast" to "fancy," and in the workplace, schools, and other institutional settings as well. There are more than 10,000 items on the shelves of today's supermarkets, and thousands more are introduced by food manufacturers every year. Consumers can save by purchasing house brands or "specials," using "cents-off" coupons, or by choosing generic or "no frills" items. These are simply packaged and perhaps "imperfect" in appearance or other indication of quality, while nutritionally comparable to higher-priced advertised brand-name items.

Work schedules for most people ensure that lunch will be the meal most frequently consumed outside the home. When their place of work does not provide meal service many choose fast-food restaurants, which are popular with families and teenagers as well. A growing segment of the food industry, in 1976 fast-food restaurants accounted for 25 percent of all restaurant sales and were patronized by nearly three-fourths of all American households. Typical meals at these establishments have relatively high energy and sodium content and tend to be low in vitamin A and crude fiber, although they provide adequate supplies of many nutrients.

A growing concern nationwide has been in relation to the health aspects of food. Vegetarianism has been growing in popularity. Many people are purchasing a variety of items from so-called "health food" stores in the belief that such foods are in some way better than the supermarket version. In particular there has been growing consumption of "organic" produce, grown without recourse to chemical fertilizer or pesticides. Concerns for personal health, for the safety and preservation of the environment, and mistrust of "big" government and industry have encouraged a growing consumerist movement.

BIBLIOGRAPHY

Appledorf, H. Nutritional analysis of foods from fast food chains. *Food Technology* 28(4):50, 1974.

Appledorf, H., and L. S. Kelly. Proximate and mineral content of fast foods. *Journal of the American Dietetic Association* 74:35, 1979.

Brewster, L., and M. F. Jacobson. *The changing American diet.* Washington, D.C.: Center for Science in the Public Interest, 1978.

Bureau of the Census. *Households and families by type: March 1977 (advance report).* Washington, D.C.: U.S. Government Printing Office, 1977.

Burros, M. Working men and women both cooking. *Boston Globe,* July 12, 1978, p. 17.

Business Week. Corporate strategies: Mars. August 14, 1978, p. 52.

Carson, R. *Silent spring.* Boston: Houghton Mifflin, 1962.

Christon, A. S. Diet soft drinks promise continued growth and profit potential. *Food Product Development,* February 1977, p. 56.

Donovan, W. P., and H. Appledorf. Fatty acid content of franchise chicken dinners. *Journal of Food Science* 37:961, 1972.

DONOVAN, W. P. AND H. APPLEDORF. Protein, fat and mineral analysis of franchise chicken dinners. *Journal of Food Science* 38:79, 1973.

Federal Register. Restaurant foods: Statements of general policy or interpretation. Vol. 41:51001, November 19, 1976.

FOOD AND DRUG ADMINISTRATION. *Food and nutrition: Knowledge and beliefs. A nationwide study among food shoppers by response analysis.* Washington, D.C.: FDA, 1974.

FOOD AND DRUG ADMINISTRATION. *Consumer nutrition knowledge survey, a nationwide study of food shopper's knowledge, beliefs, attitudes and reported behavior regarding food and nutrition: Factors related to nutrition labeling.* Washington, D.C.: FDA, 1975.

Food Product Development. Dining habits of married couples surveyed. March 1978, p. 69.

Food Product Development. We're drinking ever more beer. April 1978.

Food Product Development. Marketing product flavor. August 1978, p. 51.

Food Product Development. Snack consumption improves, new varieties "add on" volume. October 1978, p. 63.

GIFFT, H. H., M. B. WASHBON, AND G. G. HARRISON. *Nutrition, behavior, and change.* Englewood Cliffs, N.J.: Prentice-Hall, 1972.

HAUSMAN, P. Natural food myths. *Nutrition Action* 5(4):3, 1978.

ISOM, P. Nutritive value and cost of fast-food meals. *Family Economics Review,* Fall 1976, p. 10.

KEEN, S. Eating our way to enlightenment. *Psychology Today,* October 1978, p. 62.

LEE, D. Cultural factors in dietary choice. *American Journal of Clinical Nutrition* 5(2):166, 1957.

LEVERTON, R. M. Organic, inorganic: What they mean. In *1974 Yearbook of Agriculture.* Washington, D.C.: USDA, 1974.

LOWENBERG, M. E., AND B. L. LUCAS. Feeding families and children—1776 to 1976. *Journal of the American Dietetic Association* 68:207, 1976.

LOWENBERG, M. E., E. N. TODHUNTER, E. D. WILSON, J. R. SAVAGE, AND J. L. LUBAWSKI. *Food and people,* 3rd ed. New York: John Wiley, 1979.

MACDOUGALL, A. K. Natural—Is it all in the name? *Nutrition Action* 5(12):11, 1978.

MARSTON, R., AND L. PAGE. Nutrient content of the national food supply. *National Food Review* (USDA), December 1978, p. 41.

MASLOW, A. H. *Motivation and personality.* New York: Harper & Row, 1970.

MAYER, J. Can you tell the meat from the "real" thing? *Family Health* 8(9):40, 1976.

POPE, L. No name grocery products doing well. *Boston Globe,* December 13, 1978.

RICE, B. Cooking with psychophysics. *Psychology Today,* November 1978, p. 80.

SCALA, J. U.S. consumption patterns serve as indices for dietary product design. *Food Product Development,* March 1978, p. 48.

SCHAFER, R., AND E. A. YETLEY. Social psychology of food faddism. *Journal of the American Dietetic Association* 66:129, 1975.

SHAPIRO, L. J., AND D. BOHMBACH. Eating habits force changes in marketing. *Advertising Age,* October 30, 1978, p. 27.

SHAW, R. E., AND D. PINTO. Where's your next meal coming from. *The Nielsen Researcher,* No. 1, 1978.

STEPHENSON, M. The confusing world of health foods. *FDA Consumer,* July-August 1978, p. 19.

TELSER, E. Nutrition and eating: Do Americans practice what they preach? *Food Product Development,* June 1978, p. 82.

WELLS, P. Powdered martinis and other surprises coming in the future. *New York Times,* January 10, 1979, p. C-1.

WHEELER, E. F. Food choice and the U.S. dietary goals. *Journal of Human Nutrition* 32:325, 1978.

WITTY, H., AND E. S. COLCHIE. *Better than store-bought.* New York: Harper & Row, 1979.

YOUNG, E. A., E. H. BRENNAN, AND G. L. IRVING. Perspectives on fast foods. *Dietetic Currents* 5(5):1, 1978.

SUGGESTED ADDITIONAL READING

ARTHUR, C. Checking out supermarkets. *Nutrition Action* 5(7):3, 1978.

BENDER, A. E. Food preferences of males and females. *Proceedings of the Nutrition Society* 35:181, 1976.

BROWN, G. B., I. M. CELENDER, AND A. E. SLOAN. What the U.S. consumer knows, thinks—and practices when it comes to nutrition. *Food Product Development,* May 1978, p. 35.

DONOVAN, W. P., AND H. APPLEDORF. Protein, fat, and mineral analyses of franchise chicken dinners. *Journal of Food Science* 38:79, 1973.

DWYER, J., AND E. ALSTON. Nutrition in family life. *Food Product Development,* November 1976, p. 44.

FINEBERG, L. Fast food for adolescents. *American Journal of Diseases of Children* 130:362, 1976.

Food Product Development. What will consumers of 1998 demand for their food dollars? October 1978, p. 60.

GORDON, J. A., AND V. KILGORE. Planning ethnic menus. *Hospitals, J. A. H. A.,* November 1, 1971, p. 87.

GREECHER, C. P., AND B. SHANNON. Impact of fast food meals on nutrient intake of two groups. *Journal of the American Dietetic Association* 70:368, 1977.

GRIVETTI, L. E. Culture, diet and nutrition: Selected themes and topics. *BioScience* 28:171, 1978.

HARRIS, M., AND E. B. ROSS. How beef became king. *Psychology Today,* October 1978, p. 88.

HOPKINS, H. Food marketing without frills. *FDA Consumer,* November 1978, p. 6.

KATZ, D., AND M. T. GOODWIN. *Foods: Where nutrition, politics, and culture meet.* Washington, D.C.: Center for Science in the Public Interest, 1976.

MILLER, S. A. The kinetics of diet and culture. *Technology Review,* August-September 1978, p. 39.

SIMOONS, F. J. Traditional use and avoidance of foods of animal origin: A cultural historical view. *BioScience* 28:178, 1978.

Chapter 12

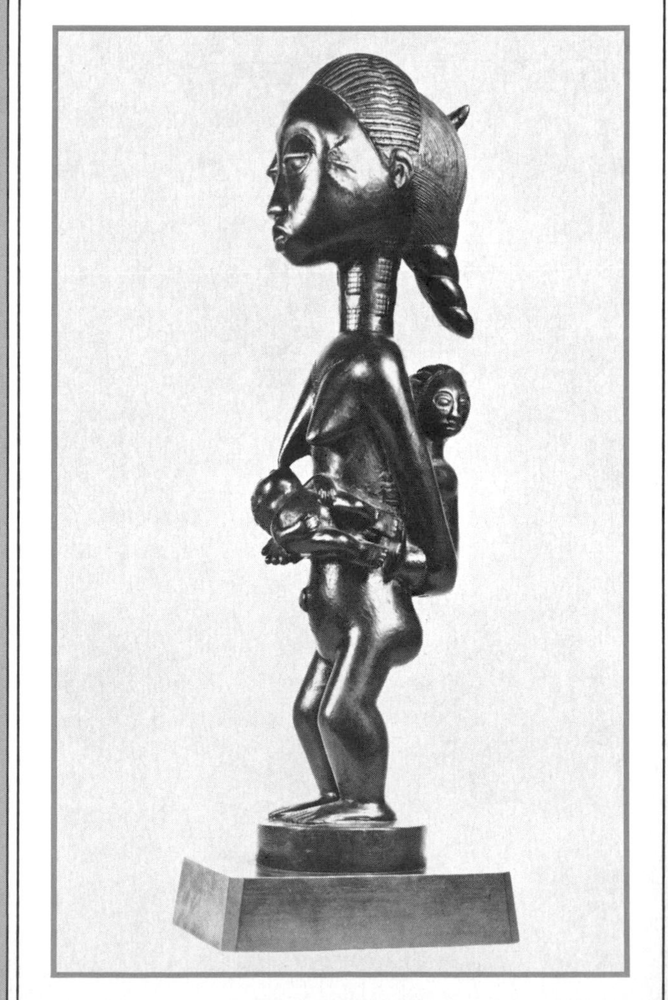

Mother and Children, Baule, Ivory Coast

Nutrition in Pregnancy and Lactation

Growing from one single cell to a complex organism with millions of cells in just the 40 weeks of pregnancy is quite a feat—but every human being has done so. The nutritional bond between a mother and her unborn child which makes that extraordinary development possible is the subject of the present chapter.

Good nutrition maintains the optimal health of the mother-to-be, ensures that her nutrient stores are not depleted by the demands of the fetus, and provides for the needs of the growing fetus at the same time. Our discussion begins with an account of fetal development and of the developmental stages of human pregnancy, including the postpregnancy period of milk production (lactation). Against this physiological background we will examine the various nutrition-related concerns for the health and well-being of both baby-to-be and mother-to-be, including the ways in which the nutritional needs of pregnant and lactating women differ from those of nonpregnant and nonlactating women, and the translation of the nutritional needs of this period into food intake patterns. The special nutritional concerns of pregnant adolescents will also be considered.

HUMAN PREGNANCY

Previous chapters have explained how foods taken into the body from the external environment provide the substrate for growth, structure, function, and regulation of the internal environment. This close interrelationship is probably most apparent during pregnancy and lactation. From the time between conception and birth, the single cell that is a fertilized egg must grow and develop into a full-sized 3 to 3.5 kilogram (6.5 to 7.5 lb) human being, capable of surviving in the outside world. Never again will growth and development proceed so rapidly. It is easy to understand why the developing fetus requires the significant amounts of energy and nutrients that must be provided by the mother.

Sequence of Prenatal Development

There are three distinct developmental stages of prenatal life. The first, *blastogenesis,* occupies the first two weeks following fertilization. The fertilized egg (zygote) immediately divides into two cells, each of which then divides into two more, and so on. The zygote soon becomes a cell-lined hollow sphere, the *blastula.* While cell division is taking place, cell enlargement does not occur because there is as yet no source of nourishment for the zygote, which remains the same overall size as the original ovum despite the rapid proliferation of cells. As the cells continue to divide, two layers are distinguished. The inner cell mass will become the *embryo,* and the outer "feeding" layer or *trophoblast* will differentiate to form the *placenta.* At this point the blastula becomes attached to the wall of the uterus. The trophoblast penetrates the uterine lining and absorbs material from the lining to provide the first nourishment for the new organism.

Meanwhile the inner cell mass is separating into two spherical forms, separated by a thin cellular disc. This disc will become the embryo itself; one of the spheres becomes a yolk sac (which in humans does not contain yolk) and the other becomes a fluid-filled sac, the amnion, which will provide a

TABLE 12-1
Development of Systems in the Embryo

System	Chronology	
Dental	4–6 months:	Hard tissue of primary teeth
Nervous	0–9 months:	Increased number of brain cells Survival reflexes present at birth
Muscles	5–6 weeks:	Development of nerve attachments to muscles
	8 weeks:	Involuntary muscles function
	16 weeks:	Muscle movement can be felt
Skin	4 months:	0.5% fat
	5 months:	6% fat
	birth:	15% fat
Eyes	7 weeks:	Nerves, eyelids, lens
	10 weeks:	Eyelids fused shut
	7–8 months:	Eyes open but not mature, even at birth
Ears	4–8 weeks:	Structure develops into final form
	16 weeks:	Assumes typical appearance
Cardiovascular	6 weeks:	First fetal organ (heart) completed
	2 months:	Circulation developed
Respiratory	6 weeks:	Trachea, bronchi, lung buds
	12 weeks:	Lungs take shape, fluid inhaled
Digestive	8 weeks:	Lip fusion
	12 weeks:	Palate fusion
	5 months:	Production of bile, digestive juices
Excretory	7 weeks:	Bladder and urethra separate
	16 weeks:	Kidneys assume final form
Reproductive	6 weeks:	Gonads first appear
	7–9 weeks:	Gonads differentiate
Skeletal	2–8 weeks:	Skeleton formation
	12 weeks:	Bone begins to replace cartilage

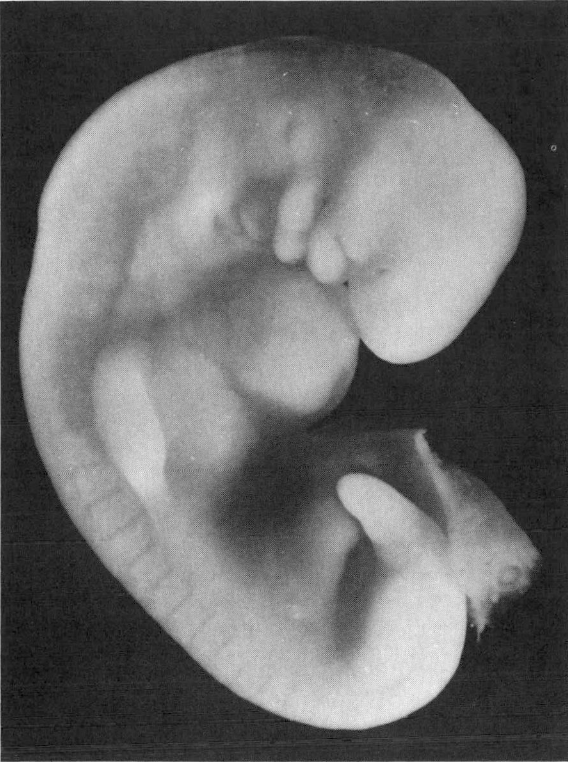

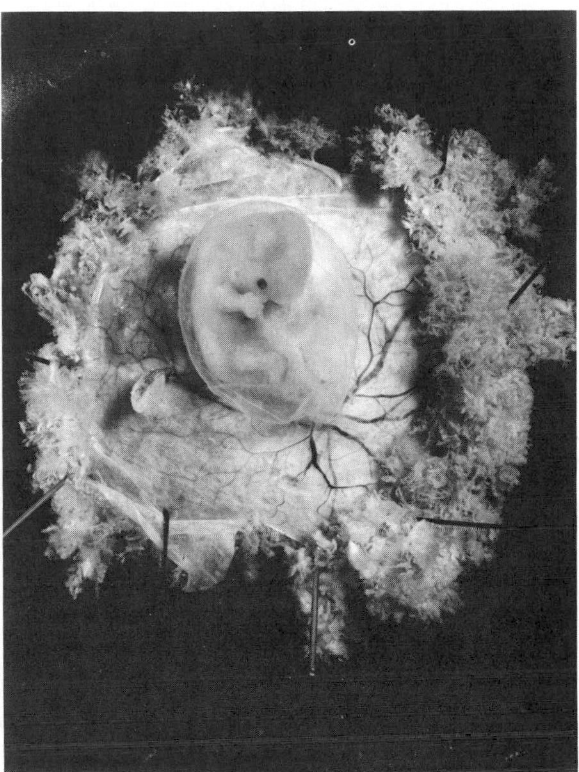

(Left) Embryo, 4 weeks. Tiny "buds" and indentations are the only suggestions of the structures—arms and legs, ears and eyes—that will develop in the next few weeks. (Carnegie Institution)

(Right) Embryo, 7 weeks, surrounded by amniotic sac, and placenta. Arms, hands, eyes and ears have taken definite shape. (Carnegie Institution)

protective environment as well as nourishment for the embryo. In the *embryonic stage* the embryonic disc begins to differentiate into three types of cells, the *germinal layers*. The *ectoderm* or outermost layer of cells will form the brain, nervous system, hair, skin, and sensory organs. The *mesoderm* or middle layer will provide the body's supporting structures—bone, muscle, connective tissue, and parts of the cardiovascular, excretory, and reproductive systems. The innermost layer or *endoderm* will form the lining of the respiratory, urinary, and digestive tracts. Sixty days (eight weeks) after fertilization the embryonic stage is completed, and many components of the skeleton, brain, eyes, ears, heart, and lungs are fully formed (see Table 12-1).

With the start of the third gestational month, the embryo is considered a *fetus*. The *fetal stage* of development, which continues until birth, is a time of rapid growth. The specialized cells continue to divide and now also begin to grow in size. What at 3 weeks had been a tiny embryo weighing only 6 grams, by 24 weeks has grown to about 30 centimeters and 640 grams. At the time of birth, the fully grown fetus will measure around 50 centimeters and weigh about 3,250 grams.

The information that guides this dramatic progression from blastocyst to newborn baby is precisely programmed in the genetic material carried by the egg and the sperm. Apparently there is a different genetic timetable for the development of each body system, and each is vulnerable to nutritional insult. Each system—muscular, skeletal, circulatory, and so on—develops at its own particular rate and pattern. Research on laboratory animals, for example, indicates that restricted maternal protein intake during a critical period of fetal nervous system development causes the offspring's brain to have fewer than the normal number of cells. The same short-term nutritional deficiency that might affect nervous system growth may have little effect on another body system that is not at a similarly critical developmental stage.

Nutrient needs during the embryonic stage are so infinitesimal that only severe malnutrition on the part of the mother would have a significant effect. Fetal nutrient requirements increase during pregnancy and are greatest during the last trimester, when expansion of both the size and the number of cells is greatest.

When nutritional deficiencies continue throughout the term of pregnancy, every body system is in some way affected. In various studies, pregnant animals placed on restricted diets have consistently produced offspring of low birth weight, reduced brain cell number and head size, and proportionate reductions in the size of various body organs. Nutrition is not the only time-specific influence on fetal development. The potentially harmful effects of drugs such as Thalidomide or illnesses such as German measles are also keyed to developmental stages of specific systems.

It would be unethical to perform deprivation experiments on human mothers and offspring. Specific data for nutritional needs in human pregnancy have accumulated as a result of a limited number of studies of aborted fetuses and studies involving natural and/or accidental disruptions to a population's food supply. Much evidence is thus circumstantial and epidemiological. The consequences of the food shortages of wartime Europe, for example, have been analyzed. The most acute famines occurred in Leningrad in 1942 and in Holland during the winter of 1944–1945. The resulting data corroborate the results of animal studies: Severe nutritional deficits early in prenatal existence increase fetal mortality rates and affect physiological development; in the later months of pregnancy the primary effect is to significantly decrease overall growth and birth weight (Smith, 1947). Similarly, autopsies of stillborn infants in the United States have shown that those from low-income families were smaller in overall size and had smaller livers, adrenal glands, and other organs than those from higher-income and presumably better-nourished families (Naeye et al., 1969).

Placental Function

The placenta, or afterbirth, which is delivered along with the newborn baby, is one pregnancy product that has always been readily available for study. Microscopic examination of placental tissues has shown that infants who experienced prenatal growth failure, or are from low-income populations, had placentas of smaller size and fewer cells than those who were better nourished (Winick, 1970).

During blastogenesis and after, the embryo and placenta develop simultaneously. After implantation in the uterine wall, part of the embryonic mesoderm attaches as a lining to the trophoblast to become the *chorion* (see Figure 12-1). The chorion sends numerous projections into the uterine lining, and from these develop the network of blood vessels that constitutes the fetal

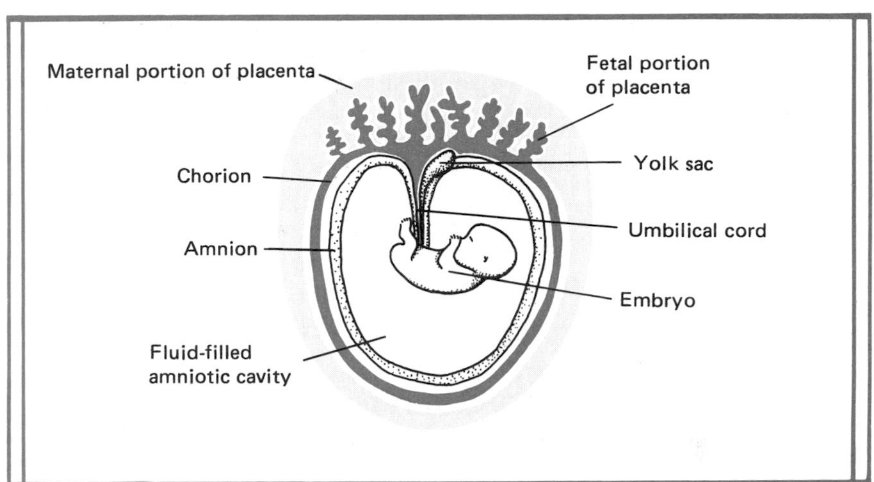

FIGURE 12-1
Intrauterine Environment of the Fetus

part of the placenta. These chorionic villi function in much the same way as the intestinal villi, providing the extensive surface area needed for nutrient transfer. While the embryonic portion of the placenta is being formed, the mother's body is responding. Glands and blood vessels within the uterine lining develop, and muscle fibers increase in size and strength.

Exchanges of nutrients and wastes take place in the placenta much as they do in the gastrointestinal tract: by passive transport, facilitated diffusion, and active transport across placental membranes. Oxygen and nutrients pass from the mother to the fetus; carbon dioxide and metabolic wastes pass in the opposite direction, to be eliminated by the mother's body. What makes these placental transfers so complex is the involvement of two separate blood supplies—one from the mother and the other from the fetus. There is no exchange of blood between the two, only an exchange of nutrients from one blood compartment to another. Maternal hemoglobin levels are vital to maintain the oxygen exchange system. Because 1.34 milliliters of oxygen are carried by each gram of hemoglobin, it is important for the mother to avoid iron deficiency, which would depress her hemoglobin levels and, consequently, reduce the supply of oxygen available to her developing child.

Water and the fat-soluble vitamins diffuse to the fetal circulation. Amino acids, glucose, the water-soluble vitamins, and such minerals as calcium, sodium, and iron are actively transported. The placental membranes have at any one time a limited carrying capacity for actively transported materials, and it has been suggested that excessive intakes of water-soluble vitamins (such as ascorbic acid) on the part of the mother may compete with transport of essential amino acids and impair growth and development (Malone, 1975). Placental membranes also assure that nutrients needed by the fetus in higher concentrations than the mother requires will not follow the concentration gradient and rush back into the mother's bloodstream.

With one exception, protein molecules do not cross the placenta, since they are too large to penetrate the cells of the placental villi. The fetus must synthesize its own proteins from the amino acids it receives from the maternal circulation. The exception is a specific maternal antibody which is structurally able to penetrate, and which provides important immunoresistance to infection that lasts until six or more months after birth.

In addition to serving as the conduit for these exchanges, the placenta supplements the mother's hormone production, becoming the primary source of progesterone and estrogen and the sole source of several hormones normally produced only during gestation: human chorionic gonadotrophin (HCG), human placental lactogen (HPL), human chorionic somatomammotrophin (HCS), and human chorionic thyrotrophin (HCT). Although much of this hormone production is stimulated by biochemical precursors produced by the fetus, the gestational hormones act primarily to regulate the mother's pregnancy and postpartum progress.

Maternal Hormones and Tissues

The normal physiological adjustment process of pregnancy causes a number of changes in the mother's body, many of which are mediated by hormones. The more than 30 hormones secreted during gestation include some that are present only during that time and others, normally present, whose rates of secretion are altered in pregnancy. They are proteins or steroids that are synthesized from amino acid and cholesterol precursors in endocrine glands throughout the body. Those hormones with the most far-reaching effects are progesterone and estrogen, both of which are present in increased supply during pregnancy.

Progesterone, which acts on smooth muscle tissue to produce relaxation, allows the uterus to expand as the fetus grows. Gastrointestinal muscles relax as well, slowing intestinal motility, with the obvious benefit to the fetus of additonal absorption time and consequent increases in serum nutrient levels. Unfortunately, maternal constipation is often a side effect of reduced motility.

Progesterone also enhances fat storage, especially in the back, thighs, and abdomen, with smaller amounts deposited in mammary tissue. Generally increased fat storage throughout the body is not only physically protective of the fetus but provides a potential energy reserve. Progesterone also heightens respiratory sensitivity, leading to hyperventilation, thus increasing the energy and oxygen supply available to the fetus and increasing the capacity to expire carbon dioxide.

Estrogen aids in expanding the uterus. By acting on components of connective tissue, it causes these tissues to become flexible enough to accommodate the shifts of bones and organs as they are displaced by the growing fetus and makes possible dilation at birth. But this same biochemical reaction also enhances fluid retention in connective tissue, which is common in pregnancy. At the same time, progesterone has a sodium-depleting effect. The combined results alter electrolyte and fluid balance to a considerable extent. However, unless water retention is associated with hypertension and proteinuria (protein in the urine), there is no cause for concern. Normal fluid retention in pregnancy may even provide some benefits: Women with mild edema tend to have larger babies and a lower rate of premature delivery. Mild edema is not by itself associated with any danger to the fetus (Williams, 1977).

Other hormones have strictly metabolic effects. Thyroxine production is increased and, by a complex series of reactions, results in increasing maternal appetite as well as speeding the rate of breathing to provide additional oxygen for energy production from ingested food. As pregnancy progresses, the action of insulin becomes less efficient. Normally this is not a problem. However, in a diabetic or prediabetic mother, the output of insulin may be so low that glucose metabolism is impaired, with potentially serious effects for both fetus and mother. Cortisone, which is involved in the maintenance of blood glucose levels by stimulating gluconeogenesis from amino acids, is produced in greater amounts during the final days of pregnancy in response to increased estrogen production.

Other changes during pregnancy involve both blood volume and composition and kidney function. Expansion of maternal blood volume facilitates the transport of nutrients and metabolic wastes between mother and fetus. The highest plasma volume is reached at 34 to 36 weeks, when the mother's body contains 50 percent more plasma than when fertilization took place. As a result of this increase, the *concentrations* of many constituents in the blood (protein, water-soluble vitamins, minerals) are somewhat diminished during pregnancy. Kidney function is altered to accommodate the greater blood volume and increased amount of waste products. More blood flows through the kidneys, and the glomerular filtration rate is increased. There is, however, no related increase in the reabsorptive capacity of the kidney tubules, and as a result substantial quantities of some water-soluble nutrients are flushed out of the mother's body along with normal metabolic wastes.

IMPACT OF NUTRITION ON THE OUTCOME OF PREGNANCY

Over the years the nutritional beliefs transmitted to pregnant women have been just as much a matter of fashion as the clothing they were expected to wear. It was long believed the fetus would draw all the sustenance it needed from the mother's body. The concept of the fetus as a "parasite" on the maternal "hostess" was, in fact, quite prominent in obstetrical textbooks and practice during the early part of the century, despite the lack of any supporting scientific evidence. It was also believed that pregnant women would instinctively choose to eat the foods required by the fetus even if the items of choice were lobster salad, pickles, or watermelon (none of which, or course, are specifically beneficial).

Most persistent was the advice to "eat for two." And, considering the increased hormonal output, the increasing demands for nutrients and energy, the need for more oxygen, and the physical demands on the mother's body of fetal growth, this advice does carry a certain logic, although it is not quantitatively exact. Then the fashion shifted, at least in the United States, as the national preoccupation with slimness led to greater concern for the mother's postnatal figure than for her pregnancy needs. Now, as fitness and health have become popular concerns, the pendulum appears to be swinging back to an emphasis on nutritional plenty. This time, however, science rather than fashion is being cited as evidence.

What is the nutritional reality? For a considerable part of its uterine life, the embryo/fetus is extremely small, and its requirements equally so. Thus, fetal development in the earliest months of pregnancy has relatively little nutritional impact on the mother. But during the growth months of pregnancy, and especially the last trimester, the mother's nutritional requirements are indeed increased. The mother's prepregnancy nutritional status has a great impact on the fetus from the moment of conception on. Women who start pregnancy with a long history of good nutrition are more likely to maintain good health and to bear healthy babies.

Determining Pregnancy Outcomes

The desired outcome of pregnancy is a healthy and well-developed baby, born with minimal difficulty to a healthy mother. Repeated studies over many years have shown that the best available measures of desirable outcome include weight at birth, fetal mortality, and maternal and infant mortality and morbidity. Consistently, low birth weight babies (under 2500 grams, or about 5½ pounds) experience a higher mortality rate and have a greater number of physical and mental handicaps than newborns of normal weight. Many studies have been done to define the maternal factors that influence the outcome of pregnancy and to examine the effect of nutritional supplementation on these parameters.

In the United States, maternal mortality and morbidity (12.0 per 100,000 live births in 1975) is largely traceable to toxemia, abortion, hemorrhage, and infection—conditions often preventable through good prenatal care. Table 12-2 shows that, although U.S. maternal mortality rates are low, they are not the lowest in the Western world; there is still much that can be done to improve pregnancy outcomes, especially in particular U.S. population groups. A "natural experiment" provided by wartime conditions in England in the 1940s gave evidence of a direct association between maternal nutrition and infant viability. Food rationing policies gave priority to pregnant and lactating women, thus improving the quality of their diets. Although there were no changes in other factors such as prenatal care or maternal age, the rate of stillbirths fell dramatically (Thomson and Hytten, 1973).

A recent study of pregnant women in a predominantly rural Wisconsin county attempted to determine the impact of maternal diet and other factors on pregnancy outcomes. It must be remembered that these are statistical correlations and not demonstrated cause-and-effect relationships. It was found that a higher birth weight of infants was associated with longer duration of pregnancy, the overall quality of the maternal diet, and greater weight gain of the mother during pregnancy; low birth weights were associated with increased numbers of cigarettes smoked per day by the mother, among other factors (Philipps and Johnson, 1977).

In another study changes in plasma levels of free amino acids, reflecting the protein intake of the mother, were measured during the last trimester of pregnancy, and positively correlated with birth weight. Mothers with low concentrations of free amino acids delivered low birth weight babies, suggestive of fetal undernutrition (McClain et al., 1978).

These and other studies make overwhelmingly clear that maternal nutri-

TABLE 12-2
Maternal Mortality Rates in Selected Countries, 1975

Country	Deaths per 100,000 Live Births
Cape Verde, Africa	130.8
Costa Rica	59.9
Bahamas	49.6
West Germany (Federal Republic)	34.8
Japan	27.6
East Germany (Democratic Republic)	23.3
Austria	16.0
Israel	15.7
Poland	14.3
United States	12.0
England and Wales	11.4
Netherlands	10.7
Switzerland	10.1
Belgium	9.2
Norway	7.1
Australia	5.6
Denmark	5.6
Puerto Rico	2.9
Sweden	2.0

Source: United Nations, Department of International Economic and Social Affairs, *Demographic yearbook 1977* (New York: United Nations, 1978), pp. 358–361.

tion is a major factor in pregnancy outcome as determined by birth weight. Other interrelated factors include the mother's age, the number of previous pregnancies, her prepregnancy weight, her socioeconomic status and race, and the extent to which she smokes, drinks alcoholic beverages, and/or uses drugs. The precise role of any particular factor is difficult to determine, and more research is needed.

Determination of the relative importance of any one factor is complicated by the fact that, overall, the physiological efficiency of human reproduction is very high, even under adverse conditions. Even among impoverished populations and in developing countries, where most women enter pregnancy with suboptimal health and marginal nutritional deficiencies, delivery of apparently healthy infants is the rule and not the exception (Thomson and Hytten, 1973). But these successful pregnancies are followed by up to 25 percent infant mortality in many geographic areas; stresses of the external environment, including poor sanitation, complicate the transition to extrauterine life. Optimal prenatal conditions would better prepare infants to withstand the stresses of the world they enter at birth.

A number of studies have sought to determine the effect of nutritional supplementation on pregnancy. Early studies of vitamin and mineral supplements on the outcome of pregnancy resulted in equivocal findings and have been criticized for incomplete evaluation of nutritional status of the mothers both before and during pregnancy. More recent studies have attempted to consider this important factor.

In Guatemala, a preindustrialized country in which women typically gain an average of 15 pounds during pregnancy and where low birth weight is a significant problem, the typical diet during pregnancy provides 40 grams of protein and 1,500 kilocalories per day. Although this protein:energy ratio is adequate, the total energy intake is not. To study the effects of nutritional intervention, Lechtig et al. (1975) provided one group of women with a supplement containing both protein and calories. Another group received a supplement providing calories but no protein. Both supplements contained vitamins and minerals. The data indicated that as the supplemental energy intake increased, infant birth weights increased and fewer low birth weight babies were delivered. Furthermore, the increased birth weights were associated with proportional increases in placental weight, suggesting that the benefit of improved maternal nutrition may be due in whole or in part to its effect on the size, and consequently functional capacity, of the placenta. It is of interest that the amount, and not the type, of supplement influenced these results. At a given level of energy intake, it did not matter whether protein was included in the supplement. These findings suggest that energy and not protein is the limiting factor in diets consumed by pregnant Guatemalan women.

Results of this Guatemalan study and others from developing nations are applicable to high-risk mothers in industrialized nations as well. In a Montreal study, dietary counseling and supplements to meet individualized needs were provided for more than 1,500 low-income pregnant women, all of whom had been at nutritional risk prior to pregnancy. The incidence of low birth weight among infants born to these women decreased to the national average and was lower than in the surrounding area; and the rate of complications was lower than in the surrounding area as well. Maternal weight gain was shown to be directly related to infant birth weight, and those women who received nutritional assistance for longer periods tended to gain more weight and have fewer low birth weight infants than those who were involved in the program for a shorter period of time (Primrose and Higgins, 1971).

In a recent study, pregnant California women were provided with three levels of supplementation: One group received a high-protein, high-energy, vitamin-and-mineral-containing beverage, a second group received a lower-protein and lower-energy version of the same beverage, and a control group received only the vitamin and mineral supplementation. None of the three levels of supplementation appeared to have any significant effects on the subsequent birth weights of infants delivered by these women (Adams et al., 1978a). Even before supplementation, however, the majority of these women were getting from 66 to 100 percent of the recommended dietary allowances for kilocalories and protein (Adams et al., 1978b) and thus would show minimal effects of supplementation.

It appears, then, that supplementation per se has no demonstrable effect on the pregnancy outcomes of otherwise adequately fed women. But evidence from a number of studies indicates that, for women who are poorly nourished in their earlier years and enter pregnancy without nutrient reserves, dietary supplementation during pregnancy can be crucial to the outcome of the pregnancy.

In 1970 the Committee on Maternal Nutrition summarized the findings of a number of studies and issued a report which included a recommendation that special dietary review and counseling be available to all pregnant women, with special attention paid to those who enter pregnancy with poor dietary habits and in an undernourished state (Committee on Maternal Nutrition,

1970). It is also apparent that, as Beal has said, "If a woman has been well nourished throughout her life, her intake during pregnancy, unless very different, is likely to have relatively little effect either on the course of pregnancy or the health and size of her infant. If she is poorly nourished during her own growing years and enters pregnancy without reserves, her diet during pregnancy becomes crucial" (1971, cited in Adams et al., 1978a). These conclusions have implications for nutritional behaviors of girls and women during their growth years.

NUTRITIONAL CONSIDERATIONS DURING PREGNANCY

The tremendous growth of maternal and fetal tissues during pregnancy substantially increases a woman's nutritional requirements. The fetus may not be a parasite, but it makes its own demands and asserts its nutritional rights. The fetus requires nutrients for all of the major metabolic processes involved in energy production, cell and tissue growth, and maintenance of structures and function. It will, to a certain extent, deplete maternal nutrient stores if necessary to supplement what is provided by the mother's food intake. The demands placed on maternal organs, and normal maintenance of the mother's health, must also be considered. Each nutrient has a role in pregnancy, but some play a more obvious role than others. Although experimentally derived data for specific physiological requirements are generally lacking, recommended dietary allowances are set higher for most nutrients during pregnancy (Table 12-3).

TABLE 12-3
Comparison of RDAs in Nonpregnant, Pregnant, and Lactating Women

Nutrients	Nonpregnant Adult	Pregnant	Lactating
Energy (kcal)	2,000	+300 = 2,300	+500 = 2,500
Protein (g)	44	+30 = 74	+20 = 64
Vitamin A (RE; IU)	800; 4,000	1,000; 5,000	1,200; 6,000
Vitamin D (μg)	5	10	10
Vitamin E (mg αT.E.)	8	10	11
Vitamin C (mg)	60	80	100
Folacin (μg)	400	800	500
Niacin (mg N.E.)	13	15	18
Riboflavin (mg)	1.2	1.5	1.7
Thiamin (mg)	1.0	1.4	1.5
Vitamin B_6 (mg)	2.0	2.6	2.5
Vitamin B_{12} (μg)	3.0	4.0	4.0
Calcium (mg)	800	1,200	1,200
Phosphorus (mg)	800	1,200	1,200
Iodine (μg)	150	.75	200
Iron (mg)	18	18+	18+
Magnesium (mg)	300	450	450
Zinc (mg)	15	20	25

Source: Food and Nutrition Board, National Research Council, *Recommended dietary allowances*, 9th ed. (Washington, D.C.: National Academy of Sciences, 1979).

Energy

As any mother will tell you, pregnancy is hard work! In addition to the demands made on her system by increased basal metabolism, for almost half of her pregnancy a woman must carry around the equivalent of a small hiking pack balanced quite firmly across her midsection. The energy cost of lugging this ever-increasing extra weight, and adjusting metabolic function accordingly, has been estimated at 80,000 kilocalories over nine months. This averages out to about 300 extra kilocalories per day, a rather small amount. This additional energy is not needed equally throughout the course of pregnancy, however; requirements generally increase as pregnancy progresses. Unlike previous estimates, current energy allowances do not assume that physical activity of the mother decreases near term. A recent study reports, in fact, that modern American women, who normally lead relatively sedentary lives, do not alter their activity appreciably during the last trimester, and thus do not "save" calories (Blackburn and Calloway, 1976). However, a woman who remains physically active will have to adjust her energy intake accordingly, perhaps to a level of 45 kilocalories per kilogram of pregnant body weight, consuming 2,500 to 2,600 kilocalories daily in the last ten weeks.

In addition, it has been shown that many women do not increase energy *intake* gradually. Instead, they maintain a constant level of energy consumption that is higher than necessary during the first trimester and less than recommended levels during the third trimester (King and Charlet, 1978). It has been suggested that the maternal fat stores deposited during the period of excessive energy intake early in the pregnancy provide a resource to be drawn on during the later weeks and, especially, during lactation. Approximately 3,500 grams of adipose tissue, representing 30,000 kilocalories, are deposited in the mother's body during pregnancy.

Those women who enter pregnancy in an underweight condition should pay particular attention to increasing energy intake levels by at least the recommended 300 kilocalories per day, so as to replenish their body stores of energy (King and Charlet, 1978).

Closely tied to recommendations for energy intake is medical opinion about optimal weight gain during pregnancy. In the late nineteenth century, when modern surgical techniques were not yet available, weight limitation was generally advised, especially for women whose pelvic cages were small (and whose babies today would be delivered by cesarean section). A fluid-restricted, low-carbohydrate, high-protein diet, the so-called Prochownick diet, named for a German physician, was prescribed to produce infants small enough to deliver easily. This remained standard practice well into the twentieth century, despite a lack of scientific verification for its value (Vermeersch, 1977). Weight control in pregnancy is, even today, a subject of confusion, often influenced by antiquated notions.

It is important to recognize that weight gain of three and even four times the weight of the newborn baby is both *normal* and *desirable*. The baby accounts for *less than half* of the total normal weight gain during pregnancy, and most of the baby's growth in size occurs in the last trimester.

As Figure 12-2 shows, the growth of the uterus and expansion of the blood supply account for most of the weight gain during the first trimester (13 weeks) of pregnancy. The recommended weight gain over this period is

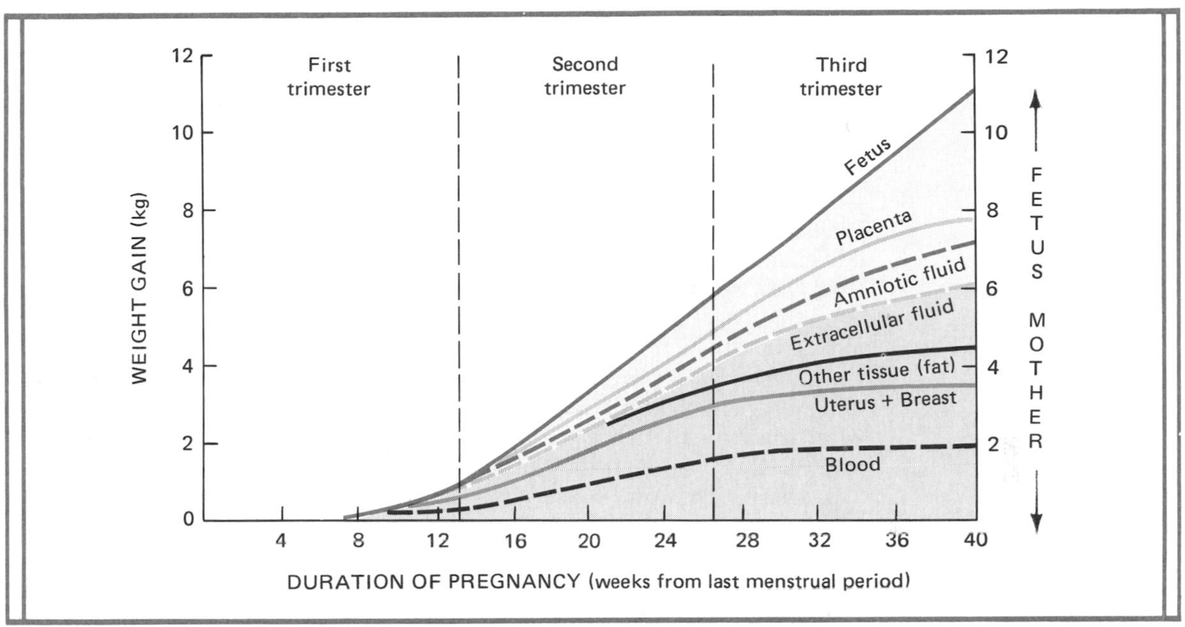

FIGURE 12-2

Components of Weight Gain during Pregnancy

Source: R. M. Pitkin, Nutritional support in obstetrics and gynecology, *Clinical Obstetrics and Gynecology* 19(3):489, 1976.

approximately 1 to 2 kilograms (2 to 4.5 lb). In the second trimester weight gain should average 0.35 to 0.4 kilograms (0.8 to 0.9 lb) per week, much of it accounted for by growth of the placenta, uterus, and breasts, and increased maternal body fluid volume. In this middle part of the pregnancy the mother's appetite and weight gain will be greatest. However, the baby's weight does not become a major component of the maternal weight gain until the third trimester. By the time of delivery, the new mother can expect to have gained *at least* 22 to 27 pounds, with first-time (primapara) or young mothers gaining somewhat more than multiparous and older women. On average, daily food intake should provide a minimum of 36 kilocalories per kilogram of pregnant body weight, or about 16 kilocalories per pound. The pattern of weight gain, however, is more significant than the total amount added. A sudden leveling off or marked increase in maternal weight may indicate a nutritional or other problem.

Warnings against excessive weight gain during pregnancy have been aimed in particular at preventing the development of fluid accumulation and hypertension (**toxemia**). However, such warnings have failed to distinguish between added weight due to normal tissue growth and that resulting from excessive fluid accumulation. There is no evidence to associate weight gain due to excess energy intake with the development of toxemia (Committee on Maternal Nutrition, 1970).

Women who are obese before becoming pregnant do face increased risks of some complications, particularly hypertension and diabetes mellitus. Even for them, however, energy-restricted food intakes are not advisable during pregnancy. Overweight women often try to restrict their weight gain during pregnancy, hoping to lose weight at the end of the nine months. But the potential interference with fetal development makes this unwise. Obese women should, however, be careful to guard against excessive weight gain during pregnancy, and they should take the opportunity to improve their eating habits by eliminating empty-calorie foods and consuming those with high nutrient density, as well as to increase their physical activity. Accumulation of excessive maternal adipose tissue should be avoided. Following the energy and nutrient RDAs should for most women result in the desirable pattern of weight gain just described. Also, an energy-restricted diet quite frequently reduces the intake of nutrients necessary for fetal well-being. In addition, a calorie-restricted diet carries the risk of catabolizing body protein stores and *necessary* fat stores, which would result in ketonemia, a maternal condition that has been correlated with mental retardation in the offspring of affected mothers (Pitkin, 1976). As some consolation for the figure-conscious, the high levels of progesterone that cause storage of added fat during pregnancy decrease rapidly after birth, and even more rapidly in lactating mothers. Most women experience a dramatic postpartum weight loss and should be back to their prepregnant weights in a few months.

Underweight women have different problems, especially if their low body weight is associated with overall low nutrient intake. Because underweight women frequently have low birth weight babies, nutritional supplementation, counseling, and careful supervision of the mother's progress during pregnancy are necessary. Underweight individuals should eat sufficient amounts of carefully selected nutritious foods to meet both energy and nutrient needs.

Protein

A normal pattern of weight gain during pregnancy indicates only that overall energy intake is adequate, but not that specific nutrient requirements are being met. In the United States, protein intake is seldom a problem. However, a study of low-income women in Oklahoma City found that their plasma levels of total free amino acids were significantly lower than normal and correlated directly with delivery of low birth weight babies (McClain et al., 1978).

Protein serves as the structural building material for synthesis of hormones, cells, and tissues in the fetus, the placenta, and the mother herself. The recommended protein allowance for nonpregnant women is 44 grams per day. There is little demand for additional protein in the early months of pregnancy. This is fortunate, since many women do not realize they are pregnant for some time, particularly if they do not experience morning sickness. By the second month of pregnancy, however, an extra 30 grams per day of protein is recommended (Food and Nutrition Board, 1979). That's the equivalent of 4 to 5 ounces of meat or fish, or 4 glasses of milk. Planning the increased protein needs for strict vegetarians requires careful consideration of complementary protein sources (see Chapter 4).

Vitamins

Because of their role in energy production, the B vitamins thiamin, riboflavin, and niacin are important components of diet during pregnancy. Thiamin is a coenzyme necessary in the last step of the metabolic pathway by which glucose is converted to pyruvic acid and then to acetyl CoA. Riboflavin and niacin are respectively components of the coenzymes flavin adenine dinucleotide (FAD) and niacin adenine dinucleotide (NAD) that produce energy by controlling the transfer of hydrogen atoms through the electron transport system. Severe deficiencies of these three B vitamins during pregnancy cause fetal death, low birth weight, and congenital malformations in laboratory animals; comparable findings have not been observed in humans (Heller et al., 1974a, 1974b).

Pyridoxine (vitamin B_6) and folic acid are needed for protein synthesis, and thus for fetal development and growth; folacin and vitamin B_{12} are involved in synthesis of red blood cells; and vitamin C is essential for the development of collagen, the important connective tissue protein. The coenzyme roles and other functions of these water-soluble vitamins were described in Chapter 7, and food sources of each were listed there as well. Recommended dietary allowances for all of these are increased during pregnancy, as shown in Table 12-3. While increases for most are moderate, the recommendation for folacin doubles to 800 micrograms per day. This reflects the importance of this vitamin in DNA and RNA synthesis, not only for red blood cell formation but for the rapid growth of fetal and placental cells as well. For cells to divide, DNA must replicate itself, transmitting the identical genetic information to the RNA templates that go into the new cell. Folacin is involved in almost every aspect of the replication process. Dietary sources of folacin are few and unreliable. Leafy green vegetables, the best source, lose up to 80 percent of their vitamin content during storage and cooking. As many as 60 percent of pregnant women studied have low serum folate levels, although few of them show deficiency symptoms, notably megaloblastic anemia. It is possible that pregnancy hormones interfere with folacin absorption and thus account for the prevalence of low serum levels. At present, there is no evidence that this common deficiency has any adverse effect on the course or outcome of pregnancy. Since the consequences of major deficiency could be serious, however, the National Research Council recommends oral supplements to provide 200 to 400 micrograms daily in the last half of pregnancy.

Also, supplementation with vitamin B_{12} should be considered by strict vegetarian women who become pregnant. As discussed in Chapter 7, there is a potential problem of severe deficiency among the nursing infants of such mothers. Early treatment of affected infants will reverse infant symptoms, but if the mother's diet is supplemented during pregnancy and lactation the problem is avoided altogether.

Folacin, vitamin B_{12}, and for non-milk drinkers vitamin D are the only vitamins for which supplementation should be considered. Although the allowance for ascorbic acid is increased during pregnancy because of fetal needs, supplementation is not desirable, and the recommended amount can easily be provided by dietary sources. Overdosage in pregnancy may cause infantile "rebound" scurvy. High vitamin C levels during gestation may cause fetal adaptation in the form of rapid catabolism of the excess. When the infant's ascorbic acid supply is decreased after birth, the high catabolic rate is still maintained, at least temporarily, and so the normally necessary quantity of the vitamin is not retained by the newborn. Since there is no significant proof of advantageous effects of high levels of vitamin C that would justify this risk to the infant, megadoses during pregnancy are definitely not advised.

The fat-soluble vitamins A, D, E, and K are also essential components of the diet of the pregnant woman. Vitamin A is necessary for the development of skin and epithelial tissue lining internal organs, while vitamin D is required for the healthy development of bones and teeth. Vitamin E helps to protect cell membranes and Vitamin K is important for the blood clotting process. Because these are present in maternal body stores, and can easily be provided in diet, supplementation is usually unnecessary. It is, in fact, ill-advised, particularly for women who drink vitamin D-fortified milk. Excesses of vitamins A and D have produced symptoms in laboratory animals and, although the implications for human beings are not clear, there is no need to run any risk. Excess vitamin D may actually produce rebound hypercalcemia in the newborn (Pitkin, 1976) and should be avoided. There is no evidence that fetuses (or their mothers) benefit from supplemental vitamin E; vitamin K is routinely administered to newborn infants.

Vitamins ingested in excess of physiological need no longer have a vitamin effect. Therapeutic doses of any substance are not warranted unless medically prescribed. Self-dosing with an excess of vitamins is no different from self-dosing with aspirin, tranquilizers, or any other substance. In pregnancy, as at any other time, a well-balanced diet is the best protection against nutrient deficiencies.

Minerals

Table 12-3 indicates increases in the recommended allowances for the minerals calcium, phosphorus, iodine, iron, magnesium, and zinc. Other trace minerals such as chromium and copper are important in reproduction, but needs for them in human pregnancy have not been evaluated, and they can be provided by consuming a diversified diet.

CALCIUM. Calcium is a vital structural component of the fetal skeleton, which will contain an average of 27.4 grams of calcium at birth (Pitkin, 1976). Most skeletal calcification takes place in the third trimester, but the calcium RDA for pregnant women has been set a constant 1,200 milligrams per day, the amount found in one quart of milk. Milk products such as yogurt, cheese, and ice cream contain lesser amounts, but meals can be planned to meet the requirement from a balance of milk and milk products. However, women who do not or cannot consume milk or milk products must rely on other sources. Since calcium present in plant sources may not be totally available for absorption, strict vegetarians may require calcium supplementation. If milk intake is clearly adequate, calcium supplementation is not necessary.

PHOSPHORUS. Phosphorus activates glucose and glycogen so that they can produce energy, aids in the transformation of many B vitamins to coenzymes, and is necessary for skeletal growth. The naturally high levels of phosphorus in animal protein foods, dairy products, snack items, and carbonated beverages ensure an adequate phosphorus supply in every diet to meet the RDA of 1,200 milligrams during pregnancy.

IODINE. As a component of thyroid hormone, iodine is essential for the regulation of basal metabolism. The RDA for iodine (175 μg) is easily supplied by the use of iodized salt; but women who avoid iodized salt—perhaps by using only sea salt or by adhering to a sodium-restricted diet—must rely on other sources (see Chapter 8).

IRON. Unfortunately, iron requirements are not as easily met. Iron is a major raw material for maintaining red blood cell synthesis in both the mother and the fetus. About 290 milligrams (mg) of iron are required for additional hemoglobin as the mother's blood volume expands. Another 134 mg are stored in the placenta, and a final 246 mg goes to the blood and body stores of the fetus. This can be a significant drain on the mother's iron stores; for even when they are adequate at conception, iron utilization increases dramatically. Some help comes from the gastrointestinal system, where slowed motility increases iron absorption from its usual 10 percent to approximately 30 percent of dietary intake. And about 120 mg of iron which would ordinarily be lost in menstruation is conserved during pregnancy. Still, the mother often comes up short—short of iron and short of breath. Her reduced hemoglobin concentration means that her body must increase its cardiac output to meet its oxygen needs and those of the fetus. So much extra cardiac work is physiologically fatiguing, and in extreme instances of severe iron deficiency, reduced hemoglobin levels can lead to cardiac arrest or death from hemorrhage during delivery.

As pointed out in Chapter 8, it is not easy to satisfy the normal iron requirements of women even with an otherwise nutritionally balanced diet. Organ meats, some shellfish, and prune juice are the only iron-rich foods. Foods normally consumed in the typical American diet yield only 6 mg of iron or 1,000 kilocalories. To meet even the RDA for nonpregnant women (18 mg), 3,000 kilocalories would have to be consumed—an unrealistically high figure even for pregnant women. And because most women have minimal iron stores and run the risk of developing anemia, the RDA during pregnancy is greater than 18 mg. Therefore, iron supplementation during pregnancy is routinely prescribed. The provision of 30 to 60 mg of iron per day (usually as 150 to 300 mg of ferrous sulfate) is recommended throughout pregnancy and for several months following delivery.

SODIUM. Although there is no RDA for sodium, recommended intakes of this mineral during pregnancy have been a source of controversy. Previous knowledge suggested that pregnancy is accompanied by sodium retention, associated with fluid accumulation, hypertension, and resultant toxemia. Therefore sodium was frequently restricted. However, recent research indicates that pregnancy is a salt-*losing* condition that may result in decreased body fluid volume and subsequent constriction of blood vessels if sodium is not provided in adequate amounts by the diet. Consequently, proponents of this theory suggest that salt intake should be *increased* during pregnancy. Pregnant women are currently advised to salt their food "to taste," to trust the body's normal renal mechanisms to maintain the optimal sodium level, and not to restrict dietary salt.

FLUID. Finally, pregnant women should maintain adequate fluid balance by consuming six to eight glasses of beverages per day. Diuretics should not be used, since they deplete the body of fluid, sodium, and frequently potassium.

General Nutrient Recommendations

When nutrients are considered individually in terms of requirements during pregnancy, the problem of meeting needs through diet seems overwhelming. But a normal and diverse diet that meets the somewhat expanded energy requirements of this period will provide adequate amounts of almost all nutrients. Folate, B_{12}, vitamin D, calcium, and iron present special problems for some women, and supplementation may be advised. Other nutrients that may be underconsumed during pregnancy, especially by adolescents, are zinc, magnesium, and vitamin B_6. Since there are abundant dietary sources of these (see Chapters 7 and 8), supplementation is usually unnecessary. Although concern is often expressed for protein and vitamin A levels, no underconsumption of these nutrients has been documented in the United States (King and Charlet, 1978). It should be kept in mind that the precise requirements for all essential nutrients are not yet known; therefore, diversity in the diet is especially crucial during pregnancy to increase the probability that all nutrients needed by the mother and fetus will be ingested in adequate amounts.

FOOD PATTERNS DURING PREGNANCY

Many women experience a significant change in their eating habits even before their first prenatal visit to a physician. Often a sudden aversion to usual early-morning favorites, such as coffee or bacon, is the first inkling of pregnancy. By the time that aversion had been translated into actual nausea or vomiting (the familiar "morning sickness"), the diagnosis was established, and the newly expectant mother was well on her way to new eating patterns. Typically, with little to eat in the morning, women reach lunch time with a ravenous appetite that is still strong at the dinner hour. The result is likely to be increased energy intake and concomitant excess weight gain in early pregnancy.

In the first trimester, the mother's increased tissue development and blood supply is the major component of weight gained. In addition, most pregnant women have a tendency to store additional body fat. This may be of concern to many weight-conscious women, but the fat deposition of early pregnancy has a purpose in the final weeks, when appetite often decreases just as fetal nutrient and energy needs sharply increase. The fat deposits of early pregnancy provide a literal and figurative "cushion" for baby to fall back upon.

Women who may have a problem regulating weight gain could add protein from relative low-calorie foods such as chicken, fish, and legumes, rather than the higher-calorie beef choices. Other good sources of protein include eggs, skim milk, and cheese. Women who are strict vegetarians should include daily an additional serving of a complementary protein combination such as legumes and rice, or peanut butter and whole grain bread, to assure supplies of the essential amino acids. Foods with high complex-carbohydrate content, such as bread, cereal, rice, and noodles, provide 2 or more grams of protein per serving; potatoes and many other vegetables are also moderate protein sources. Table 12-4 lists the foods that are needed during pregnancy to meet the nutritional demands of both mother and infant.

TABLE 12-4
Foods Needed during Pregnancy

Food	Daily amount
Milk	1 qt (or equivalent)
Eggs	1–2
Meat	2 servings (liver often)
Cheese	1–2 servings, additional snacks
Grains (whole, enriched)	4–5 slices or servings
Legumes, nuts	1–2 servings a week
Green and yellow fruits, vegetables	1–2 servings
Citrus fruit	2
Additional vitamin C foods	Frequently, as desired
Other vegetables and fruits	1–2 servings
Butter, fortified margarine	2 tbsp (or as needed)
Other foods: grains, fruits, vegetables, other proteins	As needed for energy and added vitamins and minerals
Fluid	6–8 glasses (including milk)

*Source: Adapted from S. Williams, *Handbook of maternal and infant nutrition* (Berkeley, Calif.: SRW Productions, 1976).

Dietary Cravings and Aversions

Many pregnant women experience a strong change in their food likes and dislikes. In one study 30 percent of women who regularly consumed coffee and/or alcoholic beverages before becoming pregnant found that these had little appeal during pregnancy. The number of women citing nausea or loss of a "taste" for the beverage as the reason for their aversion far outweighed the number who reduced intakes out of concern for their health or that of the fetus (Hook, 1978).

Cravings for food were more frequent than aversions and were reported for ice cream, chocolate and other candies, sweetened baked goods, and fruit juices. Fried meats and poultry, vegetables, and foods with oregano-seasoned sauces were the most common aversions in this study (Hook, 1978).

It has been hypothesized that cravings in pregnancy are a response to the increased need of the mother; the number of women in the above-cited study reporting an increased desire for ice cream and milk would seemingly support this. However, while approximately 50 percent of these women increased their intake of milk and 21 percent increased ice cream consumption, most women did not *crave* these and a few even developed aversions to them (Hook, 1978). It has also been suggested that food aversions have a biochemical basis and develop in reaction to substances released by the fetus. Research to confirm these hypotheses remains to be done. But many women will simply say, "Coffee didn't smell good any more," or "I just lost my appetite for steak." With all of the other physiological changes taking place during these eventful nine months, it is little wonder that a woman's senses of smell and taste are altered as well.

Cravings for nonfood items during pregnancy have also been described. The intentional consumption of nonfood items is known as **pica,** and it has been documented since ancient times. It is found among males and females, nonpregnant and pregnant, throughout the world and may involve the consumption of ice, various clay and earth substances, soot, wax, and even shoe polish.

It has been suggested that pica is a response to a mineral imbalance. However, studies have shown that pica may be practiced by individuals who are not nutritionally deprived. Another explanation is that clay or starch consumption may reduce nausea. The consumption of clay, laundry starch, and similar materials by southern American black women, especially during pregnancy, is a well-known phenomenon. It is clear that whatever factors may be involved, there is a large cultural, traditional component to the development of this habit (Grivetti, 1978).

SPECIAL NUTRITIONAL CONCERNS DURING PREGNANCY

For the vast majority of women, pregnancy is medically uneventful. Although there are certain predictable and inevitable discomforts, severe problems are rare in women who receive good prenatal care and who have a history of nutritional health. Too many women still do not receive adequate prenatal care, however, and many others who regularly see a physician neglect to follow nutritional advice even when it is given. At greatest risk for complications are women who are under 15 years of age; are under- or overweight; have had three pregnancies within two years; have a history of poor obstetrical performance; are economically deprived; are heavy smokers, drinkers, or drug takers; or have a chronic systemic disease such as diabetes or hypertension and require a special therapeutic diet (Task Force on Nutrition, 1978).

Nutritional Anemias

Anemia, a significant decrease in hemoglobin and red blood cells, is the most common example of a particular nutritional concern. It is diagnosed by blood tests that measure the concentration of hemoglobin and the volume (size) and number of red blood cells. Normal values for hemoglobin in healthy young women average 13.7 g/dl, with a range of 12 to 15.4 g/dl (Scott and Pritchard, 1967). But because of the increased plasma volume that occurs during pregnancy, a "physiological anemia" develops, in which a hemoglobin level of 11 g/dl is considered acceptable. A value lower than this is indicative of true anemia in pregnancy.

Anemia may be due to nutrient deficiencies (iron, protein, vitamin B_6, vitamin B_{12}, or folic acid) or to medical or hereditary conditions. Symptoms include fatigue, weakness, loss of appetite, edema, and shortness of breath. Extreme cases pose the risk of maternal and fetal mortality.

Iron deficiency accounts for more than 75 percent of the acquired anemias of pregnancy, and folic acid deficiency accounts for much of the rest. Anemias due to both of these causes can be easily treated, and even more easily avoided, through adequate intake of appropriate foods and/or supplements. Again, prior nutritional status markedly influences the probability of anemia.

Pregnancy Toxemias

Toxemia (preeclampsia and eclampsia) is a term that describes a potentially life-threatening condition occurring in a small percentage of pregnant women, usually after the twentieth week of pregnancy. Most important symptoms of preeclampsia are sudden onset of hypertension, proteinuria, and generalized edema leading to dramatic weight gain. Dizziness, headache, visual disturbances, nausea, and vomiting may also be present. When this constellation of symptoms is complicated by convulsions, eclampsia is diagnosed.

By definition, the word *toxemia* means "blood toxins," but despite significant amounts of research, no such toxins have been identified. It was once thought, for example, that sodium was the culprit because of its effects of fluid retention. The typical antidote—diuresis—unfortunately caused even more deleterious effects than the original problem. Another theory held that excess weight gain was at fault, and energy-restricted diets were recommended. But most studies do not support this hypothesis.

Other theories have been proposed, but as yet none has been proven. Because in the United States toxemia is most prevalent in low-income, nonwhite populations known to receive poor diets and poor medical care and to enter pregnancy in a debilitated state, the presently accepted approach to preventing toxemia is comprehensive prenatal care, including education about a balanced diet, adequate in all nutrients and energy content. Prenatal nutritional counseling, nutrient supplementation if needed, guidance in dealing with life stresses, and careful monitoring of pregnancy through weigh-ins and blood tests should be provided for all pregnant women and especially those from high-risk populations. Sudden weight gain, signaling edema, calls for immediate intervention. Fortunately, most cases of preeclampsia do not result in eclampsia. Because of the medical risks to both mother and infant, hospitalization and bed rest are required for eclampsia and delivery by cesarean section is usually indicated.

Gastrointestinal Disturbances

About two-thirds of pregnant women experience a nauseous feeling on arising, even before their first menstrual period is missed. Despite some assertions to the contrary, there are clear physiological reasons for this "morning sickness," related primarily to the hormonal changes of early pregnancy. Anxiety and poor dietary habits may also contribute. In some cases, morning sickness is not confined to the morning, but may recur throughout the day. The best treatment is small, frequent meals consisting of dry, easily digested, high-energy foods. Avoiding highly spiced and fatty foods at mealtime also seems to help. Drinking liquids before or after, rather than with, meals is often helpful as well. The problem usually disappears by the end of the first trimester. When it does not, or when severe persistent vomiting develops, hospitalization for intravenous feeding may be necessary to prevent dehydration. Fortunately, this is quite rare (Fairweather, 1978).

Gastrointestinal problems of one kind or another are almost universal among pregnant women. Among them are constipation due to decreased intestinal motility and as a side effect of iron supplements in some women, heartburn and abnormal fullness caused by the pressure of the enlarging uterus crowding against the stomach. All of these gastrointestinal ailments are amenable to nutritional correction. Increased intake of fluid, dietary fiber, and "natural" laxatives such as prunes and figs will do much to improve local intestinal complaints. Smaller and more frequent meals and thorough chewing will mitigate other problems. Such casual remedies as baking soda, "candy-type" antacids, and the entire gamut of nonprescription medications often resorted to for pain, tension, and sleeplessness should be avoided, as should laxative preparations in general.

Other Considerations

The thalidomide tragedy of the early 1960s awakened many physicians and patients to the risks of medication in pregnancy. Thalidomide, a widely used hypnotic (sleep-producing) agent, was often given to ease the insomnia of early pregnancy. Unfortunately, this was most ill-chosen timing; thalidomide impaired the development of fetal limbs that were forming at that precise

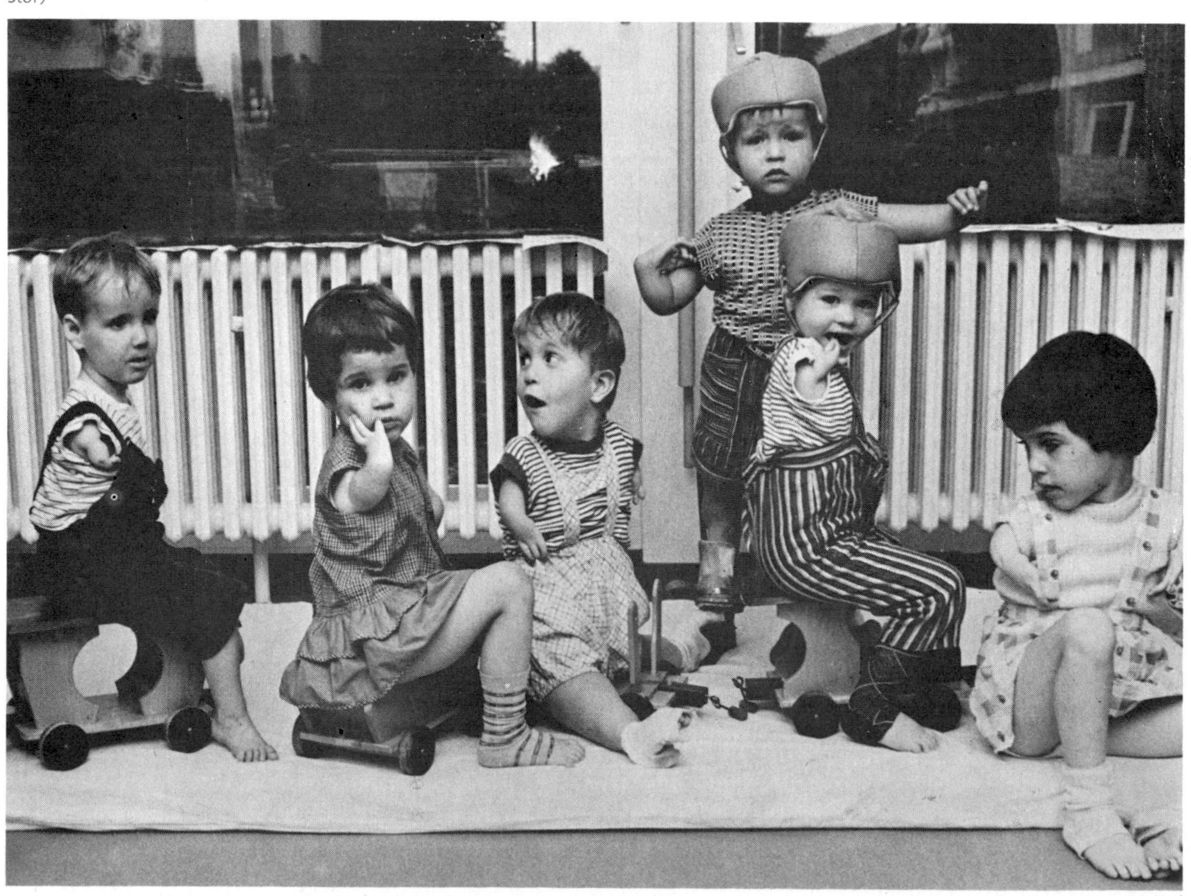

Children born to mothers who took Thalidomide during pregnancy, at an Orthopedic Clinic at the University of Heidelberg, Germany. The children, who learn through play how to make use of their stunted or artificial arms and legs, must wear helmets to protect their heads in case they fall. (Stern (Doring)/Black Star)

time. The birth of thousands of limbless or otherwise malformed "thalidomide babies," now young adults, alerted researchers and physicians to the possible consequences of casual drug-taking by women who are or may be pregnant.

MEDICATION. Even common aspirin may cause fetal damage. The same medications that may be harmless at other times may have deleterious effects on the absorption, metabolism, placental transfer, and fetal utilization of nutrients when taken during pregnancy. (Look at the labels on many over-the-counter preparations. You'll be surprised to see how many say "Not recommended for use by women who are or may be pregnant.") In fact, *no* medication should be taken by the pregnant woman without prescription. Pregnant women should, furthermore, question their physicians about medications given them. But all too often, the woman herself begs for "something so I can sleep" or "just a temporary prescription until my headaches go away." This practice should be avoided: The potential risks are too great.

CAFFEINE. Caffeine is probably the most popular and most readily available drug in the world. It occurs not only in coffee, but in tea, chocolate, cola drinks, and over-the-counter medications. Caffeine crosses the placenta, and researchers are still exploring its possible effects on the fetus. Although excessive caffeine intakes in pregnancy have been linked with cleft palate, congenital malformations, miscarriages, infertility, breech presentations during labor, and other pregnancy problems (*Nutrition Action*, 1978), supporting evidence is indeed scanty. Whether excessive caffeine intake has a demonstrated adverse effect on humans, and particularly pregnant women and their unborn children, remains to be proven.

PSYCHOACTIVE (MOOD-ALTERING) SUBSTANCES. Although there is little available data on the effects of marijuana in pregnancy, any type of smoking can affect blood carbon dioxide levels and possibly impair fetal oxygen supplies. We cannot, on the basis of present evidence, be certain that marijuana does not have long-term effects on the smoker or her babies. The active ingredient in marijuana is able to cross the placenta (Harbison and Mantilla-Plata, 1972), and reports that chronic long-term marijuana use in young adult men produces breast enlargement (Harmon and Aliapoulios, 1972) and lowered plasma testosterone levels (Kolodny et al., 1974) suggest that marijuana may indeed produce hormonal changes in the developing fetus as well. The subsequent effects are as yet unknown, but they may in fact be significant.

In addition, marijuana is known to be an appetite depressant, which may interfere with optimal food intake during pregnancy. Finally, marijuana smoke contains a known pharmacological agent—tetrahydrocannabinol, the active isomer of *Cannabis*, which is used medically as a sedative and analgesic. Its central nervous system effects are well known to satisfied users: euphoria, hallucinations, and other mental changes. How many of those effects, and frequent unwanted side effects, may be due to unknown additives or fillers in any particular marijuana supply cannot be evaluated.

The fetal effects of heroin are well known. Heroin addicts deliver low birth weight babies who are themselves addicted and must go through painful

PERSPECTIVE ON
Pregnancy in Adolescence

The risk of pregnancy complications and fetal and maternal morbidity and mortality are increased for mothers still in their teens. There are 30 percent more low birth weight infants born to all teenagers than to women from 20 to 24 years of age and more than twice as many underweight babies born to adolescents 15 years and younger (Stickle and Ma, 1975). Of babies born to mothers under 15, 6 percent of all firstborns and nearly 10 percent of second-borns die in the first year of life (USDHEW 1973a), and those that survive are from two to four times more likely to have neurological defects than babies born to women aged 20 to 24 (USDHEW, 1973b).

The social disabilities of teenage parenthood are equally dramatic. Approximately one-third (300,000) of all pregnancies of women 19 years and younger end in abortion, half of them performed on women 17 years or less (Abortion Surveillance, 1977). The overwhelming majority of teenage pregnancies occur out of wedlock; if the young parents do marry during the pregnancy, there is an estimated 50 percent chance that the marriage will end in divorce (McAnarney, 1978). In the meantime, schooling is disrupted; families are disturbed and disrupted; the potential earning capacity of the young mother (and father) is sharply reduced; a cycle of dependence on public assistance may be perpetuated or begun; and the resulting baby is likely to have poor medical care, poor emotional care, and/or spend years in a public institution or a succession of foster homes.

EFFECT OF MATERNAL AGE ON MORTALITY

Age of Mother	Maternal Deaths per 100,000 Deliveries
Under 15	46.7
15–19	11.9
20–24	9.2
25–29	13.1
30–34	26.2
35–39	44.2
40–44	78.5
45 and over	154.5

Source: Adapted from G. Stickle and P. Ma. Pregnancy in adolescents: Scope of the problem. Reprinted from *Contemporary Ob/Gyn* (New York: McGraw-Hill, 1975).

EFFECT OF MATERNAL AGE ON INFANT BIRTH WEIGHT

Age of Mother	Percent of Infants of Low Birth Weight (<2,500 grams)
Under 15	16
15–19	10
20–29	6.5
30–39	7
40 and over	9

Source: Adapted from G. Stickle and P. Ma. Pregnancy in adolescents: Scope of the problem. Reprinted from *Contemporary Ob/Gyn* (New York: McGraw-Hill, 1975).

The single leading contributor to this host of medical and social problems is the age of the mother at conception. During most of the teen years, the girl's physiological, educational, and social development are still incomplete. Although physical growth and sexual maturation proceed at varied rates in different individuals (Chapter 13), it is generally true that growth is not completed until four years after menarche (onset of menstruation) in the adolescent girl. Today, menarche occurs at about 12½ years of age on average, earlier than in previous generations; the younger the teenager is at conception, the greater is the risk of damage to both her and her infant. Girls who become pregnant during this developmental period are at biological risk because their bodies are still anatomically and physiologically immature. During this period of rapid growth, the young woman's own body requires increased amounts of nutrients and energy. If pregnancy occurs at this time, fetal nutrient needs are met to whatever extent is possible at the expense of the young mother (McGanity, 1978).

Complicating these factors, the pregnant teenager is more likely to be a member of a lower socioeconomic group, having a history of suboptimal nutritional status and lack of adequate medical care.

Even more damaging, the vast majority of such pregnancies are neither planned nor desired. In many cases, the fact of pregnancy is denied for several months until even abortion is not a viable alternative. During this denial period, most probably the worried teenager restricts her food intake, in the hopes that she will not become heavier. With typical teenage concern for fashion and figure, she may fight the increasing pangs of hunger in efforts to maintain her slender curves. By the time her pregnancy can no longer be hidden or denied and she is at last seen by an obstetrician, it may be too late to offset the damage to her health and to the development of her child.

Problems are not, however, inevitable or insuperable for the pregnant teenager. It has been shown that those who receive adequate prenatal medical attention do not as a group have any greater incidence of complications than do more mature child bearing women, and they generally have a lower rate of complications than do women over 40 (Battaglia et al., 1963). But two-thirds of teenage pregnancies and 90 percent of out-of-wedlock pregnant teenagers do not benefit from any prenatal care (Monthly Vital Statistics Report, 1977).

ESTIMATES OF DIETARY NEEDS OF PREGNANT TEENAGERS

Nutrient	Recommended intake for pregnant teenagers
Energy (kcal/kg)	45
Protein (g/kg)	1.3
Calcium (g)	1.6
Phosphorus (g)	1.6
Iron (mg)	18[a]
Magnesium (mg)	450
Iodine (μg)	140
Zinc (mg)	20
Vitamin A (IU)	5,000
Vitamin D (IU)	400
Vitamin E (IU)	14
Ascorbic acid (mg)	60
Niacin (mg)	16
Riboflavin (mg)	1.7
Thiamin (mg)	1.4
Folacin (mg)	0.8
Vitamin B_6 (mg)	2.5
Vitamin B_{12} (μg)	4

[a] Supplemental iron recommended for pregnant teenagers.
Source: Adapted from J. C. King and H. N. Jacobson. Nutrition and pregnancy in adolescence. In *The teenage pregnant girl*, ed. J. Zackler and W. Brandstadt (Charles C Thomas, Springfield, Ill., 1975).

Unfortunately, the penalties for not obtaining medical care fall more heavily upon the newborn children than upon their teenage mothers. The postnatal environment of an infant whose birth was unplanned, unwanted, and financially disastrous is unlikely to improve the prognosis for overcoming any initial medical handicaps. Those who survive the first year of life are not likely to thrive in the typical environment of unstable family life, unemployment, and welfare dependence that often follows teenage pregnancy. Eight out of ten teenagers who bear children by age 17 never finish high school and are unlikely to find remunerative employment—even if they can find a solution to the problem of child care during working hours.

It seems obvious that prevention of the undesired problem of teenage pregnancy is preferable to perpetuation of the cycle of socioeconomic problems. Education for responsible sexuality and increased availability of contraceptives and abortion are proposed as answers. But sex education courses in the schools meet with resistance in many communities and are greeted with snickers by many students. And this high-risk age group has proved unwilling to accept birth control procedures for a variety of reasons (Zelnick and Kantner, 1977). For the present, then, provision of early medical care and attention to nutritional needs represent the best hopes for teenage mothers and their babies. The pregnant teenager must be encouraged to eat balanced, regular meals, to achieve an adequate weight gain (2,400 to 2,700 kcal per day is the usual energy intake range), and take supplements when indicated. Health care professionals should pay special attention to ensure that these young patients follow the dietary advice they receive and make appropriate adjustments if resistance is encountered. Follow-up is especially important for young teenagers who enter pregnancy in a poor nutritional state, who have been on slimming regimens, and whose low socioeconomic status makes them particularly vulnerable to continued nutritional neglect.

withdrawal immediately after birth when their "regular supply" is cut off. Addicted mothers, moreover, are not likely to obtain prenatal medical care or to be conscious of the nutritional content of their diets. The combined risks to the innocent, newborn "bystander" are hard to exaggerate.

ALCOHOL. Recent studies indicate that as little as 1 ounce of alcohol per day may increase the risks of stillbirth, low birth weight, physical malformations, poor sucking ability, and numerous medical complications in the postnatal period (Ouellette et al., 1977). Damage to the fetus seems to be correlated both with the amount of alcohol intake and with how effectively the mother's body metabolizes and excretes that alcohol. Thus, it is possible that risks may be higher for some moderate drinkers than for some heavier drinkers.

Other studies on known alcoholics indicate that total alcohol consumption may not be as important as the maximum concentrations that may be reached during critical periods of infant development (USDHEW, 1978). When these "binge levels" do impinge on critical periods, Fetal Alcohol Syndrome (FAS) is the result. It is expressed in widespread neuropathologic malformations in the newborn, caused by failure of fetal brain cells to migrate to their proper location. The current incidence of FAS makes it the third leading cause of birth defects associated with mental retardation and the only one of these leading causes that is preventable. Animal studies suggest that daily consumption of more than 3 ounces may put the infant at risk for FAS. It is not necessary, however, for the pregnant woman to give up social drinking altogether during nine months; moderation is the key.

SMOKING. Numerous studies have indicated that women who smoke have a higher rate of spontaneous abortion and low birth weight babies than do nonsmokers, along with a greater likelihood of complications during labor and delivery, which is often premature. The more a woman smokes, the smaller her baby is likely to be, and those babies never seem to catch up in growth. Some of them don't have the chance—babies of smokers are more likely to die at birth or during the first year of life. The infants of women who smoke less than a pack a day have a 20 percent greater risk of mortality in the first month of life, while the infants of women who smoke more than a pack a day have a 35 percent greater risk. Children whose mothers smoke are more likely to have neurological defects, be hyperactive, and to have psychological and learning difficulties (USDHEW, 1979).

Although many of the ill effects due to smoking have been blamed on its major pharmacological component, nicotine—well known to be a nervous system stimulant at smoking dosages—the risks of smoking during pregnancy appear to be more closely related to the carbon monoxide present in cigarette smoke. The oxygen-carrying capacity of both maternal and fetal blood supplies is diminished because carbon monoxide replaces oxygen in the mother's blood, thus reducing the oxygen supply to her growing fetus. Some recent research indicates that compensation may occur in fetal red cells; postnatal hemoglobin and hematocrit levels in 10,399 neonates were found to be significantly higher for babies born to smokers than to nonsmokers (Garn et al., 1978). Nevertheless, this compensation is insufficient to prevent the fetal abnormalities that are so frequently reported.

In addition to the effects on blood oxygenation, the fetal malnutrition associated with cigarette smoking may be partially mediated by nutritional factors. Clinical and epidemiological studies have established that carbohydrate and protein metabolism is impaired in heavy smokers and that plasma levels of ascorbic acid and vitamins B_{12} and B_6 are decreased as well (USDHEW, 1979). These data have clear implications for pregnant women in particular.

LACTATION

The nine months of pregnancy are the prelude not only to childbirth, but to the nutritionally important period to come. The umbilical cord may be cut, but the nurturing bond between mother and child is not severed. A new system is ready to take over: the lactating breast.

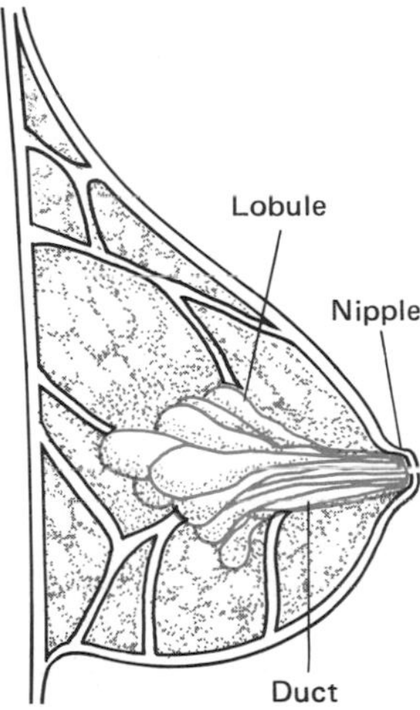

FIGURE 12-3
Development of the Mammary Gland during Pregnancy
Source: Adapted from F. L. Strand, *Physiology: A regulatory systems approach* (New York: Macmillan, 1978), p. 536.

Physiology

Many of the physiological changes occurring in the mother during pregnancy are preparation for lactation. During the first and second trimester, terminal tubules connected to the mammary milk ducts proliferate and group together to form what are known as lobules or acinar structures, in which milk will be produced (see Figure 12-3). Whether the breast is large or small, it will contain from 15 to 20 of these ducts, which connect the milk-producing centers to the nipples from which milk will be released. This is all the "equipment" that is required for successful nursing. Neither breast size nor shape has any influence on the ability of women to nurse. Almost all women who want to breast-feed can readily do so. In the next chapter we will examine the effects of breast-feeding on infants; our concern in this chapter is for the development of the capability for lactation in pregnancy.

Microscopic studies of breast tissue have shown that the milk is produced in secretory (alveolar) cells which synthesize lactose, the predominant carbohydrate in milk. Progesterone, the primary pregnancy hormone, inhibits lactose production, thereby preventing significant milk accumulation during pregnancy. After birth, however, progesterone levels fall, while levels of prolactin, the lactation hormone, rise, and the mammary alveolar cells go into full operation (see Figure 12-4). Prolactin is released by the hypothalamus in response to suckling by the infant. Suckling also stimulates production of oxytocin from the posterior pituitary gland. Circulation of oxytocin causes the musclelike cells in the breast to contract, which propels milk through the ducts for release through the nipple.

In addition to lactose, three major milk proteins are synthesized by the alveolar cells: casein, α-lactalbumin, and β-lactalbumin. Most of the amino acids contained in these proteins are taken up directly from the mother's plasma, although some of the nonessential amino acids are synthesized in the alveolar cells.

Composition of Human Milk

Constituent	Percent
Water	88
Lactose	6.8
Protein	3
Fat	3
Salts	trace

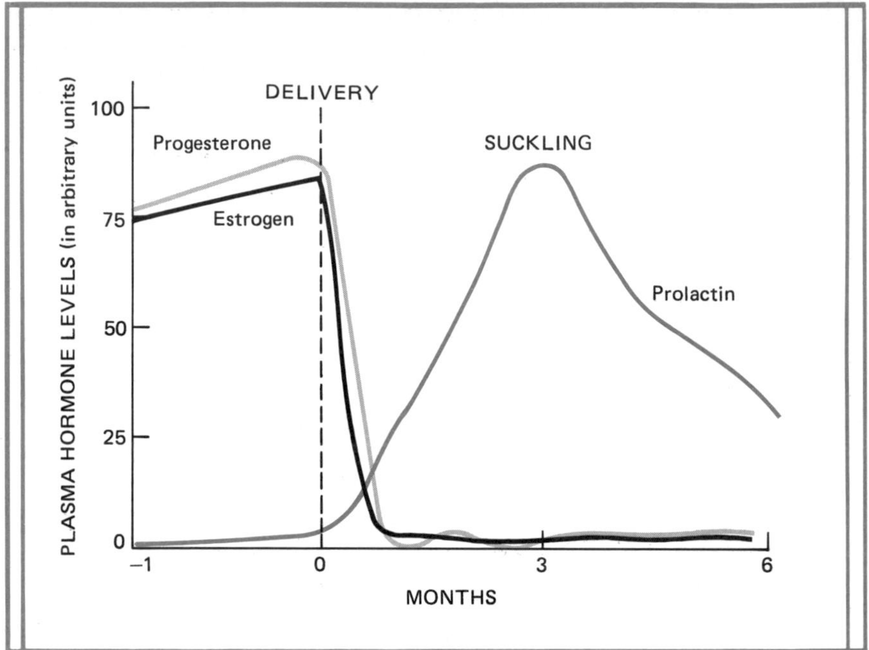

FIGURE 12-4
Hormone Production before and after Delivery

Source: Adapted from F. L. Strand, *Physiology: A regulatory systems approach* (New York: Macmillan, 1978), p. 537.

Nutritional Considerations

When she starts to nurse, the new mother has about 2 to 4 kilograms (about 4.5 to 9 lb) of new fat stores deposited during pregnancy, which serve as a kind of back-up energy supply. These fat stores may be mobilized to provide approximately 200 to 300 kcal per day for about three months. It has been calculated that, because human breast milk contains approximately 70 kcal/100 ml and maternal efficiency in converting stored energy to milk energy is at least 80 percent, the mother will need approximately 90 additional kcal for every 100 ml of milk she must produce. Thus, for 850 ml of milk, the average amount produced each day after lactation is established, the nursing mother needs nearly 800 kcal above her normal daily requirements. With 200 to 300 kcal available from existing fat stores, at least for the first three months, that will mean an additional 500 kcal per day that must be provided by their diet, or 200 kcal more than during pregnancy (see Table 12-3). If lactation continues beyond three months, energy intake must be increased by an additional 200 to 300 kcal per day (Pitkin, 1976).

A mother who does not nurse will not need this additional energy intake, and she will have to lose the accumulated adipose tissue as well. As the woman resumes her prepregnancy eating pattern and normal—or probably increased—activity following childbirth, extra fat stores will gradually be depleted.

Because the alveolar cells synthesize milk protein, and also utilize some protein from maternal plasma, the RDA for protein is 20 grams higher for lactating women than for nonlactating women (see Table 12-3). Since there is no lack of protein in the diet of most Americans, there is little concern about protein deficiency in lactating women in the United States. Even in countries where protein-energy malnutrition is common, however, protein levels in milk are not reduced, although total milk volume may be greatly diminished (Sims, 1978). The protein content of human milk remains remarkably constant despite the variations in maternal food intakes, leading to the conclusion that the essential amino acids are supplied from maternal stores when they are lacking in the mother's diet.

Breast milk also contains significant amounts of fat, mostly in the form of triglycerides, but also including small amounts of phospholipids, cholesterol, and free fatty acids. The levels of all lipids except fatty acids in breast milk appear to be independent of levels in the maternal bloodstream. Like carbohydrate and protein, the lipid content of breast milk is maintained even at the expense of maternal stores (Mellies et al., 1978).

Breast milk also contains fat-soluble vitamins A and E and small amounts of vitamin D, and calcium, iron, copper, fluoride, and other minerals. Addition of these vitamins to the mother's diet during lactation does not appear to increase their levels in breast milk. In contrast, maternal serum levels of the water-soluble vitamins and of some trace minerals are reflected in the nutritional composition of breast milk (Sims, 1978). In particular, breast milk content of ascorbic acid, thiamin, and riboflavin most closely reflect intake levels; pantothenic acid, pyridoxine (vitamin B_6), biotin, folic acid, and vitamin B_{12} content also relate to the mothers' dietary intake. The implications for cigarette smokers should be remembered.

Excessive intakes of these nutrients are not advantageous and may even be damaging. Megadoses of vitamin B_6 have been shown to suppress the elevated prolactin levels that stimulate milk secretion in the lactating breast (Greentree, 1979), and supplementation with extremely large amounts is not advised. The level of vitamin D in breast milk is not adequate for an infant's needs; supplementation of the infant's diet, not the mother's, is the solution (see Chapter 13).

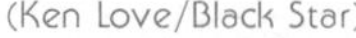
(Ken Love/Black Star)

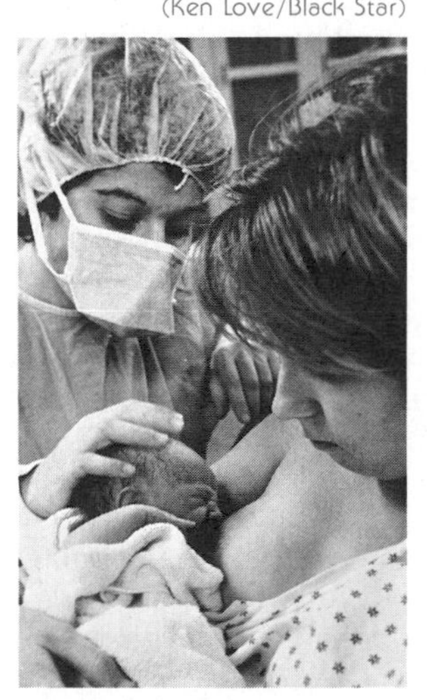

Food Patterns

Milk production is very efficient. Even in mothers with poor nutritional status, milk production is of sufficiently high quality to support a growing infant. For all of the major and many of the minor nutrients, maternal stores can be utilized. The breast milk content of calcium averages 250 to 350 milligrams daily, even when maternal intake is markedly deficient. While beneficial for the infant, significant amounts of the mother's skeletal calcium are mobilized to provide this level (Pitkin, 1976). To prevent their own stores of vital nutrients from being depleted, and to ensure that sufficient amounts of vitamins and trace minerals are available for milk production, nursing mothers require a plentiful, well-balanced diet.

Exactly what should be in that diet, however, is a matter of some debate. A recent study found little specific, well-documented information that might guide nursing mothers to sound diet planning (Sims, 1978). It was found also that physicians' recommendations to them vary widely. Some routinely prescribe nutritional supplements. Some often recommend avoidance of chocolate and spicy foods, but suggest consumption of large quantities of fluids, even including beer and wine.

Some general guidelines have been established, however. The quality of the diet should be similar to that consumed during pregnancy, with additional energy intake to maintain lactation. At least 1 quart of vitamin D-fortified milk, or its equivalent, should be consumed every day, either as a beverage or incorporated into other foods: Vitamin D will increase the maternal utilization of calcium and phosphorus. High-quality protein and liberal amounts of fruits, vegetables, and grain products will ensure adequate provision of essential amino acids, vitamins and minerals. Fluid intake is important—nursing women should consume 2 to 3 quarts of fluid per day. Supplementation practices should parallel those necessary during pregnancy, especially for strict vegetarians. Iron supplementation should be continued for several months for all women, not because of lactation requirements, but to replenish maternal iron reserves which are usually depleted during pregnancy.

Scientific data may be scanty, but nursing mothers have been providing nutritional foundations for their young since mammals appeared on earth some 200 million years ago. The biological innovation has been a success, and the limited number of studies that have been conducted demonstrate the effectiveness of the mechanism by which infant food is produced and delivered.

Some of today's concerns derive from today's living patterns, and they will be further discussed in the next chapter. For example, there is evidence that a mother's high alcohol consumption can affect nursing infants (Binkiewicz et al., 1978). The possibility of contamination of breast milk when the mother is exposed to environmental pollutants such as DDT and polychlorinated biphenyls (PCBs) has also generated some controversy. Although DDT can no longer be used, and PCB levels are decreasing due to federal regulations, they may be present in the water and food supply in some areas where they were once heavily used. Women living in such areas who desire to nurse should consult their state agricultural department and county medical society for advice.

The nursing mother needs no special foods and need avoid no foods. Increased *amounts* of food are needed, however, to provide the energy, protein, calcium and other nutrients that must be used for the infant's milk supply, and the iron to replenish the mother's own depleted reserves. Energy intake should be monitored by the mother's weight status; as the baby grows older and is gradually weaned to other foods, less milk will be taken, and the amount of energy the mother needs will decline. Unless the mother decreases her own energy intake she will experience an undesirable weight gain as lactation diminishes.

Virtually every woman who wants to nurse her baby can do so, but the lifestyle of contemporary American communities does not always facilitate this natural process. Many women have found that a support system such as that offered by the international La Leche League, or by other women who have nursed their babies, helps them to cope with the various psychological and lifestyle problems that arise.

SUMMARY

The complex growth and development process known as pregnancy requires significant amounts of nutrients and energy. Starting with the early developmental stages of blastogenesis and embryonic maturation, nutritional factors can influence the precisely programmed progression from zygote to fully formed infant. The placenta, which develops simultaneously with the embryo, serves as the transfer mechanism for conveying vital nutrients and oxygen from mother to growing fetus. If placental development is impaired, as it may be in the case of chronic maternal protein-energy malnutrition, the fetus will receive less nourishment, leading to possible fetal malnutrition, low birth weight, and subsequent morbidity or mortality.

The placenta is also the primary source of progesterone and estrogen and the unique source of several other hormones. These hormones act primarily on the mother to increase the flexibility of muscle and connective tissue, to increase fluid retention and fat storage, and to expand her blood volume. Other physiological adaptations influence kidney function and intestinal motility.

Although these and other physiological changes increase the demand for nutrients and oxygen, no radical dietary changes are required in pregnancy. If a woman is well nourished before pregnancy, she is likely to remain well nourished during pregnancy. A balanced diet is recommended, with an additional allowance of 300 kilocalories per day. Iron and folate, which are seriously depleted by the demand for increased hemoglobin as the blood volume expands and fetal development proceeds, probably should be provided in the form of supplements. Women who are lactose-intolerant may need a calcium supplement; those who are strict vegetarians should have vitamin B_{12} supplementation and pay particular attention to consumption of complementary protein foods. Women who enter pregnancy without dietary reserves and have a history of poor nutrition should have nutritional consultation, proper diet, and additional supplementation as necessary; such women are at greatest risk of developing complications during pregnancy and delivering low birth weight babies.

The most important indicator of adequate fetal growth is maternal weight gain. A pregnancy weight gain of at least 22 to 27 pounds is both normal and desirable. In the early weeks, weight gain is slow and accounted for mostly by uterine growth and expanded blood volume. During the second trimester, weight gain should average about 1 pound per week, much of it going to the placenta, uterus, and breasts. When the fetus begins to increase its growth in the last trimester, this constant weight gain should continue, even if the mother's appetite and food consumption decrease. Even if a woman is obese, this same pattern and amount of weight gain should be followed to ensure adequate supplies of nutrients and energy for herself and for proper fetal development.

Despite attention to dietary requirements, several nutrition-related complications of pregnancy may occur. Anemia, which causes fatigue, anorexia, edema, and shortness of breath, can be corrected by appropriate dietary supplementation. Pregnancy toxemias are another complication, most frequently seen in low-income populations known to have poor diet and poor medical attention. Although the exact cause and best prevention for pregnancy toxemias are not known, a nutritionally balanced and adequate diet seems to aid in their prevention. Other common, but less-serious, medical concerns of pregnancy include "morning sickness," constipation, and heartburn. In all of these conditions, simple measures usually prove effective. Drugs may be prescribed rarely, but the pregnant woman should never attempt casual self-medication. Medications and other substances—including alcoholic beverages and smoking—may have injurious effects on absorption, metabolism, placental transfer, and fetal utilization of nutrients, and on the development of the fetus.

Nutrient needs during lactation are similar to those of pregnancy, but with additional caloric requirements. Even in a malnourished woman, the quality of milk is usually quite good, but at the expense of her own meager nutrient stores. However, a mother who maintains her own good nutrition will help to maximize the quality and quantity of her milk to meet her baby's needs. Iron supplements should be continued after delivery to replenish maternal reserves.

Additional attention to nutritional needs is required during pregnancy and lactation for certain high-risk groups, including very young (teenage) mothers, diabetics, hypertensives, and others with chronic or genetically transmitted disorders.

BIBLIOGRAPHY

ABORTION SURVEILLANCE. *Annual summary, 1975.* Atlanta: Center for Disease Control, 1977.

ADAMS, S. O., G. D. BARR, AND R. L. HUENEMANN. Effect of nutritional supplementation in pregnancy. I. Outcome of pregnancy. *Journal of the American Dietetic Association* 72:144, 1978a.

ADAMS, S. O., R. L. HUENEMANN, W. H. BRUVOLD, AND G. E. BARR. Effect of nutritional supplementation in pregnancy. II. Effect on diet. *Journal of the American Dietetic Association* 73:630, 1978b.

BATTAGLIA, F. C., T. M. FRAZIER, AND A. E. HELLEGERS. Obstetric and pediatric complications of juvenile pregnancy. *Pediatrics* 32:902, 1963.

BINKIEWICZ, A., M. J. ROBINSON, AND B. SENIOR. Pseudo-Cushing syndrome caused by alcohol in breast milk. *Journal of Pediatrics* 93:965, 1978.

BLACKBURN, M. W., AND D. H. CALLOWAY. Energy expenditure and consumption of mature, pregnant, and lactating women. *Journal of the American Dietetic Association* 69:29, 1976.

COMMITTEE ON MATERNAL NUTRITION, FOOD AND NUTRITION BOARD, NATIONAL RESEARCH COUNCIL. *Maternal nutrition and the course of pregnancy.* Washington, D.C.: National Academy of Sciences, 1970.

FAIRWEATHER, D. V. I. Nausea and vomiting during pregnancy. In *Obstetrics and gynecology annual,* ed. R. M. Wynn. New York: Appleton-Century-Crofts, 1978.

FOOD AND NUTRITION BOARD, NATIONAL RESEARCH COUNCIL. *Recommended Dietary Allowances,* 9th ed. Washington, D.C.: National Academy of Sciences, 1979.

GARN, S. M., H. A. SHAW, AND K. D. MCCABE. Effect of maternal smoking on hemoglobins and hematocrits of the newborn. *American Journal of Clinical Nutrition* 31:557, 1978.

GREENTREE, L. B. Dangers of vitamin B_6 in nursing mothers. *New England Journal of Medicine* 300(3):141, 1979.

GRIVETTI, L. E. Culture, diet, and nutrition: Selected themes and topics. *BioScience* 28(3):171, 1978.

HARBISON, R. D., AND B. MANTILLA-PLATA. Prenatal toxicity, maternal distribution and placental transfer of tetrahydrocannabinol. *Journal of Pharmacology and Experimental Therapeutics* 180:446, 1972.

HARMON, J., AND M. ALIAPOULIOS. Gynecomastia in marihuana users. *New England Journal of Medicine* 287:936, 1972.

HELLER, S., R. M. SALKELD, AND W. F. KORNER. Vitamin B_1 status in pregnancy. *American Journal of Clinical Nutrition* 27:1221, 1974a.

HELLER, S., R. M. SALKELD, AND W. F. KORNER. Riboflavin status in pregnancy. *American Journal of Clinical Nutrition* 27:1125, 1974b.

HOOK, E. B. Dietary cravings and aversions during pregnancy. *American Journal of Clinical Nutrition* 31:1355, 1978.

KING, J. C., AND S. CHARLET. Current concepts in nutrition—Pregnant women and premature infants. *Journal of Nutrition Education* 10(4):158, 1978.

KOLODNY, R. C., W. H. MASTERS, R. M. KOLODNER, AND G. TORO. Depression of plasma testosterone levels after chronic intensive marihuana use. *New England Journal of Medicine* 290:872, 1974.

LECHTIG, A., H. DELGADO, R. LASKY, C. YARBROUGH, R. E. KLEIN, J.-P. HABICHT, AND M. BEHAR. Maternal nutrition and fetal growth in developing countries. *American Journal of Diseases of Childhood* 129:553, 1975.

MCANARNEY, E. R. Adolescent pregnancy—A national priority. *American Journal of Diseases of Children* 132(2):125, 1978.

MCCLAIN, P. E., J. METCOFF, W. M. CROSBY, AND J. P. COSTILOE. Relationship of maternal amino acid profiles at 25 weeks of gestation to fetal growth. *American Journal of Clinical Nutrition* 31:401, 1978.

MCGANITY, W. J. Testimony of William J. McGanity, M.D., Professor and Chairman of the Department of Obstetrics and Gynecology, University of Texas Medical Branch: Hearings before the Nutrition Subcommittee of the Committee on Agriculture, Nutrition, and Forestry. U.S. Senate, 95th Congress, 2nd session, April 4, 1978.

MALONE, J. I. Vitamin passage across the placenta. *Clinical Perinatology* 2:295, 1975.

MELLIES, M. J., T. T. ISHIKAWA, P. GARTSIDE, K. BURTON, J. MACGEE, K. ALLEN, P. M. STEINER, D. BRADY, AND C. J. CLARK. Effects of varying maternal dietary cholesterol and phytosterol in lactating women and their infants. *American Journal of Clinical Nutrition* 31:1347, 1978.

Monthly Vital Statistics Report. Natality statistics from the National Center for Health Statistics: Teenage childbearing: United States, 1966–1975. USDHEW Publication No. (HRA) 77-1120. Vol. 26, No. 5 (Supplement), 1977.

NAEYE, R. L., M. M. DIENER, AND W. S. DELLINGER. Urban poverty: Effects on prenatal nutrition. *Science* 166:1026, 1969.

Nutrition Action. Caffeine: What doctors say. November 1978, p. 8.

OUELLETTE, E. M., H. L. ROSETT, N. P. ROSMAN, AND L. WEINER. Adverse effects on offspring of maternal alcohol abuse during pregnancy. *New England Journal of Medicine* 297(10):528, 1977.

PHILIPPS, C., AND N. E. JOHNSON. The impact of quality of diet and other factors on birth weight of infants. *American Journal of Clinical Nutrition* 30:215, 1977.

PITKIN, R. M. Nutritional support in obstetrics and gynecology. *Clinical Obstetrics and Gynecology* 19(3):489, 1976.

PRIMROSE, T., AND A. HIGGINS. A study of human prepartum nutrition. *Journal of Reproductive Medicine* 7:257, 1971.

SCOTT, D. E., AND J. A. PRITCHARD. Iron deficiency in healthy young college women. *Journal of the American Medical Association* 199:897, 1967.

SIMS, L. S. Dietary status of lactating women. I. Nutrient intake from food and from supplements. *Journal of the American Dietetic Association* 73:139, 1978.

SMITH, C. A. Effects of maternal undernutrition upon the newborn infant in Holland. *Journal of Pediatrics* 30:229, 1947.

Stickle, G., and P. Ma. Pregnancy in adolescents: Scope of the problem. Reprinted from *Contemporary Ob/Gyn*. New York: McGraw-Hill, 1975.

Task Force on Nutrition. *Assessment of maternal nutrition*. Chicago: American College of Obstetricians and Gynecologists, 1978.

Thomson, A. M., and F. E. Hytten. Nutrition during pregnancy. *World Review of Nutrition and Dietetics* 16:22, 1973.

USDHEW. Teenage childbearing, extent and circumstances: Consortium on early childbearing. Washington, D.C.: Maternal and Child Health Service, 1973a.

USDHEW. *The women and their pregnancies: The collaborative perinatal study of the National Institute of Neurological Diseases and Stroke*. DHEW Publication No. (NIH) 73-379. Washington, D.C.: U.S. Government Printing Office, 1973b.

USDHEW. *The third special report to the U.S. Congress on alcohol and health*. Rockville, Md.: National Institute on Alcohol Abuse and Alcoholism, 1978.

USDHEW. *Surgeon General's report on smoking and health*. Washington, D.C.: U.S. Government Printing Office, 1979.

Vermeersch, J. Maternal nutrition and the outcome of pregnancy. In *Nutrition in pregnancy and lactation*, eds. B. S. Worthington, J. Vermeersch, and S. R. Williams. St. Louis: C. V. Mosby, 1977.

Williams, S. R. Nutritional therapy in special conditions of pregnancy. In *Nutrition in pregnancy and lactation*, eds. B. S. Worthington, J. Vermeersch, and S. R. Williams. St. Louis: C. V. Mosby, 1977.

Winick, M. Fetal malnutrition. *Clinics in Obstetrics and Gynecology* 13:537, 1970.

Zelnik, M., and J. F. Kantner. Sexual and contraceptive experience of young unmarried women in the United States, 1976 and 1971. *Family Planning Perspectives* 9:55, 1977.

SUGGESTED ADDITIONAL READING

Ashe, J. R., F. A. Schofield, and M. R. Gram. The retention of calcium, iron, phosphorus, and magnesium during pregnancy: The adequacy of prenatal diets with and without supplementation. *American Journal of Clinical Nutrition* 32:286, 1979.

Bruhn, C. M., and R. M. Pangborn. Reported incidence of pica among migrant families. *Journal of the American Dietetic Association* 58:417, 1971.

Bunker, M. L., and M. McWilliams. Caffeine content of common beverages. *Journal of the American Dietetic Association* 74:28, 1979.

Burke, B. S., V. A. Beal, S. B. Kirkwood, and H. C. Stuart. The influence of nutrition during pregnancy upon the condition of the infant at birth. *Journal of Nutrition* 25:569, 1943.

Burke, B. S., V. V. Harding, and H. C. Stuart. Nutrition studies during pregnancy. IV. Relation of protein content of mother's diet during pregnancy to birth length, birth weight, and condition of infant at birth. *Journal of Pediatrics* 23:506, 1943.

Chopra, J. G. Effect of steroid contraceptives on lactation. *American Journal of Clinical Nutrition* 25:1202, 1972.

Committee on Nutrition of the Mother and Preschool child, Food and Nutrition Board, National Research Council. *Laboratory indices of nutritional status in pregnancy*. Washington, D.C.: National Academy of Sciences, 1978.

Garn, S. M., K. Hoff, and K. D. McCabe. Maternal fatness and placental size. *American Journal of Clinical Nutrition* 32:277, 1979.

Hanson, J. W., K. L. Jones, and W. D. Smith. Fetal alcohol syndrome: Experience with 41 patients. *Journal of the American Medical Association* 235:1458, 1976.

MORA, J. O., B. DEPAREDES, M. WAGNER, L. DENAVARRO, J. SUESCUM, N. CHRISTIANSEN, AND M. G. HERRERA. Nutritional supplementation and the outcome of pregnancy. I. Birth weight. *American Journal of Clinical Nutrition* 32:455, 1979.

PIKE, R. L., AND D. S. GURSKY. Further evidence of deleterious effects produced by sodium restriction during pregnancy. *American Journal of Clinical Nutrition* 23:883, 1970.

POTTER, J. M., AND P. J. NESTEL. The effects of dietary fatty acids and cholesterol on the milk lipids of lactating women and the plasma cholesterol of breast-fed infants. *American Journal of Clinical Nutrition* 29:54, 1976.

SIMS, L. S. Dietary status of lactating women. II. Relation of nutritional knowledge and attitudes to nutrient intake. *Journal of the American Dietetic Association* 73:147, 1978.

SINGLETON, N. C., H. LEWIS, AND J. J. PARKER. The diet of pregnant teenagers. *Journal of Home Economics* 68:43, 1976.

WINICK, M., ed. *Nutrition and development.* New York: John Wiley, 1972.

WORTHINGTON, B. S., J. VERMEERSCH, AND S. R. WILLIAMS, eds. *Nutrition in pregnancy and lactation.* St. Louis: C. V. Mosby, 1977.

Chapter 13

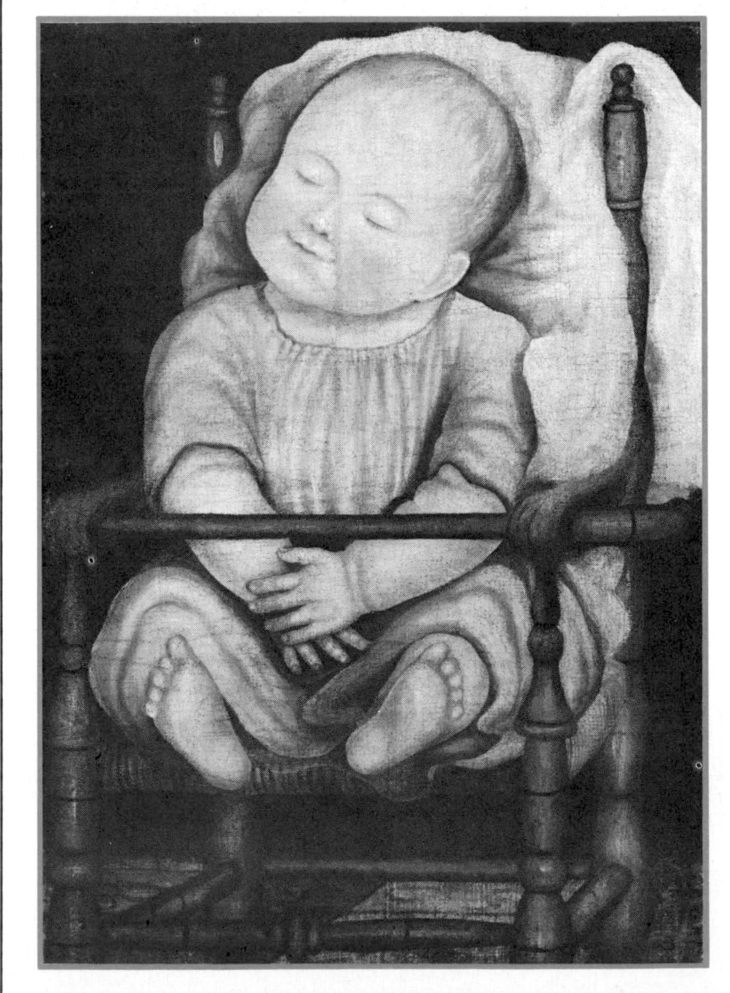

Baby in Red Chair, artist unknown

Nutrition in the Growing Years

In its declaration proclaiming 1979 as the International Year of the Child, the United Nations stated as its first principle, "The child must be given the means requisite for its normal development, both materially and spiritually," and as its second, "The child that is hungry must be fed." It is in childhood, during the growing years, that developmental patterns are established which influence both health and achievement during all the years that follow. The role of food in growth and development, from infancy (0 to 12 months) through childhood (1 to 12 years) to adolescence (13 to 19 years), is the focus of this chapter.

Growth—the gradual accumulation of tissue—and development—the maturation, regulation, and integration of the systems of the total internal environment—are two separate but closely related processes. Their interrelationship is a complex blend of genetics and environment. Only with proper support from the external environment—food, shelter, nurturing—can the body's internal physiological program unfold in the orderly manner predetermined by genetic mechanisms.

For the fetus, whose external environment is limited to the confines of the mother's uterus, internal growth and development depends almost entirely on the mother's available nutrient supply. At birth the interplay between external and internal environments becomes more complex, as the infant's external world suddenly expands. Food now begins to function not only as a substrate for physiological growth and development, but also as a stimulus for the sociocultural development that is equally vital to human functioning.

INTRODUCTION TO INFANT NUTRITION

The growth processes begun during gestation continue at a rapid rate in the first year of life. The most obvious indication of this rapid growth is weight gain. By age 4 or 5 months, birth weight is doubled; by the end of twelve months it is tripled. In respect to this rapidity of growth, infancy is an extension of prenatal life. But in other respects, it is quite different. The newborn can no longer depend on its mother's body for oxygen, temperature control, the removal of waste products. As a free-living being, it must learn to meet the needs of its internal environment and respond to changes in the external environment. The mother, continuing her role as primary caretaker, also plays a strong role in this adaptation, providing warmth, protection, cuddling, and, most important, food.

Probably no aspect of postnatal care has been scrutinized more closely than food and infant feeding practices. Current opinions on breast- versus bottle-feeding, when to introduce solid foods, desirable weight gain during infancy, and many other nutritional issues are based as much on changing social values and environmental and economic conditions as on scientific knowledge. Each of these issues will be examined from the perspective of the healthy newborn, one for whom the outcome of pregnancy was normal birth weight and normal medical status.

GROWTH AND DEVELOPMENT DURING INFANCY (0 TO 12 MONTHS)

Growth is due to increases in total cell number (hyperplasia), in cell size (hypertrophy), and in the amount of intercellular material. The rate and timing of each of these growth processes is controlled by heredity, hormonal action, and environmental impact, all of which interact to produce identifiable patterns of growth.

Patterns of Growth

Growth in body length is most rapid in the early months. Using birth length as a reference, the infant's length increases 20 percent by 3 months of age, at 1 year by 50 percent, and at 2 years by 75 percent. Somewhere between age 2 to 2½, the child reaches 50 percent of its expected adult height. If growth continued at this rapid rate, kindergarten children would be of adult size. Instead, the velocity of growth decelerates steadily throughout the early years, reaching a plateau at age 5 that will last until the growth spurt of adolescence.

Changes in body composition and differential growth patterns of various body tissues are also apparent during these years. The amount of body fat, which accounts for only about 12 percent of body weight at birth, doubles by 1 year of age. Concomitantly, body water decreases from 75 percent of body weight at birth to about 59 percent at age 1 year.

Brain growth is also most rapid in the early months; by 1½ years, brain growth is about 90 percent complete. At birth, the head accounts for one-third of an infant's length; at age 2 years, the child's head circumference is about two-thirds of its expected adult size. Nutritional deprivation during this critical period of brain growth is associated with decreased head circumference, brain weight, and brain protein content, factors that may impair intellectual functioning throughout later life.

These growth phases create the characteristic body proportions identified with infancy, childhood, and adolescence. Relative head size decreases during the infant's first year, when growth occurs mainly in the trunk (spinal column). By age 12 months, the trunk has reached approximately 60 percent of its final adult size. From then until adolescence, leg growth makes the most impressive gains, creating the typical appearance of the gangly preteenager. Trunk length increases during the adolescent growth spurt, thus balancing body proportions.

Assessment of Growth

Growth during infancy is so rapid that most mothers don't need a scale to tell them that their baby is thriving. Nevertheless, periodic measurement of weight, height, and head circumference is recommended to ensure that an infant's growth is following a normal progression. The National Center for Health Statistics has developed growth charts for infants and children that take into account the wide variability in physical growth of children for differing genetic, ethnic, and socioeconomic populations. These NCHS measures have replaced earlier standards that, although derived from studies of carefully selected children, did not reflect the wide diversity of the contemporary United States population (see Chapter 10).

Figures 13-1 and 13-2 show the NCHS percentile measures for length and weight of male and female infants from birth to 36 months. Using these charts, the appropriate values for each measure are plotted periodically, at the time of every pediatric check-up. Thus a record accumulates, indicating the developmental history of the child. Measurements between the 25th and 75th percentiles are generally interpreted as normal. More important, however, is consistency of development within a narrower percentile range. An infant who had been in the 95th percentile both for length and weight in the first 3 months of life might be suspected of having developmental problems if at 6 months her weight was in the 70th percentile while length was still in the higher percentile.

The typical well-baby examination should include length and weight measurements, a thorough clinical examination, and a review of the infant's skin tone and general appearance. Head circumference measurements are

FIGURE 13-1 (p. 502)

Weight and Height by Age for Girls from Birth to 36 Months

Source: Adapted from National Center for Health Statistics, *NCHS growth charts, 1976,* Monthly Vital Statistics Report, Vol. 25, No. 3, Supp. (HRA) 75-1120 (Rockville, Maryland: Health Resources Administration, June, 1976). Data from the Fels Research Institute, Yellow Springs, Ohio. © 1976 Ross Laboratories.

FIGURE 13-2 (p. 503)

Weight and Height by Age for Boys from Birth to 36 Months

Source: Adapted from National Center for Health Statistics, *NCHS growth charts, 1976,* Monthly Vital Statistics Report, Vol. 25, No. 3, Supp. (HRA) 76-1120 (Rockville, Maryland: Health Resources Administration, June 1976). Data from the Fels Research Institute, Yellow Springs, Ohio. © 1976 Ross Laboratories.

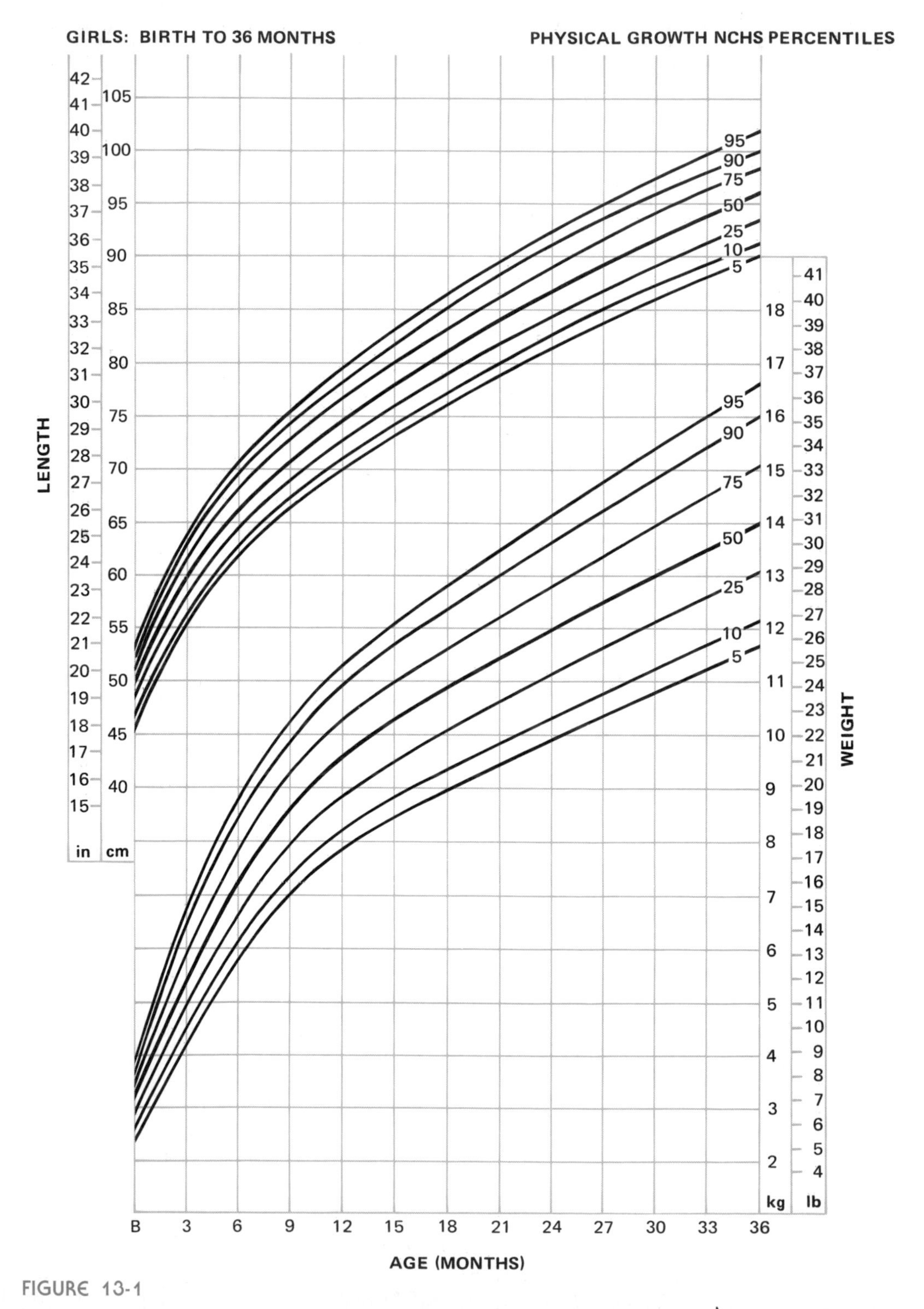

GIRLS: BIRTH TO 36 MONTHS
PHYSICAL GROWTH NCHS PERCENTILES
LENGTH
WEIGHT
AGE (MONTHS)
in
cm
kg
lb
95
90
75
50
25
10
5

FIGURE 13-1

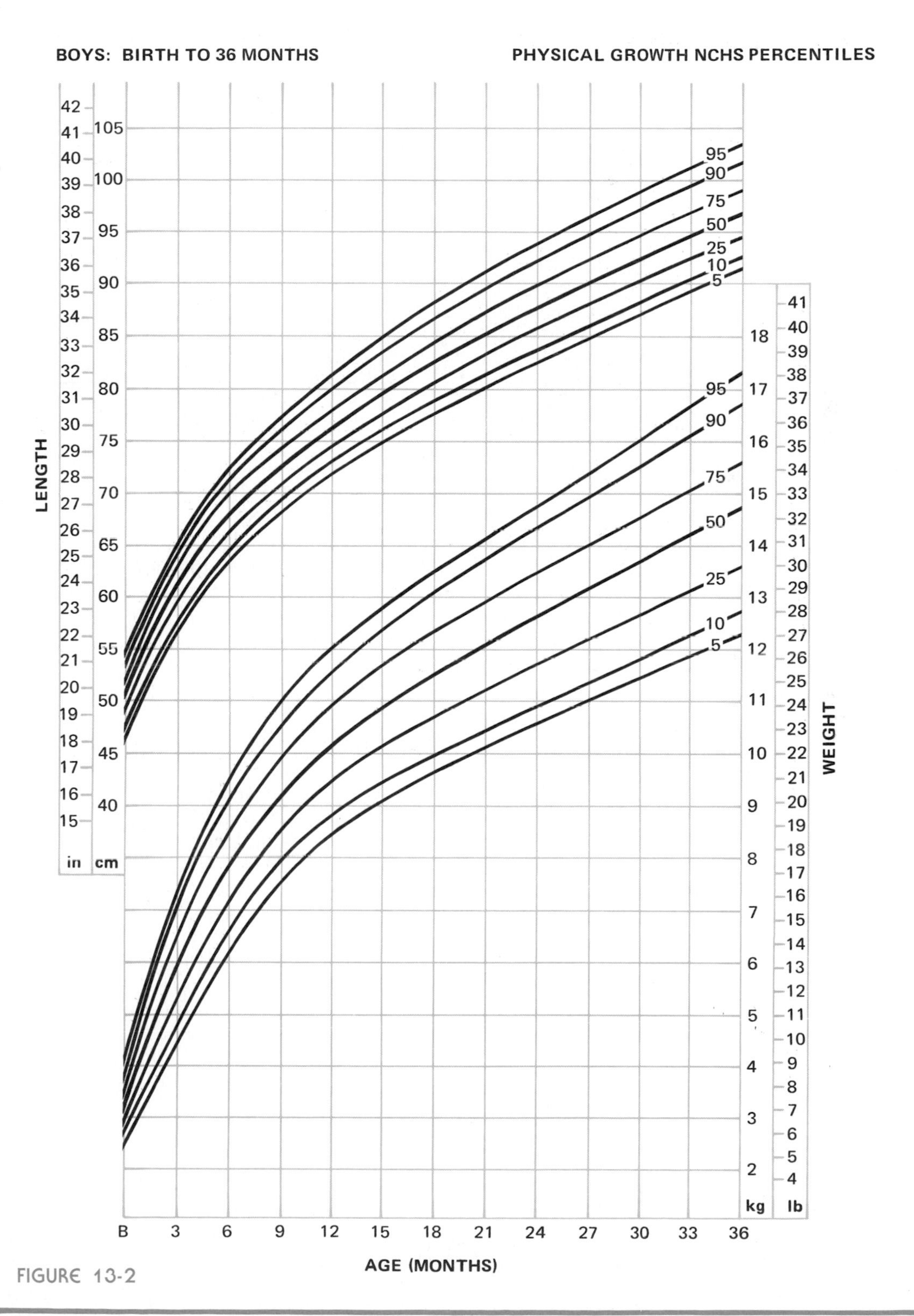
BOYS: BIRTH TO 36 MONTHS
PHYSICAL GROWTH NCHS PERCENTILES
LENGTH
in
cm
WEIGHT
kg
lb
95
90
75
50
25
10
5
B 3 6 9 12 15 18 21 24 27 30 33 36
AGE (MONTHS)

FIGURE 13-2

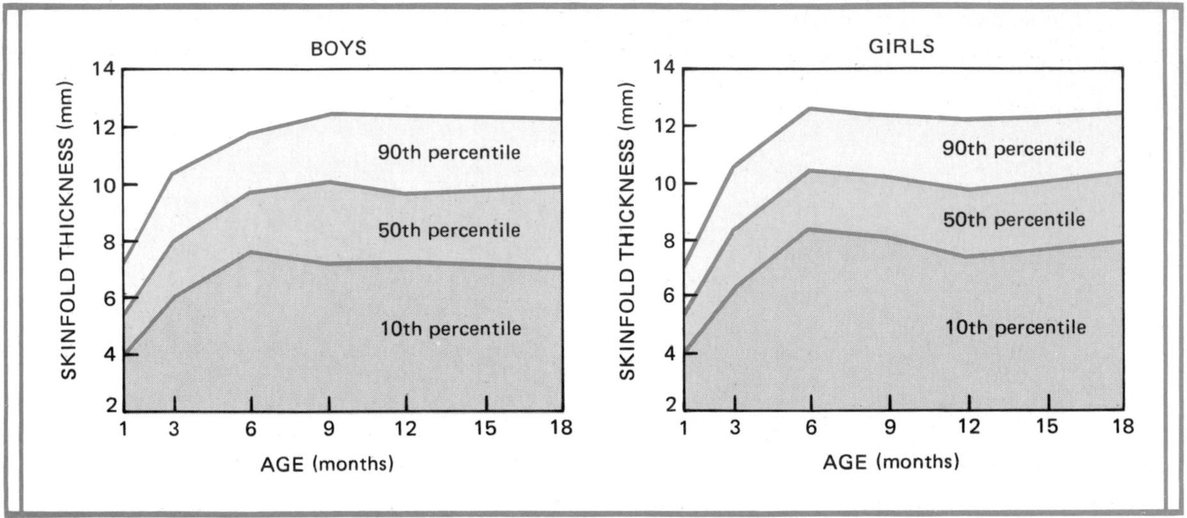

FIGURE 13-3

Curves of Skinfold Thickness

Data are from a longitudinal study of Swedish children (122 boys and 90 girls) in an urban community.

Source: P. Karlberg, I. Engstrom, and H. Lichtenstein. Development of children in a Swedish urban community. A prospective longitudinal study. III. Physical growth during the first three years of life. *Acta Paediatrica Scandinavica*, Supplement 187:48, 1968.

sometimes taken, and the National Center for Health Statistics provides a standardized graph of these as well. Generally, growth charts are best used as screening tools, not as diagnostic tools. Although in most cases they provide reassurance that the child is growing normally, they are also helpful in identifying children whose rate of maturation is abnormal, perhaps as a result of under- or overnutrition.

Because of the high incidence of anemia in infants, it has been suggested that iron status be checked by means of hematocrit and hemoglobin tests as a routine component of well-baby care. Monitoring of serum cholesterol at 3 months and 1 year of age has also been recommended, for early identification of children who may be genetically or otherwise predisposed to elevated serum cholesterol levels. Because of studies suggesting that low-cholesterol diets can reduce serum levels even in very young children, and possibly prevent later vascular and coronary problems, early identification of children at risk becomes important (Winick, 1978). Periodic caliper measurements of skinfold thickness to measure the extent of fat deposition are also advised (see Figure 13-3).

NUTRIENT REQUIREMENTS DURING INFANCY

It is widely agreed that food is the most important determinant of infant growth and development, but there is little consensus about the kinds and amount of food that are optimal. Very little is actually known about the nutrient needs of infants. In estimating recommended levels of nutrients for the first year of life, the Food and Nutrition Board relied not on experimental studies, but on the traditional view that breast milk from well-nourished women is the biologically correct standard for infant nourishment. Thus, infant RDAs assume that breast milk supplies protein, energy, minerals, vitamins, and fluid in the amounts and proportions best suited for optimal development, and that prepared formulas and food supplements must come as close as possible to duplicating these nutrient proportions.

Energy

Breast milk provides approximately 7 percent of kilocalories from protein, 55 percent from fat, and 38 percent from carbohydrate. Most commercially prepared formulas closely match these figures.

Because infants have a high rate of heat loss due to their relatively large body surface area, their energy requirements for basal metabolism are quite high, approximating 55 kcal/kg. Another 35 kcal/kg is required for growth and 10 to 25 kcal/kg for activity, yielding a total daily energy requirement of 115 kcal/kg (48 kcal/lb) during the first 6 months of life. Compared with the 35 kcal/kg recommended for adults, the high metabolic needs of infants become apparent. During the first few months of life, all energy intake can be provided by breast milk or formula. In the second six months of life, the energy requirement as a function of body weight gradually decreases to approximately 105 kcal/kg, and solid food begins to supply some of the needed energy.

Protein

The protein required for rapid muscular and skeletal growth accounts for the recommendations of 2.2 g/kg body weight for the first six months of life, and 2.0 g/kg during the second half of the first year. This compares with the 0.8 g/kg recommended for adults. To facilitate comparisons between individual nutrients and prepared formulas, nutrient allowances for infants are sometimes expressed in terms of energy intake, rather than per unit of body weight. Human milk provides about 1.5 grams of protein for every 100 kilocalories and is adequate for full term infants. Formulas should contain a minimum of 1.8 grams of protein per 100 kilocalories. This figure assumes that the proteins in prepared formulas are of high biological value, providing the essential amino acids required for protein synthesis.

Protein intakes of less than 6 percent of energy intakes are considered inadequate for optimal brain growth and general development. Excessive protein intakes (levels higher than 16 percent of energy intakes) should be avoided as well, because this quantity may overwhelm the ability of the infant's kidneys to excrete the excess nitrogen; it is in any case an inefficient and expensive way of providing energy.

Fat

In an infant's diet, fat is a significant source of energy; it is a vehicle for essential fatty acids and the fat-soluble vitamins and contributes to the feeling of satiety through which the infant learns to regulate appetite. There is no RDA for fat, but the Food and Nutrition Board recommends that at least 15 percent of kilocalories be supplied by easily digested fats, with 3 percent of total energy intake provided in the form of linoleic acid, an important precursor for prostaglandins (regulatory substances found throughout the body). The preferred intake of dietary fat is from 30 to 54 percent of total kilocalories.

Concern about obesity and heart disease has led to recommendations that infants be fed skim milk. However, its low energy density and relatively high protein content have been shown to retard normal weight gain in infants (Woodruff, 1978). For these reasons, and because it does not provide adequate essential fatty acids, skim milk should not be used for infant feeding.

Carbohydrates

Carbohydrate provides the remainder of energy intake, accounting for 35 to 65 percent of total kilocalories. Lactose, the natural sugar in both human and cow's milk, facilitates calcium absorption and is an immediate precursor of galactose. Galactose is a component of myelin in nerve fibers and of collagen in connective tissue, cartilage, and bone. Other carbohydrates (glucose, sucrose, fructose) may be used in infant formulas, and galactose is then synthesized from glucose in the liver.

Vitamins and Minerals

Recommendations for vitamin and mineral intakes during infancy are shown in Table 13-1, which presents figures of both the Food and Nutrition Board and the American Academy of Pediatrics. These two bodies have taken differing approaches, primarily because the AAP was concerned with developing standards for infant formulas. Reacting to concerns about the ability of formulas to meet the nutrient needs of infants, the AAP has suggested minimum and in some cases maximum levels of intake. The AAP points out that future research may identify other essential nutrients and their biological interactions, redefine physiological requirements, and result in re-evaluation of current recommendations. This same philosophy—new knowledge leads to better understanding—is also upheld by the FNB. Both groups agree that intakes in excess of these recommendations offer no advantage in the feeding of normal full-term infants and may in fact have adverse effects (Woodruff, 1978).

Fluid

The infant's high metabolic rate leads to the production of significant quantities of metabolic wastes, which require water for excretion. During the first year of life, an infant needs about 120 to 160 ml/kg of fluid each day. The amount of human or cow's milk needed to supply an infant's recommended daily nutrient and energy intake would also supply 150 to 200 ml/kg of fluid, which is more than sufficient except in extremely hot weather.

TABLE 13-1
Comparison of RDAs with Minimum Nutrient Recommendations in Infancy

Nutrient	NAS-NRC RDA[a]			AAP Minimum Nutrient Recommendations[b]
	0-6 mo.	*6-12 mo.*	*Units*	
Energy	115	105	kcal/kg.	100–110 kcal/kg
Protein	2.2	2.0	g/kg	1.8 g/100 kcal
Fat	—	—	—	3.3–6.0 g/kcal[c]
Vitamin A	420	400	RE	260 IU/100 kcal[d]
Vitamin D	10	10	μg	40 IU/100 kcal[e]
Vitamin E	3	4	mg αT.E[g]	0.3 IU/100 kcal[f]
Vitamin K	12	10–20	μg[h]	4.0 IU/100 kcal
Vitamin C	35	35	mg	8.1 mg/100 kcal
Folacin	30	45	μg	4.0 μg/100 kcal
Niacin	6	8	mg	250.0 μg/100 kcal
Riboflavin	0.4	0.6	mg	60.0 μg/100 kcal
Thiamin	0.3	0.5	mg	40.0 μg/100 kcal
Vitamin B_6	0.3	0.6	mg	35.0 μg/100 kcal
Vitamin B_{12}	0.5	1.5	μg	0.15 μg/100 kcal
Biotin	35	50	μg[h]	1.5 μg/100 kcal
Choline	—	—	—	7.0 mg/100 kcal
Inositol	—	—	—	4.0 mg/100 kcal
Calcium	360	540	mg	50 mg/100 kcal
Phosphorus	240	360	mg	25 mg/100 kcal
Iodine	40	50	μg	5 μg/100 kcal
Iron	10	15	mg	0.15 mg/100 kcal
Magnesium	50	70	mg	6.0 mg/100 kcal
Zinc	3	5	mg	0.5 mg/100 kcal
Copper	0.5–0.7	0.7–1.0	mg[h]	60.0 μg/100 kcal
Manganese	0.5–0.7	0.7–1.0	mg[h]	5.0 μg/100 kcal
Sodium	115–350	250–750	mg[h]	20–60 mg/100 kcal
Potassium	350–925	425–1275	mg[h]	80–200 mg/100 kcal
Chloride	275–700	400–1200	mg[h]	55–150 mg/100 kcal

[a] Food and Nutrition Board, National Academy of Sciences, *Recommended daily dietary allowances,* revised 1979 (Washington, D.C.: National Research Council, 1979).
[b] Committee on Nutrition, American Academy of Pediatrics, *Pediatrics* 57:278, 1976.
[c] Recommended intake of 300 mg linoleic acid/100 kcal.
[d] Maximum value recommended is 750 IU/100 kcal.
[e] As cholecalciferol, 10 μg cholecalciferol equals 400 IU vitamin D.
[f] Maximum value recommended is 100 IU/100 kcal.
[g] Formulas containing vegetable oils should contain 0.7 IU of vitamin E/g linoleic acid.
[h] Estimated safe and adequate daily dietary intakes, Food and Nutrition Board, 1979.

FEEDING PRACTICES IN INFANCY

For obvious ethical reasons, the nursery rarely serves as a laboratory. Relatively few data exist, therefore, to unequivocally support the use of one feeding practice over another, although observations throughout the years have resulted in a more informed basis for particular recommendations. Perhaps the central issue has been the relative benefits of breast versus formula feeding, an area colored by culture and technology.

Traditionally, infant nutrition was considered to be solely the mother's concern. In certain societies, however, it was considered inappropriate for women of the upper socioeconomic classes to nurse their infants. Also, some women could not supply breast milk for their babies due to illness or death. In these situations, another lactating woman could be hired as a wet nurse, but the outcome was often uncertain. Many wet nurses came from low socioeconomic backgrounds and carried diseases which they transmitted to the nursing infants. Similarly uncertain results were associated with feeding milk from cows, goats, or donkeys. Occasionally broths were tried. In all such cases, prognosis for the infant was quite poor.

Thus, it is not surprising that until the beginning of the twentieth century, almost all women nursed their infants. By that time, the rudimentary chemical analyses of human milk (first attempted in the mid-1800s) had become sophisticated enough to permit production of synthetic formulas for infant feeding. These new products had obvious appeal to better-educated women, who were not hard to convince that formula feeding represented a modern, scientific advance over the primitive human breast. Bottle-feeding, like other fashions, was widely written about in magazines and rapidly adopted by women throughout the country.

Breast-Feeding

The past decade has seen a reversal, with better-educated women leading the way back to breast-feeding on the basis of its being more "natural," and because of scientific support for its greater nutritional and health-promoting value. But in today's world, there are definite impediments to wide acceptance of breast-feeding. For one thing, this natural practice is embarrassing to many segments of the population. In their commentary on breast-feeding, the American Academy of Pediatrics remarked on the curious contradiction of a society that tolerates all degrees of sexual explicitness in movies, books, and other media, but continues to relegate the normal act of breast-feeding to the privacy of closed doors and drawn shades (American Academy of Pediatrics, 1978).

NUTRITIONAL CONSIDERATIONS. Human milk was designed for consumption by human infants, and under normal conditions it is best suited to their nutritional needs. Most commercially available formulas simulate mother's milk by modifying the cow's milk on which they are based. Cow's milk differs in a number of ways from human milk, particularly in regard to protein and mineral content. Table 13-2 compares the nutrient content of human and cow's milk.

ENERGY AND CARBOHYDRATE CONTENT. Cow's milk and human milk have approximately the same energy content, about 70 kilocalories per 100 milliliters. However, this energy level is achieved with different proportions of its components, with more carbohydrate (lactose) in human milk and more protein in cow's milk.

PROTEIN. Protein provides 20 percent of the kilocalories in cow's milk, in comparison with the 7 percent supplied by breast milk protein. Qualitative

TABLE 13-2
Average Composition of Mature Human Milk and Whole Cow's Milk (nutrients and energy content per 100 ml)

	Mature Human Milk	Whole Cow's Milk
Water, ml	91.0	90.6
Energy, kcal (kJ)	73(307)	63(265)
Carbohydrate, g	7.2	4.8
Protein, g	1.1	3.4
Lipid, g	4.5	3.4
Fatty acids		
saturated, g	2.09	2.14
monounsaturated, g	1.73	0.99
polyunsaturated, g	0.52	0.12
Cholesterol, mg	14.6	14.4
Ash, g	0.2	0.7
Calcium, mg	33	123
Chlorine, mg	43	103
Magnesium, mg	3	13
Phosphorus, mg	15	96
Potassium, mg	53	156
Sodium, mg	18	50
Copper, μg	40	30
Iron, μg	30	50
Zinc, μg	180	390
Ascorbic acid, mg	5.2	0.97
Thiamin, mg	0.015	0.04
Riboflavin, mg	0.037	0.17
Niacin, mg	0.18	0.09
Pantothenic acid, mg	0.23	0.32
Vitamin B_6, mg	0.01	0.04
Folacin, μg	5.2	5.2
Vitamin B_{12}, μg	0.047	0.37
Vitamin A, RE (IU)	67(251)	32(130)
Vitamin D, IU	2.2	42 (if fortified)

Source: Adapted from L. P. Posati and M. L. Orr, *Composition of foods—Dairy and egg products—Raw, processed, prepared,* USDA Agriculture Handbook 8-1 (Washington, D.C.: U.S. Government Printing Office, 1976), pp. 77, 107; and I. G. Macy and H. J. Kelly, Human milk and cow's milk in human nutrition. In *Milk: The mammary gland and its secretion,* Vol. 2, ed. S. K. Kon and A. T. Cowie (New York and London: Academic Press, 1961), pp. 265–304.

differences exist as well. Sixty percent of the protein in human milk is whey (lactalbumin); the rest is casein. In cow's milk, the distribution is 18 and 82 percent respectively. Digestibility of milk protein is affected by this ratio: Milk protein containing large amounts of casein forms a tough, hard-to-digest curd after exposure to hydrochloric acid in the stomach. The amino acid contents of the two milks also differ: Cow's milk contains a higher methionine:cystine ratio. This appears to be significant in the feeding of premature infants, who are less able to metabolize methionine (Raiha, 1974).

FAT. Although the lipid content of human and cow's milk is similar, breast milk lipids are better absorbed. Differences in fatty acid composition account for this observation. Human milk contains more unsaturated fatty acids; in addition, palmitate is found primarily in the 2-position of the glycerol molecule, which favors the absorption of monoglycerides (see Chapter 3). The

$H_2C—O—$Fatty acid
$HC—O—$Palmitate
$H_2C—O—$Fatty acid

replacement of butterfat with vegetable oils has significantly improved lipid absorption from commercial formulas and also decreased their cholesterol and saturated fatty acid content.

Controversy exists over whether this reduction in cholesterol is indeed advantageous. Some studies indicate that exogenous cholesterol may be important to nerve tissue formation and bile salt synthesis in the infant. Also of interest are studies of laboratory animals showing that ingestion of cholesterol by newborns may increase production of enzymes that more efficiently metabolize cholesterol, subsequently contributing to lowered serum levels. Additional research is needed to evaluate the effects of manipulating dietary cholesterol during the neonatal period on serum cholesterol levels in later life (American Academy of Pediatrics, 1978).

It has also been shown that the fat content of breast milk increases in the course of a feeding; this suggests that the greater amount of fat present near the end of the feeding signals satiety to the infant.

TRACE MINERALS AND VITAMINS. Recent research has focused on the micronutrient content of breast milk. Trace minerals and vitamins appear in variable amounts in human milk, a reflection at least in part of maternal intakes. As knowledge of the vitamin and trace mineral content of breast milk increases, it will facilitate the estimation of requirements for these micronutrients and the addition of appropriate amounts to commercial formulas. New information about the interrelationships and bioavailability of trace minerals, with applications to nutritional science in general, will also be derived from increased understanding of the components of breast milk (Johnson and Evans, 1978; Kirskey et al., 1979).

Both human and cow's milk have similar, but low, iron content. However, recent data suggest that about 50 percent of the iron in human milk is absorbed, whereas the iron in pasteurized cow's milk is less well utilized (Saarinen et al., 1977). Heat treatment of cow's milk formulas increases iron availability, but very young infants who receive whole cow's milk are at risk of developing an iron deficiency.

A recent report suggests that human milk meets the daily iron requirements of exclusively breast-fed full-term infants, at least until birth weight has tripled (McMillan et al., 1976). But few infants are exclusively breast-fed for that length of time, and the addition of solid food has been reported to decrease significantly the high bioavailability of breast milk iron (Saarinen and Siimes, 1979). Therefore, iron supplements are routinely prescribed for all infants, unless they are fed an iron-fortified formula.

IMMUNOLOGICAL PROPERTIES. It has been recognized for many years that human milk helps to protect newborns from infectious disease. Two iron-containing proteins found in breast milk, lactoferrin and transferrin, have antibacterial properties. Cow's milk contains a much smaller amount of lactoferrin; furthermore, its antibacterial effect is destroyed during processing. The presence of these antibacterial agents may be one of the reasons for the immunological properties that have been attributed to breast milk but not to infant formulas. Unlike cow's milk formulas, breast milk also contains leukocytes, antibody-secreting cells, and antibodies to some intestinal microorganisms. Recent attention has turned to defining the mechanisms that might explain the long-recognized clinical observation that breast-fed infants, especially in developing countries, suffer from fewer infections and allergies than do bottle-fed infants In a long-term study in Helsinki, breast-feeding for more than six months was associated with a lower incidence of a variety of allergic reactions, even in infants with a family history of such disorders (Saarinen et al., 1979).

OTHER CONSIDERATIONS. Breast milk has a lower concentration of electrolytes than does cow's milk, and the low solute load is apparently better suited to the level of kidney function of human infants. The higher sodium concentration of cow's milk can strain the capacity of the immature kidneys to excrete sodium, resulting in hypernatremia (excess sodium in blood).

Economic and psychological factors are often cited as advantages of breast-feeding. It has often been stated that breast-feeding is more expensive than formula-feeding because of the additional food the mother must consume to produce the needed milk. Generally speaking, there is no reason for the cost of the relatively small additional amount of food for the mother (see Chapter 12) to be excessively high. On the contrary, the cost of any prepared formula for infant feeding exceeds the cost of human milk, and those costs increase with the conveniences built into the manufacturer's package. Whole cow's milk is the least expensive, but it is not advised; formula prepared at home from evaporated milk, corn syrup, and water is also less expensive than breast milk but does not meet prescribed recommendations for vitamin C and iron.

Cost per Ounce of Some Milk-Based Infant Feedings

Type of Feedings	Cost
Whole milk[a]	$.0123
Home-prepared[b]	.0142
Lactation on moderate-cost maternal diet	.0180
Commercial formula[c]	
concentrated	.0238
powdered	.0258
ready-to-serve	.0291

[a]Not recommended.
[b]A 13-ounce can of evaporated milk diluted with an equal amount of water, and mixed with corn (Karo) syrup to make 28 ounces.
[c]Average of Enfamil and Similac.

Source: Adapted from E. Lamm, J. Delaney, and J. T. Dwyer, Economy in the feeding of infants, *Pediatric Clinics of North America* 24:71, 1977.

The psychological value of breast-feeding is less susceptible to quantitative measurement. There is no experimental evidence to substantiate differences in psychological or physical development in infants related to their mode of feeding. Warmth, contact, and gentleness can be achieved with bottle-feeding as much as with breast-feeding.

Under some circumstances women should not breast-feed their infants. Infectious diseases such as active pulmonary tuberculosis, which might be transmitted to the infant, are a contraindication to breast-feeding. Other chronic diseases, however, including heart disease, diabetes, hepatitis, and nephrosis, do not automatically rule out breast-feeding, particularly if they have been under medical control during a successful pregnancy. However, conditions that are being treated with anticoagulants, certain antibiotics, thyroid gland suppressants, radioactive compounds, anticancer drugs, and even large quantities of aspirin make nursing unwise, since these drugs are likely to appear in the breast milk in harmful quantities (Taylor and Worthington, 1977). Preliminary research indicates that oral contraceptives containing low levels of estrogens and other hormones are unlikely to affect male or female infants or to suppress lactation (Savage, 1977); long-term results of this practice, however, are not yet available.

Indiscriminate drug use is definitely not advised for nursing mothers. The high morbidity and mortality of babies born to narcotic-addicted mothers is related both to their incidence of withdrawal symptoms and to frequent prematurity, respiratory distress, and generally poor pre- and postnatal care. Although nursing was once recommended as the best way of treating withdrawal symptoms in addicted infants, many addicts use more than one psychoactive substance which might appear in their milk, further damaging the newborn. Tobacco and alcohol abuse, in particular, have been shown to complicate problems in such infants. In normal infants born to nonaddicted mothers, however, moderate maternal use of alcohol and nicotine (cigarettes) has not proved to be a contraindication to breast-feeding.

Unintentional exposure to environmental pollutants has caused concern for nursing mothers. In recent years, several incidents have been reported in which polychorinated biphenyls (PCBs), inhaled in industrial settings or consumed with contaminated cooking oil or other foods, were stored in maternal adipose tissue and later excreted in the fat of breast milk. Fortunately, these incidents are rare, and there appear to be no significant effects of this exposure in breast-fed infants. Some pediatricians recommend that the milk of women who may have been exposed to this pollutant be monitored to determine PCB levels.

Bottle-Feeding

Most commercially prepared formulas contain cow's milk, which is modified in several ways to make it more suitable for human infants. Protein and solute contents are reduced; carbohydrate levels are increased with the addition of sucrose, lactose, or oligosaccharides; vegetable oils are substituted for butter fat; and vitamins and minerals are added. The energy density of the finished product is about 670 kilocalories per liter (20 kcal/oz). This scientifically formulated mixture is then evaporated and canned or dried, to be reconstituted at home. It is important that instructions for dilution be followed precisely, as given by the pediatrician or on the package label. To meet the needs of modern mobility, formulas are now available in ready-to-feed bottles; only a sterile nipple cap need be attached.

Home-prepared formula can also be made from a base of canned evaporated (not sweetened condensed) milk, to which boiled (sterile) water and corn syrup are added; proportions should be recommended by a pediatrician.

Commercial formulas have also been developed for babies with special problems such as metabolic disorders, allergy to cow's milk protein, or lactose intolerancc. Somc of these special formulas are made with soy protein.Simulated formulas are important in the management of infants and children with inherited digestive defects and allergies; they are also used by parents who want their formula-fed babies to follow a vegetarian diet.

Current Recommendations

Although it is generally agreed that nutritional adequacy can be attained with either breast- or formula-feeding, the American Academy of Pediatrics and most nutritionists still conclude that breast is best. Ideally, breast milk should be the only major source of nutrients for the first five to six months of an infant's life to ensure proper growth and development. It is assumed that human milk is best able to meet the needs of the human species and that in most nursing mothers it is produced in the precise quantity required by each infant.

Quantity should not be a concern to a nursing mother. There is no way to tell if a baby at the breast has taken 3 ounces, 6 ounces, or more. This is an advantage, not a disadvantage. There is no evidence that 8 fluid ounces (standard bottle size) at every feeding is the ideal amount for every infant. Yet mothers typically persist in presenting a bottle until it is emptied, although the baby actually might not need that much. This "good to the last drop" attitude has been implicated as a possible contributor to obesity, which may be due to formation of excessive numbers of fat cells in infancy. Whereas mothers who bottle-feed may have difficulty gauging their babies' changing needs, those who breast-feed can normally assume that the baby is taking as much milk as necessary.

An infant's requirement for milk changes with age, growth, and other food intake. When milk provides the only source of energy and nutrients, average daily needs increase from 18 ounces before 1 month of age, to 21 ounces from 1 to 2 months, 24 ounces from 2 to 3 months, and 30 ounces from 3 to 6 months. It then decreases to 28 ounces from 6 to 9 months when other sources of nourishment are added to the infant diet. Breast-fed babies can easily make these adjustments: It is less likely that bottle-feeding mothers will permit their baby's changing appetite to be the sole guide of how much formula is consumed.

Often the modern world makes it difficult for a woman to achieve peace of mind about breast-feeding. Women often fear that nursing will ruin the shape of their breasts and decrease their sexual attractiveness. Similarly, as more women return to work, they may find it impossible to breast-feed and maintain their work schedules; scheduling child care and a job is usually complicated enough. But fortunately the past opposition to breast-feeding has diminished in recent years, as more and more women are returning to the "natural" method of infant feeding.

Almost every woman who wants to nurse is physiologically and psychologically able to produce sufficient milk to satisfy the nutritional needs of her newborn infant. Many women do require instruction and encouragement in learning how to breast-feed and, as breast-feeding is becoming more popular, self-help groups such as the Human Lactation Center[1] and La Leche League[2] are proliferating. These supportive groups are doing much to dispel mistaken ideas that small-breasted, nervous, or working mothers should not attempt to breast-feed.

Vitamin and Mineral Supplementation

Nutritionists believe that breast milk and modern commercial formulas come quite close to meeting all the nutrient requirements of infancy. Nevertheless, almost every new mother carrying home her tiny infant also carries a small bottle of vitamin drops. Most pediatricians recommend these vitamin preparations and most mothers use them, not because they have been proven necessary, but because they have not yet been proven unnecessary.

[1]Human Lactation Center, Ltd., 666 Sturgis Highway, Westport, Conn. 06880.
[2]La Leche League International, 9616 Minneapolis Avenue, Franklin Park, Ill. 60131.

PERSPECTIVE ON
Formula-Feeding in Developing Countries

The United States and other modernized countries have long encouraged the development of valuable natural resources in developing areas of the world, and Western technology has made much of this development possible. It is ironic, then, that these same nations also provide technology that discourages the use of one natural resource that developing countries have in abundant supply: breast milk.

Milk as a resource? It is indeed, since the cost of replacing it with a commercial product is prohibitive for most inhabitants of Third World nations. In Uganda a laborer would have to spend one-third, and in Tanzania one-half, of a day's wages to buy a day's supply of infant formula. According to figures released by the World Bank, the cost of wasted human milk is in the billions of dollars (Berg, 1977).

Yet commercial infant formula has been aggressively marketed in countries whose people cannot afford to buy it and where homes are not equipped with refrigeration, a clean water supply, or adequate heat and equipment for sterilization of bottles and water.

The facts prove that formula cannot be generally used in such circumstances. In Chile, for example, half the mothers receiving formula from the National Health Service were found to be using it incorrectly. In Mexico, diarrhea was ten times more prevalent in a group of formula-fed infants than in a group of breast-fed children, presumably because polluted water was used in preparation of the formula and because these infants were denied the immunological protection provided by breast-feeding. In San Salvador, three-fourths of the infants in one study who died between the first and fifth months of life had been breast-fed for less than 30 days (Berg, 1977). Because of its high cost, overdilution of formulas is not uncommon. While the formula lasts longer, its nutrient content has been similarly diluted, contributing to the higher mortality rates in bottle-fed infants in developing countries.

These reports have formed the basis of a number of complaints and lawsuits brought against the manufacturers and distributors of infant formula in Third World nations. Although such companies have not been enjoined by law from marketing their products, the publicity given to their sales efforts has resulted in government-sponsored pro-breast-feeding information campaigns.

It was once thought that infant formula might be an answer to protein-energy malnutrition in developing countries. Studies have repeatedly shown, however, that malnourished women nevertheless produce surprisingly high-quality milk, usually in quantities sufficient to nourish their infants (see Chapter 12). As in industrialized countries, women who are unable to nurse have benefited from the availability of commercial formulas when they received instructions in its proper preparation. But in usual circumstances, there is little evidence of any gain in infant survival when formula replaces mother's milk (Jelliffe and Jelliffe, 1978)—and any gain there may be is more than cancelled out by the fact that relatively few families in developing countries are able to afford adequate supplies of formula or have the facilities to prepare it correctly. In societies that are still largely traditional, the traditional method of providing infant nourishment is advised.

SUPPLEMENTS FOR BREAST-FED INFANTS. For the first three months of life, breast milk contains adequate amounts of all nutrients—except fluorine and vitamin D. Some research, however, suggests that breast milk supplies sufficient quantities of vitamin D in a water-soluble form. Until this is confirmed by further research, nursing infants should receive vitamin D supplements (10 μg daily), especially if they are not regularly exposed to sunlight. Fluoride must be provided as well, even when the mother is drinking from a fluoridated water supply, because this mineral is inadequately transferred to her milk. Although breast milk provides only a small amount of iron, 50 percent—a relatively high proportion—is absorbed; in combination with stores of the mineral laid down in fetal life, this should be sufficient up to 3 or 4 months of age. However, Fomon et al. (1979) recommend a daily supplement, preferably in the form of ferrous sulfate. Other supplements should be considered if the mother's diet is poor or unbalanced. Infants nursed by strict vegetarian mothers may be at risk of vitamin B_{12} deficiency and should receive supplementation (see Chapter 7).

SUPPLEMENTS FOR BOTTLE-FED INFANTS. Most commercial formulas are supplemented with added nutrients, including iron, vitamin C, and vitamin D. For this reason, mothers who feed formula must be cautioned *against* additional supplements, which may prove harmful to their newborns. Of course, if the formula chosen does not meet normal requirements for iron or other minerals or vitamins, or if the particular baby has special needs, then the pediatrician may well prescribe supplementation.

The fluoride content of formulas reflects the water supply used to manufacture or dilute the product (Tinanoff and Mueller, 1978). Because manufacturers have recently reduced the fluoride content of their infant formulas, bottle-fed infants should be given fluoride supplements, taking into account the fluoride concentration of the local water supply.

Most commercial formulas contain ascorbic acid in amounts sufficient to withstand heat processing. However, if evaporated milk formula is being prepared in the home, vitamin C supplements should be given. Because young babies are often allergic to orange juice, it is not introduced for several months, and then in dilute form and small amounts, gradually increased as the baby shows signs of tolerating it. For this reason, supplemental doses of ascorbic acid are generally given until orange juice has been added to the diet in sufficient quantity.

Introduction of Solid Foods

As the popularity of breast-feeding has waxed and waned, so too has the accepted wisdom of when to introduce solid foods.

TIMING. An infant requires solid foods when milk or formula can no longer provide the nutrients and energy necessary for optimal growth and development. A century ago, it was customary to wait until the second year of life to wean a baby from breast to solids. By the 1960s the pendulum had swung to the other extreme, and infants were commonly receiving cereal at 2 to 3 days of age and meat and vegetable combinations at 17 days. Among factors responsible for this shift were the increasing availability of commercially prepared infant foods and the popular belief that early introduction of solid foods was related somehow to better and earlier maturation and development. Most recently, solids (sometimes called *beikost*) are being introduced between 4 and 6 months of age. This timing is now considered best both from a developmental point of view and on the basis of physiological and nutritional needs.

DEVELOPMENT. Babies are not able to initiate voluntary swallowing movements until they are about 16 weeks of age. Earlier than that, swallowing is merely the final component of the sucking reflex. Thus, any solid foods that are introduced before that time cannot be handled easily and will automatically be pushed out of the baby's mouth. This is known as the extrusion reflex. Also, in the earliest months the infant has only limited ability to communicate feelings about eating. Sometime during the fourth month, however, the infant becomes able not only to draw in its upper lip to keep foods inside the mouth, but can also lean forward to express eagerness to eat, or turn aside to signal that "enough is enough." For these reasons, nutritionists believe that earlier introduction of solids runs counter to developmental patterns and may lead to overfeeding of an infant who cannot handle, but also cannot refuse, what is put into its mouth.

Physiological correlates of these developmental signs generally support this timing. The salivary enzymes necessary for digesting complex carbohydrates are not present until the second or third month of age, and kidneys do not function efficiently until the end of the second month of life.

These are average developmental stages, and any given baby may deviate from any of them by several weeks or more. The best way to tell when a baby is developmentally ready for the introduction of solid foods is to pay attention to signals given by the baby. The first appearance of drooling indicates increased salivary production. The appearance of new facial expressions, especially in the mouth area, indicate maturation of oral musculature. The most significant sign of a baby's readiness for new foods is hunger: When the baby takes 26 to 30 ounces of milk from the bottle in 24 hours, or nurses voraciously and is trying to get more after each feeding, or seems hungry after shorter intervals, an alert parent might sense that the time is right to introduce solid foods.

When solid foods are offered before the baby is ready to accept them, a negative pattern of interaction between infant and parent may be established, with negative ramifications for the acceptance of food at a later date. Many parents attempt to add solids in the early months in the belief that hunger is preventing the baby from sleeping through the night. But the ability to sleep for longer periods is developmentally independent of the need for nonmilk sources of food.

Some parents go to the other extreme and delay the introduction of solid foods past the age of 6 months in the belief that milk is the only food a baby needs. This practice tends to be associated with breast-feeding. But because of the growing appetite of the older baby, the excessive amounts of milk consumed will prevent development of an appetite for foods that are better sources of nutrients, such as iron, needed by the middle of the first year. Also, the breast-fed infant needs some protein-rich foods by this age.

CHOOSING SOLID FOODS. A wide variety of prepared foods is waiting to tempt baby's appetite—iron-fortified cereals in dry form to be mixed with formula, or milk; jars of egg yolks, meats, strained vegetables, meat-and-vegetable combinations, fruit-and-cereal combinations, cottage cheese, puddings, and more. Generally, cooked cereal is the recommended first food. It has the advantage of being able to be mixed with formula or milk to any desired consistency; typically 1 teaspoon of dried cereal mixed with 1 tablespoon of fluid should be offered by spoon before giving bottle or breast to a hungry baby.

A baby will usually look surprised at this new event, but parents should not interpret a baby's deservedly puzzled reaction to these new sensations as a negative response. If the first feeding of cereal is not readily accepted—and often it is not—they should try again the next day and the next, always when the baby is hungry. Soon the cereal will be received eagerly; only 22 out of 383 mothers reported problems, physiological or otherwise, with infant acceptance of cereals (Harris and Chan, 1969). After a while less milk can be used in proportion to dry cereal. Some parents mix a little cereal into the formula and feed it by bottle, using a nipple with an enlarged hole. Although this ensures that the cereal will be ingested and the nutritional benefits gained, it does little to acquaint the infant with the experience of eating new foods.

Once a baby has acquired the knack of eating, other foods can be tried. Usually, fruit purees are added next, then strained vegetables, vegetable and meat combinations, egg yolks, and strained meats.

Newborns apparently do not have a preference for the taste of a salt solution (Maller and Desor, 1973). Despite this, salt and monosodium glutamate were routinely added to commercial infant foods, probably to appeal to the tastes of parents. Widespread consumer concern that oversalting might predispose susceptible infants to hypertension in adulthood and condition individuals to want salty foods, and reports that monosodium glutamate caused brain malformation in young laboratory animals, led manufacturers to omit these additions in the late 1970s. Table 13-3 compares the sodium content of baby foods before and after salt was omitted. In recent years, oversweetening has been frowned upon as well. Many baby fruits and desserts today are prepared with only enough sugar to counteract the natural tartness of the fruit. New formulations of baby foods do contain some additives that were not present in earlier years, such as ascorbic acid in applesauce and other fruits to help meet infants' vitamin C requirements (Matthews and Workman, 1978). Modified starch is also added to some items to improve their texture. The USDA has recently published a handbook which reflects some of these changes in the composition of baby foods (USDA, 1978).

Some parents prefer to prepare their own baby foods, which they know will be free of additives. This practice is acceptable if sanitary conditions are maintained for all utensils and equipment used. Wooden cutting boards should not be used; only fresh and unblemished produce should be purchased; leftovers should be refrigerated or frozen promptly.

Whenever possible the baby should be fed at the same time as, and in the same room with, the other members of the family. Eating is a social experience, and the pleasure of family intimacy at mealtime enhances appetite and establishes a wholesome pattern for the future. In this setting the infant learns to welcome both new foods and new social relationships. In the second

TABLE 13-3
Sodium Content of Selected Baby Foods (mg/100 g)

Food	Agriculture Handbook 8	Revised Values
Oatmeal (dry)	437	30
Beans, green	213	88
Beef (strained)	228	140
Vegetables and lamb	269	118

Source: R. H. Matthews and M.Y. Workman, Nutrient content of selected baby foods, *Journal of the American Dietetic Association* 72:27, 1978, Table 7.

half of the first year, some finger foods can be added—a crust of bread, pieces of chicken meat, boneless fish, carrot sticks, cubes of boiled potato. The baby should be encouraged to explore these new taste and texture experiences, even at the risk of some messiness. The goal is a child who enjoys food.

Special Concerns in Infant Feeding

Not all feeding problems are of social origin. A baby who refuses foods or appears uncomfortable after eating may be suffering from a physiological problem that interferes with digestion or metabolism. In very young infants, bloating, abdominal pains, and similar symptoms are often interpreted as signs of lactose malabsorption. Studies indicate that true lactose malabsorption is quite rare in infancy even in ethnic groups previously thought to have hereditary lactase deficiency (Lebenthal, 1979) (see Chapter 2). Food allergies, however, are not so rare, and can produce similar symptoms.

ALLERGIES. Milk allergy often causes an allergic reaction in infants, largely because milk is their primary food. There may be sensitivity not to lactose but to one of the three milk proteins: lactalbumin, lactoglobulin, and casein. Lactalbumin is the most frequent culprit. When solid foods are introduced—especially egg, wheat, citrus fruit, and fish—susceptible infants may experience allergic reactions. The best treatment is to avoid the offending foods. Only one new food should be introduced at a time; then, if there is any reaction, it will be easy to identify the cause. In a family with a history of allergies, new foods should be introduced slowly and with caution. Rice and oats are less allergic than wheat and so are advisable choices as the first solid food for babies. Banana, either mashed or in dry form mixed with a little formula, is also a good early food.

FEEDING OF LOW BIRTH WEIGHT INFANTS. Other biologically based feeding problems relate to birth weight. The basal metabolic rate of low birth weight infants is lower than that of full-term infants during the first week of life, but it reaches and exceeds the full-term's level by the second week. Thus, daily energy requirements in proportion to body weight are higher for low birth weight infants. At the same time their stomachs are smaller than normal for their age and can hold less food at a time. They should receive more frequent feedings (every three hours or more often) to meet their high energy needs, and they may need more concentrated formulas to supply their energy and protein requirements (Committee on Nutrition, 1978).

OBESITY. At the other end of the scale, high birth weight infants or those who gain excess weight in early infancy may also require nutritional monitoring. Contrary to some study results, the type of milk fed to infants and the early or late introduction of solid foods may not be a significant factor in their tendency to remain overweight in childhood and in adulthood (Himes, 1979).

VEGETARIANISM. Chapters 4 and 7 mentioned some special problems of infants nursed by strict vegetarian mothers. Suggestions for supplementation of the mother's diet were given in Chapter 12. Concerns for iron and vitamin B_{12} status should not be taken lightly; severe deficiencies have been reported (Frader et al., 1978). A recent report of profound protein-energy malnutrition has come from a vegetarian community where breast-fed infants were weaned at 3 months and fed an extremely low-energy preparation of home-prepared soya milk with no foods of animal origin and no vitamin supplementation. Retarded physical development, anemia, rickets, osteoporosis, and other severe deficiency symptoms were observed. Intervention and prescription of a balanced vegetarian diet conforming to the beliefs of the parents was generally successful (Zmora et al., 1979).

NUTRITIONAL STATUS OF AMERICAN INFANTS

There have been few studies that were broad-based enough to provide adequate data for an accurate, overall appraisal of the nutritional status of American infants. A Preschool Nutrition Survey, conducted from November 1968 to December 1970, studied about 3,400 children age 1 to 6 years and was designed to provide an overview of nutritional status for that age group. At about the same time the Ten-State Nutrition Survey was being carried out to determine the extent of malnutrition in the United States, and it focused primarily on adults in poverty and near-poverty communities (see Chapter 10). Some 3,700 children under 6 years of age were included in the TSNS. The Health and Nutrition Examination Survey (HANES) of 1971–1974 was more representative of the general population and included about 3,500 children from birth to 18 years, of whom about 1,500 were 6 or younger. Designed as a continuing survey of nutritional status representative of the national population, HANES should eventually produce a sizable body of data. Preliminary material is, however, all that is available at present.

Generally, these surveys do not indicate major nutrient deficiencies in young American children. More than 30 percent of the infants in the Ten-State Nutrition Survey had iron and vitamin C intakes less than two-thirds of the RDA for those nutrients, and anemia was identified in many. Anemia has consistently been identified in more limited studies as well.

Other than widespread iron deficiency, however, few nutritional problems were found. It was apparent, though, that nutritional deficiencies were more prevalent among lower socioeconomic segments of the population. Evidence that early nutritional deficiencies may cause later abnormalities in physical and mental functioning has spurred programs to alleviate malnutrition in the young. The Women, Infants, and Children Supplemental Food Program (WIC) in particular has increased food buying power for mothers and their young children. (WIC, School Lunch Programs, and Food Stamps are discussed in Chapter 16.)

Infant Nutrition: The Final Analysis

The mother is usually the final arbiter about what, when, and how much an infant will be fed. She needs information, and considerable support, in making these decisions. Current recommendations for feeding normal infants

(Fomon et al., 1979) reflect present knowledge. As research continues in this important area, the long-term consequences of early feeding practices will emerge. This is an important goal, for a good start in the early years is the best guarantee of physical and mental health in all the growth stages that follow.

INTRODUCTION TO NUTRITION DURING CHILDHOOD

At 1 year of age, the child bears scant resemblance to the infant at 1 month. At the brink of the second year, birth weight has tripled and length has increased by 50 percent or more. The child has developed a full crop of hair and 6 to 12 teeth. In addition to this visible physical progress, there has been significant behavioral, emotional, and social maturation. The child can sit, stand, and perhaps walk and speak a few words, cry in anger and frustration rather than just because of hunger, recognize family members and other familiar faces, and charm them all with a ready smile. The typical 1-year-old has achieved a transition from breast milk or formula to solid food and whole milk and has joined the rest of the family at the dining table.

In the preschool years, attitudes toward food and eating evolve that will last throughout life. Although the child's food needs are a reflection of a changing internal environment, the eating habits and food preferences that develop are influenced by the external environment.

CHILDHOOD GROWTH PATTERNS

In comparison with the rapid growth of the first 12 months, the rate of growth decreases considerably during the childhood years. Between 2 and 10 years of age, the average height increment is about 2 to 4 inches per year, compared to the 9 or 10 inches typically added in the first year. Weight is gained at a proportionately slower rate as well. While most infants gain about 16 pounds during the first year, toddlers and older children typically gain from 4 to 8 pounds each year. (Figures 13-4 and 13-5 depict normal growth patterns during childhood and adolescence.)

The easily visible signs of growth provided by height and weight measures reflect underlying changes in the accumulation of muscle tissue, skeletal growth, and deposition of fat. Just as height and weight vary from one child to the next, differences in body composition are also apparent. Garn et al. (1975)

FIGURE 13-4 (opp. page)

Weight and Height by Age for Girls from 2 to 18 Years

Source: Adapted from National Center for Health Statistics, *NCHS growth charts, 1976.* Monthly Vital Statistics Report, Vol. 25, No. 3, Supp., (HRA) 76-1120 (Rockville, Maryland: Health Resources Administration, June, 1976). © 1976 Ross, Laboratories.

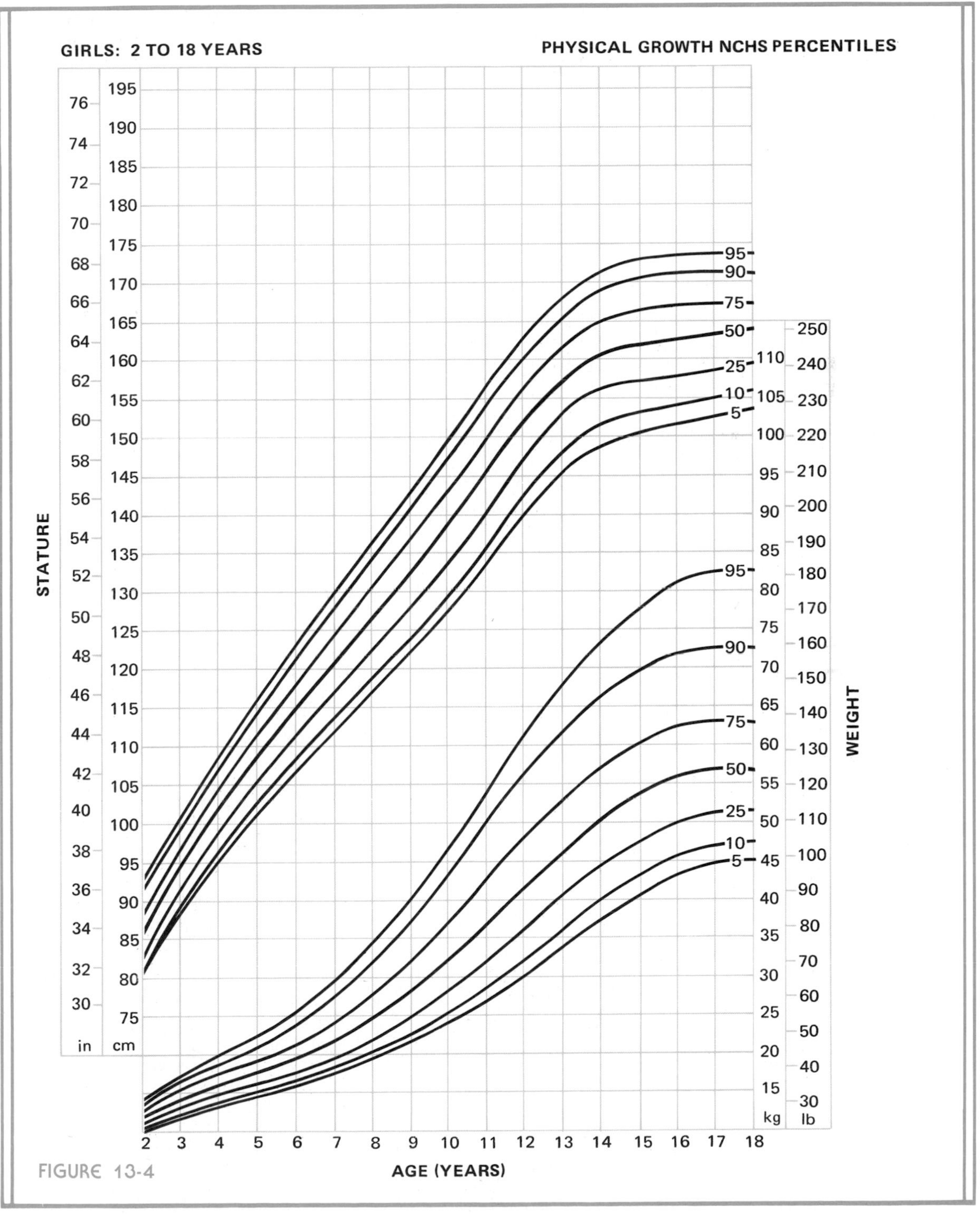
GIRLS: 2 TO 18 YEARS
PHYSICAL GROWTH NCHS PERCENTILES
STATURE
in
cm
WEIGHT
kg
lb
AGE (YEARS)
95
90
75
50
25
10
5

FIGURE 13-4

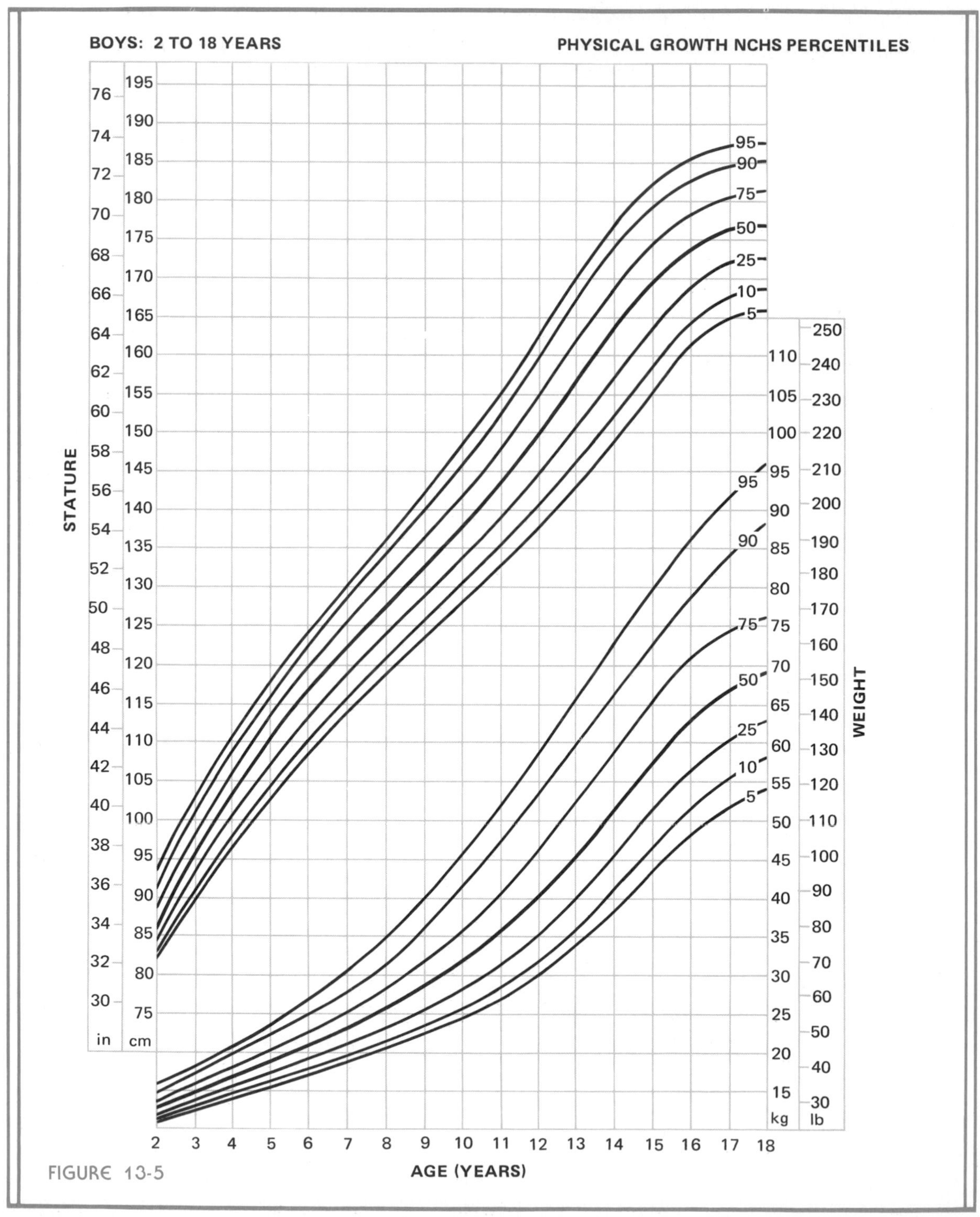
BOYS: 2 TO 18 YEARS
PHYSICAL GROWTH NCHS PERCENTILES
STATURE
WEIGHT
AGE (YEARS)
in
cm
kg
lb
95
90
75
50
25
10
5

FIGURE 13-5

FIGURE 13-5 (opp. page)

Weight and Height by Age for Boys from 2 to 18 Years

Source: Adapted from National Center for Health Statistics, *NCHS growth charts, 1976,* Monthly Vital Statistics Report, Vol. 25, No. 3, Supp. (HRA) 76-1120 (Rockville, Maryland: Health Resources Administration, June, 1976). © Ross Laboratories.

have observed that obese children are not only fatter than the nonobese, but are also taller and have relatively greater skeletal mass.

Records of height and weight are important indicators of general health in children and of nutritional health in particular. Although the effects of nutrient deprivation on weight gain are most readily apparent, linear growth is also affected by severe undernutrition. Systemic diseases that disrupt absorption, digestion, and metabolism, as well as general undernutrition, can interfere with physical growth. It is important that growth records be maintained for every child, because when abnormal signs are recognized early enough, growth deficits may be halted and even reversed.

There is apparently a developmental period in which "catch-up" growth, within genetically predetermined limits, is possible. In Europe during and after the Second World War, it was observed that average heights of young children and adolescents were generally lower than those of the prewar childhood generation, a result of wartime food shortages. Dietary supplements of milk or high-energy foods given to selected groups of undernourished children produced increases in height, weight, and skeletal maturity significantly greater than those of children whose diets were not supplemented. Similar growth spurts attributable to dietary improvements have been reported even in racial groups whose members had once been considered to be genetically small. In Japan, for example, children born since World War II have been found to be significantly taller than children of the prewar period; the increment has been ascribed to their greater intake of animal protein, although increased consumption of animal-derived foods presumably increased the energy content of their diets as well. Thus, dietary protein would be "spared" from use for energy production, and the amino acids could be used more efficiently for growth.

NUTRITIONAL NEEDS DURING CHILDHOOD

When nutrient and energy needs of children are expressed per pound or kilogram of body weight, they are actually lower than those of infants. Of course, because children are larger, their absolute nutritional needs are indeed increased. Table 13-4 shows the RDAs for children of different ages.

Energy

Energy needs in childhood, as in other stages of the life cycle, vary according to individual body size and composition, rate of growth, and physical activity. The amount of energy required just for growth in the first 12 months of life is so great that, although toddlers and youngsters are markedly more active than

TABLE 13-4 **RDAs for Children**

							Fat-Soluble Vitamins			Water-Soluble Vitamins							Minerals					
Age years	Weight kg	Weight lb	Height cm	Height in	Energy kcal	Protein gm	Vitamin A (μg RE)	Vitamin D (μg)	Vitamin E Activity (mg α T.E.)	Vitamin C (mg)	Folacin μg	Niacin mg	Riboflavin mg	Thiamin mg	Vitamin B_6 mg	Vitamin B_{12} μg	Calcium mg	Phosphorus mg	Iodine μg	Iron mg	Magnesium mg	Zinc mg
1-3	13	29	90	35	1300	23	400	10	5	45	100	9	0.8	0.7	0.9	2.0	800	800	70	15	150	10
4-6	20	44	112	44	1700	30	500	10	6	45	200	11	1.0	0.9	1.3	2.5	800	800	90	10	200	10
7-10	28	62	132	52	2400	34	700	10	7	45	300	16	1.4	1.2	1.6	3.0	800	800	120	10	250	10

Source: Food and Nutrition Board, National Academy of Sciences, *Recommended daily dietary allowances,* revised 1979 (Washington, D.C.: National Research Council, 1979).

infants, their total energy needs in proportion to body weight are actually less. Thus the recommended energy allowance for a child from ages 1 through 10 is only 85 to 100 kilocalories per kilogram compared to 105 to 115 kilocalories per kilogram of body weight during the first 12 months. Individual energy requirements, of course, must take into account the variation in physical activity from one child to the next. Observations of height, weight, and general physical appearance are the best indicators of how well a given child's energy intake is matched to needs. Tendencies toward obesity or to extreme underweight can and should be monitored and corrected promptly.

Protein

Protein Allowances for Children

Age years	Protein Requirement g/kg of body weight
1-3	1.8
4-6	1.5
7-10	1.2

Protein can provide energy, but its primary function is to supply the amino acids necessary for growth and development. As with the RDA for energy, the recommended daily protein intake for children also decreases in proportion to body weight, while increasing in absolute quantity. During the years from 1 to 10, 1.8 to 1.2 grams per kilogram of body weight is recommended; this compares with 2.0 to 2.2 grams per kilogram during the child's first year (Food and Nutrition Board, 1979).

This recommendation assumes that high-quality proteins (milk, meat, eggs, dairy products, or food combinations that provide complementary proteins) will be consumed to provide essential amino acids. Because amino acids will be deaminated and used as a source of energy when total energy intake is insufficient, they will not be available for protein synthesis if the overall diet is inadequate. On the other hand, consumption in excess of this recommendation is not needed; it is economically wasteful and nutritionally unnecessary.

Carbohydrate and Fat

There are no RDAs for carbohydrate and fat for any age group. Both of these nutrients provide energy, and fats are important as sources of essential fatty acids. From 30 to 40 percent of energy intake should be provided as dietary lipid, with 2 to 5 percent in the form of essential fatty acids (Fomon, 1974). These percentages are usually met through consumption of whole milk, meat, margarine or butter, mayonnaise, salad dressing, peanut butter, cheese, and other common foods. If there is too little fat in the diet, meals will be dry and unpalatable; there will also be an accompanying risk of essential fatty acid deficiency. Too much fat will limit the child's appetite for other foods and might contribute to obesity.

Well-publicized findings that excess fat consumption in early life may play a role in later development of coronary heart disease have caused some parents to question the need for so much fat, especially high-cholesterol foods, in children's diets. This concern has led nutritionists and pediatricians to recommend that consumption of foods high in cholesterol and with excessive quantities of fat be limited for children in familes with a history of cardiovascular disease or hyperlipidemia. But there is little or no evidence of benefit in restricting lipid intake for normal healthy children. Misplaced concern about high-cholesterol foods, particularly eggs, may cause parents to limit intake of otherwise excellent foods. Especially for children with finicky food habits, eggs can be an important source of complete protein as well as of many other nutrients.

In the United States, carbohydrates supply about 40 to 50 percent of children's energy needs. Although the Food and Nutrition Board has not established an RDA for carbohydrate, a minimum of 50 to 100 grams per day (200 to 400 kcal) has been suggested. The greatest part of carbohydrate intake should be in the form of complex carbohydrates and naturally-occurring sugars found in bananas, apples, raisins, and other fruits. Carbohydrates in the form of sucrose in candy bars and soft drinks should be consumed in moderation. The excess energy provided by these foods may contribute to obesity, and the simple sugars to dental caries. In addition, these foods limit a child's appetite for other, more nutritious, foods.

Vitamins and Minerals

Active growing children require a full complement of vitamins and minerals. Although a diversified diet usually meets these needs, supplements are useful and necessary when a child's food intake is limited by illness or quirky food habits, or if specific deficiencies have been diagnosed.

Many of the vitamins and minerals are necessary for skeletal and tissue growth, and thus are especially important for growing children. Vitamin D is of particular importance for bone growth and development. Children whose exposure to sunlight is limited should receive 10 μg of this antirachitic vitamin per day, the amount contained in a quart of fortified milk. Cod-liver oil and other supplements providing vitamins D and A are no longer considered necessary for children. Because these vitamins are fat soluble, excesses tend to accumulate in adipose tissue and may build up to toxic levels. Vitamin D supplementation is advisable for healthy children only if they get no sunshine and drink no milk, and should not exceed 10 μg per day.

DEVELOPMENT OF FOOD BEHAVIORS

After the first cry that fills the newborn's lungs with air, the next cry is likely to be a plaintive call for food. The way in which parents meet these early, instinctive food demands sets the stage for permanent eating patterns and develops the desirable motivation we know as appetite.

There is a vast difference between hunger—the unpleasant sensation of stomach pain, weakness, and general irritability—and appetite—the pleasurable anticipation that food will both assuage hunger and delight the senses. All healthy infants and children show hunger; the fact that all do not appear to show appetite is the crux of our discussion. The earliest feeding experiences are associated with comfort, contentment, and the pleasure of interpersonal closeness between mother and child. These associations are gradually extended to all other individuals who may provide food—father, relatives, babysitters, friends—and to the entire feeding environment—the chair in which the mother sits for feeding, the bottle, even the towel used for burping. Before long, the infant responds to the sight of a bottle being filled or the mother preparing food, and begins to cry. Such responses to food cues are the first signs of a developing appetite, the first signs that the infant understands the purpose of eating.

Influence of Parents and Home

Infants typically make their first chewing movements, even before a tooth has erupted, at about 6 months of age. Those who are given small pieces of hard toast or a similar food soon master the art of chewing, while those who are not given such food at this time have difficulty learning to chew (Lowenberg, 1977). The same is true for every developmental ability. As soon, therefore, as a child is able to pick up small pieces of food, to poke at and explore new foods, to hold a cup or a spoon and help in the feeding process, appropriate foods and utensils should be provided. By taking advantage of skills as they appear, parents can encourage the acquisition of the many behaviors necessary for lifelong enjoyment of food and good nutrition.

Toddlers are often in a naturally negative stage just when they should be introduced to new food experiences. They say "No-no" even though that is not what they really mean. This negativism is a universal stage of development, necessary for children to separate themselves psychologically and develop the independence required for the next stages of maturation. But parents tend to respond to what the child says, not to the underlying meanings. The more the child resists, the more anxious the parent becomes, and the more likely the child is to continue resisting. This pattern of stress and resistance creates unhappy mealtimes and poor eaters, setting a destructive pattern for years to come.

With a seat at the family dining table comes a child's-eye view of not only what parents, siblings, and guests are eating, but their attitudes about it. The adult conversation may have a strong effect. If, as one commentator has said, the purpose of grown-ups at the table is simply to make sure that the children eat (Marzollo, 1979), the children will learn early that they can get more attention by *not* eating. Negative comments about food from other family members can also have an impact, and so can special treatment accorded to another member of the family. If a father refuses to eat something, his children are not likely to want that food either. One wise mother served spinach and cucumbers—foods her husband would not accept—to her children only on nights when their father was not home in time for dinner, and both of her children have enjoyed those foods ever since. Even excessive

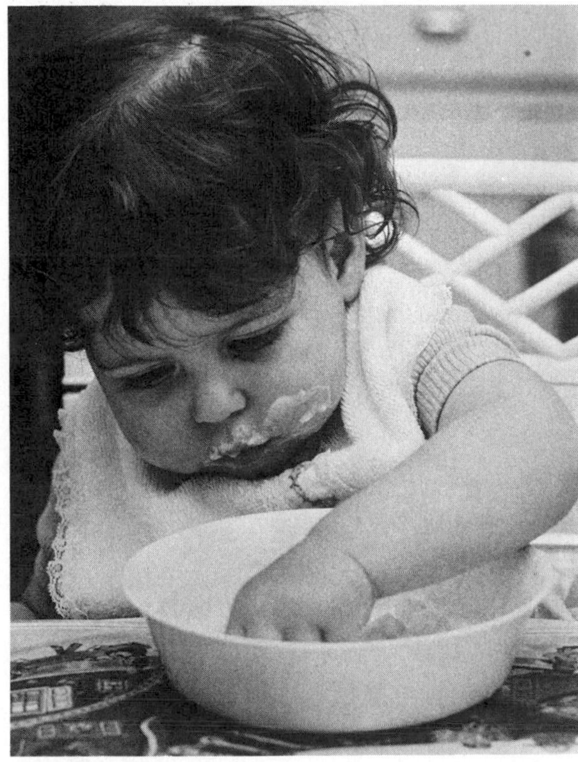

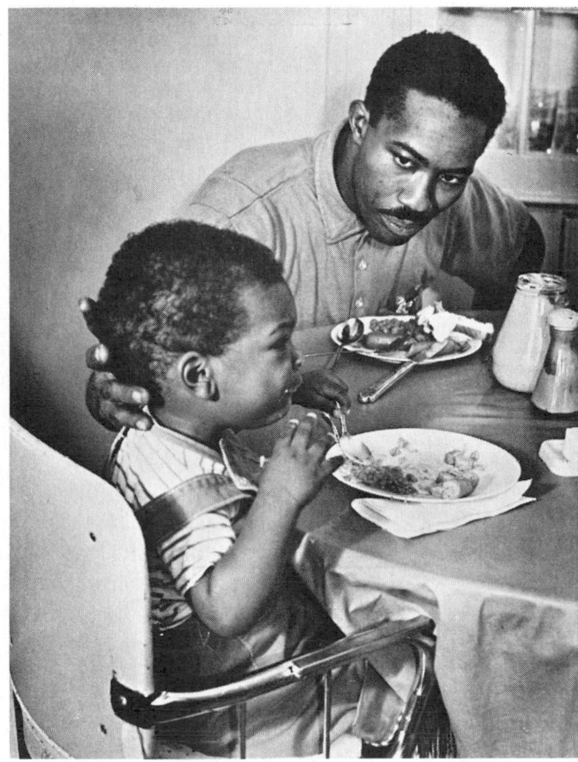

Children learn to enjoy food when they are allowed to feed themselves (even at the cost of some messiness!) and when mealtime is a shared family experience. (Left: Erika Stone, Photo Researchers, Inc. Right: Hanna W. Schreiber, Rapho/Photo Researchers, Inc.)

discussion about food—Do you like the chicken? Have some more salad. Wait 'til you taste the potatoes!—can diminish a child's appetite. And so can an overfilled plate.

Parents may be unable to avoid negative influences brought into the home by well-meaning babysitters or grandparents. The sitter who must get every last morsel into the child, and devises distracting entertainments while pushing a spoon into an unwilling mouth, has contributed to mealtime havoc in many homes. A grandparent who says "eat your fish because it's good for you" can undo many happy hours of eating fish because it tastes good.

Outside Influences: School and Friends

As more and more mothers have joined the work force, the care and feeding of many 2- and 3-year-olds is left to others. This situation often contributes to good nutritional practices. Since child care centers, and the preschools and kindergartens that serve meals, are usually licensed by agencies that mandate sound mealtime patterns and provide some foods (see Chapter 16), the child whose at-home nutrition is marginal may for the first time be introduced to well-balanced meals and a diversified diet.

In many preschool and early elementary school programs, children have an opportunity to become involved in the preparation and serving of their own meals. A class field trip to a local market to buy ingredients for vegetable soup, and then a morning spent preparing them and watching the simmering pot, may create interest in foods that, at home, do not seem appealing. Also, the activity provided in school may help the child to work up an appetite, and by lunchtime be hungry enough to eat whatever is put on the plate. Eating with other children, perhaps singing or playing a game at the table while waiting for the next course, is an enjoyable social experience that enhances appetite.

But some children who have acquired excellent attitudes at home may learn undesirable food habits by watching their peers. It may take only one small voice saying "yeccch" to the green beans to turn a former bean lover against them. No parents can completely prevent such influences; they can only hope that the positive atmosphere of the home will be strong enough to counteract any damage done by other children's poor dining habits.

As the child gets older and moves up through elementary grades, increasing influence is wielded by peers. More independent now of parents, children have some money in their pockets to use at the corner candy store or the in-school vending machine. Nutritional quality is not guaranteed by the availability of feeding programs in the schools or even by a balanced brown-bag lunch brought from home. Children seldom eat everything on their lunch trays; and many a mother would be distressed to find that the shiny red apple she packed was traded to another child for a gooey caramel bar—with obvious benefit to the child who got the apple!

Influence of the Mass Media

Parental vigilance is no match for the television set and its continual messages to "enjoy chocolatey this" or "try some finger-licking that." Children soon become aware that "chocolatey" and "finger-licking" are more important than nutritious, fresh, or well balanced. Almost all homes in the United States have at least one television set, and today's children spend more time in their preschool years watching television than they will spend in the classroom during four years of college. It has been estimated that over 20 percent of those viewing hours are spent watching commercials. And of those commercials, at least 40 percent mention food—a figure that is as high as 70 percent in the hours when children are watching. According to Federal Trade Commission studies and parental observations, much of this advertising is for presweetened cereals, candy, and fast-food products served at local "family" restaurants.

The young child is often unable to separate commercial messages from the regular program; preschoolers, it has been found, attend just as closely and receptively to commercial messages as to entertainment segments (Ward et al., 1972). Parents have been quick to realize this and have formed groups such as Action for Children's Television (ACT), which has pressured the Federal Communications Commission and the Federal Trade Commission to limit commercial interruptions during childrens' prime viewing hours.

In the mid-1970s, the National Advertising Board restricted by about 20 percent the amount of commercial time permitted during children's programs. Many television stations voluntarily limited this time even further. In addition, companies were prohibited from using stars to endorse food products and from advertising "kiddy vitamins" during children's shows.

In 1979, the Federal Trade Commission held public hearings as part of a two-year investigation into the influence of television advertising. ACT has proposed that *all* television commercials directed at children under 12 years of age be banned, but that is unlikely to occur.

By definition, the mass media comprise print as well as audio and visual materials that reach large numbers of people to provide information and entertainment. Magazines for children, radio, billboards and other forms of public placards, and even package design carry advertising messages relating to food. We cannot isolate a child from society—and it is probably not even desirable to do so. The child must interact with other children and learn to live as well as possible in the world as it is. Parents can monitor their children's television watching; but more importantly, they should not give in to pressure to buy every food or snack that is advertised.

Recommendations for Encouraging Good Food Habits

Obviously, positive nutritional patterns cannot be legislated; they must begin in the home during the formative years and be reinforced daily. A relaxed atmosphere at mealtime gives children a chance to develop at their own rate.

Few parents realize how little food a young child actually needs. A child of average size and normal rate of development can manage only about 1 tablespoon of each type of food served at each meal for each year of his or her age. In other words, a 2-year-old could be expected to consume 2 tablespoons of meat, 2 tablespoons of vegetables, and 2 tablespoons of fruit, in addition to the regular serving of milk or juice. The total food served at one meal to a 2-year-old should be just 6 tablespoons or about ⅓ cup—far less than most 2-year-olds are urged to eat. By this standard parents may realize that their "poor" eaters are actually excellent eaters, and perhaps that their "good" eaters have become overeaters! Children should be offered small servings for other reasons as well. A heaped-up plate is overwhelming and often deters appetite. And second helpings can be freely offered, allowing the child to ask for more.

Children have their likes and dislikes just as adults do, and these should be respected. Trying to force a food which a child dislikes will only stiffen the opposition and turn what is probably a temporary matter of taste into a permanent aversion. If a variety of foods is available, there should be no problem about providing nutritionally valid substitutes. A child who does not care for lettuce and tomatoes may welcome raw carrots and celery. Pineapple juice may be more acceptable than orange juice; melon preferred to grapefruit; rice chosen over potatoes.

Even good eaters go on occasional food jags, refusing some former favorites and limiting their diet to one or two foods at each meal. When parents respond with understanding—and some ingenuity—the child's erratic eating is likely to be of short duration and little nutritional significance. For a child who will eat only desserts, the ingenious parent may fix egg custards or fruit purees. When a substitute is available, a child learns to try more foods because there is always something familiar to eat if a new food doesn't work out. Sometimes a child will even say, "I think I'll like it next time," or give another clue about food readiness to an alert parent.

Children's tastes change, often with amazing rapidity. The child who consumes nothing but hamburger at the age of 4 discovers chicken at $4\frac{1}{2}$. Children's tastes may seem inconsistent: The child who cannot look at a cooked green pea on a plate may devour a bowl full of them raw. And something that might not be touched at dinnertime may appear very appetizing during a half-hour alone in the kitchen with father or mother while dinner is being prepared. This is a good time to introduce new foods: "Mommy and Daddy are going to have this; would you like to try some?"

Some children will eat only "breakfast" foods—for breakfast, lunch, and supper. But this need not be a problem. Eggs and toast can be offered at any meal, perhaps with a slice of meat or a raw vegetable on the side. Only cultural conditions dictate that chicken is for dinner and cereals for breakfast. And a cereal can be served as a side dish at dinner—cornmeal or farina are good choices, palatable with margarine or, for the more sophisticated tastes of the rest of the family, any tomato- or meat-based sauce.

An important tactic is to introduce new foods at the beginning of the meal, when the child is hungry. Hunger may win out over prejudice, and a new dish is added to the repertoire. An older child may be allowed to help plan menus; even a kindergartener can understand the Basic Food Groups and be shown how they are used to plan the dishes that appear on the family table.

As in so many other areas, parents must steer carefully between extremes when it comes to the development of food behaviors in their children. On the one hand they must set reasonable limits on a child's intake, while on the other they must encourage the development of self-control. They must teach the importance of eating a variety of foods, but they must respect the child's integrity and right to have likes and dislikes. They must teach table manners, while recognizing the slow development of those skills that make manners possible. And through it all they must keep the atmosphere at the dining table pleasant, even when stressful situations arise. This is as important as any other recommendation: Eating is supposed to be enjoyable for children . . . and for their parents, too.

NUTRITION IN CHILDHOOD

Foods for Children

Foods generally enjoyed by preschoolers include cereals, breads, crackers, crunchy raw vegetables, meats that are easy to chew, fruits, and sweet baked goods such as cookies. Many children will accept any meat that comes with a bone for a "handle," while others will eat only hamburger. Generally, because youngsters are not yet comfortable with utensils, they are happy with finger foods. Raw vegetables—garden-fresh green beans, carrots, cucumbers, and red or green peppers cut in small pieces or "sticks"—are usually welcome. The attractive colors of raw vegetables and their crunchy texture make them more appealing than most cooked vegetables.

Mild tastes also tend to please young palates. Foods are usually preferred without sauces, gravies, or strong seasonings. And most children like to see their food arranged neatly and in separate "categories" on the plate—woe to the parent who inadvertently slips a green pea into the mashed potatoes!

Children often go through phases of extreme fussiness about their food and the way it is presented. They may eat a sandwich only if it is cut into two rectangles, but not into triangles; they may not eat anything green; they may decide that two different foods cannot occupy the same plate. A parent's best recourse when these food-related compulsions appear is to take them lightly; in all probability they will go away in their own good time if no fuss is made. But a parent should avoid encouraging such behaviors and even try gently to discourage them. The favorite plate may be in the dishwasher at lunchtime one day; the sandwich can be accidentally cut on the diagonal and peanut butter will still taste the same; green food can be served appetizingly to the rest of the family, and the child will see that nothing happens to those who consume it. A sense of humor at such times goes a long way, too.

The introduction of new foods should not be anticipated with dread, even if such ventures were unsuccessful in the past. In one study, the youngest preschoolers were more accepting of new foods than were 4- and 5-year-olds (Owen et al., 1974): Apparently children too get more set in their ways as they get older, even in the earliest years. Because new foods will appear throughout life, they should be presented regularly to young children, even to those who have seldom accepted them previously. There's always a first time.

Parents should not expect that a child will eat a full portion of anything new. Usually several experimental tastes over a period of weeks are needed before a normal portion will be accepted. If a food is rejected, a parent should wait a few weeks and try again. One mother introduces new foods to her children by saying "I only have enough to give you a little taste, but if you like it I'll make more the next time." Usually by the third taste the children are hooked.

Meals should be served at regular times. This provides a necessary order in children's lives, helps their "biological clocks" to function effectively, and will also help establish regular work, sleep, and bowel habits. Children often become hungry between regular meals, however, and snacktimes can be inserted into their schedule as well. It is important to allow children to become hungry for their meals. Snacks are so widely available today that many never learn to feel hunger, although they may develop fine appetites for filling snack foods such as soft drinks, potato chips, and candy. Snacks in themselves are not harmful, and they may help a small stomach hold out until dinner time—even adults need a coffee break—but snacks substantial enough to impair eating at regular meals should be avoided. Nuts, fruits, juices, and cheese are snack foods that provide valuable nutrients and can be served in moderation.

The consumption of highly sugared foods should be minimized. It has been found that children from 1 to 5 years consume more soft drinks per unit of body weight than do older children—or indeed any other age group (Burg, 1975). Soft drinks contain large amounts of either sugar or nonnutritive sweeteners, making them particularly poor snack choices for children. Fruit-

PERSPECTIVE ON
Dental Caries

Tooth development begins long before an infant's first pearl-white incisor clinks against a spoon. During the embryonic and fetal periods, teeth and their related structures—the jaws, palate, salivary glands, and associated tissues—undergo the same genetically programmed development as other tissues and organs. The growing dental tissues require provision of nutrients first for cell proliferation and then for cell growth, and they are particularly sensitive to malnutrition, infection, and the action of drugs. At birth, the newborn possesses 20 fully formed primary teeth beneath the gum line, which will begin to erupt during the first year of life. Meanwhile, below the primary teeth, the permanent teeth are being formed.

Dental health begins with good maternal nutrition during pregnancy continues with proper diet in infancy, and later includes regular brushing and dental check-ups throughout childhood and adulthood. The need for this continuing attention and care seems surprising because teeth can withstand environmental ravages for millions of years, to be excavated up in prime condition by paleontologists. The conclusion is startling: A few short years in the harsh environment of the human mouth can be far more destructive than centuries of wind, rain, and changing seasons.

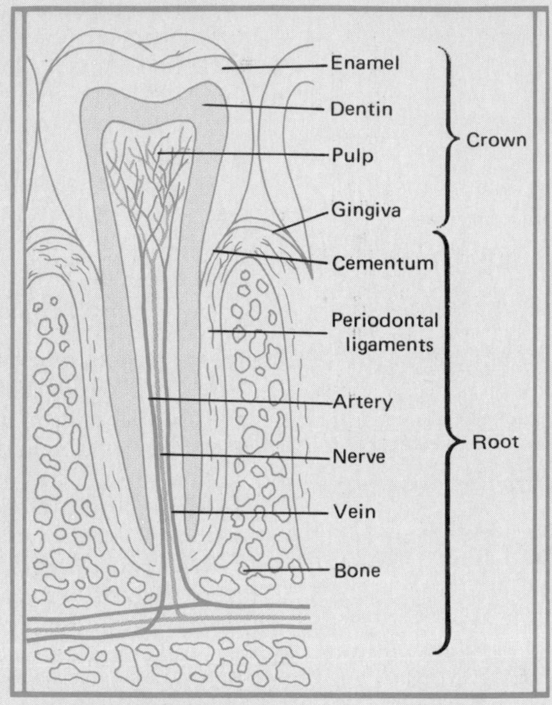

Structure of a Healthy Tooth

Tooth Structure and Development. A tooth's longevity owes much to its fortresslike structure, illustrated in the figure. The outermost wall or enamel is more than 95 percent inorganic, consisting largely of calcium, phosphorus, and magnesium. The next protective layer, dentin, is slightly softer (75 to 80 percent inorganic) and is composed primarily of calcium and phosphorus. The last mineralized layer is the cementum, which surrounds the bottom part of the tooth below the gum line, acting as an interface between the tooth and the surrounding bony jaw tissue. Periodontal ligaments or fibers extend from the cementum to the bone, attaching the teeth to the jaw. Inside these three hard outer layers is the pulp, a soft, fleshy inner tissue containing sensitive nerves and blood vessels.

In embryonic life the protein matrix for the tooth is laid down. Gradually it becomes increasingly mineralized, requiring vitamins A, C, and D, as well as calcium, phosphorus, and magnesium. Given these raw materials, an almost impenetrable tooth fortress takes shape.

Dental Caries. Some people, no matter what their diet or dental habits, have teeth that are relatively resistant to damage. But most people are more or less vulnerable to tooth decay. Three major factors contribute to the development of dental caries: The *host* is a tooth made susceptible by genetic and environmental factors including prenatal nutrition. The *agent* is the colony of oral bacteria, the mass of microbes that inhabit the mouth and cling to the surface of human teeth. The *environment*, consisting of conditions inside the mouth, is provided by dietary substrates that support bacterial growth and metabolism and also by saliva, which helps to protect teeth from dental decay.

The gelatinous plaque formed by colonies of oral bacteria keeps these organisms in close proximity to the tooth surface and prevents the cleansing and buffering action of saliva. In addition, bacteria produce a sticky polysaccharide (dextran) from ingested carbohydrate, which further increases plaque adherence to the teeth.

The carious process begins when the bacteria metabolize glucose (derived from ingested carbohydrate and dextran) to lactic and other acids. These acids demineralize the teeth, starting with the enamel and proceeding inward toward the dentin. Because this layer is softer, the process is accelerated and bacteria invade the pulp. The all-too-familiar cavity, and sometimes toothache, is the result of this invasive bacterial infection.

Prevention. Although dental caries is a complex and multifactorial disease, preventive measures can be directed against each of the three factors in its development. Control of oral bacteria and improvement of the oral environment can be accomplished by minimizing the amount of sugar in the diet and especially by avoiding sticky sugared foods that will adhere to the teeth. Studies in Vipeholm, Sweden, have demonstrated that the total amount of sugar consumed is not as much at fault in the development of caries as is the frequency of exposure to it. Subjects who consumed large quantities of sugared foods but only at mealtimes had fewer cavities than subjects who ate sugared items in smaller quantities many times during the day (Gustafson et al., 1954). Sticky foods such as caramels and hard candy keep sugars in close contact with the teeth for long periods of time, increasing the amount of damage that is done.

All aspects of carbohydrate implication in dental caries are found in "nursing bottle syndrome." This problem is commonly found in young children who receive a bottle at bedtime. The fermentable carbohydrates contained in milk, juice, or sometimes sugared water collect in the mouth and are rapidly converted to demineralizing acids. The unfortunate result is rampant tooth decay, typically affecting the upper front teeth but often extending to the back teeth as well. Since few infants and very young children are taken for dental examinations, parents may not recognize the severity of the problem until the teeth have become so painfully decayed or abscessed that foods cannot be ingested. Children with this condition may lose all their deciduous teeth by the time they are 3 or 4 years of age. Badly damaged teeth must be extracted, causing pain and anxiety for the child and expense to the parents. Dental appliances may be needed to maintain tooth spacing until the permanent teeth come in. Speech may also be impaired. Psychological distress and the inability to eat, with obvious nutritional implications, are additional consequences.

Teeth can be made less susceptible to dental decay by treatment with fluoride, provided in drinking water, toothpaste, supplements, and/or by dental treatment (see table). In many communities, these

SUPPLEMENTAL FLUORIDE DOSAGE SCHEDULE (MG/DAY)

Age	Fluoride in Drinking Water (ppm)		
	<.03	.03–0.7	>0.7
2 weeks–2 years	0.25	0	0
2–3 years	0.50	0.25	0
3–16 years	1.00	0.50	0

Source: Committee on Nutrition, American Academy of Pediatrics, Fluoride supplementation: Revised dosage schedules, Pediatrics 63:151, 1979.

With the lips held back by a plastic device, the damage of "nursing bottle syndrome" can be clearly seen. Characteristically, there is extensive damage to the upper front teeth while the lower front teeth are unaffected. (Dr. Marvin H. Berman)

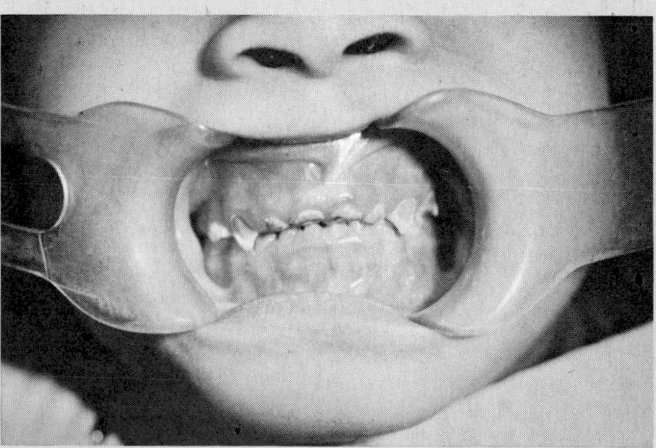

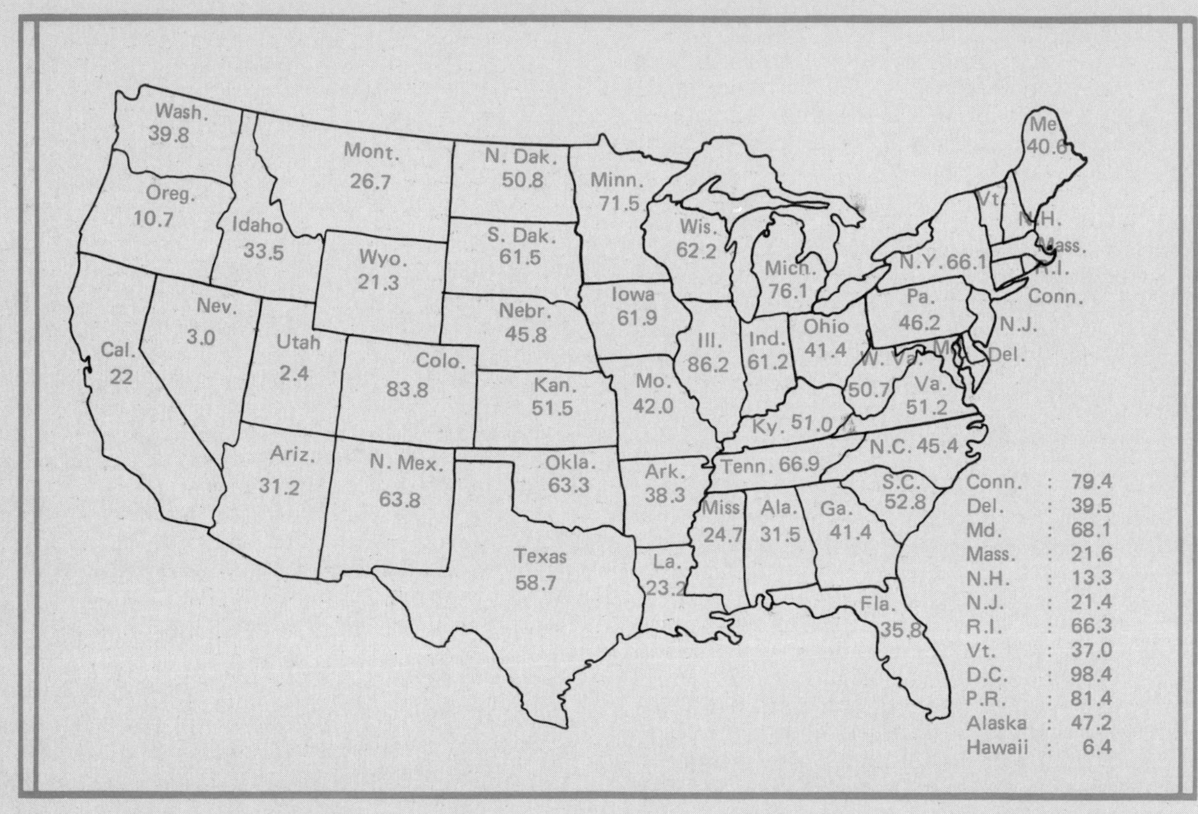

Fluoridation in the United States. The first number for each state refers to the percentage of its population on public water supplies with natural or controlled fluoridation. Source: USDHEW, ***Fluoridation census, 1975,*** Publication No. 740-116/3782 (Washington, D.C.: U.S. Government Printing Office, 1977), p. 6.

amounts are supplied in local water (see map). Current fluoridation recommendations are shown in the table. The safety of fluoridated water has been demonstrated repeatedly (see Chapter 8).

The effectiveness of water fluoridation was shown in a classic study in two neighboring New York State communities. In Newburgh, where 1 part per million (1 mg/l) of fluoride was added to the public water supply in 1945, children under 10 years of age had from 60 to 65 percent fewer decayed, missing, or filled teeth (the DMF Index) than those children in Kingston, where water had not been fluoridated. Newburgh's 12-to-14-year-olds, who had received fluoridated water since early childhood but not since birth, had 48 percent less dental damage than youngsters the same age in Kingston, and 16-year-olds 40 percent less (Ast and Fitzgerald, 1962). Apparently fluoride is most effective during the years when teeth are developing, and its effectiveness increases with longer exposures. As fluoride accumulates over time in the enamel, it makes teeth more resistant to the acid produced by bacteria.

Dentists recommend that, where water is not fluoridated, children receive daily fluoride supplements, rinse their mouths (not swallow) once weekly with fluoride rinses, receive topical fluoride treatments twice yearly in the dental office, and brush with flu-

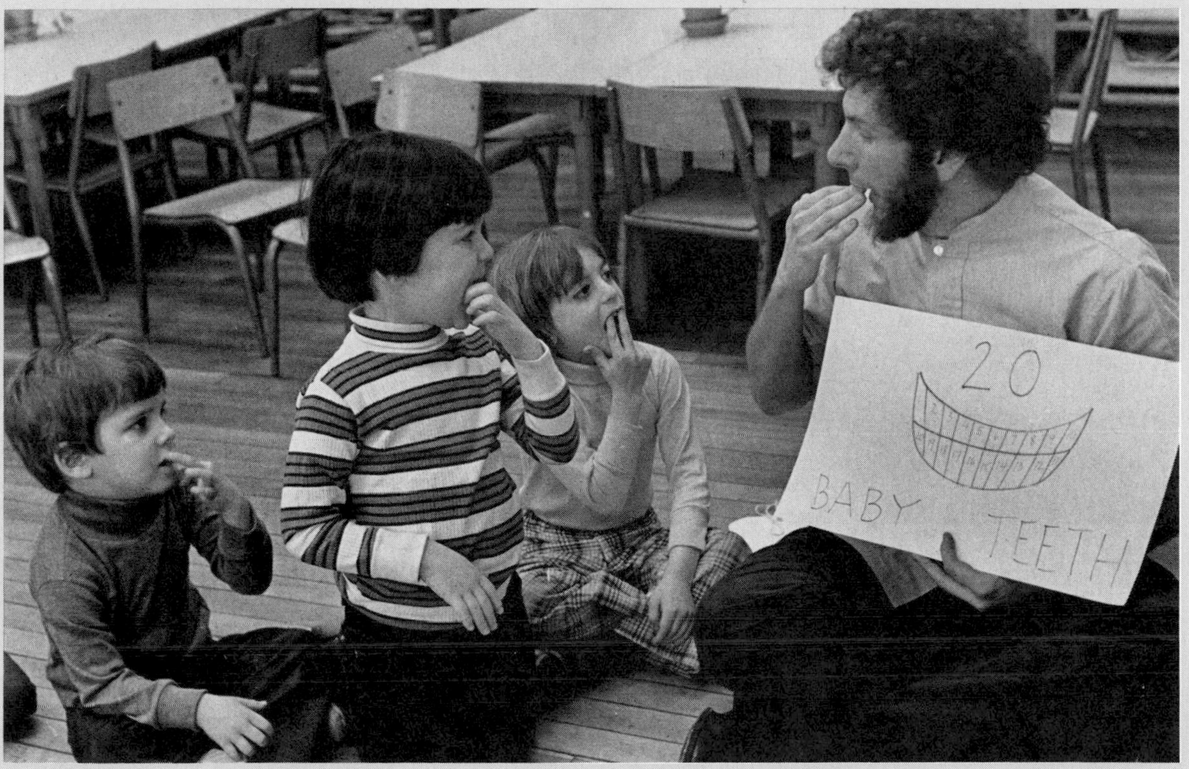

A dentist visits a kindergarten classroom to teach children how to care for their teeth. (Hanna W. Schreiber, Rapho/Photo Researchers, Inc.)

oride toothpaste. This is definitely not too much fluoride; a young child would have to take 4 or 5 milligrams per day for tooth mottling (dental fluorosis) to occur. Under 3 years, though, the maximum level is 1 milligram per day. Since one quart of fluoridated water contains only about 1 milligram, it is unlikely that a child would ingest too much. Fluoride supplements should *not* be used when a community water supply is fluoridated at a level of 1 ppm.

Dental Care for Children. Since "baby" teeth are destined to be lost anyway, many people are unconcerned about dental care for young children. But the consequences of early neglect can last a lifetime. The loss of even a single baby tooth may cause shifts in the spacing of the permanent teeth, necessitating corrective measures later on. Even when teeth are not decayed, accumulating plaque can irritate periodontal tissues and over the years destroy the gingiva or periodontal ligaments, a condition that is particularly prevalent in adulthood but which probably begins in childhood and adolescence.

The early establishment of sound dental care lays the foundation for a healthy mouth throughout life. Oral hygiene for the child should include lessons in effective brushing and the provision of a suitable toothbrush. Children should visit the dentist by the time they are 3 years old, even if they appear to be in good dental health. Early visits to a dentist can alleviate fear and anxiety and will help to interest children in the care of their own teeth.

flavored beverages are also highly sweetened, and they may present a real problem for nutritionally conscientious parents because they are often served at "juice-and-cookies time" in schools and camps. Provision only of fruit juices, milk, and water as beverages at home, however, can condition children to accept only these drinks and to reject highly sugared ones. When the importance of eating and drinking nutritious foods is emphasized in the home, even young children will learn the difference—and can take pride in their greater awareness and the higher nutritional quality of their diets.

Special Concerns for Childhood Nutrition

In childhood, dietary habits are established that will influence development, health, and the enjoyment of food throughout life. Of particular concern to nutritionists today are those children whose food intake patterns may result in illness or obesity in the growing years, and cause later problems as well. An abundance of food and an increasingly sedentary lifestyle have made obesity all too common among children as well as adults. And the proliferation among young adults of alternate eating patterns, specifically of vegetarian diets with varying degrees of limitation, is affecting the health status of increasing numbers of young children.

OBESITY. Although it is not certain that childhood obesity produces adult obesity, there is enough evidence to suggest a correlation. Childhood obesity can be difficult for parents to recognize. A plump infant or toddler is more appealing to most people than a thin, wiry one. In fact, parents of thin children are more likely to be concerned about their health than are parents of heavier children. But what appears to be cute baby fat may be the beginning of a persistent obesity problem.

Children of obese parents tend to be obese too, while those of thin parents tend to be thin. Most evidence indicates, however, that family eating patterns, and not the family genetic makeup, are the primary reason. Obese children, like obese adults, are less physically active than the nonobese; family lifestyle may be a factor in this as well.

There are apparently certain critical periods for the development of obesity. In late infancy and early childhood, when growth rate diminishes and energy requirements decrease, parents may continue to "push" foods, thus starting a pattern of overfeeding. Again, at about 6 years of age, children start school and their physical activities become limited at the same time as new eating schedules and "social snacking". And finally, just before puberty, many children get heavier before they grow taller and may decrease their physical activity even further; at the same time, social snacking becomes an important activity. Often, however, children who gain weight disproportionately at this time will assume more pleasing body proportions as their linear growth catches up. The school-age weight spurt is more serious than gains during the other two periods.

Whenever obesity develops, the strategy is the same: less energy intake and more energy expenditure. For children, however, the goal is not drastic weight *loss* but *maintenance* of the weight level to allow linear growth and normal body development as the child gains in height. Because childhood is a time of active physiological growth, intake should not be less than 1,200 to 1,400 kilocalories per day, to ensure an adequate supply of all essential nutrients. This may indeed mean a change in a child's meal and snack patterns, but a change may benefit the entire family. For most children, the substitution of fruit for cake, candy, or soft drinks and of raw or cooked green or crunchy vegetables for some of the starchy foods will suffice. Lower-fat meats are also advised; broiled chicken and lean roasted meats should replace fried chicken and several hamburgers a week. Skim milk can be substituted for whole milk after 2 years of age. At the same time, a few "special occasion" foods should be permitted, so the dieting child does not feel too deprived. But when pizza, birthday cake, or an ice cream sundae have been eaten, the following day's meals should be adjusted accordingly.

Weight control programs and diet clinics have been developed expressly for children. These group approaches introduce young people to new eating patterns and behavior changes that can help them to control their food intake. Often these groups encourage other family members to join their children, on the premise that family eating patterns are the most significant contributor to childhood obesity. Social and psychological family problems should receive appropriate counseling and other supportive services.

VEGETARIANISM. The popularity of alternative lifestyles is reflected in nontraditional food patterns, the most popular of which is vegetarianism. Unfortunately, there has been a corresponding increase in nutrition-related problems affecting children consuming vegetarian diets.

A strict vegetarian diet, excluding eggs, milk, and other dairy products, may not provide necessary levels of energy, vitamin D, vitamin B_{12}, calcium, iron, or high-quality protein required during the growth years. Rickets has been seen among children in macrobiotic vegetarian families, and dietary intake records have documented marginal consumption of calcium and phosphorus as well as of vitamin D in these children (Dwyer et al., 1979). Growth retardation in vegetarian children may result from insufficient intake of the essential amino acids needed for protein synthesis, as well as of energy. A group of breast-fed children of vegetarian mothers appeared to develop at the average rate until 6 months of age, but when other foods were introduced they grew more slowly than other children of the same age on omnivorous diets. From 18 months of age until 5 years the vegetarian children again grew at similar rates, suggesting that some catch-up growth may be possible, but that there is a period when growth in the young child is particularly vulnerable to nutrient deficits (Schull et al., 1977).

Vegetarian parents should be particularly attentive to regular health examinations for their children and to careful diet planning. A variety of different legumes, grains, nuts, oil seeds, green leafy vegetables, and fruits will provide adequate protein, most B vitamins, energy, and most other vitamins and minerals. Iron and vitamin B_{12} supplementation however (the latter from fortified soybean milk or other products) are advised. Unfortunately there has been an increase in the number of adults belonging to groups that advocate extremely restrictive diets and avoid medical services; concern for their children is growing.

PERSPECTIVE ON
Nutrition and Hyperactivity

Children who seem to be in constant motion, who need and get little sleep, whose moods change frequently, and who are inattentive and have difficulty learning, have long been a puzzle as well as a trial to their parents and teachers. The fidgety undisciplined child was once called overactive, then hyperactive, and in recent years has received a formal diagnostic status as *hyperkinetic.* This constitutes the single most common behavioral disorder seen by child psychiatrists, and it ranges in incidence from 2 to 10 percent of all elementary school children. From three to nine times as many boys as girls are so diagnosed (Harper et al., 1978).

Typically, such children are referred for diagnosis by teachers who find their classroom behavior disruptive, although their parents are usually better able to handle them. It has been suggested that many children diagnosed as hyperkinetic may actually be within the normal range of behavior, especially for boys, and that the behavioral standards in schools may discriminate against boys.

Since the 1950s, the usual treatment for hyperactivity has been medication with stimulants such as amphetamines, which paradoxically have a calming effect on these excitable children. These drugs, however, have some unwanted side effects, such as appetite depression and some growth retardation. In 1973, Dr. Benjamin Feingold, of the Kaiser Permanente Medical Center in San Francisco, reported dramatic behavioral improvement in 30 to 50 percent of the hyperkinetic children he had treated with special additive-free diets. According to Feingold, an allergist, ingestion of artificial colors and flavors, preservatives, and natural salicylates (compounds which cause allergic reactions in sensitive people) caused hyperactivity in previously normal children and made previously hyperkinetic children worse. In addition, he noted that even minute quantities of such substances were sufficient to make a calmed child regress to previous agitated behavior (Bierman and Furukawa, 1978).

Many parents, encouraged by these reports, voluntarily put their children on the food intake patterns recommended by Feingold (1974) in a popular book, and they claimed to notice improvements. Several researchers have attempted to test the effectiveness of the additive-free diet under strictly controlled conditions, but their findings have been ambiguous. In one series of experiments, most parents and teachers of previously diagnosed hyperactive children were unable to detect differences in the behavior of these children when they consumed additive-free or control diets. Even more striking, they did not detect any increase in hyperactivity when children were deliberately given foods containing artificial colors (Harley et al., 1978). In other tests, some teachers but not parents have noted behavioral improvements in boys 6 to 12 years of age when they received the additive-free diet *after* being on the control diet, but not when the additive-free diet *preceded* the control diet (Conners et al., 1976). No explanation for this limited sequence effect has been offered.

Critics argue that Feingold has not provided experimental evidence but only anecdotal evidence of the effectiveness of his program, and they suggest that the extent of family concern and involvement with the child on this program may account for the observed improvements. Behavioral improvement is, in any case, difficult to quantify. Isolated behavioral traits—talking too much, for example—may be perceived differently by parents and teachers. Controlled studies are difficult to conduct because of the subjective nature of the observations, but the few results to date are sufficiently promising that further research may identify certain children for whom the Feingold diet is effective.

A different kind of question has arisen concerning the nutritional adequacy of the original Feingold diet. Because of the omission of foods containing salicylates in natural form (apples, cucumbers, oranges, strawberries, tomatoes, among others), it was found that this intake pattern provided inadequate amounts of ascorbic acid. Parents who wish to try this diet for their children should obtain nutritional counseling; vitamin supplementation may be recommended.

Some parents of hyperkinetic children may wish to try this means of moderating behavior. Aside from the concern for nutritional adequacy over a prolonged period, the "can't hurt, might help" philosophy should provide reassurance.

NUTRITIONAL STATUS OF AMERICAN CHILDREN

The Preschool Nutrition Survey, the Ten-State Nutrition Survey, and HANES indicate that nutritional status of children at all ages is generally good, but that children at the lower end of the socioeconomic spectrum tend to have poorer intakes of several nutrients than children from middle- and upper-income families and tend to be of smaller stature as well. Obesity and low iron and calcium intakes were the most prevalent nutrition-related problems; the incidence of obesity tended to correlate with higher family income. Suboptimal vitamin A intakes were found particularly in Hispanic and black children; more than one-tenth of all children had low vitamin C intakes; and anemia was found in from 7 to 12 percent of all children in these studies (Owen and Lippman, 1977). Protein intakes, on the other hand, were consistently from 50 to 100 percent higher than RDAs.

Large numbers of young children—from 25 to 40 percent of preschoolers, according to these surveys—receive vitamin and mineral supplements. In a study of second and sixth grade children it was found that, without dietary supplements, iron, calcium, vitamin A, thiamin, and niacin intakes were unsatisfactory in significant numbers of children; fewer had to rely on supplements for ascorbic acid and riboflavin. Older children, and girls, were less likely to consume adequate levels of nutrients. Calcium intake of nearly half of the children was inadequate; and for those whose intakes met or exceeded the RDA, their mid-morning milk at school contributed a sizable proportion. These results would seem to make supplementation generally advisable (Cook and Payne, 1979). However, the best way to ensure adequate intake of all nutrients, including those which are *not* contained in dietary supplements, is to encourage consumption of a variety of nutritious foods.

A study of young children with iron-deficiency anemia has identified a number of related social and environmental factors. In comparison to a group of controls, anemic children were more likely to be the youngest in their family, have more siblings, drink more milk, and have been introduced to commercial baby foods at a later age; their mothers were more likely to be separated or divorced, be dissatisfied with the child's food habits and general abilities, and to spend less money on food for each person in the household (Czajka-Narins et al., 1978). Some of these factors may help to identify children who may be at risk and to target public information programs about child and family nutrition at young parents.

It is the responsibility of society as a whole, as well as of parents as individuals, to make sure that growing children receive an adequate nutritional foundation for their future growth. Sound nutritional practices in childhood will produce adults who enjoy meals, consume nutritionally adequate diets that are neither excessive nor scanty, who do not "use" food for emotional "blackmail" or other manipulative purposes—and who will bring up *their* children, the succeeding generation, to have positive food attitudes also. If good food habits are cultivated in childhood, there will be little need for concern about the ultimate outcomes of adolescent foodways.

INTRODUCTION TO NUTRITION DURING ADOLESCENCE

In the continuum from infancy through adulthood, the beginning of a new stage of development is seldom clearly defined. While infancy obviously starts at birth, the boundaries between infancy and childhood, and between childhood and adolescence, are not at all distinct. But while adolescence has neither a clear beginning nor a clear end, the physiological events of this period are very distinctive indeed. It is a critical period of rapid development—but in most youngsters there is a lack of synchronization between the physical, emotional, and social aspects of that development. Although the preschool and school years are recognized as being extremely important influences on the personality and behavioral traits of the mature adult, further important modifications, coming increasingly from the world outside the home and family, are made during the adolescent years.

Teenagers are neither children nor adults, and this time can be a difficult one for them as well as for their parents and teachers. Both parents and children recognize the need for, and want, increased independence for the growing young person. Yet each too often sends out confused signals to the other, leading to varying degrees of conflict. There are many areas of parent-child disagreement—cars, dating, hours, dress, study habits, and sometimes food. As teenagers try to differentiate themselves from parental beliefs, and to keep up with their peer group, their dietary habits often change. At the same time, their rapidly growing bodies require even more nutritional support than during the childhood years.

NORMAL GROWTH AND DEVELOPMENT DURING ADOLESCENCE

Of all the changes that occur during adolescence, the most obvious are increased stature, altered body composition, and sexual maturation. The rate of growth during adolescence is second only to that of early infancy. But while development in the first year of life is relatively predictable for all infants, the rate and timing of development in adolescents is highly individual. Although both female and male infants have the same developmental patterns, female and male adolescents have markedly different rates and patterns of development. A prepubertal growth spurt is characteristic only of human beings. Adolescents in developing countries do not experience the growth spurt, probably because of nutritional deprivation (McKigney and Munro, 1976). Growth patterns in adolescence are shown in Figures 13-6 and 13-7.

Height

The adolescent growth spurt for most girls occurs before the teen years and prior to menarche (the onset of menstruation). Even during grade school years, girls are often taller than boys, a situation that continues until some-

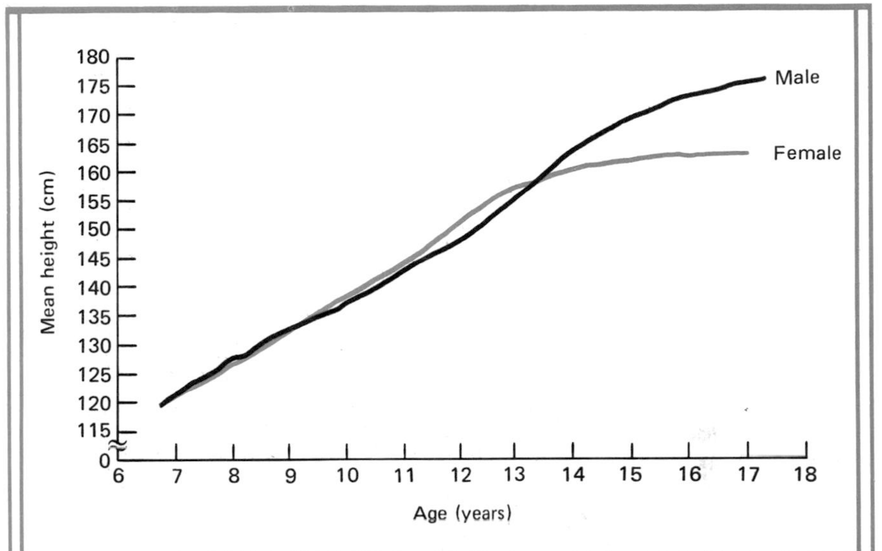

FIGURE 13-6

Growth Patterns—Height

Mean height attained by U.S. youths 6–18 years of age by quarter-year age groups.

Source: National Center for Health Statistics, *Height and weight of youths 12–17 years, United States 1966–70.* Vital and Health Statistics, Series 11, No. 124, USDHEW Pub. No. (HSM) 73-1606 (Washington, D.C.: U.S. Government Printing Office, 1973).

time between 12 and 15 when boys catch up and rapidly exceed the height of their female schoolmates. Girls who have a particularly large and early growth spurt also reach puberty at an early age. They do not, however, necessarily grow taller than later-maturing contemporaries. Once reproductive capacity is achieved by adolescent girls, the rate of growth slows dramatically.

In males the secondary sexual characteristics appear at the onset of the growth spurt. Male growth continues far longer than is generally believed; from 17 to 28 years, boys grow about 2.3 centimeters, compared with 1.2 centimeters for girls (Garn and Wagner, 1969). This prolonged growth period has implications for the nutritional requirements of young adults.

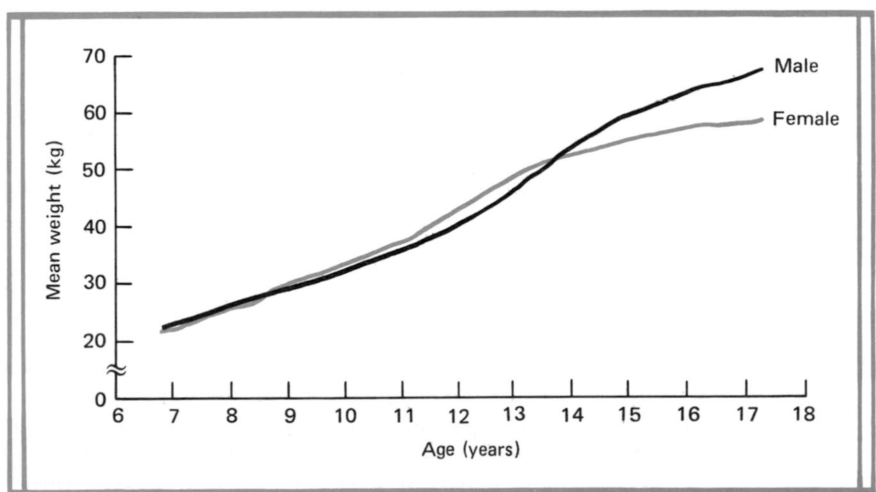

FIGURE 13-7

Growth Patterns—Weight

Mean weight attained by U.S. youths 6–18 years of age by quarter-year age groups.

Source: National Center for Health Statistics, *Height and weight of youths 12–17 years, United States 1966–70.* Vital and Health Statistics, Series 11, No. 124, USDHEW Pub. No. (HSM) 73-1606 (Washington, D.C.: U.S. Government Printing Office, 1973).

Weight

The adolescent growth spurt is related to increases in both cell number and cell size, which are paralleled by significant weight gains. Girls progress earlier than boys in this area as well. During the preadolescent years, girls store fat and may gain significant weight—as much as 10 pounds in a single prepuberty year. And because weight gain precedes the increase in height, preteens are frequently chubby. But girls who have not previously been obese normally regain their childhood proportions at the time their growth spurt begins. Boys may not lose prepuberty fat until the time of their greatest linear growth and after; loss of body fat at that time is probably related to the increased levels of testosterone and the coordinate development of upper body musculature.

Body Composition

Just as the timing of height and weight spurts differs in males and females, so does their body composition, which is markedly influenced by hormones. In girls, body fat is deposited in the hips and breast tissues. Boys have a greater lean body mass, with greater muscular and skeletal development.

Sexual Maturation

The hormonal changes that cause fat deposition in females and increased lean body mass in males are also responsible for maturation of the reproductive systems of both sexes. Menarche in girls is an obvious sign of sexual maturation, although ovulation generally does not occur with regularity until about two years later. Hormonal changes also trigger the development of secondary sex characteristics, such as the growth of pubic and body hair and the voice change and growth of facial hair in males.

Because chronological age is not the best indicator of maturation, secondary sex characteristics are used as an index of pubertal development, and they form the basis of thc sex-maturity ratings (SMR). In girls the quantity and pattern of pubic hair and the development of breasts are key indicators; in boys the growth of the penis and testes and the development of pubic hair are used. A five-point scale has been developed, with SMR 1 representing the prepubertal stage, SMR 2 indicating the first visible signs of change, SMR 3 and 4 intermediate stages of development, and SMR 5 representing adult maturation (see Table 13-5). Other developmental events can be correlated with these stages: In girls, peak growth velocity occurs at SMR 2; and menarche usually occurs at SMR 4, although it may occur at SMR 3. In boys, peak growth velocity occurs at SMR 3 and is followed by the growth of facial and body hair in SMR 4; chest hair usually does not develop until after SMR 5 (Tanner, 1962).

In industrial nations the onset of puberty has for more than a century been occurring at earlier ages, and this is often attributed to improved nutrition throughout infancy and childhood; some would include improved maternal nutrition during fetal life as a factor as well. Evidence is accumulating that the onset of menses in girls takes place only after a certain body weight and proportion of body fat has been attained (Frisch, 1972).

TABLE 13-5
Sex Maturity Ratings

Boys			
Stage	*Pubic Hair*	*Penis*	*Testes*
1	None	Preadolescent	Preadolescent
2	Scanty, long, slightly pigmented	Slight enlargement	Enlarged scrotum, pink, texture altered
3	Darker, starts to curl, small amount	Penis longer	Larger
4	Resembles adult type, but less in quantity; coarse, curly	Larger; glans and breadth increase in size	Larger, scrotum dark
5	Adult distribution, spread to medial surface of thighs	Adult	Adult

Girls		
Stage	*Pubic Hair*	*Breasts*
1	Preadolescent	Preadolescent
2	Sparse, lightly pigmented, straight, medial border of labia	Breast and papilla elevated as small mound; areolar diameter increased
3	Darker, begining to curl, increased amount	Breast and areola enlarged, no contour separation
4	Coarse, curly, abundant, but amount less than in adult	Areola and papilla form secondary mound
5	Adult feminine triangle, spread to medial surface of thighs	Mature; nipple projects, areola part of general breast contour

Source: Adapted from J. M. Tanner, *Growth at adolescence*, 2nd ed. (Oxford, England: Blackwell Scientific Publications, 1962.

The readily observed physical changes noted in the SMR system reflect the internal physiological developments of puberty, and they are much better indicators of pubertal development than is chronological age. For this reason, SMRs can be a basis for setting nutrient requirements for adolescents.

NUTRITIONAL REQUIREMENTS DURING ADOLESCENCE

Because of individual variation in adolescent growth and development patterns, the problems of establishing RDAs for this age group are greater than for any other. The RDAs are presently categorized by age and sex to reflect *average* adolescent growth patterns (see Table 13-6). It has been suggested that SMRs be used to estimate nutrient allowances for teenagers. This would be more accurate than standards based on chronological age, but

TABLE 13-6
RDAs for Adolescents

	11–14 years		15–18 years		19–22 years	
	M	*F*	*M*	*F*	*M*	*F*
Energy (kcal)	2,700	2,200	2,800	2,100	2,900	2,100
(MJ)	11.3	9.2	11.8	8.8	12.2	8.8
Protein (g)	45	46	56	46	56	44
Vitamin A (RE)	1,000	800	1,000	800	1,000	800
Vitamin D (μg)	10	10	10	10	7.5	7.5
Vitamin E (mg αT.E.)	8	8	10	8	10	8
Vitamin C (mg)	50	50	60	60	60	60
Folacin (μg)	400	400	400	400	400	400
Niacin (mg)	18	15	18	14	19	14
Riboflavin (mg)	1.6	1.3	1.7	1.3	1.7	1.3
Thiamin (mg)	1.4	1.1	1.4	1.1	1.5	1.1
Vitamin B_6 (mg)	1.8	1.8	2.0	2.0	2.2	2.0
Vitamin B_{12} (μg)	3.0	3.0	3.0	3.0	3.0	3.0
Calcium (mg)	1,200	1,200	1,200	1,200	800	800
Phosphorus (mg)	1,200	1,200	1,200	1,200	800	800
Iodine (μg)	150	150	150	150	150	150
Iron (mg)	18	18	18	18	10	18
Magnesium (mg)	350	300	400	300	350	300
Zinc (mg)	15	15	15	15	15	15

Source: Food and Nutrition Board, National Academy of Sciences, *Recommended daily dietary allowances*, revised 1979 (Washington, D.C.: National Research Council, 1979).

in terms of practicality little would be gained and some convenience would be lost. It has also been suggested that RDA tables should differentiate energy and nutrient needs by sex from the ages of 8 or 9, because of the increase in growth rate that starts before 11 years of age in most girls today (McKigney and Munro, 1976).

Energy

The demand for energy closely parallels the velocity of growth. In girls, growth velocity peaks between age 11 and 14 and then declines, while boys' growth velocity—and therefore energy requirements—are highest in the mid- and late teen years. Adolescents' natural appetites increase markedly to accompany these growth spurts—and parents are usually surprised to find their 12-year-old daughter consuming as much or more food than they do. Typically, energy expenditure is also increased, so that what may seem to be overeating is actually necessary.

Protein

Accurate experimental data on which to base protein recommendations do not exist for adolescents, and the estimates shown in the table are extrapolated from the needs of infants, taking growth velocity and body weight into account. Protein requirements for girls are highest in the years from 15 to 18, and then decrease as their growth rate declines. Adolescent males require additional protein to promote the growth of skeletal and muscle tissue; their needs remain high throughout the adult years.

Vitamins and Minerals

There are little experimental data to support specific recommendations, but the rapid rate of development and growth during the adolescent years is itself evidence of increased need for the micronutrients. Calcium and phosphorus allowances are increased by 50 percent for both boys and girls during the periods of maximum growth, to provide for rapid bone development; recommended intakes then decrease to adult levels.

Increases in blood volume and muscle mass during adolescence and the onset of menstruation in girls account for higher iron requirements in these years. The allowance for both girls and boys is 18 milligrams per day; after 18 years of age, the RDA for males decreases to the adult level of 10 milligrams per day.

ADOLESCENT EATING PATTERNS

Just as growth and appetites peak, psychological and social pressures dramatically alter the adolescent's response to food. The growing desire for independence, peer acceptance, and socializing may conflict with increased physiological needs for more food and more sleep.

Casual eating is characteristic of these years, caused by the erratic work and social schedules of young people. School activities that differ from day to day, athletic training and events, part-time jobs, and the haphazard demands of an active social life may all interfere with normal mealtimes. In early adolescence eating patterns are likely to be regular because these youngsters still spend most mealtimes at school or at home, and they are under closer parental supervision than in later years. But by the mid-teens, adolescents increasingly are somewhere other than home at mealtimes, and food availability tends to determine their food choices. When hunger strikes it's easy to get a soft drink and a packet of cookies from a vending machine or to join the crowd for pizza or a burger and fries.

Although the influence of peers is significant, a survey of nearly 400 college freshmen showed that it is modified by individual preferences as well as by the influence of family food patterns; those whose mothers had prepared breakfast for them during childhood continued to follow regular breakfast and lunch habits away from home. Changes in food selections made by these students were attributed to the difficulty in obtaining the kinds of foods, such as fruit and cheese, that were readily available in the home (Stasch et al., 1970).

In the teen years, snacking is a way of life and may account for as much as a third of total energy intake; for some teens it may represent an even greater proportion. Depending on the choice of snack foods, individual nutrients may be in short supply. The nutrient value of the usual snack choices is highly variable. Soft drinks and candy, while readily available, provide energy but few if any nutrients. Fresh fruits and vegetables are least likely to be consumed as snacks because they are usually least likely to be at hand when an imperative hunger pang is felt.

Teenagers have always been interested in their appearance, particularly at this time of rapid body change. In their desire to conform to cultural ideals of the tall, broad-shouldered male and the slim but buxom female, teenagers often fluctuate between skimping and gorging. But adolescent self-image can be wildly inaccurate: 70 percent of girls in one study thought they were too fat, although only about 15 percent were actually overweight. Of the males surveyed, 59 percent thought they were too thin, while only 25 percent were really underweight (Huenemann et al., 1966). Skipping meals to be skinny, or omitting nutritious foods like bread and milk, can be detrimental to overall health in the teen years.

Adolescent rebelliousness, peer pressure, and a new-found interest in health may actually lead to a greater emphasis on nutrition in the home. Many young people are using food as one means of asserting independence, and they have introduced new food patterns such as vegetarianism, use of organically grown foods, or adherence to kosher dietary laws into the home. For some teens these new food preferences prove to be temporary, but for others they become long lasting. As long as a wide enough variety of food items is consumed to meet the adolescent's increased nutrient and energy needs, alternate food patterns do not pose any problems.

Recently it has become socially acceptable for teenagers to consume "health" foods such as freshly prepared vegetable juices, salads, and yogurt. Students are requesting such foods from their school cafeterias, and in some instances food service managers have found it advantageous to invite student participation in menu planning. Teenagers have also become involved in the political and social issues affecting food supply; ecological concerns on a world and community level are reflected in greater attention to the quality of what is consumed by the individual. Eagerness for knowledge about nutrition and their own bodies is also characteristic of today's adolescents, and it affords an opportunity for effective nutrition education.

Foods for Adolescents: Recommendations

Teenagers should consume at least four servings of milk or milk products (cheese, ice cream, yogurt, puddings), two servings of high-protein foods (meat, fish, poultry, eggs, legumes), and four servings each from the fruits/vegetables and grain groups. Raw fruits and vegetables are often more acceptable than cooked varieties. Since surveys indicate that adolescents' diets are typically low in calcium, ascorbic acid, and vitamin A, a special effort should be made to include foods containing these nutrients in the daily meal plan. Girls should pay particular attention to including good sources of iron in their diets (see Chapter 8).

Increased portion sizes and second helpings at regular family meals will meet teenagers' increased nutrient requirements and their increased energy needs as well. Breakfast should not be skipped; the high nutrient content of breakfast foods and the energy provided by this meal are needed for the day's activities. Girls are most likely to be breakfast skippers in a misguided attempt to control their weight; they often end up snacking more as a result. Snacks can be counted upon to provide additional energy, but they should not replace foods that contribute significant nutrients as well. The availability of nutritious snacks in the family refrigerator and pantry—fruits and juices, cheese and crackers, ice cream, milk, yogurt, peanut butter, raw vegetables, whole grain cereals—will increase the probability that at least some snacks will be nutritionally valuable. For young people who make it a practice to select such items an occasional soft drink shouldn't be guilt-provoking.

Special Concerns During Adolescence

Superimposed on the increased physiological demands for energy and nutrients for the adolescent body are the many external pressures of teenage life. Because of social pressures and erratic physical development, eating patterns may not be adjusted to actual nutrient needs. Changes in physical activity may significantly increase or decrease energy needs. Both girls and boys are subject to peer pressures to participate in alcohol and drug use, which may impair food intake and nutrient metabolism.

ENERGY BALANCE. About 30 percent of teenagers are overweight, but only about 15 percent are actually obese. Teenage obesity is often a continuation of a childhood pattern, and it may even be due to adipose tissue laid down before 2 years of age. But adolescent obesity also characteristically develops in the years from 10 to 14. If the body fat deposited in early adolescence is not dissipated during the growth spurt that follows, the teenager will have to work hard to lose it in the later teen years. Otherwise an overweight future is virtually inevitable—those who remain overweight at the end of adolescence tend to be overweight throughout adult life.

Adolescent obesity may also result from dramatically lowered activity levels, especially for girls. Boys, who are generally more active, tend to lose stored adipose tissue more readily. Also, because of their greater energy requirements over a longer period of time, a moderate deficit in energy consumption will more rapidly be reflected in changed body build. But many overweight teenagers, too embarrassed to participate in sports, lose an opportunity not only to lose weight but to enhance their social lives as well. The increasing opportunity for today's young women to participate in active sports is beneficial and far more effective in weight control than crash diets and meal skipping. Habits of physical activity developed during adolescence carry over into the adult years, a further benefit.

For the overweight teenager of either sex, moderate decreases in energy intakes, while maintaining nutrient levels, can usually be achieved by reducing the number of snacks, desserts, and second portions. An occasional "treat" should be allowed, however, to avoid strong feelings of deprivation and to provide for social activities. Denying the urge to socialize at the local pizzeria may be even more difficult than denying the urge for pizza itself. However, pizza should not be a daily food indulgence for the overweight of any age. Regular meals, instead of meal skipping, will discourage binging. Fruit snacks and salad bar lunches will also help. Diet groups especially for teenagers have been formed in many communities and schools; it is particularly helpful at this socially conscious time of life to associate with others who have the same problem.

At the opposite end of the energy spectrum is anorexia nervosa, discussed in Chapter 5. Teenage girls are particularly prone to this syndrome of self-imposed starvation; those who succumb to it require medical, nutritional, and psychological support.

ALCOHOL AND DRUG USE. More teenagers have been using mood-changing substances in the last two decades. Widespread use of drugs is a relatively recent phenomenon, which seems to have peaked in the mid-1970s. Since then, however, alcohol use among adolescents has been increasing. Many drugs affect the biochemical mechanisms and physiological systems involved in nutrient metabolism, and they may alter appetite and influence food intakes as well. Alcoholic beverages contain significant amounts of energy and will contribute to weight gain if consumed regularly; because they contain few nutrients, overall nutritional status will be compromised if they replace nutritious foods.

For the increasing numbers of girls still in the growing years who are taking oral contraceptive agents, there is concern as well. Effects on nutrient metabolism of adult women have been noted (see Chapter 14), and it seems likely that younger women would be even more strongly affected.

ACNE. Skin problems, a particular trial of adolescents, are popularly ascribed to dietary causes. Nutrition often does play a role, but not the role it is popularly assigned. There is, for example, no evidence that fatty foods such as chocolate, fried chicken, and french fried potatoes, or acid foods such as pickles and vinegar, cause acne. A derivative of vitamin A may have a beneficial effect in cases of severe acne (see Chapter 6); it is being tested but is not commercially available.

DENTAL HEALTH. A direct correlation exists between consumption of snacks, especially of sticky, sugar-rich foods, and tooth decay in adolescents. A recent study has also found significantly fewer cavities in teenagers who had frequent snacks of apples, fruit juice, and sugarless gum (Clancy et al., 1977), suggesting that the issue isn't whether or not to snack, but which snacks to choose.

Adolescents' dental hygiene is often complicated by orthodontic appliances. Braces and other mouth hardware that appear almost indigenous to the teenage mouth interfere with tooth brushing and may contribute to decay, especially if the wearer consumes sticky foods that adhere to the appliances and remain in contact with the tooth surface. For this reason, and because of possible damage to the wires, orthodontists advise against chewing gum, caramels, and similar foods, and stress the importance of regular and thorough oral hygiene practices.

PREGNANCY. The demands of pregnancy at a time of unfinished growth and increased nutrient requirements for the mother creates serious competition between her needs and those of her growing baby. Combined with the typically inadequate medical supervision and poor dietary habits of those girls most at risk of incurring pregnancy, this fact almost ensures a suboptimal outcome for both mother and infant (see Chapter 12). Nutritional guidance, medical supervision, counseling, and continued schooling should all be available for the pregnant teenager.

NUTRITIONAL STATUS OF AMERICAN TEENAGERS

The Ten-State Nutrition Survey (1968–1970) found that of all age groups, adolescents had the highest prevalence of "unsatisfactory" nutritional status (Mueller, 1976). It is possible that the RDAs (1968) against which intake levels were compared were unrealistically high. In a relatively affluent Iowa population sampled in another study, the iron intake of girls was inadequate, and both boys and girls often skipped breakfast and rarely ate green vegetables. But vitamin A, riboflavin, and calcium intakes from the generous consumption of dairy products, were good in this group (Hodges and Krehl, 1965).

Generally, adolescents consistently fall below RDA levels in their intake of calcium, vitamin A, vitamin C, and iron, with these deficiencies being accentuated in girls. Boys tend to come closer to RDA levels simply because of the greater amount of food they consume to meet appetite demands and energy needs; whereas girls, whose energy needs are less, frequently diet and decrease their total food and nutrient intakes even more. Too often, energy-rich and nutrient-poor foods are chosen instead of more nutritious items. Soft drinks, coffee, tea, and alcoholic beverages may replace milk and juice consumption. Milk drinking diminishes in the teen years because it has a "kid's food" image, and it may also be a particular problem for those of nonwhite racial groups because of an acquired lactose intolerance. But ice cream, yogurt, and cheese are nutritious substitutes, and milk itself can be consumed in moderate amounts even by those who are lactose intolerant.

While surveys in the United States indicate that some nutrients are in short supply in teenage diets, the major concerns are obesity, iron deficiency, anorexia nervosa, dental caries, and pregnancy. In both the Ten-State and Iowa studies cited above, dental caries was the most common medical problem of adolescents (Hodges, 1976). Iron is the nutrient most likely to be consumed in deficient amounts by teenagers, and low ascorbic acid and calcium intakes are also concerns.

Attention should focus on defining more realistically the nutrient requirements of this age group. Nutrition education at school and for the family will give individuals the information they need to monitor and improve their own food intakes. Whether they do or not, however, depends on their degree of motivation.

Adult condemnation of the sometimes quirky food habits of teenagers will fall on deaf ears. Mere repetition of the Basic Food Groups and advice from teachers or parents to eat "because it's good for you" are just plain boring to most adolescents, who have been hearing it all since kindergarten—or think they have. But teens are a potentially receptive audience for nutrition information presented in a factual, interesting, and above all, nonpatronizing way. Teens want the facts. They want to know how their bodies work and what their bodies need. They are concerned about their health, their appearance, and their performance of school work and in athletic events. They will respond to information that can be put to use *now*.

Participating in learning activities in the classroom, sharing responsibilities for meal planning and preparation in the home, involvement in nutrition-related projects at school and in the community—all these are approaches through which young people can be reached and their food habits influenced. True learning comes with self-discovery. Given the information they need and want, teens will have their own reasons for incorporating it into their daily lives. This is a period of energy, enthusiasm, and intellectual discovery; it is an opportunity for sound nutritional education that must not be lost.

SUMMARY

From the moment of birth an individual becomes dependent on the external environment for food, shelter, and nurturing. Food does more than provide the nutrients needed for physical growth; it is part of the environment that fosters social, emotional, and behavioral development.

Growth during infancy (birth to 12 months) is very rapid—birth weight triples and height increases by 9 or 10 inches. While there is wide agreement that food is an important determinant of growth and development, actual feeding practices have been the subject of controversy—and changes of fashion—over the years. Most experts now agree that the average infant can be adequately nourished by either breast or formula milk, but the American Academy of Pediatrics has endorsed breast-feeding for normal infants.

Breast milk confers several advantages over commercial formulas, including immunological protection. Most commercially available formulas are based on cow's milk that is modified to approximate the composition of human milk. The use of unmodified cow's milk, whether whole or skim, is not appropriate during infancy.

Breast-feeding is sometimes contraindicated; if the mother has an infectious disease or is taking certain medications, bottle-feeding is the better choice. Young infants require supplementation with vitamin D, iron, and fluoride, unless these are provided in formulas.

The optimal time for introducing solid foods into the infant diet is now considered to be 4 to 6 months of age, when babies become able to initiate swallowing. Until then, milk or formula can meet their nutritional needs. Solid foods should be introduced gradually. Diversity in nutrients, tastes, and textures at this early time will be a positive influence on food preferences in later life.

Growth during childhood (1 to 12 years) is much less rapid than in infancy, averaging 2 to 4 inches and 4 to 8 pounds per year for most of this period. Height and weight records are important indicators of health and may provide the earliest signs of undernutrition, disease, or overnutrition.

Nutritional requirements during childhood reflect growth rate and physical activity. In relation to body weight they are proportionately less than during the first year of life.

Eating behaviors and food preferences are influenced by the school environment, by friends, and by the mass media. Children are better able to withstand adverse influences if appropriate eating habits are developed at home and reinforced daily. Children should not be forced to "finish everything" or to eat foods they initially reject. A relaxed mealtime atmosphere and tolerance of the child's changing tastes are important.

The growth rate during adolescence (13 to 19 years) is second only to that during infancy. The most obvious changes are increased stature, change of body composition, and sexual maturation. But unlike the relatively predictable growth of infants, the rate and timing of adolescent growth and development are highly variable.

Nutritional requirements for adolescents are as variable as their growth patterns and closely parallel the latter. Adolescents tend to have casual attitudes toward eating and are greatly influenced by peers.

BIBLIOGRAPHY

American Academy of Pediatrics. Breast-feeding. *Pediatrics* 62(4):591, 1978.

Ast, D. B., and B. Fitzgerald. Effectiveness of water fluoridation. *Journal of the American Dental Association* 65:581, 1962.

Berg, A. The crisis in infant feeding practices. *Nutrition Today*, January-February 1977, p. 18.

Bierman, C. W., and C. T. Furukawa. Food additives and hyperkinesis: Are there nuts among the berries? *Pediatrics* 61:932, 1978.

Burg, A. W. How much caffeine in a cup? *Tea Coffee Journal*, January 1975, p. 4.

Clancy, K. L., B. G. Bibby, H. J. V. Goldberg, L. W. Ripa, and J. Barenie. Snack food intake of adolescents and caries development. *Journal of Dental Research* 56:568, 1977.

Committee on Nutrition of the Mother and Preschool Child. Fetal and infant nutrition and susceptibility to obesity. *American Journal of Clinical Nutrition* 31:2026, 1978.

Conners, C. K., C. H. Goyette, D. A. Southwick, J. M. Lees, and P. A. Andrulonis. Food additives and hyperkinesis: A controlled double-blind experiment. *Pediatrics* 58:154, 1976.

Cook, C. C., and I. R. Payne. Effect of supplements on the nutrient intake of children. *Journal of the American Dietetic Association* 74:130, 1979.

Czajka-Narins, D. M., T. B. Haddy, D. J. Kallen. Nutrition and social correlates in iron deficiency anemia. *American Journal of Clinical Nutrition* 31:955, 1978.

Dwyer, J. T., W. H. Dietz, Jr., G. Hass, and R. Suskind. Risk of nutritional rickets among vegetarian children. *American Journal of Diseases of Children* 133:134, 1979.

Feingold, B. F. *Why your child is hyperactive*. New York: Random House, 1974.

Fomon, S. J. *Infant nutrition*, 2nd ed. Philadelphia: Saunders, 1974.

Fomon, S. J., L. J. Filer, T. A. Anderson, and E. E. Ziegler. Recommendations for feeding normal infants. *Pediatrics* 63:52, 1979.

Food and Nutrition Board, National Research Council. Recommended dietary allowances, revised 1979. Washington, D.C.: National Academy of Sciences, 1979.

Frader, J., B. Reibman, and D. Turkewitz. Vitamin B_{12} deficiency in strict vegetarians. *New England Journal of Medicine* 299:1319, 1978.

Frisch, R. Weight at menarche: Similarity for well-nourished and undernourished girls at differing ages, and evidence for historical constancy. *Pediatrics* 50:445, 1972.

Garn, S. M., D. C. Clark, and K. E. Guire. Growth, body composition and development of obese and lean children. In *Childhood obesity*, ed. M. Winick. New York: John Wiley, 1975.

Garn, S. M., and B. Wagner. The adolescent growth of the skeletal mass and its implications to mineral requirements. In *Adolescent nutrition and growth*, ed. F. Heald. New York: Meredith Corp., 1969.

Gustafson, B. E., C. Quensel, L. Lanke, et al. Vipeholm dental caries study. *Acta Odontologica Scandinavia* 11:232, 1954.

Harley, J. P., R. S. Ray, L. Tomasi, P. L. Eichman, C. G. Matthews, R. Chun, C. S.

CLEELAND, AND E. TRAISMAN. Hyperkinesis and food additives: Testing the Feingold hypothesis. *Pediatrics* 61:818, 1978.

HARPER, P. H., C. H. GOYETTE, AND C. K. CONNERS. Nutrient intakes of children on the hyperkinesis diet. *Journal of the American Dietetic Association* 73:515, 1978.

HARRIS, L. E., AND J. C. M. CHAN. Infant feeding practices. *American Journal of Diseases of Children* 117:483, 1969.

HIMES, J. H. Infant feeding practices and obesity. *Journal of the American Dietetic Association* 75:122, 1979.

HODGES, R. E. Vitamin and mineral requirements in adolescence. In *Nutrient requirements in adolescence,* ed. J. I. McKigney and H. N. Munro. Cambridge, Mass.: M.I.T. Press, 1976.

HODGES, R. E., AND W. A. KREHL. Nutritional status of teenagers in Iowa. *American Journal of Clinical Nutrition* 17:200, 1965.

HUENEMANN, R. L., L. R. SHAPIRO, M. C. HAMPTON, AND B. W. MITCHELL. A longitudinal study of gross body composition and body conformation and their association with food and activity in a teenage population: Views of teenage subjects on body conformation, food and activity. *American Journal of Clinical Nutrition* 18:325, 1966.

JELLIFFE, D. B., AND F. P. JELLIFFE. The volume and composition of human milk in poorly nourished communities: A review. *American Journal of Clinical Nutrition* 31:492, 1978.

JOHNSON, P. E., AND G. W. EVANS. Relative zinc availability in human breast milk, infant formulas, and cow's milk. *American Journal of Clinical Nutrition* 31:416, 1978.

KIRSKEY, A., J. A. ERNST, J. L. ROEPKE, AND T.-L. TSAI. Influence of mineral intake and use of oral contraceptives before pregnancy on the mineral content of human colostrum and of mature milk. *American Journal of Clinical Nutrition* 32:30, 1979.

LEBENTHAL, B. Lactose malabsorption and milk consumption in infants and children. *American Journal of Diseases of Children* 133:21, 1979.

LOWENBERG, M. E. The development of food patterns in young children. In *Nutrition in infancy and childhood,* ed. P. Pipes. St. Louis: C. V. Mosby, 1977.

MCKIGNEY, J. I., AND H. N. MUNRO, eds. *Nutrient requirements in adolescence.* Cambridge, Mass.: M.I.T. Press, 1976.

MCMILLAN, J. A., S. A. LANDAW, AND F. A. OSKI. Iron sufficiency in breast-fed infants and the availability of iron from human milk. *Pediatrics* 58:686, 1976.

MALLER, O., AND J. A. DESOR. Effect of taste on ingestion by human newborns. In *Oral sensation and perception,* ed. J. F. Bosma. USDHEW publication No. (NIH) 73-546. Bethesda, Md.: USDHEW, 1973.

MARZOLLO, J. Indigestible miseries of family mealtime. *New York Times,* March 28, 1979.

MATTHEWS, R. H., AND M. Y. WORKMAN. Nutrient content of selected baby foods. *Journal of the American Dietetic Association* 72:27, 1978.

MELLIES, M. J., T. T. ISHIKAWA, P. S. GARTSIDE, K. BURTON, J. MACGEE, K. ALLEN, P. M. STEINER, D. BRADY, AND C. J. GLUECK. Effects of varying maternal dietary fatty acids in lactating women and their infants. *American Journal of Clinical Nutrition* 32:299, 1979.

MUELLER, J. F. Current dietary recommendations for adolescents. In *Nutrient requirements in adolescence,* ed. J. I. McKigney and H. N. Munro. Cambridge, Mass.: M.I.T. Press, 1976.

OWEN, G., AND G. LIPPMAN. Nutritional status of infants and young children: U.S.A. *Pediatric Clinics of North America* 24:212, 1977.

OWEN, G. M., ET AL. A study of nutritional status of preschool children in the United States, 1968–1970. *Pediatrics* Supplement 53:597, 1974.

RAIHA, N. C. R. Biochemical basis for nutritional management of preterm infants. *Pediatrics* 53:147, 1974.

SAARINEN, U. M., AND M. A. SIIMES. Iron absorption from breast milk, cow's milk, and iron-supplemented formula: An opportunistic use of changes in total body iron determined by hemoglobin, ferritin, and body weight in 132 infants. *Pediatric Research* 13:143, 1979.

SAARINEN, U. M., A. BACKMAN, M. KAJOSAARI, AND M. A. SIIMES. Prolonged breast-feeding as prophylaxis for atopic disease. *The Lancet* 2(8135):163, 1979.

SAARINEN, U. M., M. A. SIIMES, AND P. R. DALLMAN. Iron absorption in infants: High bioavailability of breast milk iron as indicated by the extrinsic tag method of iron absorption and by the concentration of serum ferritin. *Journal of Pediatrics* 91:36, 1977.

SAVAGE, R. L. Drugs and breast milk. *Journal of Human Nutrition* 31:459, 1977.

SHULL, M. W., R. B. REED, I. VALADIAN, R. PALOMBO, H. THORNE, AND J. T. DWYER. Velocities of growth in vegetarian preschool children. *Pediatrics* 60:410, 1977.

STASCH, A. R., M. M. JOHNSON, G. J. SPANGLER. Food practices and preferences of some college students. *Journal of the American Dietetic Association* 57:523, 1970.

TANNER, J. M. *Growth at adolescence,* 2nd ed. Oxford: Blackwell Scientific Publications, 1962.

TAYLOR, L. E., AND B. S. WORTHINGTON. Guidance for lactating mothers. In *Nutrition in pregnancy and lactation,* ed. B. S. Worthington, J. Vermeersch, and S. R. Williams. St. Louis: C. V. Mosby, 1977.

TINANOFF, N., AND B. MUELLER. Fluoride content in milk and formula for infants. *Prevention,* January-February 1978, p. 53.

WARD, S., D. LEVINSON, AND D. WACKMAN. Children's attention to television commercials. In *Television and social behavior,* Vol. 4: *Television in day to day life: Patterns of use,* ed. E. E. Rubinstein, G. A. Comstock, and J. P. Murray. Washington, D.C.: U.S. Government Printing Office, 1972.

WINICK, M. New ideas in infant nutrition. *Current Prescribing,* August 1978. p. 73.

WOODRUFF, C. W. The science of infant nutrition and the art of infant feeding. *Journal of the American Medical Association* 240:657, 1978.

ZMORA, E., R. GORODISCHER, AND J. BAR-ZIV. Multiple nutritional deficiencies in infants from a strict vegetarian community. *American Journal of Diseases of Children* 133:141, 1979.

SUGGESTED ADDITIONAL READING

AMERICAN ACADEMY OF PEDIATRICS. Salt intake and eating patterns of infants and children in relation to blood pressure. *Pediatrics* 53:115, 1974.

BURT, J. V., AND A. A. HERTZLER. Parental influence on the child's food preference. *Journal of Nutrition Education* 10(3):127, 1978.

CALIENDO, M. A., D. SANJUR, J. WRIGHT, AND G. CUMMINGS. Nutritional status of preschool children. *Journal of the American Dietetic Association* 71:20, 1977.

D'AUGELLI, A. R., AND H. SMICIKLAS-WRIGHT. The case for primary prevention of overweight through the family. *Journal of Nutrition Education* 10(2):76, 1978.

DEPAOLA, D. P., AND M. C. ALFANO. Diet and oral health. *Nutrition Today,* May-June 1977, p. 6.

FOMON, S. J., AND R. G. STRAUSS. Nutrient deficiencies in breast-fed infants. *New England Journal of Medicine 299:356, 1978.*

FRICKER, H. S., AND S. SEGAL. Narcotic addiction, pregnancy, and the newborn. *American Journal of Diseases of Children* 132:360, 1978.

MARTIN, J. B., AND C. W. BERRY. Cariogenicity of selected processed, machine-vended, and health food snacks. *Journal of the American Dietetic Association* 75:159, 1979.

MAYER, J. Obesity during childhood. In *Childhood obesity,* ed. M. Winick. New York: Wiley, 1976.

PIPES, P. *Nutrition in infancy and childhood.* St. Louis: C. V. Mosby, 1977.

PIPES, P. When should semisolid foods be fed to infants? *Journal of Nutrition Education* 9(2):57, 1977.

Chapter 14

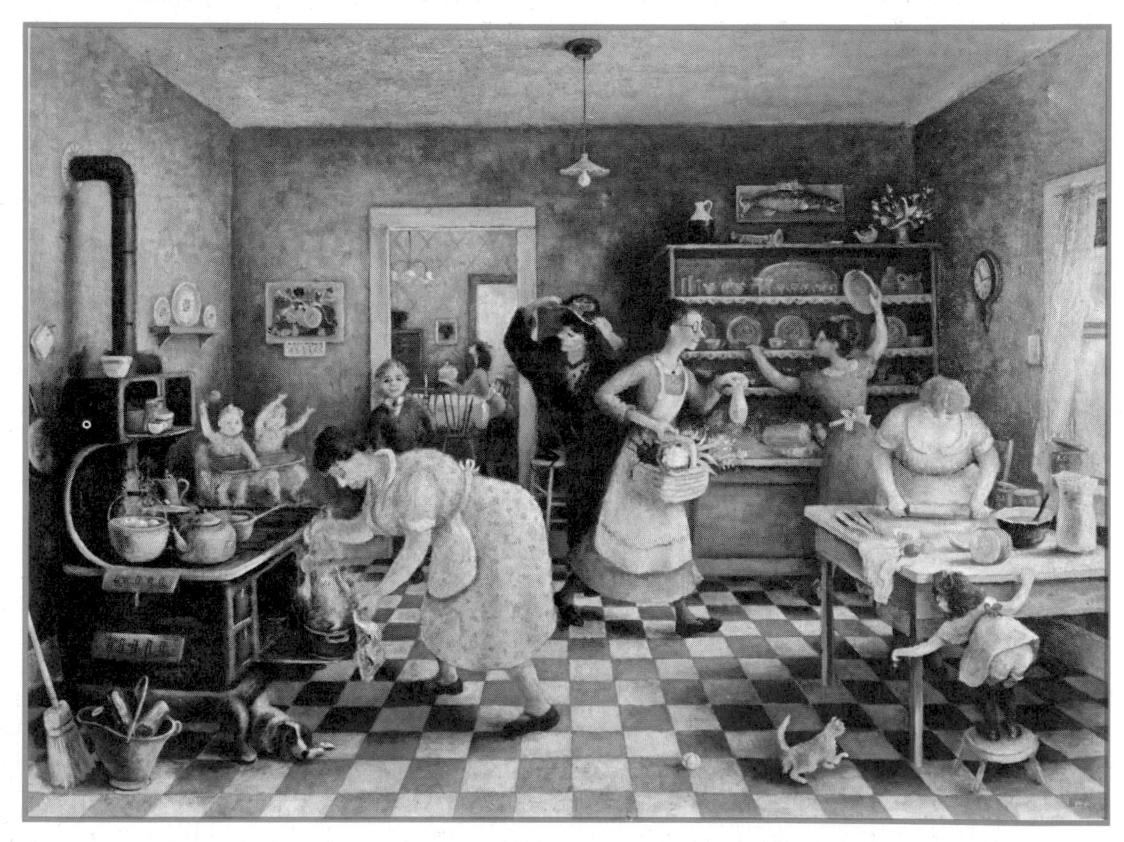

Thanksgiving, 1935, by Doris Lee

The Adult Years

Adulthood is the most creative, productive, and active stage of life. New responsibilities are assumed; a new generation is conceived and nurtured; and the ideas, goods, and services that contribute to national growth and the well-being of society are produced.

To divide the adult years into three stages—early, middle, and elderly—as is commonly done, is somewhat false and arbitrary. There is no one landmark birthday that separates early adulthood from the middle years, or maturity from older age. In our youth-oriented society, this stereotyping tends to promote an agist point of view. Most of us will become middle-aged and then elderly, a reality that should be ample motivation to change attitudes toward the older generation.

Aging characterizes all of life. It is continuous with development, and in this sense can be said to begin at the instant of conception. Although physical growth is generally complete by early adulthood, the body's tissues and cells remain in a dynamic state. Aging does not proceed at the same rate in all individuals. Differences in heredity, environment, and health care can cause wide disparities in physical condition and health status between individuals of the same age. Admittedly, there is a greater probability that older adults will be afflicted with chronic diseases that may cause discomfort and eventually result in death. But chronic ailments and other factors contributing to increased morbidity and mortality often appear in the fourth decade of life—hardly "old age," as anyone over thirty can attest.

Gerontology, a field of study that effectively began in the late 1950s and expanded rapidly in the 1970s, explores the psychosocial, physiological, economic, and medical aspects of aging. The rapid recent development of this field is related to the increasing numbers of people surviving into the seventh, eighth, and ninth decades of life. There are in the United States some 23 million people over 65 years of age, and more than 32 million over 60 years of age, representing 11 and 15 percent of the population, respectively. It is projected that by the year 2000 there will be 29 to 33 million people over 65 years, representing 20 percent of the total population (see Table 14-1). These projections can be made with confidence because the senior citizens of the first decades of the twenty-first century have already been born; the elderly of the year 2000 are in their 40s today (U.S. Bureau of the Census, 1977).

TABLE 14-1
Population Shifts in the United States, 1960–1990

Age	Population in Millions				Percent Change		
	1960	1970	1980	1990	1960–1970	1970–1980	1980–1990
Under 20	69	77	73	77	+11.1%	−5.2%	+5.7%
20–24	11	17	21	18	+54.3	+22.6	−15.4
25–34	23	26	37	42	+10.4	+46.1	+13.1
35–44	24	23	26	37	−4.5	+9.6	+45.5
45–54	21	23	22	25	+13.3	−3.9	+9.9
55–64	16	19	21	20	+19.4	+13.0	−3.4
65 and over	17	20	24	28	+20.4	+19.8	+15.4
Total	181	205	224	247	+13.4%	+9.4%	+10.0%

Source: Based on data from Bureau of the Census, *Current population reports*, Series P-25.

These projections challenge us as a nation to find new measures to ensure the quality of life for older adults. They challenge us to revise the stereotypical thinking of the past, when the truly old were few and often infirm. We can no longer perceive all older adults as impoverished, sickly, helpless, and ineffective. There are, certainly, many who conform to this description, but as more people live longer and healthier lives the inactive and incapacitated elderly become an ever-smaller proportion of the total. The needs of the helpless elderly must be met, as must the needs of the helpless of all ages. But an increasing number of today's older adults are financially comfortable, healthy, and physically and economically active.

Our concern in this chapter is with the nutrition-related health problems and the nutritional status of adults of all ages, with particular attention to the special nutritional needs of people in older age. Throughout life, cells remain active, producing energy and metabolic products to sustain the whole organism. Metabolism may slow down, but it does not cease. Nourishment is needed until the end of life.

THE AGING PROCESS

While aging continues throughout life, the physiological processes of adulthood are different from those of the growing years. Once physical growth has ceased and reproductive capacity has been attained, the catabolic rate (cell breakdown) slightly exceeds the anabolic rate (cell growth), except for women during pregnancy and lactation. As a result of this new equilibrium, there is a gradual net decrease in the number of cells in the body.

Theories of Aging

All body structures are made of molecules and all body functions depend on molecules. Yet only in the last 20 years have theories of aging been developed that take molecular changes in the body into account. Earlier theories were descriptive, predicated on observations of the external evidence of aging, such as stooped gait, gray hair, and wrinkled skin. Today's theories attempt to explain these observations in terms of events taking place at the cellular and molecular levels, ascribing the causes of aging to environmental or to genetic conditions.

Environmental theorists explain that the accumulation of external and physiological stress eventually wears out the body and its tissues, a "wear and tear" approach. Some believe that exposure to low-level radiation produces cumulative tissue damage that is ultimately fatal. Radiation causes mutations that result in cell abnormalities, ultimately damaging DNA and impeding protein synthesis so that the cell deteriorates before it can replicate or be repaired. But cellular repair mechanisms are quite efficient, and this theory is not widely accepted as a primary cause of aging.

A related theory centers on "free radicals," highly reactive compounds produced intracellularly by cosmic radiation. Free radicals induce peroxidation of unsaturated fatty acids, thereby affecting cell membranes and damaging vital cell structures such as mitochondria and the endoplasmic reticulum. Those who promote the free radical theory of aging tend to believe that vitamin E can protect against lipid peroxidation by free radicals (Tappel, 1967). Others recommend ascorbic acid and selenium as antioxidants. Whether this chain of events is the cause of aging, and whether vitamin E or any other nutrient can affect it, is subject to much debate and further research. It is, however, clear that free radical formation and related cell pathology are real events in the aging body (Weg, 1978).

A predominant genetic theory postulates a biological "time clock" that puts a natural limit to the number of times a cell can replicate itself, at least **in vitro** (Hayflick, 1976). It appears that the potential life span of some cell types is greater than that of others. According to another genetic view of aging, there may be losses of the information coded into the DNA and RNA. This may cause defective or insufficient amounts of enzymes to be produced during protein synthesis, resulting in various kinds of cell dysfunction. Other effects of changes in nucleic acids have also been suggested, among them that the body's immunologic capacity progressively decreases with advancing age; lacking this protection, the autoimmune reactions of the body increase, with the body virtually attacking itself (Rowe, 1978).

A variation of the "time clock" theory focuses on collagen, the most abundant body protein and a major constituent of connective tissue, found throughout the body. Progressive cross-linking between collagen molecules apparently is responsible for the loss of flexibility of muscle fibers (resulting in body stiffness) and the decreased efficiency of cardiac muscle contraction. While collagen cross-linkage does occur in the aging process, the extent to which it is a cause of aging is unclear.

Extensive research is needed to clarify all of these theories and others. But it seems certain that no single reason for aging will be found and that no way will be found to reverse or halt its effects. The aging process is complex and involves many factors. It is also, despite the claims of fad-diet promoters and cosmetic and drug companies, irreversible. To foster any hopes of increasing an individual's life span through use of any food, nutrient, or other substance, taken internally or applied externally, is irresponsible.

Nutritional Factors and Longevity

Because the nutrients contained in food are metabolized into body components and structures, it is tempting and rational to hypothesize that nutritional factors play a direct and decisive role in longevity. Indeed, a well-known yogurt manufacturer has taken advantage of that temptation with a television commercial in which some long-lived residents of Soviet Georgia are shown happily spooning the manufacturer's product into their mouths. There is no concrete evidence that any one food or nutrient will guarantee extra years. But nutritional status does have a great deal to do with the quality of life and may indeed have an effect on its length. Individuals who are well nourished feel healthier, have more energy, and are usually better able to withstand physiological and psychological stresses than are those on nutritionally poor diets. There also appears to be a relationship between long-term energy intake and longevity. Years ago, McCay et al. (1935) demonstrated that rats experienced a longer life span when their energy intakes were restricted from early life. More recently, Ross and his colleagues have confirmed McCay's findings: Lean and chronically undernourished rats live longer (Ross, 1976). Although these results support the observations that human obesity is associated with a shortened life, the severe experimental conditions used in these animal studies cannot be imposed on humans. Thus, direct application of these research findings to humans is not yet warranted.

Excessive intakes of some nutrients—salt, fats, sugar—as well as some nonnutrient substances have been implicated in decreasing life span by contributing to serious illnesses. Excess sodium does appear to play a part in causing hypertension in susceptible people, and a high-fat diet may contribute to coronary heart disease and certain types of cancer. Relatively few of the many food additives on the market have been found to be harmful. More research is needed to clarify the relationship of individual foods and nutrients to disease and longevity.

Physiological Changes during the Life Span

The *causes* of aging may be unknown, but all individuals experience gradually decreased and/or altered function of various physiological systems throughout their lives. The degree and rate of change vary from one individual to the next, but ultimately every human who lives long enough will experience some of these body changes.

Skin changes are among the most obvious. Changes in the molecular structure of collagen and in the activity of sebaceous glands under the skin can cause the skin to become increasingly dry and wrinkled and can produce warts and tumors. Bruise marks on the skin indicate that underlying blood vessel walls have become fragile.

Changes in bones, muscles, ligaments, and joints are responsible for body stiffness and stooped posture. Calcification and ossification of tissues cause muscles and joints to become less flexible, bones more likely to fracture, and ligaments more easily torn. There is some shrinkage in height, due to shrinkage in cartilaginous material between the bones of the spinal column. Those structural changes can affect other systems: When the body is compressed and stooped, respiration becomes more labored; weakened abdominal and pelvic muscles contribute to difficulties in urination and defecation.

Alterations in the nervous system may be reflected in tremors or changed facial expressions. Reflexes are slowed, and it may take a longer time to change position or recover balance. Short-term memory may be less efficient. Personality changes such as increased passivity, fear of anything new and unusual, possessiveness, and depression may have a physiological as well as psychological component. It is believed that changes in the blood supply to the brain as well as changes in nervous system functioning are responsible for these and other effects.

Efficiency of renal function also decreases with age, even when there is no diagnosed renal disease. This in turn alters the electrolyte and water balance in the body, which depends on highly intricate kidney functions to reabsorb water and sodium, filter out wastes, and maintain the delicate balance of body fluids (see Chapter 9).

In the cardiovascular system the diminution of muscle elasticity is demonstrated as the heart becomes less able to respond to extra work. With increased resistance to blood flow from less flexible blood vessels, higher blood pressure is common. At the same time, blood cholesterol levels decrease between age 60 and 70 (however, this could be explained by the fact that the people with higher levels are more likely to die prematurely due to atherosclerosis and subsequent vascular disease) (Rowe, 1978).

Many people find one or more of their sensory organs becoming less sensitive; sight, hearing, smell, touch, and taste may all be impaired, although not equally in all individuals. Lessened taste acuity is due to a reduction in the number of taste buds as well as to neurological changes. Diminished salivation may cause an increase in dental caries, as well as difficulty in swallowing.

Decreased secretion of hydrochloric acid, pepsin, and intrinsic factor by stomach cells will impair the efficiency of digestion and absorption, particularly of protein and vitamin B_{12}. Changes in digestive glands often affect the absorption of calcium, lactose, and the fat-soluble vitamins. There is a slowing down of the reflex muscular movements that propel nutrients and wastes through the digestive tract. Digestion and absorption become less efficient, and constipation due to slowed colonic motility is a common complaint.

Among other frequent metabolic changes are the decreases in glucose tolerance and in the basal metabolic rate. The latter change is due to the fact that, since lean body mass decreases by 10 to 15 percent after the age of 50, less energy is needed to maintain the smaller body mass. This has implications for energy requirements. All of these changes are exacerbated when disease is imposed on the aging process.

Changes in the reproductive systems are experienced by both men and women; loss of the ability to reproduce takes place earlier—usually in the late 40s or early 50s—and is more obvious in women than are corresponding changes in men. Although their physical responsiveness gradually alters, men have been able to father children even in their late 70s. In women the menopause is not physiologically associated with a loss of sexual interest or capacity, nor is it necessarily accompanied by distressing symptoms. Only 15 to 25 percent of women consult physicians because of discomfort and difficulties at this time (Todhunter, 1977).

Although none of these changes happens overnight, and indeed many people never experience them, they can adversely affect nutritional status in various ways. Individuals who are not able to breathe deeply or move easily, or whose vision, smell, or taste is impaired, are likely to experience a loss of appetite. Lack of exercise also impairs digestion. Shopping and food preparation become burdensome for those who are unable to move about readily, or who have difficulty reading signs and labels. Disturbed enzyme production and renal dysfunction affect nutrient metabolism.

The cumulative deficits of body function in older age are increasingly apparent because more and more people are living longer. Average life expectancy at birth for the population as a whole reached a record high of 73.2 years in 1977 (National Center for Health Statistics, 1979). Figure 14-1 shows the increase in life expectancy for males and females since 1930.

The generally steady increase in longevity over the years is largely due to the conquest of the communicable diseases that formerly proved fatal in earlier life. Hygienic measures, immunizations, and antibiotics have virtually removed this category of diseases from the leading causes of death during the twentieth century. Today, heart disease, cancer, and cerebrovascular diseases account for more than two-thirds of all deaths; only 2.7 percent of U.S. deaths in 1977 were caused by influenza and pneumonia (see Table 14-2), formerly significant causes of death.

NUTRITIONAL REQUIREMENTS FOR ADULTS

Younger adults too may have medical problems that interfere with food intakes and utilization and thus with nutrient requirements. Gall bladder disease often strikes people in their 30s; ulcers, hiatus hernia, and other

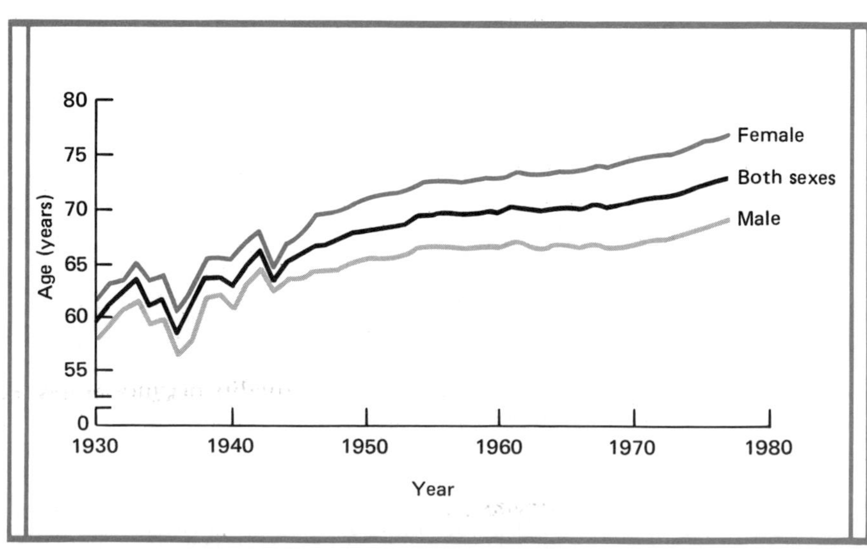

FIGURE 14-1
Life Expectancy by Sex, 1930–1977

Source: National Center for Health Statistics, Final mortality statistics, 1977, *Monthly Vital Statistics Report*, USDHEW Pub. No. (PHS) 79-1120, Vol. 28, No. 1, Supplement, May 11, 1979.

TABLE 14-2
Death Rates for 15 Leading Causes of Death, United States, 1977

Rank	Cause of death	Death Rate (per 100,000 population)	Percent of Total Deaths
	All causes	878.1	100.0
1	Diseases of heart	332.3	37.8
2	Malignant neoplasms, including neoplasms of lymphatic and hematopoietic tissues	178.7	20.4
3	Cerebrovascular diseases	84.1	9.6
4	Accidents	47.7	5.4
	Motor vehicle accidents	22.9	—
	All other accidents	24.8	—
5	Influenza and pneumonia	23.7	2.7
6	Diabetes mellitus	15.2	1.7
7	Cirrhosis of liver	14.3	1.6
8	Arteriosclerosis	13.3	1.5
9	Suicide	13.3	1.5
10	Certain causes of mortality in early infancy	10.8	1.2
11	Bronchitis, emphysema, and asthma	10.3	1.2
12	Homicide	9.2	1.0
13	Congenital anomalies	6.0	0.7
14	Nephritis and nephrosis	3.9	0.4
15	Septicemia	3.3	0.4
—	All other causes	112.0	12.8

Source: National Center for Health Statistics, Final Mortality Statistics, 1977, *Monthly Vital Statistics Report*, USDHEW Pub. No. (PHS) 79-1120, Vol. 28, No. 1, Supplement, May 11, 1979.

chronic conditions of the gastrointestinal tract may cause adults at various ages to be concerned over what and when they eat. These and other conditions require medication that often affects metabolism of one or more nutrients.

Nutrient Needs

Because of the various physiological changes throughout adult life, nutrient requirements change as well. If an individual has been maintaining a well-balanced diet through the developmental years, there needn't be dramatic changes in terms of the quality or kinds of food eaten in adulthood; the same nutrients are essential at every age, because basically the same body processes are taking place.

ENERGY. For most people, energy needs do change with age. After the growth spurt of adolescence, there is a steady decline in energy requirements.

As aging progresses and activity levels and the basal metabolic rate decline, energy requirements drop steadily. The total amount of food consumed should decrease accordingly. Most individuals will automatically and consciously reduce intakes at some point in every decade of life, starting in the mid- to late twenties. The exact ages and amounts involved, however, vary from one individual to the next; those who remain physically active after age 50 will need to consume more kilocalories than those who are less active.

Although the elderly need less energy, the need for protein, vitamins, and minerals (except iron for women) does not decline with advancing years. The RDAs for energy and nutrients in adulthood are shown in Table 14-3. It should be remembered that RDAs are designed for healthy Americans and do not provide for the special needs of individuals who are ill, under stress, or taking medication.

CARBOHYDRATES. Because of the reduced ability to metabolize glucose, consumption of simple carbohydrates should be restricted to avoid placing excessive demands on the body's ability to digest and absorb sugar. In addition, excessive sugar intake will contribute to unnecessary energy consumption. Complex carbohydrates, however, are important in the diet of all adults, and particularly for the elderly; such foods as whole grains, enriched cereals, potatoes, and dried beans should be included regularly. These foods contain B vitamins, iron, various trace minerals, and fiber, and should constitute 40 to 45 percent of the total energy intake of an adult, according to the Food and Nutrition Board. From 5 to 10 percent of energy intake may come from sugars. High-fiber foods are of particular importance for older adults because they help to maintain intestinal function and prevent constipation.

FAT. Because of research linking dietary fat to high serum cholesterol levels and atherosclerosis, it is advisable that intake of dietary fat, and particularly of saturated fat, be reduced to 30 to 35 percent of total energy intakes throughout the adult years. Serum cholesterol levels seem to peak in men between the ages of 50 and 59, and in women from 60 to 69, after which they decline. Serum triglycerides, on the other hand, increase with age for both sexes. It is not necessary or advisable, however, to completely eliminate cholesterol-containing foods from the diets of people over 65. Egg yolk, liver, and vitamin D-fortified milk are excellent sources of nutrients which may otherwise be consumed in inadequate amounts if these foods are unduly restricted. Use of polyunsaturated fats in cooking and for salad dressing, avoidance of fried foods, and trimming the visible fat from meat is advised, and this will adequately minimize intake of saturated fats for most people. Indigestion associated with fat intake can be lessened if fat is consumed in moderate amounts at every meal rather than in large quantities at one meal.

PROTEIN. A study of protein synthesis in infants, young adults, and elderly women, all consuming adequate diets, showed that the rate of protein synthesis declines with age, but that there is no marked variation in the efficiency of nitrogen utilization. Based on this study, it is estimated that the dietary protein requirements decline by approximately 30 percent between the ages of 20 and 75 (Young et al., 1975). Because of decreased protein synthesis and the decline of body protein mass with age, it would seem that

TABLE 14-3
RDAs for Adults

	Males		Females	
Nutrient	23–50 yrs	51+ years[a]	23–50 years[b]	51+ years[a]
Energy (kcal)	2,700	2,400	2,000	1,800
(MJ)	11.3	10.0	8.4	7.6
Protein (gm)	56	56	44	44
Vitamin A (RE)	1,000	1,000	800	800
Vitamin D (μg)	5	5	5	5
Vitamin E (mgαTE)	10	10	8	8
Vitamin C (mg)	60	60	60	60
Folacin (μg)	400	400	400	400
Niacin (mg NE)	18	16	13	13
Riboflavin (mg)	1.6	1.4	1.2	1.2
Thiamin (mg)	1.4	1.2	1.0	1.0
Vitamin B_6 (mg)	2.2	2.2	2.0	2.0
Calcium (mg)	800	800	800	800
Phosphorus (mg)	800	800	800	800
Iodine (μg)	150	150	150	150
Iron (mg)	10	10	18	10
Magnesium (mg)	350	350	300	300
Zinc (mg)	15	15	15	15
Vitamin K (μg)[c]	70–140	70–140	70–140	70–140
Biotin (μg)[c]	100–200	100–200	100–200	100–200
Pantothenic acid (mg)[c]	4–7	4–7	4–7	4–7
Copper (mg)[c d]	2.0–3.0	2.0–3.0	2.0–3.0	2.0–3.0
Manganese (mg)[c d]	2.5–5.0	2.5–5.0	2.5–5.0	2.5–5.0
Fluoride (mg)[c d]	1.5–4.0	1.5–4.0	1.5–4.0	1.5–4.0
Chromium (mg)[c d]	0.05–0.2	0.05–0.2	0.05–0.2	0.05–0.2
Selenium (mg)[c d]	0.05–0.2	0.05–0.2	0.05–0.2	0.05–0.2
Molybdenum (mg)[c d]	0.15–0.5	0.15–0.5	0.15–0.5	0.15–0.5
Sodium (mg)[c]	1,100–3,300	1,100–3,300	1,100–3,300	1,100–3,300
Potassium (mg)[c]	1,875–5,625	1,875–5,625	1,875–5,625	1,875–5,625
Chloride (mg)[c]	1,700–5,100	1,700–5,100	1,700–5,100	1,700–5,100

[a]For age 76 and above, the energy RDA for men is 2,050 kilocalories (8.6 mJ) and for women 1,600 kilocalories (6.7 mJ).
[b]Nonpregnant, nonlactating.
[c]Estimated safe and adequate daily dietary intakes of additional selected vitamins and minerals. Because there is less information on which to base allowances, these figures are provided in the form of ranges of recommended intakes.
[d]Trace elements. Since the toxic levels for many trace elements may be only several times usual intakes, the upper levels for the trace elements given in this table should not be habitually exceeded.

Source: Food and Nutrition Board, National Research Council, *Recommended dietary allowances*, 9th ed. (Washington, D.C.: National Academy of Sciences, 1979).

older adults would need less protein than younger adults. However, some research has indicated otherwise; it has been suggested, for example, that in older adults who are inadequately nourished, protein intake is diverted to meet energy needs, and that additional protein in older age might retard deterioration of muscle tissue (Durnin, 1968; Weg, 1978). Pending more definitive research, the RDA for protein is constant throughout the adult years (Table 14-3). Estimates of protein needs apply to healthy individuals.

Older adults who suffer from gastrointestinal problems, infection, or changed metabolic efficiency as a result of disease or medication may well require increased protein intakes.

VITAMINS. Generally, there is little experimental data on which to base requirements for the micronutrients. Recommendations are, consequently, based on observations indicating relatively widespread deficiencies of some vitamins and minerals.

The RDA for vitamin A is 1,000 RE for adult males and 800 RE for females. It has been speculated that the deficiencies frequently observed in the elderly could be the result of impaired ability to absorb or store vitamin A compounds or to convert the provitamin forms to the active vitamin. Lack of dietary fat, inadequate bile secretion, use of laxatives and antibiotics, and/or pancreatic insufficiency may all interfere with vitamin A absorption. Some clinical findings that often occur in older adults—slow adaptation of the eyes to darkness, scaly skin, and some eye lesions—have responded favorably to the administration of vitamin A.

Vitamin D is especially important in older age due to its role in the metabolism of calcium needed for bone health and maintenance. Because bone decalcification is common in the later years, daily vitamin D intake of 5 micrograms of cholecalciferol—from fortified milk or a supplement—is advisable throughout adulthood and poses no toxicity risk.

Because of its antioxidant properties, vitamin E has received a great deal of popular attention as a possible factor in retardation of the effects of aging; as yet research has not definitively supported this role. In any case, usual intakes of the vitamin appear to be adequate for most individuals, without supplementation.

Older adults may need greater amounts of some B vitamins, especially thiamin, vitamins B_6 and B_{12}, and folic acid. Inadequate intakes of vitamin B_{12} could contribute to disorientation, fatigue, and depression among the elderly. The increased need for these vitamins may result from less efficient absorption, or altered metabolism and excretion, resulting not only from physiological change but from certain medications.

MINERALS. Calcium absorption apparently decreases with age, contributing to osteoporosis or a reduction in the amount of bone, often resulting in fractures. Recent evidence suggests that increased dietary calcium leads to an improvement in this condition for some people (Lee and Johnson, 1979). The importance of maintaining adequate calcium intakes throughout adult life is underscored by the RDA of 800 milligrams. Calcium is also important for maintaining health of the oral tissues; decalcification of the jawbone may contribute to tooth loosening and periodontal disease. Adequate calcium, phosphorus, and fluoride intakes throughout life may be preventive factors.

Iron deficiency is common among the elderly, especially among those with low incomes. It may develop gradually when a diet low in iron is coupled with chronic blood loss, or be due to poor absorption or inadequate utilization by the body. Iron-rich foods should be included in the diets of all older adults. The Food and Nutrition Board recommends a daily dietary allowance of 10 milligrams of iron for all individuals over the age of 50. The iron requirements of women are higher during the years of menstruation, but after menopause women's need for iron is the same as that of men.

FLUID. Adequate fluid intake will increase the efficiency of kidney and bowel function, helping to eliminate wastes and relieve constipation. To maintain fluid balance, it is suggested that individuals over 65 should consume a minimum of 2 liters of fluid daily, 50 percent of which can come from foods. The Food and Nutrition Board recommends 1 milliliter of water for each kilocalorie of food consumed for all individuals of all ages. Drinking three to five glasses of water or other liquids per day is advised.

Effects of Medication on Nutrient Needs

If ours is an overfed society, as is often suggested, it is also an overmedicated one. The numbers and combinations of drugs—both prescription and nonprescription—that are taken by people of all ages, and especially by older adults, is astonishing. As noted in Chapter 6 and elsewhere in this book, drugs may interfere with the absorption, metabolism, and excretion of nutrients. Conversely, nutrients may interfere with drug action, thereby modifying the effectiveness of a prescribed dose. As more is learned about this fascinating subject, changes will undoubtedly be made in the practices of pharmacists, physicians, and nutritionists, and perhaps even of consumers themselves.

DRUG–NUTRIENT INTERACTIONS. The significance of the interaction between medication and nutrients in any individual depends on the previous nutritional status of that person, the dose and duration of drug use, the condition for which the medication is being used, and the particular drug or drug combination being taken. Older adults are more likely to be using multiple drugs on a routine basis than are younger people, and thus the possibility of creating a biologically significant interaction is increased in the later years. Undesired effects may be exacerbated by the probably inadequate nutritional status of an individual who is both elderly and ill.

Even in earlier adulthood, drug–nutrient interactions may be significant. People of all ages, hoping to feel better, unthinkingly down tranquilizers, amphetamines, sleeping pills, aspirin, and antihistamines—not to mention various quantities of alcohol—totally unaware that they may be upsetting their bodies' ability to absorb the very nutrients that would truly help them to feel good. Aspirin, which is widely and often indiscriminately used by people of all ages for relief of mild or chronic pain, depletes tissue levels of ascorbic acid, increases its urinary excretion, and may block the absorption of ascorbic acid into the bloodstream.

Other frequent interactions include the following:

- Hydralazine, used for moderation of hypertension, and L-dopa, a treatment for Parkinson's disease, may cause vitamin B_6 deficiency.
- Mineral oil, often used as a laxative, has an adverse effect on the absorption of all fat-soluble vitamins and can have a significant effect on vitamin A and D status.
- The antibiotic Neomycin alters the body's absorptive capacity within six hours after the first dose is ingested and diminishes production of pancreatic lipase.
- Long-term diuretic therapy for cardiac failure could result in magnesium, potassium, and zinc depletion.

In addition, drugs may cause nausea, vomiting, altered taste sensations, and loss of appetite. These effects have serious implications for nutritional status.

It is also possible for food and nutrients to interfere with the action of a drug. For example, consumption of foods high in vitamin K such as green vegetables may counteract the effects of anticoagulant medication; because vitamin K promotes blood clotting, it antagonizes the desired effect of the drug.

Food prevents rapid absorption of medication, which should generally be taken when the stomach is empty (unless the drug itself is a gastric irritant). Delayed drug absorption will decrease its effective dose in most circumstances. In addition, certain nutrients can influence the absorption of particular medications. Milk and milk products interfere with tetracycline absorption, for example (Roe, 1976).

As research continues to identify drug–nutrient interactions, professionals should provide (and consumers should expect) information about when to take drugs in relation to mealtimes and about food items to be included or restricted during drug usage to maximize drug effectiveness without compromising nutritional status.

ORAL CONTRACEPTIVE AGENTS. Few drugs are as widely and continuously used over long periods of time as are hormonal contraceptives. In the years since they were introduced, epidemiological and clinical evidence has been accumulating on their effects, including those on nutrient metabolism. But experimental data on their metabolic consequences, or the influence of nutritional status on the side effects of these contraceptives, is still scarce.

It has been observed that hormonal contraceptive use raises serum levels of triglycerides, cholesterol, phospholipids, and lecithin, and also increases the risk of some vascular conditions. Recent studies have also noted an increased risk of myocardial infarction, but it is not clear whether this is due to altered lipid metabolism or to alterations in blood clotting factors (Belsey, 1977). Contradictory effects on carbohydrate metabolism have been noted. Abnormal glucose tolerance may occur in about 10 percent of women who have taken oral contraceptives for a year or more, especially those with a family history of diabetes, who deliver high birth weight infants, or who are obese. This condition is reversible and disappears within three months after oral contraceptive use is discontinued.

Oral contraceptive hormones appear to affect protein metabolism in much the same way as the hormonal changes of pregnancy, with a decrease in blood levels of amino acids as well as of albumin; they increase the levels of many of the proteins synthesized in the liver, and especially of carrier proteins. Alterations in protein metabolism may affect the serum concentrations or metabolism of other nutrients as well. It has been suggested that the development of abnormal glucose tolerance may be related to alteration in tryptophan metabolism, which also affects vitamin B_6 status. Deficiency of this vitamin has been linked to the onset of depression in many women taking a combination-hormone type of oral contraceptive; large doses of the vitamin have been found to be therapeutic (Larsson-Cohn, 1975). Because of possible negative impacts of large amounts of pyridoxine and because not all women are equally affected, routine vitamin B6 supplementation for all women using combined oral contraceptives has not been recommended.

Plasma levels of vitamin A, iron, and copper apparently increase in women using hormonal contraception. The increases in iron may in part be due to lessened menstrual flow and consequent reduction of hemoglobin loss; an increase in carrier proteins may also account for the greater presence of these nutrients in the circulation. Increase in retinol-binding protein is associated with increased serum levels of vitamin A. Studies of the effects of oral contraceptives on ascorbic acid metabolism have produced contradictory findings (Hudiburgh and Milner, 1979). In addition, some women develop signs of folacin deficiency.

Metabolic effects of oral contraceptive agents are not uniformly experienced by women taking these drugs, and there are not yet enough data to assess their long-term effects. Especially lacking are data about the effects for women whose nutrient intakes are inadequate; this problem is currently being addressed by the World Health Organization by studies in India, Thailand, and Egypt (Belsey, 1977). Pending results and recommendations resulting from these and other studies, there is cause for concern in the United States, particularly for the many young women whose use of oral contraceptives begins during their own growth years. Additional nutrient requirements, if any, for these young women cannot be estimated at present.

HEALTH STATUS OF ADULTS

Good health is not merely the absence of disease, but a state of physical, mental, emotional, and social well-being. Young and middle-aged adults who are relatively healthy will occasionally show the effects of chronic or acute disease, undoubtedly related to an interaction between genetic and environmental factors. The environmental factors include, among others, lifestyle, exposure and reaction to stress, food-related behaviors, and economics. There is increasing evidence that the impact in the later years of at least some environmental factors can be modified by the behaviors and attitudes formed earlier in life. At any age, conditions of lifestyle and personal habits that may make one unnecessarily vulnerable to physiological stress can be changed, and preventive health measures can be instituted. If good health care habits have not been previously established, the early and middle adult years are the time to make appropriate changes.

Just as adults in the middle years plan for their financial future, so should they plan for their future health status. And today many are. More concerned than ever about health, today's adults are jogging, swimming, playing tennis, skating, and regularly participating in other forms of exercise to keep all muscles, including heart muscle, in optimum condition. They are cutting down on fat, sugar, and sodium consumption in the hopes of avoiding debilitating diseases associated with later life.

The major factors hindering adequate preventive medical care for younger adults are inconvenience and economics. Programs instituted by various governmental agencies and the corporate world are helping to overcome these problems, by bringing clinical care into the neighborhood and the workplace and through prepaid medical insurance and memberships in health maintenance organizations (HMOs) that distribute costs broadly over the years and

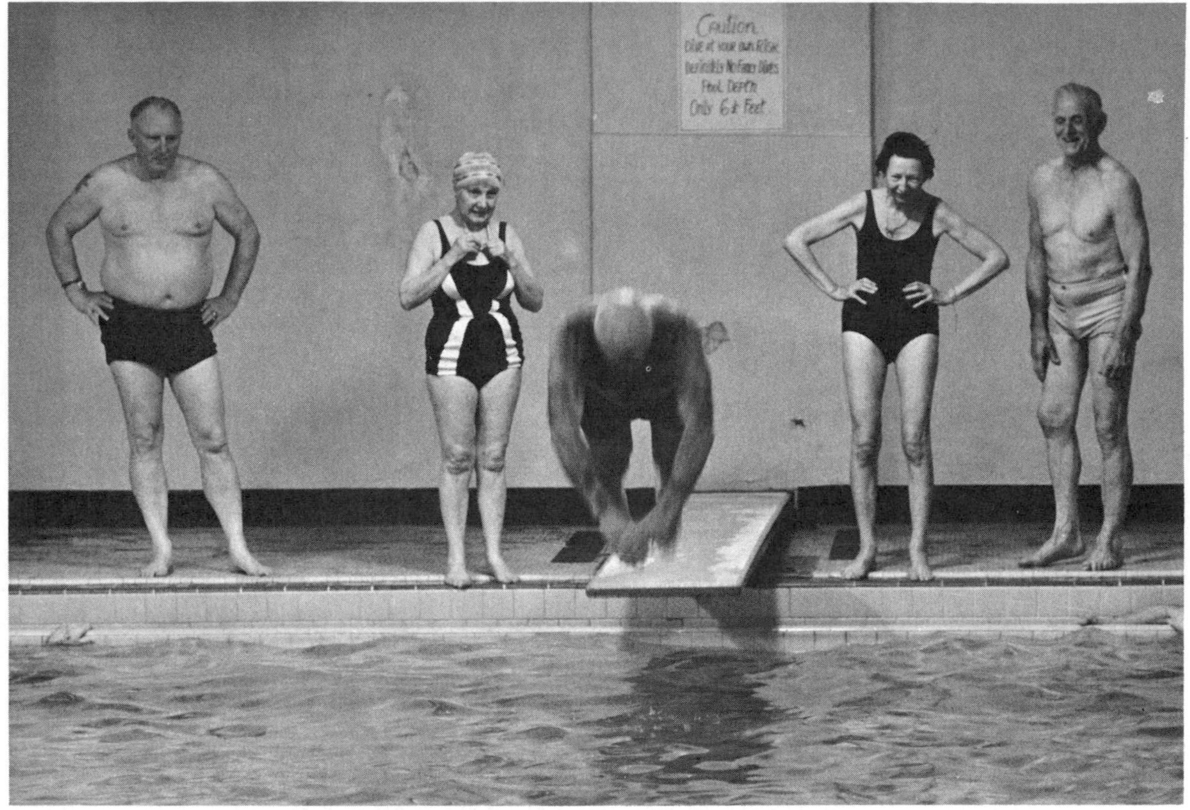

The growing awareness of the importance of physical fitness throughout adult life has resulted in many swimming classes for older adults. (Jay Lurie, Black Star)

among large groups of people. At the same time the media have increased public awareness of the role of preventive care during earlier adulthood in lessening the need for crisis intervention later on.

NUTRITIONAL CONCERNS IN THE ADULT YEARS

Although it is beyond the scope of this text to deal with the medical and nutritional management of some of the conditions associated with aging, a summary of some widespread concerns will indicate those areas that are problematic.

Energy Balance

It is estimated that from 30 to 40 percent of the adult population in the United States is moderately overweight or obese; because this third of the population is more likely to experience additional health problems, there is cause for concern. Many people simply don't realize that the eating habits they enjoyed as teenagers and young adults are inappropriate in their middle years. As life becomes more sedentary, as basal metabolic rate decreases, as the coffee klatches, cocktail parties, dinner parties, and business meetings proliferate, the chances of weight gain increase immeasurably. Women whose activity levels suddenly drop and who spend more time at home, and men over 30 who are still eating as much as when they were teenagers, are particularly susceptible to development of that roll of fat around the middle.

The problem is compounded because overweight people are less likely to exercise. Like poor eating habits, the habit of not exercising is difficult to reverse later in life. Individuals must be persuaded to reduce energy intake before it's too late and to establish an exercise routine early in life and follow it through adulthood. The evidence linking obesity to diabetes, hypertension, gall bladder disease, arteriosclerosis, and some forms of cancer is too overwhelming to be ignored.

There is, however, a sizeable number of older adults who are underweight. This may be related to an underlying disease process or to insufficient food intake. Markedly underweight individuals are particularly vulnerable when illness strikes; they literally have no reserves with which to fight back, and they can become increasingly debilitated. When steady weight loss is noticed, attempts should be made to prevent further losses and to increase energy intakes to restore reserves. When food intake is decreased, nutrient intake is also diminished, further compromising health status.

Diabetes Mellitus

Maturity-onset diabetes has been found to be highly age dependent, doubling with every decade of life and most likely to appear during the 40s. Diabetics are 17 times more prone to kidney disease than nondiabetics, 5 times more susceptible to gangrene, twice as likely to have heart disease and stroke, and 25 times more likely to become blind—the disease is now the leading cause of newly developed blindness. Diabetes has in fact been shown to have an adverse effect on virtually all systems of the body. A recent commentary suggests that because it accelerates the onset of other degenerative diseases, diabetes might be categorized as an accelerated form of aging (Kent, 1976). Maturity-onset diabetes can usually be controlled by diet, weight loss, and perhaps medication; insulin therapy is seldom necessary.

Digestive System Concerns

DENTITION. Approximately half of the population over 65 years of age have lost all their teeth. Three-quarters of those edentulous persons have satisfactory dentures, leaving one-quarter without any chewing apparatus at all. Many cannot afford the cost of dentures; others may have ill-fitting appliances that are too uncomfortable to use. If uncomfortable dentures are worn, chewing is difficult and painful. Of the 50 percent of elderly who do have their natural teeth, a great many have periodontal disease, a chronic infection of the gums with erosion of the underlying bone, followed by loosening and ultimately loss of teeth.

These dental changes affect many older adults and may limit food intake. If soft foods must be eaten as a result of dental problems, sources of many nutrients and fiber are not consumed. The blandness and lack of textural interest of most soft foods lessens appetite and thus limits intake even more.

PEPTIC ULCER. Ulcers are lesions in the lining of the gastrointestinal tract. Gastric ulcers occur in the stomach, and duodenal ulcers are located in the upper part of the small intestine. The direct cause of an ulcer is an excessively acidic gastrointestinal environment. It is not clear, however, why the acidity increases, and why the normally protective mucus secretion of the stomach and duodenum are not effective in preventing this condition. Faulty dietary habits, smoking, heavy aspirin use, and excessive consumption of coffee and cola drinks have all been implicated. So have physical and emotional stress, as well as family predisposition. No single cause has been ascertained.

Ulcers may cause gastric discomfort several hours after eating, when the stomach is empty and its excessive acid content is in direct contact with the stomach or intestinal lining. The lesion may eventually penetrate the entire mucosal wall; the result is a perforated ulcer that in turn leads to hemorrhage.

Treatment for ulcers consists of rest, antacid therapy, and regular and frequent meals; the food acts as a buffer against the acid. Meals should contain all nutrients, including moderate amounts of fat so that some food remains in the stomach for a longer period. In the past it was thought that milk was the supreme buffer for stomach acid and large quantities were recommended, but this is no longer believed to be especially helpful. Sipping milk at intervals during an acute attack may alleviate distress to some extent, but consumption of several glasses a day is unnecessary.

Recent research on laboratory animals indicates that prostaglandins (fatty acid derivatives) can reduce the secretion of stomach acid, protect cells lining the gut from damage, and help to heal ulcers that have already been formed. Clinical trials are projected.

A considerable body of folklore has built up concerning the diet for the ulcer sufferer. Studies indicate that most persons with chronic ulcers can eat almost anything. Black pepper, chili, horseradish, coffee, alcohol, and cola drinks are the exceptions—and some can tolerate even those (ADA, 1971).

GALL BLADDER DISEASE. The gall bladder is the storage organ for bile synthesized by the liver. Most gall bladder disease is due to irritation, inflammation, and obstruction caused by the formation of gallstones. These cholesterol-containing crystals can become quite large and may necessitate the removal of the gall bladder. The incidence of gall bladder disease increases with age. Women in their 40s who are overweight seem to have a tendency toward the disease, as do an increasing number of women using oral contraceptive agents.

There is no evidence that cholesterol-restricted diets will decrease gallstones, but a high-fat diet does cause discomfort to persons with the disorder. A low-fat diet is therefore recommended. Once the gall bladder has been surgically removed, most individuals can resume their normal eating habits within several months. This is possible because the liver continues to synthesize bile, which is released into the upper part of the small intestine, apparently in sufficient quantity and concentration to emulsify dietary fats, aiding digestion and subsequent absorption.

MALABSORPTION. Lactose malabsorption, due to inadequate production of lactase, occurs most frequently among adults in the nonwhite population and in certain white ethnic groups as well (see Chapter 2). Malabsorption of vitamin B_{12} and of calcium are also associated with advancing age, possibly as consequences of lower gastric acidity. Since most absorption takes place in the small intestine, intestinal diseases or removal of part of the intestine will also compromise absorptive capacity.

DIVERTICULOSIS. Diverticulosis occurs when outpouchings (diverticula) form in the intestinal wall, due to intralumenal pressure. These bulging pockets may become inflamed, a condition known as diverticulitis, which is often accompanied by considerable pain. Serious diverticular disease may affect 5 to 10 percent of the over-60 population in the United States. A lack of dietary fiber has been implicated as a contributing factor, and increased consumption of fiber-containing complex carbohydrate foods is recommended as a preventive as well as a treatment measure (see Chapter 2).

CONSTIPATION. Constipation often is a result of a diet consisting largely of processed and easy-to-chew foods and inadequate amounts of fiber-containing fruits, vegetables, whole-grain breads, and bran. It can also be aggravated by the misuse of laxatives taken to relieve the condition. Moreover, a constant use of cathartics can lead to diarrhea, vomiting, fluid loss, depletion of potassium, damage to the lining of the colon, and hemorrhoids. Medication frequently taken for "acid stomach" can also interfere with normal bowel function; constipation is a frequent side effect of antacids that contain aluminum or calcium carbonate. Anthihistamines, antidepressants, antispasmodics, muscle relaxants, and tranquilizers—all used frequently—can also retard bowel function.

The preferred treatment for constipation is consumption of high-fiber foods which increase the bulk of stools and reduce transit time through the gastrointestinal tract. Also recommended are generous fluid intake and exercise. If laxatives are required, those containing nonirritating ingredients such as cellulose derivatives should be selected. Laxatives should be used sparingly, and always accompanied by an 8-ounce glass of water.

Anemias

Nutritional anemia, often found in older adults, results from multiple deficiencies, usually of iron, protein, vitamin B_{12}, folacin, and/or ascorbic acid, along with reduced gastric acidity. The elderly are more often afflicted by the various anemias than are younger people. The Ten-State Nutrition Survey found a higher incidence of iron deficiency in adults over 60 years of age, regardless of income or race, than in younger people. Older people are particularly at risk for nutritional anemias because their lower energy requirement and lower food intakes result in lower nutrient intakes as well. Folic acid deficiency and its result, megaloblastic anemia, is particularly common in the elderly because this vitamin is not widely present in food, is easily destroyed in cooking, and may be poorly absorbed.

Atherosclerosis and Coronary Heart Disease

Obesity, stress, lack of exercise, smoking, and excess dietary cholesterol, saturated fat, and sodium have all been implicated as contributors to blood vessel and coronary heart disease. Women under 50 are less likely than men to experience CHD, but after menopause rates for women are similar to those for men of the same age. Women at younger ages are increasingly being affected as well, presumably because of the changed lifestyle of many women today. As women become full participants in the work force, they are subject to the same occupation-related stresses that men have traditionally experienced; for many this is superimposed on the stresses of managing a household, and guilt and conflict over responsibilities to husbands and children. The role of cigarette smoking in the development of cardiovascular disease is being given new attention as it has been observed that women who smoke are more susceptible than nonsmokers to heart attacks and certain kinds of cerebral hemorrhages, as well as to other noncardiovascular conditions. And more women are smoking today then ever; since 1965 there has been an 8.5 percent decrease in the number of adult men who smoke, but an 11.1 percent increase in the number of women smokers. Moreover, in comparision to men, more women are heavy smokers and more inhale.

Caffeine—found in coffee, tea, and cola beverages—has also been implicated by some recent studies as a causative factor in cardiovascular disease, but the data are contradictory. Prolonged and excessive coffee consumption—over six cups daily—may be associated with arrhythmia in a small percent of the population. It has been suggested that heavy coffee and tea consumption can exacerbate the effects of other risk factors leading to

TABLE 14-4
Black-White Ratio in Prevalence of Hypertension

Age and Weight Class	Men	Women
20–39		
Underweight	2.28	2.30
Normal weight	1.69	2.47
Overweight	1.48	1.82
All weights	1.59	2.34
40–64		
Underweight	1.65	2.19
Normal weight	1.53	1.86
Overweight	1.44	1.53
All weights	1.48	1.77

Note: Ratio is rate in blacks divided by rate in whites. Hypertension is defined here as diastolic blood pressure $\geq$95 mm Hg or reporting current use of antihypertensive medication.

Source: R. Stamler, J. Stamler, W. F. Riedlinger, G. Algebra, and R. H. Roberts, Weight and blood pressure, *Journal of the American Medical Association* 240:1607, 1978.

myocardial infarction and other cardiovascular diseases (Dawber et al., 1974). Diagnosed arteriosclerosis and heart disease respond to medication, weight loss, and nutritional management, as well as to behavioral and lifestyle changes to reduce stress and other contributing factors.

Hypertension

Hypertension, which affects at least 20 percent of the population in the United States, has been implicated as a risk factor for coronary heart disease, stroke, and renal failure. Blacks are more susceptible to hypertension than whites (Table 14-4). While there is no certain evidence that nutritional factors *cause* high blood pressure, there is evidence that blood pressure can be reduced by lowering sodium intake. Obesity is also a contributing factor; in the 20 to 39 age group, hypertension is twice as prevalent among those who are overweight as it is in the normal-weight population (Stamler et al., 1978). Weight loss in obese hypertensive adults, continued weight control with sound nutritional and exercise habits, reduction of sodium intake, and antihypertensive medication are effective treatments (see also Chapter 8.)

Bones and Joints

Arthritis, osteoporosis, and osteomalacia are all common ailments of older adulthood. Arthritis, which is painful and debilitating to millions in their middle and later years, is an inflammation of the joints, and it may afflict any movable part of the skeleton. Despite many popularly hailed theories, there is no effective nutritional therapy. Weight control to minimize the burden on the joints and aspirin to relieve pain are advised. Because those with arthritis often take large doses of aspirin daily, side effects such as gastrointestinal bleeding and decreased ascorbic acid absorption are of nutritional concern. Aspirin should be taken with food, milk, or an antacid.

Osteoporosis, or decreased bone mass, is associated with aging and is especially common in women between the ages of 40 and 60. A decrease in the calcium content of bone, accompanied by a reduction in the amount of bone, is apparently the direct cause of this disorder. Relative estrogen deficiency, physical inactivity, and perhaps inadequate calcium intake in the early and middle adult years are thought to be involved in the etiology of this disorder, which weakens bones and makes them more susceptible to fracture. A dietary regimen high in calcium and vitamin D to promote calcium absorption may be effective in preventing and/or reversing bone loss.

Osteomalacia is characterized by demineralization of bone, leaving the structure vulnerable to fracture. It is most likely to affect older adults who do not drink milk or get adequate sunlight, who have conditions interfering with calcium absorption such as liver or kidney disease, or who take anticonvulsant medication. Because osteomalacia is caused by a deficiency of vitamin D, supplements are necessary to promote calcium utilization. Calcium supplements may also be prescribed.

PERSPECTIVE ON
Nutrition and Cancer

Cancer is the second leading cause of death in the United States. It is estimated that 80 to 90 percent of all cancers are induced by environmental factors—smoking, occupational contamination, air and water pollution, and food substances—and are thus potentially preventable. These estimates are derived from epidemiological studies in which the incidence of a particular kind of cancer is associated with specific environmental factors. Association, however, does not imply causation. The causes of cancer, a complex disease, are not definitely known at present. But the process by which cancer develops is beginning to be understood.

How Cancer Develops. In the initiation stage the DNA of normal cells is altered by the action of a virus, chemical, and/or other agent. These cells become capable of multiplying more rapidly than normal, and this is what happens in the subsequent, or promotion, stage. In some tissues, areas of rapidly dividing cells constitute a firm mass known as a tumor. Not all tumors are cancerous; some are benign and confined to the local area in which they originated. Malignant tumors, on the other hand, invade surrounding tissue, releasing cells that initiate secondary tumors, metastases, in other parts of the body. Because the gastrointestinal tract provides a major route of entry into the body for numerous substances, the influence of nutritional factors on the initiation and promotion of cancer has been receiving considerable attention.

Among findings that suggest a nutritional relationship are:

- In women, cancers of the breast, gall bladder, and uterus have been associated with increased body mass or obesity (Wynder et al., 1966).
- Carcinoma of the large bowel in men, but not in women, has been associated with obesity.
- Japanese migrants to the United States had higher incidence of stomach and colon cancer than those who remained in Japan and who, presumably, consumed the traditional diet; by the third generation, the cancer mortality rate of Japanese-Americans was identical with that of native Americans.
- Seventh Day Adventists, whose diet is largely vegetarian, have had a much lower incidence of cancer than other groups.
- In Japan, when the consumption of milk and milk products increased between 1949 and 1971, there was a decrease in the incidence of stomach cancer.

Nutritional factors may affect cancer development by directly introducing carcinogenic substances into the body or by providing substrates from which the body's enzyme and other systems produce irregular cell activity. Because experimentation with human subjects is not ethically feasible, evidence from animal experiments must be relied on to support the accumulating epidemiological data. Increasingly, carcinogenic studies are being done on human cells grown in a tissue culture in a controlled environment in the laboratory. This overcomes the problems of species difference (is a compound that causes cancer in a rat equally damaging to human tissue?) but it does not compensate for the involvement of the total organism in the disease process. Despite shortcomings, human tissue culture experiments are a significant addition to the research attack on the causes of tumor growth.

Although cancer is a multifactorial disease, evidence is building for a nutritional component, which possibly acts by triggering or accelerating the activity of a virus or other carcinogenic agent. Because diet is easier for the individual to manipulate than are such factors as air pollution and heredity, it is important to understand the dietary factors which are presently implicated, in specific forms of cancer.

Breast Cancer. Among women whose diets contain little animal fat, there is a significantly lower incidence of breast cancer than in women who consume the larger amounts of animal fats typical of the American diet (Dunn, 1975). Experiments with laboratory animals have provided confirmatory evidence: High-fat and high-saturated-fat diets have increased spontaneous tumor incidence in mice (Carroll and Khor, 1975) and accelerated the development of breast tumors from known carcinogens in rats (Chan and Cohen, 1974). It is theorized that a high-fat diet causes changes in hormone balance that promote cancer development. Nonnutritional factors also are involved; low incidence of breast cancer is found, for example, in women who bear their first child at an early age (Hankin and Rawlings, 1978).

Gastrointestinal Tract Cancer. Different nutritional factors are likely contributors to colon and gastric cancer. A high-fat diet has been repeatedly associated with cancer of the large intestine. Gastric cancer, on the other hand, is correlated with low intakes of raw vegetables, milk and milk products (Gori, 1977). The role suggested for dietary fiber in preventing cancer of the colon has been discussed in Chapter 2.

Nutritional Factors as Cancer Preventatives. Research has begun to identify the possible preventive effects against cancer of some nutrients and other substances present in the food supply. In some studies with experimental animals ascorbic acid and α-tocopherol (vitamin E) were found to inhibit the formation of nitrosamines in the stomach and large intestine. Nitrosamines, which are potent carcinogens, are formed when certain amine-containing compounds react with nitrites, often used as a preservative in meats such as bacon. Other studies, however, have detected no anticancer effect of vitamins C or E; additional research is in progress.

The best defined preventive nutritional factors related to cancer are dietary lipid and fiber. Low fat and high fiber intakes are characteristic of populations in which there is a low incidence of all types of cancer; in the United States, diets with high fat and low fiber intakes have repeatedly been associated with cancer.

Nutritional Effects on Cancer Patients. Several consequences of cancer influence nutritional status: cachexia or wasting and weakness; anorexia or lack of appetite; and metabolic changes such as imbalance in iron metabolism and absorption. Anorexia may be a direct result of the weakness produced by the disease itself, or be a consequence of the radiation and chemotherapies used to treat it. Many patients report a change in taste perception, in which some foods become tasteless and animal protein foods become bitter. A result of these alterations in appetite and metabolism, and of the disease process itself, is the loss of muscle tissue and of body fat. Sudden and inexplicable loss of weight may be the first indication of tumor growth, as nutrient intake is diverted to the uses of the diseased tissue (Rose, 1978).

The cancer patient requires vigorous nutritional support during all stages; consultation of the patient and family with a nutritionist should be part of the course of treatment. Too often, cancer patients succumb not to their cancers but rather to the effects of prolonged malnutrition that accompany the disease.

As the number of cancer patients has increased, public awareness of the disease has also increased. But because it is not yet fully understood, and because response to current modes of treatment is individual and variable, cancer remains a mysterious and frightening condition. Too often people will cling to any promise of a cure, accounting for the popularity of substances such as Laetrile for which cures are claimed but unproven. Research continues to look for answers, to more clearly define causes, and to arrive at preventive measures, and useful treatments. Among research priorities are the definition of nutritional and dietary requirements, taking individual genetic and environmental factors into account, and investigation of the role of various dietary factors in prevention and disease therapy.

Based on current evidence, some recommendations can be made with assurance: Decreased intakes of animal fat and increased consumption of fiber from whole grains, fruits, and vegetables are clearly in order. Cigarette smoking apparently enhances the effect of other carcinogens and should be discontinued. The role of food additives, which has received a great deal of public attention, is not that clear; very few of the 1,200 or more food additives are possible carcinogens. Consumption of a variety of foods, in moderate amounts, and maintenance of ideal body weight are also recommended. A prudent diet, one which considers both the RDAs and the dietary goals (see Chapter 16), is recommended by most nutritionists. It is not a guarantee that cancer will not develop, however, just as restricting cholesterol and salt intakes is no guarantee against development of cardiovascular disease. Too many unknown variables are involved in the etiology of these multifactorial diseases.

FOOD PATTERNS: DETERMINANTS AND RECOMMENDATIONS

For most of the adult years, food patterns are determined by likes and dislikes, availability, lifestyle, and other environmental factors. Consumption of a diversified diet from all food groups will maximize the probability of consuming all nutrients in adequate balance.

For Most of the Adult Years

Moderate rather than excessive amounts of food will provide for energy balance without undesirable weight gain. Reduced intake of fats, and especially saturated fats, and of salt and sugar are recommended; these three substances are implicated in the etiology of chronic diseases, and sugar and fat contribute to obesity as well. As fat and sugar intakes are reduced, consumption of dietary fiber will almost automatically increase. Because obesity is associated with chronic diseases and is a major problem among the middle aged, a special effort may be needed in adulthood to achieve and maintain ideal body weight through sound dietary practices and exercise.

In Later Adulthood

Determinants of the foods desired, available, and consumed are more complex for many older adults. Both physiological and psychosocial factors are involved.

PHYSIOLOGICAL DETERMINANTS OF FOOD BEHAVIORS. The physiological changes of the later years may have a variety of impacts on the foods that are preferred, allowed, or available. The net effect of physiological factors is often a lessened overall intake or a lower nutrient intake. There are several reasons for this.

Food loses its appeal when there is poor taste and smell perception, or when bland, soft, or pureed foods are required because of illness or dental handicaps. Poor vision may interfere with shopping and with acquiring information about food quality and availability. When loss of taste perception is due to zinc deficiency and not to other causes, supplementation with 15 milligrams per day of the mineral in the form of zinc sulfate is effective (Greger and Geissler, 1978).

Physical disabilities affecting mobility, as are common in those suffering from arthritis, fractures, or other trauma, also tend to reduce the variety and quantity of the diet. Disabilities may affect the ability to feed oneself as well, and to chew and swallow some foods. Because a limited diet is often an inadequate diet, individuals with motor disabilities are likely not to get nutritional support adequate to promote healing. Foods easily purchased and prepared are relied on, and tea and toast become the boring, and nonnutritious, staples of an overall inadequate diet.

Therapeutic diets prescribed for those with heart disease, diabetes, or other chronic ailments may further limit food choices and make food selection and consumption of a nutritionally balanced diet even more difficult. Medication taken for these and other conditions may also interfere with nutritional status, by upsetting metabolism and limiting absorption of key nutrients.

PSYCHOSOCIAL DETERMINANTS OF FOOD BEHAVIORS. Economic, demographic, and attitudinal factors all interact to limit, for too many of the elderly, the quality of nutrition. Economic realities affect not only the minority of the elderly who are truly poor, but the majority who are living on fixed and minimal incomes. These millions have little leeway with which to respond to rising costs in an inflationary era. Heating and housing costs have proper claims on limited budgets. As food costs rise, the kinds and quantities of foods purchased must be restricted. It is particularly important for those on limited budgets to learn to identify relatively low-cost foods with high nutrient density.

Older adults can be active and conscientious shoppers. One study of food-buying behaviors found that when 84 percent of families with at least one member 65 years or older compared prices before buying, 72 percent favored merchants who offered senior citizens discounts, and 65 percent used advertising as a guide to product purchases. Thirteen percent or more of this group were eligible for food stamps, but only 6 percent reported using them (Mason and Bearden, 1978). Other studies have similarly indicated that a majority of older adults do not take advantage of food stamps to which they are entitled. To many of today's elderly who are strong believers in the work ethic, food stamps carry the connotation of charity. Also, many may be intimidated by the bureaucratic procedures involved in establishing eligibility.

A careful consumer reads labels and examines cans for bulges that would indicate spoilage.
(Henry Monroe, Black Star)

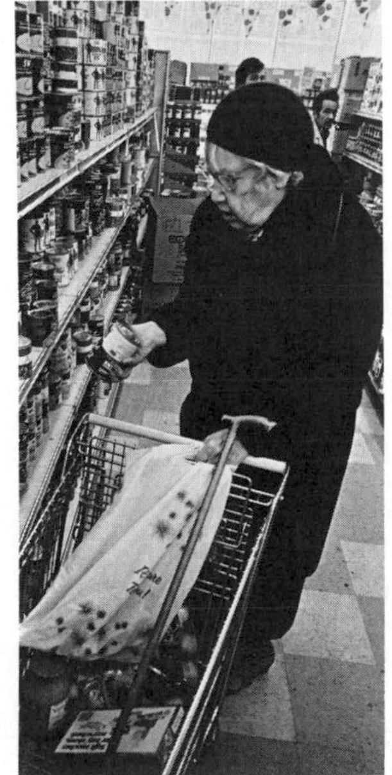

Loneliness is probably the most important determinant of food-related behaviors in older people. A meal to be eaten alone often does not seem worth the effort to prepare it. Older women who once cooked for a husband and family have difficulty cooking just for themselves; older men have had little experience in cooking, and in too many instances do not have the skills or experience required to prepare even the simplest meals. Canned and frozen foods become staples. Prewrapped supermarket packages of meat and produce seldom come in single or two-portion amounts, and higher prices per unit weight are charged for smaller-size cans and frozen foods. Food purchased and prepared in larger quantities may spoil before it is eaten. Supermarkets are stocking more single-serving items, especially in metropolitan areas, but there is still an economic penalty as well as a psychological one for those who are alone.

As young people relocate to take advantage of career opportunities elsewhere, their older parents are left at home, often in changing communities in which they do not know their new neighbors, or in a deteriorating part of an older city succumbing to urban blight. Fear of going out at night, or of leaving the home at all, may in many cases be a realistic response to an unpleasant situation. But these and other realities can produce changes in attitude and personality; and for many of the solitary elderly, fear of contact with outsiders can become a phobia.

Those who own their own homes may be unable to afford necessary heating oil and maintenance costs on fixed budgets and be unable to afford the moving and rental costs a new apartment would require. Others cannot move for psychological reasons—too many beloved possessions would have to be disposed of and too many memories would be reawakened. Yet remaining in the old house may contribute to a feeling of isolation and even to desolation and depression if it is strongly associated with memories of earlier happier times.

Many older people must, for economic reasons, live in single rooms where there may not be adequate space for food storage or facilities for food preparation. They are restricted to the purchase of nonperishable foods and perhaps a minimal amount of cooking on a hot plate. In too many communities public transportation is inadequate or lacking. Those who cannot drive (and because of the expense of maintaining a car, faltering eyesight, and other factors, this is true of many older people) or have difficulty walking must rely on others for assistance with shopping. Or they may have to patronize small neighborhood stores where the prices are higher and the selection smaller. Loneliness, isolation, boredom, and depression all can cause lack of appetite. So can a monotonous food selection due to financial limitations, ill health, or inability to shop for and prepare food. Other older adults may turn to overeating out of boredom and, instead of choosing nutrient-rich products, indulge in energy-dense, nutrient-poor foods. Those who are very set in their ways may have strong food preferences and prejudices and be reluctant to try anything new, no matter how beneficial it might be for them. Others, used to the food patterns of their ethnic heritage and prevented by chronic problems from consuming familiar foods, may find substitutions tasteless.

Fears of ill health also affect the eating habits of the elderly. They fall prey to claims made by health faddists and often, instead of purchasing nutritious and varied foods, they purchase expensive supplemental vitamins and so-called health foods.

Recommendations: Foods for the Adult Years

Consumption of a diversified diet is the best nutritional approach throughout life, including all the stages of adulthood. Problems of providing adequate diversity of foods in single-person households affect not only the elderly but the increasing numbers of single adults living alone at all ages. Young adults are postponing marriage while they establish their careers; more people who have been married are divorced and living alone. At every age, a solitary meal is likely to be an unplanned, carelessly prepared, and hurriedly gobbled snack, a hasty visit to a fast-food outlet, or a sandwich brought in from a counter delicatessen.

FOOD FOR SINGLE ADULTS. Young or old, single adults should make an effort to *dine*, even when they must dine alone. A table that is set, music or a good book for company, and a planned menu even if only for one will pay off in greater enjoyment, better digestion, and improved nutrition. Even breakfast should be given this attention as a pleasant start to a busy day. Developing an interest in cuisine and experimenting with herbs, spices, and new food items can create interest in food preparation even in single-portion quantities. Double portions can be prepared and half promptly labeled and placed in the freezer as a bonus treat for the following week. Nutrition is enhanced when social activities are planned for mealtimes; friends should be invited to dinner regularly or exchange dinner visits between two or more people planned. Dinner in a "tablecloth" or ethnic restaurant should be a regularly scheduled treat.

IRON NEEDS IN ADULTHOOD. Women who have not yet reached menopause may require iron supplementation, especially if they have had several pregnancies. Intakes of less than the RDA of 18 milligrams per day are common in this group; however, because the RDA includes a wide margin of safety to be applicable to a maximal number of people, it is probable that most adult women are consuming at or near their *individual* requirement levels of this mineral. Generally, adult men and postmenopausal women do not require iron supplementation unless a disease condition interferes with iron absorption. Only if a nutritional deficiency has been diagnosed through laboratory analysis of hemoglobin and red blood cell count should supplementation be considered, and then it should be taken under medical supervision.

RECOMMENDATIONS FOR OLDER ADULTS. Preparation of balanced meals may be a challenge for older adults for whom economic, physiological, or other factors interfere with previous food patterns. High quality protein, provided either by foods of animal origin or complementary plant proteins, is important; vitamins and minerals from whole-grain breads and cereals, fruits, and vegetables should be included as well. Fiber from these foods is particularly beneficial in keeping the digestive tract in good working order in the later years and is as effective as most laxatives in improving chronic constipation, without their side effects of reduced absorption of key nutrients.

Because bone disorders can result from lack of calcium, a special effort should be made by the elderly to include good sources of calcium daily. For those who may have difficulty in drinking adequate quantities of milk as a beverage, consumption of cheese, ice cream, yogurt, custards, and puddings will make a good contribution. Many people avoid drinking milk because they fear the gastrointestinal distress that can result from decreased production of lactase, the enzyme that digests lactose (see Chapter 2). Even those in whom lactase deficiency has been diagnostically established, however, can consume milk in moderate amounts (Marrs, 1978). In addition to providing calcium, milk is a good source of protein and, if fortified, of vitamins A and D, and is thus an important component of the diet of older adults.

Fluid intake is important too, to maintain bowel regularity and electrolyte and fluid balance. Milk, soups, cereals, and juices, as well as water, provide fluid. For most adults, soft drink consumption should be limited as should energy-dense snack foods in general: They add to energy intake without providing nutrients.

Money-saving ways to maximize nutrient intake include: saving vegetable cooking liquid for use in soups and cream sauces; combining leftover vegetables in a casserole with toasted strips of cheese; and baking or poaching apples, pears, or peaches, or sauteeing banana slices in margarine for dessert or snacks.

Those who are not able to consume an adequate quantity of food at three regular meals may be helped by eating four or five small meals, or by snacking regularly between meals. Flagging appetites can be improved with regular exercise, such as daily walking or swimming. Meals shared with friends, either at home or in a restaurant (breakfast get-togethers are inexpensive and a pleasant break in routine), are also appetite stimulants. An effort should be made to avoid monotony by trying new foods or recipes. Meals should be eaten at regular times. The overweight should avoid snacks and all energy-dense and nutrient-scarce foods.

PERSPECTIVE ON Alcoholism

Alcohol consumption has an impact on both nutrient intake and nutritional status. Drinking in moderation is not harmful, and may in fact stimulate the appetite, provide feelings of relaxation, and become a vehicle for sociability. Findings based on statistical association show that consumption of up to 2.5 ounces daily may actually decrease the incidence of coronary artery disease (Yano et al., 1977). But excessive alcohol consumption, which pervades all population subgroups, all classes, all ages, and all geographical areas of the country, is a major health problem. It is estimated that 7 percent of adults 18 years and older, or 9.3 to 10 million persons, are problem drinkers. Among young people aged 14 to 17, about 3.3 million or 19 percent are problem drinkers (Chafetz, 1979). Teenage drinking is of special concern, and especially high increases have been noted among seventh-grade boys, eighth- and ninth-grade girls, and college students. Factors associated with teenage drinking include: heavy drinking by parents; peer conformity; broken homes; unsatisfactory parent-child relationships; and personality disturbances such as a sense of alienation, low self-esteem, and a high degree of anxiety.

Drinking has increased among adult women as well, although far fewer women than men are affected. Women who have a high risk of becoming excessive drinkers are those whose roles and lifestyles are untraditional, who are divorced or separated, who are under the age of 35, and who have jobs outside the home. The report of the National Institute on Alcohol Abuse and Alcoholism (1974) found that the age group from 21 to 29 had the highest proportion of women who drank to excess.

Effects of Alcoholism. Alcohol is exceedingly destructive to the human body. It affects every system in the body, with the digestive, nervous, circulatory and endocrine systems and the muscles being most likely to sustain damage. Alcohol can produce disease states in every organ that it contacts; cancers of the mouth, the tongue, the esophagus, the pharynx, and the larynx are all associated with alcoholism. For those who both smoke and drink, the risk of cancer is greatly increased. Alcohol does not undergo digestion, but is absorbed directly into the circulation; hence the fairly speedy effects of alcohol on the brain. Small amounts are absorbed from the stomach and the remainder from the small intestine. Alcohol is oxidized in a complex series of reactions as it circulates through the body and is ultimately converted to carbon dioxide, water, and energy. Small amounts are excreted unchanged by the kidneys and through exhalation from the lungs.

Alcohol may cause food to be propelled more rapidly through the intestine, reducing absorption, particularly of calcium, thiamin, vitamin B_{12}, and amino acids. The greatest damage occurs in the liver, where alcohol disrupts the conversion of amino acids to glucose, resulting in hypoglycemia in individuals with marginal nutritional status and in an excessive breakdown of fatty acids. Alcohol also inhibits synthesis of certain blood and transfer proteins, while promoting synthesis of others, including lipoproteins, thereby tending to increase serum triglyceride levels. The alteration in fat metabolism may have a cumulative effect, resulting in the condition known as "fatty liver," a cause of liver failure and death, especially in younger alcoholics (Chafetz, 1979). Equally serious are the effects of the substitution of alcohol for intake of nutrient-containing foods.

The most common physical disorder resulting from alcoholism is cirrhosis of the liver, in which liver cells are replaced by scar tissue. Onset of cirrhosis may

Nutrition for the elderly can often be improved most readily at the source—when food is purchased. Shopping can provide both exercise and recreation. Use of a shopping cart will eliminate the need to carry heavy bundles. Ways to economize on food should not be overlooked: Some supermarkets offer senior citizens discounts on one day of the week; food coupons—but only for items one normally uses—should be clipped from newspaper and magazine advertisements. Nutritional information on package

be related to nutritional deficiencies accompanying alcoholism and to genetic and other factors, as well as to the direct effects of alcohol on the metabolic processes taking place in the liver (Chafetz, 1979). Pancreatic disorders and disruption of enzyme production also occur.

Excessive alcohol consumption causes nervous system disorders including depression and, when severe enough, anesthesia and coma. Alcoholism is an addictive disease, and withdrawal symptoms can be severe, the most dramatic being delirium tremens. Lung capacity may be reduced over a period of time, causing shortness of breath and congestive heart failure. Other disturbances of the heart and heart muscle include hypertension and irregular heartbeat (arrythmia). Nutrient deficiencies affect resistance to infection and produce a variety of secondary effects including skin infections, which may be exaggerated by thiamin and protein deficiencies, complicated by poor hygiene and neglect. A nutrition-related side effect of excessive alcohol consumption can be weight gain. Most alcoholic beverages contain "empty calories," having negligible nutrient content. Wine and beer, however, do contain some vitamins and minerals. Even moderate consumption of alcohol has been shown to decrease energy intake from foods, although in one study nutrient intakes compared favorably with the RDAs (Barboriak et al., 1978). Heavy drinking certainly curtails nutrient intakes, dulls the appetite for food, and results in expenditure of substantial amounts of money for alcoholic beverages rather than nourishing food.

Alcoholism affects not only the individual who drinks. Persons close to the alcoholic suffer verbal and physical abuse; strangers suffer accidental injuries. A pregnant woman who drinks excessively may be contributing to physical abnormalities and low birth weight in her unborn child, and she is likely to be inadequate in nurturing her child. Society as a whole pays the cost of alcoholism in work-days lost, services and emergency medical care provided, and in many other ways.

Treatment and Prevention. The best treatment for alcoholism remains to be discovered; research in this area has lagged, at least in part because of societal attitudes. On the one hand drinking is condoned, and even encouraged, as a sociable act; on the other hand, the alcoholic is considered undesirable and hopeless. While only 5 percent of all alcoholics are of the "Skid Row" variety, this archaic view of the problem has deterred the scientific community from learning how best to help the other 95 percent.

Alcoholics Anonymous is perhaps the best treatment available, and its combination of behavioral and group therapy has proved effective for many alcoholics. But a large number of heavy drinkers either avoid AA or find it doesn't work for them. Some are helped by the use of drugs, particularly Antabuse, which produces vomiting and severe gastrointestinal distress when alcohol is consumed. But because the side effects can be alarming, occasionally fatal, Antabuse therapy is far from ideal. Work therapy, in conjunction with other approaches, can be helpful to some persons who drink to assuage feelings of depression or loneliness. But the work must absorb the interest and energies of the individual. Restoration of the vitamin, mineral, and protein levels (reduced because of low intake, poor digestion, or malabsorption) is essential in the treatment of alcoholics. Nutritional support to protect against liver damage is only useful when alcohol consumption is controlled; abstinence can help to prevent additional tissue damage and even reverse some symptoms.

The best treatment for alcoholism is prevention. Young people should be taught about the effects of excessive alcohol consumption. Alcoholism is a serious health problem in our society, but one that can be avoided.

labels should be consulted. Meal plans and shopping lists should be made after consulting weekly advertisements to take advantage of advertised specials—and shopping lists should be followed. Purchased foods should be stored properly, and perishables used promptly. If a purchase is unsatisfactory for any reason, the store manager should be informed. (The role of supplementary feeding programs in nutrition for older adults is discussed in Chapter 16.)

NUTRITIONAL STATUS OF ADULTS

The major nutritional problem in adults is overweight; adult women also frequently show signs of iron deficiency. Although there are some pockets of frank malnutrition throughout the country, it is neither widespread nor of major proportions. More prevalent is undernutrition, which was shown by the Ten-State Nutrition Survey to particularly affect people from low-income population groups. Low serum levels of ascorbic acid and iron deficiency anemia were particularly prevalent, especially in women. Nutritional status of older people who live in nursing homes may differ from that of individuals in their own homes. In a 1973 study of 529 noninstitutionalized elderly of all economic backgrounds, aged 60 to 102 years, it was found that, although more than half lived alone, their diets were as adequate as those who lived with others; but many had nutrient intakes of less than two-thirds the RDA (Todhunter, 1976). Nursing homes generally have a consulting dietitian, and studies have shown that foods served in nursing homes provide nutrients in adequate amounts (Brown et al., 1977). Not all served food is consumed, however, especially by those who are ill.

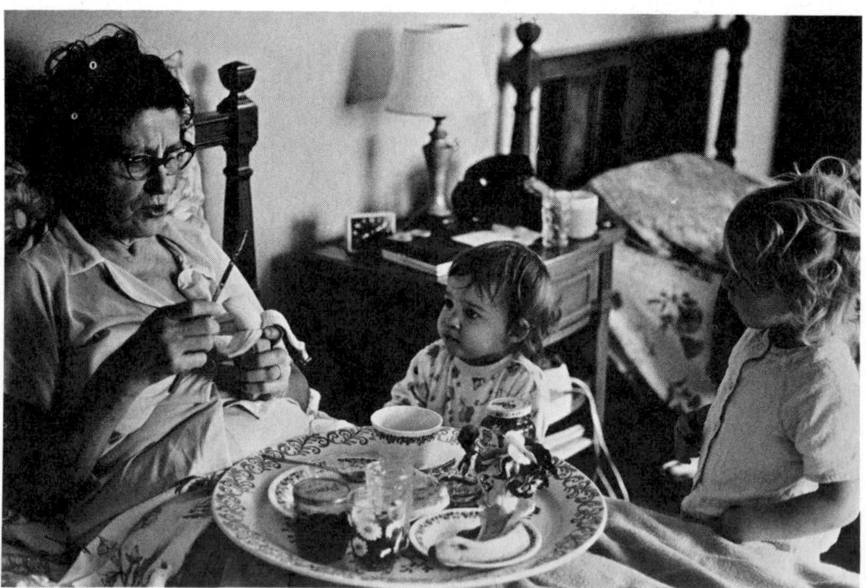

Grandma gets breakfast in bed on Mother's Day. (Sylvia Johnson Woodfin Camp 1 Associates)

In a study comparing energy intake of free-living and institutionalized individuals, the energy intakes of the independent-living subjects were significantly higher than those of the residents of nursing homes (Guthrie et al., 1972). The Ten-State Nutrition Survey found that, in general, low-income older people consumed a smaller quantity of food than those with higher income and their choice of foods resulted in a relatively lower energy intake. Vitamins A and C and calcium are the nutrients most likely to be in short supply in the diets of older adults. Because there have been few studies of the actual requirements of older adults, there is some difficulty in assessing their nutritional status by dietary means. The RDAs for this segment of the population are therefore based on extrapolation from studies on younger adults; they are set at higher levels for most nutrients than most individuals will need, to provide a substantial margin of safety.

LOOKING AHEAD

Life is a continuity, and the last part of the life cycle can be as rewarding as any other stage. If health is good, and positive habits and a variety of interests are cultivated throughout the adult years, physical and intellectual activity can be maintained through the ninth and even tenth decade, as increasing numbers of older people are demonstrating every day. Optimal health and body functioning can be achieved by maintaining ideal body weight, exercising regularly and in moderation, eating a diversified diet in moderation, and minimizing stress by creating a balance in one's life between work, friends and family, and recreational activities.

Because how one eats affects how one's life progresses, nutrition education is important, especially for young adults. They can be reached in the work place, in their children's schools, through nutritional counseling when a new baby is born, through popular publications, and as a consequence of new interests such as travel and gourmet cookery. Public education is a new and growing career area for nutritionists, who can reach a wide public through such means as advertisements and pamphlets sponsored by food-producing companies and supermarkets. Government-funded group feeding programs for older adults present a particularly good opportunity for nutrition education.

Older adults can also be reached through their various social organizations and the specialized publications targeted to this group. Patronizing tones and methods will not work with the elderly; they are not children and will resent being talked to as if they were. They are eager for information that can be put to practical use: ways to save money, interesting new recipes, and suggestions for adding nutrient content to their daily meals. Most important, in open-ended group sessions they should be given the opportunity to raise questions about their own problems, so that discussion can be targeted to their needs.

As a result of the growing numbers of older people, and the growing interest in all aspects of aging, more government funding has been made available for research as well as for social programs. Eventually this research emphasis should lead to a more satisfactory determination of actual nutrient requirements, providing more definitive data against which to assess nutritional status. These in turn will lead to more accurate and specific recommendations for food and nutrient intake, will emphasize the importance of nutrition in the later ages, and will have an impact on supplementary feeding programs.

The aging process is being studied on some 800 men and women in the Baltimore Longitudinal Study of Aging sponsored by the National Institute on Aging. A new human research institute sponsored by the USDA has been established in Boston at Tufts University to conduct research on the nutritional, physiological, and biochemical factors relating to the aging process. The goal of this Human Nutrition Laboratory on Aging is to coordinate and refine known information and to generate new data. Only continued research will provide the foundation on which recommendations and practices can build.

As the increased longevity of the population attests, nutritional improvements in the last century have benefited millions living and enjoying life in older age today. As more is learned, the quality of life for all members of this large and growing segment of our population can be enhanced. This research frontier is important to all of us at every age, for in the continuity of the life cycle we will be the older adults of the future.

SUMMARY

In the United States today more than 23 million people are over 65 years of age; by the year 2000 at least 29 million people will be in this age group. Aging, however, begins at conception and is continuous throughout life. Although physical growth is completed by early adulthood, the body's tissues and cells remain in a dynamic state, with catabolism slightly exceeding anabolism, resulting in a net decrease in the number of cells. There are wide differences between individuals in the effects of aging.

Theories variously ascribe aging to changes in DNA produced by low-level radiation, to wear and tear that ultimately depletes cell resources, to free radicals resulting from cosmic radiation oxidizing fatty acid components of cellular structures. A genetic explanation involves a biological "time clock" that naturally limits the number of times a cell can replicate itself; and some believe that information coded into DNA and RNA is progressively lost or altered over the years. Aging is probably multifactorial, resulting from the interaction of several mechanisms.

There is no concrete evidence that any one food or nutrient will increase longevity, but there is abundant evidence that the quality of nutrition throughout life is an influence on health and well-being. Obesity, excessive intakes of salt, fats, and sugar, and inadequate consumption of fiber-rich foods are all associated with chronic and severe disease conditions in the middle and later years and with higher mortality rates.

Among the many physiological changes that come with advancing years are changes in metabolism. Decreases in taste sensitivity and in the production of saliva and several digestive enzymes lead to poorer appetite and lowered efficiency of metabolism. The use of medications may also lessen nutrient absorption.

A decrease in the basal metabolic rate along with generally lower levels of physical activity reduce the need for energy intake in the later years. Since recommendations for most nutrients, however, remain at the same level throughout the adult years, it is important to maintain nutrient intakes even while energy intake is reduced. Fluid intake of 2 liters per day is also advised.

Although today's older adults are in generally better health than those of any previous generation, many are afflicted with chronic and serious disease conditions, especially toward the end of life. Among the most debilitating of these conditions are diabetes, peptic ulcers, arthritis, and osteoporosis. Various forms of cancer, atherosclerosis, coronary heart disease, and hypertension affect millions in the middle as well as later years. Those receiving treatment for any of these or other conditions should be aware that medication can interfere with nutrient utilization, and conversely, that food can decrease the effectiveness of some medications.

Especially in older age, health problems may have an adverse effect on appetite, interfere with shopping and food preparation, and make feeding oneself or chewing difficult. Economic and psychosocial factors also affect food behaviors and therefore nutritional status. Public information programs about nutrition targeted at all ages will encourage younger adults to establish positive eating and exercise habits, improve the quality of food consumed throughout life, and thus prepare the way for a healthy and well-nourished older age.

BIBLIOGRAPHY

ADA. Position paper on bland diet in the treatment of chronic duodenal ulcer disease. *Journal of the American Dietetic Association* 59:244, 1971.

Barboriak, J. J., C. B. Rooney, T. H. Leitschuh, and A. J. Anderson. Alcohol and nutrient intake of elderly men. *Journal of the American Dietetic Association* 72:493, 1978.

Belsey, M. A. Hormonal contraception and nutrition. In *Nutritional impacts in women*, eds. K. S. Moghissi and T. N. Evans. New York: Harper & Row, 1977.

Brown, P. T., J. G. Bergan, E. P. Parsons, and I. Krol. Dietary status of elderly people. *Journal of the American Dietetic Association* 71:41, 1977.

Carroll, K. K., and Khor, H. T. Dietary fat in relation to tumorigenesis. In *Progress in biochemical pharmacology: Lipids and tumors*, ed. K. K. Carroll. White Plains, N.Y.: S. Karger, 1975.

Chafetz, M. E. Alcohol and alcoholism. *American Scientist* 67:293, 1979.

Chan, P. C., and L. A. Cohen. Effect of dietary fat antiestrogen, and antiprolactin on the development of mammary tumors in rats. *Journal of the National Cancer Institute* 52:25, 1974.

Dawber, T. R., W. B. Kannel, and T. Gordon. Coffee and cardiovascular disease: Observations from the Framingham Study. *New England Journal of Medicine* 291:871, 1974.

Dunn, J. E., Jr. Cancer epidemiology in populations of the United States—with emphasis on Hawaii and California—and Japan. *Cancer Research* 35:3240, 1975.

Durnin, J. V. G. A. Energy—Requirements, intake and balance. *Proceedings of the Nutrition Society* 27:188, 1968.

Food and Nutrition Board, National Research Council. *Recommended dietary allowances*, 9th ed. Washington, D.C.: National Academy of Sciences, 1979.

Gori, G. B. Diet and cancer. *Journal of the American Dietetic Association* 71:375, 1977.

GREGER, J. L., AND A. H. GEISSLER. Effect of zinc supplementation on taste acuity of the aged. *American Journal of Clinical Nutrition* 31:633, 1978.

GUTHRIE, H. A., K. BLACK, AND J. P. MADDEN. Nutritional practices of elderly citizens in rural Pennsylvania. *Gerontologist* 12:330, 1972.

HANKIN, J. H., AND V. RAWLINGS. Diet and breast cancer. *American Journal of Clinical Nutrition* 31:2005, 1978.

HAYFLICK, L. The cell biology of human aging. *New England Journal of Medicine* 295:1302, 1976.

HUDIBURGH, N. K., AND A. N. MILNER. Influence of oral contraceptives on ascorbic acid and triglyceride status. *Journal of the American Dietetic Association* 75:19, 1979.

KENT, S. Is diabetes a form of accelerated aging? *Geriatrics*, November 1976, p. 140.

LARSSON-COHN, U. Oral contraceptives and vitamins: A review. *American Journal of Obstetrics and Gynecology* 121:84, 1975.

LEE, C. J., AND G. H. JOHNSON. Effect of supplementary calcium and calcium-rich foods on bone density of elderly females with osteoporosis. *Federation Proceedings* 38:772, 1979.

McCAY, C. M., M. F. CROWELL, AND L. A. MAYNARD. The effect of retarded growth upon the length of lifespan and upon the ultimate baby size. *Journal of Nutrition* 10:63, 1935.

MARRS, D. C. Milk drinking by the elderly of three races. *Journal of the American Dietetic Association* 72:495, 1978.

MASON, J. B., AND W. O. BEARDEN. Profiling the shopping behavior of elderly consumers. *Gerontologist* 18:454, 1978.

NATIONAL CENTER FOR HEALTH STATISTICS. Final mortality statistics, 1977. *Monthly Vital Statistics Report.* USDHEW Pub. No. (PHS) 79-1120, Vol. 28, No. 1, Supplement, May 11, 1979.

NATIONAL INSTITUTE ON ALCOHOL ABUSE AND ALCOHOLISM. Second report to U.S. Congress. Washington, D.C.: USDHEW, 1974.

ROE, D. A. *Drug induced nutritional deficiencies.* Westport, Conn.: Avi Publishing Co., 1976.

ROSE, J. C. Nutritional problems in radiotherapy patients. *American Journal of Nursing*, July 1978, p. 1194.

ROSS, N. H. Nutrition and longevity in experimental animals. In *Nutrition and aging*, ed. M. Winick. New York: John Wiley, 1976.

ROWE, D. Aging—A jewel in the mosaic of life. *Journal of the American Dietetic Association* 78:478, 1978.

STAMLER, R., J. STAMLER, W. F. RIEDLINGER, G. ALGERA, AND R. H. ROBERTS. Weight and blood pressure. *Journal of the American Medical Association* 240:1607, 1978.

TAPPEL, A. L. Where old age begins. *Nutrition Today* 2:2, 1967.

TODHUNTER, E. N. Life style and nutrient intake in the elderly. In *Nutrition and aging*, ed. M. Winick. New York: John Wiley, 1976.

TODHUNTER, E. N. Nutrition in menopausal and postmenopausal women. In *Nutritional impacts in women*, eds. K. S. Moghissi and T. N. Evans. New York: Harper & Row, 1977.

U.S. BUREAU OF THE CENSUS. Current population reports. Series 25-P, 1977.

WEG, R. B. *Nutrition and the later years.* Ethel Percy Andrus Gerontology Center. Los Angeles: University of Southern California Press, 1978.

WYNDER, E. L., G. C. ESCHER, AND N. MANTEL. An epidemiological investigation of cancer of the endometrium. *Cancer* 19:489, 1966.

YANO, K., G. G. RHOADS, AND A. KAGAN. Coffee, alcohol and risk of coronary heart disease among Japanese men living in Hawaii. *New England Journal of Medicine* 297:405, 1977.

YOUNG, V. R., W. P. STEFFEE, P. B. PENCHARZ, J. C. WINTERER, AND N. S. SCRIMSHAW. Total human body protein requirements at various ages. *Nature* 253:192, 1975.

SUGGESTED ADDITIONAL READING

American Journal of Clinical Nutrition. Symposium: Oral contraceptives and nutrients. 28:371, 1975.

ANWAR, M. Nutritional hypervitaminosis D and the genesis of pteoralacia in the elderly. *Journal of the American Geriatrics Society* 26:309, 1978.

DUKES, G. E., J. G. KUHN, AND R. P. EVANS. Alcohol in pharmaceutical products. *American Family Physician* 16:97, 1977.

GRAHAM, D. M. Caffeine—Its identity, dietary sources, intake and biological effects. *Nutrition Reviews* 36(4):97, 1978.

GROTKOWSKI, M. L., AND L. S. SIMS. Nutritional knowledge, attitudes, and dietary practices of the elderly. *Journal of the American Dietetic Association* 72:499, 1978.

HARTLEY, H. National conference on nutrition in cancer. *Nutrition Today*, September-October 1978, p. 6.

KRITCHEVSKY, D. Diet, lipid metabolism and aging. *Federation Proceedings* 38:2001, 1979.

LIEBER, C. S. Alcohol and nutrition. *Nutrition News*, October 1976, p. 9.

MOGHISSI, K. S., AND T. N. EVANS, EDS. *Nutritional impacts in women throughout life with emphasis on reproduction.* New York: Harper & Row, 1977.

MUNRO, H. N. Tumor-host competition for nutrients in the cancer patient. *Journal of the American Dietetic Association* 71:380, 1977.

Nutrition Reviews. Special Report: Food and cancer. 36(10):313, 1978.

STIEDEMANN, M., C. JANSEN, AND I. HARRILL. Nutritional status of elderly men and women. *Journal of the American Dietetic Association* 73:132, 1978.

TROLL, L. E. Eating and aging. *Journal of the American Dietetic Association* 59:456, 1971.

WINICK, M., ED. *Nutrition and aging.* New York: John Wiley, 1976.

WYNDER, E. L. The dietary environment and cancer. *Journal of the American Dietetic Association* 71:385, 1977.

YOUNG, V. R. Diet as a modulator of aging and longevity. *Federation Proceedings* 38:1994, 1979.

Chapter 15

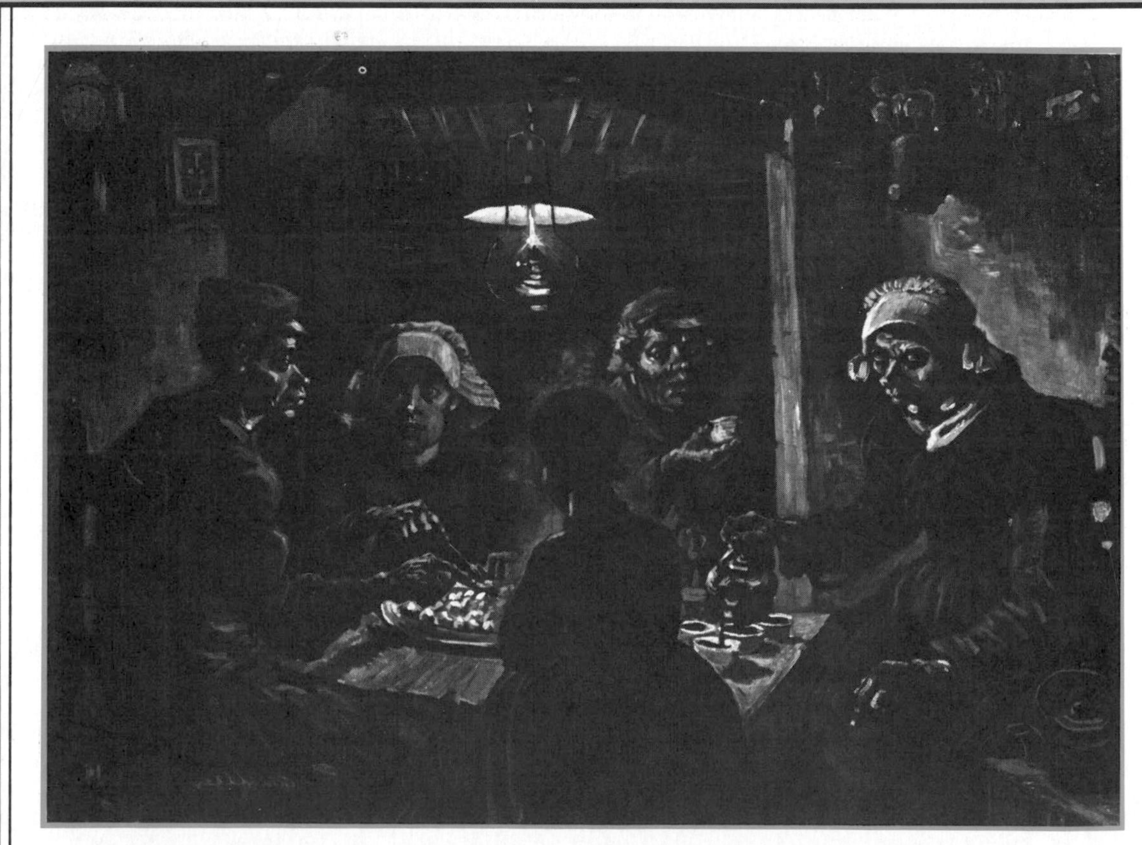

The Potato Eaters by Vincent van Gogh

International Nutrition—Issues, Problems, Strategies

Nowhere is the interaction between the external and internal environments more evident than in the relationship between food production and health. In some of the world's nations, nutrient needs far exceed nutrient availability, and widespread malnutrition harshly impairs the quality of life. Yet in countries such as the United States, that benefit from optimal climate, technological development, stable government, and efficient distribution systems, malnutrition also exists, frequently in the form of overnutrition, but too often as undernutrition among poverty-level population subgroups. Food stamps, surplus food distribution, and other nutrition programs help to eradicate these small pockets of malnutrition in the Westernized countries. But similar programs on an international scale make scarcely a dent in the devastating problem of malnutrition in developing countries around the globe. In times of war, floods, earthquakes, and other disasters the international community effectively bands together to provide emergency feeding; meanwhile it is unable to eliminate the epidemic levels of hunger, suffering, and death that are chronic in deprived areas. The causes of world hunger are varied; personal poverty, national underutilization of both natural and human resources, unstable political, social, and economic conditions—all these play a role.

For most Americans, starvation is an abstract concept. Although we may have collected pennies for UNICEF at Halloween, or listened to parental pleas to "Think of the hungry children in India" as we dawdled over our string beans, the reality of starvation is difficult to grasp. Starvation is a complex and very real problem of imbalance in the world's food production and food distribution systems that is particularly evident in the developing nations. What factors cause it? What are the results? What is being done to avoid it? What is the outlook for the future?

INTERNATIONAL SURVEILLANCE POLICIES

In comparing eating patterns, food choices, and nutrient intakes in various countries, it is necessary to have some kind of standard against which widely varied diets can be judged. Our examination of world food problems begins with a discussion of some of the current international standards and the types of surveys from which these standards were derived.

Dietary Standards

The dietary standards developed by the United States and referred to throughout this text are, of course, the RDAs. Other nations and international organizations have also developed dietary standards. Table 15-1 presents selected values from several of these. Most are calculated by age and sex, with increased intakes specified for pregnancy and lactation. As with the standard developed in the United States, the purpose of standards of other nations and agencies is to prescribe a general level of nutrient intake that will promote and maintain health for most of the population.

From the obvious differences between each country's standards, it is apparent that needs, and estimation of those needs, vary widely. Genetic and environmental differences affect nutritional requirements from country to country. In extremely hot climates, for example, people do not require as many kilocalories to maintain body heat as they do in temperate or cool climates. General patterns of physical activity—which vary markedly throughout the world—also influence recommendations for energy intake. The abundance of sunshine and the extent to which people spend their time out of doors in subtropical areas might lessen the need for dietary vitamin D. Indigenous dietary patterns also play a role. Because high protein intakes appear to reduce calcium retention, the need for dietary calcium may be higher in countries such as the United States, where meat consumption is high. These many differences are reflected most obviously in the FAO/WHO figures in Table 15-1; since these figures are meant to be international, rather than national in scope, they are designed to cover a wide span of countries, lifestyles, activity levels, and food patterns and supplies.

The first attempt to produce international standards was made by the

TABLE 15-1 Comparison of Dietary Standards

Country	Sex	Age	Weight kg	Energy kcal	Protein[a] gm	Calcium mg	Iron mg	Vitamin A RE	B_1 mg	B_2 mg
Canada	F	19–35	56	2,100	41	700	14	800	1.1	1.3
	M	19–35	70	3,000	56	800	10	1,000	1.5	1.8
Colombia	F	20–29	55	1,900	60	400–500	15	1,000	0.8	1.1
	M	20–29	65	2,850	68	400–500	10	1,000	1.1	1.7
FAO/WHO	F	20–39	55	2,200	41	400–500	19	750	0.9	1.3
	M	20–39	65	3,000	53	400–500	6	750	1.3	1.8
United States[d]	F	23–50	55	2,000	44	800	18	800	1.0	1.2
	M	23–50	70	2,700	56	800	10	1,000	1.4	1.6

[a]Assume Net Protein Utilization (NPU) of 70.
[b]As niacin equivalents (preformed niacin plus 60 mg tryptophan: 1 mg niacin)
[c]As free folacin, except for USA values, where total folacin (free plus bound) is considered.
[d]Recommended Dietary Allowances, Revised 1979.

Niacin[b] mg	Folacin[c] μg	Vitamin C mg
14	200	30
20	200	30
12.5	—	50
13.8	—	50
15.2	200	30
21.1	200	30
13	400	60
18	400	60

League of Nations' Technical Commission on Nutrition in 1938. Recommendations were given for energy and 11 nutrients: calcium, phosphorus, iron, iodine, vitamin A, thiamin, riboflavin, vitamin C, vitamin D, protein, and fats. Recommendations for energy and 10 nutrients came from the British Medical Association in 1950, and for energy and 11 nutrients from FAO/WHO in 1974; in 1974 the United States and Canada included vitamin E, pyridoxine, vitamin B_{12}, magnesium, and zinc. In 1975 the Deutsche Gesellschaft für Ernährung showed recommended intakes for 24 nutrients including water, essential fatty acids, sodium, chloride, potassium, pantothenic acid, and fluoride.

The diversity in recommendations by these groups reflect different points of view concerning standards. Some are set at or near a theoretical average need; others are designed to provide generously for the vast majority of the population by adding a margin of safety to the estimated average. Truswell (1976) has recently reviewed the history of dietary standards.

Nutritional Surveys

Many nations and several international agencies have undertaken nutrition assessment surveys to document existing problems, the categories of persons affected, specific deficiencies, and to identify the reasons for them. The same kinds of biochemical, anthropometric, clinical, and dietary tools used in nutrition surveys in the United States (see Chapter 10) have been employed by other countries. The Food and Agriculture Organization (FAO) of the United Nations has conducted international food and nutrition surveys since World War II, as has the United States Department of Agriculture. A United States agency, the Inter-Departmental Committee of Nutrition for National Defense (later called National Development) (ICNND) developed a methodology for such surveys; the ICNND has been succeeded by the Nutrition Program of the U.S. Public Health Service, which conducts surveys for and in cooperation with more than 30 countries. These surveys, taken from 1956 to 1969, included medical, biochemical, and dietary assessment, and evaluated food production, processing, and distribution methods (Caliendo, 1979). Other countries have also been active. Since 1949 Japan has conducted annual national nutrition surveys to obtain data for programs designed to improve food supplies and dietary habits. In 1968 the Nutrition Canada survey was begun.

Why should countries spend so much time and effort on nutritional surveillance? They do it primarily because of a growing recognition that the nutritional status of individuals and population groups affects the medical and socioeconomic health of the entire country. Good nutrition is a vital national resource and, as such, deserves to be cultivated, protected, and monitored. National nutrition assessments are aimed at:

- Identifying the nature, extent, and development of nutritional problems
- Specifying nutritionally vulnerable subgroups and community needs
- Establishing a baseline against which future assessments can be measured
- Recognizing changing nutitional trends and predicting future needs
- Establishing priorities for food and nutrition policies to meet current and projected needs (Christakis, 1973).

Nutrition Canada, for example, was designed to generate data regarding the prevalence of nutritional diseases in various segments of the Canadian population and to determine the quantities and types of foods consumed throughout the country. Methods used included anthropometric measurements, blood and urine analyses, dental histories, and dietary interviews of more than 19,000 subjects. A special effort was made to acquire data about Indians living on reservations and Eskimos in the northern territories.

Among the problems identified were overweight, found in large numbers of adults; iron deficiency and low serum folate levels in men, women, and children; suboptimal protein intakes during pregnancy, and subsequent protein and/or energy deficit in many children under age 5; low intakes of calcium and vitamin D in infants, children, and adolescents; inadequate thiamin intakes in adults, especially pregnant women; vitamin C deficiency in the Eskimo and Indian populations; moderate vitamin A deficiency in pregnant Indians and Eskimos; and moderate enlargement of the thyroid in significant numbers of all Canadians.

Despite this surprisingly large compendium of nutritional problems, Canadian nutritionists believe that the true incidence of deficiencies is even greater, since those who participated in the survey were more likely to be aware of nutrition and its importance. Based on that assumption, guidelines were proposed for the addition of nutrients to foods and for nutrition education programs (Nutrition Canada, 1973).

Limited studies in war-torn South Vietnam have identified a variety of nutritional problems. In 1971, Vietnamese army physicians studied 40 families from 21 villages. They found average intakes of less than 1,950 kilocalories per day; the average need was estimated to be 2,100 kilocalories. Adequate protein intake was provided by seafood, pork, and the concentrated fish sauce nuoc mam, used as a condiment. Calcium and vitamin A intakes were low, but iron—largely from nuoc mam and leafy vegetables—was high. Intakes of thiamin and riboflavin were adequate where hand-milled rice was used, but inadequate where polished rice was the staple (Kaufman, 1979). More recent studies in Vietnam have identified numerous deficiency-related conditions, as years of warfare and political instability have taken a severe toll on the production and distribution of foods. A 1978 study by a team of American nutritionists and other health professionals heard Vietnamese government officials blame unfavorable weather conditions—typhoons, drought, and unusually cold weather during the growing season—for food shortages of between 1 and 2 million tons a year, leading to rationing of staple items and exhorbitant market prices. Caloric deficits were reported to be apparent even to the casual observer; kwashiorkor, marasmus, and xerophthalmia were observed in clinical settings, and a high rate of infectious diseases testified to markedly lowered resistance (Kaufman, 1979).

THE PROBLEMS OF UNDERNUTRITION

As these few examples indicate, the results of nutrient deficiencies can be quite varied, and range from minor to moderate to severe. Among the most devastating are stunted physical and mental development, nutritional deficiency diseases, decreased wound-healing ability, general tissue breakdown, impaired metabolism, and consequent increases in morbidity and mortality. Affected populations typically show decreased activity levels and impaired mental functioning which in turn decreases their productivity and lessens the chance that they will be able to improve their own lifestyle. Because of their rapid growth rate and concomitant need for energy and nutrients, children are particularly vulnerable to all these effects and under such conditions seldom achieve their genetic potential for physical or intellectual development.

Scope of the Problem

Various estimates of the worldwide prevalence of malnutrition suggest that from 400 to 500 million persons are affected. Malnutrition may be due to a simple lack of one or more essential nutrients, resulting in a specific deficiency disease, or to a general shortage of food. Protein and energy deficits cause listlessness, muscle wastage, growth failure, and ultimately kwashiorkor, marasmus, or—usually—combined protein-energy malnutrition (PEM).

The basic cause of undernutrition is a severe shortage of food. In developing countries, traditional methods of food production and distribution cannot provide enough food for an ever-increasing population. The result is a chronically inadequate food supply.

In some parts of the world malnutrition is an episodic event, due to a sudden and temporary but major disruption in food availability. Famine caused by warfare and drought have been the primary causes of this kind of malnutrition, producing starvation when there is simply little or no food to be had. The sudden onset of protein-energy malnutrition, with associated secondary symptoms such as infectious disease, is accompanied by a sharp and widespread increase in mortality rates. In Biafra in the late 1960s and in Cambodia in the late 1970s, civil strife led tens of thousands to flee their homes and farms, bringing food production to a halt and causing mass starvation.

Undernutrition and Its Effects

The specific impairments seen in malnourished populations depend on the specific nutrients that are lacking in the diet.

PROTEIN-ENERGY MALNUTRITION. Protein-energy malnutrition (PEM) is the most prevalent type of undernutrition in the developing countries of the world. PEM has two principal forms, kwashiorkor and marasmus. Kwashiorkor results from a diet in which energy intake is adequate but protein content is not. It is characterized by edema, which gives a bloated, pot-bellied appearance to its victims, usually young children who have been weaned from breast milk to an inadequate diet consisting primarily of starchy or sugary liquid gruels. These children are also likely to have depigmented skin which looks patchy and gray and depigmented reddish hair.

Marasmus, on the other hand, results from severe energy deficits caused by overall food deprivation. It is common in poverty-level infants who are not breast-fed and in children of any age who have a markedly insufficient diet. Children with marasmus do not have edema or pot belly but appear to be all skin and bones. Although protein intakes may on the surface appear to be adequate, protein is diverted from its usual anabolic role to meet energy needs, and tissue wastage is the consequence.

In reality, the etiology of these two conditions is often indistinguishable, because diets deficient in protein are generally characterized by insufficient energy content as well. It is not clear why one child develops kwashiorkor while another suffers from marasmus. Recent research has suggested that individual differences in adaptation to nutritional stress may explain this confusing phenomenon (Rao, 1975). Because of the overlapping causes and effects of kwashiorkor and marasmus, and because essentially the same nutritional therapy is applied for both conditions, it is more convenient to consider them as two sides of the same coin, protein-energy malnutrition. In the past, kwashiorkor was treated with protein-enriched diets, but because of the new thinking about PEM all manifestations of this condition are treated with overall increased quantities of food of balanced nutrient content. Without treatment the disease is fatal. With treatment the prognosis is good; symptoms can be reversed in a matter of months. The extent of lasting effects depends on the stage of physical development during which the deficiency occurred, the length of time and severity of the condition, and the stage of development at which therapy was instituted.

OTHER NUTRITIONAL DEFICIENCY DISEASES. PEM is not the only nutritional deficiency disorder prevalent in developing nations. Nutritional anemias, endemic goiter, ariboflavinosis, and a variety of dental conditions are widespread. Vitamin A deficiency results in blindness for large segments of these populations, and rickets afflicts many as well. Pellagra, beriberi, and scurvy are found in some areas.

The International Congress of Nutrition, meeting in Hamburg in 1966, recommended that the international community address the nutritional deficiencies of the developing world in terms of priorities, with PEM deserving of primary attention because of the large numbers of victims, the high mortality rates, and the extensive physical and mental disabilities that result. Vitamin A deficiency, responsible for xerophthalmia and a high mortality rate in children as well as extensive blindness throughout whole populations, was given the next priority. Nutritional anemias and endemic goiter are widespread but can be halted by relatively simple means (Bengoa, 1967).

NUTRITION AND INFECTION. One of the first published reports to call international attention to the synergistic relationship between malnutrition and infection was issued by the World Health Organization in the late 1960s (Scrimshaw et al., 1968). Since then, many studies have concurred that undernourished children are more susceptible to infections and, conversely, that infection worsens nutritional status. Undernourished Mexican populations, for example, suffer a fatality rate from measles that is 180 times higher than in the United States (Caliendo, 1979). Multiple nutritional deficiencies inhibit the body's ability to produce antibodies and other mechanisms to protect against infectious disease. Thus, undernourished individuals will have less resistance than well-nourished ones with which to fight off disease.

The relationship may not be that simple, however. In one recent study it was found, for example, that undernourished children from one small village in India were actually less susceptible to measles infection than the better nourished children when body weight was used as the criterion for nutritional status. Only 40 percent of the village children classified below the 25th percentile for weight contracted the disease during an epidemic, while 57 to 69 percent of those with weights between the 25th and 75th percentiles did develop measles (Sinha, 1977). Much remains to be learned about the biochemical relationship between malnutrition and susceptibility to infection.

The effect of infection on nutrition is more clear. Bacterial and viral infections deplete the body's nitrogen content. Diseases that produce vomiting, sweating, or diarrhea cause fluid, protein, energy, and general electrolyte and nutrient losses. At the same time, infection is often accompanied by loss of appetite. Furthermore, cultural traditions often dictate the use of enemas or purgative treatment for diarrhea, and restrict intake to teas or weak broths, all of which reduce nutrient intake and absorption just when it is most needed.

Some researchers have concluded that diarrheal diseases cannot be eradicated in underdeveloped nations, where poor sanitation and contaminated water supplies are constant environmental hazards. But in one study of preschool children living in a poor area of Colombia, the introduction of piped water and flush toilets did not seem to affect the prevalence of diarrhea. When feeding programs were instituted to improve the children's nutritional status, however, the frequency of diarrheal disease dropped significantly, and the decrease was greatest among those who were most severely malnourished at the start of the study. While malnutrition is not directly responsible for intestinal infections, improving nutrition does appear to be the most readily available and cost-effective method of increasing resistance to infectious disease (Wray, 1978).

NUTRITION AND BEHAVIOR. The apathy, irritability, and inattention so common in malnourished children have led nutritionists to postulate a direct link between dietary deficiency and behavior. This hypothesis has received strong support from many animal studies, in which malnourished rats demonstrated behavioral and learning difficulties that persisted even after refeeding and rehabilitation; these abnormalities even appeared to be transmitted to succeeding generations whose prenatal nutrient supplies were sufficient (Crowley and Griesel, 1963). Attempts to confirm these effects in humans are complicated by the fact that malnutrition rarely occurs in isolation from other factors which are known to affect behavior. Studies have repeatedly documented associations between childhood malnutrition and lower socioeconomic status, poor housing, unemployment, broken homes, and recurrent illness. Do the frequently observed emotional or learning problems in these children result from inadequate nutrition, unstimulating environment, or a family's preoccupation with economic and/or personal problems? What are the roles of poor maternal nutrition or lack of prenatal medical care? A number of studies have demonstrated a clear association between malnutrition and retarded mental development in school-age children. On the other hand, Dutch women who were pregnant during the famine of World War II delivered low birth weight babies of normal intelligence (Stein et al., 1975). What was the role of the mother's prepregnancy nutritional status and of the gradual improvement in diet during the early years of these children's lives?

And what was the contribution of the generally middle-class lifestyle of their families? From this perspective, malnutrition is only one of the several concomitants of poverty that predisposes to impaired intellectual and behavioral development.

Biochemical evidence demonstrates a significant role for nutritional effects on the central nervous system. The quantity of neurotransmitter substances, the activity of brain enzymes, and even the size and composition of brain cells are adversely affected by severe malnutrition. Some of these changes depend on the timing of deprivation, since the brain is most vulnerable to nutritional insult during periods of growth. Studies of brain components in Ugandan children who died between the ages of 1 day and 15 years have found lower than normal brain weights at every age in those who were malnourished (Brown, 1966). But it has been suggested that there is potential for catch-up growth and development, and even that central nervous system changes may be reversible at early stages.

Obviously, additional research is needed before conclusions can be drawn. Some current studies indicate that learning problems among poorly nourished urban children in the United States and elsewhere may be deficits in performance rather than intellect and due to a variety of interacting factors (Read, 1973; Brozek, 1978).

Factors Contributing to Malnutrition

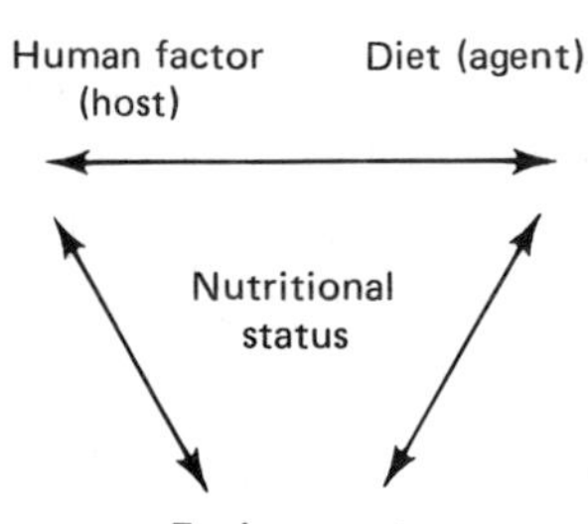

Nutrient deficiencies do not exist in a vacuum. Lack of food to eat is related to inadequate production and distribution. Environmental factors influence the choice of diet and the availability of food and its component nutrients. These are in turn influenced by individual human differences in nutrient needs and utilization. Human factors affect the means of production as well. These three factors—environment, diet, and host—form an epidemiological triangle, interacting to determine the incidence of nutritional disease. The dietary determinants of malnutrition are varied; the environmental and individual factors are equally complex.

ENVIRONMENTAL FACTORS AFFECTING FOOD PRODUCTION. Unfavorable climatic events—droughts, flooding, cold spells—can cause widespread famine, while favorable temperatures and adequate rainfall ensure a long-term abundance of crops. Generally, weather conditions are unpredictable and uncontrollable, but meteorological methods are improving and long-range predictions are aided by cameras and other instruments placed on space satellites. It is possible to buffer some climatic events and environmental conditions by cloud seeding, irrigation, and cultivation of selected, hardy crops, but it is not possible to change climates from unfavorable to favorable, or to outwit devastating storms. Worldwide weather conditions appear to be changing. The north temperate zones may be becoming colder, while some tropical areas such as India and Pakistan are receiving less rainfall.

Careful management of available water supplies is important not only for agriculture, but for human survival. Although three-fourths of the earth is water, only 2.5 percent of that is nonoceanic; of the limited fresh water, more than 70 percent is located in glaciers and ice caps where it is unavailable for productive purposes. Rain and snow recirculate the world's water resources and help to increase local supplies, but it is estimated that only 0.007 percent of the earth's water falls back as precipitation, of which two-thirds evaporates or is transpired by plants. According to a recent report of the International Institute for Environmental Development, 70 percent of the world population is without safe, dependable water supplies (Agency for International Development, 1977). Overpopulation, a growing problem, further depletes these scarce supplies.

Overpopulation also threatens to diminish available land resources, and when land is scarce, people go hungry. Land is necessary not only for agricultural use, but for grazing, housing, energy production, and transportation. Land for these purposes is usually taken from the best growing areas, because that is where the population centers are. Moreover, cropland is constantly being lost through erosion, diversion of irrigation water to nonfarming uses, and overcultivation. As a result, expanding deserts are depriving increasing numbers of people of their means of food production and, potentially, of a means of survival; one in every seven of the world's people now lives in areas classified as arid or semiarid (Brown, 1978).

AGRICULTURAL PRACTICES. Fertilizers, pesticides, crop rotation, and irrigation increase crop yields, providing not only more food, but more nutritious food from plants that have absorbed valuable soil nutrients. But these agricultural aids are not available in many parts of the world. Lack of knowledge, of adequate technology, and of financial resources all contribute to poor crop yields, with an obvious nutritional effect on local farmers and their families.

ECONOMICS. The costs of seed, fertilizer, farm machinery, and labor vary throughout the world; in proportion to purchasing power, these costs are greatest in developing nations. Many farmers are unable to purchase products they need to produce food and generate income. Economic conditions in other lands may have a greater impact than local events. Inflationary price increases have made the costs of manufactured goods too high for many developing nations. Countries paying for supplies with American currency found that the decreased purchasing power of the dollar contributed to a 14 percent increase in the cost of imported goods in 1978 (New York Times, 1979).

ENERGY. Energy is needed to move water for irrigation, to mechanize farm operations, to transport farm supplies and harvested produce, and to manufacture fertilizers, herbicides, and pesticides. Higher prices for fuel and petroleum products and for producing other energy sources have also affected farm production around the world. An indirect effect of the energy crisis on food availability exists: As the newly-rich oil producing and exporting countries (OPEC) have demanded more food imports, the cost of food to poorer nations has increased. In Mexico newly discovered oil reserves may bring relief from long-term malnutrition and underdevelopment, but Mexico's increased purchasing power will channel food supplies away from other countries that will no longer be able to afford them (*New York Times*, 1979).

PRODUCTIVITY AND THE HUMAN FACTOR. Acceptability of a new timetable for planting may depend on whether women or men do the planting, and what other cultural customs such as dance ceremonies or puberty rites are tied into the agricultural calendar. Introduction of new equipment may require a shift from female to male involvement at a certain stage of the production process, with ramifications throughout community life. Increased productivity, however, may well prove to be a strong motivating factor for change.

CONCLUSIONS: FACTORS AFFECTING PRODUCTIVITY. Increased agricultural production is essential for the developing nations, but it will not be achieved without a massive assault on the multiple factors that influence productivity. In these countries agriculture is the primary sector of the economy. The health and well-being of a population, and therefore its future productivity, is strongly tied to improved food production. For these reasons, no economic development will be possible unless first attention is paid to improving crop yields and variety. The development of an advanced industrial economy necessitates a whole new pattern of life and cannot be achieved without high technological development in the agricultural sector. Lack of synchrony between agricultural, industrial, and social advances is a key reason for the failure of so many "five-year plans."

FOOD DISTRIBUTION: THE HUMAN FACTOR. Food distribution, like production, is influenced by environmental and human factors. If a nation is able to increase its food supply while stabilizing its population, the average amount of food available for distribution to each person then increases. This principle has worked in developed countries, where food production has increased while population growth has slowed and even halted. But in developing countries population gains have absorbed nearly all production increases. Although the rate of world population growth has slowed in recent years, there is still an annual net increase of about 80 million persons (U.S. Bureau of the Census, 1978). Meanwhile, although the poorest countries have the greatest rate of population increase, their food production per capita has improved only slightly (see Figure 15-1).

Population dynamics are complex. Although lack of food decreases the population by contributing to infant, maternal, and childhood morbidity and mortality, it is certainly not a humane method of population control. But improvements in food supplies and social and economic conditions tend to create new problems of excess population by increasing infant survival. It has been suggested that programs to limit fertility (birth control) in developing countries will not succeed until parents can be assured that their children will survive (Wyon and Gordon, 1971). Without improved nutrition, the latter event is unlikely. The relationship between fertility and nutrition is indeed complex.

Cultural and religious practices often limit food usage. No culture utilizes all available potential foods. In our own culture, although there is no specific religious or other taboo for most of us, insects and horseflesh are viewed with repugnance; rabbit is consumed by only a few, usually from a cultural tradition such as that of Germany or France where this is an accepted food item. Often foods are permitted to some members of the community but forbidden to others. Children or pregnant women are frequently prevented

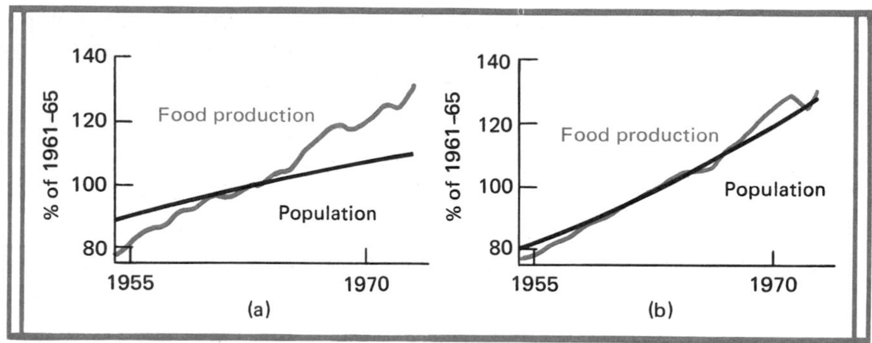

FIGURE 15-1

Food Production and Population for (a) Developed and (b) Developing Countries

Food production has increased in both developed and developing countries at a comparable, steady rate over the past two decades. The population increases in the developing countries, however, have far outstripped the increase in food production, resulting in less food per capita.

Source: M. A. Caliendo, *Nutrition and the world food crisis* (New York: Macmillan, 1979), p. 185.

from eating eggs, because "the baby will cluck like a hen" (Jamaica) or the newborn child will be a girl (Liberia) (Caliendo, 1979). Even where there is no food taboo, people are generally reluctant to add newly introduced strange things to their diets. Food surpluses delivered to nations which need them may be refused because they are unfamiliar.

In some cultures, men receive choice foods and receive them first, with the less nutritious "pickings" left for women and children. In Alor, Indonesia, meat is distributed to each household according to the number of males living there (Simoons, 1961). In other areas, cultural traditions demand that food be shared only with certain relatives or only with individuals from similar caste groups. These and other social and cultural practices may prevent distribution of food according to needs.

Individual characteristics such as age, sex, prior nutritional status, psychological and physiological development, activity level, genetic inheritance, and the presence of pregnancy, lactation, or disease help to determine each person's need for specific nutrients. Ability to adapt to decreased caloric and nutrient intake also differs from person to person. A diet that may be adequate for one individual may lead to malnutrition in another. Individual psychological differences also determine what foods will be eaten, and in what quantities. Personal likes and dislikes, habits, and traditions are nonnutritive aspects of food behavior that often originate in childhood and are important determinants of actual intakes.

ECONOMICS AND FOOD DISTRIBUTION. No matter how much food is produced, people who can't afford to buy it will remain malnourished. Although improved productivity will result in additional purchasing power on a national as well as an individual level, the increased mechanization needed to add to productivity may have the unwanted effect of promoting unemployment. Increased demand by newly developing nations drives prices up

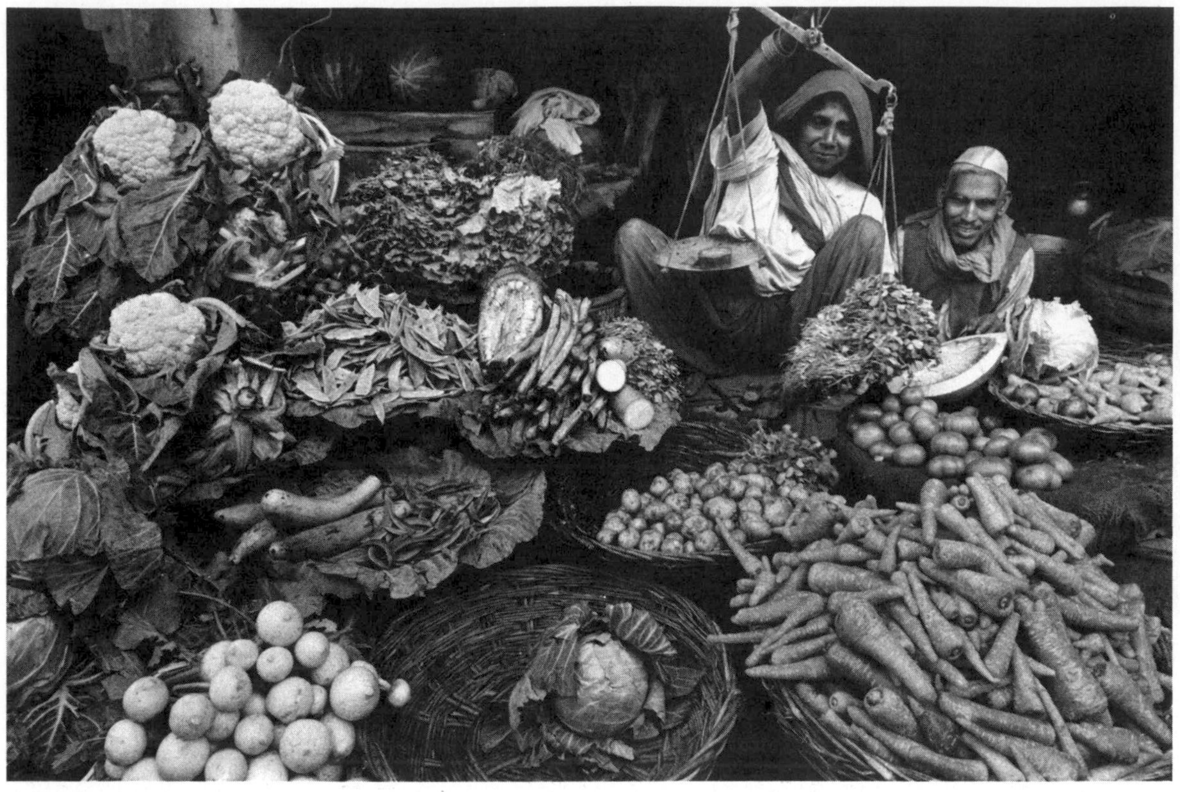

In the developing nations, food distribution systems depend on independent merchants such as these men whose vegetable stand is located in the main food market in Patna, Bihar, India. (Bernard Pierre Wolff, Photo Researchers, Inc.)

on the international market and may further deprive poorer peoples. Recent price raises related to purchases by China and the wealthy OPEC nations have increased costs to the least developed nations, who have fewer commodities to trade on the world market. On the other hand, additional demand on the world market may be a spur to production. In the United States, for example, production of soybeans and soybean oil increased by over 255,000 tons per year from 1965 to 1977, 90 percent of it for export (Holz, 1979). On a national level, the shift from a traditional, largely barter economy to a money economy produces a whole range of economic and social dislocations.

International trade agreements and food laws limit what can be shipped to needy nations and what prices must be paid. Health and sanitary regulations set by some countries prohibit the importation of foods treated with certain additives and pesticides. During the "lemon war" of 1975, "fought" between Japan and the United States, Japan banned the importation of citrus fruit treated with the fungicide orthophenylphenol (OPP), a chemical that was approved by all other major shipping and marketing countries of the world. American citrus growers suffered tremendous financial losses, a problem of little concern to Japanese citrus growers. Although Japan finally relented on OPP, a similar war is presently raging over American use of another fungicide, thiabendazole (Fayans, 1979). While these conflicts did not affect urgently needed foods, other trade policies have done so. Large Chinese orders for

American grain during 1979, for example, provided the impetus for American price-support programs that encouraged farmers to store grain rather than release it for export to other countries. Fortunately, India, Southern Asia, Russia, and Western European countries enjoyed good growing seasons and did not require as large quantities of American grain as they had in previous years, thus reducing pressure on the American supply (Robbins, 1979).

PROCESSING TECHNIQUES. The ability to preserve perishable foods and to store excess foods for use in time of need provides a significant buffer against malnutrition. The improvement in nutritional status enjoyed by most Americans in the twentieth century is due as much to improved processing and transportation facilities as to improved farm productivity. Processing makes it possible for foods that are plentiful in one area to be shipped to other areas where they are scarce. In addition, processing techniques can provide an entry to world markets, even for traditionally poor nations. Mexico, for example, increased its budget for fisheries by over 50 percent in 1979, much of that money going to processing centers which prepare frozen fish products for export (*New York Times*, 1979).

TRANSPORTATION. In developing countries, many of which consist of mountainous or desert areas, roads and rails are sadly lacking. Even where transportation systems are available, the high costs of motor vehicles and fuel tend to curtail distribution of food and supplies. Lack of adequate transportation also affects a country's ability to export goods and to distribute food imports. Stories of flour and rice shipments rotting at the docks while inland peoples starve are common.

STRATEGIES FOR CHANGE

Technology can serve as a buffer against changes in weather, population, and economic conditions. Technology can make possible increased crop yields, better storage, and more efficient distribution. What technology can't do, however, is to prevent major natural disasters, stabilize political unrest, or convince individuals to select nutritionally beneficial foods. Recent decades have seen recurrent energy crises, growing Third World populations, unstable governments on every continent, and large gaps between "have" and "have not" nations and individuals.

An integrated approach combining better production and distribution with curtailed population growth, better and more available health care, and improved sanitation is needed. The goal is getting food to the people who need it, at a price they can afford. To do this, technology must be tempered with regard for personal needs and values so that people will not be displaced suddenly from their accustomed jobs; deprived of the salaries that give them purchasing power, nutritional status will deteriorate even further. Nutrition education programs must be tailored to local customs and beliefs. Only a broad range of strategies will accomplish the far-ranging changes that are required to improve nutritional status and health for all the world's peoples.

Increasing Food Production and Distribution

The question facing developing nations is not only *how* to increase food supplies, but *what* food supplies to increase. Everywhere, as income levels rise, people seek out better food. People at the lowest socioeconomic level consume diets high in starch from rice, corn, and root crops. With higher incomes protein-rich foods such as meat are added to the menu. Finally luxury items such as refined foods and out-of-season fruits and vegetables make their appearance. New foods have been found to be most acceptable if they are introduced in the sequence of this "food ladder"; this nearly universal human tendency must be considered in the development of new food sources and planning of food distribution programs.

In industrialized nations there has been considerable controversy over meat-centered diets, which are resource-expensive. Many people believe that using grain to feed cattle is quite wasteful, when that same grain could be used directly as food, contributing to world food supplies. Others argue that the grazing lands used for cattle could not be efficiently transformed into growing lands, that meat products contribute to general nutritional health and serve as "buffers" during temporary periods of bad weather and crop shortages.

This is a complex question and is related to the efficiency of the so-called **food chain.** The food chain starts with the inorganic materials provided in soil—minerals, nitrogen, and water—and carbon dioxide from the atmosphere. Energized by the sun, plants synthesize sugar and starch, releasing oxygen to the air; they incorporate nitrogen and minerals into other plant materials. Plants are consumed by animals, including humans. In turn, humans consume some animals. In their life processes animals (including

FIGURE 15-2
The Food Chain

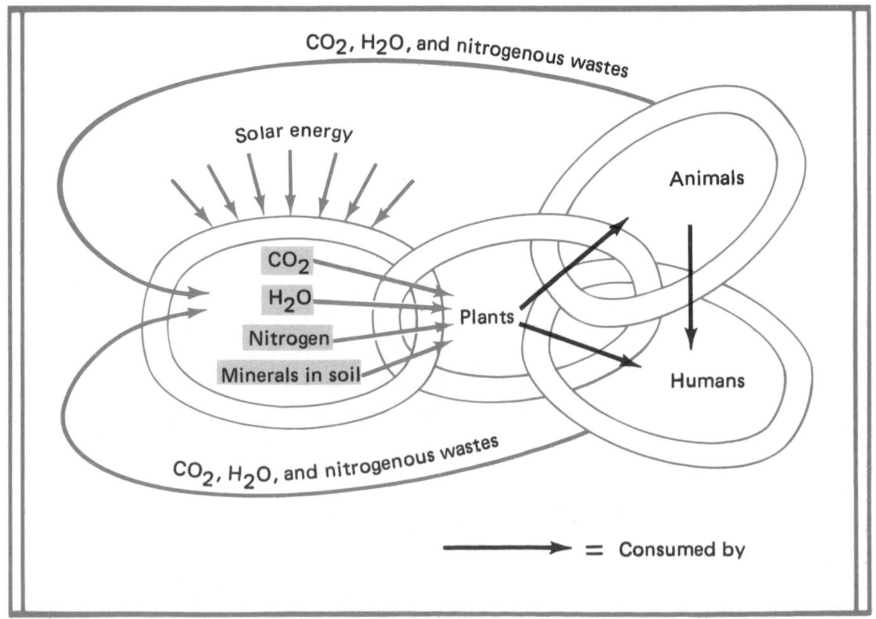

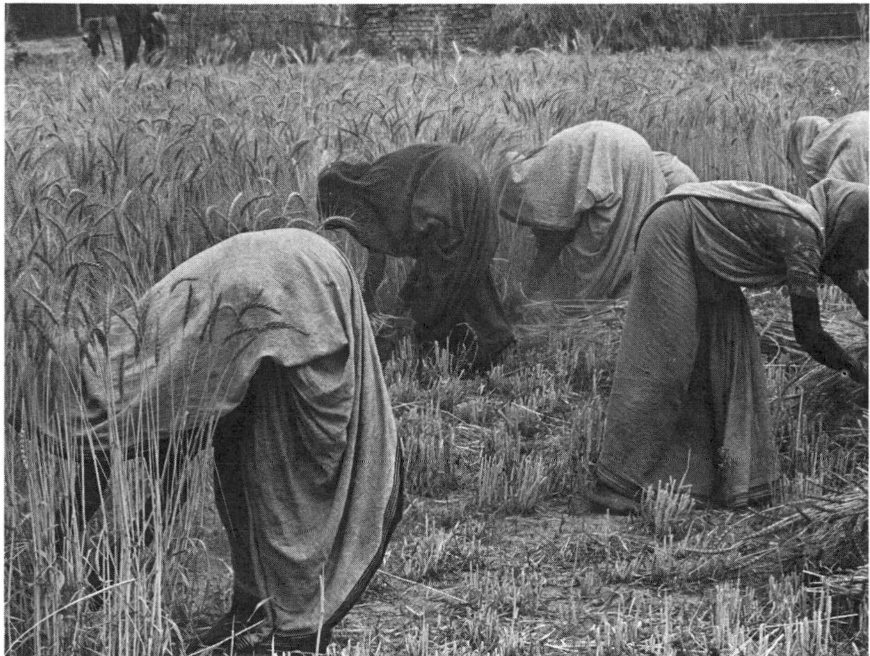

Women in Bihar, India, harvesting a crop of high-yielding wheat, grown after the local irrigation system was renovated. The irrigation improvement program was a project of the Indian government, assisted by the United Nations Food and Agriculture Organization World Food Program. (WFP/FAO photo by Peyton Johnson)

humans) utilize oxygen and release carbon dioxide, water, and nitrogenous wastes, which are recycled back to the beginning of the food chain (see Figure 15-2). The food sources found in every environmental setting (or ecological niche, as environmentalists and others term it) follow this general pattern. In any given ecological niche the interactions between plants and animals may be quite complex, with important economic and nutritional implications.

THE HISTORICAL FRAMEWORK. Until about the middle of this century, most of the world's wealthier nations had a direct, albeit colonial, responsibility for most of the underdeveloped nations and territories. The result of several centuries of history, this responsibility was formalized after World War I through mandates and other policies of the League of Nations. Nutrition aid programs, when they existed at all, consisted of the distribution of surplus grains and other commodities in response to an emergency situation such as drought or flooding. After World War II, colonial empires were disbanded as nationalist movements flourished throughout the world. But malnutrition increased as expanding populations put pressure on the resources of new nations just beginning modernization programs. What little was produced by a combination of traditional and new methods had to be stretched even further. Governments and economists as well as nutritionists and health care personnel began to be concerned about providing adequate nutritious food for the world's people.

DEFINITION OF GOALS. The goals of food supply planners are to increase agricultural productivity and make a sufficient and nutritionally balanced diet available at a cost that can be afforded by all people. The Food and Agriculture Organization of the United Nations believes that nutrition, as an integral part of national development, must be promoted through three related strategies:

1. Plans for development should stress increased food production and more equitable distribution of income among populations, especially in rural areas.
2. Processing, marketing, and distribution of foods to all parts of a population should be improved by altering agricultural customs and patterns and the types of foods being produced.
3. Population subgroups most at risk of poor health and nutritional status should receive multifaceted intervention.

Strategies directed toward these ends must consider available human and environmental resources and the sociocultural values of the people concerned (Food and Agriculture Organization, 1976).

New Food Sources

Many believe that agriculture alone, even enhanced by modern technology, can never provide enough food for all of the world's people. Believing that protein deficits were the greatest problem, many food technologists turned to industrial synthesis of new protein foods. The list of such foods reads like alphabet soup: TVP, FPC, SCP. Other strategies rely on fortifying foods and exploring locally available items not generally used for food.

TVP. Texturized vegetable proteins (TVP) were developed from a soybean base during World War II, and soybeans were soon being incorporated into many protein foods as "extenders." Although this was a new food item for most Americans and Europeans, the Chinese and Japanese have been consuming a variety of soybean products for centuries. During the beef shortages of the 1970s, TVP became a familiar "stretcher" for hamburger meat. It has also become a popular item at vegetarian and "health bar" restaurants, served as a "steak" with mushroom sauce, for example, or as a "mock hamburger" sandwich. Texturized vegetable protein is also used to simulate other meat products as well. By one estimate, soya consumption rose 50 percent during 1977 alone (Scrimgeour, 1978).

FPC. With the success of vegetable proteins, the United States Bureau of Commercial Fisheries became interested in the possibility of extracting protein from "trash" fish that were judged unfit for human consumption. By the late 1960s the first production plant was built. But as a result of start-up costs and inflation, the first fish protein concentrate (FPC) cost $5.08 per pound, rather than the originally projected 25 to 35 cents. Then it was discovered that FPC products were culturally unacceptable in societies unused to eating fish. Finally, there were shortages in the supplies of suitable fish. The only FPC factory in the United States was forced to close, and planners came to realize that high-protein food substitutes were not a panacea for all food problems (Pariser et al., 1978).

SCP. The FPC experience has not deterred the search for new protein sources. Among the most promising new products are single-cell proteins (SCP), a wide classification that includes protein derived from bacteria, yeasts, molds, and algae, which are grown on decaying oil wastes, sewage, molasses, and even petroleum. A particular advantage of SCP production is that microbial growth is extremely rapid, doubling in less than an hour. Moreover, SCP contains other nutrients, including vitamins, minerals, lipids, and carbohydrates. The use of microbes *as* food, or to *produce* food, is not a complete innovation. Beer, bread, sauerkraut, yogurt, and cheese are familiar foods produced by fermenting microorganisms. SCP is also familiar in many Third World countries. The Aztecs gathered algae from the surface of lakes in ancient Mexico, and in Africa Lake Chad provides algae for regional peoples today (Scrimgeour, 1978). Unfortunately, some forms of SCP precipitate gastrointestinal and kidney problems in humans. Palatability of most forms is a major problem as well. Consequently, most SCP products have been introduced for use as animal feed, substituting for grains which then become available for human use.

In a village in Sumatra, Indonesia, a volunteer health worker weighs a child who has been consuming a nutritionally-enriched diet. Funding and expertise from the Save the Children Foundation introduced soybeans to the village as a cash crop, and taught the people how to grow them and manufacture soybean curd. Health workers were trained to instruct mothers in using the new food in their children's diets. Mothers saw the dramatic improvement in their children's growth and development after monthly weighings. (Kenneth Phillips/Save the Children).

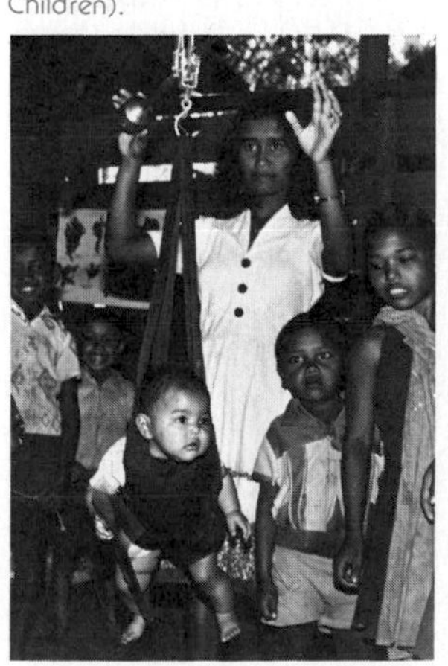

LOCALLY AVAILABLE FOODS. When a mule-train expedition of botanists recently discovered an extremely hardy perennial variety of corn in the remote mountainous regions of Sierra de Manantlan in Mexico, hopes were raised that it might provide genetic material to transform traditional corn into a low-cost, self-perpetuating perennial crop. At present, a substantial part of the cost of cultivating corn arises from the need to plow under old crops and sow new ones every year. The discovery of *Zea diploperennis* surprised scientists, but it was no news to Mexican natives of that region. They were accustomed to grinding the seeds of the wild variety with those of their regular corn, but only in times of hardship (Sullivan, 1979).

The problem of cultural preferences has plagued nutrition programs for years. When "foreign" foods are accepted by local populations, they are often misused. In stores throughout the Third World, American cookies and crackers are sold one by one, and sugared cereals are scooped from the box for purchase by the cupful, often at high prices (Lappé and Collins, 1977). To avoid misuse of food materials new food programs have tried to promote local self-sufficiency. Home-made food combinations or indigenous mixes have become an important part of nutrition programs in India (where groundnuts, wheat, and chickpeas are combined) and Zambia (soya, maize, and wheat). Typically such mixes are in flour form, to be used as or added to doughs (Pellet, 1976).

FORMULATED, FORTIFIED, AND SUPPLEMENTAL FOODS. A related approach involves fortification of locally available foods. The addition of vitamins D and A to milk is a common practice in the United States; the addition of niacin to flours was in part responsible for the control of pellagra. Similar efforts have been tried in countries where specific vitamin and mineral deficiencies are widespread. Synthesized forms of vitamin A have been added to such foods as margarine, milk, tea leaves, cereal grains, rice, sugar, and salt in various parts of the world (Bauernfeind, 1979). Iodized salt has been introduced in areas where goiter is prevalent. Iron and thiamin are other nutrients used in fortification efforts. Foods chosen for fortification must be

PERSPECTIVE ON
The Green Revolution

In the quarter century following 1950, the total grain produced by developing nations increased 78 percent, although land under cultivation expanded by only 35 percent. Yield per acre increased by more than a third. The reason was the Green Revolution, the development of new high-yielding varieties (HYV) of food grains that are more weather-resistant and mature in less time than traditional varieties.

The new seeds are hybrids, developed after intensive effort in agricultural research laboratories. The first evidence that these techniques could work came from Mexico in the late 1940s; wheat yields doubled in a decade, and doubled again during the 1960s. The same techniques were applied to rice and, by the early 1970s, 17 million hectares of land in Asia and North Africa were planted with HYV wheat, 16 million hectares in HYV rice (Economic Research Service, 1975). (One hectare equals approximately 2.5 acres.) The potential effect of intensive crop production on previously cultivated land appeared limitless.

Limitations of the Green Revolution. But high-yielding grain seeds alone do not a revolution make. Also required are generous supplies of water, fertilizer, and pesticides. In their absence yields fall sharply. Sustained drought in the Soviet Union, Argentina, Australia, the Philippines, India, Southeast Asia, and parts of Africa during 1972 caused a sudden and unexpected drop in the world's food output—the first decline in 20 years. Then oil prices soared, boosting the cost of pesticides, herbicides, and nitrogen-based fertilizers, all products whose manufacture requires petroleum. The Green Revolution wilted.

Water availability depends not only on rainfall but on the extent and kind of irrigation. The new seed varieties require well-controlled irrigation systems. Development of suitable irrigation networks and control mechanisms are often beyond the technological and capital investment capabilities of developing nations.

Availability of pesticides, fertilizer, and machinery to produce and process the new grains also depends on capital investment, on the marketing and distribution systems in these countries, and on the size of producing farms. Subsistence farmers cannot afford cash outlays. In developing nations those farmers who have larger holdings of land under cultivation and can afford the investment in related materials are the most likely to adopt the new

centrally supplied and consumed widely, especially by children and other vulnerable members of the population.

Special food products (termed "commerciogenic nutritious foods," or CNF) have also been formulated to meet local needs (Popkin and Latham, 1973). Protein beverages such as Yoo Hoo (U.S. and Iran), Puma (Guyana), Saci (Brazil), and Milpro (India) have been among the most successful CNF products. Professional advertising and marketing campaigns have made these beverages successful competitors of name brand soft drinks. Hong Kong provides a market for over 120 million bottles annually of the local Vitasoy drink (Pellet, 1976).

CNF products also include milk-based foods for infants, high-protein snack foods, and enriched cereal products. Incaparina is a high-protein mixture of maize and cottonseed flour widely advertised and available throughout Latin America. But in Guatemala, where Incaparina is well known and accepted, sales account for only about 3 kilograms per family per year, too little to counteract malnutrition. The problem with this and other CNF products sold in local markets is that those who need them most can't afford to buy them. It has been suggested that CNF be distributed free to the poor and grains, because they can afford the investment and because they stand to gain the most. Thus the discrepancy between haves and have nots is perpetuated (Cleaver, 1972).

For related reasons, the new agriculture will tend to have a regional base, as economic conditions in a limited area favor its adoption. Because in developing countries storage and distribution facilities are not adequate on nationwide levels, the gains realized from the Green Revolution are not equitably distributed throughout the society. In India, nearly half of the HYV wheat was planted in two states and two-thirds of the rice in two other states (Economic Research Service, 1975).

Traditional production methods and distribution systems are nearly everywhere closely tied to social customs. Reorganizing into larger holdings, as has been done in Eastern Europe and China, creates long-range dislocations and may not improve overall productivity.

Still another problem is the vulnerability of HYVs to pests and disease. Because HYVs are genetically more uniform than native varieties, they have not adapted to local ecological conditions. Consequently they are more vulnerable to crop disease caused by pests and insects against which they have no natural defenses. Moreover, the more rapidly HYV is adopted in a region, the more completely is the traditional grain variety displaced; genetic diversity and ecological immunity go with it. Also displaced are other nongrain traditional crops such as legumes, important sources of protein and iron in the largely nonmeat diets of most inhabitants of developing countries (Berg, 1973).

Prospects. The problems mentioned above are real, and many critics have relegated the Green Revolution to the back burner. But as the developing nations move toward more integrated economies with more diversified productivity, as communications develop within these countries to make it possible to reach the people through public information programs, and as political stability is realized, many of the problems presently faced in the introduction of HYVs will be resolved. As social customs change to accommodate political and economic realities, wider adoption of these techniques will become possible. Government planning can allocate land equitably between the new and traditional crops so that ecological and nutritional balances are maintained. The Green Revolution has not proved to be a panacea, but it is among the best prospects for bringing food production on a regional basis into balance with a population's food needs; it also points out that a single approach will not solve the world food crisis.

needy, in the same manner as foods have been distributed for many years by international agencies such as UNICEF and CARE, with an emphasis on feeding hungry children. Such programs have in the past utilized surplus foods. As surplus supplies dwindle, the idea of substituting CNF products becomes attractive. However, the high cost of production and distribution and the lack of long-term benefit to needy nations argue against this type of supplementary feeding, except in emergency famine situations. It has been observed that large supplementary feeding programs permit governments to postpone coping with malnutrition by dealing only with the symptoms and delaying work on the causes (Berg, 1973).

NEW ENERGY SOURCES AND APPROPRIATE TECHNOLOGY. Wood, plant matter, and animal dung are used as fuels in many parts of the world because commercial fuels and the equipment to use them are too expensive. It is estimated that wood fuel provides a third of the energy from nonanimal sources in Asia, two-thirds in Africa, a fifth in Latin America, and 6 percent in the Near East (Arnold and Jongma, 1978). As supplies of wood fuel diminish, more animal dung is used, thus reducing the supply of an inexpensive, widely available natural fertilizer. Crop yields would then be expected to diminish.

Efforts are being made to improve methods of extracting energy from other natural resources, using materials that are readily available in these lands. A solar heater to purify water made of burned-out fluorescent tubes is the product of a research community of Colombia, where highly trained technicians devise simple, low-cost hardware and processes for use in developing areas. This is "appropriate technology," or "A.T.," which concentrates on small-scale, energy-efficient means that can be used at the family or village level. Results include a pedal-powered grinding machine that can process as much yucca root in a day as traditionally done by hand in two months, transforming this South American dietary staple into an export crop; a windmill, powered by breezes of as little as 5 miles an hour, to pump water for irrigation and drinking was also designed. Small-scale farm machinery and low-cost housing materials and techniques are other products of the A.T. approach (Rensberger, 1979).

A related idea has been the development of fuel derived from wood alcohol, or "gasahol," which can substitute for high-cost gasoline as a fuel for motor vehicles. Brazil is pioneering this technology, largely utilizing sugar cane. Available technology also substitutes insects for industrial pesticides, using them as natural predators; 30 million wasps and 20 gallons of ladybugs were exported from California to Peru for this purpose (Lappé and Collins, 1977).

Contribution of Nutritional Anthropology

The influences of tradition on food production, distribution, and consumption patterns have been repeatedly cited throughout this discussion. Human behaviors, individual and cultural, influence whether food available in the external environment will be assimilated into the internal environment of the body. Human and cultural elements make the difference when food policies, usually well-intended, fall short of their goals.

How can new foods be introduced to people whose diet, reinforced by religious practices, has been unchanged for centuries? How can nutritious products be marketed to an undernourished population too poor to purchase them? A productive approach to these and related problems is contributed by **nutritional anthropology.** This new discipline is concerned with patterns of food acquisition and consumption and the health and nutritional status of human beings within a cultural and ecological context.

Participant observation, living with the group being studied, is the basic research method of traditional anthropology. To study food behaviors, nutritional anthropologists record the kinds and amounts of foods gathered, raised, exchanged, purchased, prepared, and consumed, and they observe the human behaviors and interactions involved in all of these processes. To analyze their data and determine nutritional status, the assessment tools of clinicians and nutritional scientists are used as well (see Chapter 10).

IDENTIFICATION OF FOOD SOURCES. Through this combination approach food sources that are used by a people, and additional sources available to them, can be identified. Strategies can then be devised for taking

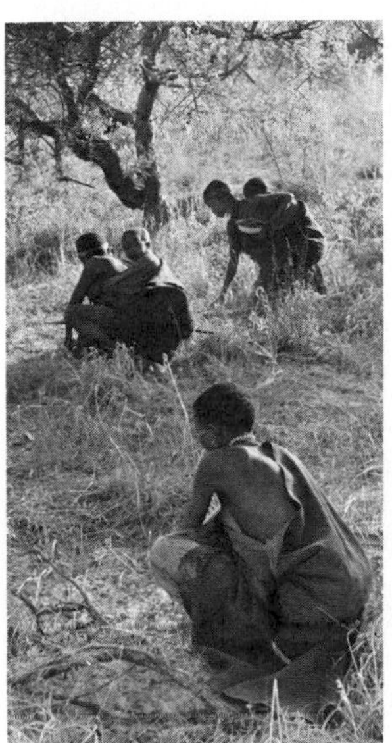

San women dig for tubers amid the dry brush of the Kalihari desert in Africa. (Shostak/Anthro-Photo)

the best advantage of the resources of an area. Small changes in food-related behaviors can often make a big difference in nutritional status. When it was observed that one tribe had a high incidence of xerophthalmia while a group sharing the same semidesert area and having similar social patterns was free of the disease, an anthropologist was consulted. It was discovered that the disease-free group gathered seedling shoots in the early morning, when there was just enough dampness from dew to produce them; after a few hours the seedlings withered. The disease-ridden tribe did not make use of this food resource, which was a source of sufficient carotene to prevent deficiency (Robson, 1978).

Nutritional anthropologists analyze the food patterns of a people to determine the nutrient content of their diet, often revealing considerable wisdom in the food choices of native peoples. In Malaysia, small sun-dried fish are consumed, bones and all, twice daily, providing substantial amounts of calcium and the essential amino acids needed to complement protein in rice, the dietary staple. Similarly, the Latin American custom of soaking maize in a solution of lime (calcium carbonate) before pounding it into meal has been shown to add dietary calcium and to convert the niacin content of the corn into a biologically available form, thus acting as a pellagra preventive (Wilson, 1978).

The anthropological approach also relates foodways to other aspects of daily life. The San Bushmen are hunter-gatherers of the Kalahari desert of southern Africa. Great seasonal variation in rainfall and temperatures leads to sharp fluctuations in their natural food supply. Weight losses of as much as 6 percent were observed in the dry season, and analysis of birth data indicated that this was the period of lowest fertility for San women. Birth data for a neighboring people whose diets were supplemented with cultivated food showed a more even distribution of fertility. These findings led to the hypothesis that the diminished food intake of San women in the dry season sharply reduces production of the steroid hormones that maintain fertility. The seasonal fluctuation of the natural food supply provides a natural cyclic method of population control, and introduction of supplemental food resources may contribute to an increase in birth rates (Wilmsen, 1978).

DEVELOPING STRATEGIES FOR CHANGE. Nutritional anthropology is an offshoot of applied anthropology, which aims to use research findings to improve human living conditions. An important nutritional application lies in the development of strategies for dietary change among peoples consuming marginal or inadequate diets. In one early attempt, a multidisciplinary medical team worked with the Zulus of South Africa. In discussions the Zulu recalled long-forgotten vegetable-eating customs of their pastoral ancestors, and this made possible the subsequent introduction of vegetable cultivation. They had a strong taboo against drinking milk from cows that did not belong to their family of origin; as a result, married women who lived with their husbands' families did not drink milk. Powdered milk, which could not be identified as coming from the cows of any family, was accepted. Over the ten-year period of this project, infant mortality dropped from 276 to 96 per thousand live births (Cassel, 1955).

Such results are dramatic evidence of the effectiveness of an approach to nutritional problems that takes sociocultural factors into consideration.

Because their accomplishment requires considerable expense, time, and patience, it is not feasible to institute such intensive programs on a broad scale. The insights provided by nutritional anthropology can, however, be incorporated in related fields where they will enhance the usefulness of other programs.

Health and Education Programs

Education is a slow process. Food habits are deeply embedded in cultural traditions and fulfill many human needs. Changes should ideally be compatible with existing cultural traditions and not disrupt traditional values and practices. It isn't sufficient to *tell* East African women, who believe bone marrow will cause frequent head colds in their infants, that it is a good source of nutrients and will do no harm. They must be convinced, through patient explanation and repeated creative examples.

In 1964 a public health team set up "mothercraft centers" in a number of villages in Haiti. Each center was in a typical community home with local furnishings (no stoves, refrigerators, or ovens), and staffed by Haitian women who were given two months of special training. The program was targeted at preschool children who showed signs of PEM and at their mothers. The children stayed at the center daily for several months, and the mothers for at least one day a week. Sanitary care and improved feeding methods were provided and demonstrated, but no medical treatment was offered. Recipes were devised using traditional food items to provide complementary proteins and balanced nutrient content, and these were demonstrated to the mothers. Resources for family planning and community development were discussed with the men as well. Typically, improvements were seen in the children in as little as three months (King et al., 1978).

Improved feeding practices by themselves can do little to improve life when infection and poor hygiene remain constant. Many of the world's people have little concept of the association between sanitation and health; the germ theory of disease is unknown to them. The period of weaning is the time when infants are most vulnerable to disease spread through poor hygiene and also the time when they are suddenly exposed to bacteria, viruses, parasites, and insects. Undernutrition, repeated bouts of infection, and "weanling diarrhea" are widespread throughout the Third World (Brown, 1978). Sanitary intervention and broad-scaled health care education must be part of any effort to improve nutritional status.

PLANNING AND POLICY MAKING

Strategies for improving nutritional status of the people in developing nations must address the entire range of problems that cause undernutrition. Planning should be preceded by thoughtful fact-finding by means of thorough surveys. The resulting data and other relevant factors should be analyzed by a multidisciplinary team including health care specialists, nutritionists, anthropologists, political scientists, and economic planners.

Supplemental food programs have been sponsored by a number of agencies, including UNICEF, the Peace Corps, the WHO/FAO, and numerous religious and private groups. Simple food distribution can alleviate starvation in an emergency but has no lasting effects. As a tool for reducing chronic malnutrition, such programs have proved inadequate. Programs of two kinds have generally been tried. In central feeding programs meals are served in a specific location; in take-home programs food items are periodically distributed to individuals for preparation at home.

Central meal programs tend to disrupt daily life patterns and do not provide for those unable to travel to the distribution site because of ill health, weather, or family and occupational responsibilities. Take-home programs are usually intended to provide supplemental foods for pregnant women and young children who are most likely to be inadequately nourished. It has been found, however, that these food supplies are often used as substitutes for regular food items and are diverted from their intended purpose and used to bolster the diets of older children and men. In some families, 30 to 50 percent of the supplements were not consumed at all. Elsewhere the supplementary food was sold to others in the community. The investigators were left with the disturbing question of whether a rigorous program of nutrition education would have been more beneficial than their attempt at food distribution (*Nutrition Reviews*, 1978).

Widespread drought, poor harvests, and declining surpluses of the early 1970s helped to raise the world's food consciousness. The World Food Conference of 1974 created a new $1 billion International Fund for Agricultural Development and resolved to establish better procedures for emergency food aid and an internationally coordinated system of food aid stocks targeted at 10 million tons. But in the years that followed little was accomplished, as inflation, recession, and the energy crisis diverted government attention.

Intervention strategies must reflect the specific conditions of the target area. Although many problems are widespread throughout the developing world, the specific human and ecological details vary from one nation, and even one community, to the next. Not everybody needs more protein at the expense of an increase in total available food volume. And an increase in food production and availability through new technology or other means is of little use if economic dislocations and underemployment do not provide people with the incomes with which to purchase it. Education programs must help people to make use of new food resources as their local economy changes. Cultures do change, or acculturate, over time—but there is often a substantial time lag before cultural institutions adapt to economic changes. The factors tending toward widespread undernutrition in developing nations have, if anything, intensified during recent years. Only a concerted attack by international agencies and national governments will do the job that remains to be done (see Figure 15-3).

OUTLOOK

Each day, the world grows by approximately 190,000 people, more than two-thirds of whom are born in developing nations. About 12 percent will die in infancy, and the majority of those that live will suffer from hunger and malnutrition. Must this be so?

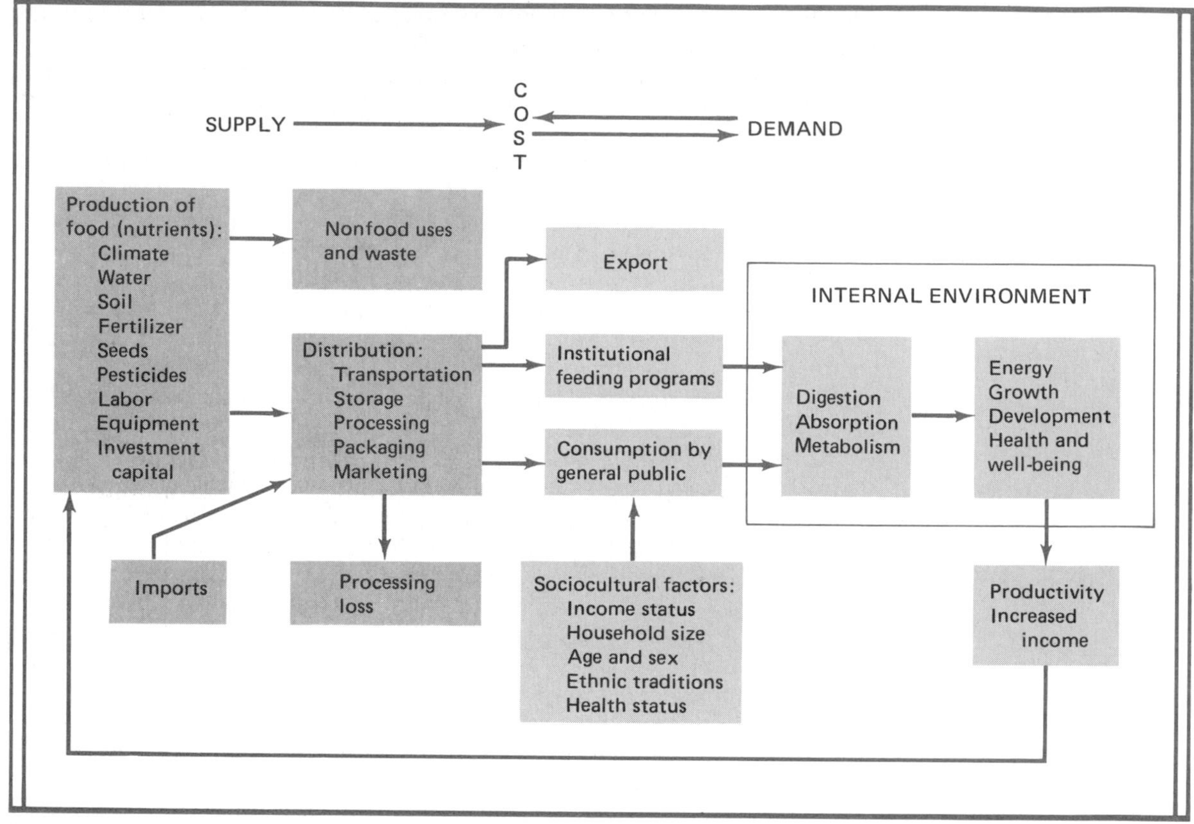

FIGURE 15-3

Strategies and Consequences of Effective Nutrition Planning

Source: Adapted from J. M. Pines, A systematic approach to nutrition planning, *Professional Nutritionist*, Fall 1976, pp. 13–14.

Pessimists fear a bleak future for world food production. Although current weather conditions have been favorable, a major weather-related crop shortfall in the United States, the Soviet Union, or any other key country could seriously threaten available food supplies. In time of short supply, assistance might have to be channeled selectively only to countries which seem likely to survive with some aid, rather than to those whose people are in more desperate straits. The necessity for the "triage" approach is questioned by more optimistic observers who believe that accelerated agricultural development is within the grasp of subsistence farmers. They cite numerous instances of successful "forced-pace agricultural and rural development" in areas given access to modern techniques for managing land, water, seeds, fertilizer, pesticides, roads, markets, and prices (Wortman and Cummings, 1978).

As the success of American agribusiness proves, the world does, in fact, possess the capability to feed all of its inhabitants. What is needed is a commitment on the part of leaders in developing and wealthy nations alike, to make that capability a reality for everyone, whether alive today or yet to be born.

SUMMARY

Malnutrition results from an imbalance between nutrient needs and nutrient intake. It can be traced most often to an imbalance between the world's food production and food distribution systems that is particularly evident in economically disadvantaged nations.

Diagnosing malnutrition requires nutritional and health standards against which widely varied diets and widely varied growth patterns can be judged. Nutritional surveys of many population groups have been used to identify normal growth and development and to select groups who require medical and nutritional assistance. Using these standards, nutritionists have estimated that malnutrition affects from 400 to 500 million people. Problems range from simple deficiencies of one or more essential nutrients, to chronic deficiencies of protein and energy, which cause listlessness, muscle wastage, growth failure, infection, and, often, death. Because of their high growth rate and increased need for nutrients, infants and children are particularly vulnerable to these problems. They typically develop kwashiorkor or marasmus, conditions characterized by impairment in growth and mental functioning.

Dealing with the causes of malnutrition requires attention to environmental factors that affect food *production* (climate, water supply, land availability, agricultural technology, economic costs, energy requirements, local customs); *distribution* (economic purchasing power, population densities, trade agreements, processing techniques, transportation systems, cultural practices); and *human* characteristics (age, sex, nutritional history, activity level, genetic inheritance, pregnancy, lactation, disease states, metabolism, psychological and cultural conditioning). Any programs devised to correct malnutrition must recognize these interrelated factors and attempt to deal with their full scope, rather than emphasizing only one link in the nutritional chain. Multifaceted programs that introduce new technology, new food sources, economic growth, and nutritional and health education programs, within the context of local culture and ecology, will prove most successful in improving health and nutritional status of the people in the developing world.

BIBLIOGRAPHY

AGENCY FOR INTERNATIONAL DEVELOPMENT. Water: A world problem. *War on Hunger* 11(7):1, 1977.

ARNOLD, J. E. M., AND J. JONGMA. Wood, fuel, and charcoal in developing countries. *Unasylva* 29(118):2, 1978.

BAUERNFEIND, J. Nutrification technology alleviates deficiency problems in underdeveloped countries. *Food Product Development*, March 1979, p. 66.

BENGOA, J. M. Priorities in public health nutrition problems. In *Proceedings of the Seventh International Congress of Nutrition, 1967*, Vol. 4. Hamburg: Wieweg, 1967.

BERG, A. *The nutrition factor*. Washington, D.C.: Brookings Institute, 1973.

BROWN, L. Worldwatch Paper 24: The worldwide loss of cropland. Worldwatch Institute, 1978.

BROWN, R. Organ weight in malnutrition with special reference to brain weight. *Developmental Medicine and Child Neurology* 8:512, 1966.

BROZEK, J. Malnutrition and behavior. A decade of conferences. *Journal of the American Dietetic Association* 72:17, 1978.

CALIENDO, M. A. *Nutrition and the world food crisis*. New York: Macmillan, 1979.

CASSEL, J. A comprehensive health program among South African Zulus, In *Health, culture, and community*, ed. B. D. Paul. New York: Russell Sage Foundation, 1955

CHRISTAKIS, G. Nutritional assessment in health programs. *Journal of the American Public Health Association* 63 (Supplement), November 1973.

CLEAVER, H. M. The contradictions of the Green Revolution. *American Economic Review* 62(2):177, 1972.

CROWLEY, J. J., AND R. D. GRIESEL. The development of second generation low protein rats. *Journal of Genetic Psychology* 103:233, 1963.

ECONOMIC RESEARCH SERVICE. *The world food situation and prospects to 1985.* Washington, D.C.: U.S. Department of Agriculture, 1975.

FAYANS, H. B. Impact of food laws, regulations, and standards on world food supply. *Food Technology,* June 1979, p. 76.

FOOD AND AGRICULTURE ORGANIZATION. Food and nutrition strategies in national development. *Ninth Report of the Joint FAO/WHO Expert Committee on Nutrition.* Tech. Rept. Series 584. Geneva: World Health Organization, 1976.

HOLZ, A. E. Fats and oils—Future impact of economic and political trends. *Food Technology,* June 1979, p. 74.

KAUFMAN, M. Vietnam, 1978: Crisis in food, nutrition, and health. *Journal of the American Dietetic Association* 74:310, 1979.

KING, K. W., W. FOUGERE, R. E. WEBB, G. BERGGREN, W. L. BERGGREN, AND A. HILIARE. Preventive and therapeutic benefits in relation to cost. Performed over 10 years of Mothercraft Centers in Haiti. *American Journal of Clinical Nutrition* 31:679: 1978.

LAPPÉ, F. M., AND J. COLLINS, WITH C. FOWLER. *Beyond the myth of scarcity.* Boston: Houghton Mifflin, 1977.

New York Times. World's top economic news of 1978. New York Times International Economic Survey. February 4, 1979, p. 79.

NUTRITION CANADA. *Nutrition: A national priority.* 1973.

Nutrition Reviews. How useful are supplementary feeding programs? Vol. 36(9):278, 1978.

PARISER, E. R., M. B. WALLERSTEIN, C. J. CORKERY, AND N. L. BROWN. *Fish protein concentrate: Panacea for protein malnutrition?* Cambridge: M.I.T. Press, 1978.

PELLET, P. L. Role of food mixtures in combating childhood malnutrition in developing countries. In *Nutrition in the community,* ed. D. McLaren. London: John Wiley, 1976.

POPKIN, B. M., AND M. C. LATHAM. The limitations and dangers of commerciogenic nutritious foods. *American Journal of Clinical Nutrition* 26:1015, 1973.

RAO, K. S. Jaya: Evolution of kwashiorkor and marasmus. *Lancet* 1:709, 1975.

READ, M. S. Malnutrition, hunger and behavior. I. Malnutrition and learning. *Journal of the American Dietetic Association* 63:379, 1973.

RENSBERGER, B. Technology spreading in third world. *New York Times,* April 10, 1979.

ROBBINS, W. Dilemma in food: Getting it to the hungry. New York Times International Economic Survey. *New York Times* February 4, 1979, p 18.

ROBSON, J. R. K. Contribution of anthropology to the assessment of nutritional status. *Federation Proceedings* 37:47, 1978.

SCRIMGEOUR, M. Unconventional sources of protein. *Journal of Human Nutrition* 32:439, 1978.

SCRIMSHAW, N. S., C. E. TAYLOR, AND J. E. GORDON. *Interactions of nutrition and infection.* Geneva: World Health Organization, 1968.

SIMOONS, F. J. *Eat not this flesh. Food avoidances in the old world.* Madison, Wisc.: University of Wisconsin Press, 1961.

SINHA, D. P. Measles and malnutrition in a West Bengal village. *Tropical and Geographical Medicine* 29:125, 1977.

STEIN, Z., M. SUSSER, G. SAENGER, AND F. MAROLLA. *Famine and human development: The Dutch hunger winter of 1944–1945.* London: Oxford University Press, 1975.

SULLIVAN, W. Hope for creating perennial corn raised by a new plant discovery. *New York Times*, February 5, 1979, p. 1.

TRUSWELL, A. S. Symposium on some aspects of diet and health. *Proceedings of the Nutrition Society* 35:1, 1976.

U.S. BUREAU OF THE CENSUS. *World population: 1977—Advance summary*. Washington, D.C.: Population Division, Bureau of the Census, 1978.

WILMSEN, E. N. Seasonal effects of dietary intake on Kalahari San. *Federation Proceedings* 37:65, 1978.

WILSON, C. S. Contributions of nutrition science to anthropological research. *Federation Proceedings* 37:73, 1978.

WORTMAN, S., AND R. W. CUMMINGS. *To feed this world: The challenge and the strategy*. Baltimore: Johns Hopkins, 1978.

WRAY, J. D. Direct nutrition intervention and the control of diarrheal diseases in preschool children. *American Journal of Clinical Nutrition* 31:2073, 1978.

WYON, J. B., AND J. E. GORDON. *The Khanna study*. Cambridge: Harvard University Press, 1971.

SUGGESTED ADDITIONAL READING

BAKER, S. J., AND E. M. DEMAEYER. Nutritional anemia: Its understanding and control with special reference to the work of the World Health Organization. *American Journal of Clinical Nutrition* 32:368, 1979.

BERG, A., N. S. SCRIMSHAW, AND D. L. CALL, EDS. *Nutrition, national development and planning*. Cambridge: M.I.T. Press, 1973.

BROWN, R. E. Weaning foods in developing countries. *American Journal of Clinical Nutrition*, 31:2066, 1978.

CHANDRA, R. K. Antibody formation in first and second generation offspring of nutritionally deprived rats. *Science* 190:289, 1975.

COX, G. W. Famine symposium—The ecology of famine: An overview. *Ecology of Food and Nutrition* 6:207, 1978.

Dairy Council Digest. Nutrition and anthropology. Vol. 49(5):1, 1978.

FORD, B. *Alternative protein for the year 2000*. New York: William Morrow, 1978.

Journal of the American Dietetic Association. Nutritional anthropology. Vol. 71:13, 1977.

MAYER, J. The dimensions of human hunger. In *Food and agriculture*, ed. *Scientific American*. San Francisco: Freeman, 1976.

PREMA, K., N. NAIDU, AND S. N. KUMARI. Lactation and fertility. *American Journal of Clinical Nutrition* 32:1298, 1979.

READ, M. S. Malnutrition, hunger and behavior. II. Hunger, school feeding programs and behavior. *Journal of the American Dietetic Association* 63:386, 1974.

READER, J. Microcosm of a continental force: Tribalism in Kenya. *Smithsonian* 10:40, 1979.

SOLON, F. S., T. L. FERNANDEZ, M. C. LATHEM, AND B. M. POPKIN. Planning, implementation, and evaluation of a fortification program: Control of vitamin A deficiency in the Philippines. *Journal of the American Dietetic Association* 74:112, 1979.

Chapter 16

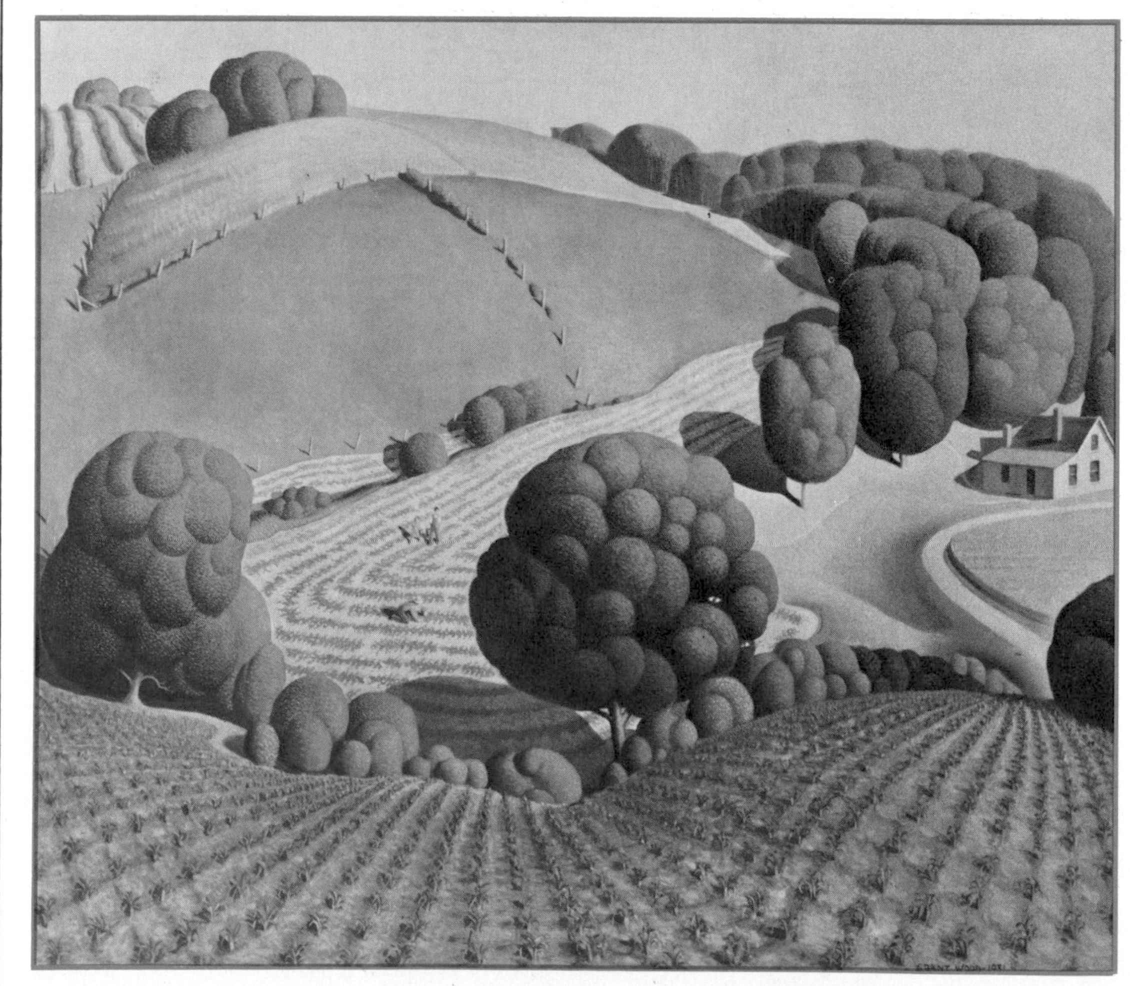

Young Corn by Grant Wood

Toward a National Food and Nutrition Policy

Human nutritional needs should play a primary role in agriculture, food, and health policies. Nutritional concerns have prompted legislation throughout the years, but there is not yet a national nutrition policy in the United States. Such a policy would coordinate food, agriculture, and health policies, and would result in a specific plan of action.

In the early 1900s it began to be realized that nutritional deficiencies could be the cause of disease, and during the 1920s and 1930s research was directed toward elucidating the structure and metabolic function of the vitamins. By 1940, the 40 odd nutrients (except for vitamin B_{12} and folic acid) needed to ensure a nutritionally adequate diet had been isolated and chemically characterized. During the 1940s nutritional research was geared to wartime needs and in 1943 the Food and Nutrition Board of the National Academy of Sciences—National Research Council established desired standards of nutrient intake.

Food availability had been a concern during the depression years, when President Franklin D. Roosevelt saw "one-third of a nation ill clothed, ill housed and ill fed." But production soon expanded to meet wartime needs. Throughout the 1950s and part of the 1960s the emphasis was on food production, surpluses, and farm income rather than nutritional health. It was simply assumed that we were a well-fed and healthy people with a plentiful supply of all the foods we needed. And then in 1968 a CBS television documentary, "Hunger in America," exploded the myth: There on the screen was shocking evidence that hunger and malnutrition still existed throughout the country.

In 1968 the United States Department of Agriculture published the results of its Food Consumption Survey: food supply and food consumption patterns in the United States were going through some disturbing changes. In 1969, the White House Conference on Food, Nutrition, and Health presented further proof of inadequate nutrition, and proposed governmental actions to deal with the problems.

The economic, social, and political changes of the 1970s brought a new awareness of nutritional problems, not only at home but abroad. Poor harvests around the world, huge grain sales to the Soviet Union, starving children in Biafra, the energy crisis, and widespread inflation accompanied by

TABLE 16-1
Goals of a National Nutrition Policy

1. To assure an adequate wholesome food supply at reasonable cost to meet the needs of all segments of the population, this supply being available at a level consistent with the affordable life style of the era
2. To maintain food resources sufficient to meet emergency needs and to fulfill a responsible role as a nation in meeting world food needs
3. To develop a level of sound public knowledge and responsible understanding of nutrition and foods that will promote maximal nutritional health
4. To maintain a system of quality and safety control that justifies public confidence in its food supply
5. To support research and education in foods and nutrition with adequate resources and reasoned priorities to solve important current problems and to permit exploratory basic research

Source: National Nutrition Consortium, Inc., Guidelines for a national nutrition policy, *Nutrition Reviews* 32:153, 1974.

higher domestic food prices, all contributed to a growing awareness that there was indeed a food crisis. In 1974 the National Nutrition Consortium issued guidelines for a national nutrition policy (see Table 16-1). The results of two national nutrition surveys were published and a Select Committee of the U.S. Senate issued the Dietary Goals in 1977.

Today many federal agencies are involved with agriculture, food, and health programs. It is recognized that research, education, and food assistance programs should be coordinated in order to be cost-effective and to reach more people. There is awareness that government, consumers, academicians, health-care providers, and the food and agriculture industries should be involved in the development, implementation, and evaluation of national nutrition policies and programs. This chapter will examine the nutritional issues in the United States, the factors that contribute to them, and existing and proposed strategies to address and overcome them.

NUTRITIONAL CONCERNS TODAY

In the past, emphasis was placed on prevention of nutritional deficiencies. The HANES and the Ten-State Nutrition Surveys showed that this concern has remained valid for certain population groups and individuals in the United States (see Chapter 10). Undernutrition in the United States, moreover, is a minor problem compared to its extent and severity in developing countries. Today, however, the major concern of physicians and nutritionists in this country is not undernutrition but overnutrition. The American diet, high in energy-dense foods, fats, sugar, and salt may be as damaging to the human body as a vitamin-deficient diet, albeit in different ways. Coronary heart disease, hypertension, cancer of the colon and breast, dental caries, and diabetes are all prevalent in industrialized nations and have been linked to dietary factors.

In a technological society such as ours, individual control over the kinds of foods available is minimal. The food supply for over 200 million Americans, plus a surplus for export, is produced by only 4 percent of the population. This stands in sharp contrast to the early years of our nation, when approximately 98 percent of Americans were food producers. One consequence of the centralization of food production is increased waste: In 1977, 20 percent of the food produced in the United States was lost or wasted. The General Accounting Office estimates the loss at 137 million tons, with a value of $31 billion. Of that amount, about 60 million tons, worth $5 billion, was simply left in fields and orchards because there was no commercial market for it. GAO statisticians estimated that in one recent year, the amount of food wasted during production and distribution could have fed 49 million people (Prial, 1979). These figures do not even account for consumer waste.

Also of concern are the effects of today's agricultural practices and processing methods on the quality and safety of food products and the effects of processing, storage and transport on the nutrient content of foods. Not only nutrients, but nonnutrients in our food supply are of concern. What are the long-term results of the chemical additives used to maintain and improve the flavor, appearance, and safety of foods? These and other questions are subject to debate, and most importantly, extensive research.

THE COST AND CONTENT OF OUR FOOD SUPPLY

The United States is an affluent society, and the types and amounts of food consumed by the American public reflect that affluence. Compared to that of other nations, our food supply is plentiful and inexpensive, and most of us have become accustomed to its variety and abundance. Many Americans, however, cannot share in that abundance for economic reasons, and are thus at a nutritional risk. Their very serious plight aroused national concern and became the primary focus of those interested in developing a national food policy. While undernutrition of any extent should be a matter of concern, in the United States this condition affects relatively few individuals. The focus is therefore widening to include the nutritional problems of the substantially larger, more affluent segment of the population.

Our heightened awareness of the problems of overnutrition is due to a combination of political, economic, and social factors. A growing interest in health, the consumer movement, and the greater sophistication of the public concerning medical issues have made many people aware that they must control their own lives and bodies. As a result, traditional policy creators—the farm and food industry lobbies, legislators, and the USDA—have had to consider the positions of consumer groups, organized labor, foreign policy specialists, physicians, dietitians, and nutrition scientists. The continued vigorous involvement of the latter groups will ensure that the nation's nutritional health will be a paramount factor in the establishment of food and agricultural policies.

Economic and Related Factors

Our society is complex, the origins of its problems are complex, and solutions will also be complex. All factors affecting the availability—not necessarily the quality—of our food supply are related to economic issues. As the costs of growing, processing, transporting, and distributing food increase, the price that must be paid by consumers increases also. The cost of food to the consumer rises when fuel prices go up, and when the cost of purchasing pots and pans or stoves and refrigerators is increased. The kinds of foods we can purchase depend on weather, the balance between imports and exports, subsidies to farmers, energy costs, and labor issues such as transport strikes.

The basic economic influence is the push-pull effect of supply and demand. Simple economic theory explains that when supply exceeds demand, prices fall, and when demand exceeds supply prices increase. But the effects of supply and demand are no longer as simple as that. The 1979 bumper crop of wheat made farmers smile, but consumers groaned. The huge harvest came as prices worldwide were rising, because a poor harvest in the Soviet Union was expected to stimulate world demand. American farmers put their crops in storage, awaiting the ever higher prices they expected from exports. The result was an even higher price to the American consumer (Robbins, 1979).

American production of sugar is facing increased foreign competition. Most foreign producers can grow sugar more cheaply than United States

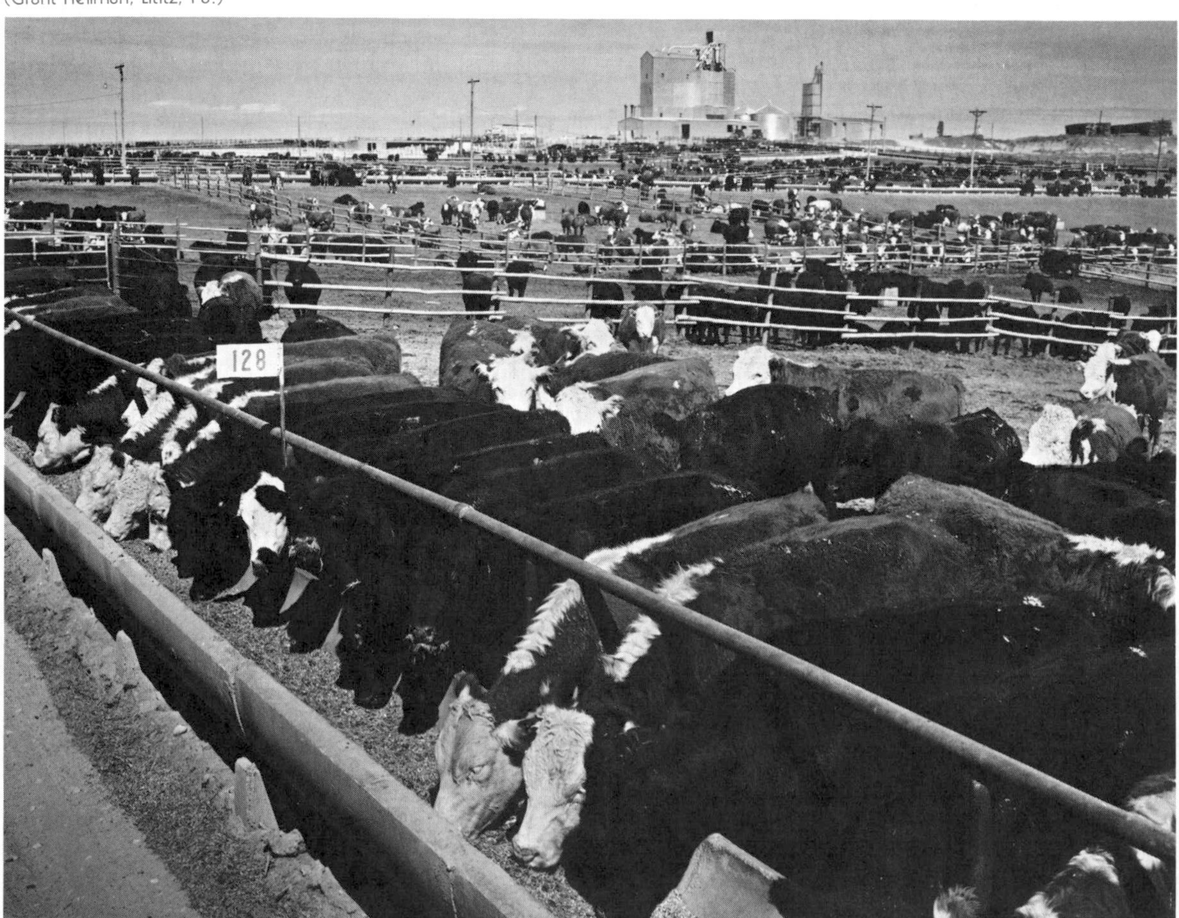

Cattle are fattened at a commercial feedlot—a key stage in the production of beef. (Grant Heilman, Lititz, Pa.)

growers can, and deliver it to United States ports at about two-thirds the cost of the domestic product. American growers are lobbying for increased government support and restriction of imports. The result would be greater prosperity for sugar beet growers, and higher prices for consumers. An increase of one cent a pound in the price of raw sugar can add $224 million a year to the nation's food bill, and raise the costs of the Coca-Cola Company, the country's largest buyer of sugar (2 billion pounds a year), as much as $20 million.

Government support for the agriculture industry may be in the form of subsidies or of price supports. Due to the high cost of labor and technology, growing costs are higher in the United States than in most other countries. To compensate for this difference, farmers receive direct payments or subsidies. Price supports, on the other hand, provide an alternative to the sale of produce. They enable growers to borrow capital in return for depositing crop surpluses as collateral. In a recent year, for example, sugar growers participating in price support programs could receive 14.73 cents per pound for raw sugar, more than they could get on the open market. They had the option of repaying the loan and reclaiming their crop, or keeping the loan and forfeiting the crop. As a result, sugar was not sold at a lower rate to any customer, and the government accumulated a substantial surplus: In early 1979 there was $122 million worth of 1977 sugar in government warehouses; storage expenses were extra (Robbins, 1979).

Decrease in U.S. Beef Shipments to Slaughterhouses

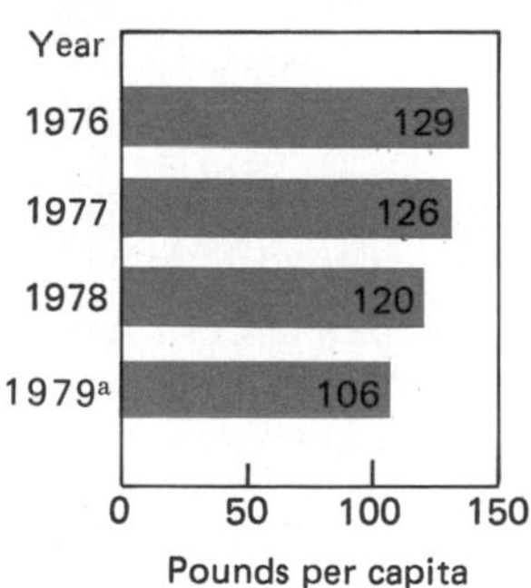

ªProjected.
Source: Cattle-Fax

Equal complexities enter into the costs of meat. One-third of America's food dollars are spent for meat. The sharply increased cost of beef (which rose 50 percent from March 1977 to March 1979) is due not only to general inflation, but also to cattle raisers deliberately holding back the supply to maintain higher prices. This practice dates back to the consumer meat boycott of 1973—demand went down, supply increased, and prices fell. A consumer victory, but not for long. Cattle raisers continued to hold back stock in hopes of a rise in beef prices. The increase didn't come and the cattle had to be sent to market anyway. The market was glutted and retail prices fell. Then the cost of feed corn doubled in six months (due primarily to the sale of reserves to the Soviet Union), and cattle raisers reduced their feed bills by sending more heifers to market. Consumers benefited from lower beef prices—but only temporarily. What they didn't know was that cattle breeding was reduced sharply and they were consuming the inventory. It was only a matter of months before demand would exceed supply, and beef prices would soar (Figure 16-1). Although the demand for beef continues, pork and poultry raisers are benefiting from the higher beef prices. These meats can be produced faster than cattle—it takes 5½ years to ready a heifer for market, 2½ years for a hog, and a few weeks for a broiler—and thus the supply can be more nearly adjusted to the demand, and prices kept more stable.

Every winter the United States population consumes about $200 million worth of tomatoes, cucumbers, squash, and eggplant from Mexico. Vegetable growers in Florida demand a limit on imports so that they can market their own produce at higher prices. If imports are restricted, the consequences could be more far-reaching than simply increased cost of a few items: Mexican growers will cut back on production and lay off workers, who will then join the stream of illegal aliens who enter the United States in hope of employ-

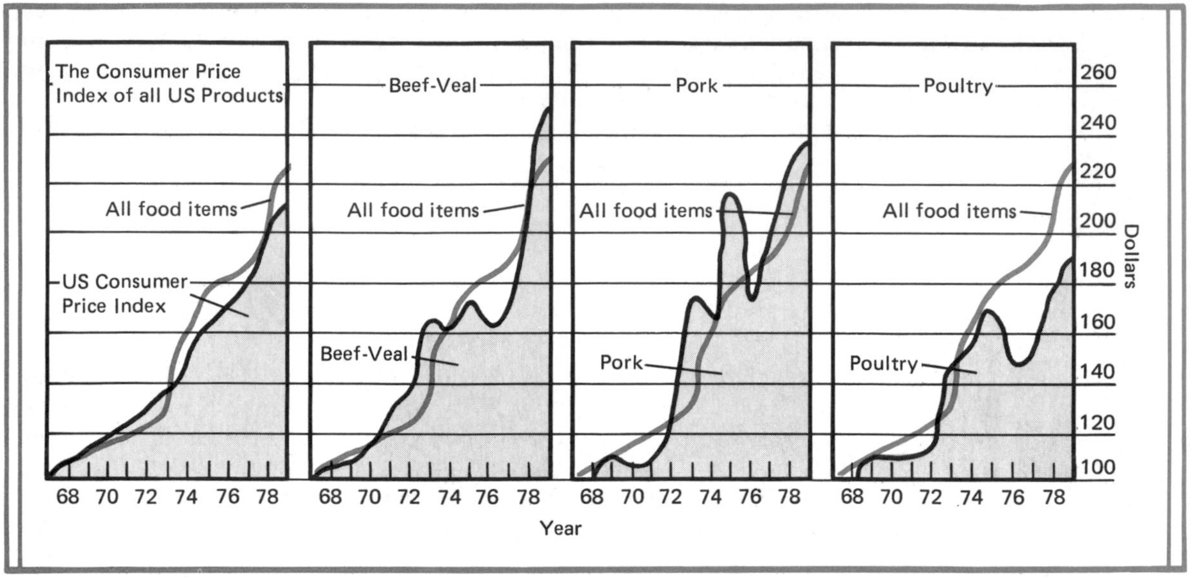

FIGURE 16-1

Comparison of the Consumer Price Index of All U.S. Products, of All Foods, and of Selected Meats

Source: Bureau of Labor Statistics
The Consumer Price Index for all food items includes beef and veal, poultry, pork, fruits and vegetables, and dairy, cereal and bakery products.

ment as migrant farm workers. Here, the low-cost migrant labor may offset any income gains for American farm workers, as well as increasing the need for various services including government surveillance of border areas and costs of deportation. Restrictions would also antagonize a hemisphere neighbor, economic and political ally, and potential oil supplier. This illustrates well the complex interaction of economic considerations involved in only one segment of the food supply.

Labor problems also affect cost and availability of our food. The efforts to unionize farm workers in California in recent years have led to boycotts of grapes and lettuce by sympathetic consumers throughout the nation, and to higher prices at supermarkets (and wine dealers) as well. A trucker's strike in 1979 doubled the cost of produce in many sections of the country. While Californians could buy four canteloupes for a dollar, Bostonians were shelling out 77 cents for one. Bing cherries, selling for 49 cents a pound on the West Coast, were advertised as "specials" at 69 cents on the East Coast.

Although labor is a key factor it is not the only one involved in food production and distribution. Weather conditions can produce bumper crops, or reduce farm output sharply. Unexpected infestation by a new insect variety can virtually obliterate a crop, as happened in 1978 when the tobacco budworm rampaged through the lettuce crop in California's Imperial Valley.

Another factor contributing to food prices is built into the structure of the food industry. Relatively few companies control a disproportionate share of the market. In 1976 the Federal Trade Commission (FTC) charged that a "tacit conspiracy" among the four major cereal-producing companies had caused millions of dollars in overcharges to customers (*Business Week*, 3/20/78). Between them these four giants controlled 95 percent of cereal sales in the United States. In such a situation it is not even necessary to directly fix prices; the lack of open competition in the industry effectively prevents lower costs to the consumer.

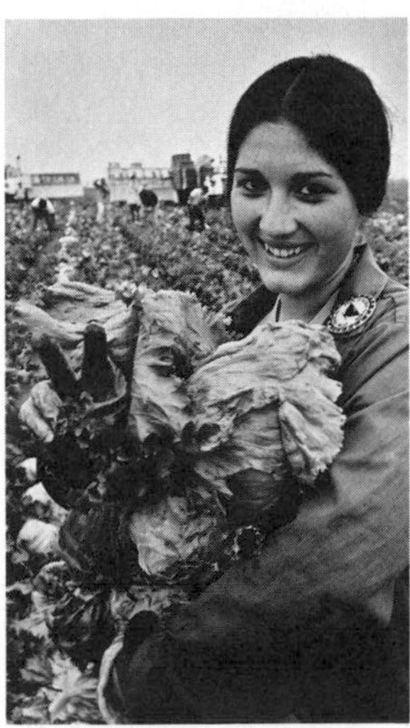

A lettuce picker and member of the United Farmworker's Organizing Committee in Salinas, California, gives the "V for Victory" sign after her union achieved recognition. (Bob Fitch, Black Star)

The general inflation of the 1970s would have raised food prices even without special crises. The high rates of unemployment nationwide, and especially for certain regional and population subgroups, have decreased purchasing power even more. As the 1970s drew to a close, Americans for the first time were contemplating a future of resource scarcity and lack of their accustomed abundance.

Energy

A key resource in these considerations, and an influence on every aspect of life, is energy. As one author stated in 1974:

> *The past year may represent a turning point in history. Numerous developments including the energy crisis, inflation, rising food costs, and depletion of our food reserves have convinced many knowledgeable people that we are now entering an era which will be characterized by a shortage of resources including food. The high energy cost of producing food makes it clear that food and the energy supply are inextricably linked. For the first time, the capacity of the United States to feed itself and meet its world food commitments is being seriously questioned. A world food crisis exists at this time, and this will have serious repercussions in this country.*
>
> —HEGSTED, 1974

Those words could have been written every year since. Since 1974 the demand for energy has increased. The price of imported oil rose steadily in the 1970s. In 1979, when the oil-producing countries raised the cost of crude oil to an average of $20 a barrel, it was the biggest increase in five years. But more price hikes were to follow. The United States, as one of the largest importers of oil (it has 6 percent of the world's population and uses 30 percent of the world's energy) is particularly vulnerable. The spiraling costs affect everything in the economy—directly, through the cost of fuel needed to power farm equipment and produce fertilizer; and indirectly, through costs of transportation, processing, and manufacturing, and through increased overhead (lighting, heating, refrigeration) in supermarkets. In the spring of 1979 distribution of food was halted nationwide as many truckers went on strike to protest restricted supplies of diesel fuel.

At the same time that consumers pay for all this, they must spend more to run their cars and heat their homes, leaving proportionately less with which to purchase more expensive food. And the cost of all other goods and services—from hairdressers to hospitals—rises as well.

What's in Our Food

The increased consumption of fabricated and processed foods presents two separate issues. In the course of processing, foods lose some of the nutrients naturally contained in them, and so manufacturers add the very vitamins and minerals that have been removed. Trace minerals present in the original product are also partly lost through processing but they are not added, because there are not enough data to determine a level that might be safely

PERSPECTIVE ON
Additives

A food additive is any substance or mixture of substances that becomes part of a food during any stage of production, processing, storage, or packaging. Additives are of two types, direct and indirect. Direct additives, of which there are approximately 2,800, are added deliberately to maintain or improve nutritional value, to maintain freshness and product quality, to help in processing or preparation, and to make foods more appealing. Some examples include sodium bicarbonate, which is added to control acidity, methyl cellulose, which imparts and maintains a desired consistency, and food colors.

Indirect additives, of which there are some 10,000, are present in foods in trace quantities as an unintentional result of some phase of production, processing, storage, or packaging. Some of these are pesticide residues, minute amounts of drugs fed to animals, and chemical substances that migrate from plastic packaging materials.

Food additives are not a new invention. Humans have always tried to preserve their food. Salt was probably used long before recorded history to preserve meat and fish; herbs and spices have always been added to foods to enliven the taste, and often in the past to conceal evidence of spoilage.

Today's extensive use of additives accompanied the shift from an agricultural to an urbanized society. There was a need for foods that could be mass-produced, distributed over long distances, stored for considerable periods of time, and be made available at reasonable prices. The sheer size of the nation and the growing distance between rural producer and metropolitan consumer added to the requirements for storage and transport. As merchandising shifted from the local produce market to the interstate supermarket chain, shelf storage and packaging needs became evident. As women left the home and joined the labor force, the demand for more prepared convenience foods increased. As purchasing power grew and tastes became more sophisticated, people wanted year-round availability of seasonal products. And as population expanded there was a bigger market to be reached. As a result of these pressures, there are more additives in foods than there have ever been before.

Food is certainly safer now than at the turn of the century when it was almost impossible to keep things from spoiling, and when manufacturers freely used toxic pigments as food coloring. But recently people have begun to wonder if we need all those chemicals. Some have been implicated as carcinogens, and people wonder how safe others may be. How valid are these worries? What should be done?

First, everything is made up of chemicals—including "natural" foods and our own bodies. Some of the chemicals naturally present in foods are extremely toxic. Carrots, for example, contain carotatoxin, a fairly potent nerve poison, and myristicin, a hallucinogen. The chemicals in onions include a mixture of disulfides and trisulfides, which exhibit antithyroid or goitrogenic activity (Hall, 1977). Nothing that we eat is free of chemicals—and many of those chemicals would be far from harmless, except that we consume them in minute quantities. Fear of all chemicals is clearly unrealistic.

But if perfectly "healthy" foods contain toxic substances, what do we know about the chemicals intentionally added to foods? How well have they been tested?

Until 1958, there were no laws specifically regulating food additives. The government had the authority to remove from the market foods that were obviously adulterated, spoiled or toxic. But in 1958, the Food Additive Amendment was enacted, according to which no additive could be

and usefully added. Excess consumption of processed foods may, therefore, present a risk of suboptimal intake of some nutrients.

Overconsumption of fortified foods may also present a problem. Cereals, candy bars, doughnuts, and other items, including many energy-dense foods, are fortified with vitamins and minerals, in part because consumers want them, in part because manufacturers perceive this as a selling point. That used until it was proved safe. With this and the 1960 Color Additive Amendment, the burden of proof shifted from the government to the manufacturer. The laws empowered the FDA to regulate additives only on the basis of safety. The agency could not limit the number of additives used, approve or judge the quality of a substance, or determine whether the additive was really needed.

The testing of an additive can take several years. First it must go through a battery of chemical tests, and then it is tested on two species of laboratory animals, usually rodents and dogs. Finally, the FDA approves its safety and regulates its use in food. A basic rule is that only one one-hundredth of the maximum amount of an additive that has been found *not* to produce any harmful effects in test animals may be used. The Delaney Clause, a special provision of the 1958 and 1960 amendments, states that a substance shown to cause cancer in animals or humans may not be added to food in any amount.

Some additives are not subject to testing. The Food Additive Amendment exempted two major categories: Some 700 additives, "generally recognized as safe" (GRAS), had been used extensively over the years with no known harmful effects. Others had been specifically approved before 1958 by the FDA or the USDA. But increasing concern over additives has brought the GRAS substances under scrutiny. A group called the Select Committee on GRAS Substances (SCOGS) is systematically reviewing some 450 additives that are considered GRAS. In addition, FDA is reviewing the safety of 2,100 flavoring agents.

Two commonly used additives have come under particular scrutiny. Nitrite and saccharin have both been found to cause cancer in test animals. According to the Delaney Clause both should be removed from the market. The saccharin story has been told in Chapter 2. There are some who claim that the government was too hasty in characterizing nitrite as a cancer-causing agent. Many caution that omission of nitrite would result in botulism, a deadly form of food poisoning. Repeal of the Delaney Amendment has been suggested by those who believe the benefits of saccharin and nitrites far outweigh the very small incidence of cancers they produce in laboratory animals; they call for a more flexible law that would permit risk-benefit assessment.

In its 1979 report on food safety, the National Academy of Sciences concluded that present law was inflexible and therefore unrealistic. A national food safety system that would encourage reasonable goals for reduction of risks in the food supply, regulate substances comprehensively taking risk levels into consideration, and permit a variety of regulatory procedures was proposed. Decision-making responsibility should incorporate the best scientific information and enlist full expression of informed public opinions (National Academy of Sciences, 1979). But it is difficult to quantify risks and benefits, particularly because they are often influenced by individual or group value judgments. Certain additives, used only for esthetic appeal, could be removed from use if consumers would accept products with an unfamiliar appearance. Most risk-benefit equations, however, are not that simple.

It is not possible to prove that a food—or anything else for that matter—is absolutely safe at all times for all people. Testing must continue—and be extended. At this time, more is known about chemical additives than about the chemicals in the natural foods we eat.

The subject of additives continues to be controversial, and investigations are continuing to determine additive safety. The best protection against toxic effects from any food chemical is consumption of a diversified diet, which will also help to provide an adequate intake of all essential nutrients. And consumers must choose which food qualities—appearance, convenience, storage time, or freedom from additives—mean the most to them.

means that many people are ingesting some nutrients in amounts two to four times greater than actual need. It is not yet known whether the long-term effects will be beneficial, harmful, or of no consequence. At the same time, people who eat fortified foods may develop a false sense of security: they frequently believe they need not consume other items which would provide a broader spectrum of micronutrients, accompanied by fewer kilocalories.

The New Challenges: Inflation and Health

As prices rise, consumers will at some point be forced to restrict food purchases and consumption. By reversing our present tendency toward overconsumption, this could well prove to be a blessing in disguise. Since most young adults perceive chronic diseases as remote possibilities, they have not been well enough motivated by health considerations to make dietary changes. Perhaps economic considerations will be a stronger influence.

An inflationary spiral challenges us all to eat better for less, and particularly challenges nutritionists to educate the public in how to get the best nutritional value for less money. Part of their task will be to clear up some misconceptions concerning sugar, fat, cholesterol, and salt and their relationship to disease. Reports seen by the general public have often become excessively alarmist, although the technical literature is sometimes contradictory. In the absence of clear-cut answers, it's little wonder that people often take the path of least resistance, saying they might as well "eat and enjoy." People eat what is available and what they have developed a taste for—the sweet, salty, and fatty foods provided by the food industry and kept visible in their living rooms by television.

GOVERNMENT AGENCIES CONCERNED ABOUT FOOD

A variety of factors, including consumer attitudes, economics, food availability, and the nature of our food system contribute to undernutrition on the one hand, and overnutrition on the other. A national nutrition policy must deal with both of these problems, improving the nutritional status of those in need while encouraging moderation of the food habits of affluence. In a complex society, many groups and individuals must play a role in solving food and nutrition problems. The federal government has thus far assumed a major role in addressing problems of a nutritional nature. Increasingly visible roles must be taken by others to ensure that a nutritionally adequate, safe, health-promoting, and affordable food supply is available to and consumed by Americans.

A number of different agencies within the federal government are involved in nutrition-related research, educational, regulatory, and food-assistance programs. The Departments of Agriculture and of Health, Education, and Welfare have the major roles in formulating and carrying out national food policies; other government agencies act in specific areas.

The Department of Agriculture

The Department of Agriculture (USDA) inspects meat and poultry shipped interstate, and inspects animal and food plant sanitation. As a service to food companies, upon request it grades fruit, vegetables, bread, and dairy products. The USDA has a tradition of success in consumer education. It funds the

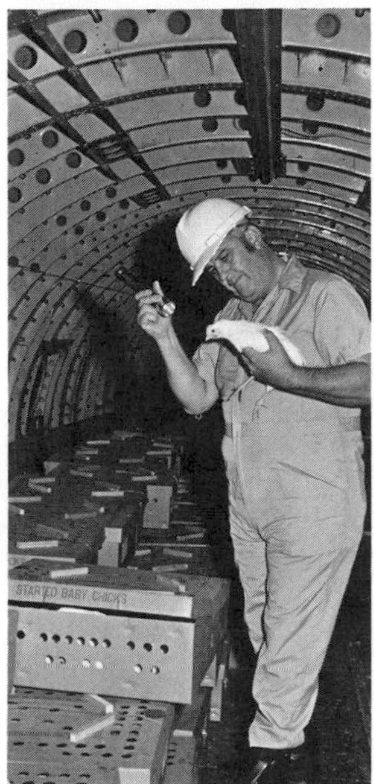

A representative of the Animal Plant Health Inspection Service of the U.S. Department of Agriculture inspects poultry during transport. (USDA-APHIS)

Expanded Food and Nutrition Education Program (EFNEP) which utilizes nutrition aides, trained homemakers from the target community, who demonstrate and explain nutritional precepts in a home-visit context.

The USDA also conducts research through its Science and Education Administration. A Human Nutrition Center coordinates research projects at a number of laboratories throughout the country. Areas under investigation include: determination of the nutrient composition of foods, and of the effects of agricultural, processing, and cooking practices on nutrient content of foods; monitoring of nutritional status, research into food preferences and habits, and development of consumer educational techniques to improve food choices and nutritional status.

The USDA also administers several food assistance programs through its Food and Nutrition Service. These include food stamps, school food programs, and the Special Supplemental Food Program for Women, Infants, and Children (WIC).

FOOD STAMPS. The Food Stamp Act was enacted in 1964 to enable low-income households to buy more food in greater variety. The stamps are coupons that can be used like money at the grocery store. Those eligible for them are given an Authorization to Participate (ATP) Card each month. With the ATP card and a Food Stamp Identification Card, an individual can get the stamps at a bank or at another licensed outlet.

To be eligible for food stamps a person must be in a low-income bracket—whether due to complete unemployment, only part-time employment, full-time employment at low wages, subsistence on welfare or other assistance payments, old age, or disability—*and* have limited financial assets. Distribution of food stamps to individuals is inversely proportional to household income, and increases with household size.

Food stamps can be used to buy any kind of food, as well as seeds or plants to grow food. They cannot be used for tobacco products, alcoholic beverages, pet food, or household supplies such as paper goods, soap, or cleaning agents.

In 1977 Congress made a major revision in the Food Stamp Act. The intention was to expand benefits for the very poor by reducing the benefits for those who were less needy. When the Food Stamp Act was first enacted, recipients had to purchase their stamps; if they did not have available cash they were unable to acquire the stamps that could save them money. The 1977 law ended the cash requirement, but eligibility standards were modified and required that able adult recipients actively seek employment. It was anticipated that the new rules would eliminate 3.5 million of the 30.8 million people eligible to receive stamps, but make possible participation for some 4 million whose poverty had previously prevented them from purchasing stamps.

Inflation, however, upset official calculations. On the basis of a projected inflation rate of 3 to 4 percent a year for food, a limit of $6.1 billion had been set on spending for the 1978–1979 fiscal year. But by the middle of that year, food prices had risen 22 percent in the two years since the law was passed, and Congress was under pressure to remove the spending limit. At the same time, because eligibility requirements and stamp allotments are revised periodically to adjust benefits to inflation, the higher-than-anticipated rate of inflation meant that increased numbers of people were eligible for benefits and were entitled to greater benefits. Where 2.4 million new recipients had been expected to enroll, 3.4 million were newly eligible. The greatest increment occurred in rural areas where the cash requirement had been a greater barrier than the government realized.

In monetary terms, what are food stamps worth to a family? As of July 1979, a family of four with a maximum net income of $596 per month (gross income minus a standard deduction—presently $70 per month—and certain specified deductions) was eligible for $61 worth of food stamps per month. Each household's allotment is based on a calculation using their net monthly income and the cost of USDA's Thrifty Food Plan (one of four Agriculture Department food plans that estimate what it will cost to obtain a nutritionally adequate diet at various levels of food expenditures). More than half the households receiving food stamps have annual incomes below $3,600, and 95 percent of the recipients have financial assets of less than $1,500. There is little doubt that food stamps are needed by those eligible to receive them. Concern has been raised that some recipients, such as students and those on strike, are not truly needy; but less than 1 percent of food stamp benefits go to persons in these categories.

There is more concern over the nutritional status of those who are eligible but who are not, for a variety of reasons, participants in the program. In 1978, before the change in the purchase requirement, it was found that in 16 states less than a third of the eligible population was benefiting; an equal number of states had at least 50 percent participation, although few had participation much higher than that.

SCHOOL FOOD PROGRAMS. Under the School Feeding Program, lunches and breakfasts are provided free or at reduced prices to children from low-income families. The 1946 National School Lunch Act evolved from the recognition that the economic and agricultural crisis of the 1930s had resulted in malnutrition of significant numbers of young people. At the same time, food surpluses were beginning to accumulate following World War II.

The School Lunch Program provided a nutrition program to reach all children based on tested nutritional research. A "Type A" lunch was planned to provide approximately one-third of a school-age child's RDAs for nutrients and energy. The lunch was to consist of:

- 8 oz of fluid fresh milk
- 2 oz of meat, eggs, poultry, fish, or cheese *or* ½ cup cooked dried peas or beans *or* 4 tbsp peanut butter
- ¾ cup of at least 2 vegetables and fruits
- 1 slice whole grain or enriched bread
- 1 tsp butter or fortified margarine as a spread or in food preparation

A recently published study by the USDA found that most "Type A" lunches as served provided less than one-third of the RDA for iron, thiamin, and energy. This loss is magnified when plate waste is considered; vitamin A, phosphorus, calcium, and protein also often fall below the recommended standard when this factor is taken into account.

In 1966 the Child Nutrition Act reached out to more children through a pilot School Breakfast Program, and with meals for preschoolers and for poverty-area children in summer recreation and other nonschool group situations. This expansion, originating in the context of the first national commitment to preschool education through Operation Head Start and the beginnings of a national day care program, led to further expansion through a number of amendments in the 1970s. The School Breakfast Program was formally added in a 1973 amendment.

Today the school nutrition program makes available breakfast, lunch, and additional milk; serves preschoolers in addition to school-age children; provides meal service within some recreation programs during the summer; sponsors nutrition education in schools and for the training of personnel; and serves three meals daily to children in full day care programs. By 1978 the school lunch program was available in 93,000 schools, reaching 90 percent of all elementary and secondary school students. The expanded breakfast service was available in nearly 23,000 schools; more than 20,000 preschool centers served lunches; and more than 84,000 schools utilized the Special Milk Program. Twenty-eight million meals were being served daily, at an annual cost of nearly $4 billion. Nationwide, the nonprofit school food service employed some 350,000 individuals (Martin, 1978).

A major continued problem with all foods served for children is plate waste, which can be substantial especially at younger ages. Small capacity, reluctance to try new foods, and the quirky eating patterns of many children are responsible. So are such factors as limited time allotted for lunch, a noisy or otherwise unpleasant lunchroom atmosphere, unpleasant serving staff, uncomfortable seating arrangements, peer pressure, and lack of choice (Jansen and Harper, 1978). Plate waste translates into lost nutrient intake, and defeats the whole idea.

The National School Lunch and Child Nutrition Amendments of 1977 proposed changes in the meal pattern to reduce portion sizes served to younger children, and permit second helpings for older students; to allow enriched or whole-grain rice and pasta products as bread alternatives; and to moderate the use of fat, sugar, and salt in meals, among other provisions (Table 16-2). It also recommended that students, teachers, and parents be involved in meal planning and other food service activities.

Some schools have involved students in meal planning, either informally or as part of school nutrition councils, for many years. Results are encouraging: When students plan menus, their choices are more likely to be eaten, and they learn the principles of nutrition at the same time. One particularly effective way to involve older students is through a food service council that might undertake such projects as food preference surveys, menu and product development and testing, and working with school authorities or outside experts in recommending architectural and decorating changes. For younger students lunchroom experiences can be integrated into other subject matter in the classroom. Social studies curricula about neighborhoods or producers and consumers, for example, provide many ways to relate occupations and raw foods to what is being served for lunch.

In April 1978, the Department of Agriculture proposed that foods which compete with the school lunch and breakfast programs could not be offered for sale in schools until after all lunch periods. Such "competitive foods," frequently dispensed by vending machines, include candy, soft drinks, frozen desserts, and chewing gum. The reason for the proposed ban was that

TABLE 16-2 School Lunch Pattern Requirements: Minimum amounts of foods listed by food components to serve children of various ages and grades

	Preschool Children		Elementary School Students		Secondary School Students
Food Components	*Group I age 1-2*	*Group II age 3-4*	*Group III grades K-3 age 5-8*	*Group IV grades 4-6 age 9-11*	*Group V grades 7-12 age 12 and up*
Meat and meat alternates[a]	1 oz	1½ oz	1½ oz	2 oz	3 oz
A serving (edible portion as served) of cooked lean meat, poultry, or fish, or meat alternates:					
The following meat alternates may be used alone or in combination to replace 1 oz. cooked lean meat:[b]					
Cheese, 1 oz					
Eggs, 1 large					
Cooked dry beans or peas, ½ cup[c]					
Peanut butter, 2 tbsp					
Vegetables and fruits[c]	½ c	½ c	½ c	¾ c	¾ c
Two or more servings consisting of vegetables or fruits or both. A serving of full-strength vegetable or fruit juice can be counted to meet not more than half the total requirement.					
Bread and bread alternates[d]	5 sl/wk	8 sl/wk	8 sl/wk	8 sl/wk	10 sl/wk
A serving (1 slice) of enriched or whole-grain bread, or bread alternates:					
The following bread alternates may be used to replace 1 slice bread:					
A serving of biscuits, rolls, muffins, etc., made with whole-grain or enriched meal or flour					
A serving (½ c) of cooked enriched or whole-grain rice, macaroni, noodles, or other pasta products[e]					
Milk, fluid[f]	½ c	¾ c	¾ c	½ p (1 c)	½ p (1 c)
Two types of milk must be offered, one of which must be unflavored fluid low-fat, skim, or buttermilk. The choice of the other is at state or local option.					

[a] It is recommended that in schools not offering a choice of meat/meat alternates each day, no one form of meat (ground, sliced, pieces,. etc.) or meat alternate be served more than 3 times per week. Meat and meat alternates must be served in a main dish, or in a main dish and one other menu item.

[b] When it is determined that the serving size of a meat alternate is excessive, the particular meat alternate shall be reduced and supplemented with an additional meat/meat alternate to meet the full requirement.

[c] Cooked dry beans or dry peas may be used as the meat alternate *or* as part of the vegetable/fruit component, but not as both food components in the same meal.

[d] One-half or more slices of bread or an equivalent amount of bread alternate must be served with each lunch with the total requirement being served during a 5-day period. Schools serving lunch 6 or 7 days per week should increase this specified quantity for the 5-day period by approximately 20 percent (⅕) for each additional day.

[e] Enriched macaroni products with fortified protein may be used as part of a meat alternate or as a bread alternate, but not as both food components in the same meal.

[f] One-half pint of milk may be used for all age/grade groups if the lesser specified amounts are determined by the school food authority to be impractical.

Source: Rules and regulations, school lunch pattern requirements. *Federal Register* 43, (163), August 22, 1978.

youngsters were spoiling their appetites for lunch by snacking on "junk food" all morning long. The proposal brought forth 2,000 comments, 82 percent in favor of some kind of ban and many who would extend it to cookies, potato chips, and so on. Many parents and school officials, however, felt that the federal government should not intervene in what they considered to be a matter for local jurisdiction. There was concern about losing vending machine revenues used for band uniforms and other expenses of extracurricular activities. Also protesting were companies and industry associations; the Hershey Foods Corporation presented data showing its candy bars to contain more nutrients than saltines, crackers, raisins, and doughnuts.

In July 1979, the USDA proposed that foods sold in competition with federally funded school meals would have to meet a nutritional standard: foods would have to provide a minimum of 5 percent of the U.S. RDA for at least one of eight specific nutrients—protein, vitamin A, vitamin C, niacin, riboflavin, thiamin, calcium, and iron. As a result, some foods—candy bars with nuts, ice cream sandwiches, or snacks with raisins—would now be permitted for sale. These new guidelines represent the Agriculture Department's first effort to evaluate food by a nutritional standard. But some nutritionists and consumers are still dissatisfied. While the proposed rule is an effort to limit foods that do not promote good nutritional practices, it does not establish standards for limiting the amount of sugar, fat, or salt content. In addition, many feel that this rule, if enacted into law, will encourage the fortification of otherwise minimally nutritious foods.

WIC. The Special Supplemental Food Program for Women, Infants, and Children began as a consequence of the findings of the Ten-State Nutrition Survey and other surveys of the nutritional status of the poor between 1968 and 1970. All showed that, although there was little evidence of vitamin deficiencies or severe protein-energy malnutrition, a great number of infants and children were smaller than average, and about half the children age 1 to 2 years showed a dietary deficiency of iron. It was also clear that the extent of undernourishment increased in direct proportion to the poverty of the family, and that the undernutrition was due to an overall inadequate intake and not to an inappropriate diet (Mauer, 1979).

In 1972, Congress authorized a two-year pilot program to provide food supplements for low-income pregnant and lactating women, infants, and children under 5 years. In 1974 the program was extended and given increased funding for four more years; continued funding was provided in 1978.

Funds are channeled to state health departments or comparable state agencies; to Indian tribes or groups recognized by the Department of the Interior; or to the Indian Health Service of the Department of Health, Education, and Welfare. These agencies distribute funds to participating local agencies.

Local agencies may participate if they provide continuous medical care and treatment to residents of a low-income area; if they serve a population of women, infants, and children at nutritional risk; if their staff includes professionals competent to interview and examine patients receiving health services; and if they have the personnel and equipment necessary to perform the required evaluative measurements, tests, and data collection. Funds received must be used for specific foods, and to pay specified administrative and nutrition education costs. Food is distributed directly or by voucher, home delivery, or a combination of systems. Local agencies are directed to utilize paraprofessionals and to provide nutrition education programs in culturally appropriate form, for instance through teaching and printed materials in the language of the ethnic group served.

Recipients of supplemental foods in the WIC program must be certified by professionals as being at risk because of inadequate nutrition, medical history, and low income. Infants receive iron-fortified formulas, iron-fortified cereal, and fruit juice which is high in vitamin C. Infants 6 months of age or older may receive vitamin D-fortified whole fluid (or evaporated) milk instead of iron-fortified infant formula. Participating women and children receive vitamin D-fortified milk and/or cheese, eggs, hot or cold cereal which is high in iron, and fruit or vegetable juice which is high in vitamin C.

Currently some 70 agencies sponsor WIC programs in 49 states and in Puerto Rico and the Virgin Islands, providing aid to about 1.12 million women, infants, and children; but an estimated 8.3 million eligible low-income individuals are not reached by the program.

Although it is generally agreed that the WIC program is valuable, there has not yet been adequate appraisal and interpretation of its effects. Evaluation was mandated in the original enabling legislation, but for a variety of reasons uniform data collection was not carried out. Evaluation of some individual local programs has been encouraging, but more thorough study is needed. Another concern is that restriction of eligibility in the most recent legislation could change the focus of the program from preventive intervention to remedial treatment.

The Department of Health, Education and Welfare

The mission of the Department of Health, Education, and Welfare (DHEW) is to protect and advance the health and well-being of the nation's people. Several agencies within DHEW play significant roles relating to foods and nutrition.

ADMINISTRATION ON AGING. The Administration on Aging (AoA) is a branch of the Office of Human Development Services. AoA was established by the Older Americans Act of 1965, and is the principal agency charged with its implementation. The AoA, in addition to supporting research on aging and training professionals to work in this field, implements the national nutrition program for this segment of the population.

The Older Americans Act established research and demonstration nutrition projects, the results of which led to the creation of a Nutrition Program for the Elderly in March 1972. Known as Title VII, this program provided funding for at least one meal a day plus supportive services in a congregate setting, for persons 60 years of age and older and their spouses. Congregate meal programs are administered by health centers and senior citizens and church groups in the community. Their goal is to offer a social experience along with a hot meal providing one-third of the adult RDAs for key nutrients. Meals may be provided by a contracting caterer or prepared on-site.

Educational and/or recreational activities may be added; crafts, lectures, exercise, dance, and poetry writing are among activities that attract older individuals for most of the day. Social workers are often available to provide counseling and referral to other agencies if necessary. A modest contribution—generally 50 cents or a dollar per meal—is requested from those who can afford it; food stamps may also be used.

The quality of food served, the services provided by a given community's program, and the extent to which the target population is reached by the congregate meal programs of Title VII vary widely. One limited evaluation based on data from 91 meal sites has found that individuals who are already more socially active are most likely to participate, perhaps because the sponsoring local agency is already familiar to them (as it would be if it were a church regularly attended, as is often the case) or because they already know other participants. It was hoped that this program would particularly reach members of low-income and minority groups, and findings show that nearly two-thirds of all participants earn less than $4,000 and about one-fourth belong to an ethnic minority. Most participants live alone and are involuntarily isolated, as through the death of a spouse (*CNI Weekly Report*, 1/11/79).

Problems of transportation in a number of communities undoubtedly prevent many older people from taking advantage of congregate meals. Pilot projects in providing transportation are being funded by the Office on the Aging in scattered localities. Other innovative approaches that will ultimately make congregate meals more widely available include the recycling of old buildings, such as unneeded schools, for senior citizen and community centers, and incorporation of part-time jobs for older people as drivers and food service aides within these programs. In these approaches funding is provided by AoA and by other agencies from the Departments of Labor or Housing and Urban Development, for example.

A related program funded by several agencies is Meals on Wheels (MOW) in which food is transported to homebound elderly people several times a week. It is designed for those who are unable to purchase or prepare their own food. Some recipients pay for the services, while others receive the meals free or at reduced cost. Food stamps may be used as payment. MOW transportation must be provided by local organizations such as a church group.

THE U.S. PUBLIC HEALTH SERVICE. The U.S. Public Health Service (USPHS) is another major branch of DHEW. It encompasses several agencies which also have specific responsibilities in food and nutrition.

The Food and Drug Administration (FDA) has primary responsibility for protecting the safety of the American food supply. Its job is to inspect food processing plants; to approve food additives for safety; to determine and set standards for foods made according to a standardized recipe (peanut butter or mayonnaise, for example) and to test such products to assure they meet these "standards of identity"; to obtain samples of foods after they are offered for sale, testing them to make sure they are safe for consumer use; and to develop regulations for food package labeling.

Until the twentieth century there were no national food laws or regulations in the United States. In 1902 the Bureau of Chemistry of the USDA began to test foods for possible toxicity. Much was found wrong with the food supply and the public was alerted. By 1906 public pressure forced the passage of the Pure Food and Drug Act, the basis of all subsequent safety regulations. The USDA was given responsibility for ascertaining the safety of all foods in interstate commerce, and assuring that any chemical added to foods was safe and had a useful purpose. But the USDA was given only the right to inspect food processing plants and to publish the results of its investigations of food products; it did not have the power to impose fines or penalties.

The FDA was created within the USDA in 1931, but was not effective until the passage of the Federal Food, Drug, and Cosmetic Act in 1938; this legislation gave the FDA power to fine and imprison those found guilty of misbranding and adulterating foods. The burden of proof was on the government, which had to investigate and prosecute alleged violators. The FDA and its powers were reassigned to the DHEW in 1953. Only meat inspection remained under the jurisdiction of the USDA.

In 1954, the Miller Pesticide Amendment, specifying maximum levels of pesticides that could remain on foods once they entered the marketplace, was added to the 1938 Food, Drug, and Cosmetic Act. The Food Additive Amendment of 1958 defined additives and for the first time placed responsibility for proving the safety and efficacy of an additive on the food industry rather than on the government. The Delaney Clause prohibiting the addition of carcinogenic substances to food was a rider attached to this act.

Another amendment, added in 1960, specified that synthetic coloring agents had to be tested and certified by the government before they could be used in foods. The Fair Package and Labeling Act of 1966 gave the FDA specific authority over the content of package labels.

The FDA has been quite visible in recent years in several areas of contemporary public concern, among them the safety of food additives and fortification of foods. The FDA has also played a prominent role in consumer education via labeling of food products. Present regulations regarding ingredient and nutrition information on foods (except for alcoholic beverages) come from FDA.

Recently the FDA, in conjunction with USDA and the Federal Trade Commission (FTC), which is responsible for the regulation of food advertising practices, held hearings in five U.S. cities to find out what consumers want package labels to tell them. There was overwhelming consumer demand for complete and specific disclosure of ingredients, and for quantitative information for total salt, total sugar, and specific fat content. There were many suggestions for dating and nutrient information to be more clearly presented, possibly through use of a graphic device (Figure 16-2 shows one solution to these problems). There was strong support for the regulation of food fortification.

The hearings also brought to light many consumer attitudes. Repeatedly, these opinions—some valid, some not—were offered: Consumers have a "right to know" what is in the food they eat; the American public needs protection from the food industry; increased processing negatively affects food quality and positively affects corporate profits; all additives are bad; much current food advertising undermines consumer efforts to select the most nutritious food possible; the FDA could immediately impose any publicly beneficial regulation; more nutritious foods can be regulated into existence; the FDA is slow to act and often responds to the interests of industry as opposed to consumers.

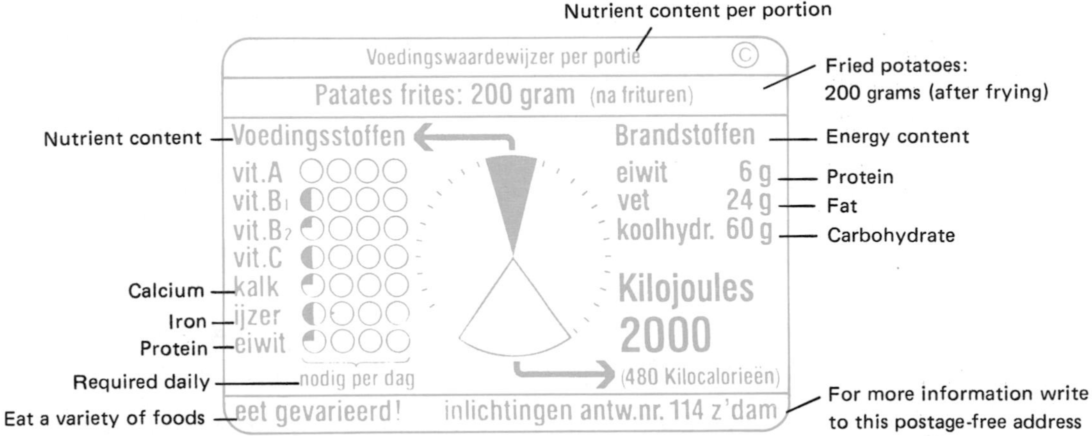

FIGURE 16-2

Graphic Nutrient Labeling.

This is the nutrient label on a potato chip package in use by a Dutch supermarket chain.

Source: H. E. Nelson, Consumer attitudes and trends. In *Plant and animal products in the U.S. food system* (Washington, D.C.: National Research Council, 1978), p. 163.

The concerned agencies are continuing to study the recommendations that came out of the hearings. Policies and legislation are expected to extend the nutritional labeling law, present guidelines for fortification of foods (specifying level of fortification and kinds of foods), and require some kind of dating system on food products.

Some regulations taking these and related concerns into account have already been proposed. In September 1978 the FDA issued "tentative final regulations" for vegetable protein products, to establish terminology for processed vegetable proteins made into or used in food products and for such food products intended as protein food substitutes. Descriptive names for vegetable proteins and derived products would indicate the protein content and its vegetable source (for example, soy flour, which is less than 65 percent protein, could not be labeled as "protein," but a soy product of 65 to 90 percent protein could be labeled "soy protein concentrate") (Hutt and Sloan, 1979). And as of July 1981, foods containing Yellow Dye No. 5 must be so identified on the ingredient statement. As many as 100,000 Americans are allergic to this coloring agent.

Further changes in labels are inevitable. Consumers want more information. Government regulatory agencies recognize that the present requirements are inadequate. But the problems of determining what data to include and in what form are enormous. There is only so much space on any label. Manufacturers are concerned that more detailed disclosure of ingredients would provide competitors with a product recipe. Moreover, extremely detailed labeling requirements would prevent minor recipe change. Such changes are often necessary to take advantage of food availability and market conditions, as when one oil is substituted for another. Consumers counter that, for various health reasons, it is important to know whether soybean or corn oil, for example, is used in the crackers or other foods they are buying.

Compromises will have to be made. It is probable that label space now devoted to advertising will have to be relinquished as information is added. Decisions will have to be made concerning the most useful data for the majority of the population. Additional information can be provided in other forms for those who want or need it; perhaps product information sheets can be posted at the point of sale or made available from manufacturers. A separate index of all food ingredients, including their chemical names, might be published. The ingenuity to provide needed information in usable form, and to make labels more relevant and accessible to all of us, should not be beyond the capacity of government or industry.

Another agency of the Public Health Service is the National Institutes of Health (NIH), consisting of 11 research institutes including the National Cancer Institute, the National Institute on Aging, and the National Institute of Dental Research. Through these and other institutes, NIH is the nation's major supporter of nutrition research, both in its own laboratories and other facilities. It also funds research and training programs in academic institutions.

Other Government Agencies

The Federal Trade Commission (FTC) regulates food advertising and the application of antitrust laws. The role of this agency in hearings regarding television advertising directed at children has been discussed in Chapter 13. One of the FTC's major missions is to protect consumers from false and misleading advertising. The agency has proposed regulations affecting food advertising: Advertising claims of "food energy" would have to be accompanied by energy content in kilocalories, and could not promise increased vigor or alertness due to the food. The terms "natural" and "organic" would be restricted and the term "health food" banned altogether. Discussion of fat, fatty acids, and cholesterol would be permitted only if actual content of saturated fat, cholesterol, and total fat is given. FTC has also recommended that restaurants making nutritional claims on their menus provide the same documentation that other food advertisers must give.

The Bureau of Alcohol, Tobacco, and Firearms (BATF) is responsible for ingredient labeling of alcoholic beverages. BATF's responsibility for this area came about in 1972 when consumer advocates noticed that no ingredients were listed on beer cans. All foods were required to have ingredient listings, and a check of the lawbooks revealed that no exception had been made for wine, beer, and distilled spirits. Subsequently, BATF agreed to require full ingredient labeling on all alcoholic beverages; by early 1979, this regulation had been scheduled to take effect on January 1, 1983.

Industry opposition to full disclosure is at the heart of the delay. Producers of wine and distilled spirits argue that labeling would be too expensive, that trade secrets would be divulged, and that consumers don't really want or need all that information. They have brought suit—another source of delay—against the FDA, which offered a labeling proposal. Within the government, FDA and BATF dispute the authority to write the final regulations. While the bureaucratic tangle continues, the only substance in alcoholic beverages whose presence and amount must be specified on the label is—alcohol.

CONGRESS AND NUTRITION. Congress plays an important role in determining food and nutrition policy. It makes laws the regulatory agencies cannot make, and it appropriates—broadly—the monies they and other enforcement agencies have to spend. Congressional concerns vary. In recent years Congress has acted on saccharin, and future action is expected on nitrites. Appropriations have been provided for Food Stamps, feeding pro-

TABLE 16-3
Some Congressional Committees and Subcommittees Concerned with Food and Nutrition Policy

HOUSE—Committees/Subcommittees
Agriculture
Domestic Marketing, Consumer Relations, and Nutrition
Science and Technology
Domestic and International Scientific Planning and Coordination (DISPAC)
Education and Labor
Elementary, Secondary, and Vocational Education
Interstate and Foreign Commerce
Health and the Environment
Government Operations
Intergovernmental Relations and Human Needs
Appropriations
Agriculture and Related Agencies; Labor—Health, Education, and Welfare
Select Committee on Aging
SENATE—Committees/Subcommittees
Agriculture, Nutrition, and Forestry
Nutrition; Agricultural Research and General Legislation; Foreign Agricultural Policy
Human Resources
Health and Scientific Research
Government Affairs
Intergovernmental Relations
Appropriations
Agriculture and Related Agencies; Labor—Health, Education, and Welfare
Select Committee on Aging

Source: K. W. McNutt, A Nutrition perspective from the Hill, *Nutrition News* 41 No. 4 (Rosemont, Illinois: National Dairy Council, 1978) p. 13.

grams for school children and the elderly, and WIC.

Both houses of Congress are concerned with matters related to food and nutrition. Through its various committees and subcommittees (See Table 16-3) Congress acquires information on which to base legislation and appropriations. Private citizens have the right and responsibility to let their senators and representatives know where they stand on issues and how they want their tax dollars spent.

Select Committees are sometimes established by Congress to conduct investigations of particular topics. They cannot propose legislation, and their reports do not require congressional approval. Select Committees may hold hearings to receive input from the public and/or from those with knowledge of and concern for the subject under investigation. *Dietary Goals for the United States* is a report prepared by the staff of the Senate Select Committee on Nutrition and Human Needs. It is not legislation. It is intended, however, to provide guidelines for development of a national nutrition policy.

The Senate Select Committee is now defunct, its responsibilities having been taken over by a subcommittee of the Agriculture, Nutrition, and Forestry Committee. Before its demise, the Committee recommended that the General Accounting Office (GAO) review all federal activity in human nutrition research. In preparing its report, the GAO solicited comments from

PERSPECTIVE ON Dietary Goals for the United States

The Senate Select Committee on Nutrition and Human Needs, under the leadership of Senator George McGovern (Democrat, S.D.), was established in 1968 to reconcile the food and farm orientation of the Agriculture Committee with the health, welfare, and research concerns of the Labor and Public Welfare Committees. Work by this committee has been responsible for expansion of the food stamp, school lunch, summer feeding, and school breakfast programs, and for establishment of the WIC program.

By 1975 the Committee had become concerned over the role of overnutrition in the etiology of, particularly, coronary heart disease, obesity, cancer, and stroke. A series of hearings and expert testimony led committee members to conclude that the U.S. government should have an overall nutrition policy, so that legislation affecting agriculture, the food industry, and the public could specifically implement this policy.

Early in 1977, *Dietary Goals for the United States* were issued (see table), and controversy immediately followed. The American Medical Association asserted that the widespread problems of obesity and iron-deficiency anemia, among others, were not addressed, and that the guidelines seemed to be directed more toward prevention of certain diseases than to general improvement of nutritional status. Other critics took issue with the specific recommendations. The 3 gram prescription for salt, for example, was widely held to be unrealistic and probably unnecessary. It was also pointed out that as guidelines for a national nutrition policy they failed to deal constructively with the major nutritional problems of the nation (Harper, 1977).

Proponents, on the other hand, emphasized the need for such goals, and stressed that the general principles represented were of greater importance than the actual numbers and provisions; that these guidelines may indeed be beneficial to large numbers of people and would certainly not be harmful to anyone; that present food intakes are contributing to disease conditions, and that this must be recognized. The goals were seen as a limited approach, not a panacea, and as a tentative, long-overdue, and potentially useful first step toward a national food and nutrition policy (Latham and Stephenson, 1977).

DIETARY GOALS FOR THE UNITED STATES
FIRST EDITION, FEBRUARY 1977

1. Increase carbohydrate consumption to account for 55 to 60 percent of energy intake.
2. Reduce overall fat consumption from approximately 40 to 30 percent of energy intake.
3. Reduce saturated fat consumption to account for about 10 percent of total energy intake; and balance that with polyunsaturated and monounsaturated fats, which should account for about 10 percent of energy intake each.
4. Reduce cholesterol consumption to about 300 mg a day.
5. Reduce sugar consumption by about 40 percent to account for about 15 percent of total energy intake.
6. Reduce salt consumption by about 50 to 85 percent to approximately 3 g (1.2 g sodium) a day.

Source: Select Committee on Nutrition and Human Needs, U.S. Senate. Dietary Goals for the United States. February, 1977.

Further hearings resulted in publication of a second edition (see table) that presented modified guidelines in terms of ranges, not absolute numbers; specifically mentioned the importance of maintaining ideal body weight; adjusted the salt recommendation; specifically excluded children, pregnant women, and the elderly from some of the recommendations; and dealt with alcohol as a source of energy intake. The final report included recommendations for achieving the dietary goals: that funds be appropriated for a public education program based on these (or a similar set of) goals; that nutrient content labeling be required on all foods; that the USDA and DHEW be funded for joint research and pilot projects in food processing to re-

DIETARY GOALS FOR THE UNITED STATES
SECOND EDITION, DECEMBER 1977

1. To avoid overweight, consume only as much energy (calories) as is expended; if overweight, decrease energy intake and increase energy expenditure.
2. Increase the consumption of complex carbohydrates and "naturally occurring" sugars from about 28 percent to about 48 percent of energy intake.
3. Reduce the consumption of refined and other processed sugars by about 45 percent to account for about 10 percent of total energy intake.
4. Reduce overall fat consumption from approximately 40 percent to about 30 percent of energy intake.
5. Reduce saturated fat consumption to account for about 10 percent of total energy intake and balance that with polyunsaturated and monounsaturated fats, which should account for about 10 percent of energy intake each.
6. Reduce cholesterol consumption to about 300 mg per day.
7. Limit the intake of sodium by reducing the intake of salt (sodium chloride) to about 5 g per day (2 g sodium).

Source: Select Committee on Nutrition and Human Needs, U.S. Senate. Dietary Goals for the United States, ed 2. December 1977.

duce risk factors in the diet; and that these two departments should receive increased funding for human nutrition research and coordinate their research efforts, and form a joint committee to periodically review nutritional concerns and their effects on agricultural policy (Woodruff, 1979).

Implementation of the Goals would require the following changes in food selection and preparation:

1. Increase consumption of fruits and vegetables and whole grains.
2. Decrease consumption of meat and increase consumption of poultry and fish.
3. Decrease consumption of foods high in fat and partially substitute polyunsaturated fat for saturated fat.
4. Except for young children, substitute nonfat milk for whole milk.
5. Decrease consumption of butterfat, eggs, and other high cholesterol sources.
6. Decrease consumption of sugar and foods high in sugar content.
7. Decrease consumption of salt and foods high in salt content.

The Dietary Goals cannot be used to plan diets; they must be used in conjunction with RDAs. The RDAs focus on what is in a nutritionally adequate diet (providing a margin of safety) while the Goals focus on moderation. The RDAs have limitations, but because they serve a useful purpose and are the best tool presently available, they have been widely accepted as reasonable guidelines. Periodic revision takes new data into account, and increases their usefulness. The same approach should be extended to the Goals. They are a first step, and nutritionists must take a strong stand here and assume responsibility for demonstrating their usefulness.

Diets based on the Dietary Goals and RDAs have been devised so that individuals can adjust their food intake patterns accordingly. For an adult male, the Goals would translate into a diet consisting of two-thirds more grain products; one-fourth more vegetables and fruits; one-twelfth more legumes, nuts, and milk; one-third *less* meat, poultry, and fish; one-fourth *less* fats and oils; half as many eggs; and half as much refined sugar and sweets (Peterkin et al., 1979). It will be difficult to devise actual meal plans to take all Goals into account, and maintain, at least initially, consumers' satisfaction with their meals.

In addition to assessing the Goals' effects on personal and national health, we cannot overlook their impact on economics. The agricultural industry is a big one, and changed consumer attitudes toward certain food items, such as beef, may have profound effects on our national economy, at least temporarily. There is no guarantee that a diet based on the Goals will prevent cancer or heart disease, although there is little doubt of the value of moderating intakes of fat, sugar, salt, total energy, and cholesterol while consuming a still diverse diet. By changing the American public's—and especially young people's—attitudes toward food, the potential effects of the Goals can be significant.

TABLE 16-4
GAO Report, March 1978

I. Gaps in present knowledge:
- Knowledge of dietary nutrients required to promote or maintain growth, development, or well-being under various stages and conditions of life.
- Information on the composition of the current U.S. food supply and the extent that nutrients are biologically available.
- Evaluation of long-term health consequences of the modern diet.
- Assessment of the nation's current nutritional status in terms of dietary excesses, imbalances, as well as deficiencies.

II. Research needs for responding to knowledge gaps:
- Long-term studies of human subjects across the full range of both health and disease.
- Comparative studies in populations of different geographic, cultural, and genetic backgrounds.
- Basic investigation of the functions and interactions of dietary components.
- Updated and expanded food composition data.
- Improved techniques for assessing long-term toxicological risks.

Source: General Accounting Office, Report to Congress, *Federal human nutrition research needs a coordinated approach to advance nutrition knowledge* (Washington, D.C.: U.S. Government Printing Office, 1978), p. ii.

32 people in the nutritional field, representing nutritional scientists, academicians, government, professional organizations, and industry, asking them to identify barriers to progress in this area. Lack of coordination of research, a shortage of nutrition scientists, and the uncertainty of federal funding for nongovernment research were repeatedly cited. In its report to Congress in March 1978, the GAO identified research gaps and needs (see Table 16-4) and called for the establishment of a centralized government-wide agency to plan and coordinate human nutrition research, define the areas of such research and the roles of various agencies, and assess the need for regional research centers to work with colleges and universities that have comprehensive departments of nutrition.

As a result of these suggestions and the Food and Agriculture Act of 1977 which designated the USDA as the major agency for human nutrition, the USDA established the Human Nutrition Center as a component of its Science and Education Administration. It also created a position within USDA to coordinate human nutrition activities within the agency and to serve as liaison to other federal agencies and various organizations involved in human nutrition. With such a center, ongoing research is reinforced and not overly duplicated—although some duplication is inevitable and indeed useful to verify findings or offer an alternative approach (General Accounting Office, 1978).

Extent of Government Influence

The Federal government influences nutrition through education and research, and by regulation of the food industry. It sets priorities for intervention. To address actual needs effectively, these efforts must be coordinated; programs and regulations must be designed in response to consumer as well as agricultural, industrial, and scientific concerns. Policies on nutrition, energy, inflation, health care, unemployment, agriculture, and international trade—and more—are all involved in providing nutritionally adequate and enjoyable diets for the American people.

Many programs are federally funded but, as in the case of Food Stamps, WIC, and congregate meals for the elderly, administered through state and local agencies. State and local governments have a role in nutritional policy through such agencies as state departments of public health and education, local nutrition resource centers, feeding programs, and inspection services. State and local governments can also have an impact on federal policy.

THE ROLE OF THE FOOD AND AGRICULTURE INDUSTRIES

The development of new strategies to encourage nutritional health will not be possible without participation by the food and agriculture industries. Industry's responsibilities to the public include:

- Provision of an adequate supply of wholesome, nourishing, and safe food
- Education through advertising
- Research to develop new food products and improve existing items
- Efficient use of land, energy, and other resources
- Maintenance of safety and quality

Over the years industry has shown that it can be responsive to the needs of the consumer, and that it can be innovative and creative in providing products that appeal to consumers, whether for taste, lifestyle, or health reasons. Salt and sugar have been removed from baby and many other foods. Nitrite-free bacon and frankfurters and low-cholesterol egg and cream substitutes have been developed. Texturized vegetable proteins have been incorporated into sausages, hamburger extenders, and other products. Peanut butter with emulsifiers, protein-enriched spaghetti, fiber-enriched bread, and vitamin- and mineral-fortified cereals and candy bars are all available.

Agriculture: Where the Food Supply Originates

Farming today is very different from what it was in the past. Increasingly, farmers are at the mercy of events and conditions over which they have little or no control. Farmers have always had to deal with severe weather conditions and pest infestations, but the centralization of our agricultural system tends to amplify their effects. The technological demands of high-intensity farming; the capital needed for land, supplies, and equipment; the need for adequate storage facilities; and the high cost of labor drive up farmers' costs. National and international events increasingly influence the economy quickly, with prices seeming to defy the law of supply and demand. Moreover, farmers appear not to be receiving their proportionate share of the food dollar. As the price of food skyrockets, farmers contend that the so-called "middleman" is reaping the profits, and have called on the government for financial and regulatory aid.

There are no easy answers to these problems. More efficient use of land, development of new crops and animal breeds, new uses for old products, a comprehensive energy policy, and support of local agriculture and marketing systems—long ago abandoned as our cities grew—are some of the approaches that should be examined.

The development of alcohol-based fuel, "gasahol," as an alternative source of energy, could have a positive effect on the food supply. Alcohol fuels can be produced from grain crops; surplus sugar is another potential source of gasahol, the development of which was cited by President Carter as a goal of a national energy program in the summer of 1979. Whether gasahol production will have a positive effect on either our energy or food problems remains to be seen.

A prime concern of consumers today is the use of chemicals by the agriculture industry for pest control, fertilizer, and to enhance the growth and health of livestock. One promising approach is known as Integrated Pest Management (IPM). Former methods of pest control left chemical residues on foods, and scattered spray in unintended directions; meanwhile the bugs developed resistance to the pesticides. IPM uses some chemicals, but also utilizes simple changes in farming practices or biological control techniques to achieve the same effect. Making insects' accustomed food supply unavailable when they need it, by planting a crop variety that matures at a different time, may be sufficient to outwit infestation. Use of natural predators and parasites is also desirable. More innovative are such techniques as using the distinctive scent of the male of the species to falsely lure females away from farmland, or releasing sterile male insects into the breeding population.

The USDA began subsidizing IPM programs in 1972. In 1975, it reported that yields had increased in 18—and profits in 24—of 25 programs applying IPM to cotton, peanuts, and tobacco. The USDA estimates that by 1986 IPM may be in use on more than 100 million acres of American cropland, which could result in annual pesticide savings of some $1 billion (Chasan, 1979).

The massive use of antibiotics in animal feed, according to the report of a congressional agency, is making bacteria more resistant with some risk to human health. At stake is the effectiveness of such drugs as penicillin and tetracycline, both widely used in animal feed for their contribution to the disease resistance and weight gain of cattle, pigs, chickens, and other farm animals. A choice will have to be made between safeguarding the effectiveness of these medications and the larger yields and greater profits of the livestock industry. The choice will perhaps be eased by the knowledge that safe alternatives exist to most of the antibiotics presently used in livestock feeds. A related issue arose a few years ago, when diethylstilbesterol (DES), used to fatten animals, was prohibited when residues were found in meat products. The action was taken because DES, used to prevent miscarriages in pregnant women during the 1940s and 1950s, has been linked to the vaginal cancers that later developed in some of their daughters.

From Farm to Market

When our food leaves the farm, it must be transported several times, processed, preserved, and packaged. Our food system depends on these practices to maintain quality (safety, appearance, and taste) and nutritional value. Methods of food processing (canning, freezing, dehydrating, freeze-drying, fermenting, and baking) have become technologically advanced, to maximize both nutritional content and freshness. In fact, many processed foods maintain higher nutritional quality than "fresh produce"—particularly if the latter is subjected to rough handling, transportation delays, or lack of refrigeration. The food industry carries a tremendous responsibility to provide food that is wholesome and nutritious, at reasonable cost. It must continue to do so—through continued testing of food additives, research to refine processing techniques which remove as few nutrients as possible from our foods, and consumer education.

At the Point of Sale

The retail segment of the food industry can influence the practices of its suppliers as well as the food habits of consumers. One chain has protested price increases that it considered excessive and unjustified; some price rollbacks were the result.

Several chains have advertised to shoppers that purchases of certain items which were "overpriced" should be avoided. Retailers have also made lower-cost substitutes for higher-priced items available, and used newspaper advertising and point-of-sale posters to explain the uses of such low-cost substitutes as ground turkey.

Supermarkets can also participate in nutrition education efforts. A Washington, D.C., chain is involved in a one-year pilot campaign in cooperation with the National Heart, Blood, and Lung Institute (NHBLI) to alert shoppers to "heart health and nutrition issues." Pamphlets are available in the more than 90 area stores, along with posters and other in-store materials, and provide information about cardiovascular disease, cholesterol, and sugar and salt consumption. Information about fat, cholesterol, and energy content of foods is displayed in the stores, and radio and newspaper advertising is being used to support the campaign, which will be evaluated by NHBLI for changes in consumer knowledge and food selection.

Consumer concern on a community level can influence the individual retailer and the chain, because retailers depend on their repeat customers for their livelihood. The place where food is purchased is perhaps the best place in which to provide food-related information for effective use by consumers. When they are shopping, customers' minds are on food and on getting the best nutritional value for their food dollars. In-store lectures and demonstrations, take-home flyers and pamphlets, seminars, store tours, effective displays and special promotions can all provide nutrition information where it is most needed and wanted. Supermarkets and alternative retail outlets such as cooperatives also play a role in maintaining nutritional quality of foods. Adequate refrigeration, freezing, and stock rotation are necessary to protect the freshness and quality of the food supply.

OTHER AGENTS FOR CHANGE

Other segments of our society provide opportunities for improving nutritional knowledge and practices. Foremost among these are the educational system and health care professionals.

Educational Institutions

At every educational level, from preschool to continuing education, opportunity exists to present nutrition information, and to carry out nutrition-related research. Nutrition education should be incorporated into classes for young children, and should certainly be a component of the school lunch program. Even greater opportunities exist at the college, university, and community education levels.

In the past there were problems of presenting information in interesting ways to boys as well as girls, who traditionally learned about nutrition in home economics courses; there were also too few qualified teachers to present nutritional material accurately. Recent federal legislation now provides the impetus for school systems to incorporate nutrition education into their curricula, and offers an opportunity for innovative programming through grant awards. State education departments are establishing nutrition curricula and encouraging the development of inservice courses to prepare teachers to present this material. Nutrition education materials and workshops for teachers are provided by the National Dairy Council and other food industry associations, and by the American Dietetic Association and other professional organizations (see list of resources in Appendix, Table I.).

Research, both basic and applied, must continue and expand. The knowledge gaps and research goals identified by the GAO report (see Table 16-4) present challenges to members of numerous disciplines—nutrition, economics, political science, biology, chemistry, engineering, sociology, psychology, and anthropology—in the academic community. Professional and student research can make substantial contributions in these areas.

Health Care Providers

Health care professionals are becoming increasingly aware that nutritional status is related to prevention of disease as well as to treatment. Pediatricians and obstetricians have long been concerned about the nutritional status of their patients as growth and development were affected. But too often the actual nutrition knowledge of even these professionals has been inadequate.

In the past, nutrition was ignored in medical and dental school curricula. It has recently begun to be included, largely because today's students are interested and have requested it. But an isolated course is not adequate; nutrition practice must be incorporated into the preclinical and clinical phases of medical training as well.

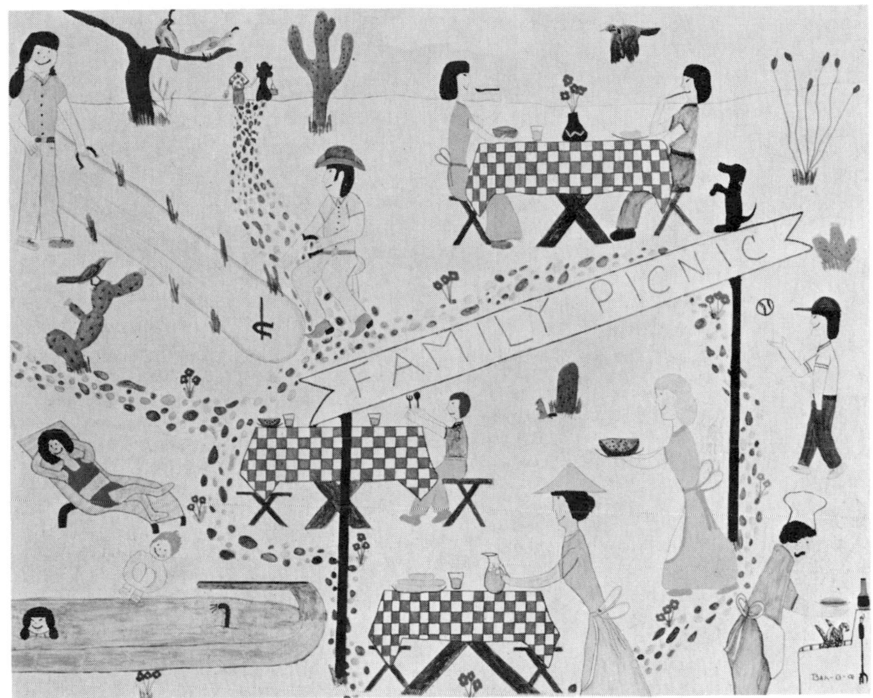

A family picnic, as seen through the eyes of an 11-year-old. (UNICEF)

All health professionals (and paraprofessionals) should be educated in nutrition, and be aware of the special expertise that can be contributed by nutritionists and dietitians. Too often the dietitian has been thought of as "the lady who puts food on the tray," rather than as the person—for gender has nothing to do with it—who is both educator and formulator of normal and special purpose diets.

Professional nutrition counseling should be available to hospitalized people and their families to provide guidance for health maintenance at home. Counseling services should also be available at community health care centers and from HMOs. Problems related to nutrition during pregnancy and for those suffering from chronic diseases could be handled through such services; prevention as well as therapy is the goal. The eagerness with which the public has greeted pronouncements on nutrition and health from the popular press and nonprofessionals indicates the extent of the need for such information from an accurate, dependable source.

Dietitians must continue to update their knowledge through educational programs and by keeping up with the current literature. And they must share their knowledge with other health care professionals. Dietitians should become activists in their communities, initiating public information programs, and letting their legislators know of their concerns. As the public interest in and concern about food and nutrition expands, the voices of the professionals in this field must be heard.

The Role of the Consumer

Consumers have an important role in defining strategies for change. There are many things individuals can do: participate in state consumer councils and other groups that are concerned with food and nutrition; become aware of the community's education programs in nutrition; learn by reading and taking courses from qualified people; write to state and federal legislators about concerns; write to food industry executives for more information about their products, or to protest improper practices or poor quality. Support of local agriculture can increase the local food supply and reduce food costs. Customer opinions can influence the kinds of foods available from retailers. It should not be assumed that Congress is influenced only by the farm lobby or the food industry; both retailers and Congress have been affected by consumer action.

Consumers have the ultimate responsibility for maintaining the quality and safety of the food supply. From the time it is purchased, throughout preparation, and until it is served, food can lose its nutritional value and become the transmitter of serious, even fatal, illness. Food safety in the home should be a key component of nutrition education for the public.

Toward a National Nutrition Policy

A national nutrition policy must involve all sectors of our population. We must learn to be economically self-sufficient, healthy, and to use our tax dollars wisely. Comprehensive policies require input from nutritional and other research. Food safety policies must involve the Food and Drug Administration, the Department of Agriculture, and the Environmental Protection Agency. Continuation of Food Stamps, School Food Service, WIC, and other feeding programs will improve nutritional status and knowledge for those most at risk of the consequences of under- and overnutrition. Nutrition education in schools at every level, in extension programs, and for community groups will produce a more knowledgeable and better nourished people.

SUMMARY

Many federal agencies are involved in agriculture, food, and health policies. There is greater recognition than ever before that research, education, and food assistance programs must be coordinated to be fully effective and to reach all sectors of the population.

Over the years, nutritional concerns have changed. For a long time, undernutrition was the focus of national food programs, but in recent years there has been increased awareness of problems associated with overnutrition, a consequence of the affluent lifestyle of most Americans. The typical diet of the population contains large amounts of energy-dense foods, fats, sugar, and salt, and may in its own way be as damaging to the human body as a vitamin-deficient diet.

Determining the nutrient content of processed foods, the value of vitamin-

and mineral-fortification, and the potential for damage of additives requires continued research. Government is addressing these concerns with renewed vigor. Carcinogenic additives are being removed from the market, and additives previously considered safe are being looked at critically. Chemical substances per se, however, are neither harmful nor beneficial; further research is needed to identify those that are useful and not potentially dangerous.

Government agencies concerned with food and nutrition include the Department of Agriculture (USDA), which administers the Food Stamp Program, school lunch programs, and WIC; the Department of Health, Education, and Welfare, which sponsors the Administration on Aging, the Food and Drug Administration, the National Institutes of Health. Congress makes laws, assigns responsibilities to agencies, and appropriates the funding for many of these programs.

The U.S. Dietary Goals, proposed in 1977 by the Senate Select Committee on Nutrition and Human Needs, may have been a turning point in the role of government in determining human nutrition priorities for the nation.

A national nutrition policy must involve every sector of the population if it is to be truly effective—the food and agriculture industries, educational institutions, health care providers, and last but not least, consumers. We are all collaborators in the effort to make the best and most nutritious use of the nation's food supply.

BIBLIOGRAPHY

Business Week. Too many cereals for the FTC. March 20, 1978, p. 166.

Chasan, D. J. How ya gonna keep bugs down (on the farm)? *Smithsonian*, January 1979, p. 78.

CNI Weekly Report. Study says AoA Program improves diet of aged. Vol. 9(2):5, 1979.

General Accounting Office. Report to the Congress. *Federal human nutrition research needs a coordinated approach to advance nutrition knowledge*. Washington, D.C.: U.S. Government Printing Office, 1978.

Hall, R. L. Safe at the plate. *Nutrition Today*, November-December 1977, p. 6.

Harper, A. E. U.S. dietary goals: Against. *Journal of Nutrition Education* 9(4):154, 1977.

Hegsted, D. M. Toward a national nutrition policy. Preface to the Report of the National Nutrition Consortium. *Nutrition Reviews* 32(5):153, 1974.

Hutt, P. B., and A. E. Sloan. FDA regulations of vegetable protein products. *Nutrition Policy Issues*, January 1979.

Jansen, G. R., and J. M. Harper. Consumption and plate waste of menu items served in the National School Lunch Program. *Journal of the American Dietetic Association* 73:395, 1978.

Latham, M. C., and L. S. Stephenson. U.S. dietary goals: For. *Journal of Nutrition Education* 9(4):152, 1977.

Martin, J. School nutrition programs in perspective. *Journal of the American Dietetic Association* 73:389, 1978.

Mauer, A. M. The WIC Program or 'The Perils of Pauline.' *American Journal of Diseases of Children* 133:478, 1979.

National Academy of Sciences. Report on Food Safety. Washington, D.C., 1979.

Peterkin, B. B., C. J. Shore, and R. L. Kerr. Some diets that meet the Dietary

Goals for the United States. *Journal of the American Dietetic Association* 74:423, 1979.

PRIAL, F. J. Efforts increase to aid groups that salvage 'unwanted' food. *New York Times*, July 10, 1979, p. C10.

ROBBINS, W. Wheat at $4: Squeezing food costs. *New York Times*, June 24, 1979.

WOODRUFF, C. W. Dietary goals for the United States. *American Journal of Diseases of Children* 133:371, 1979.

SUGGESTED ADDITIONAL READING

CHANG, A., S. KAYMAN, E. McCOY, AND L. PARZIALE. Nutrition services in child day care centers. *Journal of the American Dietetic Association* 74:356, 1979.

CULLEN, R. W., A. PAULBITSKI, AND S. M. OACE. Sodium, hypertension, and the U.S. Dietary Goals. *Journal of Nutrition Education* 10:59, 1978.

DWYER, J. Challenge of change—Nutrition and policy. *Journal of Nutrition Education* 9:54, 1977.

FOOD AND NUTRITION BOARD. Special report: Perspectives on food safety. *Nutrition Reviews* 37:29, 1979.,

GALLAGHER, C. R., AND V. M. VIVIAN. Nutrition concepts essential in the education of the medical student. *American Journal of Clinical Nutrition* 32:1330, 1979.

GUTHRIE, H. A. Effect of a flavored milk option in a school lunch program. *Journal of the American Dietetic Association* 71:35, 1977.

HARRIS, R. S., AND E. KARMAS. Nutritional evaluation of food processing, 2nd ed. Westport, Conn.: AVI Publishing Co., 1975.

HEGSTED, D. M. Food and nutrition policy: Probability and practicality. *Journal of the American Dietetic Association* 74:534, 1979.

JELLIFFE, D. B., AND E. F. P. JELLIFFE. National policy and young child nutrition. *American Journal of Clinical Nutrition* 31:1421, 1978.

McNUTT, K. W. An analysis of *Dietary goals for the United States, 2nd ed. Journal of Nutrition Education* 10(2):61, 1978.

MANUFACTURING CHEMISTS ASSOCIATION. Food Additives: Who needs them? Washington, D.C.: Manufacturing Chemists Association, 1978.

MAYER, J., ED. *U.S. nutrition policies in the seventies.* San Francisco: Freeman, 1973.

QUELCH, J. A. The resource allocation process in nutrition policy planning. *American Journal of Clinical Nutrition* 32:1058, 1979.

RICHMOND, F. W. The role of the federal government in nutrition education. *Journal of Nutrition Education* 9:150, 1977.

RUSOFF, I. I. Nutrition labeling from the industrial point of view. *Food Technology* 32:32, 1978.

STUMPH, S. E. Culture, values and food science. *BioScience* 28:186, 1978.

In Retrospect III

Nutritional science, and its application to people, is a complex discipline. It is important to understand how the internal environment of the body affects nutritional requirements, upon which recommendations for an adequate diet are based. But this is not enough. Nourishment is derived from food. The external environment—technology, physical surroundings, economics, politics, and cultural traditions—influences the foods that are available and acceptable for consumption.

The science of nutrition has provided some of the answers about the need for individual nutrients, but there is much more still to be learned. What is known, however, is that a diversified diet is the best insurance that adequate nutrients will be consumed. And although more data are needed about optimal intakes, present knowledge is sufficient to recommend that all nutrients, and energy, be consumed in moderation. Indeed, diversity and moderation appear to be the key concepts involved in the maintenance of nutritional health. These concepts will most likely withstand the test of time.

Nutrition has become everybody's business, and rightfully so. Scientists—biologists, chemists, physicists, engineers, and mathematicians—are expanding the knowledge base about nutritional biochemistry and food composition, production, and safety. Social scientists—economists, sociologists, anthropologists, psychologists, and political scientists—are identifying factors in the external environment which can be manipulated to increase the consumption of nutritious foods. Educators, media specialists, and health professionals are translating the scientific principles of the discipline into realistic plans for consumer food intakes. And government agencies and the food industry have responsibilities to ensure a food supply that is nutritious, safe, and available to the entire population.

But regardless of scientific knowledge and the resources and methods used to communicate that information to the consumer, the real choice belongs to the individual. The mere possession of knowledge does not automatically produce a change in behavior. But it is hoped that an understanding of the basic principles of nutrition will encourage people to place the importance of good nutritional behaviors into perspective in their own lives. Although consumption of a diversified, balanced, nutritionally adequate diet, with neither too much nor too little food, does not guarantee freedom from disease, it undoubtedly provides a buffer against the stresses of the external world, giving the body the substances it needs to maintain homeostasis.

The foundations for health and achievement in later life are laid in the growing years, which include the prenatal period. Conscientious attention to nutritional needs and the cultivation of positive attitudes toward food, eating, and physical activity are important parenting roles for both fathers and mothers. As adolescents enter their adult years, they become the backbone of society; most will assume parenting responsibilities as well, thereby ensuring the continuity of the life cycle. Proper nutrition for young adults can do much to make their later life a time of continued productivity, fulfillment, and health.

The science of nutrition will continue to evolve. Although this course may be your last formal exposure to the discipline, your learning need not stop. Your basic knowledge of the principles of nutrition should enable you to evaluate new information, associate new facts with those you have already learned, make informed choices about the foods you eat, and enhance the quality of your life.

Glossary

ABSORPTION The movement of digested food substances from the lumen of the intestine into intestinal cells, and from there into the bloodstream for distribution to other parts of the body.

ACETYL COENZYME A (ACETYL COA) An important metabolic intermediate that provides energy for cellular function, and is used for the synthesis of cholesterol, fatty acids, and other biological compounds.

ACID Any substance that will release hydrogen ions in solution.

ACTH (ADRENOCORTICOTROPIC HORMONE) A pituitary hormone which regulates the secretion of hormones from the adrenal cortex.

ACTIVE TRANSPORT An energy-requiring process by which certain nutrients are "pumped" from one compartment to another against a concentration gradient.

ADENOSINE TRIPHOSPHATE (ATP) A high-energy compound produced in metabolic pathways and the electron transport system; needed for cellular activity.

ADIPOCYTE Cell that stores fat.

ADIPOSE-CELL THEORY The theory that the number of adipocytes in an individual is determined by his/her earliest feeding habits.

AEROBIC PATHWAY A metabolic pathway requiring oxygen; final pathway of carbohydrate, lipid and protein metabolism, producing CO_2, water and energy; also known as the Krebs cycle, tricarboxylic acid cycle, or citric acid cycle.

ALBUMIN A water-soluble protein that increases the solubility of fatty acids in the blood, and plays a role in maintaining blood volume.

ALDOSTERONE An adrenal hormone that plays a major role in the regulation of sodium and potassium metabolism.

AMINATION The addition of an amino group ($—NH_2$) to a molecule.

AMINO ACID Any one of a large group of organic acids characterized by an amino group ($—NH_2$). Structural unit of proteins.

ANABOLISM The energy-requiring metabolic processes in which body substances are synthesized from simpler substances.

ANAEROBIC PATHWAY A set of energy-producing reactions that can proceed in the absence of oxygen. Also known as *glycolysis,* or the *Embden-Meyerhof pathway.*

ANIMAL MODEL An animal used as an experimental system in research. Rats are the animal model most widely used in nutritional studies.

ANION A negatively charged atom (i.e., an atom that has gained one or more electrons).

ANOREXIA NERVOSA A condition characterized by a profound aversion to food, resulting in extreme weight loss and sometimes death.

ANTIOXIDANT A substance that delays or prevents oxidation.

APPETITE The desire for food; influenced by external (nonphysiological) stimuli.

-ASE A suffix used to indicate an enzyme.

ATHEROSCLEROSIS A disease process in which the lumen of an artery is gradually reduced in size by the accumulation of fatty deposits on the inner walls of the artery.

ATOM The basic structural unit of all substances. All matter in the known universe consists of some 100 distinct types of atoms (i.e., elements). Atoms consist of protons, neutrons, and electrons.

BASAL METABOLIC RATE The amount of energy expended for involuntary functions of the body per unit of time: measured under standard conditions; affected by age, sex, size, shape of the body, and physiological state.

BASE Any substance that will release hydroxyl (—OH) ions.

BILE Digestive fluid produced by the liver and stored in the gall bladder. Aids in fat digestion and absorption.

BIOAVAILABILITY The extent to which any nutrient in food is available for utilization by the body.

BIOLOGICAL VALUE An index of protein quality that reflects the percentage of absorbed dietary nitrogen utilized by the body.

BOMB CALORIMETER A device used to measure the amount of heat produced by a weighed sample of food, and thus the food's energy value.

BRUSH BORDER The collective term for the numerous microvilli that cover the villi and epithelial cells of the small intestine.

CALORIE The amount of heat necessary to raise the temperature of one liter of water from 15°C to 16°C; a kilocalorie; 1 kilocalorie = 1 Calorie = 1000 calories = 4.184 kilojoules.

CALORIMETRY The measurement of heat change in an individual or system. As used in nutritional studies, the measurement of heat expenditure. (See *direct calorimetry; indirect calorimetry.*)

CARBOHYDRATE An organic compound containing carbon, hydrogen, oxygen, and sometimes nitrogen and sulfur; a major nutrient class which provides a major source of energy in the human diet; sugars and starches.

CARBOHYDRATE LOADING A dietary sequence of reduced carbohydrate intake followed by three or four days of high intake. This "loading" maximizes the storage of muscle glycogen and is used by many marathon runners, for example, in preparing for a race.

CARRIER MOLECULE Specialized protein molecule that enables large molecules to be transported across cell membranes.

CATABOLISM The energy-releasing metabolic processes in which body substances are broken down into simpler substances.

CATALYST Any substance that speeds up a chemical reaction. Although necessary for a reaction to occur, a catalyst (e.g., an enzyme) is the same in quantity and structure after the reaction as it was before.

CATION A positively charged atom (i.e., an atom that has lost one or more of its electrons).

CELL The basic structural and functional unit of living organisms.

CELLULOSE The most abundant of plant polysaccharides, and for humans, an indigestible carbohydrate; a component of dietary fiber.

CHEMICAL EQUATION An equation that uses chemical formulas and other symbols to represent the changes of bonding that occur between atoms involved in a chemical reaction.

CHEMICAL FORMULA The symbol or combination of symbols used by chemists to represent the composition of an element or compound (e.g., O_2, H_2O, NaCl).

CHEMICAL SCORE An index of protein quality; compares the essential amino acid content of a test protein with that of a standard protein.

CHEMICAL STRUCTURE In general terms, the arrangement of atoms in a molecule, or of molecules in a compound.

CHEMICAL SYMBOL The letter or letters used by chemists to represent an element (e.g., H and Ca for hydrogen and calcium, respectively).

CHOLESTEROL The chief sterol synthesized in the human body and present in all tissues; precursor of steroid hormones and vitamin D; dietary cholesterol is found primarily in egg yolks, liver and organ meats.

CHROMOSOME A giant molecule of DNA and protein located in the cell nucleus; it contains the genes and functions in heredity.

CHYME Semifluid thick mass consisting of food broken down by the digestive action of gastric juices in the stomach; passes into the small intestine.

CIS FORM A term indicating that certain atoms or groups of atoms, relative to a double bond between two carbon atoms, are on the "same side" of a molecule.

CODON A three-nucleotide unit that represents the code for the production of a specific amino acid in the process of protein synthesis.

COENZYME A nonprotein compound that functions to activate an enzyme.

COMPLETE PROTEIN A term for dietary protein that contains all of the essential amino acids in amounts sufficient for growth and maintenance.

COMPOUND A substance composed of two or more different elements (e.g., CO_2, H_2O).

CONDENSATION REACTION A chemical reaction in which two or more molecules combine.

CONTROLLED EXPERIMENT An experiment characterized by a "test group" and a "control group." Experimental conditions are identical for both groups except for a single condition or factor (e.g., a food item). Comparison of results of the test group with those of the control group should reveal the effect (if any) of the test factor or condition.

CRYSTALLINE Resembling a crystal (a solid body in which atoms are arranged in a symmetrical pattern).

CULTURE A patterned set of reactions, habits, customs, and ways of life that are characteristic of a particular group of people.

CYTOPLASM The viscous fluid surrounding the cell nucleus and containing cellular organelles.

DEAMINATION Removal of an amino group ($—NH_2$) from a molecule. Some amino acids can be converted to glucose in a process that begins with deamination.

DECARBOXYLATION Removal of a single carbon (in the form of CO_2) from a molecule. Decarboxylation reactions play an important part in the metabolism of glucose.

DEFICIENCY As used in nutrition, a term for inadequate dietary intake of a nutrient. The effect of a dietary deficiency depends on the degree of deficiency and on the function of the nutrient in the body.

DENATURATION The disruption of the structural arrangement of the atoms in a protein molecule.

DEOXYRIBONUCLEIC ACID (DNA) The hereditary material found in chromosomes.

DESCRIPTIVE EVIDENCE A set of facts that "describes" or summarizes a phenomenon. Also called "anecdotal evidence," it consists essentially of casual impressions rather than recorded data. (Compare *epidemiological evidence; experimental evidence.*)

DIABETES MELLITUS A disease resulting from impaired production of insulin. Hyperglycemia is one of its distinguishing symptoms.

DIET The food and drink an individual usually consumes; (2) A food regimen.

DIETARY RECALL A technique of dietary evaluation in which subjects are asked for specific details of their diet during the preceding 24 hours.

DIFFUSION The passive movement of substances from an area of high concentration to one of low concentration. Water and certain water-soluble nutrient molecules enter the cells of the intestinal lining via diffusion.

DIGESTION The process by which food substances are broken down into smaller units—mechanically and chemically—for absorption into the body.

DIGESTIVE SYSTEM The specific group of organs responsible for the digestion and absorption of food substances. Major organs of this system include the esophagus, stomach, and intestine.

DIGLYCERIDE A glycerol ester having two fatty acids; a lipid.

DIRECT CALORIMETRY Determination of the amount of heat released by the body.

DISACCHARIDE A sugar molecule formed by a condensation reaction between two monosaccharides.

DISACCHARIDASE One of a group of enzymes that hydrolyze disaccharides. Found in the cells of the brush border.

EDEMA Tissue swelling caused by an excess of fluid in the interstitial space; seen in thiamin and protein deficiency, as well as some other medical conditions.

ELECTROLYTE A substance that in solution is capable of conducting an electric current.

ELECTRON Negatively charged particle that revolves about the nucleus of an atom. Its mass is negligible, but its negative charge exactly balances the single positive charge of one proton.

ELEMENT A substance consisting of only one kind of atom (e.g., oxygen, iron, carbon, hydrogen).

EMBDEN-MEYERHOF PATHWAY Glycolysis; also known as the anaerobic pathway.

EMULSIFICATION Any process by which a water-insoluble substance is made more soluble. An emulsifier contains both water- and fat-soluble groups. It thus acts as a "bridge" between two substances that would not otherwise mix.

ENDOCRINE SYSTEM The system of organs (glands) that secrete hormones into the blood.

ENDOPEPTIDASE One of a group of enzymes that hydrolyze dietary proteins by breaking internal peptide bonds.

ENDOPLASMIC RETICULUM (ER) An intracellular system of membranous channels that transport materials throughout the cell. Smooth ER has no ribosomes attached to it; rough ER does.

ENERGY The capacity to do work. Energy is measured in terms of kilocalories or kilojoules. 4.184 joules = 1 calorie; 4.184 kilojoules = 1 kilocalorie (1 Calorie).

ENTEROHEPATIC CIRCULATION The return of bile components to the circulation and the liver from the intestine.

ENZYME A specialized protein molecule that catalyzes a biochemical reaction.

EPIDEMIOLOGICAL EVIDENCE Evidence based on the occurrence and distribution of a factor or factors associated with a particular phenomenon in a population (e.g., the association of heart disease and obesity).

EPINEPHRINE An important hormone produced by the adrenal glands. Under conditions of stress it stimulates the autonomic nervous system and glycogenolysis. (Also known as adrenalin.)

ESOPHAGUS The muscular canal through which food passes from the mouth to the stomach.

ESSENTIAL As applied to nutrition, an essential substance is one that the body requires for growth and maintenance but cannot synthesize in adequate amounts.

ESTER A compound resulting from the combination of an alcohol and an acid. Lipids are esters formed from alcohols and fatty acids.

ESTERIFICATION The process of forming an ester from an alcohol and an acid.

ETIOLOGY The origins or causes of a disease.

EVIDENCE Facts and information that support or refute a hypothesis. (See *descriptive evidence; epidemiological evidence; experimental evidence.*)

EXPERIMENTAL EVIDENCE Evidence derived from controlled experiments designed to test the validity of a scientific hypothesis.

EXPERIMENTAL MODEL A nonhuman system used in research studies. The most common such models in nutritional research are animals. (See *animal model.*)

EXTERNAL ENVIRONMENT The environment in which an organism exists (i.e., the environment outside an organism). (See *internal environment.*)

EXTRACELLULAR COMPARTMENT The approximately 40 percent of total body water that is found outside of cells. Consists of intravascular, interstitial, and transcellular fluids.

FATS Mixture of glycerides (esters of glycerol and fatty acids); commonly, lipids that are solid at room temperature (e.g., butter).

FAT-SOLUBLE VITAMINS Vitamins A, D, E, and K. Because of their chemical nature, they may accumulate in the body.

FATTY ACID An organic molecule; consists of a carbon and hydrogen chain with a carboxyl (acid) group at one end.

FIBER The indigestible remnant of dietary carbohydrate; dietary fiber.

FILTRATION (HYDROSTATIC PRESSURE) Fluid pressure in the blood vessels generated by the pumping action of the heart.

FOOD A collection of nutrients in a form which is eaten, digested, and metabolized to provide energy and materials that build and maintain the structure and regulate the function of the body.

FOOD CHAIN A scheme or sequence of feeding relationships that link member species of a biological community (e.g.: grass, zebra, lion).

FOODWAY A stylized food habit that has evolved as an adaptation to the physical and social environment.

FREE FATTY ACID A fatty acid released from adipose tissue by hydrolysis of a triglyceride.

FRUCTOSE A 6-carbon monosaccharide found in many fruits. Also known as levulose, or fruit sugar.

FUNCTIONAL GROUP An atom or group of atoms that determine or greatly influence the chemical behavior of the molecule to which it is attached.

GALACTOSE A 6-carbon monosaccharide; major component of lactose, or milk sugar.

GASTRIC JUICES The mixture of hydrochloric acid and digestive enzymes secreted by the glands in the lining of the stomach.

GLUCAGON A pancreatic hormone that triggers the breakdown of glycogen stored in the liver and other tissues.

GLUCONEOGENESIS Synthesis of glucose from a noncarbohydrate precursor.

GLUCOSE A 6-carbon monosaccharide also known as dextrose, or corn sugar. Found in sweet fruits and certain vegetables.

GLYCERIDE A glycerol ester formed from glycerol and a fatty acid. Mono-, di-, and triglycerides contain one, two, and three fatty acids, respectively. Glycerides constitute a major class of lipids.

GLYCEROL An important molecule (derived from glucose metabolism) from which glycerides are formed by combination with a fatty acid. (See *ester.*)

GLYCOGEN The only polysaccharide of animal origin. Stored as an energy source in some tissues; manufactured during glucose metabolism in humans.

GLYCOGENESIS The production of glycogen in the body. Glycogen is the storage form of carbohydrate in animals.

GLYCOLYSIS The production of energy from the anaerobic breakdown of glucose. Also known as the anaerobic pathway.

GOLGI BODY Cell organelle that functions in the "packaging" and storage of chemical substances before they are secreted.

GRADIENT A progressive change (either an increase or a decrease) in a physical quantity (e.g., concentration) over a specific distance.

HEME The iron-containing complex of the hemoglobin molecule.

HEXOSE A monosaccharide that contains six carbons (e.g., glucose).

HOMEOSTASIS The maintenance of a constant internal environment; the set of physiological mechanisms that maintains this environment as a constant.

HORMONE A specialized chemical substance secreted into the blood by an organ or by specific cells of an organ and which has a specific effect on "target" cells at some distance from the secreting organ.

HOUSEHOLD SURVEY In nutritional studies, a method of dietary evaluation in which a trained interviewer visits the home to obtain information about household use of foods.

HUNGER The sensation produced by the physiological need for food.

HYDROCARBON An organic compound that contains only the elements hydrogen and carbon.

HYDROGENATION A process of adding hydrogen to polyunsaturated oils to solidify them. Margarine, for example, contains hydrogenated vegetable oils.

HYDROLYSIS A reaction in which a chemical bond is split by the addition of a molecule of water.

HYPERGLYCEMIA A higher-than-normal concentration of glucose in the blood.

HYPERVITAMINOSIS Any condition resulting from the consumption (or administration) of excessive amounts of a vitamin.

HYPOGLYCEMIA A lower-than-normal concentration of glucose in the blood.

HYPOTHESIS Explanation advanced to account for an observation. In scientific research a hypothesis must be confirmed by at least one controlled experiment before it can be accepted as a valid explanation.

INCOMPLETE PROTEIN Dietary protein that contains less than the optimal amounts of essential amino acids.

INDIRECT CALORIMETRY Measurement of the amount of oxygen consumed (which is an index of the amount of energy liberated as heat).

IMINO ACID Organic acid having an imino group (—NH). (Compare *amino acid,* NH_2.)

INSULIN A pancreatic hormone that plays a crucial role in glucose metabolism. Any interference with the production or function of this hormone will produce symptoms of diabetes mellitus.

INTERNAL ENVIRONMENT The set of conditions, processes, and substances that are found inside an organism. The nutritional health of an organism is largely a function of the interaction between the internal and the external environment.

INTERNATIONAL UNITS (IU) A standard unit that represents the biologic activity of a nutrient.

INTERSTITIAL FLUID Together with transcellular fluids accounts for 80 percent of all extracellular fluid in the body (e.g., fluids that bathe all cells, saliva, etc.)

INTESTINAL LIPASE An enzyme that hydrolyzes medium- and short-chain triglycerides to glycerol plus short- and medium-chain fatty acids.

INTRACELLULAR COMPARTMENT The approximately 60 percent of body water that is contained in cells.

INTRAVASCULAR FLUID The liquid component of the blood; constitutes 20 percent of the extracellular fluid in the body.

IN VITRO Literally "on glass;" a reference to experiments performed outside the living organism.

ION Any atom that has lost one or more electrons (becoming a positively charged cation) or gained one or more electrons (becoming a negatively charged anion).

ISOMER One of two or more compounds that are identical in chemical composition but differ in structure.

JOULE A unit of energy measurement. 4.184 joules = 1 calorie; 4.184 kilojoules = 1 kilocalorie.

KETONE BODIES Fatty-acid derivatives that can function as energy-sources.

KETOSIS Excessive accumulation of ketone bodies caused by accelerated rate of tissue lipolysis.

KILOCALORIE The basic unit of energy in nutrition. The amount of energy (heat) required to raise the temperature of 1 liter of water from 15 to 16 degrees Celsius.

KREBS CYCLE The aerobic pathway for oxidation of carbohydrate, protein, and lipid to CO_2, H_2O, and energy.

LACTASE An enzyme required for the digestion of lactose (milk sugar).

LACTEAL A specialized lymph vessel in a villus.

LACTOSE Milk sugar; a disaccharide produced from the condensation of glucose and galactose. It is the only significant dietary carbohydrate of animal origin.

LEAN BODY MASS A measure of body composition; fat-free body weight.

LECITHIN Any of group of phospholipids. An important emulsifier.

LIPID One of a major class of nutrients; any one of a group of fats or fat-like substances.

LIPOGENESIS The process by which lipids are synthesized in the body.

LIPOLYSIS The breakdown of triglycerides to glycerol and fatty acids.

LIPOPROTEIN A molecule consisting of a lipid and a protein; involved in lipid transport in the blood.

LYSOSOME Cell organelle. A membrane-bound vesicle containing digestive enzymes that break down intracellular products and debris.

MACRONUTRIENT A nutrient substance or element required in large quantity (100 milligrams or more per day).

MAJOR (MACRO-) MINERALS Dietary minerals required in amounts of 100 milligrams or more per day. (See *trace mineral.*)

MALTOSE A disaccharide consisting of two glucose units. It is an intermediate product formed in the breakdown of starch in human digestion.

MATTER Anything that occupies space and has mass (or weight).

MEDIUM The substance or material in which anything moves or acts.

MEGAVITAMIN THERAPY Consumption or administration of vitamins in dosages exceeding RDAs by a factor of 10 or more.

MENARCHE The onset of menstruation in girls; the first occurrence of menstruation.

METABOLIC DISTURBANCE Any disruption of the normal processes of anabolism or catabolism.

METABOLIC WASTES The unusable endproducts of anabolic and catabolic processes which are excreted from the body.

METABOLISM A term that refers to all the chemical processes that occur in the body from the time nutrients are absorbed until they are utilized or excreted. (See *anabolism; catabolism.*)

METRIC SYSTEM A system of quantitative units based on multiples of 10.

MICELLE A specialized aggregate of monoglycerides, fatty acids, cholesterol, phospholipids, and bile.

MICRONUTRIENT A vitamin or mineral required in trace amounts for health and growth.

MICROVILLI Cylindrical outgrowths from villi and surrounding epithelial cells. They constitute the brush border, and function in absorpiton.

MINERALS A group of inorganic nutrients that includes Na, K, P, S, Ca, and Fe.

MITOCHONDRION (plural: mitochondria). Cell organelle that functions as the site of respiratory reactions involved in energy production.

MOLECULE A particle consisting of two or more atoms. The atoms may be the same element (as in O_2) or different elements (as in H_2O and CO_2).

MONOGLYCERIDE A glycerol ester containing one fatty acid.

MONOSACCHARIDE Any "simple sugar"—i.e., a sugar of the general formula $C_n (H_2O)_n$. Classes of monosaccharides are distinguished by the number of carbons they contain (e.g., hexoses all contain six carbons).

MONOUNSATURATED FATTY ACID A fatty acid with one double bond.

NATURAL FOOD As defined by the Federal Trade Commission, any food that is minimally processed and contains no artifical ingredients.

NET PROTEIN UTILIZATION (NPU) Proportion of dietary nitrogen that is retained by the body; an index of protein quality.

NEUTRON Electrically neutral particle located in the nucleus of the atom.

NONFASTING REACTIVE HYPOGLYCEMIA The most common form of hypoglycemia. Symptoms appear two to five hours after meals and are short-lived.

NORMOGLYCEMIA The condition of having normal levels of blood glucose.

NUCLEIC ACIDS DNA (deoxyribonucleic acid) and RNA (ribonucleic acid) found in the cell nucleus.

NUCLEOTIDE The basic structural unit of nucleic acid; consists of a purine or pyrimidine base combined with a sugar and phosphoric acid.

NUCLEUS, ATOMIC The central core of any atom, containing one or more protons and (except for hydrogen) one or more neutrons, contains almost all of the mass of the atom.

NUCLEUS, CELL A membrane-bound cluster of materials that functions to regulate the major activities of the cell; contains the chromosomes and the nucleolus.

NUTRIENTS Nutritional substances found in food. These are: four classes of organic compounds (carbohydrates, proteins, lipids, and vitamins), minerals, and water.

NUTRITION A term that has two meanings: (1) nutritional science, or the study of nutritional processes; (2) the overall process in which food substances are taken into the body and there transformed and utilized for the proper functioning of the body.

NUTRITIONAL ANTHROPOLOGY A new discipline concerned with patterns of food acquisition and consumption.

OBESITY An accumulation of body fat such that actual body weight exceeds ideal body weight by 20 percent or more.

OIL A lipid that is liquid at room temperature (e.g., corn oil).

OLIGOSACCHARIDE A term sometimes used in referring to a carbohydrate consisting of two to ten monosaccharide units.

ORGAN A part of an organism, consisting of one or more tissues organized to perform a specific function.

ORGANELLE Subcellular structure that performs a specialized function in a cell (e.g., ribosome).

ORGANIC CHEMISTRY The chemistry of carbon-containing compounds.

ORGANIC COMPOUND Carbon-containing compound. Four classes of such compounds are major nutrients: carbohydrates, proteins, lipids, and vitamins.

ORGANIC FOODS A general term for foods grown by methods that do not use pesticides or chemical fertilizers.

ORGANISM A living thing capable of performing all life processes; may be unicellular (bacteria) or multicellular (plants and animals).

ORTHOMOLECULAR MEDICINE A term used to describe treatment based on large amounts of naturally occurring substances (e.g., vitamins). Not an accepted medical practice.

-OSE A suffix indicating a carbohydrate.

OSMOSIS The movement of water molecules through a membrane.

OSMOTIC PRESSURE The pressure that develops when two solutions with different concentrations of solute are separated by a membrane that is permeable only to the solvent.

OSSIFICATION The process of bone formation.

OXIDATION A chemical reaction that involves the addition of oxygen or the removal of hydrogen or electrons.

PASSIVE TRANSPORT A process of diffusion by which substances move from one compartment to another down a concentration gradient; does not require energy.

PENTOSE A monosaccharide containing five carbon atoms.

PEPSIN The primary digestive enzyme produced in the stomach; a proteolytic enzyme.

PERISTALSIS Rhythmic contraction of muscles of the gastrointestinal tract that aid in propelling through the digestive system.

PH A chemical measure of relative acidity. A pH value of less than 7 is acidic; more than 7, basic. Physiological pH is 7.4.

PHOSPHOLIPID A glyceride with fatty acids and a phosphate-containing group (e.g., lecithin).

PHYTATE A phosphate-containing compound found in the outer husk of certain cereals; reduces the absorption of calcium and other minerals.

PICA A craving for nonfood items (e.g., clay).

PLASMA MEMBRANE The membrane surrounding the cell. It functions to regulate the passage of substances into and out of the cell.

POLYMERS A general term for a large molecule consisting of many smaller molecules (or monomers) that are identical or may be of several different types. Polysaccharides are polymers, as are plastics.

POLYPEPTIDE A chain of amino acids linked by peptide bonds.

POLYSACCHARIDE A carbohydrate containing more than ten monosaccharides; also termed a "complex carbohydrate," in contrast to a simple sugar.

POLYUNSATURATED FATTY ACID (PUFA) A fatty acid with two or more double bonds.

PRECURSOR In chemistry, a precursor of substance X is a compound that is transformed into X by one or several chemical reactions. (e.g., B-carotene is a precursor of vitamin A.).

PRIMARY DEFICIENCY A nutrient deficiency condition resulting directly from inadequate dietary intake.

PROTEIN One of six major classes of nutrients; an organic compound consisting of amino acids linked by peptide bonds. Proteins perform a wide variety of structural and functional roles in the body.

PROTEIN EFFICIENCY RATIO (PER) Biologic method of estimating protein quality; defined as weight gain per amount of protein consumed.

PROTEIN-ENERGY MALNUTRITION (PEM) A condition caused by insufficient protein and energy intake; characterized by retarded growth, weight loss, listlessness.

PROTEIN QUALITY A measure of the biologic efficiency of dietary protein; depends on the kinds and amounts of amino acids contained in the protein.

PROTEIN TURNOVER A term for the breakdown and replacement of protein.

PROTON Positively charged particle located in the nucleus of the atom.

PTYALIN An enzyme, found in saliva, that breaks down starch to simple sugars. Also known as salivary amylase.

PYRUVATE A metabolic intermediate formed from glucose in glycolysis, and from the deamination of alanine.

RESPIRATORY QUOTIENT The ratio of the volume of CO_2 exhaled to the amount of O_2 inhaled.

RESPIROMETER An instrument used to measure CO_2 exhaled and O_2 inhaled.

RIBONUCLEIC ACID (RNA) A nucleic acid which plays an important role in protein synthesis (messenger, ribosomal and transfer RNA).

RIBOSOME Small cellular organelle that functions as the site for protein synthesis. Ribosomes are found free in the cytoplasm and attached to the endoplasmic reticulum.

RING STRUCTURE As used in this text, a diagram for conveniently representing certain large, complex molecules.

SATURATED FATTY ACID A fatty acid all of whose carbon atoms are bound to four other atoms with single bonds (containing no double bonds).

SCIENTIFIC METHOD A general term for the steps and procedures that scientists follow in developing and testing an explanation (or hypothesis) of observed phenomena. Involves experimentation leading to evidence.

SECONDARY DEFICIENCY A nutrient deficiency caused by some factor other than inadequate ingestion of nutrients (e.g., result of malabsorption or effect of medication).

SIMPLE CARBOHYDRATE A general term for a monosaccharide or a disaccharide.

SKINFOLD THICKNESS An index of body-fat accumulation, determined by measuring the thickness of a fold of skin.

SOLUTE A substance dissolved in another substance (known as the solvent).

SOLVENT A substance in which another substance (known as the solute) is dissolved.

SPECIFIC DYNAMIC EFFECT (SDE) The increase in metabolic rate observed after the digestion, absorption, and metabolism of food.

STEATORRHEA Excess lipid in the feces. May be caused by any of several factors which impair fat digestion and absorption.

SUBSTRATE Any substance on which an enzyme acts chemically.

SUCROSE Table sugar; a disaccharide produced by condensation of glucose and fructose. A widely distributed plant sugar.

SUPERNUTRITION Any dietary regimen of specialized foods and nutritional supplements designed to increase the quality of body functioning, especially in athletic contests. Usually not necessary.

TARGET ORGAN An organ whose metabolic function responds to a hormone in a specific way.

TISSUE An aggregation of cells of the same type, such as muscle tissue, epithelial tissue, and nerve tissue.

TOXEMIA Any condition in which the blood contains toxic substances; toxemia of pregnancy is a condition characterized by edema, high blood pressure, and protein in the urine (albuminuria).

TRACE MINERALS Dietary minerals required in amounts no greater than a few milligrams per day.

TRANSCELLULAR FLUID Together with interstitial fluid accounts for 80 percent of all extracellular fluid in the body (e.g., fluids that bathe all cells, saliva, etc.).

TRANS FORM A term indicating that certain atoms or groups of atoms relative to a double bond between two carbon atoms, are on "opposite sides" of the molecule.

TRIGLYCERIDE A glycerol ester containing three fatty acids.

UNSATURATED FATTY ACID A fatty acid that contains one or more double bonds.

UREA The endproduct of protein metabolism that is excreted in urine.

VALENCE SHELL The "shell" of an atom that contains those electrons involved in reactions with other atoms. The outermost electron shell.

VEGETARIANISM The practice of consuming a diet consisting exclusively or almost exclusively of plant foods and plant products.

VILLI (SING.: VILLUS) Small, finger-like projections that line the small intestine. Function in absorption of nutrients into the body.

VITAMINS A major class of nutrients, consisting of two types—fat-soluble and water-soluble.

WATER An important nutrient containing hydrogen and oxygen.

WATER INTOXICATION A potentially fatal condition caused by an intake of fluid that exceeds the maximum rate of urinary flow.

WAX A lipid with a high melting point; composed of esters of fatty acids with an alcohol other than glycerol.

APPENDIX

APPENDIX A

Recommended Dietary Allowances[a]

	Age (years)	Weight (kg)	Weight (lbs)	Height (cm	Height (In)	Energy needs (kcal)[b]	Protein (g)	Fat-Soluble Vitamins: Vitamin A (μg RE)[c]	Vitamin D (μg)[d]	Vitamin E (mg α T.E.)[e]
Infants	0.0-0.5	6	13	60	24	kg x 115	kg x 2.2	420	10	3
	0.5-1.0	9	20	71	28	kg x 105	kg x 2.0	400	10	4
Children	1-3	13	29	90	35	1300	23	400	10	5
	4-6	20	44	112	44	1700	30	500	10	6
	7-10	28	62	132	52	2400	34	700	10	7
Males	11-14	45	99	157	62	2700	45	1000	10	8
	15-18	66	145	176	69	2800	56	1000	10	10
	19-22	70	154	177	70	2900	56	1000	7.5	10
	23-50	70	154	178	70	2700	56	1000	5	10
	51-75	70	154	178	70	2400[i]	56	1000	5	10
Females	11-14	46	101	157	62	2200	46	800	10	8
	15-18	55	120	163	64	2100	46	800	10	8
	19-22	55	120	163	64	2100	44	800	7.5	8
	23-50	55	120	163	64	2000[j]	44	800	5	8
	51-75	55	120	163	64	1800	44	800	5	8
Pregnant						+300	+30	+200	+5	+2
Lactating						+500	+20	+400	+5	+3

[a] The allowances are intended to provide for individual variations among most normal persons as they live in the United States under usual environmental stresses. Diets should be based on a variety of common foods in order to provide other nutrients for which human requirements have been less well defined.

[b] Energy allowances for children through age 18 are based on median energy intakes of children these ages followed in longitudinal growth studies. The energy allowances for younger adults are for men and women doing light work. Over age 51 the allowances represent mean energy needs, allowing for a 2% decrease in basal (resting) metabolic rate per decade and a reduction in activity. At any age there is a variation in energy needs.

[c] Retinol equivalents, 1 Retinol equivalent = 1 μg retinol or 6 μg βcarotene.

[d] As cholecalciferol. 10 μg cholecalciferol = 400 I.U. vitamin D.

[e] α tocopherol equivalents, 1 mg d-α-tocopherol = 1α T.E.

[f] 1 N.E. (niacin equivalent) is equal to 1 mg of niacin or 60 mg of dietary tryptophan.

Estimated Safe and Adequate Daily Dietary Intakes of Additional Selected Vitamins and Minerals[a]

	Age (years)	Vitamins: Vitamin K (μg)	Biotin (μg)	Pantothenic Acid (mg)	Copper (mg)	Manganese (mg)
Infants	0 - 0.5	12	35	2	0.5 - 0.7	0.5 - 0.7
	0.5 - 1	10 - 20	50	3	0.7 - 1.0	0.7 - 1.0
Children	1 - 3	15 - 30	65	3	1.0 - 1.5	1.0 - 1.5
and	4 - 6	20 - 40	85	3 - 4	1.5 - 2.0	1.5 - 2.0
Adolescents	7 - 10	30 - 60	120	4 - 5	2.0 - 2.5	2.0 - 3.0
	11+	50 - 100	100 - 200	4 - 7	2.0 - 3.0	2.5 - 5.0
Adults		70 - 140	100 - 200	4 - 7	2.0 - 3.0	2.5 - 5.0

[a] Because there is less information on which to base allowances, these figures are provided here in the form of ranges of recommended intakes.

[b] Since the toxic levels for many trace minerals may be only several times usual intakes, the upper levels for the trace minerals given in this table should not be habitually exceeded.

Water-Soluble Vitamins							Minerals					
Vitamin C (mg)	*Thiamin (mg)*	*Riboflavin (mg)*	*Niacin (mg N.E.)*[f]	*Vitamin B_6 (mg)*	*Folacin*[g] *(μg)*	*Vitamin B_{12} (μg)*[h]	*Calcium (mg)*	*Phosphorus (mg)*	*Magnesium (mg)*	*Iron (mg)*	*Zinc (mg)*	*Iodine (μg)*
35	0.3	0.4	6	0.3	30	0.5	360	240	50	10	3	40
35	0.5	0.6	8	0.6	45	1.5	540	360	70	15	5	50
45	0.7	0.8	9	0.9	100	2.0	800	800	150	15	10	70
45	0.9	1.0	11	1.3	200	2.5	800	800	200	10	10	90
45	1.2	1.4	16	1.6	300	3.0	800	800	250	10	10	120
50	1.4	1.6	18	1.8	400	3.0	1200	1200	350	18	15	150
60	1.4	1.7	18	2.0	400	3.0	1200	1200	400	18	15	150
60	1.5	1.7	19	2.2	400	3.0	800	800	350	10	15	150
60	1.4	1.6	18	2.2	400	3.0	800	800	350	10	15	150
60	1.2	1.4	16	2.2	400	3.0	800	800	350	10	15	150
50	1.1	1.3	15	1.8	400	3.0	1200	1200	300	18	15	150
60	1.1	1.3	14	2.0	400	3.0	1200	1200	300	18	15	150
60	1.1	1.3	14	2.0	400	3.0	800	800	300	18	15	150
60	1.0	1.2	13	2.0	400	3.0	800	800	300	18	15	150
60	1.0	1.2	13	2.0	400	3.0	800	800	300	10	15	150
+20	+0.4	+0.3	+2	+0.6	+400	+1.0	+400	+400	+150	i	+5	+25
+40	+0.5	+0.5	+5	+0.5	+100	+1.0	+400	+400	+150	i	+10	+50

[g] The folacin allowances refer to dietary sources as determined by *Lactobacillus casei* assay after treatment with enzymes ("conjugases") to make polyglutamyl forms of the vitamin available to the test organism.

[h] The RDA for vitamin B_{12} in infants is based on average concentration of the vitamin in human milk. The allowances after weaning are based on energy intake (as recommended by the American Academy of Pediatrics) and consideration of other factors such as intestinal absorption.

[i] Over age 75,2050 kcal.

[j] Over age 75,1600 kcal.

[k] The increased requirement during pregnancy cannot be met by the iron content of habitual American diets nor by the existing iron stores of many women; therefore the use of 30-60 mg of supplemental iron is recommended. Iron needs during lactation are not substantially different from those of non-pregnant women, but continued supplementation of the mother for 2-3 months after parturition is advisable in order to replenish stores depleted by pregnancy.

Source: Recommended Dietary Allowances, Revised 1979. Food and Nutrition Board, National Academy of Sciences-National Research Council, Washington, D.C.

Trace Minerals[b]						
Fluoride (mg)	*Chromium (mg)*	*Selenium (mg)*	*Molybdenum (mg)*	*Sodium (mg)*	*Potassium (mg)*	*Chloride (mg)*
0.1 - 0.5	0.01 - 0.04	0.01 - 0.04	0.03 - 0.06	115 - 350	350 - 925	275 - 700
0.2 - 1.0	0.02 - 0.06	0.02 - 0.06	0.04 - 0.08	250 - 750	425 - 1275	400 - 1200
0.5 - 1.5	0.02 - 0.08	0.02 - 0.08	0.05 - 0.1	325 - 975	550 - 1650	500 - 1500
1.0 - 2.5	0.03 - 0.12	0.03 - 0.12	0.06 - 0.15	450 - 1350	775 - 2325	700 - 2100
1.5 - 2.5	0.05 - 0.2	0.05 - 0.2	0.1 - 0.3	600 - 1800	1000 - 3000	925 - 2775
1.5 - 2.5	0.05 - 0.2	0.05 - 0.2	0.15 - 0.5	900 - 2700	1525 - 4575	1400 - 4200
1.5 - 4.0	0.05 - 0.2	0.05 - 0.2	0.15 - 0.5	1100 - 3300	1875 - 5625	1700 - 5100

Source: Recommended Dietary Allowances, Revised 1979. Food and Nutrition Board, National Academy of Sciences-National Research Council, Washington, D.C.

APPENDIX B

Dietary Standards for Canada

Age (years)	Sex	Weight (kg)	Height (cm)	Energy[a] (kcal)	Protein (g)	Fat soluble vitamins: Vit. A (μg RE)[b]	Fat soluble vitamins: Vit. D (μg cholecalciferol)[c]	Fat soluble vitamins: Vit. E (mg α-tocopherol)	Thiamin (mg)
0.0–0.5	Both	6	—	kg x 117	kg x 2.2 (2.0)[g]	400	10	3	0.3
0.5–1	Both	9	—	kg x 108	kg x 1.4	400	10	3	0.5
1-3	Both	13	90	1400	22	400	10	4	0.7
4-6	Both	19	110	1800	27	500	5	5	0.9
7-9	M	27	129	2200	33	700	2.5[j]	6	1.1
	F	27	128	2000	33	700	2.5[j]	6	1.0
10-12	M	36	144	2500	41	800	2.5[j]	7	1.2
	F	38	145	2300	40	800	2.5[j]	7	1.1
13-15	M	51	162	2800	52	1000	2.5[j]	9	1.4
	F	49	159	2200	43	800	2.5[j]	7	1.1
16-18	M	64	172	3200	54	1000	2.5[j]	10	1.6
	F	54	161	2100	43	800	2.5[j]	6	1.1
19-35	M	70	176	3000	56	1000	2.5[j]	9	1.5
	F	56	161	2100	41	800	2.5[j]	6	1.1
36-50	M	70	176	2700	56	1000	2.5[j]	8	1.4
	F	56	161	1900	41	800	2.5[j]	6	1.0
51+	M	70	176	2300[k]	56	1000	2.5[j]	8	1.4
	F	56	161	1800[k]	41	800	2.5[j]	6	1.0
Pregnant				+300[l]	+20	+100	+2.5[j]	+1	+0.2
Lactating				+500	+24	+400	+2.5[j]	+2	+0.4

Source: Canadian Council on Nutrition: *Dietary standards for Canada,* Can. Bull. Nutr. 6.1, 1964 (suppl. 1974).

[a] Recommendations assume characteristic activity pattern for each age group.

[b] One μg retinol equivalent (1 μg RE) corresponds to a biological activity in humans equal to 1 μg of retinol (3.33 IU) and 6 μg of β-carotene (10 IU).

[c] One μg cholecalciferol is equivalent to 40 IU vitamin D activity.

[d] Approximately 1 mg of niacin is derived from each 60 mg of dietary tryptophan.

[e] Recommendations are based on the estimated average daily protein intake of Canadians.

[f] Recommendation given in terms of free folate.

[g] Recommended protein allowance of 2.2 g/kg of body weight for infants age 0 to 2 mo and 2.0 g/kg of body weight for those age 3 to 5 mo. Protein recommendation for infants, 0 to 11 mo, assumes consumption of breastmilk or protein of equivalent quality.

Water-soluble vitamins						Minerals					
Niacin[d] *(mg)*	*Riboflavin (mg)*	*Vit.* B_6[e] *(mg)*	*Folate*[f] *(μg)*	*Vit.* B_{12} *(μg)*	*Ascorbic acid (mg)*	*Ca (mg)*	*P (mg)*	*Mg (mg)*	*I (μg)*	*Fe (mg)*	*Zn (mg)*
5	0.4	0.3	40	0.3	20[h]	500[i]	250[i]	50[i]	35[i]	7[i]	4[i]
6	0.6	0.4	60	0.3	20	500	400	50	50	7	5
9	0.8	0.8	100	0.9	20	500	500	75	70	8	5
12	1.1	1.3	100	1.5	20	500	500	100	90	9	6
14	1.3	1.6	100	1.5	30	700	700	150	110	10	7
13	1.2	1.4	100	1.5	30	700	700	150	100	10	7
17	1.5	1.8	100	3.0	30	900	900	175	130	11	8
15	1.4	1.5	100	3.0	30	1000	1000	200	120	11	9
19	1.7	2.0	200	3.0	30	1200	1200	250	140	13	10
15	1.4	1.5	200	3.0	30	800	800	250	110	14	10
21	2.0	2.0	200	3.0	30	1000	1000	300	160	14	12
14	1.3	1.5	200	3.0	30	700	700	250	110	14	11
20	1.8	2.0	200	3.0	30	800	800	300	150	10	10
14	1.3	1.5	200	3.0	30	700	700	250	110	14	9
18	1.7	2.0	200	3.0	30	800	800	300	140	10	10
13	1.2	1.5	200	3.0	30	700	700	250	100	14	9
18	1.7	2.0	200	3.0	30	800	800	300	140	10	10
13	1.2	1.5	200	3.0	30	700	700	250	100	9	9
+2	+0.3	+0.5	+50	+1.0	+20	+500	+500	+25	+15	+1[m]	+3
+7	+0.6	+0.6	+50	+0.5	+30	+500	+500	+75	+25	+1[m]	+7

[h] Considerably higher levels may be prudent for infants during the first week of life to guard against neonatal tyrosinemia.

[i] The intake of breast-fed infants may be less than the recommendation but is considered to be adequate.

[j] Most older children and adults receive enough vitamin D from irradiation but 2.5 μg daily is recommended. This recommended allowance increases to 5.0 μg daily for pregnant and lactating women and for those who are confined indoors or otherwise deprived of sunlight for extended periods.

[k] Recommended energy allowance for age 66+ years reduced to 2000 for men and 1500 for women.

[l] Increased energy allowance recommended during second and third trimesters. An increase of 100 kcal per day is recommended during first trimester.

[m] A recommended total intake of 15 mg daily during pregnancy and lactation assumes the presence of adequate stores of iron. If stores are suspected of being inadequate, additional iron as a supplement is recommended.

APPENDIX C
United States Recommended Daily Allowances (U.S. RDA)[a]

	Adults and children 4 or more years of age[b]	Infants	Children under 4 years of age[c]	Pregnant or lactating women[c]
Nutrients which must be declared on the label (in the order below)				
Protein[d]	45 g "high quality protein" 65 g "proteins in general"		—	—
Vitamin A	5000 IU	1500 IU	2500 IU	8000 IU
Vitamin C (or ascorbic acid)	60 mg	35 mg	40 mg	60 mg
Thiamin (or vitamin B_1)	1.5 mg	0.5 mg	0.7 mg	1.7 mg
Riboflavin (or vitamin B_2)	1.7 mg	0.6 mg	0.8 mg	2.0 mg
Niacin	20 mg	8 mg	9 mg	20 mg
Calcium	1.0 g	0.6 g	0.8 g	1.3 g
Iron	18 mg	15 mg	10 mg	18 mg
Nutrients which may be declared on the label (in the order below)				
Vitamin D	400 IU	400 IU	400 IU	400 IU
Vitamin E	30 IU	5 IU	10 IU	30 IU
Vitamin B_6	2.0 mg	0.4 mg	0.7 mg	2.5 mg
Folic acid (or folacin)	0.4 mg	0.1 mg	0.2 mg	0.8 mg
Vitamin B_{12}	6 μg	2 μg	3 μg	8 μg
Phosphorus	1.0 g	0.5 g	0.8 g	1.3 g
Iodine	150 μg	45 μg	70 μg	150 μg
Magnesium	400 mg	70 mg	200 mg	450 mg
Zinc	15 mg	5 mg	8 mg	15 mg
Copper[e]	2 mg	0.5 mg	1 mg	2 mg
Biotin[e]	0.3 mg	0.15 mg	0.15 mg	0.3 mg
Pantothenic acid[e]	10 mg	3 mg	5 mg	10 mg

[a] The U.S. RDA values chosen are derived from the highest value within an age category for each nutrient given in the 1968 NAS-NRC tables except for calcium and phosphorus.

[b] For use in labeling conventional foods and also for "special dietary foods."

[c] For use only with "special dietary foods."

[d] "High quality protein" is defined as having a protein efficiency ratio (PER) equal to or greater than that of casein; "proteins in general" are those with a PER less than that of casein. Total protein with a PER less than 20% that of casein are considered "not a significant source of protein" and would not be expressed on the label in terms of the U.S. RDA but only as amount per serving.

[e] There are no NAS-NRC RDAs for biotin, pantothenic acid, zinc, and copper.

APPENDIX D
Desirable Weights for Adults 25 Years of Age and Over[a]

Women[b]				
Height with shoes on (2-inch heels)				
Feet	*Inches*	*Small frame*	*Medium frame*	*Large frame*
4	10	92-98	96-107	104-119
4	11	94-101	98-110	106-122
5	0	96-104	101-113	109-125
5	1	99-107	104-116	112-128
5	2	102-110	107-119	115-131
5	3	105-113	110-122	118-134
5	4	108-116	113-126	121-138
5	5	111-119	116-130	125-142
5	6	114-123	120-135	129-146
5	7	118-127	124-139	133-150
5	8	122-131	128-143	137-154
5	9	126-135	132-147	141-158
5	10	130-140	136-151	145-163
5	11	134-144	140-155	149-168
6	0	138-148	144-159	153-173

Men				
Height with shoes on (1-inch heels)				
Feet	*Inches*	*Small frame*	*Medium frame*	*Large frame*
5	2	112-120	118-129	126-141
5	3	115-123	121-133	129-144
5	4	118-126	124-136	132-148
5	5	121-129	127-139	135-152
5	6	124-133	130-143	138-156
5	7	128-137	134-147	142-161
5	8	132-141	138-152	147-166
5	9	136-145	142-156	151-170
5	10	140-150	146-160	155-174
5	11	144-154	150-165	159-179
6	0	148-158	154-170	164-184
6	1	152-162	158-175	168-189
6	2	156-167	162-180	173-194
6	3	160-171	167-185	178-199
6	4	164-175	172-190	182-204

[a] Weight in pounds, according to frame (in indoor clothing).
[b] For women between 18 and 24 years of age, subtract 1 pound for each year under 25.

Source: Metropolitan Life Insurance Company, **How to control your weight.** New York, 1960 supplement. Based on Build and Blood Pressure Study, 1959. (N.B.: Data from the 1979 Build and Blood Pressure Study of the Association of Life Insurance Medical Directors and the Society of Actuaries are not available as this volume goes to press; for more information write the Society at 208 South LaSalle Street, Chicago, IL 60604.)

APPENDIX E

Obesity Standards Based on Skin-Fold Thickness for Caucasian Americans

Triceps Skin-Fold Thickness Indicating Obesity (mm)					
Age (years)	*Males*	*Females*	*Age (years)*	*Males*	*Females*
5	12	14	18	15	27
6	12	15	19	15	27
7	13	16	20	16	28
8	14	17	21	17	28
9	15	18	22	18	28
10	16	20	23	18	28
11	17	21	24	19	28
12	18	22	25	20	29
13	18	23	26	20	29
14	17	23	27	21	29
15	16	24	28	22	29
16	15	25	29	22	29
17	14	26	30-50	23	30

Source: Seltzer, C. C. and J. Mayer, *A simple criterion of obesity.* Postgraduate Medicine 38: A-101, 1965.

APPENDIX F

Metric Conversion Factors Commonly Used in Nutrition

Unit	Multiply by
Length:	
centimeters to inches	0.394
centimeters to meters	0.010
foot to centimeters	30.480
foot to meter	0.305
inches to centimeters	2.540
meters to inches	39.370
meters to feet	3.281
Weight:	
grams to micrograms	1 million
grams to milligrams	1000
grams to ounces	0.035
grams to pounds	0.002
kilograms to pounds	2.2
ounces to grams	28.350
pounds to kilograms	0.454
Volume:	
milliliter to fluid ounce	0.034
fluid ounce to milliliter	29.574
liter to quart	1.057
quart to liter	0.946
Energy:	
kilocalorie to kilojoule	4.184
kilocalorie to megajoule	0.004
kilojoule to kilocalorie	0.239
megajoule to kilocalorie	239

Temperature

Fahrenheit to Centigrade (Celsius):
F° − 32°, multiply by 5/9
Centigrade (Celsius) to Fahrenheit:
Multiply C° by 9/5, add 32°
Examples:
32° F or 0° C (freezing temperature)
212° F or 100° C (boiling temperature)
98.6° F or 37.0° C (body temperature)

Abbreviations commonly used in Nutrition

kcal	= kilocalorie	dl	= deciliter
kJ	= kilojoule	qt	= quart
MJ	= megajoule	pt	= pint
kg	= kilogram	c	= cup
g	= gram	tbsp (T)	= tablespoon
mg	= milligram	tsp (t)	= teaspoon
μg (mcg)	= microgram	m	= meter
lb	= pound	cm	= centimeter
oz	= ounce	ft	= foot
l	= liter	in	= inch
ml	= milliliter		

APPENDIX G
Exchange Lists for Meal Planning

Meals are planned by figuring menus to include a selection from all exchange groups that adds up to an individual's daily energy requirement in kilocalories. Consumption of some foods will use exchanges in more than one group; a glass of whole milk, for example, represents 1 milk exchange plus 2 fat exchanges. Exchange Lists are discussed in Chapter 5.

Exchange lists are groups of measured foods that have approximately the same carbohydrate, protein, fat, and energy content, and can therefore be substituted for one another.

1. Milk Exchanges

One Milk Exchange equals 12 g carbohydrate, 8 g protein, trace fat, 80 kilocalories.

One Milk Exchange is the equivalent of 1 cup skim milk.

	One Milk Exchange
Nonfat fortified milk	
Skim or nonfat milk	1 cup
Powdered (nonfat dry, before adding liquid)	1/3 cup
Canned, evaporated-skim milk	1/2 cup
Buttermilk made from skim milk	1 cup
Yogurt made from skim milk (plain, unflavored)	1 cup
Low-fat fortified milk	
1% fat fortified milk (plus 1/2 Fat Exchange)	1 cup
2% fat fortified milk (plus 1 Fat Exchange)	1 cup
Yogurt made from 2% fortified milk (plain, unflavored) (plus 1 Fat Exchange)	1 cup
Whole milk (plus 2 Fat Exchanges)	
Whole milk	1 cup
Canned, evaporated whole milk	1/2 cup
Buttermilk made from whole milk	1 cup
Yogurt made from whole milk (plain, unflavored)	1 cup

2. Vegetable Exchanges

One Vegetable Exchange equals 5 g carbohydrate, 2 g protein, 25 kilocalories.

One vegetable exchange is 1/2 cup of the following:

Asparagus	Greens:
Bean sprouts	Mustard
Beets	Spinach
Broccoli	Turnip
Brussels sprouts	Mushrooms
Cabbage	Okra
Carrots	Onions
Cauliflower	Rhubarb
Celery	Rutabaga
Cucumbers	Sauerkraut
Eggplant	String beans, green or yellow
Green pepper	Summer squash
Greens:	Tomatoes
Beet	Tomato juice
Chard	Turnips
Collards	Vegetable juice cocktail
Dandelion	Zucchini
Kale	

The following vegetables may be eaten in any amount:

Chicory	Lettuce
Chinese cabbage	Parsley
Endive	Radishes
Escarole	Watercress

Note: starchy vegetables are listed under *Bread Exchanges.*

3. Fruit Exchanges

One Fruit Exchange equals 10 g carbohydrate, 40 kilocalories.

	One Fruit Exchange
Apple	1 small
Apple juice	1/3 cup
Applesauce (unsweetened)	1/2 cup
Apricots, fresh	2 medium
Apricots, dried	4 halves
Banana	1/2 small
Berries	
Blackberries	1/2 cup
Blueberries	1/2 cup
Raspberries	1/2 cup
Strawberries	3/4 cup
Cherries	10 large
Cider	1/3 cup
Dates	2
Figs, fresh	1
Figs, dried	1
Grapefruit	1
Grapefruit juice	1/2 cup
Grapes	12
Grape juice	1/4 cup
Mango	1/2 small
Melons	
Cantaloupe	1/4 small
Honeydew	1/8 medium
Watermelon	1 cup
Nectarine	1 small
Orange	1 small
Orange juice	1/2 cup
Papaya	3/4 cup
Peach	1 medium
Pear	1 small

Persimmon, native	1 medium
Pineapple	1/2 cup
Pineapple juice	1/3 cup
Plums	2 medium
Prunes	2 medium
Prune juice	1/4 cup
Raisins	2 tablespoons
Tangerine	1 medium

Cranberries have negligible carbohydrate and energy content if no sugar is added.

4. Bread Exchanges

(Includes bread, cereals, and starchy vegetables.)
One Bread Exchange equals 15 g carbohydrate, 2 g protein, 70 kilocalories.

	One Bread Exchange
Bread:	
White (including French and Italian)	1 slice
Whole wheat	1 slice
Rye or pumpernickel	1 slice
Raisin	1 slice
Bagel, small	1/2
English muffin, small	1/2
Plain roll, bread	1
Frankfurter roll	1/2
Hamburger bun	1/2
Dried bread crumbs	3 tablespoons
Tortilla, 6"	1
Crackers:	
Arrowroot	3
Graham, 2-1/2" square	2
Matzoth, 3" x 6-1/2"	1/2
Oyster	20
Pretzels, 3-1/8" long x 1/8" diameter	25
Rye wafers, 2" x 3-1/2"	3
Saltines	6
Soda, 2-1/2" square	4
Grains and Cereals:	
Bran flakes	1/2 cup
Other ready-to-eat-unsweetened cereal	3/4 cup
Puffed cereal (unfrosted)	1 cup
Cereal (cooked)	1/2 cup
Grits (cooked)	1/2 cup
Rice or barley (cooked)	1/2 cup
Pasta (cooked), spaghetti, noodles, macaroni	1/2 cup
Popcorn (popped, no fat added)	3 cups
Cornmeal (dry)	2 tablespoons
Flour	2-1/2 tablespoons
Wheat germ	1/4 cup
Dried Beans, Peas, and Lentils:	
Beans, peas, lentils (dried and cooked)	1/2 cup
Baked beans, no pork (canned)	1/4 cup
Starchy vegetables:	
Corn	1/3 cup
Corn on cob	1 small
Lima beans	1/2 cup
Parsnips	2/3 cup
Peas, green (fresh, canned or frozen)	1/2 cup
Potato, white	1 small
Potato, mashed	1/2 cup
Pumpkin	3/4 cup
Winter squash (acorn or butternut)	1/2 cup
Yam or sweet potato	1/4 cup
Prepared foods:	
Biscuit 2" diameter (plus 1 Fat Exchange)	1
Cornbread 2" x 2" x 1" (plus 1 Fat Exchange)	1
Corn muffin, 2" diameter (plus 1 Fat Exchange)	1
Crackers, round butter type (plus 1 Fat Exchange)	5
Muffin, plain small (plus 1 Fat Exchange)	1
Potatoes, French fried, length 2" to 3-1/2" (plus 1 Fat Exchange)	8
Potato or corn chips (plus 2 Fat Exchanges)	15
Pancake, 5" x 1/2" (plus 1 Fat Exchange)	1
Waffle, 5" x 1/2" (plus 1 Fat Exchange)	1

5. Meat Exchanges

Meat Exchanges are based on lean meat. One Lean Meat Exchange equals 7 g protein, 3 g fat, 55 kilocalories.

Lean Meat	*One Lean Meat Exchange*
Beef: baby beef (very lean), chipped beef, chuck, flank steak, tenderloin, plate ribs, plate skirt steak, round (bottom, top), all cuts rump, spare ribs, tripe	1 ounce
Lamb: leg rib, sirloin, loin (roast and chops), shank, shoulder	1 ounce
Pork: leg (whole rump, center shank), ham, smoked (center slices)	1 ounce
Veal: leg, loin, rib, shank, shoulder, cutlets	1 ounce
Poultry: meat without skin of chicken, turkey, cornish hen, guinea hen, pheasant	1 ounce
Fish:	
Any fresh or frozen	1 ounce

Canned salmon, tuna, mackerel, crab and lobster	1/4 cup
Clams, oysters, scallops, shrimp	5 or 1 ounce
Sardines, drained	3
Cheeses containing less than 5 percent butterfat	1 ounce
Cottage cheese, dry and 2 percent butterfat	1/4 cup
Dried beans and peas (plus 1 Bread Exchange)	1/2 cup

Medium-Fat Meat

One Medium-fat Meat Exchange equals 1 Lean Meat Exchange plus 1/2 Fat Exchange:

	One Medium-Fat Meat Exchange
Beef: ground (15 percent fat), corned beef (canned), rib eye, round (ground commercial)	1 ounce
Pork: loin (all cuts tenderloin), shoulder arm (picnic), shoulder blade, Boston butt Canadian bacon, boiled ham	1 ounce
Liver, heart, kidney, and sweetbreads	1 ounce
Cottage cheese, creamed	1/4 cup
Cheese: mozzarella, ricotta, farmer's	1 ounce
cheese, neufchatel, parmesan, grated	3 tablespoons
Egg	1 large
Peanut butter (plus 2 additional Fat Exchanges)	2 tablespoons

High-fat Meat

One High Fat Meat Exchange equals 1 Lean Mean Exchange plus 1 Fat Exchange:

	One High-Fat Meat Exchange
Beef: brisket, corned beef (brisket), ground beef (more than 20 percent fat), hamburger (commercial), chuck (ground commercial), roast (rib), steaks (club and rib)	1 ounce
Lamb: breast	1 ounce
Pork: spare ribs, loin (back ribs), pork (ground), country style ham, deviled ham	1 ounce
Veal: breast	1 ounce
Poultry: capon, duck (domestic), goose	1 ounce
Cheese: cheddar types	1 ounce
Cold cuts	4-1/2″ x 1/8″ slice
Frankfurter	1 small

6. Fat Exchanges

One Fat Exchange equals 5 g fat, 45 kilocalories.

	One Fat Exchange
Margarine, soft, tub, stick[a]	1 teaspoon
Avocado (4″ in diameter)[b]	1/8
Oil: corn, cottonseed, safflower, soy, sunflower	1 teaspoon
Oil, olive[b]	1 teaspoon
Oil, peanut[b]	1 teaspoon
Olives[b]	5 small
Almonds[b]	10 whole
Pecans[b]	2 large whole
Peanuts[b]	
Spanish	20 whole
Virginia	10 whole
Walnuts	6 small
Nuts, other[b]	6 small
Margarine, regular stick	1 teaspoon
Butter	1 teaspoon
Bacon fat	1 teaspoon
Bacon, crisp	1 strip
Cream, light	2 tablespoons
Cream, sour	2 tablespoons
Cream, heavy	1 tablespoon
Cream cheese	1 tablespoon
French dressing[c]	1 tablespoon
Italian dressing[c]	1 tablespoon
Lard	1 teaspoon
Mayonnaise[c]	1 teaspoon
Salad dressing (mayonnaise type)[c]	2 teaspoons
Salt pork	3/4″ cube

[a] Made with corn, cottonseed, safflower, soy or sunflower oil only.
[b] Fat content is primarily monounsaturated.
[c] If made with corn, cottonseed, safflower, soy or sunflower oil can be used on fat-modified diet.

"Free" List

The following foods have negligible protein, carbohydrate, fat, and energy content:

Diet calorie free beverage	Salt and pepper	Mustard
Coffee	Red pepper	Chili powder
Tea	Paprika	Onion salt or powder
Bouillon without fat	Garlic	Horseradish
Unsweetened gelatin	Celery salt	Vinegar
Unsweetened pickles	Parsley	Mint
	Nutmeg	Cinnamon
	Lemon	Lime

Source: Exchange Lists for Meal Planning, prepared by Committees of the American Diabetes Association, Inc., and The American Dietetic Association in cooperation with The National Institute of Arthritis, Metabolism and Digestive Diseases and the National Heart and Lung Institute, National Institutes of Health, Public Health Service, U.S. Department of Health, Education, and Welfare, 1976.

APPENDIX H
Nutrient Composition of Foods*

Food	Amount	Weight g	Water g	Energy kcal	Protein g	Fat g	Total Carbohydrate g	Minerals: Calcium mg	Iron mg	Magnesium mg	Phosphorus mg	Potassium mg	Sodium mg	Vitamins: Vitamin C mg	Thiamin mg	Riboflavin mg	Niacin mg	Vitamin B_6 mg	Folacin µg	Total Vitamin A I.U.
Baby Foods																				
Cereal, barley, dry	1 tbsp	2.4	0.20	9	0.30	0.10	1.80	19.0	1.80	3.0	11.0	9	1	0.10	0.066	0.065	0.864	0.009	0.7	—
Mixed, dry	1 tbsp	2.4	0.20	9	0.30	0.10	1.80	18.0	1.52	2.0	9.0	10	1	0.10	0.059	0.065	0.833	0.005	1.0	—
Mixed, w/bananas, dry	1 tbsp	2.4	0.10	9	0.30	0.10	1.90	17.0	1.62	2.0	9.0	16	3	0.10	0.091	0.085	0.493	0.010	nd	3
Oatmeal, dry	1 tbsp	2.4	0.10	10	0.30	0.20	1.70	18.0	1.77	3.0	12.0	11	1	0.10	0.069	0.063	0.863	0.004	0.8	—
Rice, dry	1 tbsp	2.4	0.20	9	0.20	0.10	1.90	20.0	1.77	5.0	14.0	9	1	0.10	0.063	0.053	0.750	0.011	0.6	—
Dessert, Apple Brown Betty, strained	1 oz[a]	28.0	22.70	20	0.10	0	5.60	5.0	0.05	nd	nd	14	3	9.80	0.004	0.010	0.013	nd	0.1	5
Fruit, strained	1 oz[a]	28.0	23.70	17	0.10	0	4.50	2.0	0.06	1.0	2.0	27	4	0.70	0.005	0.003	0.041	0.010	0.9	71
Vanilla custard pudding	1 oz[a]	28.0	22.60	24	0.40	0.60	4.60	16.0	0.07	2.0	13.0	19	8	0.20	0.003	0.023	0.011	0.006	1.7	18
Dinner, beef & noodle, strained	1 oz[a]	28.0	25.10	15	0.60	0.50	2.00	3.0	0.12	2.0	8.0	13	8	0.30	0.010	0.012	0.205	0.014	1.4	233
Mixed vegetable, strained	1 oz[a]	28.0	25.20	11	0.30	0	2.70	6.0	0.09	nd	nd	34	2	0.80	0.004	0.009	0.142	nd	2.3	773
Vegetables & beef, strained	1 oz[a]	28.0	25.10	15	0.60	0.60	2.00	3.0	0.11	2.0	12.0	29	6	0.30	0.006	0.008	0.143	0.015	1.3	337
Vegetables & lamb, strained	1 oz[a]	28.0	25.10	15	0.60	0.60	2.00	3.0	0.10	2.0	14.0	27	6	0.30	0.005	0.010	0.150	0.013	1.0	566
Vegetables, noodles & chicken	1 oz[a]	28.0	24.70	18	0.60	0.70	2.20	8.0	0.10	nd	9.0	16	6	0.20	0.009	0.014	0.115	0.006	0.9	402
Fruit, applesauce, strained	1 oz[a]	28.0	25.10	12	0.10	0	3.10	1.0	0.06	1.0	2.0	20	1	10.90	0.003	0.008	0.017	0.009	0.5	5
Bananas with tapioca	1 oz[a]	28.0	23.80	16	0.10	0	4.30	1.0	0.06	3.0	2.0	25	3	4.70	0.003	0.009	0.052	0.033	1.6	12
Peaches, strained	1 oz[a]	28.0	22.70	20	0.10	0	5.40	2.0	0.07	2.0	3.0	46	2	8.90	0.003	0.009	0.173	0.004	1.1	46
Pears & pineapples	1 oz[a]	28.0	25.10	12	0.10	0	3.10	3.0	0.07	2.0	2.0	33	1	7.80	0.006	0.008	0.059	0.005	0.8	8
Juice, apple	1 fl oz	31.0	27.30	14	0	0	3.60	1.0	0.18	1.0	2.0	28	1	18.00	0.002	0.005	0.026	0.009	0	6
Orange	1 fl oz	31.0	27.40	14	0.20	0.10	3.20	4.0	0.05	3.0	3.0	57	0	19.40	0.014	0.009	0.074	0.017	8.2	17
Meat, beef, strained	1 oz[a]	28.0	22.90	30	3.90	1.50	0	2.0	0.42	5.0	24.0	62	23	0.60	0.003	0.040	0.808	0.040	1.6	52
Chicken, strained	1 oz[a]	28.0	22.00	37	3.90	2.20	0	18.0	0.40	4.0	27.0	40	13	0.50	0.004	0.043	0.923	0.057	2.9	38
Lamb, strained	1 oz[a]	28.0	22.80	29	4.00	1.30	0	2.0	0.42	4.0	27.0	58	18	0.30	0.005	0.057	0.829	0.043	0.6	24
Liver, strained	1 oz[a]	28.0	22.50	29	4.10	1.10	0.40	1.0	1.50	4.0	58.0	64	21	5.50	0.014	0.514	2.361	0.097	95.7	10,811
Egg yolks, strained	1 oz[a]	28.0	20.00	58	2.80	4.90	0.30	22.0	0.78	2.0	81.0	22	11	0.40	0.020	0.075	0.007	0.045	26.1	355
Vegetables, beans, green, strained	1 oz[a]	28.0	26.10	7	0.40	0	1.70	11.0	0.21	7.0	6.0	45	1	1.50	0.007	0.024	0.098	0.011	9.8	127
Carrots, strained	1 oz[a]	28.0	26.20	8	0.20	0	1.70	6.0	0.10	3.0	6.0	56	11	1.60	0.007	0.011	0.131	0.021	4.2	3249
Mixed, strained	1 oz[a]	28.0	25.40	11	0.30	0.10	2.30	4.0	0.09	3.0	6.0	36	4	0.50	0.006	0.007	0.093	0.016	1.1	1132
Peas, strained	1 oz[a]	28.0	24.80	11	1.00	0.10	2.30	6.0	0.27	4.0	12.0	32	1	1.90	0.023	0.017	0.289	0.020	7.4	160
Squash, strained	1 oz[a]	28.0	26.30	7	0.20	0.10	1.60	7.0	0.08	3.0	4.0	51	1	2.20	0.003	0.016	0.100	0.018	4.4	574
Zwieback	1 piece	7.0	0.30	30	0.70	0.70	5.20	1.0	0.04	1.0	4.0	21	16	0.40	0.015	0.017	0.092	0.006	nd	4
Beverages (except milk or fruit & vegetable products)																				
Alcoholic																				
Beer, 4.5% alcohol by volume	12 fl oz	360.0	332.00	151	1.10	0	13.70	18.0	trace	36.0	108.0	90	25	0	0	0.110	2.200	0.216	0	0
Gin, Rum, Whiskey, Vodka 80-proof	1 jigger (1.5 fl oz)	43.0	28.00	97	0	0	trace	3.0	trace	0	4.0	1	0	0	0	0	0	0	0	0
90-proof	1 jigger (1.5 fl oz)	43.0	26.00	110	0	0	trace	3.0	trace	0	4.0	1	0	0	0	0	0	0	0	0

100-proof	1 jigger (1.5 fl oz)	43.0	24.00	124	0	0	trace	3.0	trace	0	4.0	1	0	0	0	0	0	0	0	0
Wines, dessert 18.8% alcohol by volume	2 fl oz	60.0	46.00	82	0.10	0	4.60	5.0	0.20	3.0	6.0	45	2	0	0.010	0.010	0.100	0.024	0	0
Table 12.2% alcohol by volume	3.5 fl oz	100.0	86.00	85	0.10	0	4.20	9.0	0.40	8.0	10.0	92	5	0	0	0.010	0.100	0.040	0	0
Non Alcoholic																				
Carbonated																				
Cola type	12 fl oz	339.0	305.00	132	0	0	33.90	27.0	1.40	3.0	51.0	0	20	0	0	0	0	0	0	0
Cream soda	12 fl oz	371.0	330.00	160	0	0	40.80	—	—	—	—	—	—	0	0	0	0	0	0	0
Fruit flavored	12 fl oz	372.0	327.00	171	0	0	44.60	—	—	—	—	—	—	0	0	0	0	0	0	0
Ginger ale	12 fl oz	339.0	312.00	105	0	0	27.10	27.0	1.40	3.0	51.0	0	20	0	0	0	0	0	0	0
Root beer	12 fl oz	370.0	331.00	152	0	0	38.90	—	—	—	—	—	—	0	0	0	0	0	0	0
Soda, club	12 fl oz	355.0	355.00	0	0	0	0	—	—	—	—	—	—	0	0	0	0	0	0	0
Soda, quinine	12 fl oz	366.0	337.00	113	0	0	29.30	—	—	—	—	—	—	0	0	0	0	0	0	0
Coffee, instant (2 oz powder in water)	1 cup=6 fl oz	180.0	176.00	2	trace	trace	trace	4.0	0.20	9.0	7.0	65	2	0	0	trace	0.500	0.018	0	0
Tea, instant	1 cup=6 fl oz	180.0	179.00	3	0	0	0.70	0	0	4.0	0	45	0	0	0	0.02	0	0	0	0
Cereals and Grains																				
Barley, uncooked, pearled, light	1/2 cup	100.0	11.00	349	8.20	1.00	78.80	16.0	2.00	37.0	189.0	160	3	0	.120	.050	3.100	—	—	0
Biscuits	1	28.0	21.00	103	2.10	4.80	12.80	34.0	0.40	6.0	49.0	33	175	trace	0.060	0.060	0.500	0.011	2.0	trace
Bran Flakes	1 cup	35.0	1.00	106	3.60	0.60	28.20	19.0	12.40	—	125.0	137	207	12.00	0.410	0.490	4.100	0.100	6.0	1650
Breads																				
Boston Brown	1 slice	45.0	20.00	95	2.50	0.60	20.50	41.0	0.90	—	72.0	13*	113	0	0.050	0.030	0.500	—	—	0
French	1 slice	35.0	11.00	102	3.20	1.10	19.40	15.0	0.80	8.0	30.0	32	203	trace	0.100	0.080	0.900	0.018	3.0	trace
Submarine Roll	1	135.0	41.00	392	12.30	4.10	74.80	58.0	3.00	—	115.0	122	783	trace	0.380	0.300	3.400	—	—	trace
Italian	1 slice	30.0	10.00	83	2.70	0.20	16.90	5.0	0.70	5.0	23.0	22	176	0	0.090	0.060	0.800	0.020	3.0	0
Raisin	1 slice	25.0	9.00	66	1.70	0.70	13.40	18.0	0.30	6.0	22.0	58	91	trace	0.010	0.020	0.200	.009	4.0	trace
Rye, American	1 slice	25.0	9.00	61	2.30	0.30	13.00	19.0	0.40	10.0	37.0	36	139	0	0.050	0.020	0.400	0.023	9.0	0
White Enriched	1 slice	25.0	9.00	68	2.20	0.80	12.60	21.0	0.60	6.0	24.0	26	127	trace	0.060	0.050	0.600	0.009	4.0	trace
Whole Wheat	1 slice	25.0	9.00	61	2.60	0.80	11.90	25.0	0.80	10.0	57.0	68	132	trace	0.060	0.030	0.700	0.041	9.0	trace
Brownies w/nuts	1¾"x1¾"x 7/8"	20.0	2.00	97	1.30	6.30	10.20	8.0	0.40	—	30.0	38	50	trace	0.040	0.020	0.100	—	—	40
Buckwheat flour	1 cup	98.0	12.00	326	11.50	2.50	70.60	32.0	2.70	48.0	340.0	—	—	0	0.570	0.150	2.800	—	—	0
Bulghur, dry	1 cup	170.0	17.00	602	19.0	2.60	128.70	49.0	6.30	—	575.0	389	—	trace	0.480	0.240	7.700	—	—	trace
Cakes – made from mix																				
Angel Food	1/12 cake	53.0	18.00	137	3.00	0.10	31.50	50.0	0.20	8.0	63.0	32	77	0	trace	0.060	0.100	0.006	1.0	0
Coffee	1/6 cake	72.0	22.00	232	4.50	6.90	37.70	44.0	1.20	11.0	125.0	78	310	trace	0.130	0.120	1.000	0.030	6.0	120
Cupcake without icing	1	25.0	6.00	88	1.20	3.00	14.00	40.0	0.10	—	59.0	21	113	trace	0.010	0.030	0.100	—	—	40
Cupcake w/choc. icing	1	36.0	8.00	129	1.60	4.50	21.30	47.0	0.30	—	71.0	42	121	trace	0.010	0.040	0.100	—	—	60
Devil's Food w/choc. icing	1/12 cake	92.0	22.00	312	4.00	11.30	53.60	54.0	0.70	22.0	97.0	120	241	trace	0.030	0.070	0.300	0.045	30.0	140
Gingerbread	1/9 cake	63.0	23.00	174	2.00	4.30	32.20	57.0	1.00	—	63.0	173	192	trace	0.020	0.060	0.500	—	—	trace
White w/choc. icing	1/12 cake	95.0	20.00	333	3.70	10.20	59.70	94.0	0.50	—	170.0	110	216	trace	0.020	0.080	0.200	—	—	60
Yellow w/choc. icing	1/12 cake	92.0	24.00	310	3.80	10.40	53.00	84.0	0.60	18	167.0	100	209	trace	0.020	0.070	0.200	0.036	7.5	130
Cakes—home recipe																				
Boston Cream Pie	1/12 cake	69.0	24.00	208	3.50	6.50	34.40	46.0	0.30	—	70.0	61	128	trace	0.020	0.080	0.100	—	—	140
Fruit, dark	1 slice	15.0	3.00	57	0.70	2.30	9.00	11.0	0.40	2.0	17.0	74	24	trace	0.020	0.020	0.100	0.012	trace	20
Pound	1 slice	30.0	5.00	142	1.70	8.90	14.10	6.0	0.20	4.0	24.0	18	33	0	0.010	0.030	0.100	0.012	2.0	80
Sponge	1/12 cake	66.0	21.00	196	5.00	3.80	35.70	20.0	0.80	—	74.0	57	110	trace	0.030	0.090	0.100	—	—	300
Cereals																				
Corn Flakes, plain	1 cup	25.0	1.00	97	2.00	0.10	21.30	1.7	0.60	4.0	9.0	30	251	9.00	0.290	0.350	2.900	0.020	1.0	1180
Corn, puffed	1 cup	20.0	0.70	80	1.60	0.80	16.20	4.0	2.30	—	18.0	—	233	7.00	0.230	0.280	2.300	—	—	940
Farina, quick cooking	1 cup	245.0	218.00	105	3.20	0.20	21.80	147.0	12.30	8.0	162.0	25	466	0	0.120	0.070	1.000	0.024	0	0
Oats, cooked oatmeal	1 cup	240.0	208.00	132	4.80	2.40	23.30	22.0	1.40	58.0	137.0	146	523	0	0.190	0.050	0.200	0.048	26.0	0
Rice, oven popped	1 cup	30.0	1.00	117	1.80	0.10	26.30	6.0	0.80	—	28.0	29	283	11.00	0.350	0.420	3.500	—	—	1410
Rice, puffed	1 cup	15.0	6.00	60	0.90	0.10	13.40	3.0	0.30	—	14.0	15	trace	0	0.070	0.010	0.700	0.010	1.0	0
Wheat & Barley	1 cup cooked	245.0	196.00	196	7.40	0.70	39.40	22.0	2.20	76.0	201.0	trace	250	0	0.170	0.050	—	0.200	16.0	0
Wheat Flakes, added sugar vitamins	1 cup	30.0	1.00	106	3.10	0.50	24.20	12.0	3.50	27.0	83.0	81	310	11.00	0.350	0.420	3.500	0.081	5.0	1410
Wheat, puffed	1 cup plain	15	0.50	54	2.30	0.20	11.8	4	0.60	—	48	51	1	0	0.080	0.030	1.200	—	—	0
Wheat, shredded	1 large biscuit	25	1.60	89	2.50	0.50	20.0	11	0.90	33.0	97	87	1	0	0.060	0.030	1.100	0.050	2.0	0

[a]Approximately 1¾ – 2 tbsp.

*Sources and general notes for this table will be found at the end of the table, on page 681.

Food	Amount	Weight g	Water g	Energy kcal	Protein g	Fat g	Total Carbo-hydrate g	Minerals						Vitamins						
								Cal-cium mg	Iron mg	Mag-nesium mg	Phos-phorus mg	Potas-sium mg	Sod-ium mg	Vitamin C mg	Thia-min mg	Ribo-flavin mg	Niacin mg	Vitamin B_6 mg	Folacin µg	Total Vitamin A I.U.
Cookies																				
Butter	5 cookies 2" diam.	25.0	1.10	115	1.60	4.20	18.00	32.0	0.20	—	24.0	15	105	0	0.010	0.020	0.100	—	—	115
Chocolate Chip	5 cookies 2¼" diam.	52.0	1.40	248	2.90	11.10	36.60	21.0	1.00	—	60.0	71	211	trace	0.020	0.040	0.200	—	—	65
Fig Bars	4 cookies 1½"x1¾"x½"	56.0	7.60	200	2.20	3.10	42.20	44.0	0.60	14.0	34.0	111	141	trace	0.020	0.040	0.200	0.052	6.0	60
Ginger Snaps	5 cookies 2" diam.	35.0	1.10	147	2.00	3.10	28.00	26.0	0.80	—	17.0	162	200	trace	0.020	0.020	0.200	—	—	25
Macaroons	2 cookies 2¾" diam.	38.0	1.70	181	2.00	8.80	25.10	10.0	0.30	—	32.0	176	13	0	0.020	0.060	0.200	—	—	0
Oatmeal with raisins	4 cookies 2-5/8" diam.	52.0	1.40	235	3.20	8.00	38.20	11.0	1.50	—	53.0	192	84	trace	0.060	0.040	0.300	—	—	30
Peanut (sandwich type)	4 cookies 1¾" diam.	49.0	1.10	232	4.90	9.40	32.80	21.0	0.40	—	57.0	86	85	trace	0.030	0.040	1.400	—	—	100
Sandwich	4 cookies 1¾" diam.	40.0	0.80	198	1.90	9.00	27.70	10.0	0.30	—	96.0	15	193	0	0.020	0.020	0.200	—	—	0
Sugar	5 cookies 2¼" diam.	40.0	3.20	178	2.40	6.70	27.20	31.0	0.60	—	41.0	31	127	trace	0.070	0.070	0.500	—	—	45
Corn Bread, southern style	1 piece 2½"x2½"x1½"	78.0	4.00	161	5.80	5.60	22.70	94.0	0.90	—	165.0	122	490	1.00	0.100	0.150	0.500	—	—	120
Cornmeal, whole ground	1 cup	122.0	15.00	433	11.20	4.80	89.90	24.0	2.90	129.0	312.0	346	1	0	0.460	0.130	2.400	—	—	620
Cornstarch	1 tbsp.	8.0	1.00	29	trace	trace	7	0	0	trace	0	trace	trace	0	0	0	0	—	—	0
Crackers																				
Animal	10	26.0	0.80	112	1.70	2.40	20.80	14.0	0.10	—	30.0	25	79	trace	0.010	0.030	0.100	—	—	30
Butter	5	16.0	0.70	75	1.20	3.00	11.10	25.0	0.10	—	43.0	19	180	0	trace	0.010	0.200	—	—	35
Cheese	5	17.2	0.70	83	2.00	3.70	10.40	58.0	0.20	—	53.0	19	178	0	trace	0.020	0.200	—	—	trace
Graham, Sugar/Honey	1 large	14.2	0.50	58	1.00	1.60	10.00	12.0	0.20	7.0	47.0	38	72	0	trace	0.020	0.100	0.010	3.0	—
Saltines	4	11.0	0.50	48	1.00	1.30	8.00	2.0	0.10	4.0	10.0	13	123	0	trace	trace	0.100	0.008	2.0	0
Peanut Butter & Cheese	4	28.0	0.70	139	4.30	6.80	15.90	16.0	0.20	—	51.0	64	281	0	0.010	0.020	1.000	—	—	10
Donut, Plain	1	42.0	10.00	164	1.90	7.80	21.60	17.0	0.60	7.0	80.0	38	210	trace	0.070	0.070	0.500	0.017	3.0	30
Macaroni																				
Cooked, plain	1 cup	130.0	83.00	192	6.50	0.70	39.10	14.0	1.40	25.0	55.0	103	1	0	0.230	0.130	1.800	0.030	5.0	0
and cheese	1 cup	200.0	116.00	430	16.80	22.20	40.20	362.0	1.80	58.0	322.0	240	1086	trace	0.200	0.400	1.800	0.090	13.0	860
Muffins																				
Blueberry	1	40.0	16.00	112	2.90	3.70	16.80	34.0	0.60	10.0	53.0	46	253	trace	0.060	0.080	0.500	0.020	3.0	90
Bran	1	40.0	14.00	104	3.10	3.90	17.20	57.0	1.50	—	162.0	172	179	trace	0.060	0.100	1.600	—	—	90
Corn	1	40.0	13.00	126	2.80	4.00	19.20	42.0	0.70	20.0	68.0	54	192	trace	0.080	0.090	0.600	—	—	120
Plain	1	40.0	15.00	118	3.10	4.00	16.90	42.0	0.60	10.0	60.0	50	176	trace	0.070	0.090	0.600	0.020	3.0	40
Noodles																				
Egg, cooked	1 cup	160.0	113.00	200	6.60	2.40	37.30	16.0	1.40	36.0	94.0	70	3	0	0.220	0.130	1.900	0.032	4.0	110
Chow Mein, canned	½ cup	22.0	0.20	110	3.00	5.30	13.00	—	—	—	—	—	—	—	—	—	—	—	—	—
Pancakes																				
Home Recipe	4" diameter	27.0	13.00	62	1.90	1.90	9.20	27.0	0.40	4.0	38.0	33	115	trace	0.050	0.060	0.400	0.100	2.0	30
Mix, buckwheat	4" diameter	27.0	16.00	54	1.80	2.50	6.40	59.0	0.40	—	91.0	66	125	trace	0.030	0.040	0.200	—	—	60
mix, plain	4" diameter	27.0	14.00	61	1.90	2.00	8.70	58.0	0.30	4.0	70.0	42	152	trace	0.040	0.060	0.200	0.100	2.0	70
Pies, 9" diam.[a]																				
Apple	1/8 pie	118.0	56.00	302	2.60	13.10	45.00	9.0	0.40	5.0	26.0	94	355	1.00	0.020	0.020	0.500	0.047	5.0	40
Blueberry	1/8 pie	118.0	60.00	286	2.80	12.70	41.20	13.0	0.70	5.0	27.0	77	316	4.00	0.020	0.020	0.400	0.050	3.0	40
Cherry	1/8 pie	118.0	55.00	308	3.10	13.30	45.30	17.0	0.40	—	30.0	124	359	trace	0.020	0.020	0.600	—	—	520
Custard	1/8 pie	114.0	66.00	249	7.00	12.70	26.70	109.0	0.70	—	129.0	156	327	0	0.060	0.180	0.300	—	—	260
Lemon Meringue	1/8 pie	105.0	50.00	268	3.90	10.70	39.60	15.0	0.50	—	51.0	53	296	3.00	0.030	0.080	0.200	—	2.0	180
Mince	1/8 pie	118.0	51.00	320	3.00	13.60	48.60	33.0	1.20	—	45.0	210	529	1.00	0.080	0.050	0.500	—	—	trace
Pecan	1/8 pie	103.0	20.00	431	5.30	23.60	52.80	48.0	2.90	—	106.0	127	228	trace	0.160	0.070	0.300	—	—	160
Pumpkin	1/8 pie	114.0	67.00	241	4.60	12.80	27.90	58.0	0.60	7.0	79.0	182	244	trace	0.030	0.110	0.600	0.046	5.0	2819
Rhubarb	1/8 pie	118.0	56.00	299	3.00	12.60	45.10	76.0	0.80	—	31.0	188	319	4.00	0.020	0.050	0.400	—	—	60
Popovers	1	40.0	22.00	90	3.50	3.70	10.30	38.0	0.60	—	56.0	60	88	trace	0.060	0.100	0.400	—	—	130
Rice, added salt																				
brown, cooked	1 cup	195.0	137.00	232	4.90	1.20	49.70	23.0	1.00	58.0	142.0	137	550	0	0.180	0.040	2.700	0.300	15.0	0

White, cooked	1 cup	205.0	149.00	223	4.10	0.20	49.60	21.0	1.80	16.0	57.0	57	767	0	0.230	0.020	2.100	0.075	1.5	0
Parboiled	1 cup	175.0	128.00	186	3.70	0.20	40.80	33.0	1.40	—	100.0	75	627	0	0.190	0.020	2.100	—	—	0
Rolls and Buns																				
Danish Pastry	1	65.0	14.00	274	4.80	15.30	29.60	33.0	0.60	15.0	71.0	73	238	trace	0.040	0.100	0.500	—	5.0	200
Hard Roll	1 round	50.0	13.00	156	4.90	1.60	29.80	24.0	1.20	15.0	46.0	49	313	trace	0.130	0.120	0.140	—	6.0	trace
Frankfurter or Hamburger	1	40.0	13.00	119	3.30	2.20	21.20	30.0	0.80	10.0	34.0	38	202	trace	0.110	0.070	0.900	—	5.0	trace
Brown and Serve	1	26.0	7.00	84	2.20	1.90	14.20	20.0	0.50	10.0	23.0	25	136	trace	0.070	0.060	0.600	0.010	4.0	trace
Rye Flour	1 cup	88.0	10.00	308	10.00	1.50	65.80	24.0	2.30	64.0	231.0	179	1	0	0.260	0.110	2.200	—	—	0
Sesame Seeds	1 tbsp	8.0	0.40	47	1.50	4.30	1.40	9.0	0.20	1.0	47.0	—	—	0	0.010	0.010	0.400	—	5.0	—
Spaghetti																				
Plain, cooked	1 cup	130.0	83.00	192	6.50	0.70	39.10	14.0	1.40	17.0	85.0	103	1	0	0.230	0.130	1.800	0.026	3.0	0
Tomato sauce w/cheese	1 cup	250.0	192.00	260	8.80	8.80	37.00	80.0	2.30	30.0	135.0	408	955	13.00	0.250	0.180	2.300	0.100	2.0	1080
Meatballs w/tomato sauce	1 cup	248.0	174.00	332	18.60	11.70	38.70	124.0	3.70	42.0	236.0	665	1009	22.00	0.250	0.300	4.000	0.113	15.0	1590
Tortilla, corn, lime-treated	1 average 6" diam.	30.0	14.00	63	1.50	0.60	13.50	60.0	0.90	32.0	42.0	5	33	0	0.040	0.020	0.300	0.021	0	6
Waffles																				
Home-recipe	¼ of whole	50.0	21.00	140	4.70	4.90	18.80	57.0	0.90	—	87.0	73	238	trace	0.090	0.130	0.700	—	—	170
Frozen	1 waffle	22.0	9.00	56	1.60	1.40	9.20	27.0	0.40	—	46.0	35	142	trace	0.040	0.040	0.300	—	—	30
From mix	¼ of whole	50.0	21.00	138	4.40	5.30	18.10	120.0	0.70	13.0	172.0	98	343	trace	0.070	0.120	0.500	—	—	120
Wheat Flour																				
Whole	1 cup	120.0	14.00	400	16.00	2.40	85.20	49.0	4.00	136.0	446.0	444	4	0	0.660	0.140	5.200	0.400	35.0	0
White, all-purpose enriched	1 cup	137.0	16.00	499	14.40	1.40	104.30	22.0	4.00	34.0	119.0	130	3	0	0.600	0.360	4.800	0.080	22.0	0
Unenriched	1 cup	137.0	16.00	499	14.40	1.40	104.30	22.0	1.10	34.0	119.0	130	3	0	0.080	0.070	1.200	0.080	22.0	0
Wheat Germ, toasted	1 tbsp	6.0	0.20	23	1.80	0.70	3.00	3.0	0.50	20.0	70.0	57	trace	1.00	0.110	0.050	0.300	0.055	18.0	10
Dairy Products and Eggs																				
Cheeses																				
Blue	1 oz	28.0	12.02	100	6.07	8.15	0.66	150.0	0.09	7.0	110.0	73	396	0	0.008	0.108	0.2880	0.047	10.0	204
Brie	1 oz	28.0	13.73	95	5.88	7.85	0.13	52.0	0.14	—	53.0	43	178	0	0.020	0.147	0.108	0.067	18.0	189
Cheddar	1 oz	28.0	10.42	114	7.06	9.40	0.36	204.0	0.19	8.0	145.0	28	176	0	0.008	0.106	0.023	0.021	5.0	300
Cottage, creamed	1/2 cup	105.0	82.91	108	13.12	4.74	2.82	63.0	0.15	6.0	138.0	88	425	trace	0.022	0.171	0.130	0.070	13.0	171
Cottage, dry curd	1/2 cup	72.0	57.84	62	12.52	0.31	1.34	23.0	0.16	3.0	76.0	24	10	0	0.018	0.103	0.112	0.060	11.0	22
Cottage, 2% fat	1/2 cup	113.0	89.62	102	15.53	2.18	4.10	77.0	0.18	7.0	170.0	109	459	trace	0.027	0.209	0.163	0.086	15.0	79
Cream	1 oz	28.0	15.24	99	2.14	9.89	0.75	23.0	0.34	2.0	30.0	34	84	0	0.005	0.056	0.029	0.013	4.0	405
Edam	1 oz	28.0	11.78	101	7.08	7.88	0.40	207.0	0.12	8.0	152.0	53	274	0	0.010	0.110	0.023	0.022	5.0	260
Feta	1 oz	28.0	15.66	75	4.03	6.03	1.16	140.0	0.18	5.0	96.0	18	316	0	—	—	—	—	—	—
Gouda	1 oz	28.0	11.75	101	7.07	7.78	0.63	198.0	0.07	8.0	155.0	34	232	0	0.009	0.095	0.018	0.023	6.0	183
Gruyère	1 oz	28.0	9.41	117	8.45	9.17	0.10	287.0	—	—	172.0	23	95	0	0.017	0.079	0.030	0.023	3.0	346
Mozzarella	1 oz	28.0	15.35	80	5.51	6.12	0.63	147.0	0.05	5.0	105.0	19	106	0	0.004	0.069	0.024	0.016	2.0	225
Mozzarella, part skim	1 oz	28.0	15.25	72	6.88	4.51	0.78	183.0	0.06	7.0	131.0	24	132	0	0.005	0.086	0.030	0.020	2.0	166
Parmesan, grated	1 tbsp	5.0	0.88	23	2.08	1.50	0.19	69.0	0.05	3.0	40.0	5	93	0	0.002	0.019	0.016	0.005	trace	35
Provolone	1 oz	28.0	11.61	100	7.25	7.55	0.61	214.0	0.15	8.0	141.0	39	248	0	0.005	0.091	0.044	0.021	3.0	231
Ricotta, whole milk	1/2 cup	124.0	88.91	216	13.96	16.10	3.77	257.0	0.47	14.0	196.0	130	104	0	0.016	0.242	0.129	0.053	—	608
Romano	1 oz	28.0	8.76	110	9.02	7.64	1.03	302.0	—	—	215.0	—	340	0	—	0.105	0.022	—	2.0	162
Roquefort	1 oz	28.0	11.16	105	6.11	8.69	0.57	188.0	0.16	8.0	111.0	26	513	0	0.011	0.166	0.208	0.035	14.0	297
Swiss	1 oz	28.0	10.55	107	8.06	7.78	0.96	272.0	0.05	10.0	171.0	31	74	0	0.006	0.103	0.026	0.024	2.0	240
American, pasteurized process	1 oz	28.0	11.10	106	6.28	8.86	0.45	174.0	0.11	6.0	211.0	46	406	0	0.008	0.100	0.020	0.020	2.0	343
Swiss, pasteurized process	1 oz	28.0	12.00	95	7.01	7.09	0.60	219.0	0.17	8.0	216.0	61	388	0	0.004	0.078	0.011	0.010	—	229
Cream																				
Half and Half	1 tbsp	15.0	12.08	20	0.44	1.72	0.64	16.0	0.01	2.0	14.0	19	6	0.13	0.005	0.022	0.012	0.006	trace	65
Light	1 tbsp	15.0	11.06	29	0.40	2.90	0.55	14.0	0.01	1.0	12.0	18	6	0.11	0.005	0.022	0.009	0.005	trace	108
Medium	1 tbsp	15.0	10.28	37	0.37	3.75	0.52	14.0	0.01	1.0	11.0	17	6	0.11	0.004	0.020	0.008	0.005	trace	141
Heavy	1 tbsp	15.0	8.66	52	0.31	5.55	0.42	10.0	trace	1.0	9.0	11	6	0.09	0.003	0.016	0.006	0.004	1.0	220
Whipped topping, pressurized	1 tbsp	3.0	1.84	8	0.10	0.67	0.38	3.0	trace	trace	3.0	4	4	0	0.001	0.002	0.002	0.001	—	27
Sour	1 tbsp	12.0	8.51	26	0.38	2.52	0.51	14.0	0.01	1.0	10.0	17	6	0.10	0.004	0.018	0.008	0.002	1.0	95
Eggnog	1 cup	254.0	188.90	342	9.68	19.00	34.39	330.0	0.51	47.0	278.0	420	138	3.81	0.086	0.483	0.267	0.127	2.0	894
Ice Cream, Vanilla, 10% fat	1/2 cup	66.0	40.43	135	2.40	7.16	15.86	88.0	0.06	9.0	67.0	128	58	0.35	0.026	0.164	0.067	0.031	1.5	272
Ice Milk, vanilla	1/2 cup	66.0	44.94	92	2.58	2.82	14.48	88.0	0.09	10.0	65.0	132	52	0.38	0.038	0.174	0.059	0.042	1.5	107
Sherbert, orange	1/2 cup	96.0	63.76	135	1.08	1.91	29.36	51.0	0.16	8.0	37.0	99	44	1.93	0.016	0.045	0.066	0.012	7.0	92
Coffee Whitener, liquid	1/2 fl oz	15.0	11.59	20	0.15	1.50	1.71	1.0	trace	trace	10.0	29	12	0	0	0	0	0	0	13
Whitener, powdered	1 tsp	2.0	0.04	11	0.10	0.71	1.10	trace	0.02	trace	8.0	16	4	0	0	0.003	0	0	0	4
Milk																				
Whole	1 cup	244.0	214.70	150	8.03	8.15	11.37	291.0	0.12	33.0	228.0	370	120	2.29	0.093	0.395	0.205	0.102	12.0	307

[a]Unenriched flour used for crust.

Food	Amount	Weight g	Water g	Energy kcal	Protein g	Fat g	Total Carbo-hydrate g	Minerals						Vitamins						
								Cal-cium mg	Iron mg	Mag-nesium mg	Phos-phorus mg	Potas-sium mg	Sod-ium mg	Vitamin C mg	Thia-min mg	Ribo-flavin mg	Niacin mg	Vitamin B_6 mg	Folacin μg	Total Vitamin A I.U.
(Milk, whole) 2% Fat	1 cup	244.0	217.67	121	8.12	4.68	11.71	297.0	0.12	33.0	232.0	377	122	2.32	0.095	0.403	0.210	0.105	12.0	500[a]
2% Fat, & milk solids	1 cup	245.0	217.71	125	8.53	4.70	12.18	313.0	0.12	35.0	245.0	397	128	2.45	0.098	0.424	0.220	0.110	13.0	500[a]
1% Fat	1 cup	244.0	219.80	102	8.03	2.59	11.66	300.0	0.12	34.0	235.0	381	123	2.37	0.095	0.407	0.212	0.105	12.0	500[a]
1% Fat & milk solids	1 cup	245.0	220.03	104	8.53	2.38	12.18	313.0	0.12	35.0	245.0	397	128	2.45	0.098	0.424	0.220	0.110	13.0	500[a]
Skim	1 cup	245.0	222.46	86	8.35	0.44	11.88	302.0	0.10	28.0	247.0	406	126	2.40	0.088	0.343	0.216	0.098	13.0	500[a]
Skim & milk solids	1 cup	245.0	221.43	90	8.75	0.61	12.30	316.0	0.12	36.0	255.0	418	130	2.47	0.100	0.429	0.223	0.113	13.0	500[a]
Buttermilk	1 cup	245.0	220.82	99	8.11	2.16	11.74	285.0	0.12	27.0	219.0	371	257	2.40	0.083	0.377	0.142	0.083	—	81
Dry, non-fat	1/4 cup	30.0	0.95	109	10.85	0.23	15.59	377.0	0.10	33.0	290.0	538	161	2.03	0.124	0.465	0.285	0.108	15.0	11
Condensed, sweetened	1 fl oz	38.2	10.38	123	3.02	3.32	20.78	108.0	0.07	10.0	97.0	142	49	0.99	0.034	0.159	0.080	0.019	4.0	125
Evaporated, whole	1 fl oz	31.5	23.32	42	2.14	2.38	3.16	82.0	0.06	8.0	64.0	95	33	0.59	0.015	0.100	0.061	0.016	2.0	77
Chocolate, whole	1 cup	250.0	205.75	208	7.92	8.48	25.85	280.0	0.60	33.0	251.0	417	149	2.28	0.092	0.405	0.313	0.100	12.0	302
Chocolate, 2% fat	1 cup	250.0	208.95	179	8.02	5.00	26.00	284.0	0.60	33.0	254.0	422	150	2.30	0.092	0.410	0.315	0.102	12.0	500[a]
Goat, whole	1 cup	244.0	212.35	168	8.69	10.10	10.86	326.0	0.12	34.0	270.0	499	122	3.15	0.117	0.337	0.676	0.112	1.0	451
Shake																				
Chocolate, thick	11 oz	300.0	216.60	356	9.15	8.10	63.45	396.0	0.93	48.0	378.0	672	333	0	0.141	0.666	0.372	0.075	15.0	258
Vanilla, thick	11 oz	313.0	233.03	350	12.08	9.48	55.56	457.0	0.31	37.0	361.0	572	299	0	0.094	0.610	0.457	0.131	2.10	357
Yogurt																				
Plain	8 oz	227.0	199.53	139	7.88	7.38	10.58	274.0	0.11	26.0	215.0	351	105	1.20	0.066	0.322	0.170	0.073	17.0	279
Plain, lowfat & milk solids	8 oz	227.0	193.11	144	11.92	3.52	15.98	415.0	0.18	40.0	326.0	531	159	1.82	0.100	0.486	0.259	0.111	25.0	150
Plain, skim milk & milk solids	8 oz	227.0	193.47	127	13.01	0.41	17.43	452.0	0.20	43.0	355.0	579	174	1.98	0.109	0.531	0.281	0.120	28.0	16
Fruit, lowfat & milk solids	8 oz	227.0	170.93	225	9.04	2.61	42.31	314.0	0.14	30.0	247.0	402	121	1.36	0.077	0.368	0.195	0.084	19.0	111
Egg																				
Chicken, whole raw	1 egg	50.0	37.28	79	6.07	5.58	0.60	28.0	1.04	6.0	90.0	65	69	0	0.044	0.150	0.031	0.060	32.0	260
Chicken, white raw	1 egg	33.0	29.06	16	3.25	trace	0.41	4.0	0.01	3.0	4.0	45	50	0	0.002	0.094	0.029	0.001	5.0	0
Chicken, yolk, raw	1 egg	17.0	8.29	63	2.79	5.60	0.04	26.0	0.95	3.0	86.0	15	8	0	0.043	0.074	0.012	0.053	26.0	313
Chicken, fried w/butter	1 egg	46.0	33.06	83	5.37	6.41	0.53	26.0	0.92	5.0	80.0	58	144	0	0.033	0.126	0.026	0.050	22.0	286
Chicken, hard-cooked	1 egg	50.0	37.28	79	6.07	5.58	0.60	28.0	1.04	6.0	90.0	65	69	0	0.037	0.143	0.030	0.057	24.0	260
Chicken, omelet w/fat & milk	1 egg	64.0	48.83	95	5.96	7.08	1.37	47.0	0.93	8.0	97.0	85	155	0.13	0.039	0.156	0.042	0.058	22.0	311
Duck, whole raw	1 egg	70.0	49.58	130	8.97	9.64	1.02	45.0	2.70	12.0	154.0	156	102	0	0.109	0.283	0.140	0.175	56.0	930
Substitute, frozen	1/4 cup	60.0	43.86	96	6.77	6.67	1.92	44.0	1.19	—	43.0	128	120	—	0.072	0.232	—	0.080	—	810
Substitute, liquid	1.5 fl oz	47.0	38.89	40	5.64	1.56	0.30	25.0	0.99	—	57.0	155	83	0	0.052	0.141	0.052	—	—	1015
Substitute, powder	0.35 oz	10.0	0.38	44	5.49	1.29	2.16	32.0	0.31	—	47.0	74	79	0.07	0.022	0.174	0.057	—	—	122
Fast Foods																				
Burger Chef																				
Big Shef	1	186.0	nd	542	23.00	34.00	35.00	189.0	3.40	nd	278.0	384	622	2.00	0.340	0.350	5.400	nd	nd	282
Cheeseburger	1	104.0	nd	304	14.00	17.00	24.00	156.0	2.00	nd	198.0	220	535	1.00	0.220	0.230	3.200	nd	nd	266
French Fries	1 serving	68.0	nd	187	3.00	9.00	25.00	10.0	0.90	nd	76.0	581	4	14.00	0.090	0.050	2.100	nd	nd	trace
Rancher Platter	1	316.0	nd	640	30.00	38.00	44.00	57.0	5.10	nd	326.0	1370	444	24.00	0.300	0.370	8.700	nd	nd	367
Burger King																				
Cheeseburger	1	nd	nd	305	17.00	13.00	29.00	141.0	2.00	nd	229.0	219	562	0.50	0.010	0.020	2.200	nd	nd	195
Hamburger	1	nd	nd	252	14.00	9.00	29.00	45.0	2.00	nd	119.0	208	401	0.50	0.010	0.010	2.200	nd	nd	21
Whopper	1	nd	nd	606	29.00	32.00	51.00	37.0	6.00	nd	205.0	653	909	13.00	0.020	0.030	5.200	nd	nd	641
French Fries	1 serving	nd	nd	214	3.00	10.00	28.00	12.0	1.00	nd	87.0	666	5	16.00	0.010	0.010	2.420	nd	nd	0
Hot Dog	1	nd	nd	291	11.00	17.00	23.00	40.0	2.00	nd	117.0	170	841	0	0.040	0.020	2.000	nd	nd	0
Dairy Queen																				
Big Brazier Deluxe	1	213.0	nd	470	28.00	24.00	36.00	111.0	5.20	45.0	262.0	nd	920	2.50	0.340	0.370	9.600	0.380	nd	nd
Big Brazier Regular	1	184.0	nd	457	27.00	23.00	37.00	113.0	5.20	42.0	223.0	nd	910	2.00	0.370	0.390	9.600	0.340	nd	nd
Big Brazier w/cheese	1	213.0	nd	553	32.00	30.00	38.00	268.0	5.20	47.0	359.0	nd	1435	2.30	0.340	0.530	9.500	0.350	nd	495
Brazier Onion Rings	1 serving	85.0	nd	300	6.00	17.00	33.00	20.0	0.40	16.0	60.0	nd	nd	2.40	0.090	trace	0.400	0.080	nd	trace
Brazier Regular	1	106.0	nd	260	13.00	9.00	28.00	70.0	3.50	23.0	114.0	nd	576	1.00	0.280	0.260	5.000	0.130	nd	nd
Fish Sandwich	1	170.0	nd	400	20.00	17.00	41.00	60.0	1.10	24.0	200.0	nd	nd	trace	0.150	0.260	3.000	0.160	nd	trace
Fish Sandwich w/cheese	1	177.0	nd	440	24.00	21.00	39.00	150.0	0.40	24.0	250.0	nd	nd	trace	0.150	0.260	3.000	0.160	nd	100
Super Brazier Dog	1	182.0	nd	518	20.00	30.00	41.00	158.0	4.30	37.0	195.0	nd	1552	14.00	0.420	0.440	7.000	0.170	nd	trace
Super Brazier Chili Dog	1	210.0	nd	555	23.00	33.00	42.00	158.0	4.00	48.0	231.0	nd	1640	18.00	0.420	0.480	8.800	0.270	nd	nd
Buster Bar	1	149.0	nd	390	10.00	22.00	37.00	200.0	0.70	60.0	150.0	nd	nd	trace	0.090	0.340	1.600	0.120	nd	300
DQ Chocolate Dipped Cone, med.	1	156.0	nd	300	7.00	13.00	40.00	200.0	0.40	24.0	150.0	nd	nd	trace	0.090	0.340	trace	0.080	nd	300
DQ Chocolate Malt, med	1	418.0	nd	600	15.00	20.00	89.00	500.0	3.60	60.0	400.0	nd	nd	3.60	0.120	0.600	0.800	0.200	nd	750
DQ Chocolate Sundae, med	1	184.0	nd	300	6.00	7.00	53.00	200.0	1.10	32.0	150.0	nd	nd	trace	0.060	0.260	trace	0.080	nd	300
DQ Cone, med	1	142.0	nd	230	6.00	7.00	35.00	200.0	trace	24.0	150.0	nd	nd	trace	0.090	0.260	trace	0.080	nd	300

DQ Float	1	397.0	nd	330	6.00	8.00	59.00	200.0	trace	nd	200.0	nd	nd	trace	0.120	0.170	trace	nd	nd	100
DQ Freeze	1	397.0	nd	520	11.00	13.00	89.00	300.0	trace	nd	250.0	nd	nd	trace	0.150	0.340	trace	nd	nd	200
DQ Sandwich	1	60.0	nd	140	3.00	4.00	24.00	60.0	0.40	8.0	60.0	nd	nd	trace	0.030	0.140	0.400	trace	nd	100
Hot Fudge Brownie Delight	1	266.0	nd	570	11.00	22.00	83.00	300.0	1.10	40.0	250.0	nd	nd	trace	0.450	0.430	0.800	0.160	nd	500
Kentucky Fried Chicken																				
Original Recipe Dinner	1 dinner	425.0	nd	830	52.00	46.00	56.00	150.0	4.50	nd	nd	nd	2285	27.00	0.380	0.560	15.000	nd	nd	750
Extra Crispy Dinner	1 dinner	437.0	nd	950	52.00	54.00	63.00	150.0	3.60	nd	nd	nd	1915	27.00	0.380	0.560	14.000	nd	nd	750
Individual Pieces, Original																				
Recipe, Drumstick	1	54.0	28.60	136	14.00	8.00	2.00	20.0	0.90	nd	nd	nd	nd	0.60	0.040	0.120	2.700	nd	nd	30
Keel	1	96.0	50.30	283	25.00	13.00	6.00	nd	0.90	nd	nd	nd	nd	1.20	0.070	0.130	nd	nd	nd	50
Rib	1	82.0	37.70	241	19.00	15.00	8.00	55.0	1.00	nd	nd	nd	nd	1.00	0.060	0.140	5.800	nd	nd	58
Thigh	1	97.0	48.30	276	20.00	19.00	12.00	39.0	1.40	nd	nd	nd	nd	1.00	0.080	0.240	4.900	nd	nd	74
Wing	1	45.0	19.10	151	11.00	10.00	4.00	nd	0.60	nd	nd	nd	nd	1.00	0.030	0.070	nd	nd	nd	nd
Long John Silver's																				
Breaded Clams	5 oz	nd	nd	465	13.00	25.00	46.00	nd	nd	nd	nd	nd	nd	nd	nd	nd	nd	nd	nd	nd
Cole Slaw	4 oz	nd	nd	138	1.00	8.00	16.00	nd	nd	nd	nd	nd	nd	nd	nd	nd	nd	nd	nd	nd
Corn on Cob	1 piece	nd	nd	174	5.00	4.00	29.00	nd	nd	nd	nd	nd	nd	nd	nd	nd	nd	nd	nd	nd
Fish with Batter	2 pieces	nd	nd	318	19.00	19.00	19.00	nd	nd	nd	nd	nd	nd	nd	nd	nd	nd	nd	nd	nd
Hush Puppies	3 pieces	nd	nd	153	1.00	7.00	20.00	nc	nd	nd	nd	nd	nd	nd	nd	nd	nd	nd	nd	nd
Ocean Scallops	6 pieces	nd	nd	257	10.00	12.00	27.00	nc	nd	nd	nd	nd	nd	nd	nd	nd	nd	nd	nd	nd
Shrimp with Batter	6 pieces	nd	nd	269	9.00	13.00	31.00	nc	nd	nd	nd	nd	nd	nd	nd	nd	nd	nd	nd	nd
Treasure Chest	2 pc fish 2 peg legs	nd	nd	467	25.00	29.00	27.00	nc	nd	nd	nd	nd	nd	nd	nd	nd	nd	nd	nd	nd
Mc Donald's																				
Egg McMuffin	1	132.0	65.30	352	18.00	20.00	26.00	187.0	3.20	25.0	265.0	222	914	1.60	0.360	0.600	4.300	0.140	nd	361
Hot Cakes w/butter & syrup	1 serving	206.0	95.90	472	8.00	9.00	89.00	54.0	2.40	30.0	404.0	264	1071	2.10	0.310	0.430	4.000	0.060	nd	255
Big Mac	1	187.0	86.40	541	26.00	31.00	39.00	175.0	4.30	38.0	215.0	386	962	2.40	0.350	0.370	8.200	0.220	nd	327
Cheeseburger	1	114.0	51.40	306	16.00	13.00	31.00	158.0	2.90	24.0	134.0	244	725	1.60	0.240	0.300	5.500	0.100	nd	372
Filet O Fish	1	131.0	55.90	402	15.00	23.00	34.00	105.0	1.80	29.0	158.0	293	709	4.20	0.280	0.280	3.900	0.080	nd	152
French Fries	1 serving	69.0	27.80	211	3.00	11.00	26.00	10.0	0.50	23.0	49.0	570	113	11.00	0.150	0.030	2.900	0.010	nd	52
Hamburger	1	99.0	44.60	257	13.00	9.00	30.00	63.0	3.00	21.0	88.0	234	526	1.80	0.230	0.230	5.100	0.110	nd	231
Quarter Pounder	1	164.0	81.20	418	26.00	21.00	33.00	79.0	5.10	38.0	179.0	442	711	2.30	0.310	0.410	9.800	0.250	nd	164
Quarter Pounder w/cheese	1	193.0	94.20	518	31.00	29.00	34.00	251.0	4.60	43.0	257.0	472	1209	2.90	0.350	0.590	15.100	0.250	nd	683
Apple Pie	1	91.0	38.30	300	2.00	19.00	31.00	12.0	0.60	7.0	23.0	39	414	2.70	0.020	0.030	1.300	0.080	nd	69
Cherry Pie	1	92.0	38.60	298	2.00	18.00	33.00	12.0	0.40	8.0	23.0	57	456	1.30	0.020	0.030	0.400	0.020	nd	213
McDonaldland Cookies	1 serving	63.0	1.90	294	4.00	11.00	45.00	10.0	1.40	10.0	51.0	58	330	1.40	0.280	0.230	0.800	0.020	nd	48
Chocolate Shake	1	289.0	207.00	364	11.00	9.00	60.00	338.0	1.00	51.0	292.0	656	329	2.90	0.120	0.890	0.800	0.120	nd	318
Vanilla Shake	1	289.0	216.00	323	10.00	8.00	52.00	346.0	0.20	35.0	266.0	499	250	2.90	0.120	0.660	0.600	0.120	nd	346
Pizza Hut																				
Thin'N Crispy																				
Beef	½ of 10" pizza	nd	nd	490	29.00	19.00	51.00	350.0	6.30	nd	nd	nd	nd	1.20	0.300	0.600	7.000	nd	nd	750
Cheese	½ of 10" pizza	nd	nd	450	25.00	15.00	54.00	450.0	4.50	nd	nd	nd	nd	1.20	0.300	0.510	5.000	nd	nd	750
Pepperoni	½ of 10" pizza	nd	nd	430	23.00	17.00	45.00	300.0	4.50	nd	nd	nd	nd	1.20	0.300	0.510	6.000	nd	nd	1000
Supreme	½ of 10" pizza	nd	nd	510	27.00	21.00	51.00	350.0	7.20	nd	nd	nd	nd	2.40	0.380	0.680	7.000	nd	nd	1250
Thick'N Chewy																				
Beef	½ of 10" pizza	nd	nd	620	38.00	20.00	73.00	400.0	7.20	nd	nd	nd	nd	1.20	0.680	0.600	8.000	nd	nd	750
Cheese	½ of 10" pizza	nd	nd	560	34.00	14.00	71.00	500.0	5.40	nd	nd	nd	nd	1.20	0.680	0.680	7.000	nd	nd	1000
Pepperoni	½ of 10" pizza	nd	nd	560	31.00	18.00	68.00	400.0	5.40	nd	nd	nd	nd	3.60	0.680	0.680	8.000	nd	nd	1250
Supreme	½ of 10" pizza	nd	nd	640	36.00	22.00	74.00	400.0	7.20	nd	nd	nd	nd	9.00	0.750	0.850	9.000	nd	nd	1000
Taco Bell																				
Bean Burrito	1 serving	166.0	nd	343	11.00	12.00	48.00	98.0	2.80	nd	173.0	235	272	15.20	0.370	0.220	2.200	nd	nd	1657
Beef Burrito	1 serving	184.0	nd	466	30.00	21.00	37.00	83.0	4.60	nd	288.0	320	327	15.20	0.300	0.390	7.000	nd	nd	1675
Beef Tostado	1 serving	184.0	nd	291	19.00	15.00	21.00	208.0	3.40	nd	265.0	277	138	12.70	0.160	0.270	3.300	nd	nd	3450
Burrito Supreme	1 serving	225.0	nd	457	21.00	22.00	43.00	121.0	3.80	nd	245.0	350	367	16.00	0.330	0.350	4.700	nd	nd	3462
Combination Burrito	1 serving	175.0	nd	404	21.00	16.00	43.00	91.0	3.70	nd	230.0	278	300	15.20	0.340	0.310	4.600	nd	nd	1666
Pintos'N Cheese	1 serving	158.0	nd	168	11.00	5.00	21.00	150.0	2.30	nd	210.0	307	102	9.30	0.260	0.160	0.900	nd	nd	3123
Taco	1 serving	83.0	nd	186	15.00	8.00	14.00	120.0	2.50	nd	175.0	143	79	0.20	0.090	0.160	2.900	nd	nd	120
Tostada	1 serving	138.0	nd	179	9.00	6.00	25.00	191.0	2.30	nd	186.0	172	101	9.70	0.180	0.150	0.800	nd	nd	3152
Fruits																				
Apples																				
Fresh	1	180.0	152.00	96	0.30	1.00	24.00	12.0	0.50	9.0	17.0	182	2	7.00	0.050	0.030	0.200	0.054	4.0	150
Apple Juice	6 oz	186.0	163.00	87	0.20	trace	22.10	11.0	1.10	8.0	17.0	188	2	2.00	0.020	0.040	0.200	0.054	0	—
Apple Sauce (sweetened)	½ cup	128.0	97.00	116	0.20	0.20	30.40	5.0	0.60	5.0	7.0	83	2	2.00	0.020	0.020	0.050	0.039	3.0	50
Apricots																				
Canned in syrup	3 halves	85.0	65.00	73	0.50	0.10	18.70	9.0	0.30	6.0	13.0	199	1	3.00	0.020	0.020	0.300	0.043	—	1480
Dried sulfured	5 halves	18.0	4.00	46	0.90	0.10	11.60	12.0	1.00	11.0	19.0	172	5	2.00	trace	0.030	1.200	0.030	2.0	3820
Nectar	6 oz	188.0	159.00	107	0.60	0.20	27.40	17.0	0.40	7.0	23.0	284	trace	6.00	0.020	0.020	0.400	0.060	—	1790
Avocado, raw	½	125.0	92.00	188	2.40	18.50	7.10	11.0	0.70	44.0	47.0	680	5	16.00	0.120	0.230	1.800	0.525	37.0	330

[a]Values based on addition of Vitamin A to level of 2,000 I.U. per quart.

Food	Amount	Weight g	Water g	Energy kcal	Protein g	Fat g	Total Carbo-hydrate g	Minerals						Vitamins						
								Cal-cium mg	Iron mg	Mag-nesium mg	Phos-phorus mg	Potas-sium mg	Sod-ium mg	Vitamin C mg	Thia-min mg	Ribo-flavin mg	Niacin mg	Vitamin B_6 mg	Folacin μg	Total Vitamin A I.U.
Bananas	1 med	175.0	132.00	101	1.30	0.20	26.40	10.0	0.80	37.0	31.0	440	1	12.00	0.060	0.070	0.800	0.380	32.0	230
Blackberries, fresh	1 cup	144.0	122.00	84	1.70	1.30	18.60	46.0	1.30	43.0	27.0	245	1	30.00	0.040	0.060	0.600	0.080	4.0	290
Blueberries, fresh	1 cup	145.0	121.00	90	1.00	0.70	22.20	22.0	1.50	8.0	19.0	117	1	20.00	0.040	0.090	0.700	0.100	4.0	150
Cherries																				
Canned, in water, sweet	½ cup	135.0	117.00	60	1.10	0.30	14.80	19.0	0.40	12.0	16.0	162	1	4.00	0.030	0.030	0.200	0.020	4.0	75
Raw, sweet	10	75.0	60.00	47	0.90	0.20	11.70	15.0	0.30	10.0	13.0	129	1	7.00	0.030	0.040	0.300	—	—	70
Cranberries																				
Raw	1 cup	95.0	83.00	44	0.40	0.70	10.30	13.0	0.50	8.0	10.0	78	2	10.00	0.030	0.020	0.100	—	—	40
Juice	6 oz	190.0	158.00	124	0.20	0.20	31.40	10.0	0.60	—	6.0	19	2	30.00	0.020	0.020	0.100	—	—	trace
Sauce	1 cup	277.0	172.00	404	0.30	0.60	103.90	17.0	0.60	5.0	11.0	83	3	6.00	0.030	0.030	0.100	0.080	—	60
Dates, Pitted	5	40.0	9.00	110	0.90	0.20	29.20	24.0	1.20	23.0	25.0	259	1	0	0.040	0.040	0.900	0.050	5.0	20
Fruit Cocktail, canned in syrup	1 cup	255.0	203.00	194	1.00	0.30	50.20	23.0	1.00	18.0	31.0	411	13	5.00	0.050	0.030	1.000	0.020	—	360
Grapefruit																				
Canned, sweetened	1 cup	254.0	206.00	178	1.50	0.30	45.20	33.0	0.80	28.0	36.0	343	3	76.00	0.080	0.050	0.500	—	—	30
Fresh	½ of 3½" diam.	184.0	163.00	40	0.50	0.10	10.30	16.0	0.40	9.0	16.0	132	1	37.00	0.040	0.020	0.200	0.030	2.0	80
Juice, canned, unsweetened	6 oz	185.4	165.00	78	1.20	trace	18	12.0	0.60	12.0	24.0	300	trace	66.00	0.060	0.060	0.600	0.018	2.0	trace
Grapes																				
Concord	10	40.0	33.00	18	0.30	0.30	4.10	4.0	0.10	5.0	3.0	42	1	1.00	0.010	0.010	0.100	0.040	2.0	30
Grape Juice, canned	6 oz	190.0	158.00	125	0.40	trace	31.50	21.0	0.60	22.0	23.0	220	4	trace	0.080	0.040	0.400	0.040	4.0	—
Lemons																				
Fresh	¼	40.0	36.00	7	0.30	0.10	2.20	7.0	0.20	—	4.0	38	1	14.00	0.010	0.010	trace	—	—	10
Juice	1 tbsp	15.2	14.00	4	0.10	trace	1.20	1.0	trace	1.0	2.0	21	trace	7.00	trace	trace	trace	0.008	0	trace
Lemonade Concentrate, diluted	6 oz	185.0	164.00	81	0.10	trace	21.10	2.0	0.10	1.0	2.0	30	1	13.00	0.010	0.010	0.100	0.017	4	10
Limes	1	80.0	71.00	19	0.50	0.10	6.40	22.0	0.40	—	12.0	69	1	25.00	0.020	0.010	0.100	—	—	10
Limeade Concentrate, diluted	6 oz	185.0	164.00	76	0.10	trace	20.40	2.0	trace	—	2.0	24	trace	4.00	trace	trace	trace	—	—	trace
Mangos	1	300.0	261.00	152	1.60	0.90	38.80	23.0	0.90	54.0	30.0	437	16	81.00	0.120	0.120	2.500	—	—	11,090
Melons																				
Cantelope 5" diam.	½ melon	477.0	435.00	82	1.90	0.30	20.40	38.0	1.10	76.0	44.0	682	33	90.00	0.110	0.080	1.600	0.300	150.0	9240
Honeydew	1/10 melon	226.0	205.00	49	1.20	0.40	11.50	21.0	0.60	—	24.0	374	18	34.00	0.060	0.040	0.900	—	—	60
Watermelon	1/16 melon	926.0	857.00	111	2.10	0.90	27.30	30.0	2.10	70.0	43.0	426	4	30.00	0.130	0.130	0.900	0.600	16.0	2510
Nectarines	1	150.0	123.00	88	0.80	trace	23.60	6.0	0.70	19.0	33.0	406	8	18.00	—	—	—	—	—	2280
Oranges																				
Fresh	1	180.0	155.00	64	1.30	0.30	16.00	54.0	0.50	14.0	26.0	263	1	66.00	0.130	0.050	0.500	0.082	61.0	260
Juice, concentrate, diluted	6 oz	187.0	163.00	92	1.30	0.20	21.70	19.0	0.20	19.0	32.0	378	2	90.00	0.170	0.030	0.700	0.054	7.0	410
Juice, dehydrated, reconstituted	6 oz	186.0	164.00	86	1.10	0.40	20.10	19.0	0.40	—	30.0	388	1.5	82.00	0.150	0.050	0.800	—	—	375
Juice, fresh	6 oz	186.0	164.00	84	1.30	0.40	19.40	20.2	0.40	20.0	32.0	372	2	93.00	0.170	0.050	0.800	0.070	65.0	375
Papaya, raw	1 cup	140.0	124.00	55	0.80	0.10	14.00	28.0	0.40	—	22.0	328	4	78.00	0.060	0.060	0.400	—	—	2450
Peaches																				
Canned, sweetened	1 cup	256.0	202.00	200	1.00	0.30	51.50	10.0	0.80	16.0	31.0	333	5	8.00	0.030	0.050	1.500	0.050	28.0	1100
Dried, sulphured	5 halves	65.0	16.00	170	2.00	0.50	44.40	31.0	3.90	31.0	76.0	618	11	12.00	0.010	0.120	3.500	0.060	—	2535
Fresh	1,2½" diam	115.0	102.00	38	0.60	0.10	9.70	9.0	0.50	11.0	19.0	202	1	7.00	0.020	0.050	1.000	0.020	11.0	1330
Pears																				
Canned, sweetened	1 cup	255.0	203.00	194	0.50	0.50	50.00	13.0	0.50	12.0	18.0	214	3	3.00	0.030	0.050	0.300	0.034	15.0	10
Fresh, Barlett	1,2½" diam	180.0	150.00	100	1.10	0.70	25.10	13.0	0.50	13.0	18.0	213	3	7.00	0.030	0.070	0.200	0.030	9.0	30
Pineapple																				
Canned, sweetened	1 cup	255.0	204.00	189	0.80	0.30	49.50	28.0	0.80	19.0	13.0	245	3	18.00	0.200	0.050	0.500	0.175	5.0	130
Fresh	1 slice, ¾" thick	84.0	72.00	44	0.30	0.20	11.50	14.0	0.40	10.0	7.0	123	1	14.00	0.080	0.030	0.200	0.072	1.0	60
Juice, canned unsweetened	6 oz	187.0	162.00	96	0.70	0.10	24.00	21.0	0.60	22.0	15.0	254	2	24.00	0.130	0.040	0.400	—	—	20
Plums																				
Canned, sweetened	1 cup	272.0	210.00	214	1.00	0.30	55.80	23.0	2.30	14.0	26.0	367	3	5.00	0.050	0.050	1.000	0.080	—	3130
Raw	1, 1" diam	11.0	9.00	7	0.10	trace	1.80	1.8	0.10	1.0	1.7	30	trace	—	0.010	0.010	0.100	0.006	trace	30

Pomegranates	1, 3-3/8" diam	275.0	226.00	97	0.80	0.50	25.30	5.0	0.50	—	12.0	399	5	6.00	0.050	0.050	0.500	—	—	trace
Prunes																				
Dried, uncooked	10	75.0	21.00	164	1.40	0.40	43.50	33.0	2.50	30.0	51.0	448	5	2.0	0.060	0.110	1.000	—	—	1030
Juice	6 oz	192.0	154.00	148	0.80	0.20	36.50	27.0	7.90	19.0	38.0	451	4	4.0	0.020	0.020	0.800	—	—	—
Raisins, seedless	½ oz	14.0	2.00	40	0.40	trace	10.80	9.0	0.50	4.0	14.0	107	4	trace	0.020	0.010	0.100	0.034	1.5	trace
Raspberries, black, fresh	1 cup	134.0	108.00	98	2.00	1.90	21.00	40.0	1.20	40.0	29.0	267	1	24.00	0.040	0.120	1.200	—	—	trace
Strawberries																				
Fresh	1 cup whole berries	149.0	134.00	55	1.00	0.70	12.50	31.0	1.50	18.0	31.0	244	1	88.00	0.040	0.100	0.900	0.090	22.0	90
Frozen, sweetened	1 cup sliced	255.0	182.00	278	1.30	0.50	70.90	36.0	1.80	23.0	43.0	286	3	135.00	0.050	0.150	1.300	0.105	22.0	80
Tangerines	1 med	116.0	100.90	39	0.70	0.20	10.00	34.0	0.30	—	15.0	108	2	27.00	0.050	0.020	0.100	—	—	360
Herbs and Spices																				
Allspice, ground	1 tsp	1.9	0.16	5	0.12	0.17	1.37	13.0	0.13	3.0	2.0	20	1	0.75	0.002	0.001	0.054	—	—	10
Anise Seed	1 tsp	2.1	0.20	7	0.37	0.33	1.05	14.0	0.78	4.0	9.0	30	trace	—	—	—	—	—	—	—
Basil, ground	1 tsp	1.4	0.09	4	0.20	0.06	0.85	30.0	0.59	6.0	7.0	48	trace	0.86	0.002	0.004	0.097	—	—	131
Bay Leaf	1 tsp	0.6	0.03	2	0.05	0.05	0.45	5.0	0.26	1.0	1.0	3	trace	0.28	trace	0.003	0.012	—	—	37
Caroway Seed	1 tsp	2.1	0.21	7	0.42	0.31	1.05	14.0	0.34	5.0	12.0	28	trace	—	0.008	0.008	0.076	—	—	8
Celery Seed	1 tsp	2.0	0.12	8	0.36	0.50	0.83	35.0	0.90	9.0	11.0	28	3	0.34	—	—	—	—	—	1
Chili Powder	1 tsp	2.6	0.20	8	0.32	0.44	1.42	7.0	0.37	4.0	8.0	50	26	1.67	0.009	0.021	0.205	—	—	908
Cinnamon, ground	1 tsp	2.3	0.22	6	0.09	0.07	1.84	28.0	0.88	1.0	1.0	11	1	0.65	0.002	0.003	0.030	—	—	6
Cloves, ground	1 tsp	2.1	0.14	7	0.13	0.42	1.29	14.0	0.18	6.0	2.0	23	5	1.70	0.002	0.006	0.031	—	—	11
Coriander Seed	1 tsp	1.8	0.16	5	0.22	0.32	0.99	13.0	0.29	6.0	7.0	23	1	—	0.004	0.005	0.038	—	—	—
Cumin Seed	1 tsp	2.1	0.17	8	0.37	0.47	0.93	20.0	1.39	8.0	10.0	38	4	0.16	0.013	0.007	0.096	—	—	27
Curry Powder	1 tsp	2.0	0.19	6	0.25	0.28	1.16	10.0	0.59	5.0	7.0	31	1	0.23	0.005	0.006	0.069	—	—	20
Dill Seed	1 tsp	2.1	0.16	6	0.34	0.31	1.16	32.0	0.34	5.0	6.0	25	trace	—	0.009	0.006	0.059	—	—	1
Dill Weed, dried	1 tsp	1.0	0.07	3	0.20	trace	0.56	18.0	0.49	5.0	5.0	33	2	—	0.004	0.003	0.029	0.0150	—	—
Fennel Seed	1 tsp	2.0	0.18	7	0.32	0.30	1.05	24.0	0.37	8.0	10.0	34	2	—	0.008	0.007	0.121	—	—	3
Garlic Powder	1 tsp	2.8	0.18	9	0.47	0.02	2.04	2.0	0.08	2.0	12.0	31	1	—	0.013	0.004	0.019	—	—	—
Ginger, ground	1 tsp	1.8	0.17	6	0.16	0.11	1.27	2.0	0.21	3.0	3.0	24	1	—	0.001	0.003	0.093	—	—	3
Mace, ground	1 tsp	1.7	0.14	8	0.11	0.55	0.86	4.0	0.24	3.0	2.0	8	1	—	0.005	0.008	0.023	—	—	14
Marjoram, dried	1 tsp	0.6	0.05	2	0.08	0.04	0.36	12.0	0.50	2.0	2.0	9	trace	0.31	0.002	0.002	0.025	—	—	48
Nutmeg, ground	1 tsp	2.2	0.14	12	0.13	0.80	1.08	4.0	0.07	4.0	5.0	8	trace	—	0.008	0.001	0.029	—	—	2
Onion Powder	1 tsp	2.1	0.11	7	0.21	0.02	1.69	8.0	0.05	3.0	7.0	20	1	0.31	0.009	0.001	0.014	—	—	—
Oregano, ground	1 tsp	1.5	0.11	5	0.17	0.15	0.97	24.0	0.66	4.0	3.0	25	trace	—	0.005	—	0.093	—	—	104
Paprika	1 tsp	2.1	0.20	6	0.31	0.27	1.17	4.0	0.50	4.0	7.0	49	1	1.49	0.014	0.037	0.322	—	—	1273
Parsley, dried	1 tsp	0.3	0.03	1	0.07	0.01	0.15	4.0	0.29	1.0	1.0	11	1	0.37	0.001	0.004	0.024	0.003	—	70
Pepper																				
Black	1 tsp	2.1	0.22	5	0.23	0.07	1.36	9.0	0.61	4.0	4.0	26	1	—	0.002	0.005	0.024	—	—	4
Red or Cayenne	1 tsp	1.8	0.14	6	0.22	0.31	1.02	3.0	0.14	3.0	5.0	36	1	1.38	0.006	0.017	0.157	—	—	749
White	1 tsp	2.4	0.27	7	0.25	0.05	1.65	6.0	0.34	2.0	4.0	2	trace	—	0.001	0.003	0.005	—	—	—
Poppy Seed	1 tsp	2.8	0.19	15	0.50	1.25	0.66	41.0	0.26	9.0	24.0	20	1	—	0.024	0.005	0.027	0.012	—	—
Poultry Seasoning	1 tsp	1.5	0.14	5	0.14	0.11	0.98	15.0	0.53	3.0	3.0	10	trace	0.18	0.004	0.003	0.045	—	—	39
Rosemary, dried	1 tsp	1.2	0.11	4	0.06	0.18	0.77	15.0	0.35	3.0	1.0	11	1	0.74	0.006	—	0.012	—	—	38
Saffron	1 tsp	0.7	0.08	2	0.08	0.04	0.46	1.0	0.08	—	2.0	12	1	—	—	—	—	—	—	—
Sage, ground	1 tsp	0.7	0.06	2	0.07	0.09	0.43	12.0	0.20	3.0	1.0	7	trace	0.23	0.005	0.002	0.040	—	—	41
Savory, ground	1 tsp	1.4	0.13	4	0.09	0.08	0.96	30.0	0.53	5.0	2.0	15	trace	—	0.005	—	0.057	—	—	72
Sesame Seed	1 tsp	2.7	0.13	16	0.71	1.48	0.25	4.0	0.21	9.0	21.0	11	1	—	0.019	0.002	0.126	0.004	—	2
Tarragon, ground	1 tsp	1.6	0.12	5	0.36	0.12	0.80	18.0	0.52	6.0	5.0	48	1	—	0.004	0.021	0.143	—	—	67
Thyme, ground	1 tsp	1.4	0.11	4	0.13	0.10	0.89	26.0	1.73	3.0	3.0	11	1	—	0.007	0.006	0.069	—	—	53
Turmeric, ground	1 tsp	2.2	0.25	8	0.17	0.22	1.43	4.0	0.91	4.0	6.0	56	1	0.57	0.003	0.005	0.113	—	—	—
Meat, Poultry and Seafood																				
Bacon																				
Cooked	2 med slices	15.0	1.00	86	3.80	7.80	0.50	2.0	0.50	4.0	34.0	35	153	—	0.080	0.05	0.8	.016	0	0
Canadian, cooked	1 slice 3-3/8" diam	21.0	10.00	58	5.70	3.70	0.10	3.0	0.90	5.0	46.0	91	537	—	0.190	0.04	1.1	—	—	0

Food	Amount	Weight g	Water g	Energy kcal	Protein g	Fat g	Total Carbo-hydrate g	Minerals: Cal-cium mg	Iron mg	Mag-nesium mg	Phos-phorus mg	Potas-sium mg	Sod-ium mg	Vitamins: Vitamin C mg	Thia-min mg	Ribo-flavin mg	Niacin mg	Vitamin B_6 mg	Folacin µg	Total Vitamin A I.U.
Bass																				
Striped, fried	1 fillet, ½ lb	200.0	122.00	392	43.00	17.00	13.40	—	—	—	—	—	—	—	—	—	—	—	—	—
Beef																				
Ground, 21% fat	1 Patty 3" diam, ¼ lb	87.0	47.00	235	19.80	16.60	0	9.0	2.60	18.0	159.0	221	49	—	0.070	0.17	4.4	0.390	4.0	30
Round Steak, 19% fat	3 oz	85.0	46.00	222	24.30	13.10	0	10.0	3.00	25.0	213.0	272	60	—	0.070	0.19	4.8	0.300	3.0	20
Corn Beef, Hash, w/potato	1 cup	220.0	148.00	398	19.40	24.90	23.50	29.0	4.40	40.0	147.0	440	1188	—	0.020	0.20	4.6	0.160	—	—
Roast, chuck	3 oz	85.0	34.20	363	19.00	31.20	0	9.0	2.50	13.0	94.0	152	33	—	0.040	0.140	3.000	—	3.0	60
Roast, rib	3 oz	85.0	34.00	374	16.90	33.50	0	8.0	2.20	17.0	158.0	189	41	—	0.050	0.130	3.100	0.300	3.0	70
Steak, flank	¼ lb	113.0	69.70	222	34.60	8.30	0	16.0	4.30	—	170.0	276	60	—	0.060	0.260	5.200	—	—	12
Steak, sirloin	3 oz	85.0	49.90	176	27.40	6.50	0	11.0	3.30	18.0	222.0	307	67	—	0.070	0.210	5.400	—	3.0	10
Blue Fish, cooked	1 fillet, 1/3 lb	155.0	105.00	246	40.60	8.10	0	45.0	1.10	—	445.0	—	161	—	0.170	0.16	2.9	—	—	80
Chicken without skin																				
Light meat, Roasted	2 pieces 2½"x1-7/8"x ¼"	50.0	32.00	83	15.80	1.70	0	6.0	0.70	10.0	133.0	206	32	—	0.020	0.05	5.8	0.350	2.0	30
Dark meat, Roasted	4 pieces 1-7/8" x 1" x ¼"	40.0	26.00	70	11.20	2.50	0	5.0	0.70	6.0	92.0	128	34	—	0.030	0.09	2.2	0.250	2.0	60
Pot Pie	1/3 of a 9" pie	232.0	131.00	545	23.40	31.30	42.50	70.0	3.00	—	232.0	343	594	5	0.260	0.26	4.2	—	—	3090
Chili Con Carne w/beans, canned	1 cup	255.0	185.00	339	19.10	15.60	31.10	82.0	4.30	66.0	321.0	594	1354	—	0.080	0.18	3.3	0.260	23.0	150
Clams																				
Canned, drained	1 cup minced	160.0	123.00	157	25.30	4.00	3.00	—	—	180.0	—	—	—	—	—	—	—	0.130	5.0	—
Raw	4–5	70.0	56.00	56	7.80	0.60	4.10	48.0	5.30	—	106.0	218	144	—	—	—	—	—	—	—
Cod, broiled	1 fillet, 1/6 lb	65.0	42.00	111	18.50	3.40	0	20.0	0.7	18.0	178.0	265	72	—	0.050	0.07	2.0	0.180	6.0	120
Crab																				
Canned, king	1 cup, drained	135.0	104.00	136	23.50	3.40	1.50	61.0	1.10	46.0	246.0	149	1350	—	0.110	0.11	2.6	0.400	trace	—
Cooked, flaked	1 cup	125.0	98.00	116	21.60	2.40	0.60	54.0	1.00	42.0	219.0	—	—	2	0.200	0.10	3.5	—	—	2710
Fish Cakes, fried	5 small 1¼" diam	60.0	40.00	103	8.80	4.80	5.60	—	—	—	—	—	—	—	—	—	—	—	—	—
Fish Sticks																				
Breaded, cooked	4 sticks	112.0	74.00	200	18.80	10.00	7.20	12.0	0.40	20.0	188.0	—	—	—	0.040	0.08	2.0	0.060	18.0	0
Flounder, baked	1 fillet, 1/6 lb	57.0	33.00	115	17.00	4.70	0	13.0	0.80	17.0	196.0	335	135	1.00	0.040	0.05	1.4	0.097	—	—
Goose, roasted	3 oz	85.0	47.00	198	28.80	8.30	0	12.0	1.40	—	235.0	514	105	—	0.090	0.14	7.9	—	—	—
Haddock, fried	1 fillet, 1/3 lb	110.0	73.00	182	21.60	7.00	6.40	44.0	1.30	30.0	272.0	383	195	2.00	0.040	0.08	3.5	0.157	17.0	—
Halibut, broiled	1 fillet, 1/3 lb	125.0	83.00	214	31.50	8.80	0	20.0	1.00	29.0	310.0	656	168	—	0.060	0.090	10.400	0.425	20.0	850
Herring,																				
Pickled	1 piece 1¾"x7/8"x½"	15.0	8.9	33	3.10	2.30	0	—	—	—	—	—	—	—	—	—	—	—	—	—
Smoked	1 small fillet	20.0	12.00	42	4.40	2.60	0	13.0	0.30	—	51.0	—	—	—	—	0.060	0.700	0.040	—	10
Kidney Beef, cooked	1 cup, slices ¼" thick	140.0	74.00	353	46.20	16.80	1.10	25.0	18.30	25.0	342.0	454	354	trace	0.710	6.750	15.000	0.560	84.0	1610
Lamb, cooked																				
Chop, loin	2.3 oz	65.0	40.00	122	18.30	4.90	0	8.0	1.30	13.0	142.0	205	45	—	0.100	0.180	4.000	0.2	1.0	—
Chop, rib	2 oz	57.0	34.00	120	15.50	6.00	0	6.0	1.10	11.0	121.0	174	38	—	0.090	0.150	3.400	—	—	—
Leg	3 oz	85.0	53.00	158	24.40	6.00	0	11.0	1.90	19.0	202.0	273	60	—	0.140	0.260	5.300	0.272	3.0	—
Liver, cooked																				
Beef	3 oz	85.0	48.00	195	22.40	9.00	4.50	9.0	7.50	19.0	405.0	323	156	23	0.220	3.560	14.000	0.569	250.0	45,390
Calf	3 oz	85.0	44.00	222	25.10	11.20	3.40	11.0	12.10	6.0	456.0	385	100	31	0.200	3.540	14.000	0.570	—	27,800
Chicken	1 liver	25.0	16.00	41	6.60	1.10	0.80	3.0	2.10	—	40.0	38	15	4	0.040	0.670	2.900	—	—	3080
Pork	3 oz	85.0	46.00	205	25.40	9.80	2.10	13.0	24.70	20.0	458.0	336	94	19	0.290	3.710	19.000	0.552	188.0	12,670
Lobster																				
Cooked	1 cup	145.0	111.00	138	27.10	2.20	0.40	94.0	1.20	32.0	278.0	261	305	—	0.150	0.100	—	—	—	—
Newburg	1 cup	250.0	160.00	485	46.30	26.50	12.80	218.0	2.30	—	480.0	428	573	—	0.180	0.280	—	—	—	—
Ocean Perch, fried	3 oz	84.0	50.00	192	16.20	11.40	5.70	27.0	1.20	—	192.0	243	129	—	0.090	0.090	1.500	—	—	—
Oysters																				
Eastern, raw	2–3	28.0	24.00	19	2.40	0.50	1.00	27.0	1.60	9.0	41.0	34	21	—	0.040	0.050	0.700	.014	3.0	90

Cured Baked Ham	3 oz	85.0	53.00	159	21.50	7.50	0	9.0	2.70	17.0	170.0	241	770	—	0.490	0.200	3.800	0.340	9.0	0
Fresh Baked Ham	3 oz	85.0	51.00	184	25.20	8.50	0	11.0	3.20	25.0	262.0	282	62	—	0.540	0.250	4.800	0.380	2.0	0
Loin	3 oz	85.0	47.00	216	25.00	12.10	0	11.0	3.20	—	264.0	280	61	—	0.92	0.260	5.500	—	—	0
Chops	1 chop[a]	56.0	29.00	151	17.10	8.60	0	7.0	2.20	14.0	181.0	192	42	—	0.630	0.180	3.800	—	—	0
Spareribs, Cooked	yield from ½ lb	90.0	35.70	396	18.70	35.00	0	8.0	2.40	—	109.0	150	33	—	0.390	0.190	3.100	—	—	0
Salmon																				
Canned Sockeye	½ can	110.0	74.00	188	22.40	10.20	0	285.0	1.30	32.0	378.0	378	574	—	0.040	0.180	8.100	0.300	10.0	255
Fresh, broiled	3 oz	85.0	54.00	156	23.10	6.30	0	—	0.90	35.0	351.0	378	99	—	0.150	0.060	8.400	0.255	6.0	150
Smoked	1 oz	28.0	16.00	50	6.10	2.60	0	4.0	—	9.0	69.0	—	—	—	—	—	—	0.198	2.0	—
Sardines Canned in oil	1 can	92.0	57.00	187	22.10	10.20	—	402.0	2.70	36.0	459.0	543	757	—	0.030	0.180	5.000	0.164	29.0	200
Sausage, Cold Cuts, & Luncheon Meats																				
Bologna	1 slice 4½" diam	28.0	16.00	86	3.40	7.80	0.30	2.0	0.50	—	36.0	65	369	—	0.050	0.060	0.700	0.030	1.0	—
Brown & Serve Sausage	1 patty 2-3/8"x1-7/8"x½"	23.0	9.00	97	3.80	8.70	0.60	—	—	—	—	—	—	—	—	—	—	—	—	—
	1 link 3-7/8"x5/8"	17.0	7.00	72	2.80	6.40	0.50	—	—	—	—	—	—	—	—	—	—	—	—	—
Deviled Ham, cooked	1 tbsp	13.0	6.00	46	1.80	4.20	0	1.0	0.30	—	12.0	—	—	—	0.020	0.010	0.200	—	—	0
Frankfurters	1 5"x¾" diam	45.0	25.00	139	5.60	12.40	0.80	3.0	0.90	4.0	60.0	99	495	—	0.070	0.090	1.200	0.049	2.0	—
Liverwurst	1 slice	28.0	15.00	87	4.60	7.30	0.50	3.0	1.50	7.0	68.0	—	—	—	0.060	0.370	1.600	0.279	2.0	1800
Salami	1 slice 3-1/8"x1/16"	10.0	3.00	45	2.40	3.80	0.10	1.0	0.40	—	28.0	—	—	—	0.040	0.030	0.500	0.013	0.3	—
Scrapple	1 slice 2¾"x2-1/8"x¼"	25.0	15.00	54	2.20	3.40	3.70	1.0	0.30	—	16.0	—	—	—	0.050	0.030	0.500	—	—	—
Scallops, steamed	¼ lb	114.0	83.00	127	26.30	1.60	—	130.0	3.40	—	383.0	540	300	—	—	—	—	—	22.0	—
Shrimp																				
Fried	¼ lb	113.0	64.00	255	23.00	12.20	11.40	82.0	2.30	69.0	216.0	260	211	—	0.050	0.090	3.000	0.068	2.0	—
Boiled	3 oz	85.0	66.00	80	17.80	0.70	0.40	66.0	1.40	36.0	177.0	173	107	9	0.020	0.030	2.800	0.042	2.0	34
Swordfish Broiled	1 piece 1/3 lb	145.0	93.70	237	38.20	8.20	0	37.0	1.80	—	375.0	—	—	—	0.050	0.070	14.900	—	—	2790
Tongue, beef	1 slice 3"x2"x1/8"	20.0	12.00	49	4.30	3.30	0.10	1.0	0.40	3.0	23.0	33	12	—	0.010	0.060	0.700	0.033	—	—
Tuna																				
Canned in oil	1 cup drained	160.0	97.00	315	46.10	13.10	0	13.0	3.00	43.0	374.0	—	—	—	0.080	0.190	19.000	0.688	3.0	130
Canned in water	3½ oz	99.0	69.00	126	27.70	0.80	0	16.0	1.60	25.0	188.0	276	41	—	—	0.090	12.200	0.400	8.0	—
Turkey, cooked																				
Light meat w/o skin	2 slices 3 oz 4"x2"x¼"	85.0	53.00	150	28.00	3.30	0	—	1.00	20.0	—	349	70	—	0.040	0.120	9.400	0.300	3.0	—
Dark meat w/o skin	4 pieces 2½"x1-5/8"x¼"=3 oz	85.0	56.00	173	25.50	7.10	0	—	2.00	20.0	—	338	84	—	0.030	0.200	3.600	0.300	7.0	—
Turkey Giblets, Simmered	1 cup	145.0	88.00	338	29.90	22.30	2.30	—	—	—	—	—	—	—	—	3.940	—	—	—	—
Turkey Pot Pie	1/3 of 9" pie	232.0	130.00	550	24.10	31.30	42.90	63.0	3.20	—	234.0	459	633	5	0.260	0.300	5.800	—	—	3090
Veal, cooked																				
Cutlet	3 oz	85.0	51.00	184	23.00	9.40	0	9.0	2.70	20.0	196.0	258	56	—	0.060	0.210	4.600	0.300	15.0	—
Loin	3 oz	85.0	50.00	199	22.40	11.40	0	9.0	2.70	—	191.0	251	55	—	0.060	0.210	4.600	—	—	—
Stew meat	3 oz	85.0	50.00	200	23.70	10.90	0	10.0	3.00	16.0	128.0	190	41	—	0.080	0.250	5.400	—	—	—
Vegetables																				
Alfalfa Sprouts, raw	1 cup packed	100.0	90.00	40	5.00	0.6	5.00	30.0	1.40	—	—	—	—	15.00	0.1	0.2	1.5	—	—	—
Artichokes, cooked	1	300.0	260.00	10-53	3.40	0.20	11.90	61.0	1.30	—	83.0	361	36	10.00	0.080	0.050	0.800	0.300	—	180
Asparagus, fresh, cooked	4 spears	60.0	56.00	12	1.30	0.10	2.20	13.0	0.40	12.0	30.0	110	1	16.00	0.100	0.110	0.800	0.125	37.0	540
Bamboo Shoots	½ cup	76.0	69.00	20	2.00	0.20	3.90	10.0	0.40	—	45.0	403	—	3.00	0.110	0.050	0.400	—	—	15
Beans																				
Navy, cooked	½ cup	95.0	131.00	112	7.40	0.60	20.20	48.0	2.60	37.0	141.0	395	7	0	0.140	0.060	0.600	0.140	8.0	0
w/Pork & Tomato Sauce	1 cup	255.0	180.00	311	15.60	6.60	48.50	138.0	4.60	70.0	235.0	536	1181	5.00	0.200	0.080	1.500	0.950	24.0	330
Red Kidney, cooked	1 cup	185.0	128.00	218	14.40	0.90	39.60	70.0	4.40	70.0	259.0	629	6	—	0.200	0.110	1.300	0.800	20.0	10
Lima, cooked	½ cup	85.0	60.00	95	6.40	0.50	16.80	40.0	2.20	55.0	103.0	358	1	15.00	0.160	0.080	1.100	0.100	16.0	240
Mung, Sprouts	½ cup	52.0	46.00	19	2.00	0.10	3.50	10.0	0.70	—	34.0	117	3	10.00	0.070	0.070	0.400	—	—	10
Green, fresh, cooked	½ cup	62.0	58.00	16	1.00	0.20	3.40	32.0	0.40	14.0	23.0	95	3	8.00	0.050	0.050	0.300	0.039	3.0	340
Yellow, fresh, cooked	½ cup	62.0	58.00	14	0.90	0.20	2.90	32.0	0.40	—	23.0	95	4	8.00	0.050	0.050	0.300	—	—	145

[a]Three chops to the pound.

Food	Amount	Weight g	Water g	Energy kcal	Protein g	Fat g	Total Carbo-hydrate g	Minerals						Vitamins						
								Cal-cium mg	Iron mg	Mag-nesium mg	Phos-phorus mg	Potas-sium mg	Sod-ium mg	Vitamin C mg	Thia-min mg	Ribo-flavin mg	Niacin mg	Vitamin B_6 mg	Folacin µg	Total Vitamin A I.U.
Beets																				
Canned	½ cup sliced	85.0	76.00	32	0.90	0.10	7.50	16.0	0.60	12.0	16.0	142	200	3.00	0.010	0.030	0.100	0.040	16.0	15
Greens, cooked	½ cup	72.0	68.00	41	3.80	0.50	7.50	225.0	4.30	76.0	56.0	753	172	34.00	0.160	0.340	0.700	0.080	—	11,565
Broccoli, frozen, cooked	3 stalks	90.0	82.00	24	2.70	0.30	4.20	36.0	0.60	31.0	51.0	198	12	66.00	0.060	0.090	0.600	0.150	19.0	1710
Brussels Sprouts, cooked	1 cup	155.0	138.00	51	5.00	0.30	10.10	33.0	1.20	25.0	95.0	457	22	126.00	0.120	0.160	0.900	0.680	25.0	880
Cabbage																				
Chinese	1 cup	75.0	71.00	11	0.90	0.10	2.30	32.0	0.50	10.0	30.0	190	17	19.00	0.040	0.030	0.500	—	—	110
Cooked, shredded	1 cup	145.0	136.00	29	1.60	0.30	6.20	64.0	0.40	16.0	29.0	236	20	48.00	0.060	0.060	0.400	0.190	16.0	190
Raw, shredded	1 cup	90.0	83.00	22	1.20	0.20	4.90	44.0	0.40	12.0	26.0	210	18	42.00	0.050	0.050	0.300	0.140	48.0	120
Red, raw, shredded	1 cup	90.0	81.00	28	1.80	0.20	6.20	38.0	0.70	—	32.0	241	23	55.00	0.080	0.050	0.400	—	—	40
Spoon, pakchoy, cooked	1 cup	170.0	161.00	24	2.40	0.30	4.10	252.0	1.00	—	56.0	364	31	26.00	0.070	0.140	1.200	—	—	5270
Carrots																				
Cooked	½ cup diced	72.0	66.00	23	0.70	0.20	5.20	24.0	0.50	5.0	23.0	161	24	5.00	0.040	0.040	0.400	0.023	2.0	7615
Raw	1, 7½" long	81.0	71.00	30	0.80	0.10	7.00	27.0	0.50	13.0	26.0	246	34	6.00	0.040	0.040	0.400	0.112	12.0	7930
Cauliflower																				
Cooked	1 cup	125.0	116.00	28	2.90	0.30	5.10	26.0	0.90	16.0	53.0	258	11	69.00	0.110	0.100	0.800	0.200	4.0	80
Raw	1 cup	100.0	91.00	27	2.70	0.20	5.20	25.0	1.10	24.0	56.0	295	13	78.00	0.110	0.100	0.700	0.125	37.0	60
Celery, raw	1 stalk	40.0	38.00	7	0.40	trace	1.60	16.0	0.10	9.0	11.0	136	50	4.00	0.010	0.010	0.100	0.025	2.0	110
Chard, Swiss	1 cup	175.0	164.00	32	3.20	0.40	5.80	128.0	3.20	114.0	42.0	562	151	28.00	0.070	0.190	0.700	—	—	9450
Chick Peas (Garbanzos)	1 cup cooked	200.0	21.00	720	41.00	9.60	122.00	300.0	13.8	—	662.0	1594	52	—	0.620	0.300	4.000	0.250	11.0	100
Chicory	1 cup	90.0	86.00	14	0.90	0.10	2.90	16.0	0.50	12.0	19.0	164	6	—	—	—	—	—	—	trace
Collards, cooked	1 cup	190.0	170.00	63	6.80	1.30	9.70	357.0	1.50	72.0	99.0	498	—	144.00	0.210	0.380	2.300	0.340	40.0	14,820
Corn																				
Canned, cream style	1 cup	256.0	195.00	210	5.40	1.50	51.20	8.0	1.50	50.0	143.0	248	604	13.00	0.080	0.130	2.600	0.504	6.0	840
Canned, kernel	1 cup	210.0	158.00	174	5.30	1.10	43.10	6.0	1.10	43.0	153.0	204	496	11.00	0.060	0.130	2.300	0.425	5.0	740
Cob	1 ear	140.0	104.00	70	2.50	0.80	16.20	2.0	0.50	67.0	69.0	151	trace	7.00	0.090	0.080	1.100	—	—	310
Frozen, cooked	1 cup	165.0	127.00	130	5.00	0.80	31.00	5.0	1.30	36.0	120.0	304	2	8.00	0.150	0.100	2.500	—	—	580
Cow Peas, immature (Black-Eyed), cooked	½ cup	85.0	61.00	92	6.90	0.70	15.40	20.0	1.80	16.0	124.0	322	1	14.00	0.250	0.090	1.200	0.042	22.0	297
Cucumbers																				
Pared, 6-3/8" long	½	79.0	76.00	11	0.50	0.10	2.60	14.0	0.30	9.0	14.0	127	5	9.00	0.030	0.030	0.200	0.030	12.0	trace
Egg Plant, cooked, Drained	1 cup diced	200.0	189.00	38	2.00	0.40	8.20	22.0	1.20	32.0	42.0	300	2	6.00	0.100	0.080	1.000	0.160	4.0	20
Kale, fresh, cooked	1 cup	110.0	96.00	43	5.00	0.80	6.70	206.0	1.80	41.0	64.0	243	47	102.00	0.110	0.200	1.800	0.400	50.0	9130
Lentils, cooked	½ cup	100.0	72.00	106	7.80	trace	19.30	25.0	2.10	20.0	119.0	498	—	0	0.140	0.120	1.200	—	5.0	40
Lettuce																				
Boston, shredded	1 cup	55.0	52.00	8	0.70	0.10	1.40	19.0	1.10	10.0	14.0	145	5	4.00	0.030	0.030	0.200	0.030	30.0	530
Iceberg, shredded	1 cup	55.0	52.00	7	0.50	0.10	1.60	11.0	0.30	6.0	12.0	96	5	3.00	0.030	0.030	0.200	0.033	111.0	180
Mushrooms																				
Fresh	1 cup	70.0	63.00	20	1.90	0.20	3.10	4.0	0.60	9.0	81.0	290	11	2.00	0.070	0.320	2.900	0.080	14.0	trace
Canned, solids & liquids	½ cup	100.0	93.00	17	1.90	0.10	2.40	6.0	0.50	8.0	68.0	197	400	2.00	0.020	0.250	2.000	0.060	8.0	0
Onions																				
Green	2 medium	30.0	26.00	14	0.30	0.10	3.20	12.0	0.20	3.0	12.0	69	2	8.00	0.020	0.010	0.100	—	12.0	trace
White, sliced	½ cup	58.0	52.00	22	0.90	0.10	5.00	16.0	0.30	7.0	21.0	90	6	6.00	0.020	0.030	0.100	0.071	6.0	25
Parsley, raw	10 sprigs 2½" long	10.0	8.5	4	0.4	0.1	0.9	20.0	0.60	4.0	6.0	73	5	17.00	0.010	0.030	0.100	0.020	4.0	850
Parsnips																				
Diced, cooked	1 cup	155.0	127.00	102	2.30	0.80	23.10	70.0	0.90	45.0	96.0	587	12	16.00	0.110	0.120	0.200	—	—	50
Peas, green, canned, cooked	½ cup	125.0	103.00	82	4.40	0.40	15.60	25.0	2.10	16.0	82.0	120	294	11.00	0.110	0.060	1.100	0.062	19.0	560
Fresh, cooked	½ cup	80.0	65.00	57	4.30	0.30	9.70	19.0	1.50	—	79.0	157	1	16.00	0.230	0.090	1.800	—	—	430
Frozen, cooked	½ cup	80.0	66.00	54	4.10	0.20	9.40	15.0	1.50	17.0	69.0	108	92	11.00	0.220	0.070	1.400	0.104	12.0	480
Peppers																				
Sweet, green	½ cup	40.0	37.00	9	0.50	0.10	1.90	4.0	0.30	7.0	9.0	85	5	51.00	0.030	0.030	0.400	0.10	2.0	170
Sweet, red	½ cup	40.0	36.00	13	0.60	0.10	2.90	5.0	0.20	—	12.0	—	—	82.00	0.030	0.030	0.200	—	10.0	1780

Potatoes																				
Baked	1 large	202.0	152.00	145	4.00	0.20	32.80	14.0	1.10	33.0	101.0	782	6	31.00	0.150	0.070	2.700	0.300	18.0	trace
French Fries	10 strips	50.0	22.00	137	2.20	6.60	18.00	8.0	0.70	9.0	56.0	427	3	11.00	0.070	0.040	1.600	0.090	5.0	trace
Mashed w/milk & fat	1 cup	210.0	168.00	197	4.40	9.00	25.80	50.0	0.80	28.0	101.0	525	695	19.00	0.170	0.110	2.100	0.180	24.0	360
Scalloped w/cheese	1 cup	245.0	174.00	355	13.00	19.40	33.30	311.0	1.20	—	299.0	750	1095	25.00	0.150	0.290	2.200	—	—	780
Sweet Potato, baked	1	146.0	93.00	161	2.40	0.60	37.00	46.0	1.00	17.0	66.0	342	14	25.00	0.100	0.080	0.800	0.238	27.0	9230
Canned	1 cup	200.0	144.00	216	4.00	0.40	49.80	50.0	1.60	36.0	82.0	400	96	28.00	0.100	0.080	1.200	0.140	38.0	15,600
Salad	1 cup	250.0	190.00	248	6.80	7.00	40.80	80.0	1.50	—	160.0	798	1320	28.00	0.200	0.180	2.800	—	—	350
Radishes	5	25.0	23.00	4	0.20	trace	0.80	7.0	0.20	1.5	7.0	72	4	6.00	0.010	0.010	0.100	0.015	5.0	trace
Sauerkraut, canned	1 cup	235.0	218.00	42	2.40	0.50	9.40	85.0	1.20	—	42.0	329	1755	33.00	0.070	0.090	0.500	0.400	—	120
Soy Beans																				
Cooked	1 cup	180.0	128.00	234	19.80	10.30	19.40	131.0	4.90	377.0	322.0	972	4	0.00	0.380	0.160	1.100	0.078	73.0	50
Curd (Tofu)	1 piece 2½"x2¾"x1"	120.0	102.00	86	9.40	5.00	2.90	154.0	2.30	133.0	151.0	50	8	0.00	0.070	0.040	0.100	—	—	0
Spinach																				
Raw	1 cup	55.0	50.00	14	1.80	0.20	2.40	51.0	1.70	30.0	28.0	259	39	28.00	0.060	0.110	0.3	0.152	40.0	4460
Fresh, cooked	1 cup	180.0	165.00	41	5.40	0.50	6.50	167.0	4.00	120.0	68.0	583	90	50.00	0.130	0.250	0.9	0.400	120.0	14,580
Frozen, cooked	1 cup	190.0	174.00	46	5.50	0.60	7.40	200.0	4.80	120.0	84.0	688	93	53.00	0.150	0.270	1.0	0.350	120.0	15,390
Squash																				
Summer, cooked[a]	1 cup, cubed	210.0	200.00	29	1.90	0.20	6.50	53.0	0.80	31.0	53.0	296	2	21.00	0.110	0.170	1.7	0.126	4.0	820
Winter, cooked[b]	1 cup, baked	205.0	166.00	129	3.70	0.80	31.60	57.0	1.60	34.0	98.0	945	2	27.00	0.100	0.270	1.4	0.200	—	8610
Winter, frozen	1 cup, cooked	240.0	213.00	91	2.90	0.70	22.10	60.0	2.40	28.0	77.0	497	2	19.00	0.070	0.170	1.2	—	—	9360
Succotash, frozen	1 cup, cooked	170.0	126.00	158	7.10	0.70	34.90	22.0	1.70	—	145.0	418	65	10.00	0.150	0.090	2.2	—	—	510
Tomatoes																				
Canned	1 cup	241.0	226.00	51	2.40	0.50	10.40	14.0	1.20	26.0	46.0	523	313	41.00	0.120	0.070	1.7	0.216	62.0	2170
Fresh	1, 2-3/5" diam	135.0	126.00	27	1.40	0.20	5.80	16.0	0.60	17.0	33.0	300	4	28.00	0.070	0.050	0.9	0.126	23.0	1110
Juice	6 fl oz	182.0	170.00	35	1.60	0.20	7.80	13.0	1.60	18.0	33.0	413	364	29.00	0.090	0.050	1.5	0.300	18.0	1460
Paste	6 oz can	170.0	128.00	139	5.80	0.70	31.60	46.0	6.00	32.0	119.0	1510	65	83.00	0.340	0.200	5.3	0.650	32.0	5610
	1 tbsp	14.0	11.00	12	0.50	0.10	2.60	4.0	0.50	3.0	10.0	126	5	7.00	0.030	0.020	0.4	0.050	3.0	468
Turnip, cooked	1 cup cubed	155.0	145.00	36	1.20	0.30	7.60	54.0	0.60	22.0	37.0	291	53	34.00	0.060	0.080	0.5	0.108	2.0	trace
Turnip, greens, cooked	1 cup	145.0	135.00	29	3.20	0.30	5.20	267.0	1.60	40.0	54.0	—	—	100.00	0.220	0.350	0.9	1.400	—	9140
Vegetable Juice Cocktail	6 fl oz	182.0	171.00	31	1.60	0.20	6.60	22.0	0.90	—	40.0	402	364	16.00	0.090	0.050	1.5	—	—	1270
Vegetables, mixed, Frozen	1 cup cooked	182.0	150.00	116	5.80	0.50	24.40	46.0	2.40	42.0	115.0	348	96	15.00	0.220	0.130	2.0	0.170	26.0	9010
Water chestnuts, raw	1 lb	454.0	355.00	276	4.90	0.70	66.40	14.0	2.10	54.0	227.0	1747	70	14.00	0.490	0.700	3.5	—	—	0
Watercress	1 cup, whole	35.0	33.00	7	0.80	0.10	1.10	53.0	0.60	7.0	19.0	99	18	28.00	0.030	0.060	0.3	0.040	70.0	1270
Miscellaneous																				
Condiments																				
Barbeque Sauce	1 cup	250.0	202.00	228	3.80	17.30	20.00	53.0	2.00	—	50.0	435	2038	13.00	0.030	0.030	0.8	—	—	900
Horseradish, prepared	1 tsp	5.0	4.00	2	0.10	trace	0.50	3.0	trace	2.0	2.0	15	5	—	—	—	—	—	—	—
Mustard																				
Brown	1 tsp	5.0	4.00	5	0.30	0.30	0.30	6.0	0.10	2.0	7.0	7	65	—	—	—	—	—	—	—
Yellow	1 tsp	5.0	4.00	4	0.20	0.20	0.30	4.0	0.10	2.0	4.0	7	63	—	—	—	—	—	—	—
Olives																				
Green	10 large	46.0	36.00	45	0.50	4.90	0.50	24.0	0.60	7.0	7.0	21	926	—	—	—	—	0.011	7.0	120
Ripe	10 giant	80.0	64.00	89	0.80	9.50	1.80	58.0	1.10	—	11.0	23	559	—	trace	trace	—	—	—	40
Pickles																				
Dill	1 medium	65.0	61.00	7	0.50	0.10	1.40	17.0	0.70	1.0	14.0	130	928	4.00	trace	0.010	trace	0.006	2.0	70
Sour	1 medium	65.0	62.00	7	0.30	0.10	1.30	11.0	2.10	—	10.0	—	879	5.00	trace	0.010	trace	—	—	70
Sweet	1 small	15.0	9.00	22	0.10	0.10	5.50	2.0	0.20	0	2.0	—	—	1.00	trace	trace	trace	0.001	0.7	10
Relish	1 tbsp	15.0	9.00	21	0.10	0.10	5.10	3.0	0.10	—	2.0	—	107	—	—	—	—	—	—	—
Salt	1 tsp	5.5	0.01	0	0	0	0	14.0	trace	6.0	—	trace	2132	0	0	0	0	0	0	0
Soy Sauce	1 tbsp	18.0	11.00	12	1.00	0.20	1.70	15.0	0.90	—	19.0	66	1319	0	trace	0.050	0.1	—	—	0
Tartar Sauce	1 tbsp	14.0	5.00	74	0.20	8.10	0.60	3.0	0.10	—	4.0	11	99	trace	trace	trace	trace	—	—	30
Tomato Catsup	1 tbsp or 1 packet	15.0	10.00	16	0.30	0.10	3.80	3.0	0.10	4.0	8.0	54	156	2.00	0.010	0.010	0.2	0.019	5.0	210
Tomato Chili Sauce, bottled	1 tbsp	15.0	10.00	16	0.40	trace	3.70	3.0	0.10	—	8.0	56	201	2.00	0.010	0.010	0.2	—	—	210
Vinegar																				
Cider	1 tbsp	15.0	14.00	2	trace	0	0.90	1.0	0.10	trace	1.0	15	trace	—	—	—	—	—	—	—
White distilled	1 tbsp	15.0	14.00	2	—	—	0.80	—	—	—	—	2	trace	—	—	—	—	—	—	—

[a]Acorn, butternut, hubbard.

[b]Crookneck, zucchini, scalloped varieties.

								Minerals						Vitamins						
Food	Amount	Weight g	Water g	Energy kcal	Protein g	Fat g	Total Carbo-hydrate g	Cal-cium mg	Iron mg	Mag-nesium mg	Phos-phorus mg	Potas-sium mg	Sod-ium mg	Vitamin C mg	Thia-min mg	Ribo-flavin mg	Niacin mg	Vitamin B_6 mg	Folacin µg	Total Vitamin A I.U.
Fats and Oils																				
Butter																				
Regular, salted	1 pat	5.0	0.80	36	0.040	4.10	trace	1.0	0.01	trace	1.0	1	41	0	trace	0.002	0.002	trace	trace	153
Salted, whipped	1 pat	3.8	0.60	27	0.03	3.08	trace	1.0	0.01	trace	1	1	31	0	trace	0.001	0.002	trace	trace	116
Lard	1 tsp	13.0	0	117	0	13.00	0	0	0	0	0	0	0	0	0	0	0	0.003	0	0
Margarine	1 pat	5.0	0.80	36	trace	4.00	trace	1.0	0	trace	1.0	1	50	0	0	0	0	0	0	160
Oils																				
Corn, Cotton-seed, Safflower, Sesame, Soy	1 tbsp	14.0	0	120	0	14.00	0	0	0	0	0	0	0	0	0	0	0	0	0	—
Olive, Peanut	1 tbsp	14.0	0	119	0	13.50	0	0	0	0	0	0	0	0	0	0	0	0	0	—
Salad Dressing																				
Blue Cheese																				
Regular	1 tbsp	15.0	5.00	76	0.7	7.80	1.10	12.0	trace	—	11.0	6	164	trace	trace	0.020	trace	—	—	30
Low Fat	1 tbsp	15.0	13.00	12	0.5	0.90	0.70	10.0	trace	—	8.0	5	177	trace	trace	0.010	trace	—	—	30
French																				
Regular	1 tbsp	16.0	6.00	66	0.1	6.20	2.80	2.0	0.10	2.0	2.0	13	219	—	—	—	—	—	—	—
Low Fat	1 tbsp	16.0	12.00	15	0.1	0.70	2.50	2.0	0.10	—	2.0	13	126	—	—	—	—	—	—	—
Italian																				
Regular	1 tbsp	15.0	4.00	83	trace	9.00	1.00	2.0	trace	1.0	1.0	2	314	—	trace	trace	trace	0	0	trace
Low Fat	1 tbsp	16.0	14.00	8	trace	0.70	0.40	trace	trace	—	1.0	2	118	—	trace	trace	trace	0	0	trace
Mayonnaise	1 tbsp	14.0	2.00	101	0.2	11.20	0.30	3.0	0.10	0	4.0	5	84	—	trace	0.010	trace	0	0	40
Mayonnaise-type Salad Dressing	1 tbsp	15.0	6.00	65	0.2	6.30	2.20	2.0	trace	0	4.0	1	88	—	trace	trace	trace	0	0	30
Thousand Island																				
Regular	1 tbsp	16.0	5.00	80	0.1	8.00	2.50	2.0	0.10	—	3.0	18	112	trace	trace	trace	trace	—	—	50
Low Fat	1 tbsp	15.0	10.00	27	0.1	2.10	2.30	2.0	0.10	—	3.0	17	105	trace	trace	trace	trace	—	—	50
Nuts and Snacks																				
Almonds, roasted, salted	22	28.0	0.10	178	5.3	16.40	5.50	67.0	1.30	84.0	143.0	219	56	0	0.010	0.260	1.0	0.030	14.0	0
Brazil Nuts, shelled	6–8	28.0	1.30	185	4.1	19.00	3.10	53.0	1.00	65.0	196.0	203	trace	—	0.270	0.030	0.5	0.050	trace	trace
Cashews	18	28.0	1.50	159	4.9	13.00	8.30	11.0	1.10	80.0	106.0	132	4	—	0.120	0.070	0.5	0.120	8.0	30
Peanuts, roasted, salted	½ cup	72.0	1.00	421	18.7	35.80	13.60	54.0	1.50	120.0	288.0	486	301	0	0.230	0.100	12.4	0.288	19.0	—
Peanut Butter	1 tsp	16.0	0.30	94	4.0	8.10	3.00	9.0	0.30	28.0	61.0	100	97	0	0.020	0.020	2.4	0.005	2.0	—
Pecans, shelled	½ cup	54.0	2.00	371	5.0	38.40	7.90	40.0	1.30	77.0	156.0	325	trace	1.00	0.460	0.070	0.5	0.09	7.0	70
Pistachio Nuts	½ cup	76.0	4.00	449	14.6	40.60	14.40	99.0	5.50	120.0	378.0	735	—	0	0.500	—	1.1	—	—	173
Popcorn with oil, salt	1 cup	9.0	0.30	41	0.90	2.00	5.30	1.0	0.20	12.0	19.0	—	175	0	—	0.010	0.2	0.014	0	—
Potato Chips	10	20.0	0.40	114	1.10	8.00	10.00	8.0	0.40	8.0	28.0	226	[a]	3.00	0.040	0.010	1.0	0.036	2.0	trace
Pretzels, 3-Ring	10	30.0	1.00	117	2.90	1.40	22.80	7.0	0.50	—	39.0	39	504	0	0.010	0.010	0.2	0.010	—	0
Walnuts, shelled																				
Black	½ cup	62.0	2.00	392	12.80	37.00	9.20	trace	3.80	118.0	356.0	288	2	—	0.140	0.070	0.4	—	—	190
English	½ cup	50.0	2.00	326	7.40	32.00	7.90	50.0	1.60	66.0	190.0	225	1	1.00	0.160	0.070	0.4	0.360	30.0	15
Soups[b]																				
Canned																				
Bean with pork	1 cup	250.0	211.00	168	8.00	5.80	21.80	63.0	2.30	—	128.0	395	1008	3.00	0.130	0.080	1.0	—	—	650
Beef Noodle	1 cup	240.0	224.00	67	3.80	2.60	7.00	7.0	1.00	—	48.0	77	917	trace	0.050	0.070	1.0	—	—	50
Chicken Noodle	1 cup	240.0	224.00	62	3.40	1.90	7.90	10.0	0.50	10.0	36.0	55	979	trace	0.020	0.020	0.7	0.071	0	50
Clam Chowder (Manhattan)	1 cup	245.0	225.00	81	2.20	2.50	12.30	34.0	1.00	—	47.0	184	938	—	0.020	0.020	1.0	—	8.0	880
Cream of Mushroom	1 cup	240.0	215.00	134	2.40	9.60	10.10	41.0	0.50	—	50.0	98	955	trace	0.020	0.120	0.7	—	—	70
Split Pea	1 cup	245.0	209.00	145	8.60	3.20	20.60	29.0	1.50	14.0	149.0	270	941	1.00	0.250	0.150	1.5	0.120	2.0	440
Tomato	1 cup	245.0	223.00	88	2.00	2.50	15.70	15.0	0.70	17.0	34.0	230	970	12.00	0.050	0.050	1.2	0.048	9.0	1000
Vegetarian Vegetable	1 cup	245.0	225.00	78	2.20	2.00	13.20	20.0	1.00	—	39.0	172	838	—	0.050	0.050	1.0	—	—	2940
Dehydrated																				
Chicken Rice	1 cup	240.0	228.00	48	1.20	1.00	8.40	7.0	trace	—	10.0	10	622	—	trace	trace	0.2	—	—	trace
Onion	1 cup	240.0	230.00	36	1.40	1.20	5.50	10.0	0.20	—	12.0	58	689	2.00	trace	trace	trace	—	—	trace

Candy																			
Butterscotch	1 oz	28.0	0.40	113	trace	1.00	26.90	5.0	0.40	—	2.0	1	19	0	0	trace	trace	—	—	40
Caramels	1 oz	28.0	2.00	113	1.10	2.90	21.70	42.0	0.40	—	35.0	54	64	trace	0.010	0.050	0.1	trace	—	trace
Chocolate																			
Milk, plain	1 oz	28.0	0.20	147	2.20	9.20	16.10	65.0	0.30	16.0	65.0	109	27	trace	0.020	0.100	0.1	trace	1	80
Semi-sweet	1 oz	28.0	0.30	144	1.20	10.10	16.20	9.0	0.70	—	43.0	92	1	trace	trace	0.020	0.1	—	—	10
Sweet	1 oz	28.0	0.20	150	1.20	10.00	16.40	27.0	0.40	30.0	40.0	75	9	trace	0.010	0.040	0.1	—	—	trace
Fudge	1 oz	28.0	2.00	113	0.80	3.50	21.30	22.0	0.30	—	24.0	42	54	trace	0.010	0.030	0.1	—	—	trace
Gum Drops	1 oz	28.0	3.00	98	trace	0.20	24.80	2.0	0.10	—	trace	1	10	0	0	trace	trace	—	—	0
Jelly Beans	10	28.0	2.00	104	trace	0.10	26.40	3.0	0.30	—	1.0	trace	3	0	0	trace	trace	—	—	0
Marshmallows	1 large	7.0	1.00	23	0.10	trace	5.80	1.0	0.10	—	trace	trace	3	0	0	trace	trace	—	0	0
Honey, strained	1 tbsp	21.0	4.00	64	0.10	0	17.30	1.0	0.10	1.0	1.0	11	1	trace	trace	0.010	0.1	0.004	1.0	trace
Icings																			
Chocolate	1 cup[a]	275.0	39.00	1034	8.80	38.20	185.40	165.0	3.30	—	305.0	536	168	1	0.060	0.280	0.6	—	—	580
White, boiled	1 cup	94.0	17.00	297	1.30	0	75.50	2.0	trace	—	2.0	17	134	0	trace	0.030	trace	—	—	0
Jams and Preserves	1 tbsp	20.0	6.00	54	0.10	trace	14.00	4.0	0.20	1.0	2.0	18	2	trace	trace	0.010	trace	0.01	1.0	trace
Jellies	1 tbsp	18.0	5.00	49	trace	trace	12.70	4.0	0.30	1.0	1.0	14	3	1	trace	0.010	trace	0.006	0	trace
Marmalade, citrus	1 tbsp	20.0	6.00	51	0.10	trace	14.00	7.0	0.10	1.0	2.0	7	3	1	trace	trace	trace	—	—	—
Molasses																			
Light	1 tbsp	20.0	5.00	50	—	—	13.00	33.0	0.90	9.0	9.0	183	3	—	0.010	0.010	trace	—	—	—
Medium	1 tbsp	20.0	5.00	46	—	—	12.00	58.0	1.20	16.0	14.0	213	7	—	—	0.020	0.2	0.040	2.0	—
Blackstrap	1 tbsp	20.0	5.00	43	—	—	11.00	137.0	3.20	52.0	17.0	585	19	—	0.020	0.040	0.4	—	—	—
Sugar																			
Brown	½ cup, packed	110.0	2.00	410	0	0	106.00	94.0	3.80	0	21.0	378	33	0	0.010	0.040	0.2	0	0	0
White, granulated	1 tsp	4.0	0.02	15	0	0	4.00	0	trace	0	0	0	trace	0	0	0	0	0	0	0
	1 lump	5.0	0.03	19	0	0	5.00	0	trace	0	0	0	trace	0	0	0	0	0	0	0
White, powdered	1 tbsp	8.0	0.04	31	0	0	8.00	0	trace	0	0	0	trace	0	0	0	0	0	0	0
Syrups																			
Maple	1 tbsp	20.0	6.00	50	—	—	12.80	20.0	0.20	—	2.0	35	2	0	—	—	—	0	0	—
Table blends																			
Corn	1 tbsp	20.0	5.00	59	0	0	15.40	9.0	0.80	0	3.0	1	14	0	0	0	0	0	0	0
Cane and Maple	1 tbsp	20.0	6.00	50	0	0	12.80	3.0	trace	—	trace	5	trace	0	0	0	0	—	—	0
Other																			
Baking Powder	1 tsp	3.0	0.05	4	trace	trace	0.90	58.0	—	—	87.0	5	329	0	0	0	0	—	—	0
Boullion Cube	1	4.0	0.2	5	0.80	0.10	0.20	—	—	2.0	—	4	960	—	—	—	—	0	0	—
Chewing Gum, Candy coated	¾"x½"x¼" piece	1.7	0.06	5	—	—	1.60	—	—	—	—	—	—	0	0	0	0	—	—	—
Cocoa, plain, dry	1 tbsp	5.0	0.10	15	0.90	1.00	3.00	5.0	0.60	20.0	35.0	80	trace	0	0.010	0.02	0.1	—	—	—
Cocoa Mix w/non fat dry milk	1 tbsp	7.0	0.20	27	0.70	0.70	5.20	19.0	0.10	26.0	20.0	42	27	0	0.010	0.03	0	0.001	6.0	1
Gelatin, dry	1 envelope	7.0	0.90	23	6.00	trace	0	—	—	2.0	—	—	—	—	—	—	—	0	0	—
Gelatin Dessert, plain	1 cup	240.0	202.00	142	3.60	0	33.80	—	—	4.0	—	—	122	—	—	—	—	0	0	—
Gravy, meat, brown	¼ cup	72.0	48.00	164	1.20	14.00	8.00	0	0.40	1.0	8.0	76	720	0	0.040	0.03	0	0.036	1.0	0
Puddings with milk	½ cup	130.0	91.00	161	4.40	3.90	29.60	133.0	0.40	30.0	123.0	177	168	0	0.030	0.19	0.1	0.065	9.0	169
Yeast																			
Bakers, compressed	1 pkg	18.0	13.00	15	2.20	0.10	2.00	2.0	0.90	11.0	71.0	110	3	trace	0.130	0.30	2.0	—	—	trace
Bakers, dry active	1 pkg	7.0	0.04	20	2.60	0.10	2.70	3.0	1.10	3.0	90.0	140	4	trace	0.160	0.38	2.6	0.10	7.0	trace
Brewers, debittered	1 tbsp	8.0	0.04	23	3.10	0.10	3.10	17.0	1.40	18.0	140.0	152	10	trace	1.250	0.34	3.0	0.10	8.0	trace

[a]Sodium content varies; may be 1000 mg per 100 g. [b]Prepared with water according to package directions. [a]Enough to frost 1 9" diam cake layer.

Sources:
Adams, C. F. Nutritive Value of American Foods in Common Units, *Agriculture Handbook No. 456*. Agricultural Research Service, USDA. Washington, D.C. 1975.
Pennington, J.A. *Dietary Nutrient Guide*. Westport, Conn.: AVI Publishing Company, Inc., 1976.
Watt, B. K. and A. L. Merrill (with assistance of R. K. Pecot, C. F. Adams, M. L. Orr, and D. F. Miller). Composition of Foods—Raw, processed, prepared. *Agriculture Handbook No. 8*, Agricultural Research Service, USDA. Washington, D.C. 1963, reprinted 1975.
Young, E. A., E. H. Brennan, and G. L. Irving. Perspectives on fast foods. *Public Health Currents*. Ross Laboratories, Columbus, Ohio. Jan., Feb., 1979.
Church, C. F. and H. N. Church. Food values of portions commonly used, 12th edition. Philadelphia: J. B. Lippincott Co., 1975.
Posati, L. P. and M. L. Orr. Composition of Foods. Dairy and egg products; raw, processed, prepared. *Agriculture Handbook No. 8-1*; Agricultural Research Service, USDA. Washington, D. C., 1976.
Marsh, A. C., M. K. Moss, and E. W. Murphy. Composition of Foods. Spices and herbs. Raw, processed, prepared. *Agriculture Handbook No. 8-2*; Agricultural Research Service, USDA. Washington, D. C., 1977.
Gebhardt, S. E., R. Cutrufelli, and R. H. Matthews. Composition of Foods. Baby Foods. Raw, processed, prepared. *Agriculture Handbook No. 8-3*; Agricultural Research Service, USDA. Washington, D. C., 1978.

Notes:
Unless otherwise indicated, enriched flour is used in all products containing wheat flour.
— indicates lack of reliable data for a nutrient believed to be present.
nd indicates no data.
Amino acid content of foods may be found in the article *"Amino acid content of foods and biological data on proteins." FAO*. No. 24, Rome, 1970.
Fatty acid content of foods may be found in the appropriate *Handbooks No. 8* (revised editions), *Handbook 456*, and in the *Journal of the American Dietetic Association* series cited in Chapter 3.

APPENDIX I
Selected Nutrition Resources

American Dental Association
222 E. Superior Street
Chicago, IL 60611

American Diabetes Association
18 E. 48th Street
New York, NY 10017

American Dietetic Association
430 N. Michigan Avenue
Chicago, IL 60611

American Egg Board
P. O. Box 358
Northfield, IL 60093

American Heart Association
44 East 23rd Street
New York, NY 10010

American Home Economics Association
Division of Public Affairs
2010 Massachusetts Avenue, NW
Washington, DC 20036

American Institute of Nutrition
9650 Rockville Pike
Bethesda, MD 20014

American Medical Association
Council on Foods and Nutrition
535 N. Dearborn Street
Chicago, IL 60610

American Public Health Association
1015 18th Street, NW
Washington, DC 20036

Consumer Information
Public Documents Distribution Center
Pueblo, CO 81009

Food and Agriculture Organization of America, Inc.
Information Office
1776 F Street NW
Washington, DC 20437

Food and Agricultural Organization of the United Nations
(publications available from UNIPUB)

UNIPUB Inc.
P.O. Box 433
New York, NY 10016

Food and Drug Administration (FDA)
Parklane Building
5600 Fishers Lane
Rockville, MD 20852

Food and Nutrition Board
National Academy of Sciences
2101 Constitution Avenue
Washington, DC 20418

Food and Nutrition Information and Educational Materials Center
National Agricultural Library Rm 304
Beltsville, MD 20705

League for International Food Education
1155 16th St. NW Rm. 705
Washington, DC 20036

Institute of Food Technologists
221 North LaSalle Street
Chicago, IL 60601

National Foundation—March of Dimes
Health Information Department
P. O. Box 2000
White Plains, NY 10602

National Dairy Council
6300 North River Road
Rosemont, IL 60018

National Livestock & Meat Board
444 North Michigan Avenue
Chicago, IL 60611

Nutrition Foundation, Inc.
888 17th Street, NW.
Washington, DC 20006

Nutrition Today Society
P. O. Box 773
Annapolis, MD 21404

Public Affairs Committee, Inc.
381 Park Avenue South
New York, NY 10016

Society for Nutrition Education
2140 Shattuck Avenue Suite 1110
Berkeley, CA 94704

Superintendent of Documents
U.S. Government Printing Office
Washington, DC 20402

Food and Nutrition Service (federal programs including Extension Service and School Lunch)
U.S.D.A.
500 12th Street SW
Washington, DC 20250

U.S. Department of Agriculture
Nutrition Program
Agricultural Research Service
Hyattsville, MD 20782

U.S. Department of Health Education and Welfare
330 Independence Avenue SW.
Washington, DC 20201

U.S. Department of Health Education and Welfare
Maternal and Child Health Services
Health Services Administration
Rockville, MD 20852

World Health Organization
777 United Nations Plaza
New York, NY 10017

Periodicals and Magazines

CNI Weekly Report
Contemporary Nutrition
Daily Council Digest
Nutrition Action
Nutrition Today
Professional Nutritionist

Professional Journals

American Journal of Clinical Nutrition
American Journal of Public Health
Food Technology
Journal of the American Dental Association
Journal of the American Dietetic Association
Journal of the American Medical Association
Journal of Clinical Investigation
Journal of Food Science
Journal of Home Economics
Journal of Nutrition
Journal of Nutrition Education
Metabolism
New England Journal of Medicine
Nutrition Reviews
School Food Service Journal
Science
The Lancet

Index